GOODMAN'S BASIC MEDICAL ENDO

FIFTH EDITION

GOODMAN'S BASIC MEDICAL ENDOCRINOLOGY

FIFTH EDITION

ELIZABETH H. HOLT

Associate Professor of Medicine, Endocrinology, Yale School of Medicine, New Haven, CT, United States

BEATRICE LUPSA

Assistant Professor of Medicine, Endocrinology, Yale School of Medicine, New Haven, CT, United States

GRACE S. LEE

Assistant Professor of Medicine, Endocrinology, Yale School of Medicine, New Haven, CT, United States

Endocrinologist, VA CT Healthcare System, West Haven, CT, United States

HANAN BASSYOUNI

Clinical Associate Professor, Cumming School of Medicine; Faculty of Medicine, Department of Medicine; Section of Endocrinology and Metabolism, University of Calgary, Calgary, AB, Canada

HARRY E. PEERY

The Karl Riabowol Laboratory, Arnie Charbonneau Cancer Research Institute and Department of Biochemistry and Molecular Biology, Cumming School of Medicine, University of Calgary, Calgary, AB, Canada

Program in Pharmaceutical Bioengineering, Department of Bioengineering, School of Medicine and College of Engineering, University of Washington, Seattle, WA, United States

Founding Director and Research Director, The Anti-NMDA Receptor Encephalitis Foundation, Inc., Ottawa, Ontario, Canada

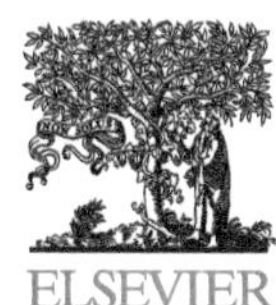

ELSEVIER

Elsevier
Radarweg 29, PO Box 211, 1000 AE Amsterdam, Netherlands
The Boulevard, Langford Lane, Kidlington, Oxford OX5 1GB, United Kingdom
50 Hampshire Street, 5th Floor, Cambridge, MA 02139, United States

Notices
Knowledge and best practice in this field are constantly changing. As new research and experience broaden our understanding, changes in research methods, professional practices, or medical treatment may become necessary.

Practitioners and researchers must always rely on their own experience and knowledge in evaluating and using any information, methods, compounds, or experiments described herein. In using such information or methods they should be mindful of their own safety and the safety of others, including parties for whom they have a professional responsibility.

To the fullest extent of the law, neither the Publisher nor the authors, contributors, or editors, assume any liability for any injury and/or damage to persons or property as a matter of products liability, negligence or otherwise, or from any use or operation of any methods, products, instructions, or ideas contained in the material herein.

British Library Cataloguing-in-Publication Data
A catalogue record for this book is available from the British Library

Library of Congress Cataloging-in-Publication Data
A catalog record for this book is available from the Library of Congress

ISBN: 978-0-12-815844-9

For Information on all Elsevier publications
visit our website at https://www.elsevier.com/books-and-journals

Printed in the United States of America

Last digit is the print number: 9 8 7 6 5 4 3 2

Publisher: Stacy Masucci
Acquisitions Editor: Tari Broderick
Editorial Project Manager: Kristi Anderson
Production Project Manager: Kiruthika Govindaraju
Cover Designer: Christian Bilbow

Typeset by MPS Limited, Chennai, India

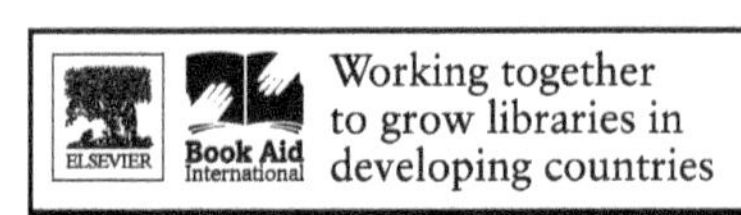

Dedications

We dedicate this book to patients with endocrine disorders and to our colleagues in the clinics and laboratories who are working to understand and treat those disorders.

Elizabeth H. Holt:
To my patients

Grace S. Lee:
To my loving husband and children.

Beatrice Lupsa:
To my father, Mircea who inspired me to be a physician.

Hanan Bassyouni:
To my Parents, husband and boys for always supporting and loving me. And to my friends, patients and students as I would not be who I am today without you.

Harry E. Peery:
To my wife, Susan B. Peery, and to our children, grandchildren, friends, students and colleagues who have supported me over the years and to the memory of Betty Noling who taught me how to write at Far Hills Country Day School.

Advice to Future Colleagues:

"Plan ahead.
Always be concerned about the dangers of mural dyslexia: The inability to read the writing on the wall."

- Lloyd H.(Holly) Smith, late renowned endocrinologist, internal medicine educator, administrator and author.

Contents

Preface

It has been 33 years since Maurice Goodman put pen to paper and wrote his Basic Medical Endocrinology in 1988, mainly for the medical students he had been teaching for 25 years but also for graduate students and upper division undergraduates. At that time, almost all medical schools still had the basic sciences taught by PhDs as part of the first 2 years (preclerkship years) of medical school.

Fast forward to 2008, when the fourth edition introduced color to the book. By that time—20 years after the first edition—interest in 2 years of basic sciences for medical students was waning. More and more, it was the clinical specialist who was teaching those courses with an emphasis on clinical examples rather than on the biochemical basis of the subject matter. This approach was accelerated even more when the basic sciences became more interested in molecular biology, genetics, and epigenetics rather than clinical applications. Yet, Dr. Goodman's text was still being appreciated at the graduate and upper division undergraduate levels.

Moving forward another 13 years, and we find that in 2021 this is still true, but now many medical schools are eliminating the basic sciences altogether and focusing on clinicians teaching only background information that is clinically relevant. As a result, these new medical programs are usually shortened by a year with an emphasis on educating family physicians rather than research physicians.

During those intervening years since the fourth edition, Dr. Goodman retired from both teaching and writing. We were invited by the publisher to take over the fifth edition of this venerable work. It was a challenge for two reasons. First, to fill Dr. Goodman's shoes and retain and expand on the molecular aspects of endocrinology and, second, to recapture some of the medical markets that evaporated when basic sciences stopped being taught by nonclinicians.

To this end, board-certified endocrinologists at leading universities in the United States and Canada were invited to provide case studies and to add some clinically related material throughout the book. At the same time, the molecular aspects of the field were updated by a respected professional in the basic sciences who teaches in the United States and Canada.

While much of the book retains the original work of Dr. Goodman—for whom we are deeply indebted—there has also been extensive updating. To begin with, we added many illustrations to depict the molecular aspects of endocrinology. These were mainly taken from other Elsevier medical publications, although some were drawn specially for this text. We also added clinical illustrations—again from Elsevier's extensive medical library of journals and textbooks.

We have also added new information—such as the putative role of oxytocin in males—and condensed other areas so that the text could still fit in a relatively small volume. While we hope these changes will meet with approval, we are always open to suggestions from the users of our book. Feel free to contact any one of the authors.

The cover image is the molecular structure of the estrogen receptor, present in both males and females. We chose this because it is the same structure in both genders, which helps underscore the promotion of equality and respect in the sciences and in medicine—and in life.

Last but not least, we want to thank our acquisition editor, Tari Broderick, our development editor, Kristi Anderson and production editor, Kiruthika Govindaraju, at Elsevier, all of whom patiently and expertly helped us in every aspect of this project. We also want to thank our spouses, who had to live a very lonely existence while we crafted our manuscript. We are deeply indebted to them for their understanding.

Elizabeth H. Holt[1], Beatrice Lupsa[1], Grace S. Lee[1], Hanan Bassyouni[2] and Harry E. Peery[2]

[1]Yale School of Medicine, Yale University, New Haven, CT, United States [2]Cumming School of Medicine, University of Calgary, Calgary, AB, Canada

CHAPTER

1

Introduction

Case Study: Giantism

Normally, cells communicate with other cells in an orderly fashion. However, in 1918 this did not happen with growth hormone in Robert Wadlow (Fig. 1.1). Did he have a tumor or did something happen to the cells that stimulated the release of growth hormone? We will never know. We do know that he began to grow very fast as a child (Table 1.1).

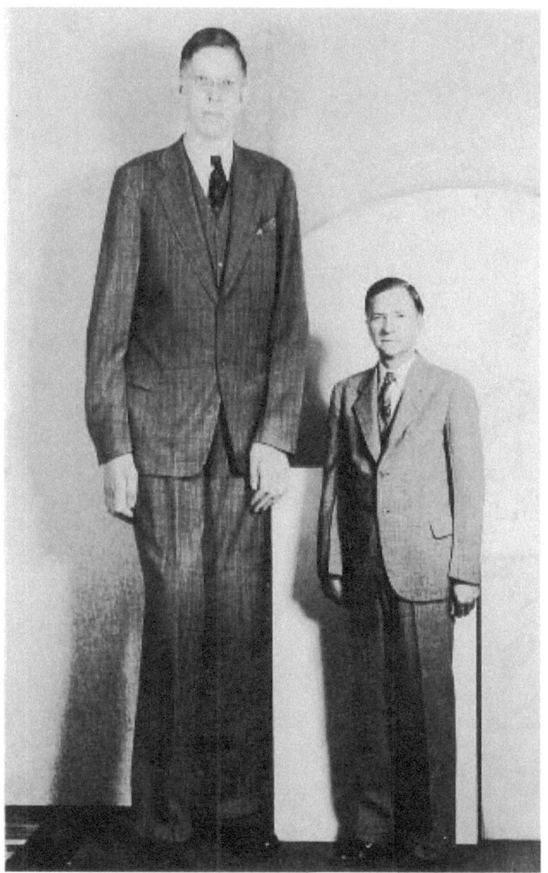

FIGURE 1.1 From a postcard showing Robert Wadlow—over 8 ft. 9 in. in this picture—with his father, who is 5′11″. Source: Wikipedia.

Goodman's Basic Medical Endocrinology.
DOI: https://doi.org/10.1016/B978-0-12-815844-9.00001-4

(cont'd)

TABLE 1.1 Growth chart of Robert Wadlow.

Age	Height	Weight	Notes	Size of	Year
Birth	1 ft. 8 in. (0.51 m)	8 lb 6 oz (3.8 kg)	Normal height of weight.	Average	February 22, 1918
6 months	2 ft. 10.5 in. (0.88 m)	30 lb (14 kg)		2 year old	August 22, 1918
1 year	3 ft. 6 in. (1.07 m)	45 lb (20 kg)	When he began to walk at 11 months, he was 3 ft. 3.5 in. (1.00 m) tall and weighed 40 lbs.	5 year old	February 22, 1919
18 months	4 ft. 3 in. (1.30 m)	67 lb (30 kg)		8 year old	August 22, 1919
2 years	4 ft. 6 in. (1.37 m)	75 lb (34 kg)		10 year old	1920
3 years	4 ft. 11 in. (1.50 m)	89 lb (40 kg)		12 year old	1921
4 years	5 ft. 3 in. (1.60 m)	105 lb (48 kg)		14 year old	1922
5 years	5 ft. 6.5 in. (1.69 m)	140 lb (64 kg)	At 5 years of age, attending kindergarten, Robert was 5′ 6 1/2" tall. He wore clothes that would fit a 17-year-old boy.	15 year old	1923
6 years	5 ft. 7 in. (1.70 m)	146 lb (66 kg)		15 year old	1924
7 years	5 ft. 10 in. (1.78 m)	159 lb (72 kg)		Height of adult male	1925
8 years	6 ft. 0 in. (1.83 m)	169 lb (77 kg)			1926
9 years	6 ft. 2 in. (1.88 m)	180 lb (82 kg)	Weighing 180 lb, he was strong enough to carry his father (who was sitting in a living room chair) up the stairs to the second floor.		1927
10 years	6 ft. 5 in. (1.96 m)	210 lb (95 kg)			1928
11 years	6 ft. 11 in. (2.11 m)	241 lb (109 kg)			1929
12 years	7 ft. 2 in. (2.18 m)	287 lb (130 kg)			1930
13 years	7 ft. 4 in. (2.24 m)	301 lb (137 kg)	World's tallest Boy Scout, averaging a growth of 4 in. (10 cm) per year since birth and wearing size 19 (US) shoes.		1931
14 years	7 ft. 5 in. (2.26 m)	331 lb (150 kg)			1932
15 years	7 ft. 10 in. (2.39 m)	354 lb (161 kg)			1933
16 years	8 ft. 1.5 in. (2.48 m)	374 lb (170 kg)			1934
17 years	8 ft. 3 in. (2.51 m)	382 lb (173 kg)	Graduated from high school on January 8, 1936 and was 8 ft. 3 in. (2.51 m).	Height of Sultan Kosen, the tallest living man	1935
18 years	8 ft. 4 in. (2.54 m)	391 lb (177 kg)			1936
19 years	8 ft. 6 in. (2.59 m)	480 lb (220 kg)			1937
20 years	8 ft. 7 in. (2.62 m)	488 lb (221 kg)			1938
21 years	8 ft. 8 in. (2.64 m)	492 lb (223 kg)			1939

(Continued)

(*cont'd*)

TABLE 1.1 (Continued)

Age	Height	Weight	Notes	Size of	Year
22.4 years	8 ft. 11.1 in. (2.72 m)	439 lb (199 kg)	At death, he was the world's tallest man according to the Guinness World Records.		June 27, 1940

His height would increase until he died. He was not well during the last year of life and so lost weight. No medical cause for his ill-health was ever given.

His condition is called giantism and is due to the overproduction of growth hormone. He was producing so much growth hormone that it competed with the receptors for insulin, causing him to develop diabetes mellitus (type II diabetes). Through processes that are not yet understood, he developed peripheral neuropathy that is the loss of sensation in his feet, legs, hands, and arms because of the diabetes.

Growth was so fast that his bones could not develop quickly enough to hold his weight. This was especially true of his legs. He had to walk with braces on his legs, use a cane, and lean on objects when standing still (Fig. 1.2).

In 1940 he developed a blister on his leg from a new brace. It became infected and, since this was before the era of antibiotics, he died of septicemia at the age of 22. He was still growing at the time of his death.

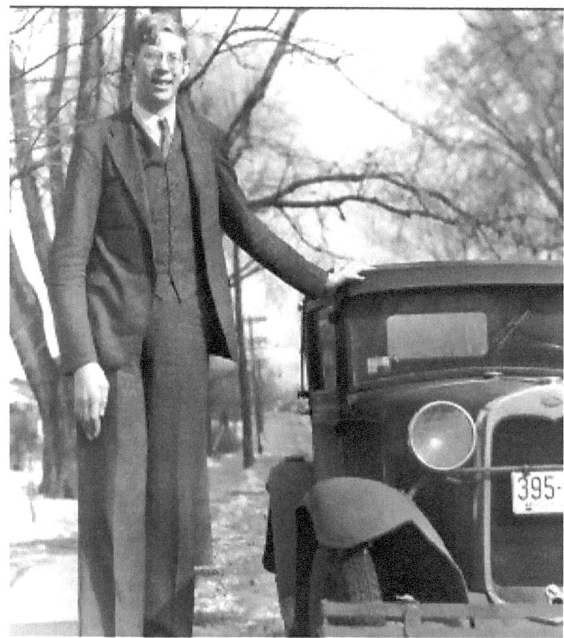

FIGURE 1.2 RobertWadlow leaning on a 1932 Ford.

Types of chemical messengers

Chemical messengers, such as growth hormone in Robert Wadlow, are one-way by which cells communicate with each other in a multicellular organism. This type of communication is slower but more sustained than the lightening-like response of the nervous system to potentially life-threatening stimuli from a body surface or viscera.

Evolutionarily, cells needed to communicate with other cells in a multicellular organism. Many of these chemical messengers have been conserved so that the mating factor receptor in primitive plants such as baker's yeast (*Saccharomyces cerevisiae*) is also to be found in animals although slightly transformed.

Types of intercellular chemical messengers include (1) autocrines—released by the cell as a self-regulator; (2) paracrines—released by neighboring cells to regulate a larger group of cells; (3) endocrines (hormones)—substances released from a distance and which strictly speaking travel part of the way in blood to reach their target tissues (however, the term is often used to mean any substance traveling in extracellular fluid); and, (4), pherocrines—substances released from one organism and passing through the environment (air or water) to affect other organisms. (Perfumes have as their base a pherocrine-like substance from either plants or animals.) Fig. 1.3 summarizes these concepts.

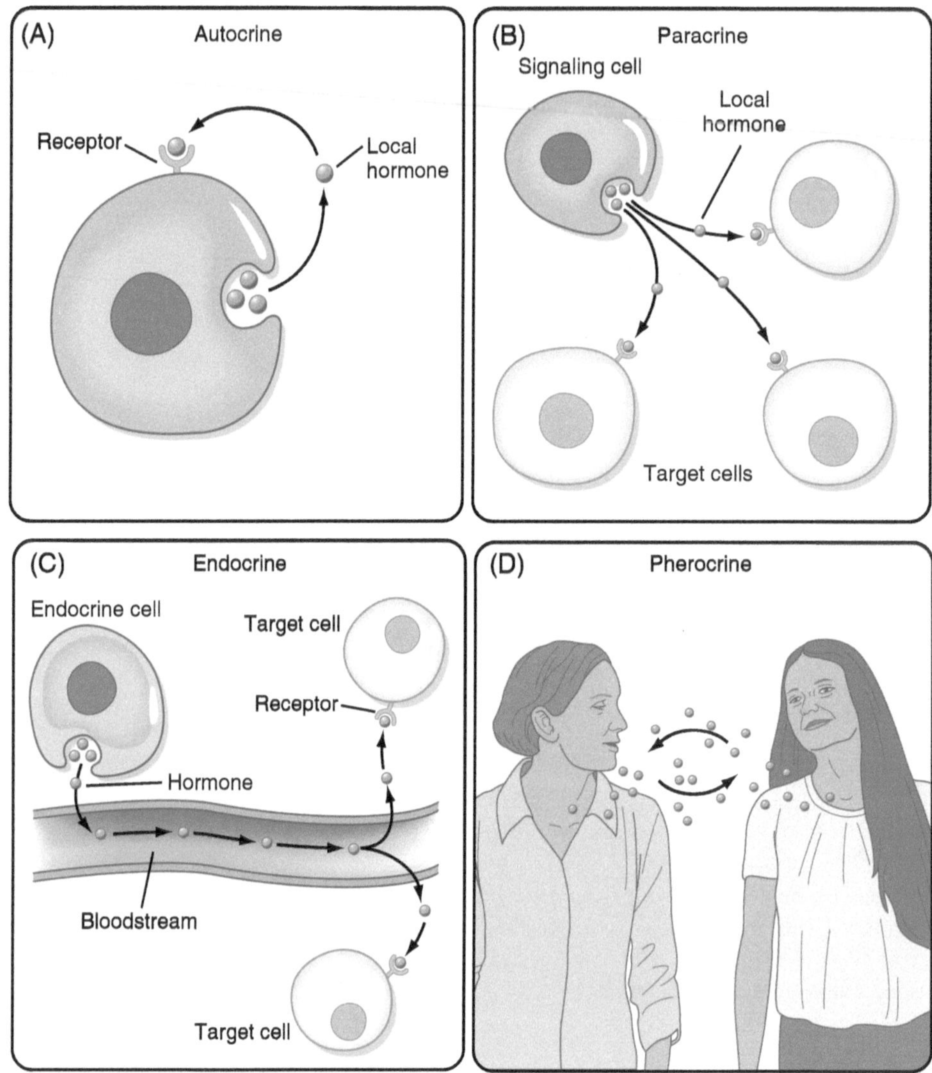

FIGURE 1.3 Types of chemical communication. (The fourth type needs to be illustrated.) Source: *From Figure 3.3 in Koeppen B. M., & Stanton B. W. (2018).* Berne and Levy's physiology *(7th ed.). Elsevier, p. 38.*

Paracrines and hormones are the most common form of intercellular communication, and while there are similarities, there are also differences as seen in Fig. 1.4.

Endocrine substances from specific glands are traditionally called hormones because they travel in the blood for at least part of their journey. Most tissues in the body produce endocrine substances and these substances are, by virtue of their traveling in the blood, also called hormones. This text will primarily be concerned with hormones of clinical importance that are produced by specialized glands. However, it will also discuss those produced by the brain, heart, and gastrointestinal tract.

Hormones are either modified proteins or steroid structures derived from cholesterol. Those that are protein usually interact with cell surface receptors and do not penetrate the cell (an exception is thyroid hormone) while those that are steroid enter the cell and combine with receptors in the nucleus as is illustrated by the effect of progesterone (a steroid), insulin-like growth factor-1, and luteinizing hormone (a protein) (Fig. 1.5).

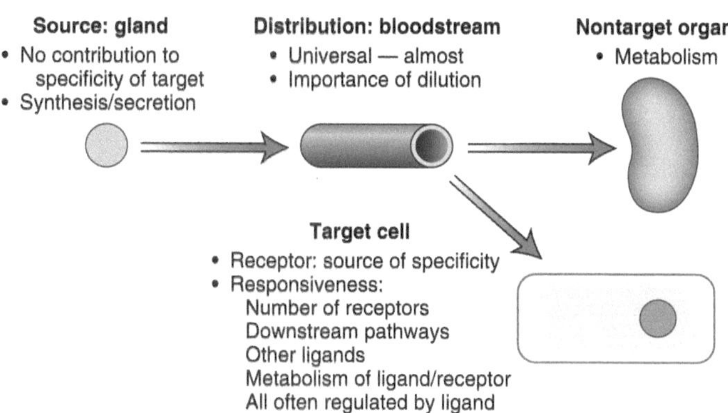

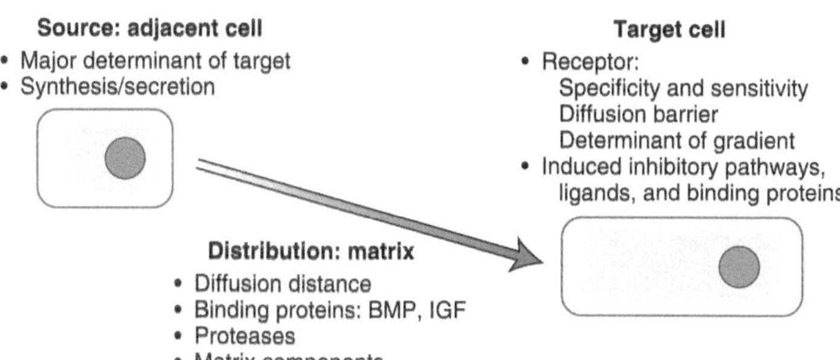

FIGURE 1.4 Hormone and paracrine signaling. Source: *From Figure 1.1, Melmed, S., Polonsky, K. S., Larson, P. R., & Kronenberg, H. M. (2016).* William's textbook of endocrinology *(13th ed.). Elsevier, p. 2.*

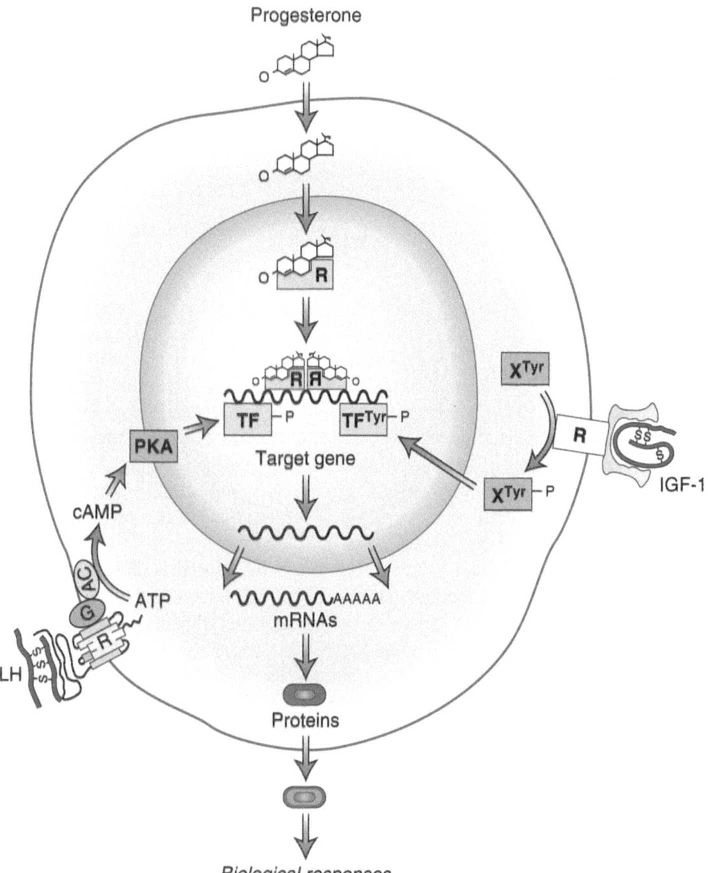

FIGURE 1.5 Showing proteins interacting with surface receptors and steroids interacting with receptors in nucleus. *AC,* Adenylate cyclase; *G,* heterotrimeric G-protein; *mRNAs,* messenger RNAs; *PKA,* protein kinase A; *R,* receptor molecule; *TF,* transcription factor; *Tyr,* tyrosine found in protein X; *X,* unknown protein substrate. Source: *From Figure 1.2, Melmed, S., Polonsky, K. S., Larson, P. R., & Kronenberg, H. M. (2016).* William's textbook of endocrinology *(13th ed.). Elsevier, p. 6.*

At the molecular level (boxed material for additional information)

Biosynthesis of hormones

Many small molecules, including nitric oxide and derivatives of amino acids and fatty acids, function as neurotransmitters or paracrine signals, but usually are not considered to be hormones, and so are discussed only when pertinent to the actions of hormones. Hormone synthesis and storage, particularly for the amino acid and steroid hormones, are presented later. A brief review of these steps also provides an opportunity for a general consideration of gene expression and protein synthesis and provides some background for understanding hormone actions.

Protein and peptide hormones are encoded in genes on the DNA (deoxyribonucleic acid) (Figs. 1.6–1.10) with each hormone usually represented only once in the genome. Information determining the amino acid

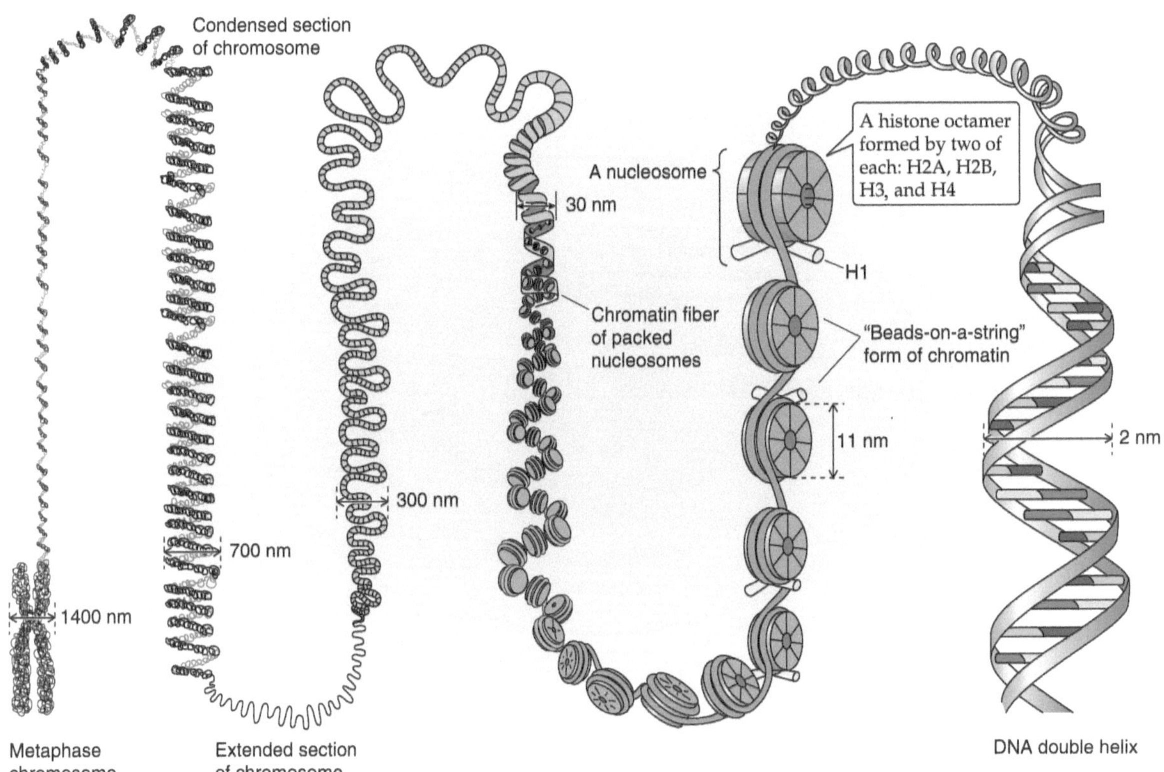

FIGURE 1.6 The organization of nuclear DNA. At the light microscopic level, the nuclear genetic material is organized into dispersed, transcriptionally active euchromatin or densely packed, transcriptionally inactive heterochromatin. Chromatin can also be mechanically connected with the nuclear membrane, and nuclear membrane perturbation can, thus, influence transcription. Chromosomes (as shown) can only be visualized by light microscopy during cell division. During mitosis, they are organized into paired chromatids connected at centromeres; the centromeres act as the locus for the formation of a kinetochore protein complex that regulates chromosome segregation at metaphase. The telomeres are repetitive nucleotide sequences that cap the termini of chromatids and permit repeated chromosomal replication without the loss of DNA at the chromosome ends. The chromatids are organized into short "P" (petite) and long "Q" (next letter in the alphabet) arms. The characteristic banding pattern of chromatids has been attributed to relative GC content (less GC content in bands relative to interbands), with genes tending to localize to interband regions. Individual chromatin fibers comprise a string of nucleosomes—DNA wound around octameric histone cores—with the nucleosomes connected via DNA linkers. Promoters are noncoding regions of DNA that initiate gene transcription; they are on the same strand and upstream of their associated gene. Enhancers are regulatory elements that can modulate gene expression over distances of 100kB or more by looping back onto promoters and recruiting additional factors that are needed to drive the expression of pre-mRNA species. The intronic sequences are subsequently spliced out of the pre-mRNA to produce the definitive message that is translated into protein—without the 3′- and 5′-UTR. In addition to the enhancer, promoter, and UTR sequences, noncoding elements are found throughout the genome; these include short repeats, regulatory factor binding regions, noncoding regulatory RNAs, and transposons. *UTR*, Untranslated regions. Source: *From Figure 4-3 in Kumar V., Abbas A.K., & Aster J.C. (2015).* Robbins and Cotran pathologic basis of disease *(9th ed.). Elsevier, p. 2.*

(*cont'd*)

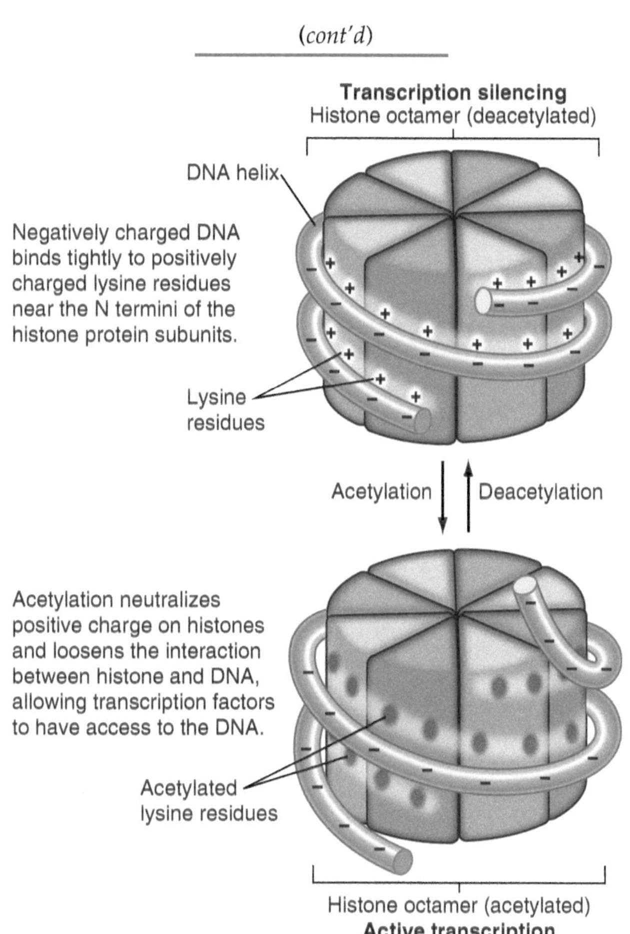

FIGURE 1.7 The ability to transcribe a region of DNA depends on whether the histone is acetylated or not. The reverse can also take place: a gene may be silenced if the histone is not acetylated. *DNA*, Deoxyribonucleic acid. Source: *Redrawn from Figure 4-17 in Boron, W. F., & Boulpaep, E. L. (2017).* Medical physiology *(3rd ed.). Elsevier, p. 95.*

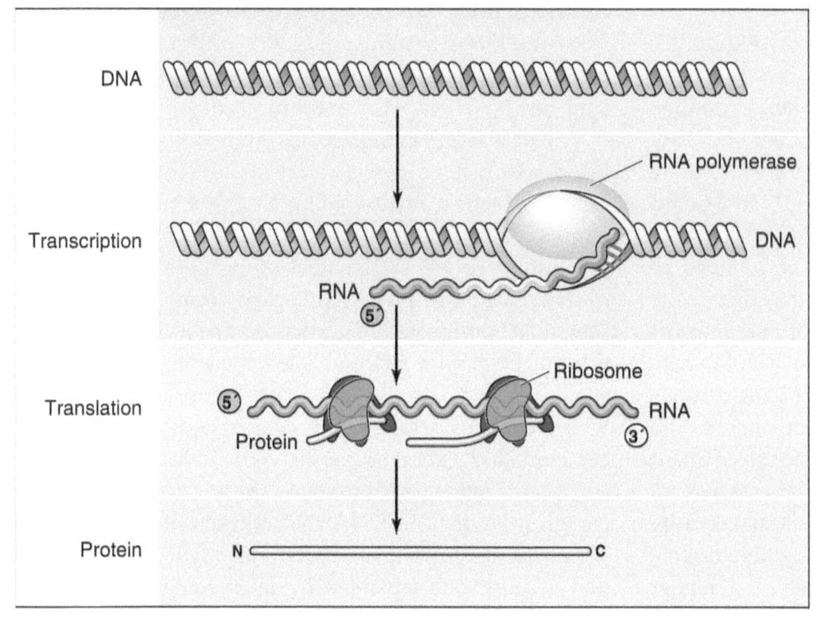

FIGURE 1.8 Summary of steps from DNA to protein. *DNA*, Deoxyribonucleic acid. Source: *From Figure 4-1 in Boron, W. F., & Boulpaep, E. L. (2017).* Medical physiology *(3rd ed.). Elsevier, p. 74.*

(*cont'd*)

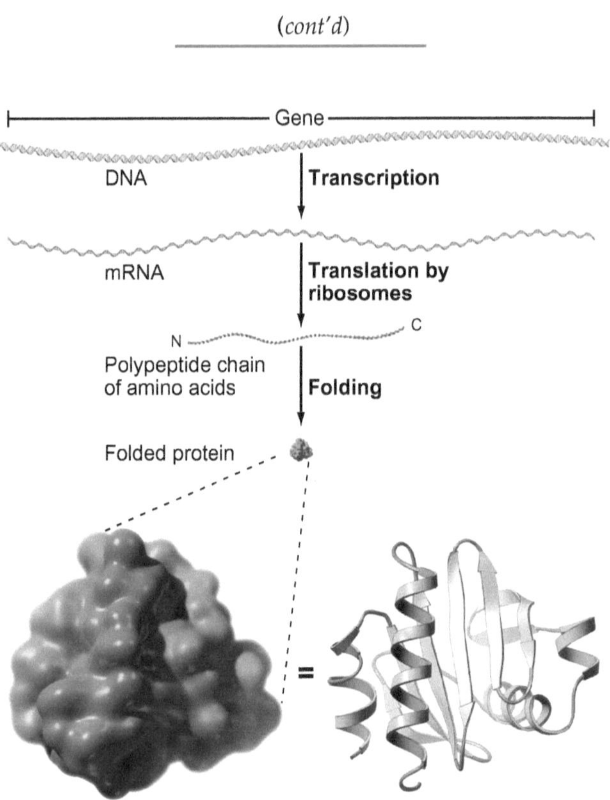

FIGURE 1.9 The steps in the synthesis of a protein. Source: *From Figure 1-4 in Pollard et al. (2017). Cell Biology (3rd ed.), Elsevier, p. 5.*

sequence of proteins is encoded in the nucleotide sequence of DNA (Fig. 1.11).

Nucleotides in DNA consist of a five-carbon sugar, deoxyribose, in ester linkage with a phosphate group, and attached in *N*-glycosidic linkage to one of four organic bases: adenine (A), guanine (G), thymidine (T), or cytidine (C). The ability of the purine bases (A) and (G) to form complementary pairs with the pyrimidine bases (T) and (C), respectively, on an adjacent strand of DNA is the fundamental property that permits accurate replication of DNA and transmission of stored information.

A single strand of DNA is a chain of millions of nucleotides linked by phosphate groups that form ester bonds with hydroxyl groups at carbon 3 of one deoxyribose and carbon 5 of the next deoxyribose. The DNA in each chromosome is present as a pair of long strands oriented in opposite directions and is organized into nucleosomes, each of which consists of a stretch of about 180 nucleotides tightly wound around a complex of eight histone molecules. The nucleosomes are linked by stretches of about 30 nucleotides, and the whole double strand of nucleoproteins is tightly coiled in a higher order of organization to form the chromosomes (Fig. 1.6).

The coiled DNA can be silenced or activated depending on whether the histone is acetylated (see Fig. 1.7).

Instructions for protein structure are transmitted from the DNA to ribosomes, the cytoplasmic sites of protein synthesis by using a messenger ribonucleic acid (mRNA) template, are summarized in Fig. 1.8.

All RNAs differ in structure from DNA only in having ribose instead of deoxyribose as its sugar and uridine (U) instead of thymidine as one of its pyrimidine bases. The nucleotide sequence of the mRNA precursor is complementary to the nucleotide sequence of DNA. mRNA synthesis proceeds linearly from an upstream "start site" designated by a particular sequence of nucleotides in DNA in a process called transcription. The start site is located downstream from the promoter region, which contains sequences to which regulatory proteins can bind, and a short sequence where RNA polymerase II and a large aggregate of proteins, the general transcription complex, binds. The DNA that is transcribed comprises segments that encode structural and regulatory information called exons separated by intervening sequences of

(*cont'd*)

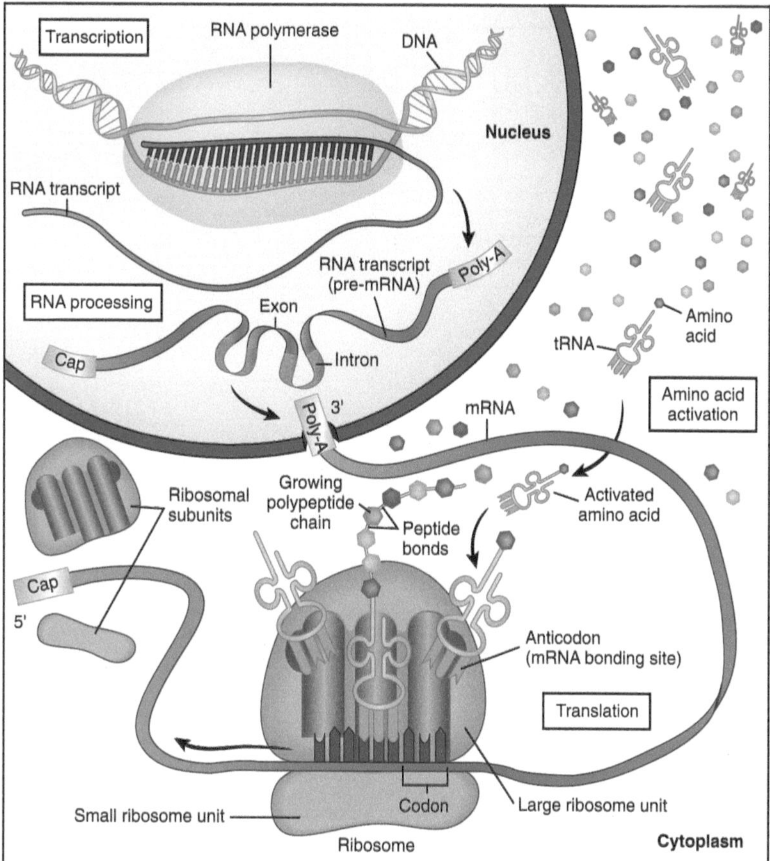

FIGURE 1.10 Summary of transcription. Source: *From Figure 4-9 in McCance and Huether, Mosby (2019). Pathophysiology (8th ed.), p. 141.*

DNA with no coding function, called introns (Fig. 1.9) and the process is summarized in Fig. 1.10.

Transcription is regulated by nuclear proteins called transcription factors or transactivating factors, which bind to regulatory sites that are usually upstream from the promoter and stimulate or repress gene transcription. These proteins form complexes with multiple other transcription factors and proteins called coactivators or corepressors, which not only govern attachment and activity of the general transcription complex but also control the "tightness" of the DNA coil and hence the accessibility of genes to the transcription apparatus. Transcription proceeds from the start site through the introns and exons and a downstream flanking sequence where a long polyadenine tail is added. A special "cap" structure containing methylated guanosine added to the opposite end of the RNA transcript permits its export from the nucleus after it is modified further by removal of the introns and attachment of the exons to each other in a process called splicing. Under some circumstances the splicing reactions may bypass some exons or parts of exons, which are then omitted from the final mRNA transcript. Because of such alternate splicing, a single gene can give rise to more than one mRNA transcript, and hence more than one protein product (Figs. 1.11 and 1.12).

Multiple mRNA transcripts may also be produced from some genes that have more than one site at which transcription can start.

Upon export from the nucleus, the mRNA transcripts attach to ribosomes where they are translated into protein. Ribosomes are large complexes of RNA and enzymes that "read" the mRNA code in triplets of nucleotides called

(cont'd)

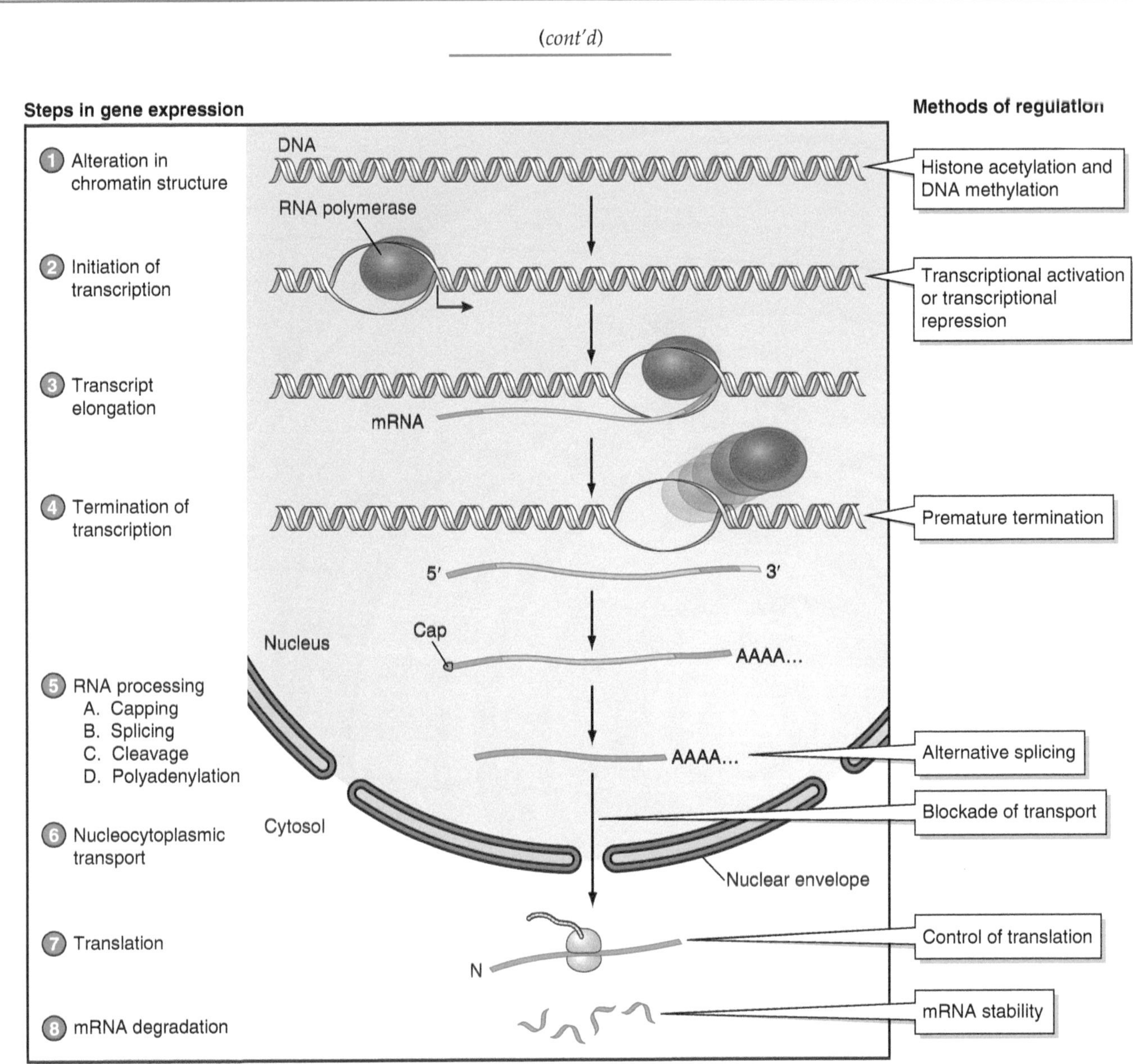

FIGURE 1.11 Steps in gene expression. Each of these steps can be altered leading to an endocrine imbalance or disorder. Source: *Redrawn from Figure 4-4 in Boron, W. F., & Boulpaep, E. L. (2017).* Medical physiology *(3rd ed.). Elsevier, p. 77.*

codons. The translation initiation site begins with the codon for methionine. Each codon designates a specific amino acid. Triplets of complementary nucleotides (anticodons) are found in small RNA molecules called transfer RNA (tRNA) each of which binds a particular amino acid and delivers it to the ribosome. Alignment of amino acids in the proper sequence is achieved by the complementary pairing of anticodons in the tRNA with codons in the mRNA (Fig. 1.12).

The tRNA thus delivers the correct amino acid to the carboxyl terminus of the growing peptide chain and holds it in position so that ribosomal enzymes can release it from the tRNA and link it to the peptide. Once the peptide bond is formed, the empty tRNA is released and the ribosome moves down the mRNA to the next codon where the next tRNA molecule charged with its amino acid waits to bind to its complementary codon. Elongation of the chain continues until the ribosome reaches a "stop" codon at which time it dissociates from the mRNA. As each ribosome moves down the mRNA, other ribosomes attach behind it to repeat the process. In this way a single mRNA molecule may be translated many times before it is degraded.

(*cont'd*)

Protein and peptide hormones are synthesized as larger molecules (prohormones and preprohormones) than the final secretory product. Proteins destined for secretion have a hydrophobic sequence of 12–30 amino acids at their amino terminals. This signal sequence is recognized by a special structure that directs the growing peptide chain through a protein channel in the endoplasmic reticular membrane (see Fig. 1.13) and into the cisternae of the endoplasmic reticulum.

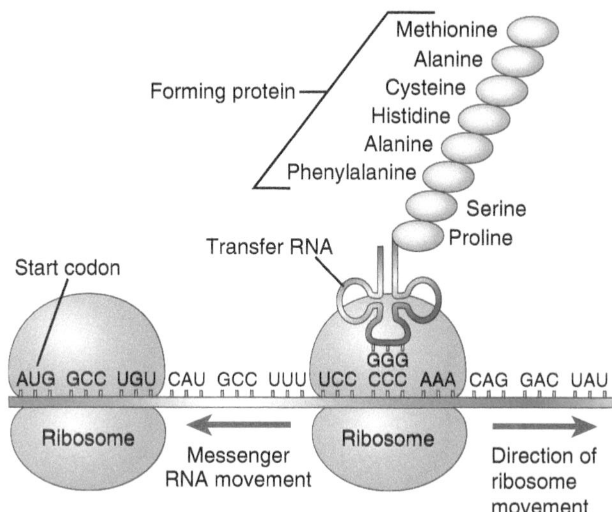

FIGURE 1.12 Translation. AUG codes for methionine, which always starts the translation of any protein. Source: *Modified from Figure 3.9 in J. E. Hall. (2016).* Guyton and Hall's textbook of medical physiology *(13th ed.). Elsevier, p. 32.*

Postsynthetic processing begins in the endoplasmic reticulum and continues as hormone precursors are translocated to the Golgi apparatus for final processing and packagingfor export. Processing begins even as the peptide chain is still elongating and includes cleavage to remove the signal peptide (Fig. 1.13). Interactions with intrinsic endoplasmic reticulum proteins facilitate proper folding and catalyze the formation of disulfide bonds linking cysteine residues. Other processing of peptide hormones may include glycosylation (addition of carbohydrate chains to asparagine residues) or coupling of subunits that are products of different genes, as seen with the pituitary glycoproteins (see Chapter 2: Pituitary Gland). Glycosylation begins in the endoplasmic reticulum and is completed in the Golgi complex, but final processing of peptide chains takes place in the secretory granules (Fig. 1.14).

The hormones, along with trypsin-like peptidases called hormone convertases, carboxypeptidase, amidating enzymes, and other peptide processing enzymes, are packaged into immature secretory vesicles that bud off from the *trans* face of the Golgi stacks (see Figs. 1.15 and 1.16).

Other proteins that are incorporated into secretory vesicles include one or more proteins of the family of

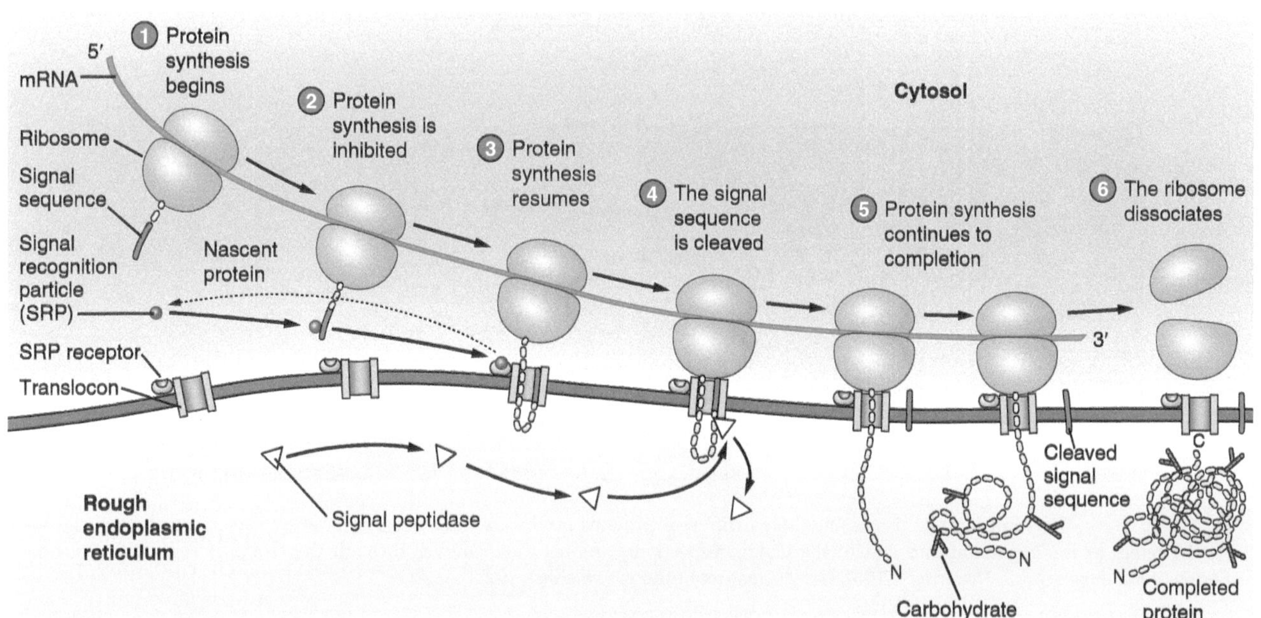

FIGURE 1.13 Synthesis and translocation into the rough endoplasmic reticulum cisterna of a protein hormone. Source: *Redrawn from Figure 2-15 in Boron, W. F., & Boulpaep, E. L. (2017).* Medical physiology *(3rd ed.). Elsevier, p. 29.*

(cont'd)

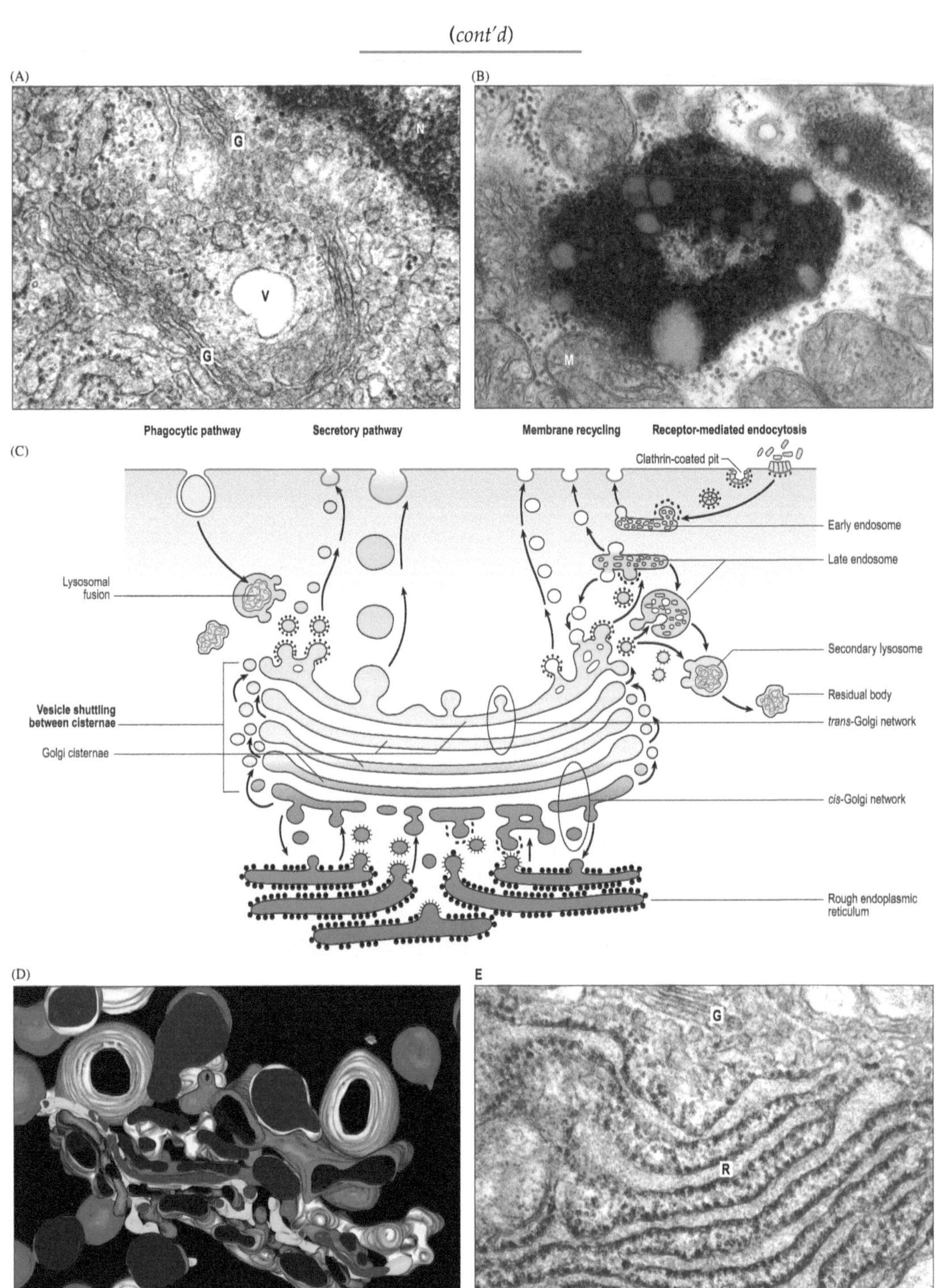

FIGURE 1.14 Posttranslational processing. Many different proteins go through the Golgi apparatus. The *cis* and *trans* Golgi networks refers to the beginning and end of the Golgi, respectively. As a protein moves through the Golgi, it is modified further. Source: *From Figure 1.5 S. Standring. (2016).* Gray's anatomy *(41st ed.). Elsevier, p. 6.*

secretogranins. These large acidic proteins contribute to the sorting of hormone into the immature vesicles, facilitate cleavage reactions at appropriate sites in the prohormone, and organize condensation of the hormone and associated proteins into dense granules. Proton pumps in the vesicle membrane acidify vesicular fluid, which

(cont'd)

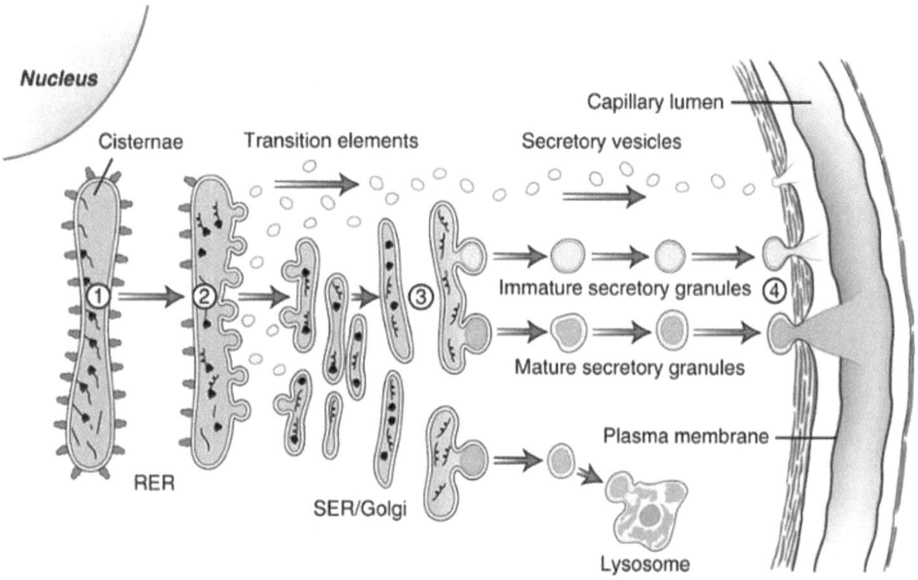

FIGURE 1.15 Steps in the posttranslational production of protein hormones. *RER*, Rough endoplasmic reticulum; *SER/Golgi*, smooth endoplasmic reticulum/Golgi apparatus. Source: *From Figure 3-1 in Melmed, S., Polonsky, K. S., Larson, P. R., & Kronenberg, H. M. (2016).* William's textbook of endocrinology *(13th ed.). Elsevier, p. 20.*

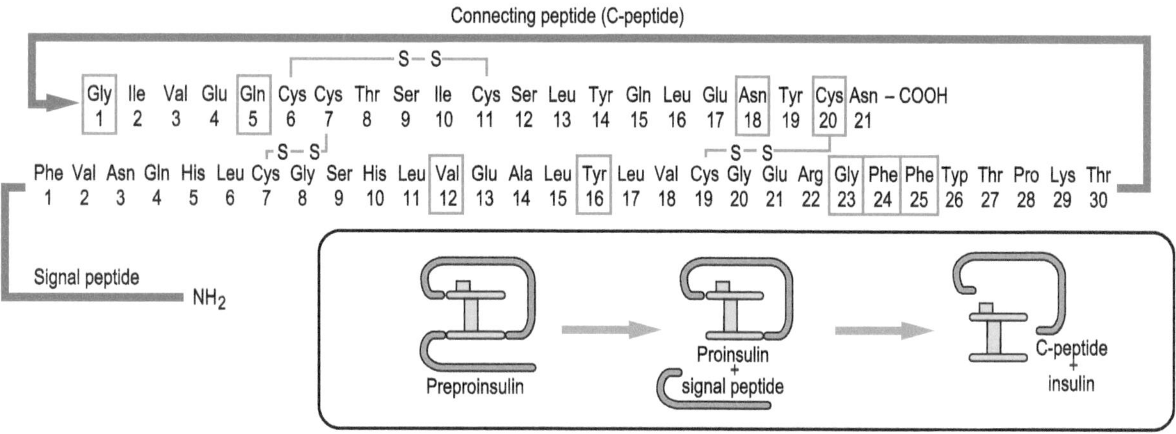

FIGURE 1.16 Showing posttranslational modification of preproinsulin. Boxes around amino acids indicate those involved in binding to the insulin receptor. Source: *From Figure 21.2. J. W. Baynes, & M. H. Dominiczak. (2019).* Medical biochemistry *(5th ed.). Elsevier, p. 445*

activates convertases and promotes extrusion of water. Cleavage of the prohormones removes those amino acid sequences that may have functioned to target the peptides to the secretory granules or to orient folding of the molecule so that disulfide bridges form in the right places. Cleavage of the prohormones by hormone convertases may yield more than one biologically active peptide from a single precursor, as seen with the adrenal corticotropic hormone and glucagon families of hormones (see Chapter 2: Pituitary Gland,

(*cont'd*)

and Chapter 6: Hormones of the Gastrointestinal Tract). Amidation of the carboxyl terminus using glycine as the amino donor is a common feature of the final maturation of many hormones. Because these processing reactions take place in secretory granules, peptide fragments, enzymes and fragments of the secretogranins, and other molecules are secreted along with the hormone. Incompletely processed or intact prohormones also escape into the circulation, sometimes in large amounts. This situation may be indicative of hyperactivity of endocrine cells or even aberrant production of hormone by nonendocrine tumor cells. Some prohormones have biological activity, and their effects may be the first manifestation of neoplasia. Some rare inherited diseases are attributable to defects in processing of normal precursor molecules. Fig. 1.16 shows the posttranslational modification of insulin.

Postsynthetic processing to the final biologically active form is not limited to the peptide hormones. Other hormones may be formed from their precursors after secretion. Postsecretory transformations to more active forms may occur in liver, kidney, fat, or blood, as well as in the target tissues themselves. For example, thyroxine, the major secretory product of the thyroid gland, is converted extrathyroidally to triiodothyronine, which is the biologically active form of the hormone (see Chapter 3: Thyroid Gland). Testosterone, the male hormone, is converted to the more active dihydrotestosterone within some target tissues and may even be converted to the female hormone, estrogen, in other tissues (see Chapter 12: Hormonal Control of Reproduction in the Male). These peripheral transformations, besides confounding the student of endocrinology, are additional sites that are vulnerable to derangement and hence must be considered as possible causes of endocrine disease.

Storage and release of hormones

Protein-derived hormones are stored in large amounts in their gland of origin so they can be released in large quantities in emergencies. While slower to have an effect than a purely nervous system response, their effect is more sustained so will continue after the immediate emergency has passed. This provides insurance against resurgence of the emergency need. Some of these protein hormone-secreting glands are neuron-derived and so the hormones are often thought of as modified neurotransmitters. Oxytocin, vasopressin, epinephrine, and norepinephrine are examples. Norepinephrine is a common neurotransmitter in the nervous system. But as a product of the adrenal medulla, it is released into the extracellular space and diffuses from there into the capillaries and so is considered a hormone. Epinephrine, too, can be found as a neurotransmitter in some parts of the brain but is considered a hormone when released from the adrenal medulla.

Some protein-derived hormones, such as thyroxin and triiodothyronine, collectively called thyroid hormone, are transported in the blood bound to proteins in the albumin fraction. Others, such as epinephrine and norepinephrine, are water-soluble and are not bound to a carrier protein.

Steroid hormones are derived from cholesterol that is either taken up from the blood or synthesized de novo within the gland or tissue. Once formed, the steroid hormones are released instead of being stored. Being insoluble in water, steroid hormones are transported in blood proteins. Hormones of the adrenal cortex, ovary, and testes fall into this category.

An exception to single endocrine gland synthesis is calcitriol, also known as vitamin D hormone, which is synthesized in a series of steps involving multiple organs (Fig. 1.17).

The first step is in the skin in the presence of a band of the ultraviolet spectrum of sunlight, in which cholecalciferol is produced from 7-dehydrocholesterol. This is transported in the blood to the liver where a hydroxy (–OH) group is added to form 25-hydroxycholecalciferol. This travels in the blood to the kidneys where, in the presence of parathormone from the parathyroid glands, a second hydroxy group is enzymatically added to form 1,25-dihydroxycholecalciferol, better known as calcitriol or vitamin D hormone. This acts on intestinal epithelial cells to take up calcium and on osteocytes to cause the reabsorption of noncrystallized (labile) bone, resulting in calcium being released into the blood. If parathormone is not present in the kidney, then 24,25-dihydroxycholecalciferol is formed. Just placing the –OH group at the 24 instead of the 1 position makes the steroid virtually inactive.

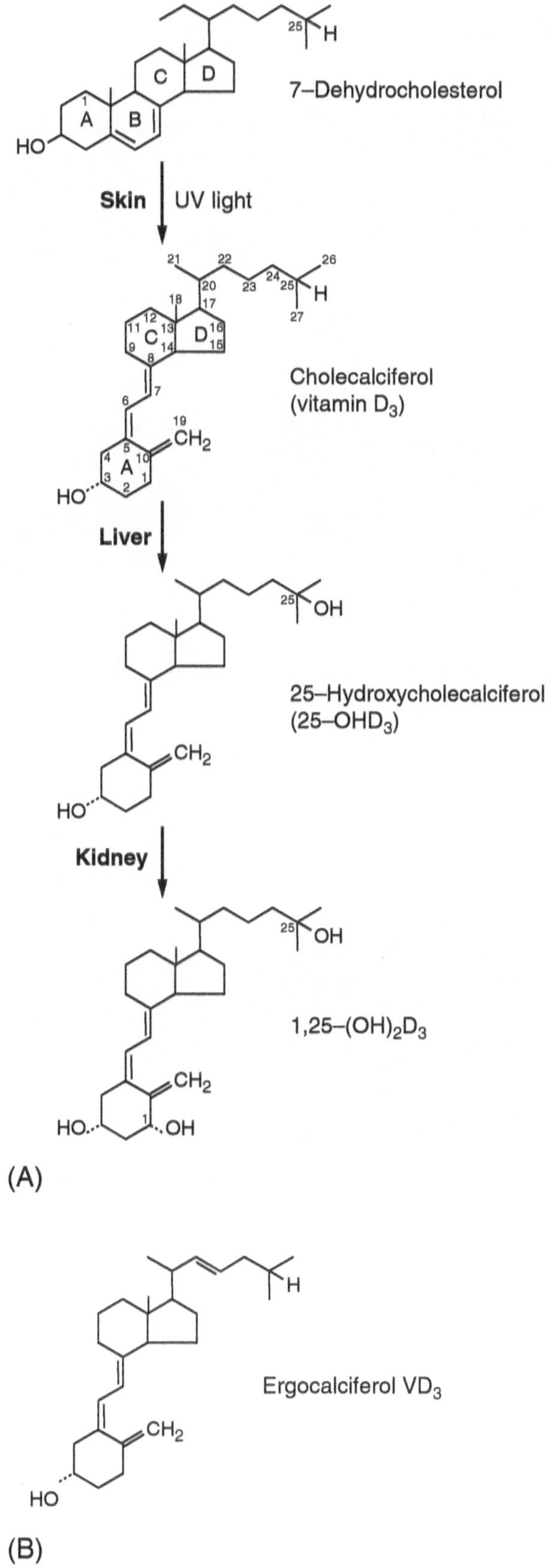

FIGURE 1.17 The stepwise synthesis of calcitriol (vitamin D hormone) from 7-dehyrocholesterol. Source: *Redrawn from Figure 52-9 in Boron, W. F., & Boulpaep, E. L. (2017).* Medical physiology *(3rd ed.). Elsevier, p. 1064.*

At the molecular level (boxed material for additional information)

Release of hormones

Protein and peptide hormones and the tyrosine derivatives, epinephrine and norepinephrine, are stored as dense granules in membrane-bound vesicles and are secreted in response to an external stimulus by the process of exocytosis (Fig. 1.18). Exocytosis can be considered to occur in several stages: (1) recruitment of vesicles to the plasma membrane, (2) tethering or docking to

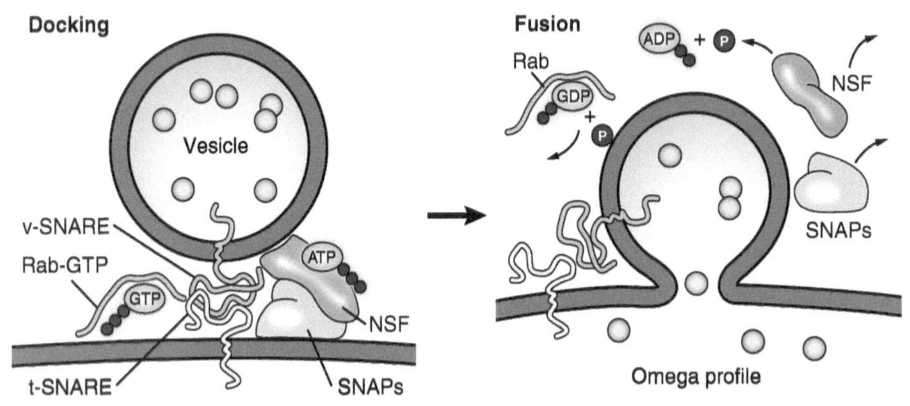

FIGURE 1.18 Exocytosis. Source: *From Figure 2-19 in Boron, W. F., & Boulpaep, E. L. (2017).* Medical physiology *(3rd ed.). Elsevier, p. 36.*

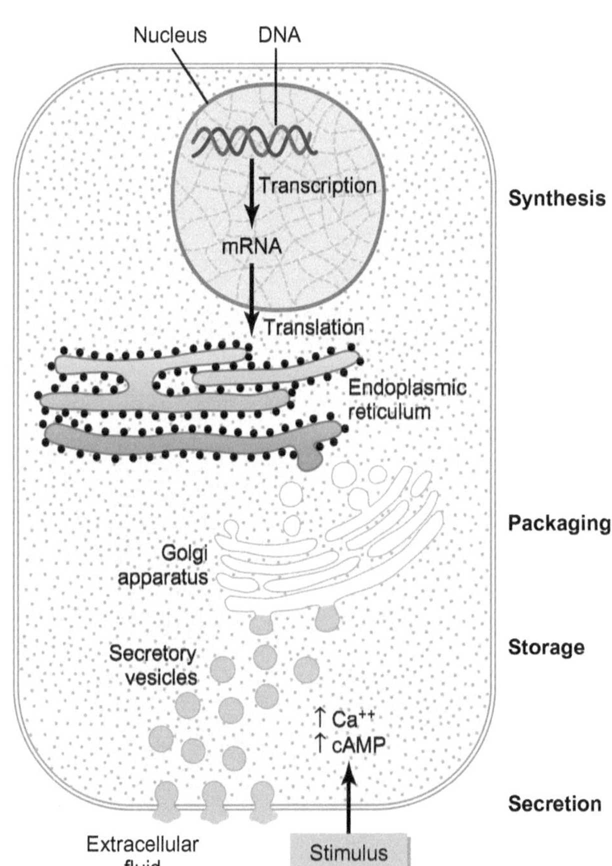

FIGURE 1.19 Exocytosis in detail. Source: *From Figure 75-2 in John E. Hall, Saunders (2016). Guyton and Hall Textbook of Medical Physiology (13th ed.), p. 926.*

(cont'd)

appropriate membrane loci, (3) priming in preparation for (4) fusion of the vesicular membrane with the plasma membrane to form a secretory pore that dilates to allow the vesicular contents to escape into the extracellular fluid, and (5) retrieval of the vesicular membrane by endocytosis to membrane by endocytosis to prevent an unsustainable increase in membrane surface that would otherwise occur.

Intrinsic proteins in the membranes of the vesicles and the plasma membranes called SNAREs (soluble *N*-ethylmaleimide-sensitive factor attachment protein receptor) govern all stages. The human genome encodes 36 SNARE proteins, which are found in all secretory cells and neurons. SNARE proteins in vesicular membranes help to target vesicles to appropriate loci in the plasma membrane. Most secretory vesicles reside deep in the cytosol and are recruited to the plasma membrane by calcium-dependent translocation along microtubules and microfilaments. A subset of secretory vesicles, called the readily releasable pool, is docked just below the plasma membranes tethered to the submembranous cytoskeleton by proteins (see Fig. 1.19). Vesicles are primed for secretion by an energy-dependent mechanism in which SNAREs in the vesicular membrane form loose attachments to partnering SNAREs in the cell membrane. A surge in intracellular free calcium, produced by the activation of calcium channels, triggers a conformational change in the SNARE complex that pulls the vesicular and plasma membranes into such close apposition that fusion occurs. As the fusion pore enlarges, the vesicle ultimately everts and unloads its cargo into the extracellular space.

Hormone transportation and fate

Most hormones circulate in blood in free solution at low, nanomolar (10−9 M) or even picomolar (10−12 M), concentrations. Steroid and thyroid hormones have limited solubility in water and so are bound to carrier proteins synthesized by the liver. Some protein and peptide hormones also circulate complexed with specific binding proteins (see Chapter 11: Hormonal Control of Growth, and Chapter 14: Hormonal Control of Pregnancy and Lactation). Bound hormones are in equilibrium with a small fraction, sometimes less than 1%, of free hormone in plasma. Only free hormones cross the capillary endothelium to reach their sites of action. Protein binding prevents renal loss of hormone by filtration and slows the rate of hormone biotransformation by decreasing cellular uptake. Bound proteins may affect hormonal responses by facilitating or impeding delivery of hormones to cells. Biological responses are related to the concentration of hormone reaching target cells, rather than the total amount present in blood. Increases in blood binding proteins during pregnancy or decreases due to liver or kidney disease can produce changes in total amounts of hormones circulating in blood even though free concentrations may be normal.

Most hormones are destroyed rapidly after secretion and have a half-life in blood of less than 10 minutes. The half-life is the time needed for its concentration to be reduced by half and depends on its rate of biotransformation (metabolism) and on the rapidity with which it can equilibrate with fluids in extravascular compartments. Epinephrine has a half-life of seconds, whereas thyroid hormone has a half-life of days. The half-life of a hormone is different from its duration of action. Some hormonal effects are produced instantaneously and may disappear as rapidly. Other hormonal effects occur after a lag time of minutes or hours, and the time of maximum response may have no relation to the hormone concentration in the blood.

The time it takes for a hormonal response to decrease may be from a few seconds to several days. Some responses persist after hormonal concentrations have returned to basal levels. Understanding a hormone dose–response curve over time and the onset and duration of action are important for an understanding of normal physiology, endocrine disease, and the limitations of hormone therapy.

In any regulatory system involving hormones or any other signal is the necessity for the signal to disappear once the appropriate information has been conveyed. Only a small amount of hormone is degraded as an aftermath to the process of signaling its biological effects. The remainder must be inactivated and excreted. Inactivation of hormones occurs enzymatically in cells, blood or intercellular spaces in the liver, kidney, and target cells. Degradation of peptide and protein hormones often involves uptake into cells by endocytosis that delivers them to cellular sites of degradation, the lysosomes and proteasomes (see Fig. 1.20). Inactivation may involve complete metabolism of the hormone so that no recognizable product appears in urine, or it

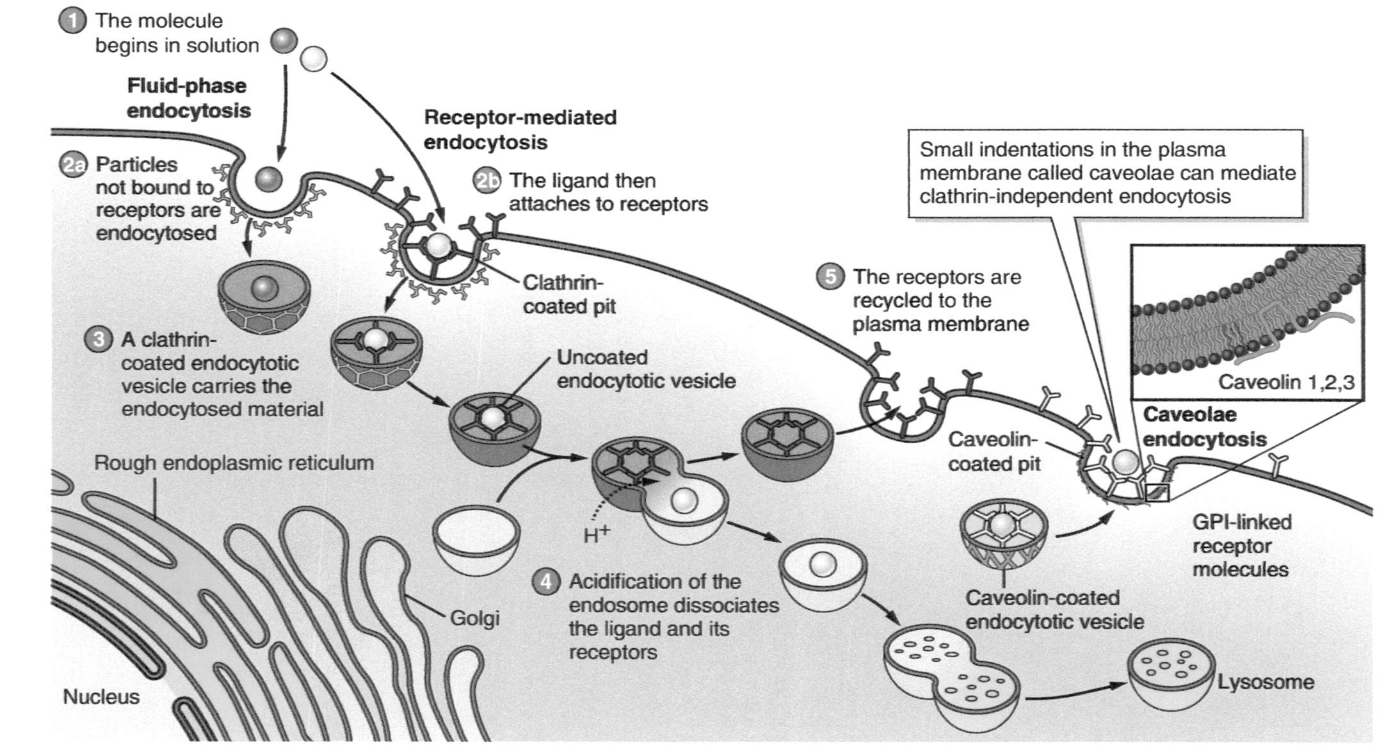

FIGURE 1.20 Endocytosis of hormones. Source: *Redrawn from Figure 2-22 in Boron, W. F., & Boulpaep, E. L. (2017).* Medical physiology *(3rd ed.). Elsevier, p. 41.*

may be limited to some simple one- or two-step process such as addition of a methyl group or glucuronic acid. In the latter cases, recognizable degradation products are found in urine and can be measured to obtain a crude index of the rate of hormone production.

The ultimate mission of a hormone is to change the activity of target cells. Cellular activity is determined by the genes that are expressed to carry out cellular functions, including cellular structure. Hormonal messages must be converted to biochemical events that influence gene expression, biochemical reaction rates, and structural changes. Conversion of a hormonal message to cellular responses is called signal transduction and the series of biochemical changes that are set in motion are described as signaling pathways, although a signaling network might be a more accurate descriptor, as pathways branch and converge only to branch again. Signal transduction is a complex topic and the focus of intense investigation in many laboratories around the world. Detailed consideration is beyond the scope of this text. Instead, only general patterns of signal transduction are considered in the following section, but the topic will be revisited where appropriate in subsequent chapters in discussing individual hormones.

Hormone specificity

Because all hormones travel in blood from their glands of origin to their target tissues, all cells are exposed to all kinds of hormones. Yet under normal circumstances, cells respond only to hormones for which the cell has a receptor. A hormone receptor is a molecule or complex of molecules inside of or on the surface of a cell that binds its hormone resulting in a molecular change, which initiates a characteristic response or group of responses. The mechanisms by which receptors operate and are regulated are not unique to endocrinology.

Hormone receptors

Characteristics of receptors

Hormone receptors are proteins or glycoproteins that are able to

- distinguish a hormone from other molecules that may have very similar structures,
- bind to the hormone (sometimes called a ligand) even when its concentration is exceedingly low (10–8–10–12 M),
- undergo a conformational change when bound to the hormone, and
- catalyze biochemical events or transmit changes in molecular conformation to adjacent molecules that produce a biochemical change.

The receptor may be a single molecule or in a subunit of a receptor complex. A hormone activates a receptor by binding to it. Any biochemical change initiated by the activated receptor is due to the properties of the receptor and not of the hormone. Under some pathophysiological conditions an aberrant antibody may react with a receptor and produce a disease state that is indistinguishable from the disease that results from the overproduction of the hormone. Hormone receptors are found on the surface, in the cytosol, or in the nucleus of target cells. Transmembrane receptors span the thickness of the cell membrane, with the hormone-binding molecule on the outer surface. Receptor molecules on the cytosolic face of the membrane communicate with other membrane or cytosolic proteins. *Trans* membrane receptors may be distributed over the entire surface or they may be confined to some microinvaginations called caveolae (Fig. 1.20).

Usually, only a few thousand receptor molecules are present in a target cell. Cells can change the number of receptors, and their responsiveness to hormones as physiological events warrant (see Chapter 5: Principles of Hormone Integration). Some receptors may be expressed only at a certain stage in the life of a cell or as a consequence of stimulation by other hormones. Often cells adjust the number of receptors they express with the amount of signal that activates them. Frequent or intense stimulation may cause a cell to downregulate (decrease) the number of receptors expressed. Conversely, cells may upregulate receptors in the face of rare or absent stimulation or in response to other signals.

Membrane receptors are internalized either alone or bound to their hormones (receptor-mediated endocytosis) and, like other cellular proteins, are broken down and replaced many times over during the lifetime of a cell. Adjustments in the relative rates of receptor synthesis or degradation may result in either up- or downregulation of receptors. Cells can also up- or downregulate receptor function through reversible covalent modifications such as adding or removing phosphate groups. Membrane-associated receptors cycle between the plasma membrane and internal membranes, and their relative abundance on the cell surface can be adjusted by reversibly sequestering them in intracellular vesicles.

Although the mammalian organism expresses literally thousands of different receptor molecules that subserve a wide variety of functions in addition to endocrine signaling, there are relatively few general patterns of signaling. Based upon the nucleotide sequence and organization of their genes and the structure of their proteins, receptors, like other proteins, can be organized into families or superfamilies that presumably arose from the same ancient progenitor gene. Even for distantly related receptors, the general features of signal transduction follow common broad outlines that are seen with families of molecules that receive and transduce signals in eukaryotic cells of species ranging from yeast to humans.

Hormonal actions mediated by intracellular receptors

The cholesterol derivatives (steroid and vitamin D hormones) are lipid-soluble and enter cells by diffusion through the lipid bilayer of the plasma membrane. Thyroid hormones, which are α-amino acids, have large nonpolar constituents and may penetrate cell membranes by diffusion, but carrier-mediated transport appears to be the primary means of entry (see Fig. 1.21).

These hormones bind to receptors that are located in the cell nucleus or cytoplasm and produce most of their effects by altering rates of gene expression. Receptors bound to steroid hormones, in turn, bind to specific nucleotide sequences in DNA (deoxyribonucleic acid), called hormone response elements (HREs), located upstream of the transcription start sites of the genes they regulate. The end result of stimulation with these hormones is a change in genomic readout, which may be expressed in the formation of new proteins or modification of the rates of synthesis of proteins already in production.

Intracellular hormone receptors belong to a very large family of transcription factors found throughout the animal kingdom. Genes for 48 members of this family have been identified in the human genome. Many of these are called orphan receptors because their ligands have not yet been identified. The most highly conserved region of nuclear receptors is a stretch of about 65–70 amino acid residues that constitutes the DNA-binding domain. This region contains one or two molecules of zinc, each coordinated with four or six cysteine residues, respectively, so that two loops of about 12 amino acids each are formed. These so-called zinc fingers can insert in a half-turn of the DNA helix and grasp the DNA at the site of the HRE (Fig. 1.22).

The hormone-binding domain, which is near the carboxyl terminus, also contains amino acid sequences that are necessary for the activation of transcription. Between the DNA-binding domain and the amino terminus is the so-called hypervariable region, which, as

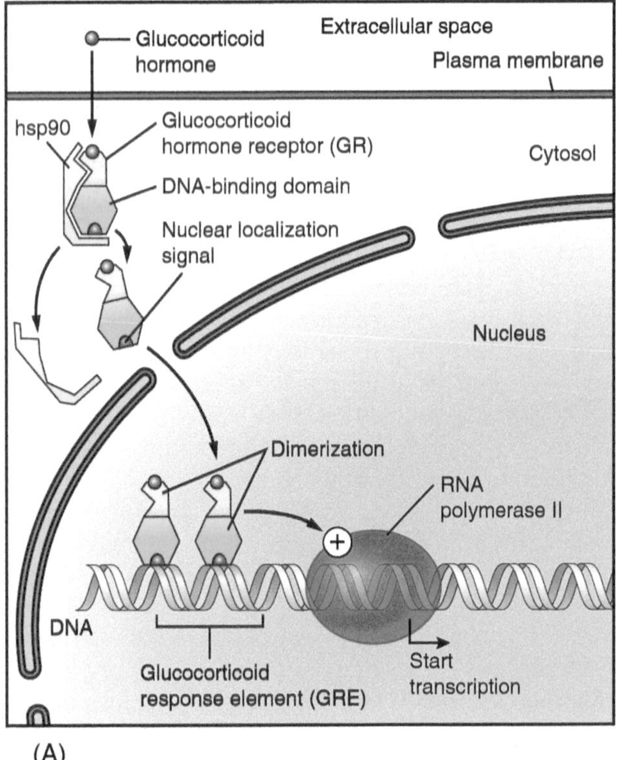

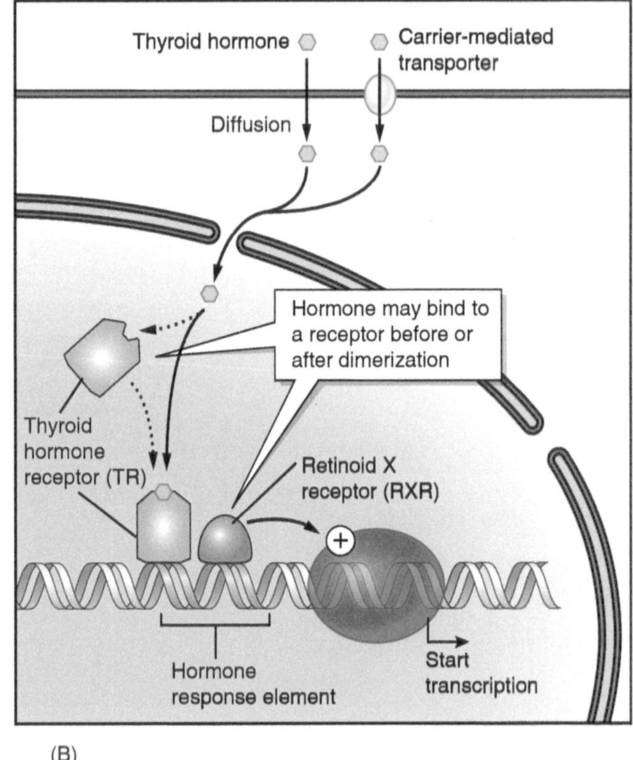

FIGURE 1.21 Transcriptional activation by a steroid and by thyroid hormone. Source: *Redrawn from Figure 4-15 in Boron, W. F., & Boulpaep, E. L. (2017).* Medical physiology *(3rd ed.). Elsevier, p. 92.*

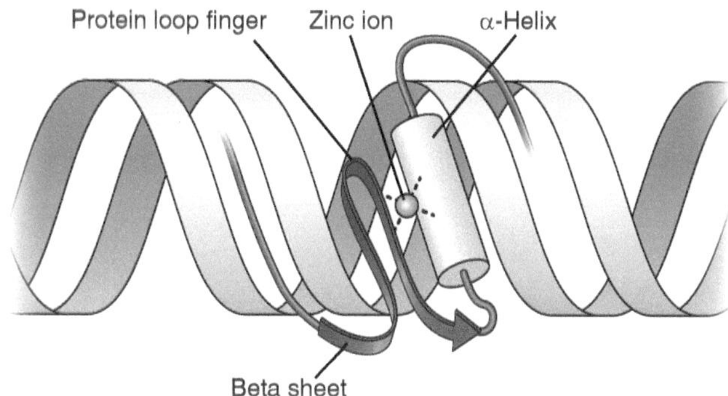

FIGURE 1.22 In this image of a zinc finger in an HRE, one zinc ion coordinates with two residues on the α-helix and two residues on the beta sheet to form the protein loop known as a finger. The finger is composed of 30 amino acids. *HRE*, Hormone response element. Source: *Redrawn from Figure 4-9 in Boron, W. F., & Boulpaep, E. L. (2017).* Medical physiology *(3rd ed.). Elsevier, p. 83.*

its name implies, differs both in size and amino acid sequence for each receptor.

The steroid hormone receptors constitute a closely related group within the family. In the unstimulated state, steroid hormone receptors are noncovalently complexed with other proteins (Fig. 1.23), including a dimer of the 90,000 Da heat shock protein (Hsp 90) that attaches adjacent to the hormone-binding domain (Fig. 1.23).

Heat shock proteins are abundant cellular proteins that are found in prokaryotes and all eukaryotic cells and are so named because their synthesis abruptly increases when cells are exposed to high temperature or other stressful conditions. These proteins are thought to keep the receptor in a configuration that is favorable for binding the hormone and incapable of binding to DNA. Binding to its hormone causes the receptor to dissociate from Hsp 90 and the other proteins. The bound receptor then forms a dimer with another liganded receptor molecule and undergoes a conformational change that increases its affinity for binding to DNA. After binding to the DNA the receptor dimers recruit other nuclear regulatory proteins, including coactivators, that facilitate uncoiling of the DNA to make it accessible to the ribonucleic acid (RNA) polymerase complex. Receptors for at least four different steroid hormones bind to the identical HRE, and yet each governs expression of a unique complement of genes. Expression of genes that are specific for each hormone is determined by which receptor is present in a particular cell, by the cohort of nuclear transcription factors, coactivators, and corepressors that are available to complex with the receptor in that cell, and by the characteristics of the regulatory components in the DNA (Fig. 1.24).

Receptors for thyroid hormone and vitamin D and compounds related to vitamin A (retinoic acid) belong to another closely related group within the same

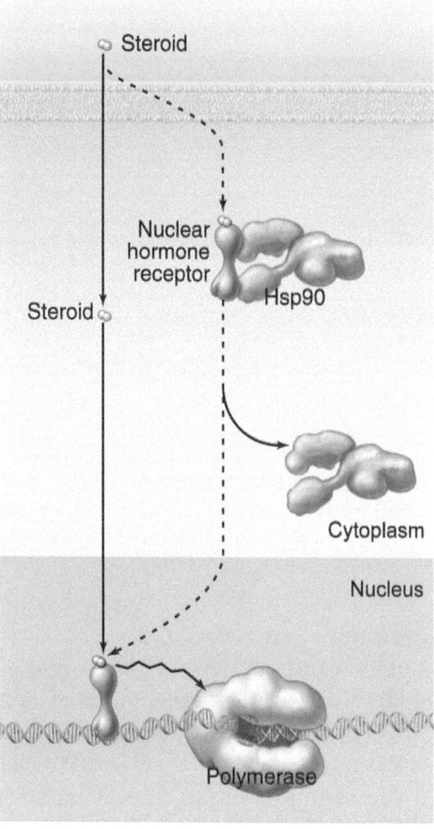

FIGURE 1.23 Steroid hormone receptors. Estrogens bind to Hsp 90, while other steroids go directly to the nucleus. Source: *From Figure 10.21 A in T. D. Pollard, et al. (2017).* Cell biology *(3rd ed.). Elsevier, p. 185.*

family of proteins as the steroid hormone receptors. Unlike the steroid hormone receptors, these receptors are bound to their HREs in DNA even in the absence of hormone and do not form complexes with Hsp 90. In further distinction from the receptors for steroid hormones, receptors for thyroid hormone and vitamin D may bind to DNA either as homodimers or as heterodimers formed with a receptor for 9-*cis* retinoic acid, often called the RXR receptor. In the absence of ligand, these DNA-bound receptors form complexes with other nuclear proteins that may promote or inhibit transcription. Upon binding its hormone, the receptor undergoes a conformational change that displaces the associated proteins and allows others to bind with the result that transcription is either activated or suppressed (Fig. 1.24).

Many steps lie between the activation of transcription and changes in cellular behavior. These include synthesis and processing of RNA, exporting it to cytosolic sites of protein synthesis, protein synthesis itself, protein processing, and delivery of the newly formed proteins to appropriate loci within the cells. These reactions necessarily occur sequentially and each takes

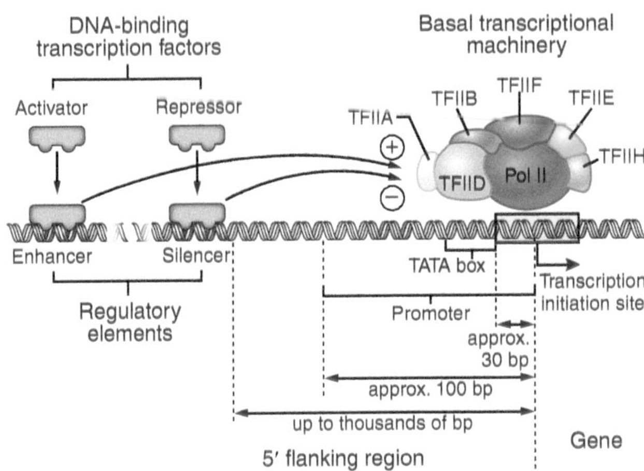

FIGURE 1.24 The basal transcriptional machinery regulates DNA transcription, showing the regulatory elements, the promotor region, and the gene itself. Pol II, RNA polymerase II. There are six general transcription factors, named TFIIA, TFIIB, TFIID, TFIIE, TFIIF, and TFIIH; transcription factors IIA, IIB, IIE, etc.; TATA, thymine/adenine box that is part of the promotor region. *DNA*, Deoxyribonucleic acid; *RNA*, ribonucleic acid. Source: *Redrawn from Figure 4-6 in Boron, W. F., & Boulpaep, E. L. (2017).* Medical physiology *(3rd ed.). Elsevier, p. 79.*

time. Transcription proceeds at a rate of about 40 nucleotides per second, so that transcribing a gene that contains 10,000 nucleotides takes almost 5 minutes. Processing the pre-RNA to mature messenger RNA (mRNA) is even slower, so that nearly 20 minutes elapse from the time RNA synthesis is initiated to the time the mRNA exits the nucleus. Protein synthesis is much faster. About 15 amino acids per second are added to the growing peptide chain. All factors considered, changes in cellular behavior that result from steroid hormone action usually are not seen for at least 30 minutes after entry of the hormone into the cells. The final protein makeup of the cell at any time thereafter is also determined by rates of RNA and protein degradation. A complete catalog of which proteins are formed in any particular cell type because of hormone action should become available soon thanks to the successful completion of the Human Genome Project and the technology that permits screening of the entire library of mRNA expressed within a cell. Gaining an understanding of the physiological role of each of these proteins will take a bit longer.

As blood levels decline, intracellular concentrations of hormone decline. Because binding is reversible, hormones dissociate from receptors and are cleared from the cell by diffusion into the extracellular fluid, usually after metabolic conversion to an inactive form. Unloaded steroid receptors dissociate from their DNA-binding sites and regulatory proteins and either recycle into new complexes with Hsp 90 and other proteins through some energy-dependent process or are degraded and replaced by new synthesis. RNA transcripts of hormone-sensitive genes are degraded usually within minutes to hours of their formation. Without continued hormonal stimulation of their synthesis, RNA templates for hormone-dependent proteins disappear, and the proteins they encode can no longer be formed. The proteins are degraded with half-lives that may range from seconds to days. Thus, just as there is delay in onset, effects of the hormones that act through nuclear receptors may persist after the hormone has been cleared from the cell.

Accumulating evidence indicates that hormones that once were thought to act only through nuclear receptors produce some rapid effects that are independent of changes in gene expression. For the most part the rapid responses that are produced are complementary to the delayed genomically mediated responses. It is likely that other, yet to be identified, receptors for these hormones are present on the cell surface or that some nuclear receptors are expressed on the cell surface as well as internally.

Hormonal actions mediated by surface receptors

The protein and peptide hormones and the amine derivatives of tyrosine cannot readily diffuse across the plasma membranes of their target cells. These hormones produce their effects by binding to receptors on the cell surface and rely on molecules on the cytosolic side of the membrane to convey the signal to the appropriate intracellular effector sites that bring about the hormonal response. There are two receptor types that involve cytoplasmic changes: G-protein-coupled receptors and catalytic receptors.

The G-protein-coupled receptors

The most frequently encountered cell surface receptors belong to a very large superfamily of proteins that couple with guanosine nucleotide-binding proteins (G-proteins) to communicate with intracellular effector molecules. This ancient superfamily of receptor molecules is widely expressed throughout eukaryotic phyla. G-protein-coupled receptors are crucial for sensing signals in the external environment such as light, taste, and odor as well as signals transmitted by hormones. G-protein-coupled receptors receive signals carried by a wide range of neurotransmitters, immune modulators, and paracrine factors. More than 1000 different G-protein-coupled receptors may be expressed in humans. About 30% of all effective pharmaceutical agents are said to target actions mediated by receptors in this superfamily and account for about two-thirds of the prescriptions written by physicians.

All G-protein-coupled receptors are composed of single strands of protein and contain seven stretches of about 25 amino acids that each form membrane-spanning α-helices (Fig. 1.25).

The single long peptide chain that constitutes the receptor thus threads through the membrane seven times creating three extracellular and three intracellular loops. For this reason, these receptors are sometimes called heptahelical receptors. The amino terminal tail is extracellular and along with the external loops may contain covalently bound carbohydrate. The carboxyl tail lies within the cytoplasm. The lengths of the loops and the carboxyl and amino terminal tails vary in characteristic ways among the different families and subfamilies of these receptors. Outward-facing components of the receptor, including parts of the α-helices, contribute to the hormone recognition and binding site. The cytosolic loops and carboxyl tail bind to specific G-proteins near the interface of the membrane and the cytosol.

G-proteins are heterotrimers that comprise α-, β-, and γ-subunits. Lipid moieties covalently attached to the α- and γ-subunits insert into the inner leaflet of the plasma membrane bilayer and tether the G-proteins to the membrane. The α-subunits are enzymes (GTPases) that catalyze the conversion of guanosine triphosphate (GTP) to guanosine diphosphate (GDP) (Fig. 1.26).

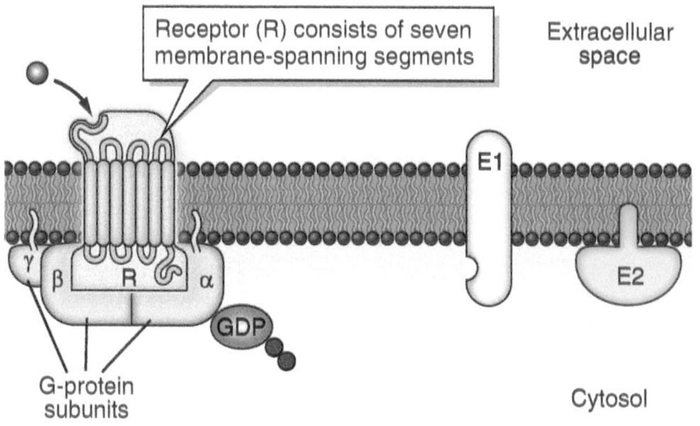

FIGURE 1.25 In step 1, this is the G-protein receptor showing the seven membrane-spanning segments and the hormone interacting with the receptor. Source: *Redrawn from Figure 3-4 in Boron, W. F., & Boulpaep, E. L. (2017).* Medical physiology *(3rd ed.). Elsevier, p. 54.*

In the inactivated or resting state, the catalytic site in the α-subunit is occupied by GDP. When the receptor binds to its hormone, a conformational change transmitted across the membrane allows its cytosolic domain to interact with the α-subunit of the G-protein in a way that causes the α-subunit to release the GDP in exchange for a molecule of GTP, and to dissociate from the βγ-subunits, which remain tightly bound to each other (Fig. 1.27).

Though tethered to the membrane, the dissociated subunits can move laterally along the inner surface of the membrane. In its GTP-bound state the α-subunit interacts

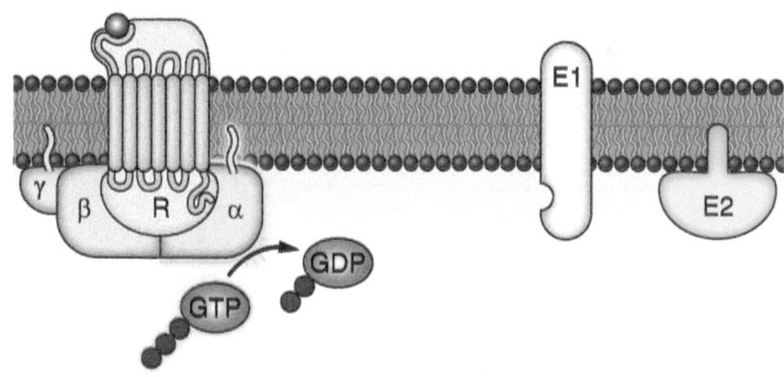

FIGURE 1.26 In step 2 the GTP is converted by GTPase (in the α-subunit) to GDP. *GDP*, Guanosine diphosphate; *GTP*, guanosine triphosphate. Source: *Redrawn from Figure 3-4 in Boron, W. F., & Boulpaep, E. L. (2017).* Medical physiology *(3rd ed.). Elsevier, p. 54.*

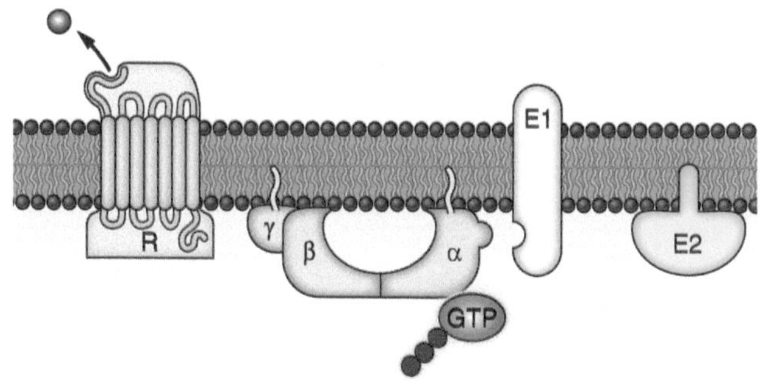

FIGURE 1.27 In step 3, the energy in GTP dissociates the G-protein from the receptor and changes its configuration. The hormone also leaves the receptor. *GTP*, Guanosine triphosphate. Source: *Redrawn from Figure 3-4 in Boron, W. F., & Boulpaep, E. L. (2017).* Medical physiology *(3rd ed.). Elsevier, p. 54.*

with and modifies the activity of membrane-associated enzymes that initiate the hormonal response (Fig. 1.28).

The liberated βγ-complex can also bind to cellular proteins and modify their activities, and both the free α-subunit and the βγ-subunits can bind to ion channel proteins and cause the channels to open or close (see Fig. 1.29).

Hydrolysis of GTP to GDP restores the resting state of the α-subunit allowing it to reassociate with the βγ-subunits to reconstitute the heterotrimer (see Fig. 1.30).

GTPase activity of the α-subunit is relatively slow. Consequently, the α-subunit may interact multiple times with effector enzymes before it returns to its resting state. In addition, because some G-proteins may be as much as one hundred times as abundant as the receptors they associate with, a single hormone-bound receptor may interact sequentially with multiple G-proteins before the hormone dissociates from the receptor. These characteristics provide mechanisms for amplification of the signal.

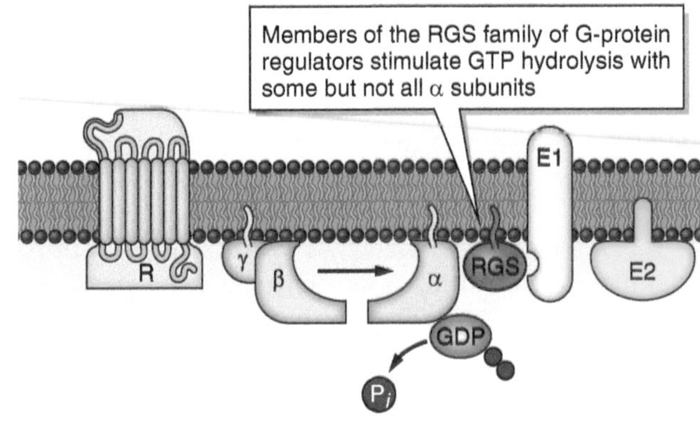

FIGURE 1.30 In step 6 (final step), inorganic phosphate is removed from GTP and the molecule becomes once again GDP. *GDP*, Guanosine diphosphate; *GTP*, guanosine triphosphate. Source: *Redrawn from Figure 3-4 in Boron, W. F., & Boulpaep, E. L. (2017).* Medical physiology *(3rd ed.). Elsevier, p. 54.*

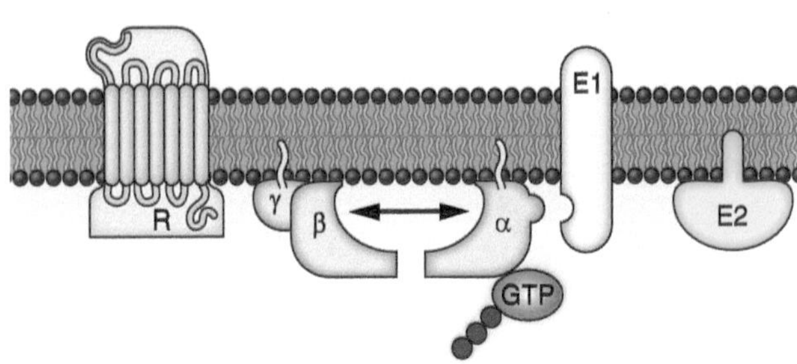

FIGURE 1.28 Instep 4, the α-GTP and the β- and γ-subunits dissociate. *GTP*, Guanosine triphosphate. Source: *Redrawn from Figure 3-4 in Boron, W. F., & Boulpaep, E. L. (2017).* Medical physiology *(3rd ed.). Elsevier, p. 54.*

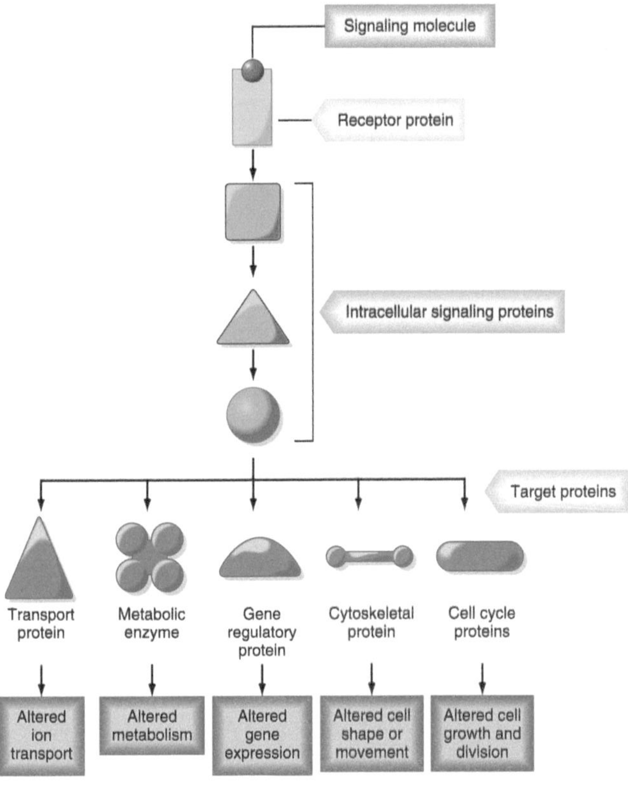

FIGURE 1.31 Diversification of the signal from a single hormone (signal molecule). Source: *From Figure 3.1 in Koeppen B. M., & Stanton B. W. (2018).* Berne and Levy's physiology *(7th ed.). Elsevier, p. 38.*

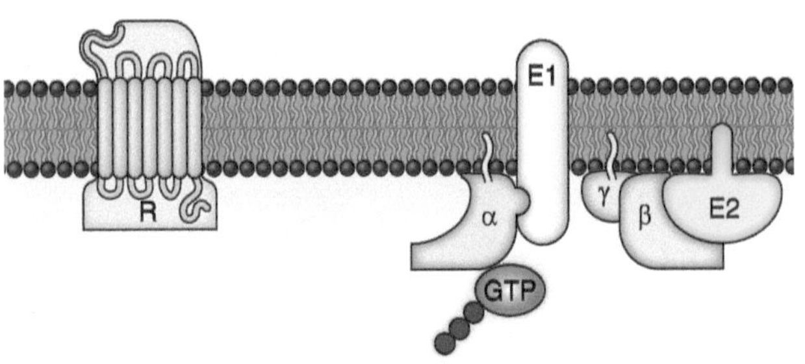

FIGURE 1.29 Step 5. Source: *Redrawn from Figure 3-4 in Boron, W. F., & Boulpaep, E. L. (2017).* Medical physiology *(3rd ed.). Elsevier, p. 54.*

The interaction of a single hormone molecule with a single receptor molecule may result in multiple signal-generating events within a cell (Fig. 1.31).

Once a signal combines with a receptor, it can be amplified and diversified within a cell so that a stronger signal with different effect can occur (Fig. 1.32).

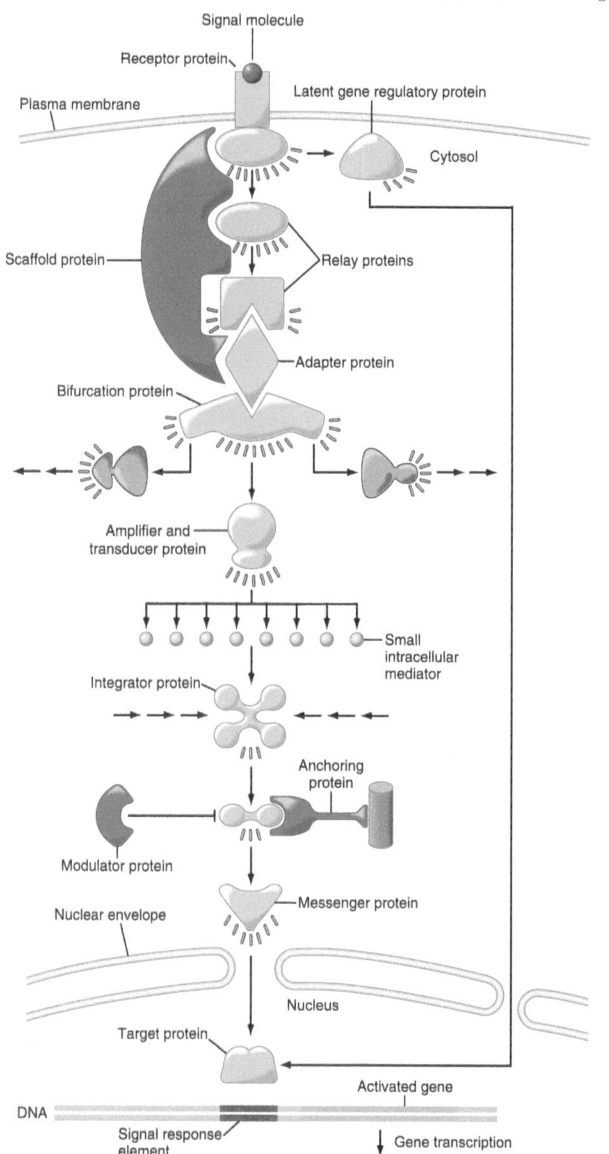

FIGURE 1.32 Illustrating different effects, with the pathway for one of those effects as a result of a hormone (signal molecule) interacting with a receptor. Source: *From Figure 3.7 in Koeppen B. M., & Stanton B. W. (2018).* Berne and Levy's physiology *(7th ed.). Elsevier, p. 43.*

Desensitization and downregulation of G-protein-coupled receptors

In addition to simple dissociation of hormone from its receptor, signaling often is terminated and receptors are desensitized to further stimulation by active cellular processes. G-protein-coupled receptors may be inactivated by phosphorylation of one of their intracellular loops catalyzed by G-protein receptor kinases. Phosphorylation uncouples the receptor from the α-subunit and promotes binding to a cytoplasmic protein of the β-arrestin family. Binding to β-arrestin may lead to receptor internalization and downregulation by sequestration in intracellular vesicles (Fig. 1.35). Sequestered receptors may recycle to the cell surface, or when cellular stimulation is prolonged, they may be degraded in lysosomes. β-Arrestins may have the additional function of serving as scaffolds for binding to a variety of other proteins, including the mitogen-activated protein (MAP) kinases (see later), and thereby provide a pathway for signaling between G-protein-coupled receptors and the nucleus (Fig. 1.35).

The second messenger concept

For a cell surface hormonal signal to be effective, it must be transmitted to the intracellular organelles and enzymes that produce the cellular response. To reach intracellular effectors, the G-protein-coupled receptors rely on intermediate molecules called second messengers, which are formed and/or released into the cytosol in response to hormonal stimulation (the first message). Second messengers activate intracellular enzymes and also amplify signals. A single hormone molecule interacting with a single receptor may result in the formation of tens or hundreds of second messenger molecules, each of which might activate an enzyme that in turn catalyzes the

At the molecular level (boxed material for additional information)

Classes of G-protein

At least three different classes of G-protein α-subunits are involved in transduction of hormonal signals. Each class includes the products of several closely related genes. α-Subunits of the "s" (stimulatory) class (Gαs) stimulate the transmembrane enzyme, adenylyl cyclase, to catalyze the synthesis of cyclic 3′,5′ adenosine monophosphate (cyclic AMP) from adenosine triphosphate, whereas α-subunits of the "i" (inhibitory) class (Gαi) inhibit the activity of adenylyl cyclase (Fig. 1.33).

α-Subunits belonging to the "q" class stimulate the activity of the membrane-bound enzyme phospholipase C-β, which catalyzes the hydrolysis of the membrane phospholipid, phosphatidylinositol 4,5-bisphosphate, to liberate inositol 1,4,5 trisphosphate (IP3) and diacylglycerol (DAG) (Fig. 1.34).

(*cont'd*)

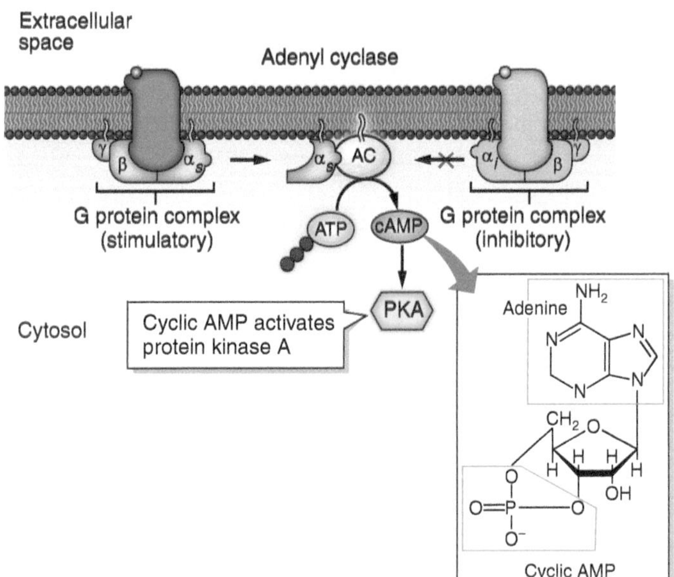

FIGURE 1.33 When α-s combines with adenyl cyclase, the effect is stimulatory; when αi combines with adenyl cyclase, the result is inhibitory. Source: *Redrawn from Figure 3-5 in Boron, W. F., & Boulpaep, E. L. (2017).* Medical physiology *(3rd ed.). Elsevier, p. 55.*

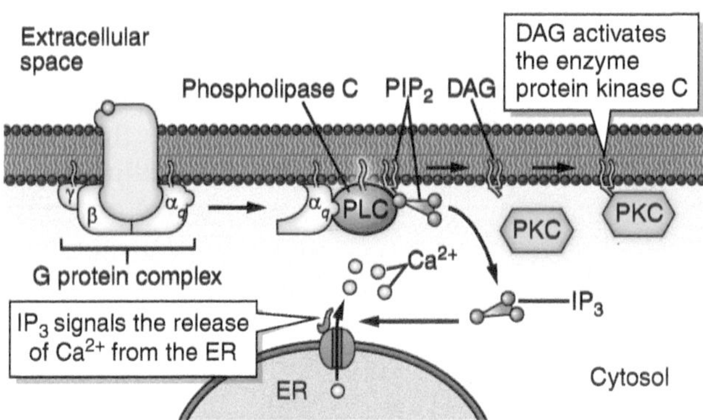

FIGURE 1.34 When αq combines with PLC, the PLC converts PIP2 to IP3 and DAG. Each of these, in turn, has different effects as illustrated, as for example, the IP3 release of calcium from the ER, the ER being the major storehouse for intracellular calcium. *DAG,* Diacylglycerol; *PIP2,* phosphatidyl inositol 4,5-bisphosphate; *PLC,* phospholipase C; *IP3,* inositol 1,4,5 triphosphate. Source: *Redrawn from Figure 3-5C in Boron, W. F., & Boulpaep, E. L. (2017).* Medical physiology *(3rd ed.). Elsevier, p. 55.*

The α-subunits of the heterotrimeric G-proteins are closely related to the small G-proteins that function as biochemical switches to regulate such processes as entry of proteins into the nucleus, sorting and trafficking of intracellular vesicles, and cytoskeletal rearrangements. There are 6 superfamilies of these small G-proteins, the most common is RAS (with over 100 members), which regulates cell proliferation. Like the α-subunits, the small G-proteins are GTPases that are in their active state when bound to GTP and in their inactive state when bound to GDP. Unlike the α-subunits, the small G-proteins do not interact directly with hormone receptors or associate with βγ-subunits. Instead of liganded receptors, the small G-proteins are activated by proteins called nucleotide exchange factors that cause them to dissociate from GDP and bind GTP. They remain activated as they slowly convert GTP to GDP, but inactivation can be accelerated by interaction with GTPase-activating proteins.

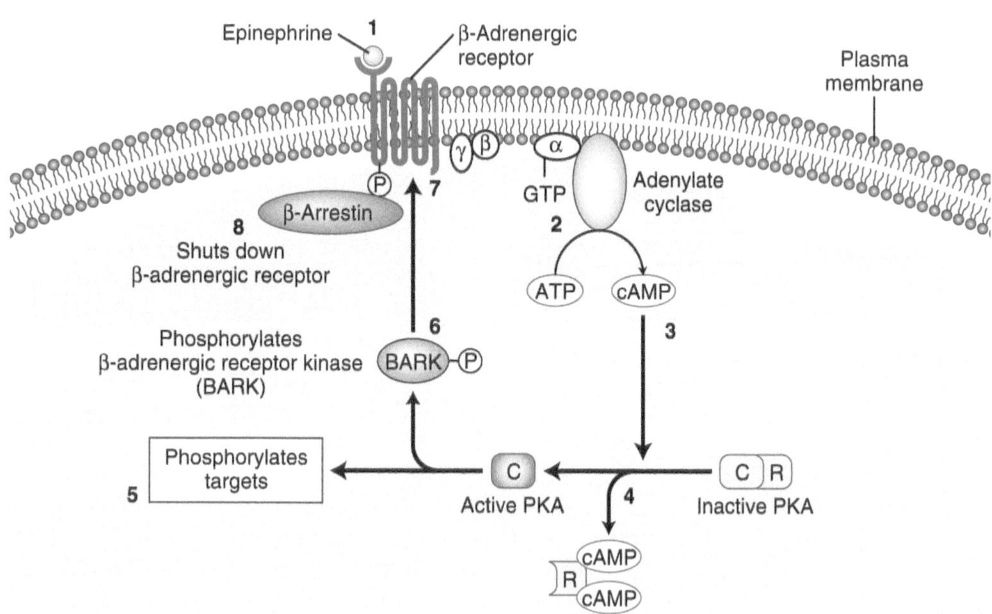

FIGURE 1.35 β-Arrestin combines with the G-protein cell receptor, inactivating it. Source: *From Figure 3-13 in Melmed, S., Polonsky, K. S., Larson, P. R., & Kronenberg, H. M. (2016).* William's textbook of endocrinology *(13th ed.). Elsevier, p. 33.*

formation of hundreds of thousands of molecules of product. Most of the responses that are mediated by second messengers are achieved by regulating the activity of enzymes in target cells, usually by adding a phosphate group. The resulting conformational change increases or decreases enzymatic activity. Therefore second messengers are responsible for specificity, diversity, and expansion or reduction in the hormone signal.

Protein kinases catalyze the transfer of the terminal phosphate from adenosine triphosphate (ATP) to a hydroxyl group in serine or threonine residues in proteins. Tyrosine kinases phosphorylate the hydroxyl groups of tyrosine residues in this way. The human genome contains about a thousand genes that encode protein kinases, but only a few are activated by second messengers. Many protein kinases are themselves activated by phosphorylation catalyzed by other protein kinases. Protein phosphatases remove phosphate groups from these residues and thus restore them to their unstimulated state. For the most part, protein phosphatases are constitutively active (i.e., are always present and active), but some specific protein phosphatases are inducible (i.e., they are directly or indirectly activated in response to hormonal stimulation).

Unlike responses that require the synthesis of new cellular proteins, responses that result from phosphorylation–dephosphorylation reactions occur very quickly, and therefore most second messenger-mediated responses are turned on and off without appreciable latency. However, second messengers can also promote the phosphorylation of transcription factors and thus regulate transcription of specific genes in much the same way as discussed for the nuclear receptors. These responses require the same time-consuming processes as are needed for nuclear receptor–mediated changes and are seen only after a delay.

Although a very large number of hormones and other first messengers act through surface receptors, only a comparatively few substances have been identified as second messengers. This is because receptors for many different extracellular signals utilize the same second messenger. When originally proposed, the hypothesis that the same second messenger might mediate different actions of many different hormones, each of which produces a unique pattern of cellular responses, was met with skepticism. The idea did not gain widespread acceptance until it was recognized that the special nature of a cellular response is determined by the particular enzymatic machinery with which a cell is endowed rather than by the signal that turns on that machinery. Thus, when activated, a hepatic cell makes glucose, and a smooth muscle cell contracts or relaxes.

Second messengers: the cyclic 3′,5′ adenosine monophosphate system

The first of the second messengers to be recognized was cyclic 3′,5′ adenosine monophosphate (cyclic AMP). Cyclic AMP transmits the hormonal signal mainly by activating the enzyme protein kinase A (PKA) (Figs. 1.36 and 1.37).

When cellular concentrations of cyclic AMP are low, two catalytic subunits of PKA are firmly bound to a dimer of regulatory subunits that keeps the tetrameric holoenzyme in the inactive state. The catalytic and regulatory subunits of PKA are products of separate genes. Reversible binding of two molecules of cyclic AMP to each regulatory subunit liberates the catalytic subunits. Cyclic AMP is degraded to 5′-AMP by a family of enzymes called cyclic AMP phosphodiesterases, which cleave the bond that links the phosphate to ribose carbon 3 to form 5′ AMP (Fig. 1.38).

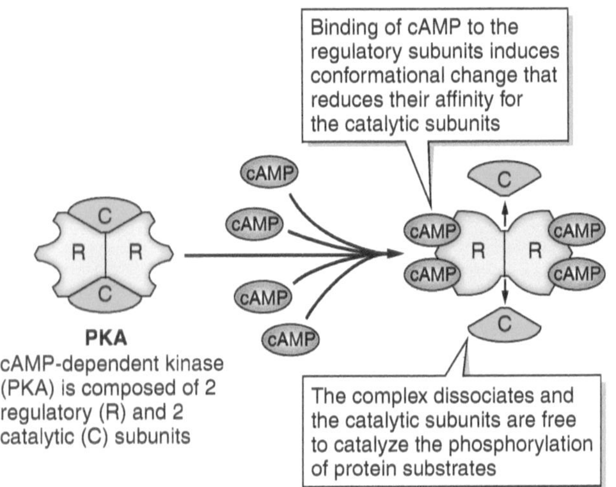

FIGURE 1.36 cAMP activates phosphate kinase. *cAMP*, Cyclic 3′,5′ adenosine monophosphate. Source: *Redrawn from Figure 3-6 in Boron, W. F., & Boulpaep, E. L. (2017).* Medical physiology *(3rd ed.). Elsevier, p. 57.*

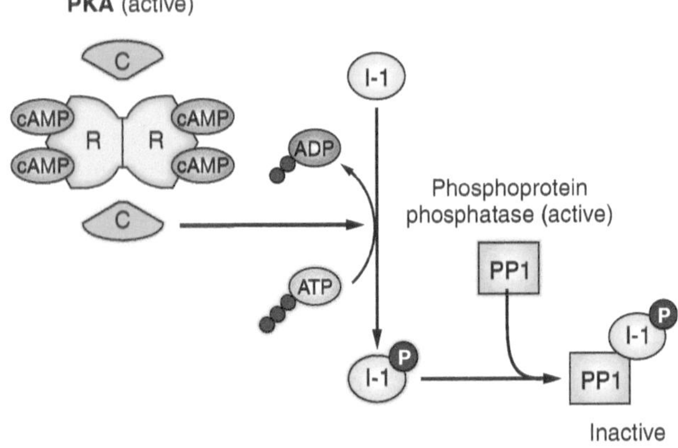

FIGURE 1.37 The activated phosphokinase phosphorylates PPI to inactivate it. *PPI*, Proton pump inhibitor. Source: *Redrawn from Figure 3-7 in Boron, W. F., & Boulpaep, E. L. (2017).* Medical physiology *(3rd ed.). Elsevier, p. 58.*

As cyclic AMP concentrations fall, bound cyclic AMP separates from the regulatory subunits, which then reassociates with the catalytic subunits restoring basal activity.

Regulatory regions of many genes contain a cyclic AMP response element (CRE) analogous to the HREs that bind nuclear hormone receptors as discussed earlier. One or more forms of CRE binding (CREB) proteins are found in the nuclei of most cells and are substrates for PKA. Dimers of phosphorylated CREB bind to the CREs of regulated genes and recruit other nuclear proteins to form complexes that regulate gene transcription in the same manner as described for the nuclear hormone receptors.

Not all the effects of cyclic AMP are mediated by PKA. Cyclic AMP can also bind to membrane channels and directly activate or inactivate them. Other actions of cyclic AMP that are independent of PKA are mediated by EPACs (exchange proteins activated directly by cyclic AMP). EPACs 1 and 2 are intracellular proteins that, upon binding cyclic AMP, interact with a small G-protein called RAP and cause it to exchange its bound GDP for GTP. Activated RAP participates in a variety of cellular functions, including ion channel and membrane transporter activity, cell–cell interactions, intracellular calcium signaling (see later), and exocytosis.

Second messengers: the calcium–calmodulin system

Calcium has long been recognized as a regulator of cellular processes and triggers such events as muscular contraction, secretion, polymerization of microtubules, and activation of various enzymes. The concentration of free calcium in cytoplasm of resting cells is very low, about one ten-thousandth of its concentration in extracellular fluid. This steep concentration gradient is maintained primarily by the actions of calcium ATPases that transfer calcium out of the cell or into storage sites within the endoplasmic reticulum and by sodium–calcium exchangers that extrude one calcium ion in exchange for three sodium ions. When cells are stimulated by some hormones, their cytosolic calcium concentration rises abruptly, increasing perhaps 10-fold or more within seconds. This is accomplished by the

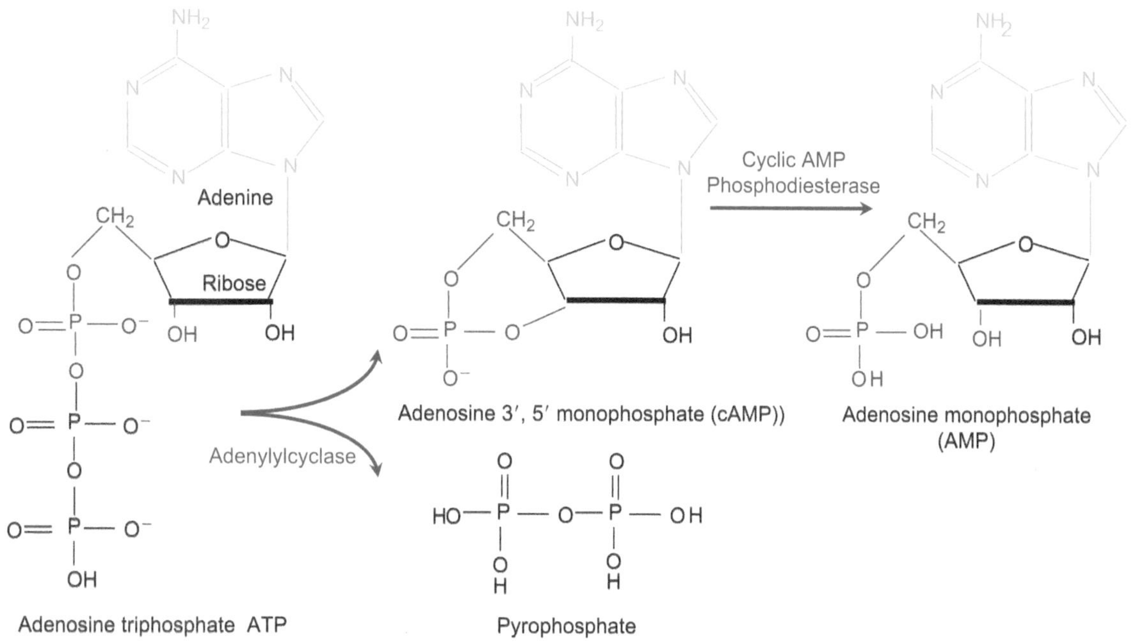

FIGURE 1.38 The conversion of ATP to cyclic AMP and degradation. *AMP*, 3′,5′ Adenosine monophosphate; *ATP*, adenosine triphosphate.

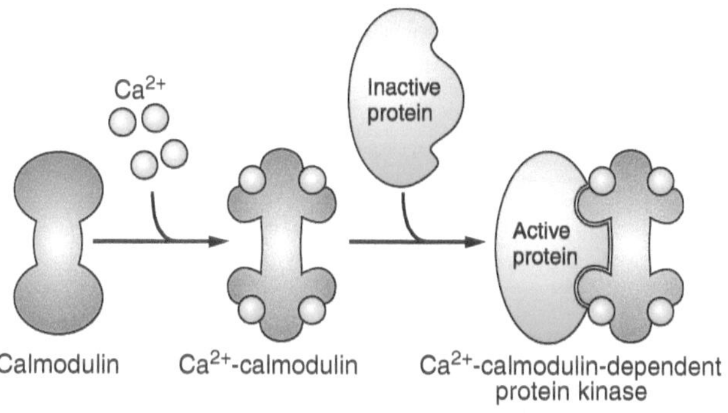

FIGURE 1.39 Calmodulin activation in the presence of calcium. Source: *Redrawn from Figure 3-9 in Boron, W. F., & Boulpaep, E. L. (2017).* Medical physiology *(3rd ed.). Elsevier, p. 57.*

release of calcium from intracellular storage sites primarily in the endoplasmic reticulum and by influx of calcium through activated calcium channels in the plasma membrane. Although calcium can directly affect the activity of some proteins, it generally does not act alone. Virtually all cells are endowed with a protein called calmodulin, which reversibly binds four calcium ions (Fig. 1.39).

When complexed with calcium, the configuration of calmodulin is modified in a way that enables it to bind to protein kinases and other enzymes and activate them. The behavior of calmodulin-dependent protein kinases is quite similar to that of PKA. Calmodulin kinase II may catalyze the phosphorylation of many of the same substrates as PKA, including CREB, and other nuclear transcription factors. Upon cessation of hormonal stimulation, calcium channels in the endoplasmic reticular and plasma membranes close, and constitutively active calcium pumps (ATPases) in these membranes restore cytoplasmic concentrations to low resting levels. A low cytosolic concentration favors the release of calcium from calmodulin, which then dissociates from the various enzymes it has activated.

Second messengers: the diacylglycerol and IP3 system

Both products of phospholipase C–catalyzed hydrolysis of phosphatidylinositol 4,5 bisphosphate, diacylglycerols (DAG) and IP3 behave as second messengers (Fig. 1.40).

IP3 diffuses through the cytosol to reach its receptors in the membranes of the endoplasmic reticulum, the Golgi apparatus, and the nucleus. Activated IP3 receptors are calcium ion channels through which these calcium-storing organelles release calcium into the cytoplasm. Operation of these channels is modulated by phosphorylation and by calcium, which is stimulatory at low concentrations and inhibitory at high concentrations.

Because of its lipid solubility DAG remains associated with the plasma membrane to which it recruits and activates another protein kinase, protein kinase C (PKC), by increasing its affinity for phosphatidylserine in the membrane. The simultaneous increase in cytosolic calcium concentration resulting from the action of IP3 complements DAG in stimulating the catalytic activity of some members of the PKC family, and conversely phosphorylation of IP3 receptors by PKC augments their calcium-releasing activity. Some members of the PKC family are stimulated by DAG even when cytosolic calcium remains at resting levels (Fig. 1.41).

IP3 is cleared from cells by stepwise dephosphorylation to inositol. DAG is cleared by addition of a phosphate group to form phosphatidic acid, which

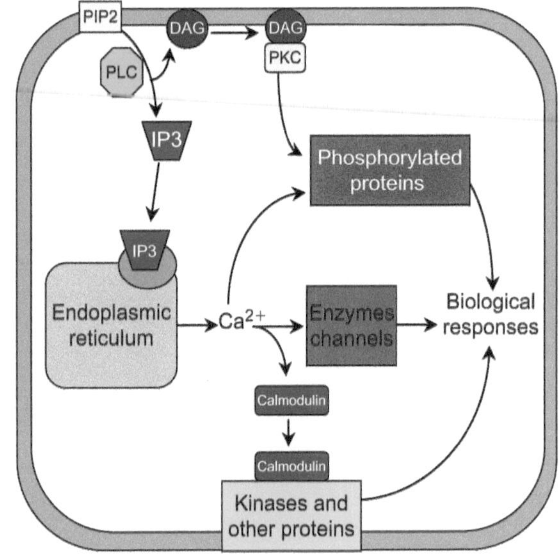

FIGURE 1.41 Signal transduction through the *IP3 DAG* second messenger system. *PIP2* is cleaved into IP3 and DAG by the action of a *PLC*. DAG activates *PKC*, which then phosphorylates a variety of proteins to produce various cell-specific effects. IP3 binds to its receptor in the membrane of the endoplasmic reticulum causing the release of Ca^{2+}, which further activates PKC, directly activates or inhibits enzymes or ion channels, or binds to calmodulin, which then binds to and activates protein kinases and other proteins. *DAG*, Diacylglycerols; *IP3*, inositol trisphosphate; *PIP2*, phosphatidyl inositol 4,5 bisphosphate; *PKC*, protein kinase C; *PLC*, phospholipase C.

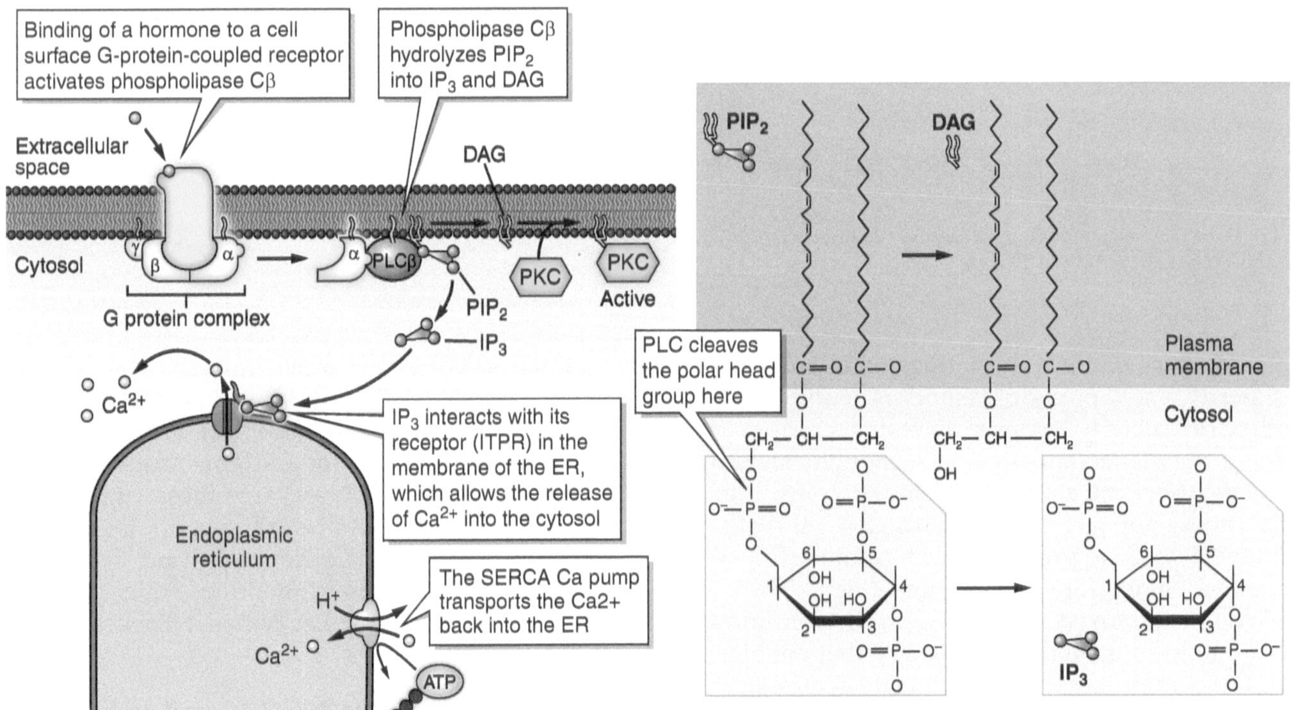

FIGURE 1.40 The production of IP3 and DAG. *DAG*, Diacylglycerol. Source: *Redrawn from Figure 3-8 A in Boron, W. F., & Boulpaep, E. L. (2017).* Medical physiology *(3rd ed.). Elsevier, p. 59.*

may then be converted to a triglyceride or resynthesized into a phospholipid. Phosphatidylinositides of the plasma membrane are regenerated by combining inositol with phosphatidic acid, which may then undergo stepwise phosphorylation of the inositol.

The phosphatidylinositol precursor of IP3 and DAG also contains a 20-carbon polyunsaturated fatty acid called arachidonic acid (Fig. 1.42).

This fatty acid typically is found in ester linkage with carbon 2 of the glycerol backbone of phospholipids and may be liberated by the action of a diacylglyceride lipase from the DAG formed in the breakdown of phosphatidylinositol. Liberation of arachidonic acid is the rate-determining step in the formation of thromboxanes, prostaglandins, and leukotrienes (see Chapter 4: The Adrenal Glands). These compounds, which are produced in virtually all cells, diffuse across the plasma membrane and behave as local regulators of nearby cells. The same hormone–receptor interaction that produces DAG and IP3 as second messages to communicate with cellular organelles frequently also results in the formation of arachidonate derivatives that inform neighboring cells that a response has been initiated. Arachidonic acid is also released from other, more abundant membrane phospholipids by the actions of the phospholipase A2 class of enzymes that can be activated by calcium, phosphorylation by PKC, and by βγ-subunits of G-proteins (Fig. 1.43).

Second messengers: cyclic guanosine 3′,5′-monophosphate

Though considerably less versatile than cyclic AMP, cyclic guanosine 3′,5′-monophosphate (cyclic GMP) plays an analogous role in many cells. Its formation from GTP is catalyzed by the enzyme guanylyl cyclase. Guanylyl cyclase and cyclic GMP–dependent protein kinase activities are present in many cells, but the activation of guanylyl cyclase is quite different from that of adenylyl cyclase. Guanylyl cyclase activity is an intrinsic property of the transmembrane receptor for atrial natriuretic hormone and is activated without the intercession of a G-protein. Guanylyl cyclase is also present in a soluble form within the cytoplasm of many cells and is activated by nitric oxide (NO). Increased formation of cyclic GMP in vascular smooth muscle is associated with relaxation and may account for vasodilator responses to the atrial natriuretic hormone (see Chapter 9: Regulation of Salt and Water Balance).

Receptors that signal through tyrosine kinase

Some hormones transmit their messages from the cell surface to intracellular effectors without the agency of second messengers. Receptors for these hormones rely on physical association between proteins (protein–protein interactions) to activate enzymes that phosphorylate transcription factors and other cytosolic proteins in much the same way as already discussed. The tyrosine kinase–dependent receptors have a single membrane-spanning region and either have intrinsic protein tyrosine kinase enzymatic activity in their intracellular domains or are associated with cytosolic protein tyrosine kinases. Receptors for insulin, the insulin-like growth factors, and the epidermal growth factor have intrinsic protein kinase activity; receptors for growth hormone, prolactin, erythropoietin, and some cytokines rely on an associated cytosolic tyrosine kinase called JAK2. Generally, the tyrosine kinase–dependent receptors are synthesized as dimers or form dimers when activated by their ligands. When a hormone binds to the extracellular domain, a conformational change in the receptor activates protein tyrosine kinases that catalyze the phosphorylation of hydroxyl groups of tyrosine residues in the cytosolic portion of the receptor itself, in the associated kinase (autophosphorylation), and in other cytosolic proteins that complex with the phosphorylated receptor.

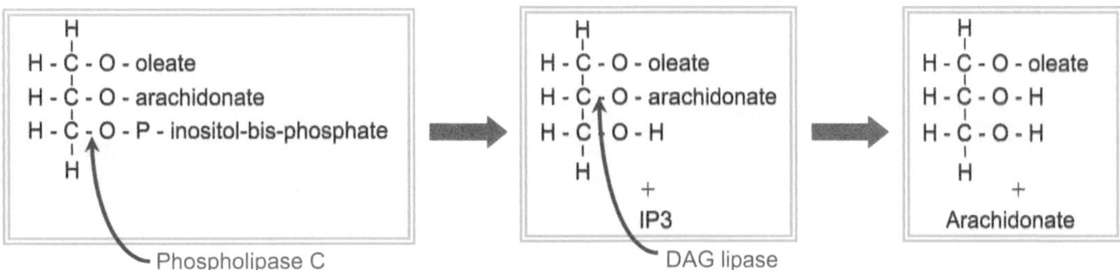

FIGURE 1.42 Arachidonate formation and the action of phospholipase C and DAG. *DAG*, Diacylglycerols.

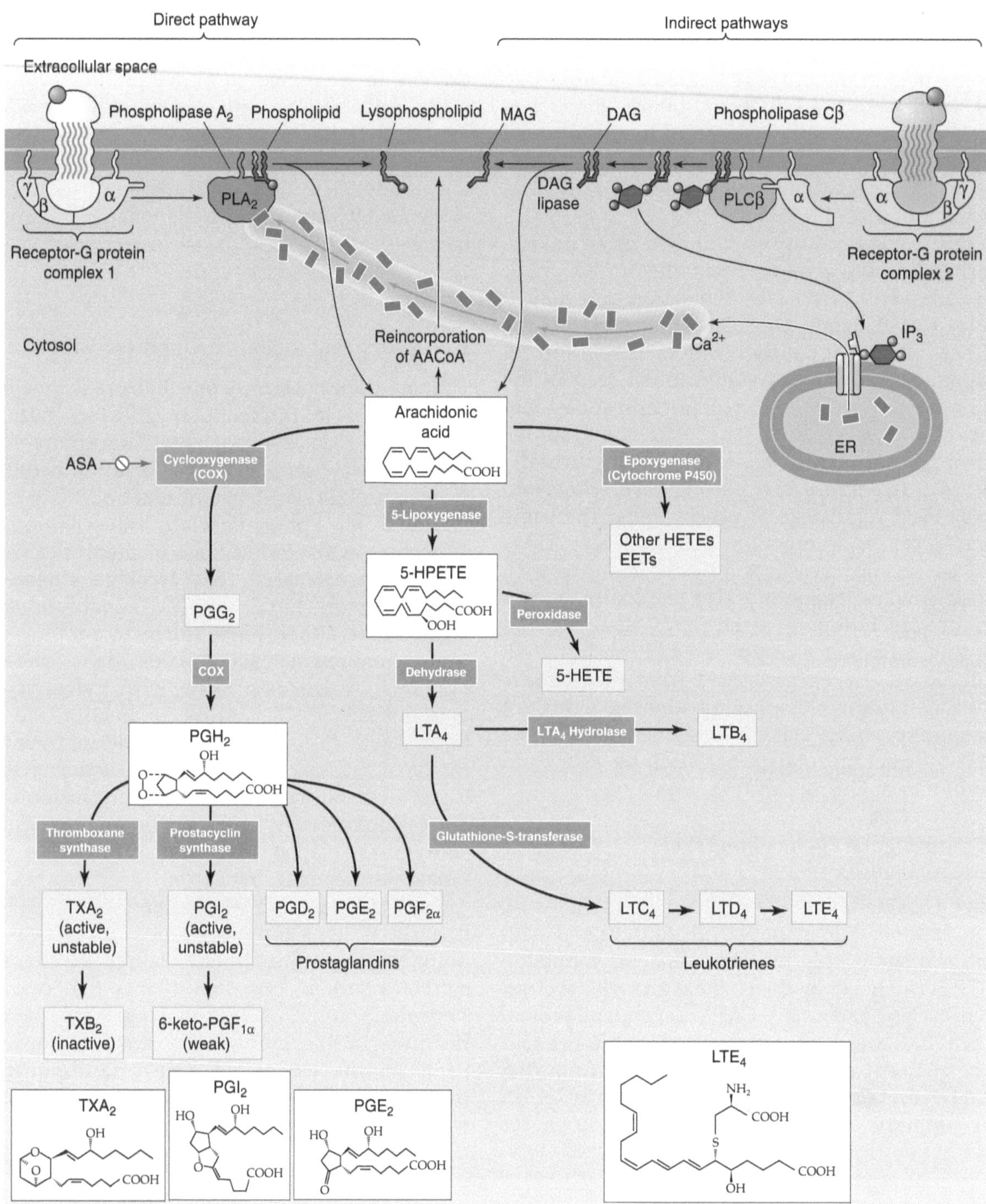

FIGURE 1.43 Formation of arachidonic acid derivatives. Source: *From Figure 3-11 in Boron, W. F., & Boulpaep, E. L. (2017).* Medical physiology *(3rd ed.). Elsevier, p. 63.*

One of the remarkable features of signaling that is particularly evident in considering the tyrosine kinase–dependent receptors is that virtually no transduction mechanism or signaling pathway is uniquely associated with expression of the actions of any one hormone. Rather, actions of the various hormones are produced through the use of many of the same pathways. For example, tyrosine phosphorylation of the insulin receptor substrates followed by the activation of phosphatidylinositol-3 kinase is a common feature of signaling by insulin, growth hormone, prolactin, leptin, several cytokines, and erythropoietin, although each hormone produces unique effects. As noted for the actions of

At the molecular level (boxed material for additional information)

Tyrosine kinases

The protein substrates for receptor-activated tyrosine kinases may have catalytic activity or may act as scaffolds to which other proteins are recruited and positioned so that enzymatic modifications are facilitated. As a result, large multiprotein signaling complexes are formed. Phosphorylated tyrosines act as docking sites for proteins that contain *src* homology 2 (SH2) domains. SH2 domains are named for the particular configuration of the tyrosine phosphate–binding region originally discovered in v-src, the cancer-inducing protein tyrosine kinase of the Rous sarcoma virus. SH2 domains represent one type of a growing list of modules within a protein that recognize and bind to specific complementary motifs in another protein. A typical SH2 domain consists of about 100 amino acid residues and recognizes a phosphorylated tyrosine in the context of the three or four amino acid residues that are downstream from the tyrosine. There are multiple SH2 groups that recognize phosphorylated tyrosines in different contexts. Typically, multiple tyrosines are phosphorylated so that several different SH2-containing proteins are recruited and initiate multiple signaling pathways. Although some responses to the activation of tyrosine kinases include modifications of cellular metabolism without nuclear participation, they often involve a change in genomic readout that promotes cell division (mitogenesis) or differentiation. One way that these receptors communicate with the genome is through the activation of the MAP kinase pathway. MAP kinase is a cytosolic enzyme that is activated by phosphorylation of both serine and tyrosine residues and then enters the nucleus where it phosphorylates and activates certain transcription factors. Activation of MAP kinase follows an indirect route that involves a small G-protein called Ras, which was originally discovered as a constitutively activated protein present in many tumors. One of the proteins that docks with phosphorylated tyrosine residues is the growth factor–binding protein 2 (Grb2). Grb2 is an adaptor protein that has an SH2 group at one end and other binding motifs at its opposite end, which enable it to bind other proteins, including a nucleotide exchange factor called SOS (Son of Sevenless[1]). By means of these protein–protein interactions, the activated receptor can thus communicate with an activate SOS, which causes Ras to exchange GTP for GDP. The effector for the Ras that is thus activated is the enzyme Raf kinase, which phosphorylates and activates the first of a cascade of MAP kinases that ultimately result in phosphorylation of nuclear transcription factors (Fig. 1.44).

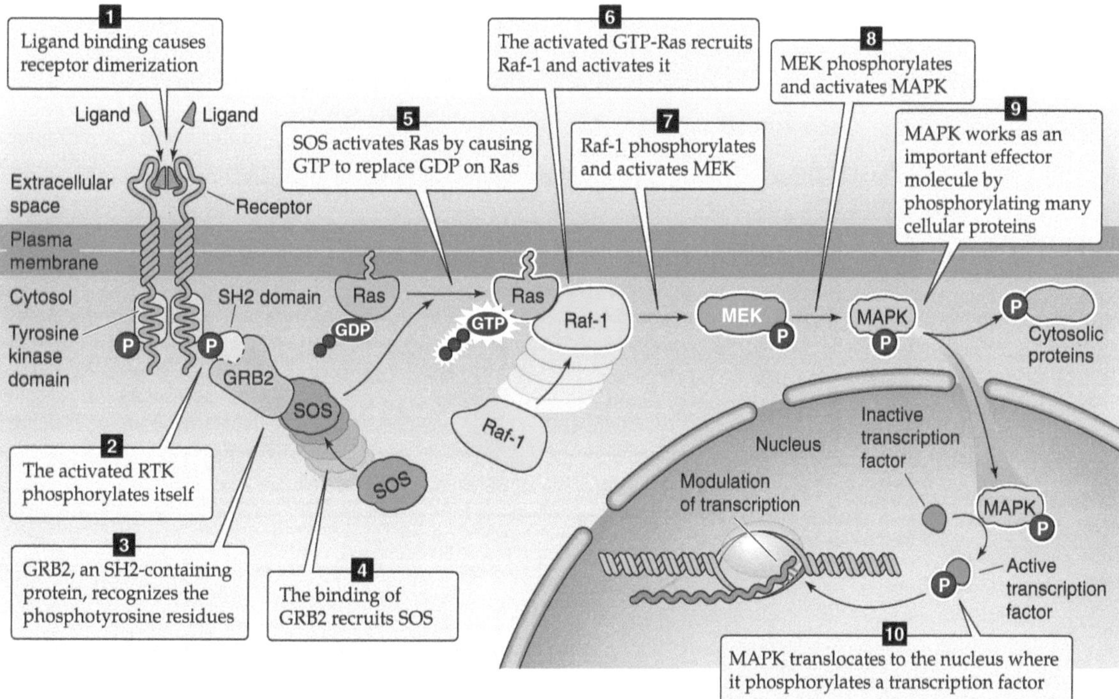

FIGURE 1.44 The Ras pathway. For details, see text. Source: *From Figure 3-13 in Boron, W. F., & Boulpaep, E. L. (2017).* Medical physiology *(3rd ed.). Elsevier, p. 69.*

(cont'd)

The gamma form of phospholipase C is another effector protein that is recruited to tyrosine phosphorylated receptors by way of its SH2 group. It is also a substrate for tyrosine kinases and is activated by tyrosine phosphorylation. Activation of this member of the phospholipase C family of proteins results in hydrolysis of phosphatidylinositol bisphosphate to produce DAG and IP3 in the same manner as already discussed for the beta forms of the enzyme associated with G-protein-coupled receptors. In this manner, tyrosine kinase–dependent receptors can stimulate cellular changes that are mediated by PKC and the calcium–calmodulin second messenger system, including phosphorylation of nuclear transcription factors by calmodulin kinase (Fig. 1.45).

Another mechanism for modifying gene expression involves the activation of a family of proteins called Stat (signal transducer and activator of transcription) proteins. The Stat proteins are transcription factors that reside in the cytosol in their inactive state. They have an SH2 group that enables them to bind to tyrosine phosphorylated proteins. When bound to the receptor/kinase complex, Stat proteins become tyrosine phosphorylated, whereupon they dissociate from their docking sites, form homodimers, and enter the nucleus where they activate transcription of specific genes (Figs. 1.46 and 1.47).

Although they were discovered as the substrates for the insulin receptor tyrosine kinase, the insulin receptor

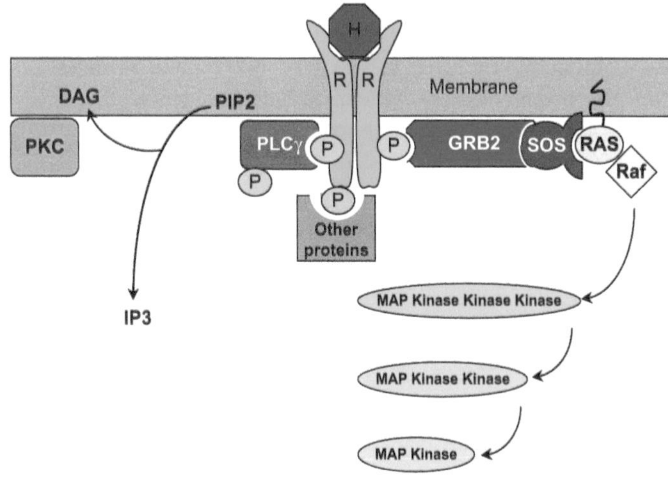

FIGURE 1.45 Phosphorylation of tyrosines on dimerized *R* following *H* binding provides docking sites for the attachment of proteins that transduce the hormonal signal. The *GRB2* binds to a phosphorylated tyrosine in the receptor and binds at its other end to the nucleotide exchange factor *SOS*, which stimulates the small G-protein *Ras* to exchange its GDP for GTP. Thus activated, Ras in turn activates the protein kinase *Raf*, which phosphorylates *MAP* kinase and initiates the *MAP* kinase cascade that ultimately phosphorylates nuclear transcription factors. The *PLC γ* docks on the phosphorylated receptor and is then tyrosine phosphorylated and activated to cleave phosphatidyl inositol 4,5 bisphosphate (*PIP2*) releasing DAG and inositol trisphosphate (*IP3*) and activating protein kinase C (*PKC*) as shown in Fig. 1.19. *DAG*, Diacylglycerols; *GDP*, guanosine diphosphate; *GRB2*, growth factor–binding protein 2; *GTP*, guanosine triphosphate; *H*, hormone; *MAP*, mitogen-activated protein; *PLC γ*, γ isoform of phospholipase C; *R*, receptors.

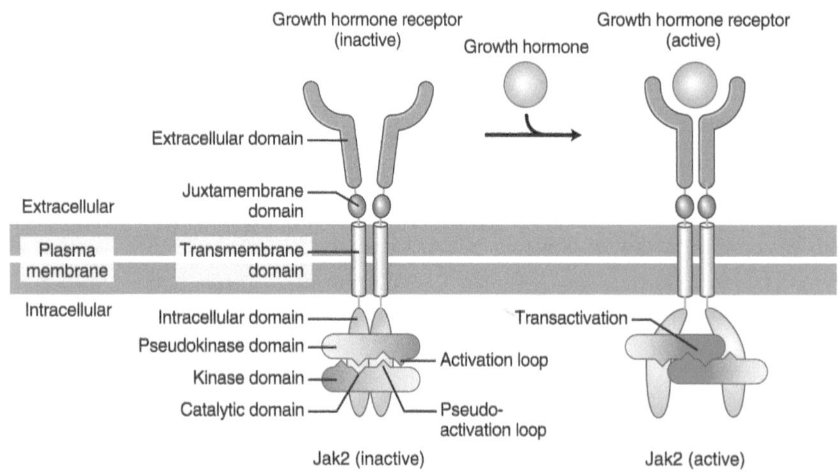

FIGURE 1.46 Scissor model for the activation of human growth hormone. Source: *From Figure 3-11 in Melmed, S., Polonsky, K. S., Larson, P. R., & Kronenberg, H. M. (2016).* William's textbook of endocrinology *(13th ed.). Elsevier, p. 31.*

(*cont'd*)

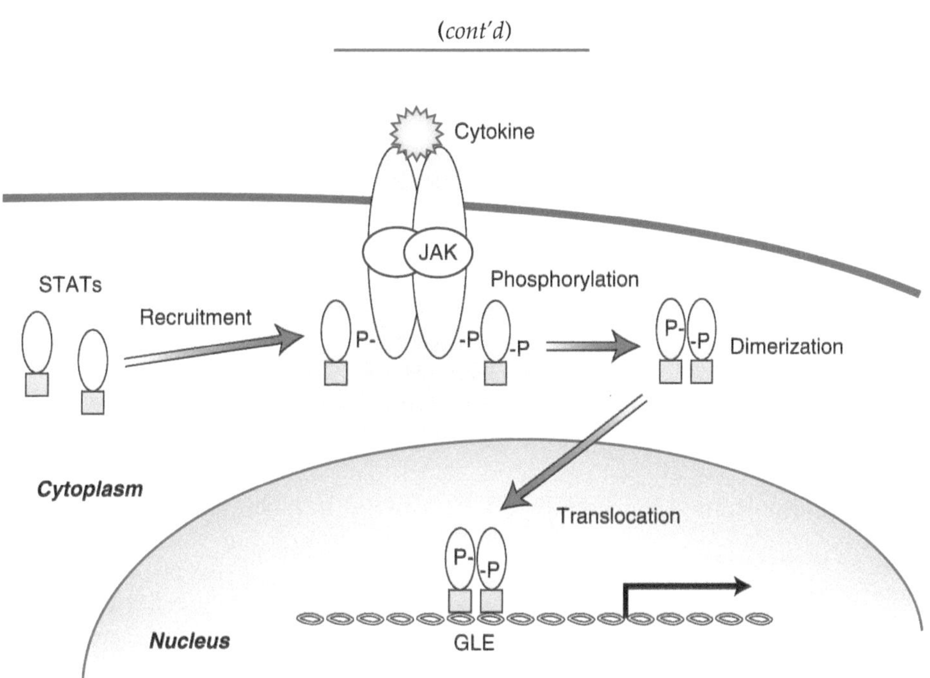

FIGURE 1.47 A continuation of Fig. 1.46 showing the effect on the nucleus. Source: *From Figure 3-12 in Melmed, S., Polonsky, K. S., Larson, P. R., & Kronenberg, H. M. (2016).* William's textbook of endocrinology *(13th ed.). Elsevier, p. 31.*

substrates (1–4) play an important role in the signaling pathways of many of the hormones and cytokines that act by way of tyrosine phosphorylation. These large proteins are phosphorylated at multiple tyrosine residues and recruit proteins that anchor other kinase-dependent signaling pathways. One of the most important of these proteins is phosphatidylinositol-3 (PI-3) kinase, which catalyzes the phosphorylation of carbon 3 of the inositol of phosphatidylinositol bisphosphate in cell membranes to form phosphatidylinositol 3,4,5 trisphosphate (PIP3). PI-3 kinase consists of a regulatory subunit that contains an SH2 domain and a catalytic subunit. Binding of the regulatory subunit to phosphorylated tyrosines of the receptor-associated complex activates the catalytic subunit. The enzymes activated by associating with PIP3 are protein kinases that regulate cellular metabolism, vesicle trafficking, cytoskeletal changes, and other responses. These responses are considered further in Chapter 7, The Pancreatic Islets, and illustrated in Fig. 7.19.

[1](In smaller case) This seemingly unusual name refers to a gene (*sev*) in the embryo of the fruit fly for the development of the R7 retina of its compound eye. If it is not present (=less), the fly cannot detect a certain band of ultraviolet light, hence R7-less or "sevenless." Proteins interacting with this gene were given whimsical names such as "son" "bride" depending on their function. These same proteins were found to be in signaling molecules in higher organisms.

the cyclic AMP-dependent hormones, the nature of the final result is a function of the particular target cell and its unique complement of enzymes and transcriptional machinery, and not the signaling pathway as shown in Fig. 1.48.

Regulation of hormone secretion

For hormones to function as carriers of critical information, their secretion must be turned on and off at precisely the right times. The organism must have some way of knowing when there is a need for a hormone to be secreted, how much is needed, and when that need has passed. As hormonal control is discussed in this and subsequent chapters, it is important to identify and understand the components of the regulation of each hormonal secretion because (1) derangements in any of the components are the bases of endocrine disease and (2) manipulation of any

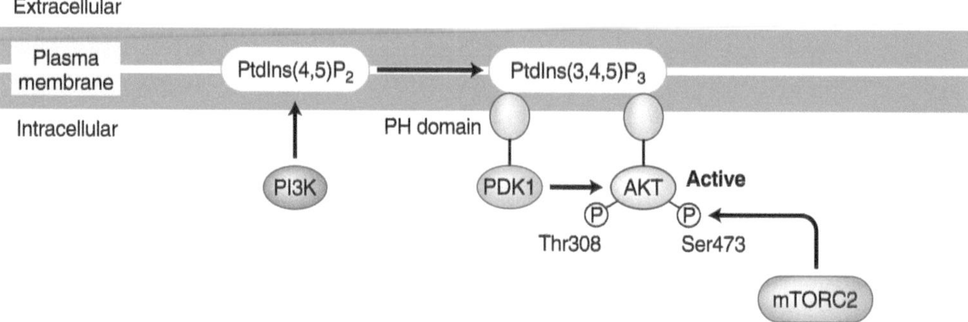

FIGURE 1.48 Activation of AKT one of the pathways in the activation of hormones. Source: *From Figure 3-15 in Melmed, S., Polonsky, K. S., Larson, P. R., & Kronenberg, H. M. (2016).* William's textbook of endocrinology *(13th ed.). Elsevier, p. 35.*

component provides an opportunity for therapeutic intervention.

Negative feedback

Secretion of most hormones is regulated by negative feedback. By negative feedback, we mean that some consequence of hormone secretion acts directly or indirectly on the secretory cell in a negative way to inhibit further secretion. A simple example from everyday experience is the thermostat. When the temperature in a room falls below some preset level, the thermostat signals the furnace to produce heat. When room temperature rises to the preset level, the signal from the thermostat to the furnace is shut off, and heat production ceases until the temperature again falls. This is a simple closed-loop feedback system and is analogous to the regulation of glucagon secretion. A fall in blood glucose detected by the alpha cells of the islets of Langerhans causes them to release glucagon, which stimulates the liver to release glucose and thereby increase blood glucose concentrations (Fig. 1.49).

With restoration of blood glucose to some predetermined level or set point, further secretion of glucagon is inhibited. This simple example involves only secreting and responding cells. Other systems may be considerably more complex and involve one or more intermediary events, but the essence of negative feedback regulation remains the same: hormones produce biological effects that directly or indirectly inhibit their further secretion.

A problem that emerges with this system of control is that the thermostat maintains room temperature constant only if the natural tendency of the temperature is to fall. If the temperature were to rise, it could not be controlled by simply turning off the furnace. This problem is at least partially resolved in hormonal systems, because at physiological set points the basal rate of secretion usually is not zero. In this example, when there is a rise in blood glucose concentration, glucagon secretion can be diminished and therefore diminish the impetus on the liver to release glucose. Some regulation above and below the set point can therefore be accomplished with just one feedback loop; this mechanism is seen in some endocrine control systems. Regulation is more efficient and precise, however, with a second, opposing loop, which is activated when the controlled variable deviates in the opposite direction. For the example with regulation of blood glucose, that second loop is provided by insulin. Insulin inhibits glucose production by the liver and is secreted in response to an elevated blood glucose level. Protection against deviation in either direction often is achieved in biological systems by the opposing actions of antagonistic control systems (Fig. 1.50).

Closed-loop negative feedback control as just described can maintain conditions only in a state of constancy. Such systems are effective in guarding against upward or downward deviations from some predetermined set point, but changing environmental demands often require temporary deviation from constancy. This can be accomplished in some cases by adjusting the set point and in other cases by a signal that overrides the set point. For example, epinephrine secreted by the adrenal medulla in response to some emergency inhibits insulin secretion and increases glucagon secretion even though the concentration of glucose in the blood may already be high. Whether the set point is changed or overridden, deviation from constancy is achieved by the intervention of some additional signal from outside the negative feedback system. In most cases, that additional signal originates with the nervous system.

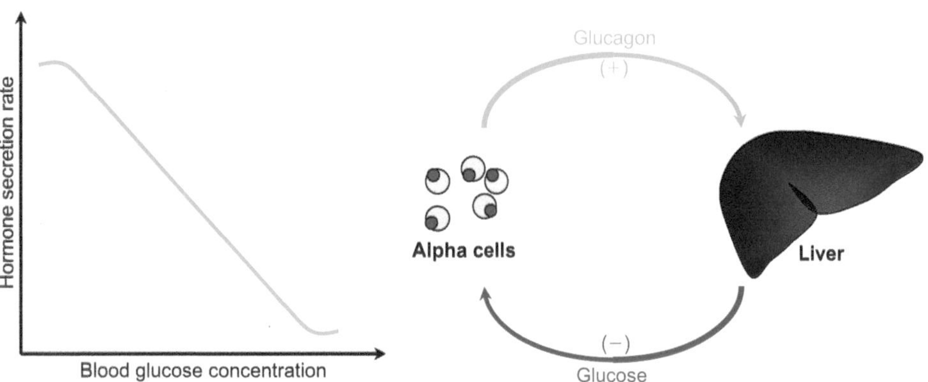

FIGURE 1.49 Negative feedback.

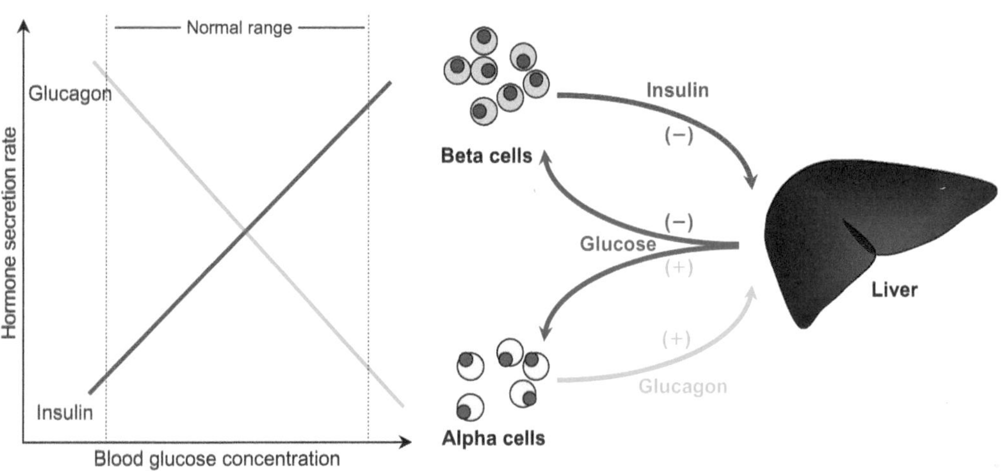

FIGURE 1.50 Negative feedback regulation of blood glucose concentration by insulin and glucagon. (−) = Inhibits, (+) = stimulates.

Hormones also initiate or regulate processes that are not limited to steady or constant conditions. Virtually all these processes are self-limiting, and their control resembles negative feedback, but of the open-loop type. For example, oxytocin is a hormone that is secreted by hypothalamic nerve cells the axons of which terminate in the posterior pituitary gland. Its secretion is necessary for the extrusion of milk from the lumen of the mammary alveoli into secretory ducts so that the infant suckling at the nipple can receive milk. In this case, sensory nerve endings in the nipple detect the signal and convey afferent information to the central nervous system, which in turn signals the release of oxytocin from axon terminals in the pituitary gland. Oxytocin causes myoepithelial cells in the breast to contract, resulting in delivery of milk to the infant. When the infant is satisfied, the suckling stimulus at the nipple ceases.

Positive feedback

By positive feedback, it is meant that some consequence of hormonal secretion acts on the secretory cells to provide an augmented drive for secretion. Rather than being self-limiting, as with negative feedback, the drive for secretion becomes progressively more intense. Positive feedback systems are unusual in biology, as they terminate with some cataclysmic, explosive event. A good example of a positive feedback system involves oxytocin and its other effect: causing contraction of uterine muscle during childbirth (Fig. 1.51). In this case the stimulus for oxytocin secretion is dilation of the uterine cervix. Upon receipt of this information through sensory nerves, the brain signals the release of oxytocin from nerve endings in the posterior pituitary gland. Enhanced uterine contraction in response to

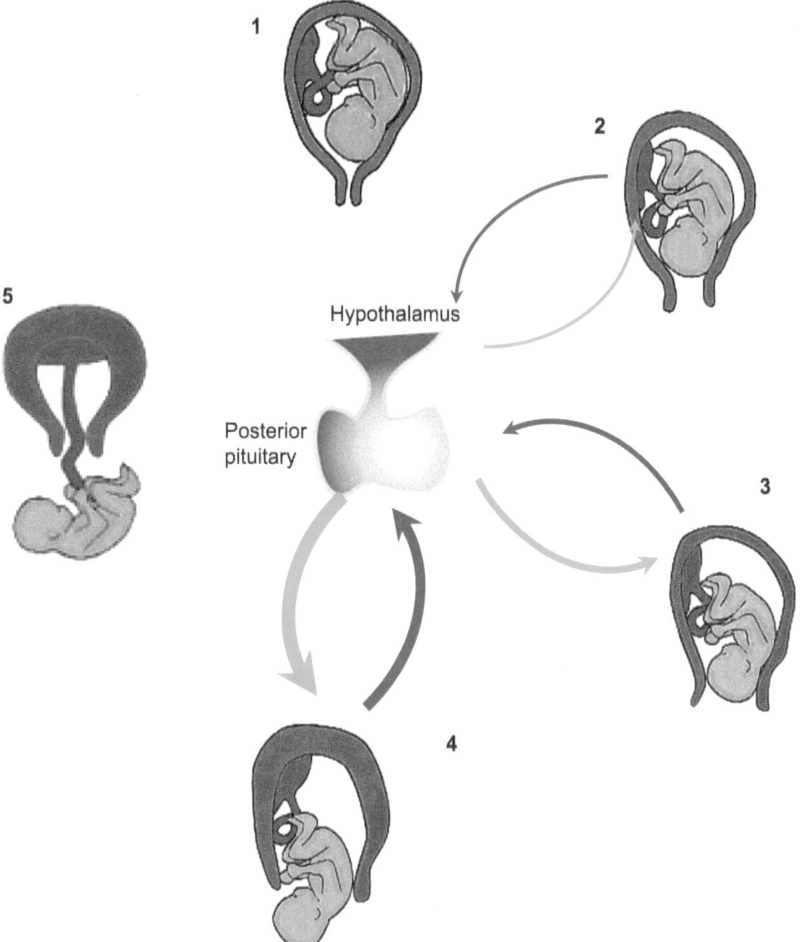

FIGURE 1.51 Positive feedback during labor and delivery.

oxytocin results in greater dilation of the cervix, which strengthens the signal for oxytocin release and so on until the infant is expelled from the uterine cavity.

Feed forward

Feed-forward controls can be considered as anticipatory or preemptive and prepare the body for an impending change or demand. For example, following a meal rich in glucose, secretory cells in the mucosa of the gastrointestinal tract secrete hormones that signal the pancreas to secrete insulin (see Chapter 6: Hormones of the Gastrointestinal Tract, and Chapter 7: The Pancreatic Islets). Having increased insulin already in the blood by the time, the glucose is absorbed thus moderates the change in blood glucose that might otherwise occur if insulin were secreted after the blood glucose concentrations started to increase. Unlike feedback systems, feed-forward systems are unaffected by the consequences of the changes they evoke and simply are shut off when the stimulus disappears.

Measurement of hormones

Whether it is for the purpose of diagnosing a patient's disease or research to gain understanding of normal physiology, it is often necessary to measure how much hormone is present in some biological fluid. Chemical detection of hormones in blood is difficult. Except for the thyroid hormones, which contain large amounts of iodine, there is no unique chemistry that sets hormones apart from other bodily constituents. Furthermore, hormones circulate in blood at minute concentrations, which further complicates the problem of their detection. Consequently, the earliest methods developed for measuring hormones were bioassays and depend on the ability of a hormone to produce a characteristic biological response. For example, induction of ovulation in the rabbit in response to an injection of urine from a pregnant woman is an indication of the presence of the placental hormone chorionic gonadotropin and is the basis for the rabbit test that was used for many years as an indicator of early pregnancy (see Chapter 14: Hormonal Control of Pregnancy and Lactation). Before hormones were identified chemically they were quantitated in units of the biological responses they produced. For example, a unit of insulin is defined as one-third of the amount needed to lower blood sugar in a 2-kg rabbit to convulsive levels within 3 hours. Although bioassays are now seldom used, some hormones, including insulin, are still standardized in terms of biological units. Terms such as milliunits and microunits are still in use.

Immunoassays

As knowledge of hormone structure increased, it became evident that peptide hormones are not identical in all species. Small differences in amino acid sequence, which may not affect the biological activity of a hormone, were found to produce antibody reactions after prolonged administration. Hormones isolated from one species were recognized as foreign substances in recipient animals of another species, which often produced antibodies to the foreign hormone. Antibodies are exquisitely sensitive and can recognize and react with tiny amounts of the foreign material (antigens) that evoked their production, even in the presence of large amounts of other substances that may be similar or different. Techniques have been devised to exploit this characteristic of antibodies for the measurement of hormones, and to detect antibody–antigen reactions even when minute quantities of antigen (hormone) are involved.

Radioimmunoassay

Reaction of a hormone with an antibody results in a complex with altered properties such that it is precipitated out of solution or behaves differently when subjected to electrophoresis or adsorption to charcoal or other substances. A typical radioimmunoassay takes advantage of the fact that iodine of high specific radioactivity can be incorporated readily into tyrosine residues of peptides and proteins and thereby permits detection and quantitation of tiny amounts of hormone. Hormones present in biological fluids are not radioactive but can compete with radioactive hormone for a limited number of antibody-binding sites. To perform a radioimmunoassay, a sample of plasma containing an unknown amount of hormone is mixed in a test tube with a known amount of antibody and a known amount of radioactive iodinated hormone. The unlabeled hormone present in the plasma competes with the iodine-labeled hormone for binding to the antibody. The more hormone present in the plasma sample, the less iodinated hormone can bind to the antibody. Antibody-bound radioactive iodine then is separated from unbound iodinated hormone by any of a variety of physicochemical means, and the ratio of bound to unbound radioactivity is determined. The amount of hormone present in plasma can be estimated by comparison with a standard curve constructed using known amounts of unlabeled hormone instead of the biological fluid samples (Fig. 1.52).

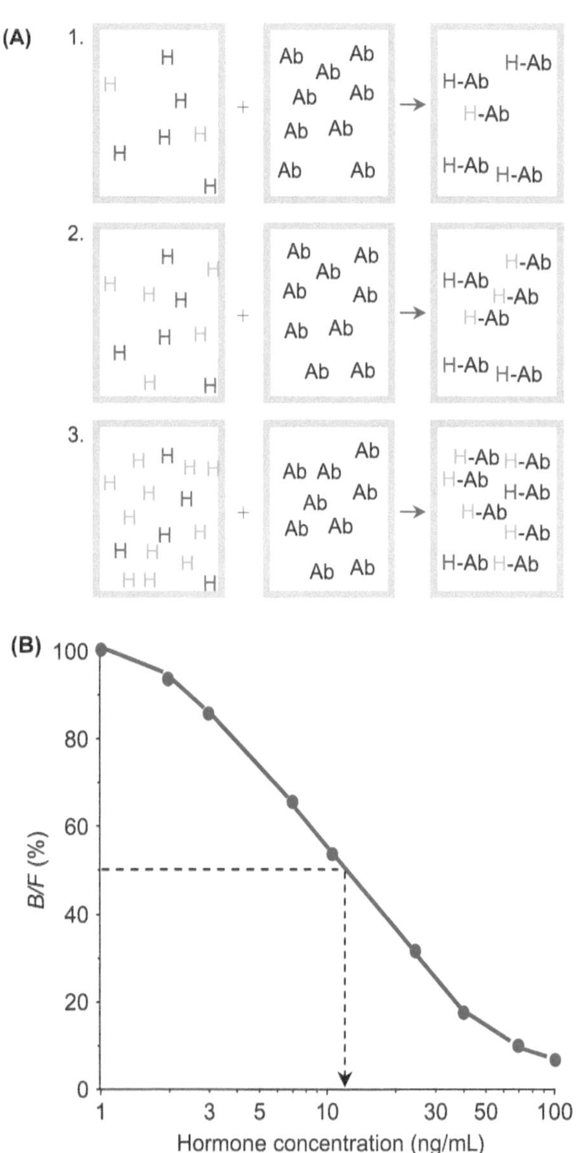

FIGURE 1.52 (A) Competing reactions that form the basis of the radioimmunoassay. Labeled hormone (*H*, shown in *red*) competes with the hormone in a biological sample (*green* H) for a limited amount of *Ab*. As the concentration of hormone in the biological sample rises (rows 1, 2, and 3), decreasing amounts of the labeled hormone appear in the *H-Ab* complex and the ratio of *B/F* labeled hormone decreases. (B) A typical standard curve used to estimate the amount of hormone in the biological sample. A *B/F* ratio of 50% corresponds to 12 ng/mL in this example. *Ab*, antibodies; *B/F*, bound/free; *H-Ab*, hormone–antibody.

Although this procedure originally was devised for protein hormones, radioimmunoassays are now available for all the known hormones. Production of specific antibodies to nonprotein hormones can be induced by first attaching these compounds to some protein, like serum albumin. For hormones that lack a site capable of incorporating iodine such as the steroids, another radioactive label can be used or a chemical tail containing tyrosine can be added. Methods are even available to replace the radioactive iodine with fluorescent tags or other labels that can be detected with great sensitivity. The major limitation of radioimmunoassays is that immunological rather than biological activity is measured by these tests, because the portion of the hormone molecule recognized by the antibody probably is not the same as the portion recognized by the hormone receptor. A protein hormone that may be biologically inactive may retain all of its immunological activity. For example, the biologically active portion of parathyroid hormone resides in the amino terminal one-third of the molecule, but the carboxyl terminal fragments formed by partial degradation of the hormone have long half-lives in blood and may account for nearly 80% of the immunoreactive parathyroid hormone in human plasma. Until this problem was understood and appropriate adjustments made, radioimmunoassays grossly overestimated the content of parathyroid hormone in plasma (see Chapter 10: Hormonal Regulation of Calcium Balance). Similarly, biologically inactive prohormones may be detected. By and large, discrepancies between biological activity and immunoactivity have not presented insurmountable difficulties and in several cases even led to increased understanding.

Immunometric assays

Even greater sensitivity and specificity in hormone detection has been attained with the development of assays that can take advantage of exquisitely sensitive detectors that can be coupled to antibodies. Such assays require the use of two different antibodies that recognize different immunological determinants in the hormone (Fig. 1.53).

One antibody is coupled to a solid support such as an agarose bead or adsorbed onto the plastic of a multiwell culture dish. The biological sample containing an unknown amount of hormone then is added under conditions in which there is a large excess of antibody so that essentially all the hormone can be bound by the antibody. The second antibody, linked to a fluorescent probe or an enzyme that can generate a colored product, then is added and allowed to bind to the hormone that is held in place by the first antibody so that the hormone is sandwiched between the two antibodies and acts to link them together. In this way the amount of antibody-linked detection system that is held to the solid support is directly proportional to the amount of hormone present in the test sample. These assays are sometimes called sandwich assays, or ELISA (enzyme-linked immunosorbent assay) when the second antibody is coupled to an enzyme that converts a substrate to a colored product.

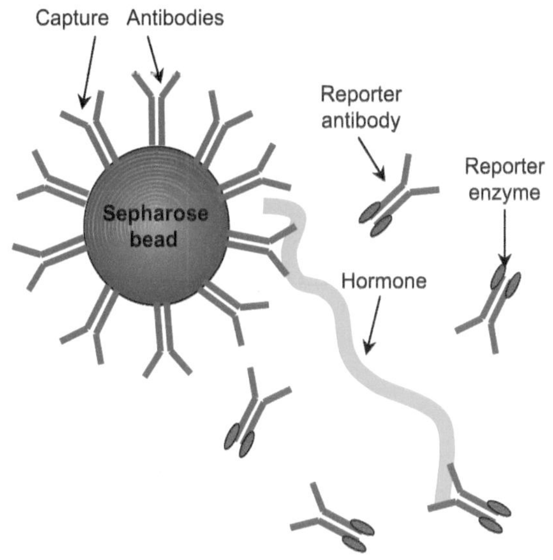

FIGURE 1.53 Sandwich type assay. The first (capture) antibody is linked to a solid support such as sepharose bead. The hormone to be measured is shown in green. The second (reporter) antibody is linked to an enzyme, which upon reacting with a test substrate gives a colored product. In this model, the amount of reporter antibody captured is directly proportional to the amount of hormone in the sample being tested.

Hormone levels in blood

It is evident now that hormone concentrations in plasma fluctuate from minute to minute and may vary widely in the normal individual over the course of a day. Hormone secretion may be episodic, pulsatile, or follow a daily rhythm (Fig. 1.54).

In most cases, it is necessary to make multiple serial measurements of hormones before a diagnosis of a hyper- or hypofunctional state can be confirmed. Endocrine disease occurs when the concentration of hormone in blood is inappropriate for the physiological situation rather than because the absolute amounts of hormone in blood are high or low. It is also becoming increasingly evident that the pattern of hormone secretion, rather than the amount secreted, may be of

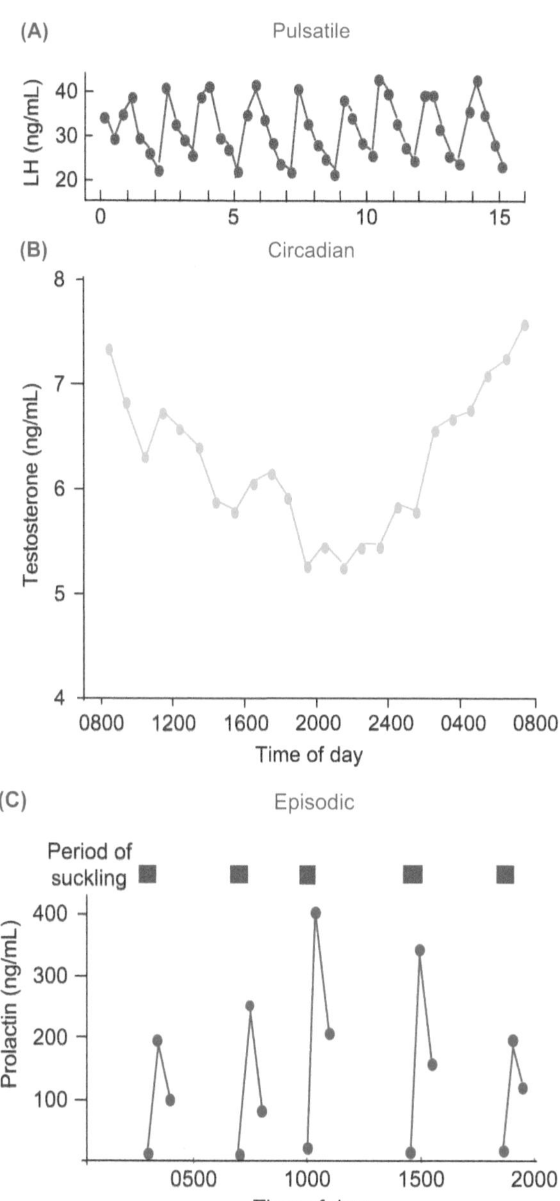

FIGURE 1.54 Changes in hormone concentrations in blood may follow different patterns: (A) daily rhythm in testosterone secretion; (B) hourly rhythm of LH secretion; and (C) episodic secretion of prolactin. *LH*, Luteinizing hormone. Source: *(A) From Bremer, et al. (1983).* The Journal of Clinical Endocrinology and Metabolism, *56, 1278; (B) From Yamaji, et al. (1972).* Endocrinology, *90, 771; and (C) From Hwang, et al. (1971).* Proceedings of the National Academy of Sciences of the United States of America, *68, 1902.*

great importance in determining hormone responses. This subject is discussed further in Chapter 12, Hormonal Control of Reproduction in the Male. It is noteworthy that for the endocrine system as well as the nervous system additional information can be transmitted by the frequency of signal production as well as by the signal itself.

Summary

The basics of cell-to-cell communication are introduced in this chapter. A review of protein synthesis from its inception in the nucleus to its final for processing in the Golgi apparatus is described in detail. The four types of intercellular chemical communication, autocrine, paracrine, endocrine, and pherocrine, are presented and explained. To receive such messages is the role of the receptor which must be selective as well as specific for the chemical message presented to it. The nature of such receptors and the different intracellular events triggered by them is explored in detail.

Suggested reading

Basic foundations

Cantley, L. (2017). Signal transduction. In W. F. Boron, & E. L. Boulpaep (Eds.), *Medical physiology* (3rd ed., pp. 47–72). Philadelphia, PA: Elsevier.

Koeppen, B. M., & Stanton, B. W. (2018). Signal transduction, membrane receptors, second messengers, and regulation of gene expression. In B. M. Koeppen, & B. W. Stanton (Eds.), *Berne and levy physiology* (7th ed., pp. 35–50). Philadelphia, PA: Elsevier. Lazar.

Lazar, M. A., & Birnbaum, M. J. (2016). Principles of hormone action. In S. Melmed, K. S. Polonsky, P. R. Larson, & H. M. Kronenberg (Eds.), *Williams textbook of endocrinology* (13th ed., pp. 18–48). Philadelphia, PA: Elsevier.

Mitchell, R. N. (2015). The cell as a unit of health and disease. In V. Kumar, A. K. Abbas, & J. C. Aster (Eds.), *Robbins and Cotran pathologic basis of disease* (9th ed., pp. 1–29). Philadelphia, PA: Elsevier.

Advanced information

Casarini, L., Santi, D., Simoni, M., & Potì, F. (2018). 'Spare' luteinizing hormone receptors: Facts and fiction. *Trends in Endocrinology & Metabolism, 29*(4), 208–217. Available from https://doi.org/10.1016/j.tem.2018.01.007.

de Kloet, E. R., Meijer, O. C., de Nicola, A. F., de Rijk, R. H., & Joëls, M. (2018). Importance of the brain corticosteroid receptor balance in metaplasticity, cognitive performance and neuro-inflammation. *Frontiers in Neuroendocrinology*. Available from https://doi.org/10.1016/j.yfrne.2018.02.003.

Fuller, P. J., Yang, J., & Young, M. J. (2017). 30 Years of the mineralocorticoid receptor: Coregulators as mediators of mineralocorticoid receptor signaling diversity. *Journal of Endocrinology, 234*(1), T23–T34. Available from https://doi.org/10.1530/joe-17-0060.

Jaiswal, B., & Gupta, A. (2018). Modulation of nuclear receptor function by chromatin modifying factor TIP60. *Endocrinology*. Available from https://doi.org/10.1210/en.2017-03190, en.2017-03190-en.02017–03190.

Kwon, O., Kim, K. W., & Kim, M.-S. (2016). Leptin signaling pathways in hypothalamic neurons. *Cellular and Molecular Life Sciences, 73*(7), 1457–1477. Available from https://doi.org/10.1007/s00018-016-2133-1.

Ong, G. S. Y., & Young, M. J. (2017). Mineralocorticoid regulation of cell function: The role of rapid signaling and gene transcription pathways. *Journal of Molecular Endocrinology, 58*(1), R33–R57. Available from https://doi.org/10.1530/jme-15-0318.

CHAPTER

2

Pituitary gland

Case study:

Pituitary mass

A 27-year-old man was snowboarding and sustained a fall in which two bones in his right hand were broken and a tendon in his right thumb was torn. His head struck the ground, but he did not lose consciousness. Upon arrival in the Emergency Department, he was complaining of a headache and a hematoma was found over the right temple. A CT scan was done and the radiologist on call read this as being normal except for the incidental finding of a 1.7 cm pituitary mass with some suprasellar extension. He was discharged and sent for further evaluation to occur 1 month later.

Signs and symptoms

His mass presented no symptoms or signs other than the mass on the CT scan.

Diagnosis

His visual fields, as determined by Goldmann kinetic perimetry, were normal.

1. What are the possible causes of the radiological abnormality? What are the most common cause and the problems to be addressed?
2. What specific points should be explored in the history?
3. What specific points should be explored on a physical exam?
4. After being informed of the relevant findings, what further investigation should be recommended?
5. Review the formal visual field testing results below and explain what is observed (insert Figs. 2.1 and 2.2).

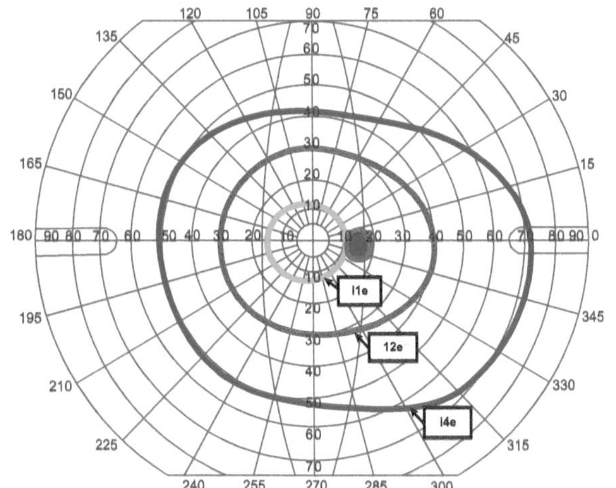

FIGURE 2.1 Goldmann kinetic perimetry is used to test the visual field. The green, red and blue lines represent the isopters in the visual field where the subject first perceived the stimulus. The colors of these lines are not indicative of these particular isopters. Different technicians can use different colors. The black scotoma is the physiological blind spot—the area of the retina where axons come together to form the ophthalmic nerve (cranial nerve II) and, as a result, there are no rods or cones. Source: *Figure 45.11 in Thurtell, M. J., Tomsak, R. L. (2016). Neuro-ophthalmology: Afferent visual system, Chapter 45. In Daroff, et al. (Ed.)* Bradley's neurology in clinical practice *(7th ed., Vol. 1, p. 580). Elsevier.*

6. What are the therapeutic options? Which should be recommended?

The most common cause of a mass this size is a non-secreting (null) pituitary adenoma, but other lesions such as craniopharyngioma and secreting tumors should also be considered.

Goodman's Basic Medical Endocrinology.
DOI: https://doi.org/10.1016/B978-0-12-815844-9.00002-6

(cont'd)

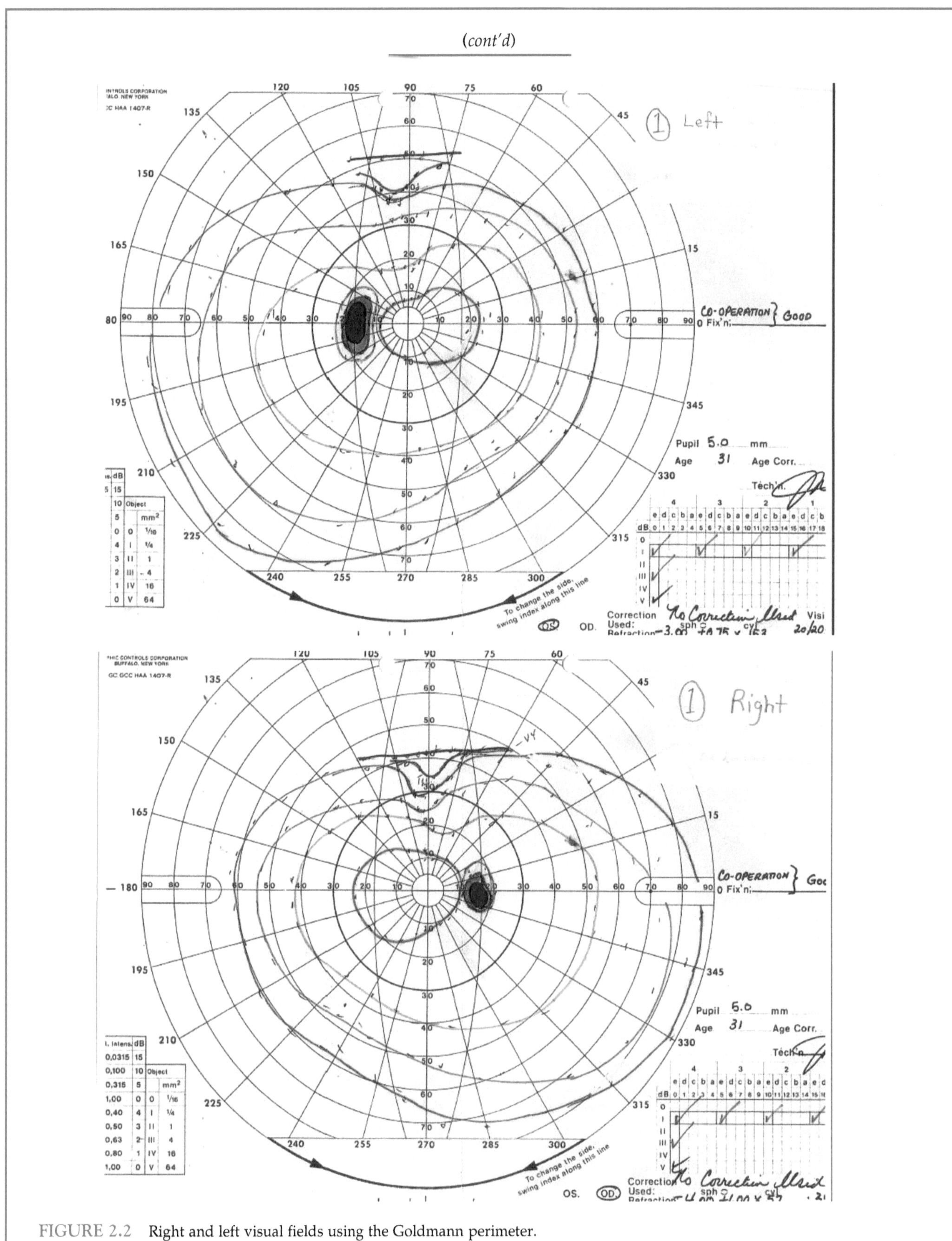

FIGURE 2.2 Right and left visual fields using the Goldmann perimeter.

(*cont'd*)

1. The potential problems to address are:
   a. Exploring for evidence of hormonal hypersecretion.
   b. Exploring for pituitary hyposecretion due to the mass effect from the tumor impinging on the surrounding normal pituitary tissue.
   c. Symptoms and signs due to the mass impinging on surrounding structures, neurological or other structures (i.e., mass symptoms).
   d. Stalk effects, that is, if the mass is extending to the suprasellar region, then one would expect to see stalk effects:
      i. Dopamine delivery down the stalk to the pituitary might be impeded leading to unopposed hyperprolactinemia.
      ii. ADH (antidiuretic hormone) delivery down the stalk to the posterior pituitary is interrupted, resulting in partial or complete diabetes insipidus due to a deficiency of ADH.
2. Hypersecretion: A history is needed to explore the possibility of prolactin (PRL), growth hormone (GH), and ACTH (adrenocorticotropic hormone) hypersecretion (those are the three commonest secreting tumors). TSH (thyroid-stimulating hormone) secreting tumors are rare. Clinically significant LH (luteinizing hormone) and FSH (follicle-stimulating hormone) secreting tumors are exceedingly rare and would result in hypogonadism due to the loss of the normal pulsatile rhythm of release. Continuous overproduction of gonadotropins ironically leads to suppression of the axis altogether.
3. Hyposecretion of any of the six anterior pituitary lobe hormones needs to be considered: ACTH, TSH, LH, and FSH. Hyposecretion of GH is not as obvious in adults and requires biochemical testing.
   PRL would typically be expected to be high rather than deficient due to the relative deficiency of dopamine which normally inhibits PRL production. Therefore one needs to ask about adrenal insufficiency symptoms, amenorrhea in women, hypogonadism in men, symptoms of hypothyroidism, etc.
4. Mass symptoms related to impinging on surrounding structures. Headaches, double vision, or loss of peripheral vision (bitemporal hemianopsia). Even postnasal drip.
   a. Stalk effects: polyuria/polydipsia (signs of DI) and galactorrhea as a sign of a relative dopamine deficiency.
5. Physical examination is again to look for the following points a–d:
   a. To look for galactorrhea, acromegaly, Cushing, and hyperthyroidism.
   b. The usual/typical order for loss of pituitary secretory function in a slowly enlarging pituitary mass is *G*H, *L*H, *F*SH, *T*SH, *A*CTH, *P*RL (i.e., GH is one of the earliest ones to go followed by gonadotropins, etc.); the easy mnemonic to use is *G*o *L*ook *F*or *T*he *A*denoma *P*lease. Look for hypothyroidism with a small soft thyroid gland, signs of hypogonadism with loss of sexual hair, small, soft testes, and loss of secondary sexual characteristics. Secondary adrenal insufficiency would be suspected clinically if blood pressure is low with postural changes etc.
   c. Mass effects of an enlarging pituitary mass will vary depending on how big the mass is and which way it grows. For example, if a tumor enlarges *superiorly*, then the structures affected are as follows:
      i. Optic chiasm (bitemporal hemianopsia)
      ii. Hypothalamus (thirst/satiety/appetite/temperature changes)
      iii. Third ventricle (obstructive hydrocephalus and papilledema)
      iv. Frontal lobe (in very large tumors) → frontal lobe dysfunction

      If a tumor enlarges *inferiorly*, then one would expect to see:

      i. A nasopharyngeal mass
      ii. CSF rhinorrhea or a postnasal drip from the CSF eroding into the sphenoidal sinus

      If a tumor enlarges laterally, then the structures affected would be:

      i. Cranial nerves 3, 4, 5, and 6 (diplopia, abnormal extraocular motion, pupillary defects, and fundoscopic exam)

(cont'd)

ii. Loss of sensation/paresthesias over V1 and V2 branches of the fifth cranial nerve distribution on the face (V3 is typically not affected)

iii. Temporal lobe (temporal lobe dysfunction/dysphasia)

d. Stalk effect: High PRL due to lack of dopamine (galactorrhea in a woman, and hypogonadism in a man). Diabetes insipidus due to ADH deficiency. (Recall that ADH is made in the supraoptic nucleus and the paraventricular nucleus, then transferred down the stalk to the posterior pituitary lobe to be stored in vacuoles until it is needed.)

6. *Case finding: the history and physical examination are both normal*

   End organ function still needs to be assessed. Assess all six hormonal axes by ordering the *end organ hormonal test.* No need to order TSH, for example, as that messenger hormone is now potentially flawed so that would have to bypass it and use the end organ hormone, that is, fT4. In this male patient, you would order a serum testosterone (free androgen index), free T4, PRL, IGF-1, and likely 8 a.m. cortisol (if equivocal, then do a dynamic stimulating test such as with an insulin tolerance test). GH could be measured at the same time as it should peak with hypoglycemia.

   Result: All of this testing is normal.

7. Case 1 shows a normal result with the expected complete range of vision represented by the full concentric circles. Note that the black central spot in the middle of the plot is the normal blind spot due to the optic nerve location in the retina. Case 1 shows a normal result with the expected complete range of vision represented by the full concentric circles. Note that the black central spot in the middle of the plot is the normal blind spot due to the optic nerve location on the retina.

Management

As this is a null adenoma, it has produced no hormones and so far is not affecting any physiological function.

1. The therapeutic options are either observation with repeat clinical and, if necessary, biochemical assessment and careful radiological and visual field monitoring every 6–12 months. Visual fields should be done by appropriate personnel. These can be arranged in specialized ophthalmology clinics to get a baseline and repeat at different intervals to assess if there is any progression in any defects. The other approach is to consider trans-sphenoidal surgery.
2. Radiotherapy can be discussed and then, if nothing else, to explain why radiotherapy is not the best initial Rx option (panhypopituitarism is a common long-term complication of radiotherapy as well as increased risk of stroke).
3. The choice of either observation or surgical therapy probably comes down to the patient's individualized case and their preferences after full discussion.

Prognosis

Complete recovery without complications is the usual outcome.

Case 2. (Summary only)

Case 2 is a patient with a large pituitary tumor and optic chiasm impingement. With Goldmann kinetic perimetry, one can see in the right visual field that there is a loss of the concentric circles of the visual field in the superior and inferior temporal range. In the left visual field, there is a loss of the concentric circles in the superior temporal range. This is the classic expected pattern of visual field involvement in a patient with a large pituitary mass. Treatment options are the same as was discussed for case 1 (Fig. 2.3).

(*cont'd*)

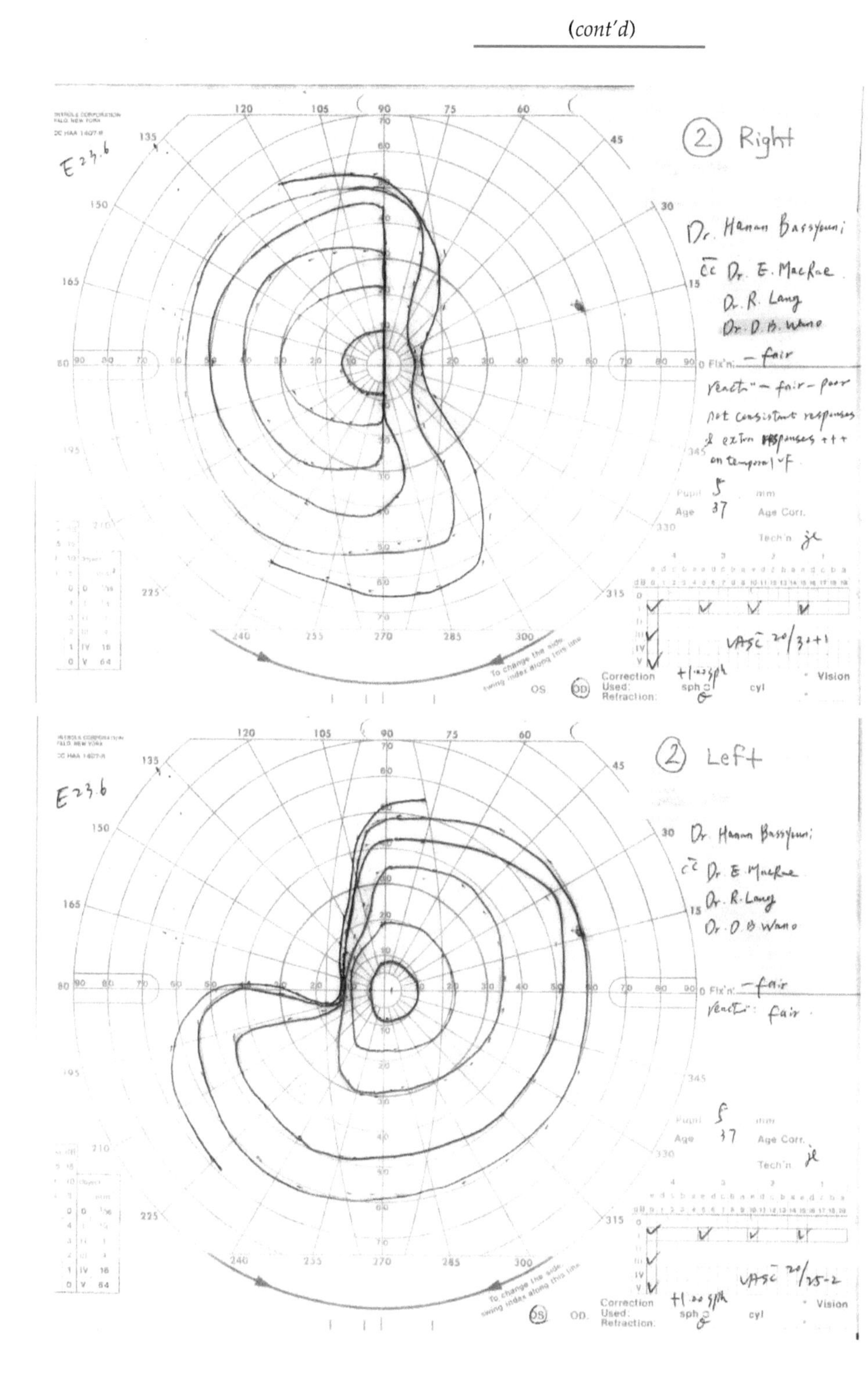

FIGURE 2.3 Case 2: Patient with large pituitary tumor impinging on the optic chiasm. Left eye visual field shows a superior temporal hemianopsia. Right eye visual field shows a superior and inferior hemianopsia.

Pituitary gland

The pituitary gland (Fig. 2.4) usually has been thought of as the "master gland" because its hormone secretions control the growth and activity of three other endocrine glands: the thyroid, adrenals, and gonads. Because the secretory activity of the master gland is itself controlled by hormones that originate in either the brain or its target glands, it is perhaps better to think of the pituitary gland as the relay between the control centers in the central nervous system and the peripheral endocrine organs. The pituitary hormones are not limited in their activity to the regulation of endocrine target glands; they also act directly on nonendocrine target tissues. Secretion of all these hormones is under the control of signals arising in both the brain and the periphery. It should be kept in mind that many of the initial findings of the actions of hormones were done in rodents and, while similar, the actions in humans can be quite different. For example, rats reproduce seasonally, while humans can reproduce all year long.

Morphology

The pituitary gland lies in a small depression in the sphenoid bone, the sella turcica, just beneath the hypothalamus, and is connected to the hypothalamus by a thin stalk called the infundibulum.

Embryology

The pituitary is a compound structure consisting of a neural or posterior lobe derived embryologically from the brainstem, and a larger anterior portion, the adenohypophysis, which derives embryologically from an outgrowth of the primitive foregut, called Rathke's pouch (Fig. 2.5).

The cells at the junction of the two lobes comprise the intermediate lobe, which is not readily identifiable as an anatomical entity in humans (Fig. 2.6).

Histology

Histologically, the anterior lobe consists of large polygonal cells arranged in cords and surrounded by a sinusoidal capillary system. Using dyes, these cells were divided into chromophils, which took up the dye, and chromophobes, which stained poorly. The chromophils were further divided into acidophils, which stained with an acidic stain, and basophils, which stained with a basic stain. The acidophils and basophils contain secretory granules, while the chromophobes are only sparsely granulated. It is now believed that the chromophobes are degranulated chromophils. Based on their characteristic staining with standard histochemical dyes and immunofluorescent stains, it is possible to identify the cells that secrete each of the pituitary hormones. It once was thought that there was

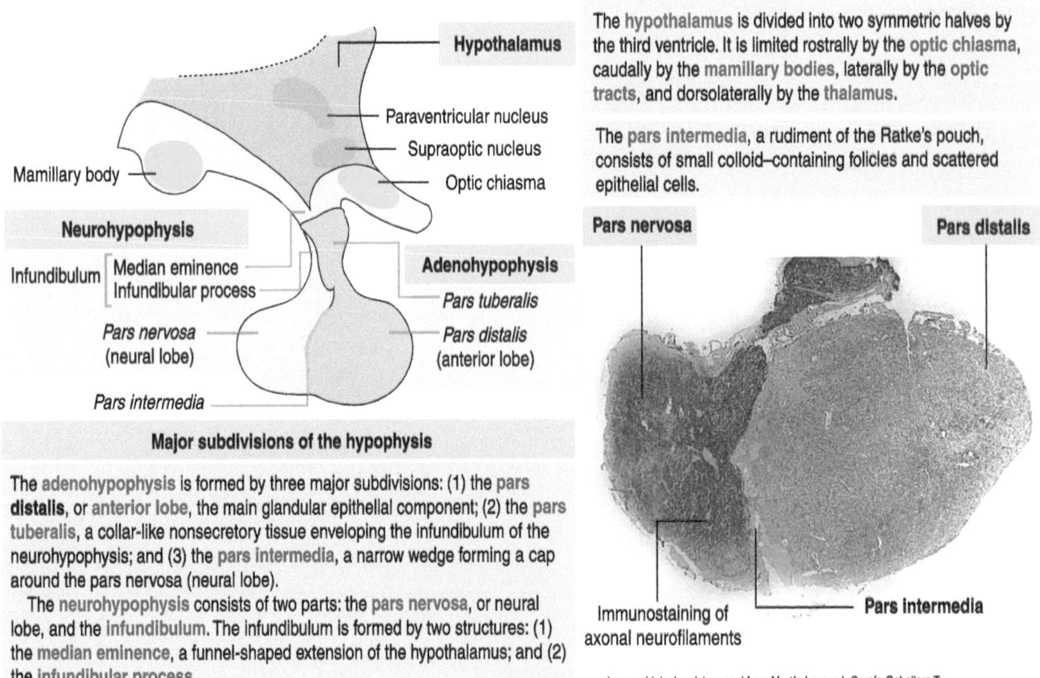

FIGURE 2.4 The pituitary gland (circle) and its relationship to the hypothalamus of the brain. Source: *From Figure 18-1 in Kierszenbaum, A. L., Tres, L. L. (2016).* Histology and cell biology: An introduction to pathology *(4th ed., p. 559). Elsevier.*

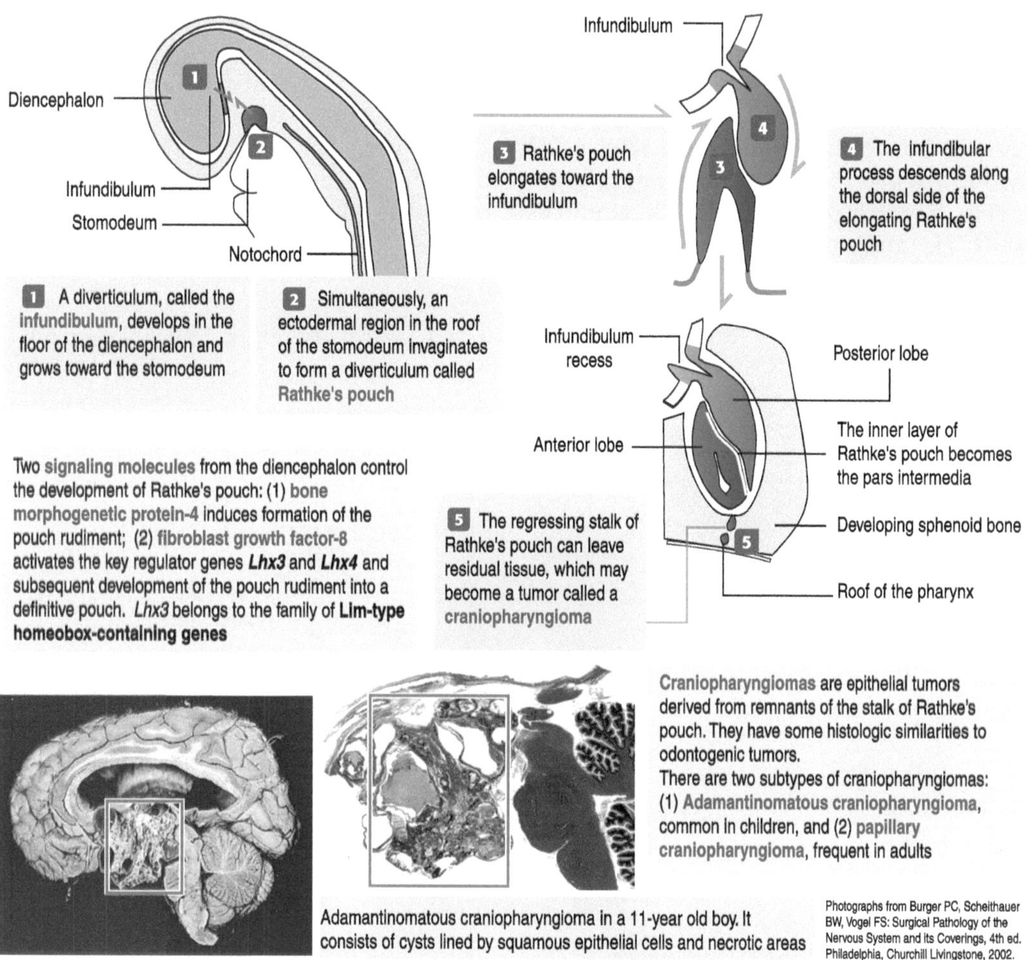

FIGURE 2.5 The embryology of the pituitary. It is formed from a downward growth from the brain and an upward invagination (Rathke's pouch) from what will be the nasopharynx. Source: *From Figure 18-2 in Kierszenbaum, A. L., Tres, L. L. (2016).* Histology and cell biology: An introduction to pathology *(4th ed., p. 560). Elsevier.*

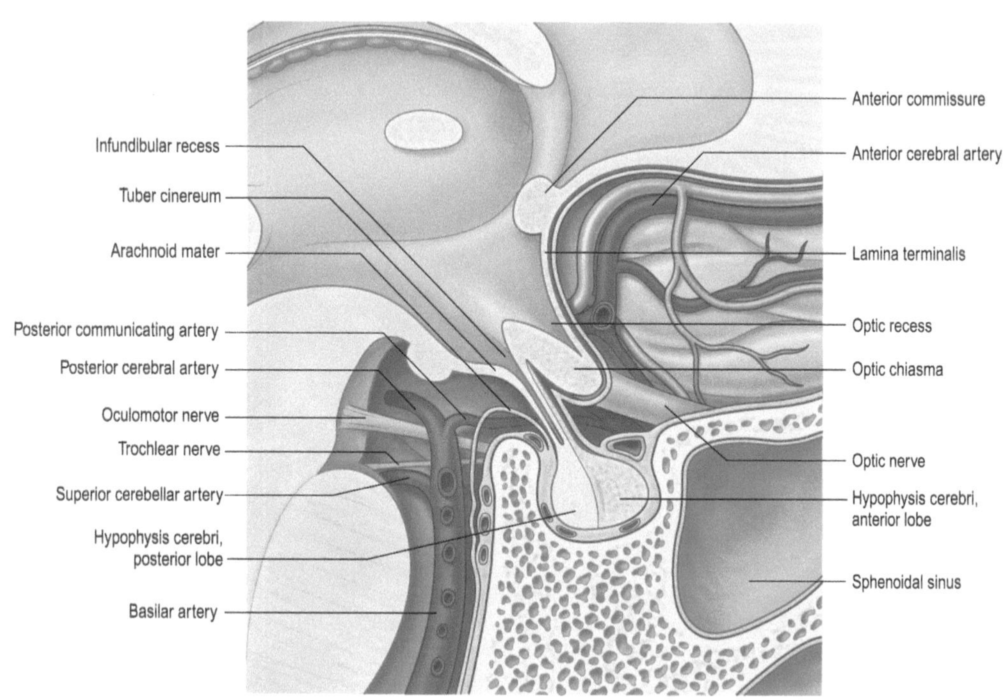

FIGURE 2.6 A cross section of the pituitary gland in the skull. Source: *From Figure 23.10 in S. Standring, et al. (Eds.). (2016).* Gray's anatomy *(41st ed., p. 360). Elsevier.*

a unique cell type for each of the pituitary hormones, but it is now recognized that some cells may produce more than one hormone. The acidophils produce GH and prolactin (PRL) while the basophils produce corticotropin (ACTH), thyrotropin (TSH), follicle stimulating hormone (FSH) and luteinizing hormone (LH). These hormones and their target structures as well as those from the posterior lobe are illustrated in Fig. 2.7.

The posterior lobe consists of two major portions: the infundibulum, or stalk, and the infundibular process, or neural lobe (Fig. 2.1). The posterior lobe is richly endowed with nerve fiber endings that contain

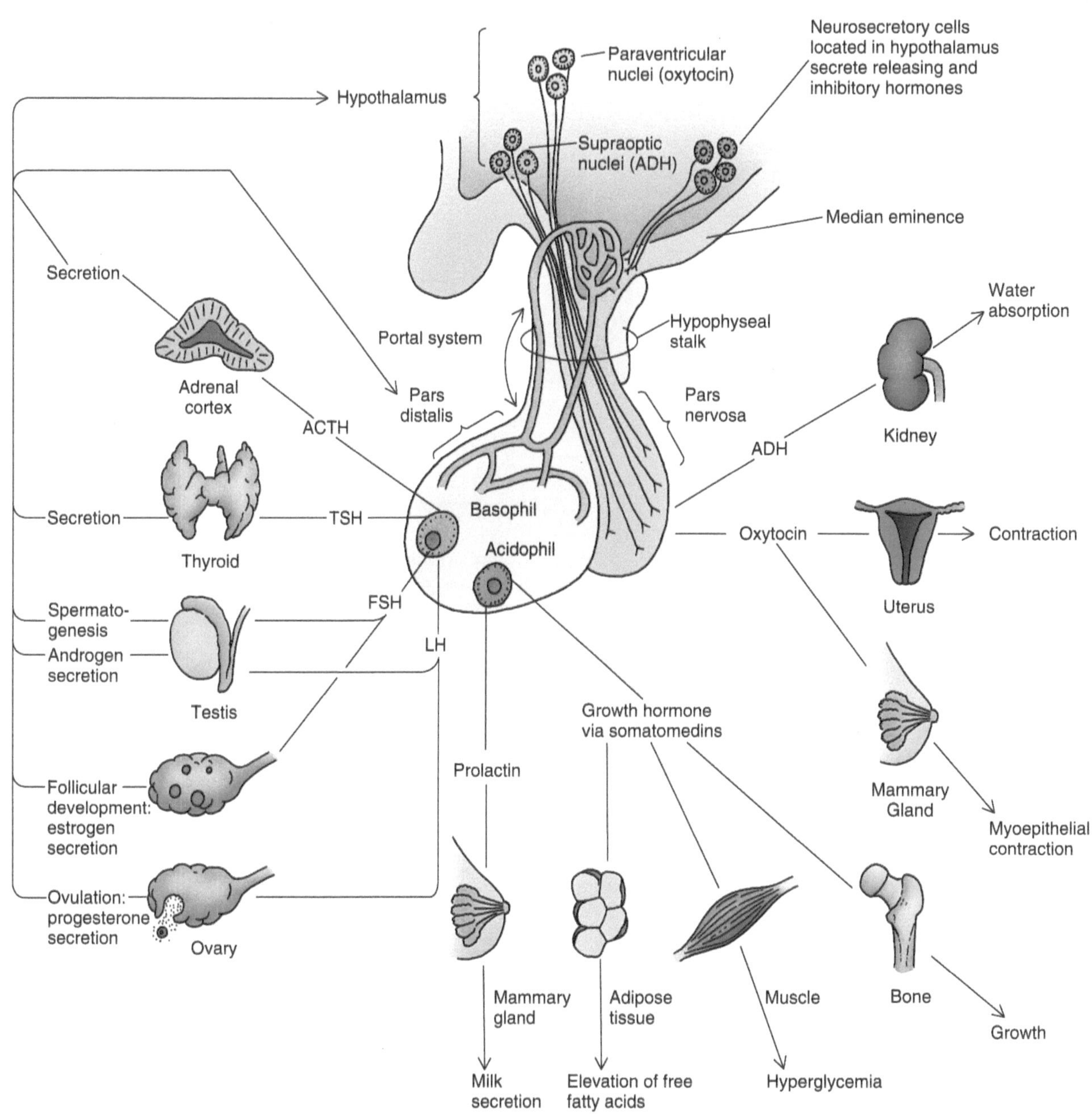

FIGURE 2.7 The origin and target structures of each of the pituitary hormones from acidophil and basophil cells. Growth hormone stimulates the liver to produce another group of hormones called somatomedins, which then act on target connective tissues. Some of the products of the target structures feed back to the hypothalamus or pituitary gland to inhibit the secretion of an additional pituitary hormone. The *pars distalis* (Latin for distal part of the anterior pituitary as opposed to the pars tuberalis that is a part of the pituitary stalk) is another term for the anterior lobe and the *pars nervosa* is another term for the posterior (neural) lobe. Source: *From Figure 13-1 in Gartner, L. P. (2017).* Textbook of histology *(4th ed., p. 348). Elsevier.*

electron-dense secretory granules. The cell bodies from which these fibers arise are in the bilaterally paired supraoptic and paraventricular nuclei of the hypothalamus. These cells are characteristically large compared to smaller, parvicellular (*parvus* is small in Latin) hypothalamic neurons and hence are called magnicellular (*magnus* means large in Latin) neurons (Fig. 2.8).

Secretory material synthesized in cell bodies in the hypothalamus is transported down the axons and stored in bulbous axon endings within the posterior lobe. They lie near the rich capillary network whose fenestrated endothelium allows secretory products to readily enter the circulation. The vascular supply and innervation of the two lobes reflect their different embryological origins and provide important clues that ultimately led to an understanding of their physiological regulation. The anterior lobe is sparsely innervated and lacks any secretomotor nerves. This fact might argue against a role for the pituitary as a relay between the central nervous system and peripheral endocrine organs, except that communication between the anterior pituitary and the brain is through vascular, rather than neural, channels.

Blood supply

The anterior lobe is linked to the brainstem by the hypothalamic–hypophyseal portal system, through which it receives most of its blood supply (Figs. 2.9 and 2.10).

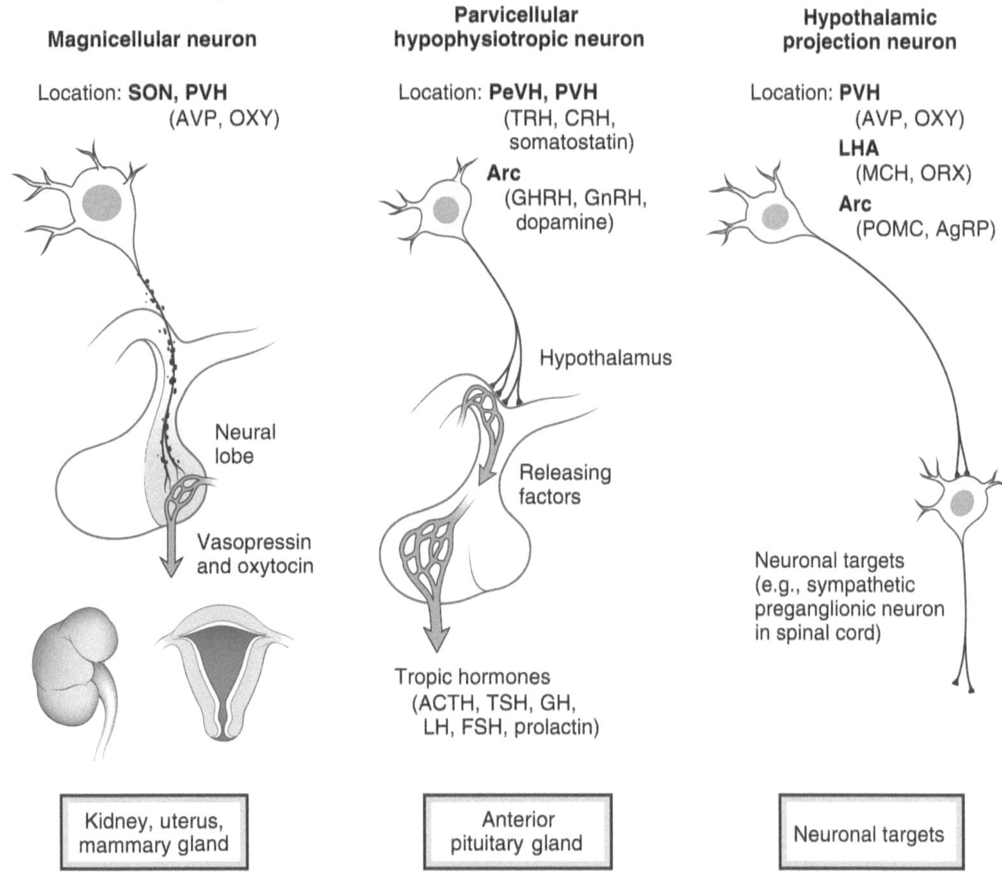

FIGURE 2.8 The magnicellular and parvicellular neurons and their secretions. These are compared to the autonomic nervous system which also has its origins in the hypothalamus, using the sympathetic system as an example. The substances they produce are AVP, OXY, TRH, CRH, GHRH, GnRH, MCH, ORX, (not covered in this textbook), POMC, AgRP, (not covered in this textbook). The tropic hormones released from the anterior pituitary gland are ACTH, TSH, GH, LH, FSH. *ACTH*, Adrenocorticotropic hormone (corticotropin); *AgRP*, agouti-related peptide; *Arc*, arcuate (infundibular) nucleus of the hypothalamus; *AVP*, arginine vasopressin (ADH); *CRH*, corticotropin-releasing hormone; *FSH*, follicle-stimulating hormone; *GH*, growth hormone (somatotropin); *GHRH*, growth hormone–releasing hormone; *GnRH*, gonadotropin-releasing hormone; *LH*, luteinizing hormone; *LHA*, lateral hypothalamic area; *MCH*, melanin-concentrating hormone; *ORX*, orexin/hypocretin; *OXY*, oxytocin; *PeVH*, periventricular hypothalamic nucleus of the hypothalamus; *POMC*, proopiomelanocortin; *PVH*, paraventricular hypothalamic nucleus; *SON*, supraoptic nucleus; *TRH*, thyrotropin-releasing hormone; *TSH*, thyroid-stimulating hormone (thyrotropin). Source: *From Figure 7-1 in Low M. J. (2016). Neuroendocrinology, Chapter 7. In S. Melmed, K. S. Polonsky, P. R. Larsen, H. M. Kronenberg. (Eds.),* Williams textbook of endocrinology *(13th ed., p. 112), Elsevier.*

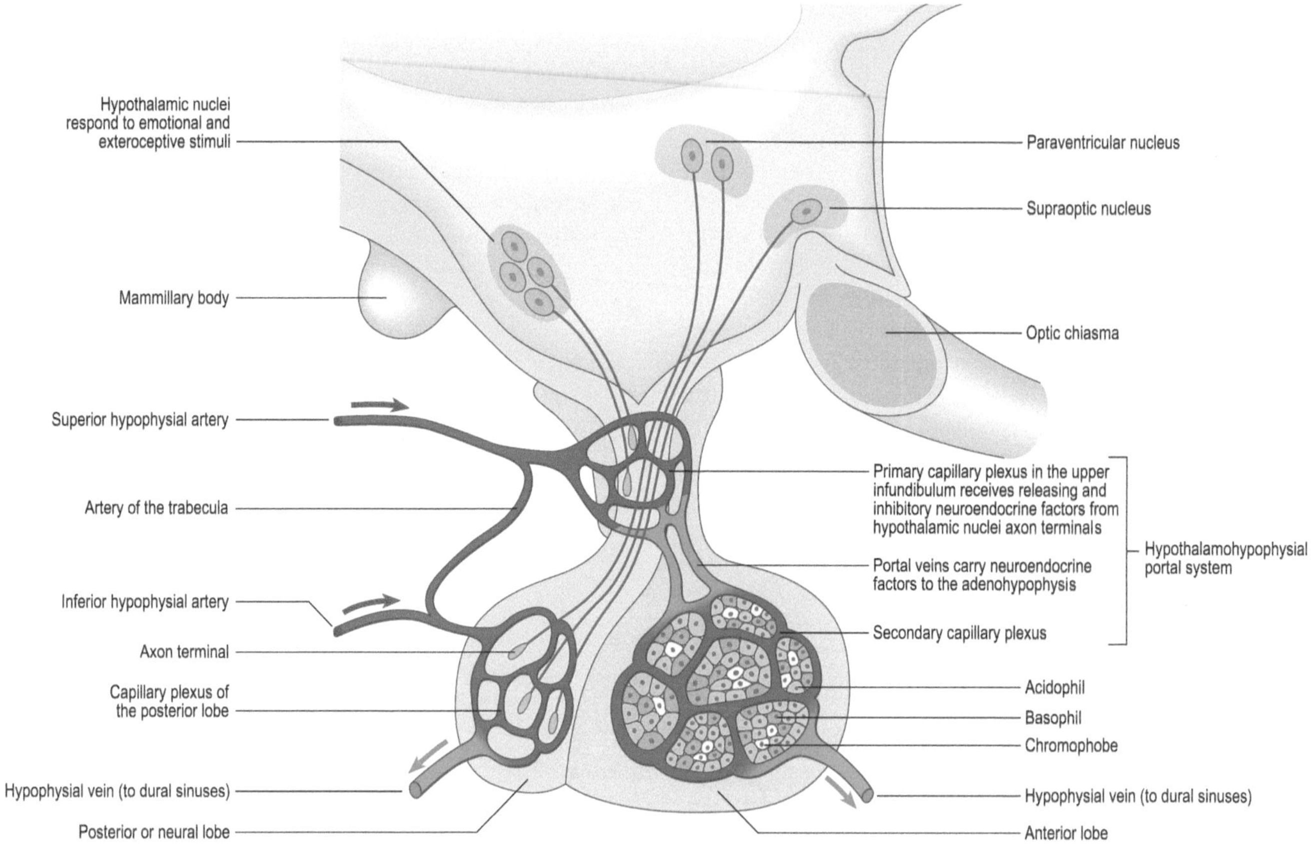

FIGURE 2.9 The blood supply to the pituitary. The venous blood from the pituitary empties into the cavernous sinus, a dural sinus which surrounds the pituitary and from there, ultimately, to the internal jugular vein. Source: *From Figure 23.11 in S. Standring, et al. (Eds.). (2016).* Gray's anatomy *(41st ed., p. 361). Elsevier.*

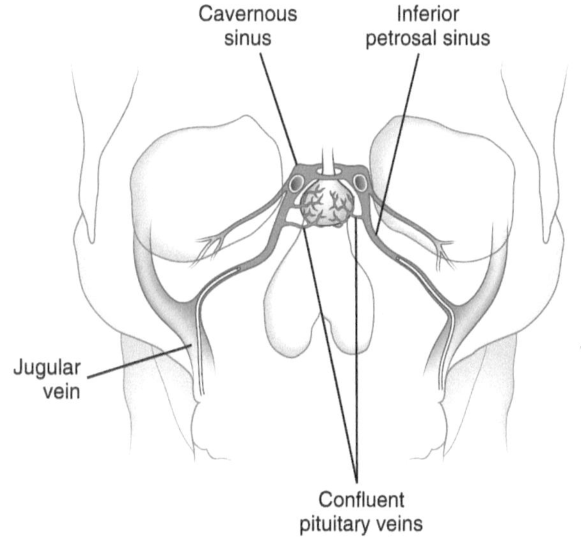

FIGURE 2.10 The venous drainage of the pituitary gland. The venous blood can be sampled and the cannula is illustrated as being inserted into the internal jugular vein. Source: *From Figure 15-24 in Stewart, P. M., Newell-Price, J. D. C. (2016). The adrenal cortex, Chapter 15. In S. Malmed, K. S. Polonsky, P. R. Larsen, H. M. Kronenberg. (Eds.),* Williams textbook of endocrinology *(13th ed., p. 519). Elsevier.*

The superior hypophyseal arteries deliver blood to an intricate network of capillaries, the primary plexus, in the median eminence of the hypothalamus. Capillaries of the primary plexus converge to form long hypophyseal portal vessels, which course down the infundibular stalk to deliver their blood to capillary sinusoids interspersed among the secretory cells of the anterior lobe. The inferior hypophyseal arteries supply a similar capillary plexus in the lower portion of the infundibular stem. These capillaries drain into short portal vessels, which supply a second sinusoidal capillary network within the anterior lobe. Nearly, all the blood that reaches the anterior lobe is carried in the long and short portal vessels. The anterior lobe receives only a small portion of its blood supply directly from the paired trabecular arteries, which branch off the superior hypophyseal arteries. In contrast, the circulation in the posterior pituitary is unremarkable. It is supplied with blood by the inferior hypophyseal arteries. Venous blood drains from both lobes through a number of short veins into the nearby cavernous sinuses.

The portal arrangement of blood flow is important because the blood that supplies the secretory cells of the anterior lobe first drains the hypothalamus. Portal blood can thus pick up chemical signals released by neurons of the central nervous system and deliver them to secretory cells of the anterior pituitary. As might be anticipated, because hypophyseal portal blood flow represents only a tiny fraction of the cardiac output, only minute amounts of neural secretions are needed to achieve biologically effective concentrations in pituitary sinusoidal blood when delivered in this way. More than 1000 times more secretory material would be needed if it were dissolved in the entire blood volume and delivered through the arterial circulation. This arrangement also provides a measure of specificity to hypothalamic secretion, as pituitary cells are the only ones exposed to concentrations that are high enough to be physiologically effective.

The anterior lobe (adenohypophysis)

Physiology

There are six anterior pituitary hormones whose physiological importance is clearly established (Fig. 2.7). They include the hormones that govern the function of the thyroid and adrenal glands, the gonads, the mammary glands, and bodily growth. They have been called "trophic" or "tropic" from the Greek *trophos*, to nourish, or *tropic*, to turn toward. Both terms are generally accepted. For example, thyrotrophin, or thyrotropin, is more accurately called TSH and stimulates the thyroid gland. Because its effects are exerted throughout the body (soma in Greek), GH has also been called somatotropic hormone, or somatotropin. Table 2.1 lists the anterior pituitary hormones and their synonyms.

The basophil cells in the anterior pituitary can also produce more than one type of hormone. Sometimes, when referring to a specific hormone, the basophil cells are named for the hormone under discussion. Thus there are thyrotropes and corticotropes—all are basophil cells—and somatotropes and lactotropes that are acidophil cells. The two gonadotropins are produced from a single basophil cell type, the gonadotrope.

All the anterior pituitary hormones are either proteins or glycoproteins. They are synthesized on ribosomes and translocated through various cellular compartments where they undergo posttranslational processing. They are packaged in membrane-bound secretory granules and secreted by exocytosis. The pituitary gland stores relatively large amounts of hormone, sufficient to meet physiological demands for many days. Over the course of many decades, these hormones were extracted, purified, and characterized. Now the structure of their genes and the intricacies of

TABLE 2.1 Hormones of the anterior pituitary gland.

Hormone	Target	Major actions in humans
Glycoprotein family		
TSH, also called thyrotropin	Thyroid gland	Stimulate synthesis and secretion of thyroid hormones
FSH	Ovary	Stimulate growth of follicles and estrogen secretion
	Testis	Act on Sertoli cells to promote maturation of sperm
LH	Ovary	Stimulate ovulation of ripe follicle and formation of corpus luteum; stimulate estrogen and progesterone synthesis by corpus luteum
	Testis	Stimulate interstitial cells of Leydig to synthesize and secrete testosterone
Growth hormone/prolactin family		
GH, also called STH	Most tissues	Promote growth in stature and mass; stimulate the production of insulin-like growth factor (IGH-I); stimulate protein synthesis; usually inhibit glucose utilization; and promote fat utilization
Prolactin	Mammary glands	Promote milk secretion and mammary growth
POMC		
ACTH, also known as adrenocorticotropin or corticotropin	Adrenal cortex	Promote synthesis and secretion of adrenal cortical hormones
β-Lipotropin	Adipose Tissue	Physiological role not established

ACTH, Adrenocorticotropic hormone; *FSH*, follicle-stimulating hormone; *GH*, growth hormone; *LH*, luteinizing hormone; *POMC*, proopiomelanocortin family; *STH*, somatotropic hormone; *TSH*, thyroid-stimulating hormone.

their synthesis and posttranslational processing are known, and we can group the anterior pituitary hormones by families.

Glycoprotein hormones

The glycoprotein hormone family includes TSH, whose only known physiological role is to stimulate secretion of thyroid hormone (Fig. 2.11), and the two gonadotropins, FSH and LH (Fig. 2.12).

Although named for their effect on the ovaries in women, both gonadotropic hormones are also crucial for the function of the testes. In women, FSH promotes the growth of ovarian follicles, and in men, it promotes formation of spermatozoa by the germinal epithelium of the testis. In women, LH induces ovulation of the ripe follicle and formation of the corpus luteum from remaining glomerulosa cells in the collapsed, ruptured follicle. It also stimulates synthesis and secretion of the

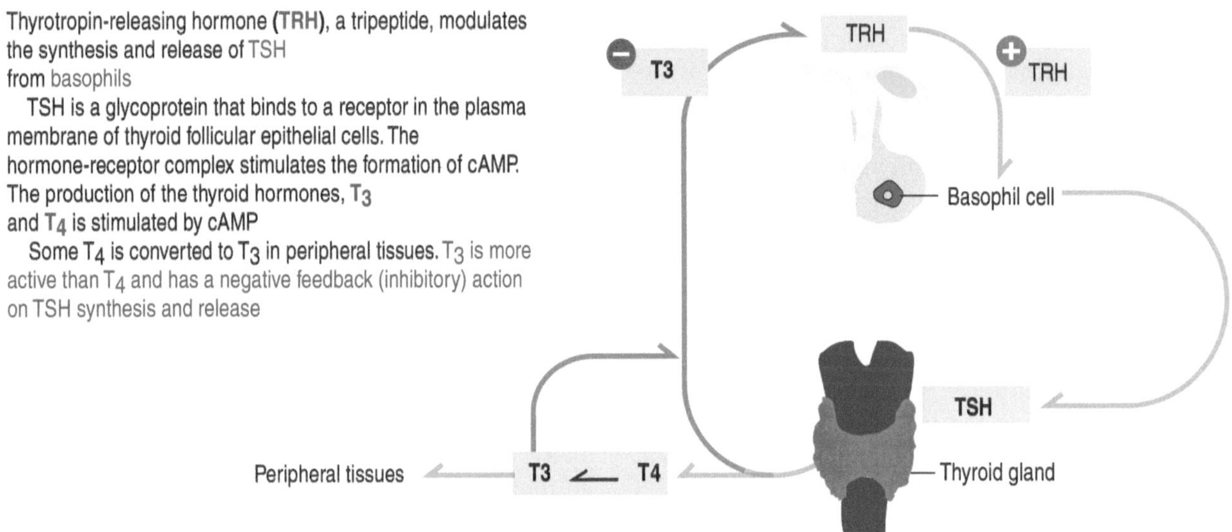

FIGURE 2.11 The production of TSH and its effect on the thyroid gland. T3 is the active form of the hormone and T4 is regarded as the storage form. Only T3 has feedback inhibition of the hypothalamus. *T3*, Triiodothyronine; *T4*, thyroxine; *TSH*, thyroid-stimulating hormone. Source: *From Figure 18-9 in Kierszenbaum, A. L., Tres, L. L. (2020).* Histology and cell biology: An introduction to pathology *(5th ed., p. 615). Elsevier.*

Neurons in the arcuate nucleus of the hypothalamus secrete GnRH (gonadotropin-releasing hormone). GnRH is secreted in pulses at 60- to 90-minute intervals and stimulates the pulsatile secretion of gonadotropins by the basophilic gonadotrophs.

In the female, FSH stimulates granulosa cells of the ovarian follicle to proliferate and secrete estradiol, inhibin, and activin. LH stimulates progesterone secretion by the corpus luteum

In the male, FSH stimulates Sertoli cell function in the seminiferous epithelium (synthesis of inhibin, activin, and androgen-binding protein). LH stimulates the production of testosterone by Leydig cells. A lack of FSH and LH in females and males leads to infertility

Kallmann's syndrome is characterized by delayed or absent puberty and anosmia (impaired sense of smell). It is clinically defined as hypogonadotropic hypogonadism (HH). Mutations in genes prevent the migration of GnRH-secreting neurons to the hypothalamic arcuate nucleus and olfactory neurons to the olfactory bulb

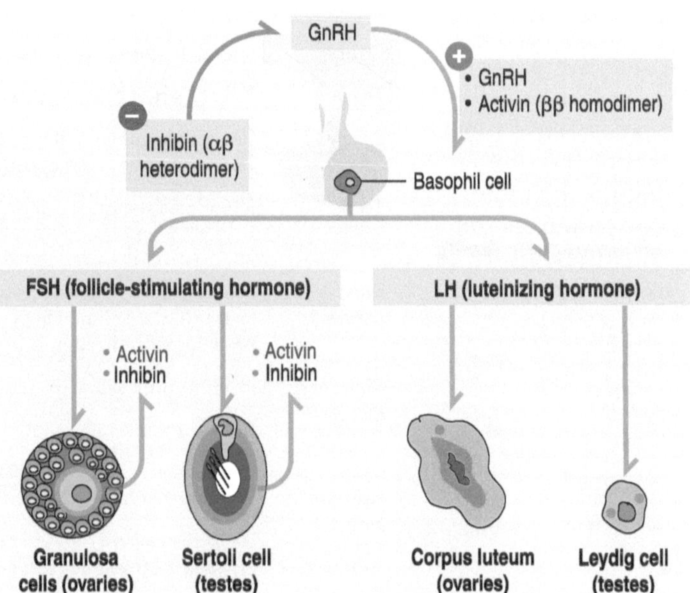

FIGURE 2.12 The synthesis of FSH and LH by the basophil cell. *FSH*, Follicle-stimulating hormone; *LH*, luteinizing hormone. Source: *Figure 18-8 in Kierszenbaum, A. L., Tres, L. L. (2016).* Histology and cell biology: An introduction to pathology *(4th ed., p. 565). Elsevier.*

ovarian hormones estrogen and progesterone. In men, LH stimulates the secretion of the male hormone, testosterone, by interstitial cells of the testis. Consequently, it has also been called interstitial cell-stimulating hormone, but this name has largely disappeared from the literature. The actions of these hormones are discussed in detail in Chapter 12, Hormonal Control of Reproduction in the Male, and Chapter 13, Hormonal Control of Reproduction in the Female: The Menstrual Cycle.

The three glycoprotein hormones are synthesized and stored in pituitary basophils and, as their name implies, each contains sugar moieties covalently linked to asparagine residues in the polypeptide chains. All three comprise two peptide subunits, designated alpha and beta, which, though tightly coupled, are not covalently linked (Fig. 2.13).

The alpha subunit of all three hormones is identical in its amino acid sequence and is the product of a single gene located on chromosome 6. The beta subunits of each are somewhat larger than the alpha subunit and confer physiological specificity. Both alpha and beta subunits contribute to receptor binding and both must be present in the receptor-binding pocket to produce a biological response. Beta subunits are encoded in separate genes located on different chromosomes: TSH β on chromosome 1, FSH β on chromosome 11, and LH β on chromosome 19, but there is a great deal of homology in their amino acid sequences. Both subunits contain carbohydrate moieties that are considerably less constant in their composition than are their peptide chains. Alpha subunits are synthesized in excess over beta subunits, and hence, it is the synthesis of beta subunits that appear to be the rate-limiting step for the production of glycoprotein hormones. Pairing of the two subunits begins in the rough endoplasmic reticulum and continues in the Golgi apparatus, where the processing of carbohydrate components of the subunits is completed. The loosely paired complex then undergoes spontaneous refolding in secretory granules into a stable, active hormone. Control of expression of the alpha and beta subunit genes is not perfectly coordinated, and free alpha and

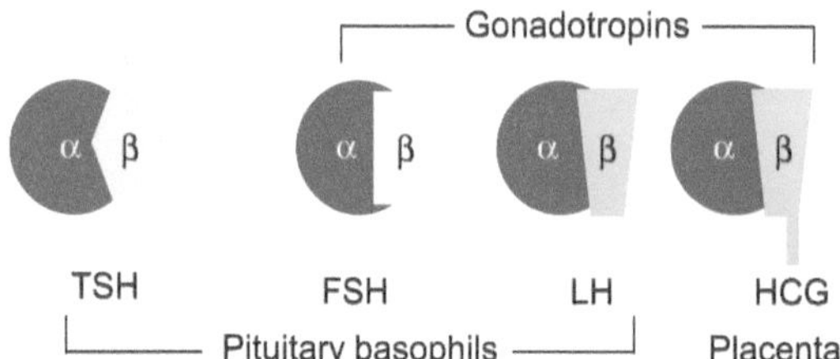

FIGURE 2.13 The glycoproteins. The three glycoproteins of pituitary origin and the placental human chorionic gonadotropin (hCG or HCG) all share a common alpha subunit.

the beta subunits of all three hormones may be found in blood plasma.

The placental hormone, human chorionic gonadotropin (hCG), is closely related chemically and functionally to the pituitary gonadotropic hormones. It, too, is a glycoprotein and consists of an alpha and a beta chain. The alpha chain is a product of the same gene as the alpha chain of pituitary glycoprotein hormones. The peptide sequence of the beta chain is identical to that of LH except that it is longer by 32 amino acids at its carboxyl terminus. Curiously, although there is only a single gene for each beta subunit of the pituitary glycoprotein hormones, the human genome contains seven copies of the hCG beta gene, all located on chromosome 19 in close proximity to the LH beta gene. Not surprisingly, hCG has biological actions that are like those of LH, as well as a unique action on the corpus luteum (Chapter 14: Hormonal Control of Pregnancy and Lactation).

Growth hormone and prolactin

GH is required for the attainment of normal adult stature (see Chapter 11: Hormonal Control of Growth) and produces metabolic effects that may not be directly related to its growth-promoting actions (Fig. 2.14).

Metabolic effects include mobilization of free fatty acids from adipose tissue and inhibition of glucose metabolism in muscle and adipose tissue. The role of GH in energy balance is discussed in Chapter 8, Hormonal Regulation of Fuel Metabolism. Somatotropes are by far the most abundant anterior pituitary cells and account for at least half the cells of the adenohypophysis. GH, which is secreted throughout life, is the most abundant of the pituitary hormones. The human pituitary gland stores between 5 and 10 mg of GH, an amount that is 20–100 times greater than other anterior pituitary hormones. Structurally, GH is closely related to another pituitary hormone, PRL, which is required for milk production in postpartum women (Chapter 14: Hormonal Control of Pregnancy and Lactation) (Fig. 2.15).

The functions of PRL in men or nonlactating women are not firmly established, but a growing body of evidence suggests that it may stimulate cells of the immune system. These pituitary hormones are closely related to the placental hormone human chorionic somatomammotropin (hCS), which has both growth-promoting and milk-producing activity in some experimental systems. Because of this property, hCS is also called human placental lactogen. Although the physiological function of this placental hormone has not been established with certainty, it may regulate maternal metabolism during pregnancy and prepare the

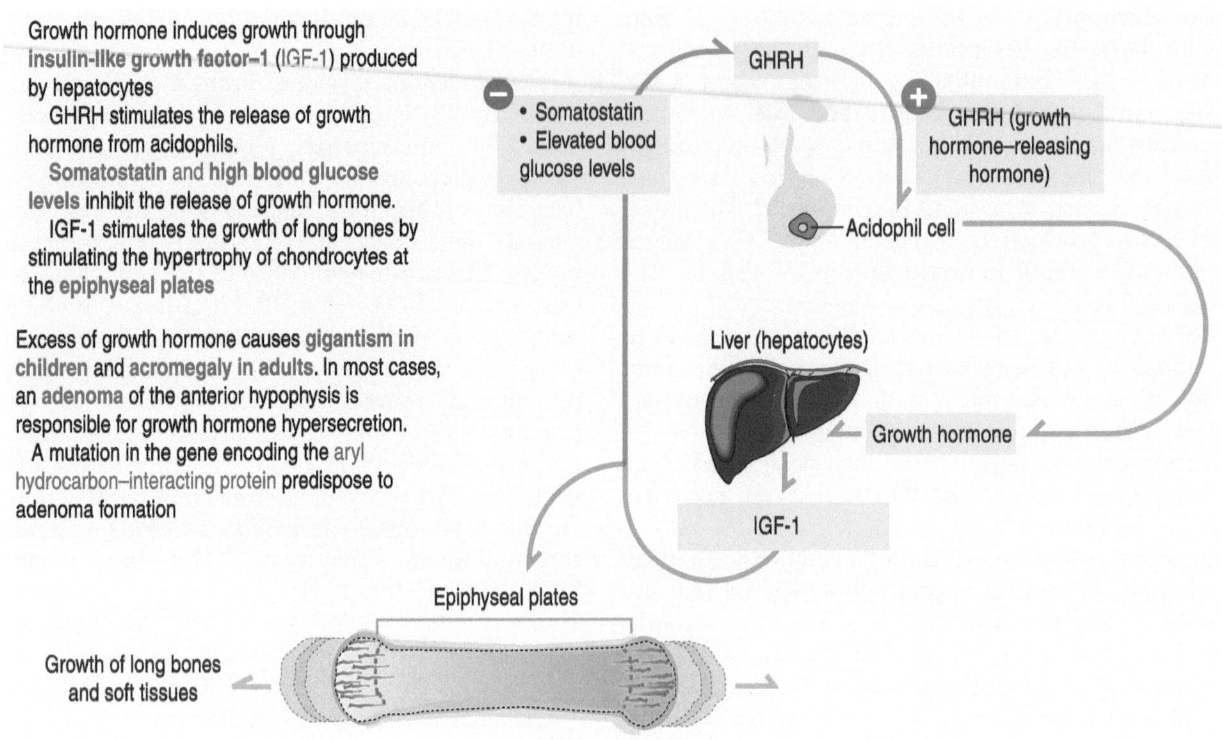

FIGURE 2.14 Growth hormone production and feedback. Growth hormone stimulates the liver to produce IGF-1, formerly called somatomedin C, which stimulates bone and other connective tissues. IGF-1 feeds back to the hypothalamus to cause the release of somatostatin which inhibits the release of more growth hormone. Source: *Figure 18-6 in Kierszenbaum, A. L., Tres, L. L. (2016).* Histology and cell biology: An introduction to pathology *(4th ed., p. 564). Elsevier.*

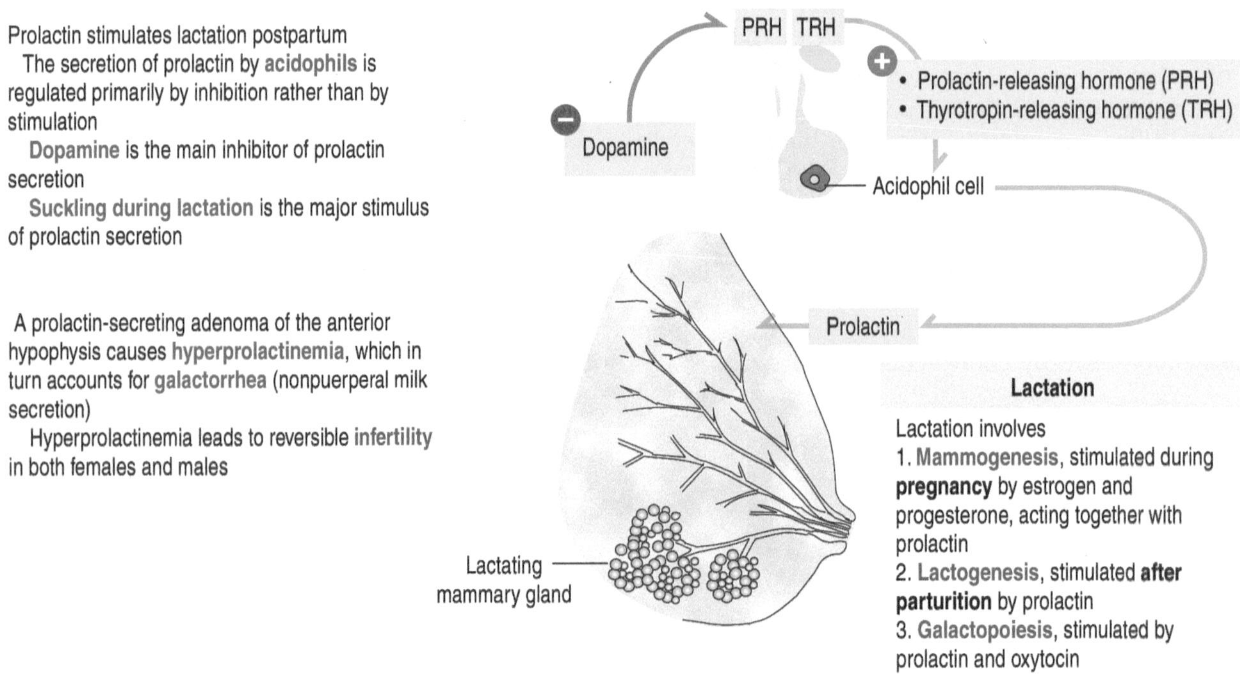

FIGURE 2.15 Prolactin production. There is no releasing hormone for prolactin. Only inhibition by dopamine. Source: *From Figure 18-7 in Kierszenbaum, A. L., Tres, L. L. (2016).* Histology and cell biology: An introduction to pathology *(4th ed., p. 564). Elsevier.*

mammary glands for lactation (Chapter 14: Hormonal Control of Pregnancy and Lactation).

GH, PRL, and hCS appear to have evolved from a single ancestral gene that duplicated several times; the GH and PRL genes before the emergence of the vertebrates, and GH and the hCS genes after the divergence of the primates from other mammalian groups. The human haploid genome contains two GH and three hCS genes all located on the long arm of chromosome 17, and a single PRL gene located on chromosome 6 (Fig. 2.16).

These genes are similar in the arrangement of their transcribed and nontranscribed portions as well as their nucleotide sequences. All comprise five exons separated by four introns located at homologous positions. All three hormones are large single-stranded peptides containing two internal disulfide bridges at corresponding parts of the molecule. PRL also has a third internal disulfide bridge. GH and hCS have about 80% of their amino acids in common, and a region 146 amino acids long is similar in hGH and PRL. Only one of the GH genes (hGH N) is expressed in the pituitary, but because of alternative splicing of the RNA transcript, two GH isoforms are produced. The larger form is the 22 kDa molecule (22K GH), which is about 10 times more abundant than the smaller, 20 kDa molecule (20K GH), which lacks amino acids 32–46. The other GH gene (hGH V) appears to be expressed only in the placenta and is the predominant form of GH in the blood of pregnant women. It encodes a protein that has the same biological actions as the pituitary hormone although it differs from the pituitary hormone in 13 amino acids and is glycosylated.

Considering the similarities in their structures, it is not surprising that GH shares some of the lactogenic activity of PRL and hCS. However, human GH also has about two-thirds of its amino acids in common with GH molecules of cattle and rats, but humans are completely insensitive to cattle or rat GH and respond only to the GH produced by humans or monkeys. This requirement of primates for primate GH is an example of species specificity and largely results from the change of a single amino acid in GH and a corresponding change of a single amino acid in the binding site in the GH receptor. Because of species specificity, human GH was in short supply until the advent of recombinant DNA technology, which made possible an almost limitless supply.

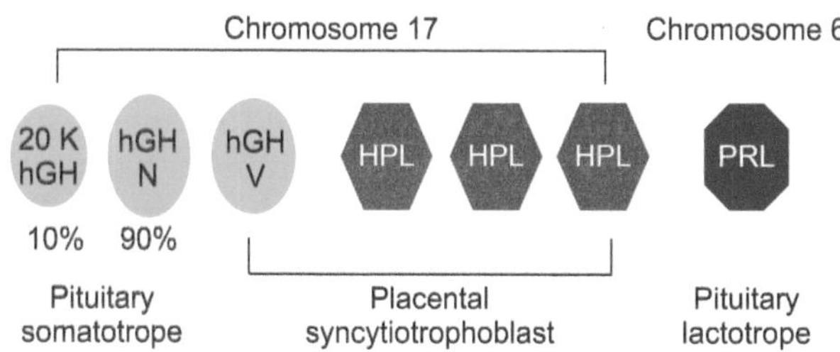

FIGURE 2.16 The growth hormone/prolactin family.

Adrenocorticotropin family

The ACTH, which is also called corticotropin or adrenocorticotropin, controls hormone production by the cortex of the adrenal glands. This family of pituitary peptides includes α-, β-, and γ-melanocyte-stimulating hormones (MSH), β- and γ-lipotropin (LPH), and β-endorphin (Fig. 2.17).

Of these, ACTH is the only product of corticotropes with an established physiological role in humans. The MSHs, which disperse melanin pigment in melanocytes in the skin of lower vertebrates, are not secreted in significant amounts by the human pituitary gland, but these compounds are produced in melanocytes and keratinocytes in the skin where they act in a paracrine or autocrine manner to affect pigmentation. However, ACTH and both β- and γ-LPH contain the sequence of seven amino acids that produce the melanocyte-stimulating effect of MSH. This likely accounts for the darkening or bronzing of the skin when these hormones are secreted in excess. α- and β-MSH also are produced by neurons in the arcuate nucleus, and play an important role in the control of food intake (Chapter 8: Hormonal Regulation of Fuel Metabolism).

β-LPH is named for its stimulatory effect on mobilization of lipids from adipose tissue in rabbits, but the physiological importance, if any, of this action in humans is uncertain. The 91-aminoacid chain of β-LPH contains at its carboxyl end the complete amino acid sequence of β-endorphin (from *end*ogenous m*orphin*e), which excites the same receptors as morphine in various cells.

The ACTH-related peptides constitute a family because of the following:

1. They contain regions of homologous amino acid sequences, which may have arisen through exon duplication.
2. Because they all are encoded in the same gene. The gene product is called proopiomelanocortin (POMC) and consists of 239 amino acids after the removal of the 26-amino acid signal peptide. The molecule contains 10 doublets of basic amino acids (arginine and lysine in various combinations), which are potential sites for cleavage by subtilisin-like endopeptidases, called prohormone convertases (PCs). At least five other enzymes produce other posttranslational modifications. Tissue-specific differences in expression of processing enzymes

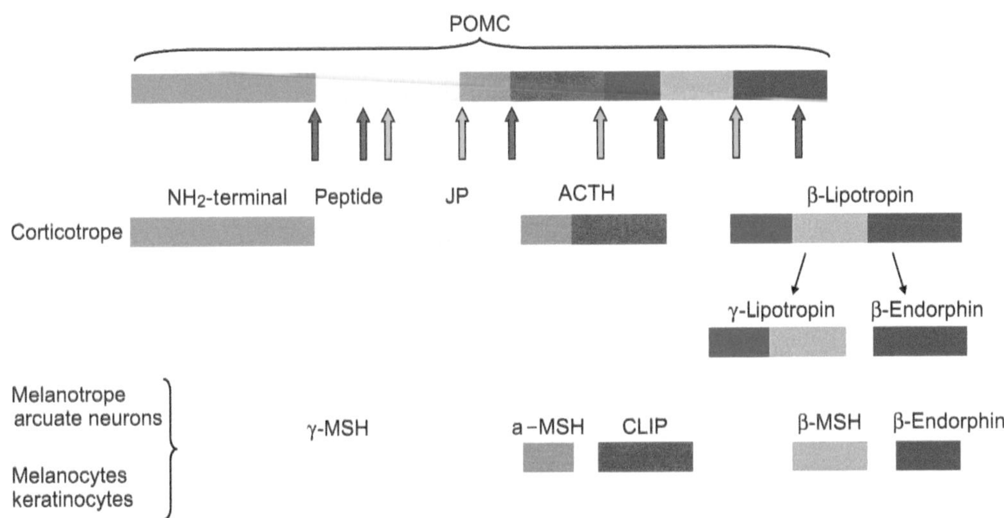

FIGURE 2.17 Proteolytic processing of POMC. Sections of the intact POMC molecule representing the different final products are shown in the various colors. Sites of cleavage by proconvertase (PC) 1 are indicated by the green arrows and by PC2 by the red arrows. Some cleavage of β-lipotropin in the corticotropes is catalyzed by PC2. Corticotropes express only PC1, but melanotropes in the rudimentary intermediate lobe, neurons, and melanocytes and keratinocytes in the skin express both PC1 and PC2. Additional posttranslational processing (not shown) includes removal of the carboxyl-terminal amino acid from each of the peptides, glycosylation, and phosphorylation of some of the peptide fragments. *CLIP*, Corticotropin-like intermediate lobe peptide; *JP*, joining peptide; *POMC*, proopiomelanocortin.

account for the differences in final secretory products of corticotropes and the other cells that express POMC. Corticotropes express PC1, whereas POMC expressing neurons and skin cells contain both PC1 and PC2. As a result, corticotropes produce fewer, but larger fragments (Fig. 2.17).

The predominant products of human corticotropes are ACTH and β-LPH. Because the final processing of POMC occurs in the secretory granule, β-LPH is secreted along with ACTH. Cleavage of β-LPH also occurs to some extent in human corticotropes, so that some β-endorphin may also be released, particularly when ACTH secretion is brisk (Fig. 2.18).

Development of the anterior pituitary gland

The various cell types of the anterior pituitary arise from a common primordium whose initial development begins when the cells of the oral ectoderm of Rathke's pouch come in contact with the cells of the developing diencephalon. Expression of several regionally specific transcription factors in different combinations appears to determine the different cellular lineages (Fig. 2.19).

Deficiencies in expression of two of these factors account for several mutant dwarf mouse strains and for the human syndromes called combined pituitary hormone deficiency syndrome. Development of thyrotropes, lactotropes, and somatotropes share a common dependence upon the homeodomain transcription factors called prop-1 and pit-1. Prop-1 appears transiently early in the development process and appears to foretell expression of the pituitary specific Pit-1, and its name derives from "prophet of Pit-1." Pit-1 is the transcription factor that is required not only for differentiation of these cell lineages but also for continued expression of GH, PRL, and the β-subunit of TSH throughout life. Pit-1 also regulates the expression of the receptor for the hypothalamic hormone that controls GH synthesis and secretion. Genetic absence of Pit-1 results in failure of the somatotropes, lactotropes, and thyrotropes to develop, and hence absence of GH, PRL, and TSH. Absence of prop-1 results in deficiencies of these three hormones as well as deficiencies in gonadotropin production. Cells destined to become corticotropes constitute a separate lineage early in pituitary differentiation and are the first to produce their cognate hormone. Corticotropes and gonadotropes depend upon expression of combinations of other transcription factors as is also true for the divergence of the pit-1 dependent cell types into their mature phenotypes. A detailed consideration of pituitary organogenesis is beyond the scope of this text.

Regulation of anterior pituitary function

Secretion of the anterior pituitary hormones is regulated by the central nervous system and hormones produced in peripheral target glands. Input from the central nervous system provides the primary drive for secretion and peripheral input plays a secondary, though vital, role in modulating secretory rates. Secretion of all the anterior pituitary hormones except PRL declines severely in the absence of stimulation from the hypothalamus as

ACTH controls predominantly the function of two zones of the adrenal cortex (**zona fasciculata** and **zona reticularis**). The zona glomerulosa is regulated by ***angiotensin II*** derived from the processing of the liver protein angiotensinogen by the proteolytic action of renin (kidneys) and converting enzyme (lungs)

ACTH stimulates the synthesis of cortisol (a glucocorticoid) and androgens. Cortisol and other steroids are metabolized in liver

Low levels of cortisol in blood, stress, and vasopressin [antidiuretic hormone (ADH)] stimulate ACTH secretion from basophils by stimulation of CRH release (positive feedback). **Cortisol is the dominating regulatory factor**

ACTH increases the pigmentation of skin. Skin darkening in **Addison's disease** and **Cushing's disease** is not determined by melanocyte-stimulating hormone (MSH), which is not normally present in human serum

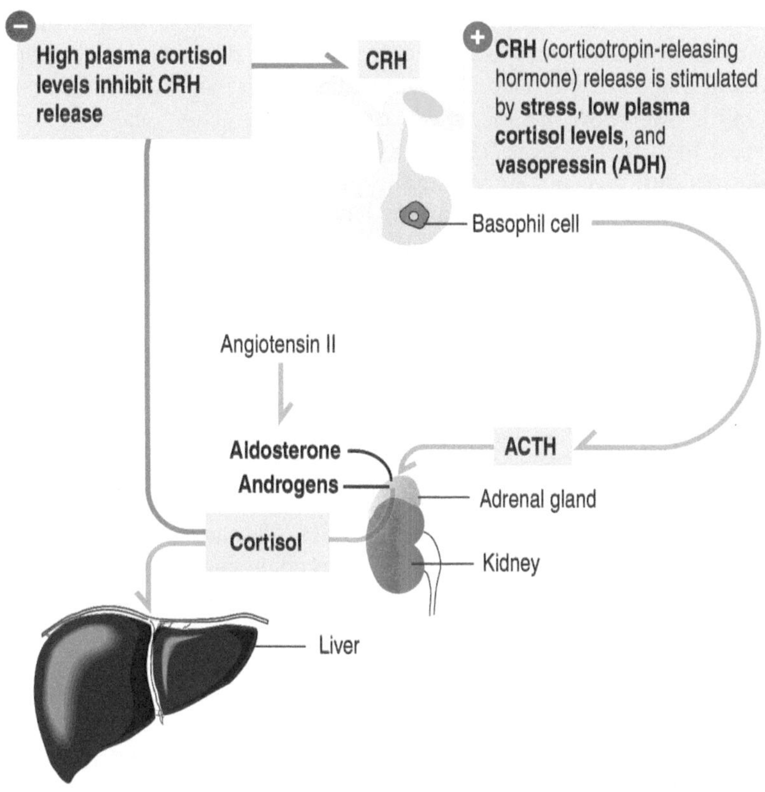

FIGURE 2.18 The production of ACTH and its effect on the adrenal gland and feedback to the hypothalamus. *ACTH,* Adrenocorticotropic hormone. Source: *From Figure 18.11 in Kierszenbaum, A. L., Tres, L. L. (2016).* Histology and cell biology: An introduction to pathology *(4th ed., p. 568). Elsevier.*

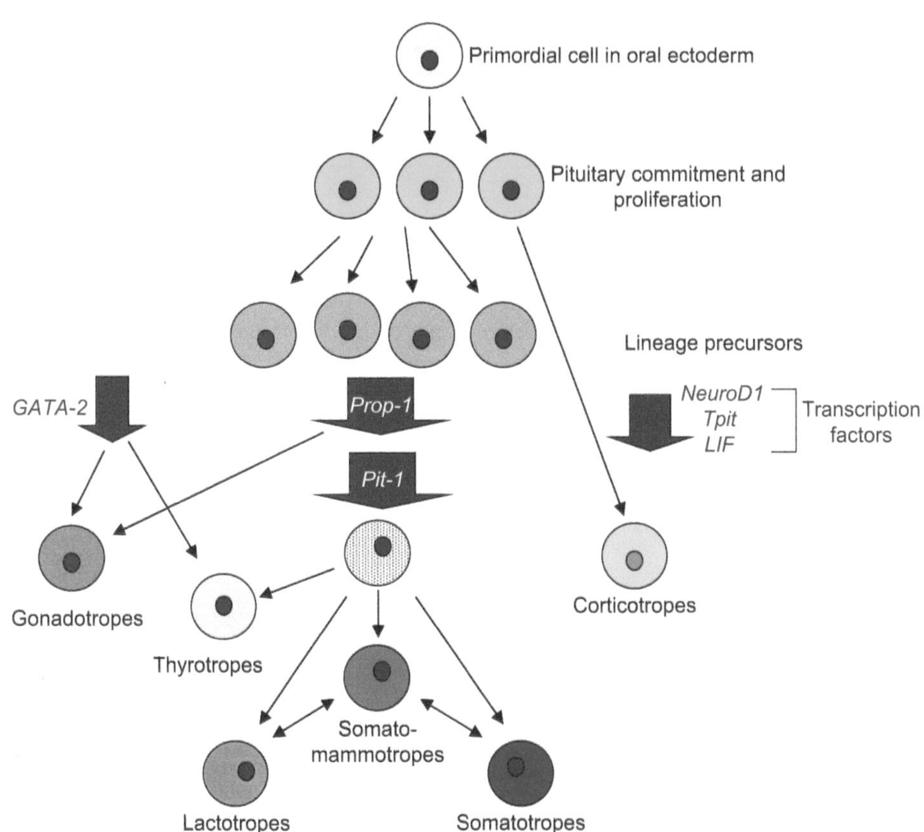

FIGURE 2.19 Development of the principal cell types of the anterior pituitary gland showing some of the critical transcription factors that give rise to each lineage. Corticotropes branch off early and form a separate lineage. Development of each of the other cell types depends on Prop-1. The lactotropes, somatotropes, and thyrotropes are derived from a common precursor until thyrotropes diverge and share a common dependence on GATA-2 with the gonadotropes.

can be produced, for example, when the pituitary gland is removed surgically from its natural location and reimplanted at a site remote from the hypothalamus. In contrast, PRL secretion is increased dramatically. The persistent high rate of secretion of PRL under these circumstances indicates not only that the pituitary glands can revascularize and survive in a new location, but also that PRL secretion is normally under tonic inhibitory control by the hypothalamus.

Secretion of each of the anterior pituitary hormones follows a diurnal pattern entrained by activity, sleep, or light-dark cycles. Secretion of each of these hormones also occurs in a pulsatile manner probably reflecting synchronized pulses of hypothalamic neurohormone release into hypophyseal portal capillaries. Pulse frequency varies widely from about 2 pulses per hour for ACTH to 1 pulse every 3 of 4 hours for TSH, GH, and PRL. Modulation of secretion in response to changes in the internal or external environment may be reflected as changes in the amplitude or frequency of secretory pulses, or by episodic bursts of secretion. In this chapter, we discuss only general aspects of the regulation of anterior pituitary function. A detailed description of the control of the secretory activity of each hormone is given in subsequent chapters in conjunction with a discussion of its role in regulating physiological processes.

Hypophysiotropic hormones

As already mentioned, the central nervous system communicates with the anterior pituitary gland by means of neurosecretions released into the hypothalamic–hypophyseal portal system.

These neurosecretions are called *hypophysiotropic hormones* and are listed in Table 2.2.

The neurons that secrete these hormones are clustered in discrete hypothalamic nuclei (Fig. 2.20).

The fact that only small amounts of the hypophysiotropic hormones are synthesized, stored, and secreted frustrated efforts to isolate and identify them for nearly 25 years. Their abundance in the hypothalamus is less than 0.1% of that of even the scarcest pituitary hormone in the anterior lobe.

The circumventricular organs

Most the brain is isolated from the rest of the body by a blood–brain barrier consisting of three parts: (1) capillary endothelial cells with tight junctions; (2) a surrounding—almost impenetrable—basal lamina secreted in part by capillary endothelial cells; and (3) a covering over the basal lamina of the foot processes of astrocytes whose cell membrane is also impermeable to many molecules. However, the brain needs to sample the environment in the rest of the body, and so there are eight areas where there is no blood–brain barrier. These areas are around the third and fourth ventricles and are thus called the circum (around) ventricular (third and fourth ventricles) organs. They are not organs in the anatomical sense (i.e., they are not composed of each of the four tissue types) but instead are structures where there is no barrier (Fig. 2.21).

TABLE 2.2 Hypophysiotropic hormones.

Hormone	Amino acids	Hypothalamic source	Physiological actions on the pituitary
CRH	41	Parvoneurons of the paraventricular nuclei	Stimulates secretion of ACTH, and β-lipotropin
GnRH, originally called LHRH	10	Arcuate nuclei	Stimulates secretion of FSH and LH
GHRH	44	Arcuate nuclei	Stimulates GH secretion
Growth hormone–releasing peptide (ghrelin)	28	Arcuate nuclei	Increases response to GHRH and may directly stimulate GH secretion
SRIF; SST	14 or 28	Anterior hypothalamic periventricular system	Inhibits secretion of GH
Prolactin-stimulating factor (?)	?	?	Stimulates prolactin secretion (?)
PIF	Dopamine	Tuberohypophyseal neurons	Inhibits prolactin secretion
TRH	3	Parvoneurons of the paraventricular nuclei	Stimulates secretion of TSH and prolactin
AVP	9	Parvoneurons of the paraventricular nuclei	Acts in concert with CRH to stimulate secretion of ACTH

ACTH, Adrenocorticotropic hormone; *AVP*, arginine vasopressin; *CRH*, corticotropin-releasing hormone; *FSH*, follicle-stimulating hormone; *GH*, growth hormone; *GHRH*, growth hormone–releasing hormone; *GnRH*, gonadotropin-releasing hormone; *LH*, luteinizing hormone; *LHRH*, luteinizing hormone–releasing hormone; *PIF*, prolactin-inhibiting factor; *SRIF*, somatotropin release–inhibiting factor; *SST*, somatostatin; *TRH*, thyrotropin-releasing hormone; *TSH*, thyroid-stimulating hormone.

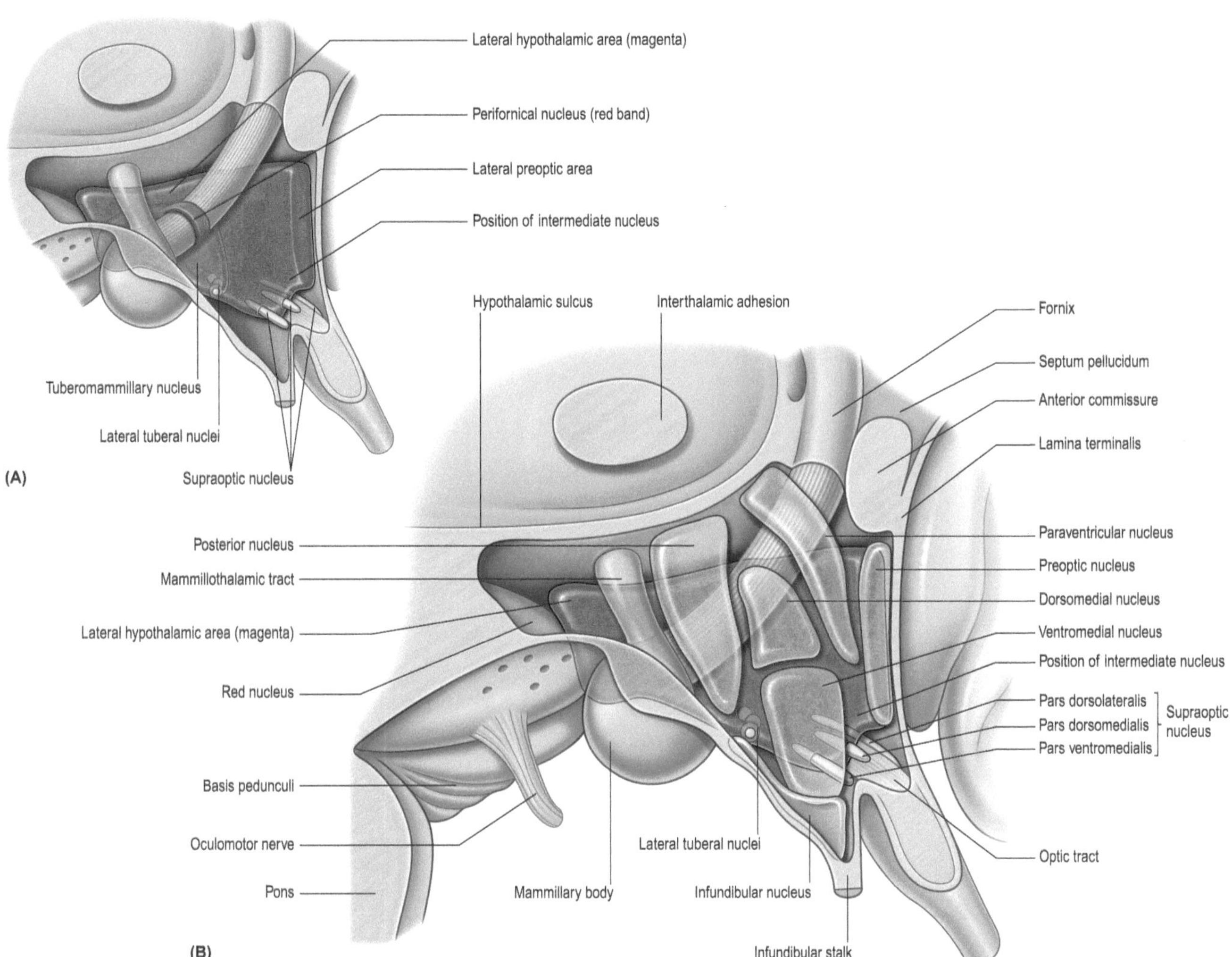

FIGURE 2.20 The hypothalamic nuclei. (A) Only the lateral groups of nuclei are shown. (B) The medial groups of nuclei have been added. Source: *From Figure 23.8 in S. Standring, et al. (Eds.). (2016).* Gray's anatomy *(41st ed., p. 357). Elsevier.*

It is these circumventricular organs that receive feedback from hormones and toxins produced elsewhere in the body. For example, monosodium glutamate influences the nuclei near the medial eminence resulting in a stimulation of appetite. Leptin, discussed later in this book, also enters the brain through this portal. The organum vasculosum lateral terminalis and subfornical organ are portals at the rostral (front) end of the third ventricle in close apposition to many nuclei that regulate numerous functions such as blood pressure, oxygenation, and levels of many hormones. The function of the portal at the subcommissural organ and pineal gland is largely unknown (the function of the pineal gland in humans is also not well understood). At the caudal end of the ventricular system lies the area postrema that can also be called the chemoreceptor trigger zone and is permeable to toxins carried in the blood from the digestive tract. These toxins will initiate a vomiting reflex carried by the vagus nerve to cause a sudden strong reverse peristalsis in the stomach and duodenum as the brain attempts to rid the body of the toxins—and the food-borne bacteria that released them. This is also an area where many baroreceptor and chemoreceptors have their CNS endings such as those from the carotid sinus via the glossopharyngeal nerve (cranial nerve IX) and the initiation of a reflex via the vagus nerve (cranial nerve X). For example, sudden pressure on the right carotid sinus will be carried into the brain on the glossopharyngeal nerve and reflexly slow down the heart rate via the vagus nerve endings to the sinus node (SA node) of the heart. This procedure is used in the ICU and ED departments to slow down a tachyarrhythmia (rapid heart rate). It should not be done without paddles nearby as sometimes the reflex is so strong that cardiac arrest ensues.

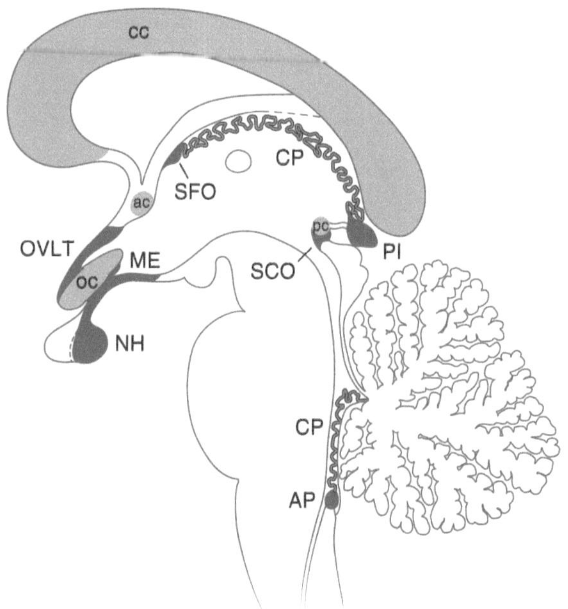

FIGURE 2.21 The eight circumventricular organs are in dark brown and are from left to right: (1) NH, (2) OVLT, (3) ME, median eminence; (4) SFO (5) CP, (6) PL, (7) SCO (8) AP, area postrema. Some anatomists do not consider the neurohypophysis to be part of the brain, so those anatomists will list only seven circumventricular organs. Light-brown structures are not part of the circumventricular organ system and are, from left to right, OC, AC, (of the corpus callosum); CC, PC (posterior commissure; of the corpus callosum). Note that the choroid plexus is in both the third and fourth ventricles. Not shown is the choroid plexus in the two lateral ventricles that also have no blood–brain barrier. *AC*, Anterior commissure; *AP*, area postrema; *CC*, corpus callosum; *CP*, choroid plexus; *NH*, neurohypophysis; *OC*, optic chiasm; *OVLT*, organum vasculosum of the lamina terminalis; *PL*, pineal gland; *SCO*, subcommissural organ; *SFO*, subfornical organ. Source: *From Figure 7-5 in Low M. J. (2016). Neuroendocrinology, Chapter 7. In S. Melmed, K. S. Polonsky, P. R. Larsen, H. M. Kronenberg. (Eds.),* Williams textbook of endocrinology *(13th ed., p. 118), Elsevier.*

Hypothalamic hormones

Thyrotropin-releasing hormone

TRH, the first of the hypothalamic neurohormones to be characterized, is a tripeptide. It was isolated, identified, and synthesized almost simultaneously in the laboratories of Roger Guillemin and Andrew Schally, who were subsequently recognized for this monumental achievement with the award of a Nobel Prize. Guillemin's laboratory processed 25 kg of sheep hypothalami to obtain 1 mg of TRH. Schally's laboratory extracted 245,000 pig hypothalami to yield only 8.2 mg of this tripeptide. The human TRH gene encodes a 242 residue preprohormone molecule that contains six copies of TRH that are released by the proteolytic activities of PC1 and PC2. TRH is synthesized primarily in parvicellular (small cell) neurons in the paraventricular nuclei of the hypothalamus and stored in nerve terminals in the median eminence. TRH also is expressed in neurons widely dispersed throughout the central nervous system and probably acts as a neurotransmitter that mediates a variety of other responses.

Actions of TRH that regulate TSH secretion and thyroid function are discussed further in Chapter 3, Thyroid Gland.

Gonadotropin-releasing hormone

Gonadotropin-releasing hormone (GnRH) was the next hypophysiotropic hormone to be isolated and characterized. Hypothalamic control over secretion of FSH and LH is exerted by a single hypothalamic decapeptide, GnRH. Endocrinologists originally had some difficulty accepting the idea that both gonadotropins are under the control of a single hypothalamic-releasing hormone because FSH and LH appear to be secreted independently under certain circumstances. Endocrinologists have now abandoned the idea that there must be separate FSH- and LH-releasing hormones as other factors can account for partial independence of LH and FSH secretion. The frequency of pulses of GnRH release determines the ratio of FSH and LH secreted. In addition, target glands secrete hormones that selectively inhibit secretion of either FSH or LH. These complex events are discussed in detail in Chapter 12, Hormonal Control of Reproduction in the Male, and Chapter 13, Hormonal Control of Reproduction in the Female: The Menstrual.

The GnRH gene encodes a 92-amino acid preprohormone that contains the 10-amino acid GnRH peptide and an adjacent 56 amino acid GnRH-associated peptide (GAP), which may also have some biological activity. GAP is found along with GnRH in nerve terminals and may be cosecreted with GnRH. Cell bodies of the neurons that release GnRH into the hypophysial portal system reside primarily in the arcuate nucleus in the anterior hypothalamus, but GnRH-containing neurons are also found in the preoptic area and project to extra-hypothalamic regions where GnRH release may be related to various aspects of reproductive behavior. GnRH also is expressed in the placenta. Curiously, humans and some other species have a second GnRH gene that is expressed elsewhere in the brain and appears to have no role in gonadotropin release.

Control of growth hormone secretion

GH secretion is controlled by the GH-releasing hormone (GHRH) and a GH release–inhibiting hormone, somatostatin, which is also called somatotropin release–inhibiting factor. In addition, a peptide called ghrelin may act both on the somatotropes to increase GH secretion by augmenting the actions of GHRH, and on the hypothalamus to increase secretion of GHRH. Ghrelin is synthesized both in the hypothalamus and the stomach. Its secretion by the stomach is thought to signal feeding behavior, and hence, ghrelin may provide a link between growth and nutrition. However, our understanding of the physiological importance of this peptide in regulating GH secretion is incomplete. Ghrelin is discussed further in Chapters 6, 8, and 11. GHRH is a member of a family of gastrointestinal and neurohormones that includes vasoactive intestinal polypeptide (VIP), glucagon (see Chapter 6: Hormones of the Gastrointestinal Tract), and the probable ancestral peptide in this family, called pituitary adenylate cyclase–activating peptide. GHRH-containing neurons are found predominantly in the arcuate nuclei, and to a lesser extent in the ventromedial nuclei of the hypothalamus. Curiously, GHRH originally was isolated from a pancreatic tumor, and normally is expressed in the pancreas, the intestinal tract, and other tissues, but the physiological role of extrahypothalamically produced GHRH is unknown.

Somatostatin was isolated from hypothalamic extracts based upon its ability to inhibit GH secretion. The somatostatin gene codes for a 118-amino acid preprohormone from which either a 14-amino acid or a 28-amino acid form of somatostatin is released from the carboxyl terminus by proteolytic cleavage. Both forms are similarly active. The remarkable conservation of the amino acid sequence of the somatostatin precursor and the presence of processed fragments that accompany somatostatin in hypothalamic nerve terminals has suggested to some investigators that additional physiological active peptides may be derived from the somatostatin gene. The somatostatin gene is widely expressed in neuronal tissue as well as in the pancreas (see Chapter 6: Hormones of the Gastrointestinal Tract) and the gastrointestinal tract. Similarly, the five isoforms of somatostatin receptors are widely distributed in the central nervous system and the periphery, consistent with a wide range of inhibitory actions of this neurohormone. The somatostatin that regulates GH secretion originates in neurons present in the preoptic, periventricular, and paraventricular nuclei, and its receptors are expressed in GHRH-containing neurons in the arcuate nucleus as well as in somatotropes. It appears that somatostatin is secreted nearly continuously by hypothalamic neurons and restrains GH secretion except during periodic brief episodes that coincide with increases in GHRH secretion. Coordinated episodes of decreased somatostatin release and increased GHRH secretion produce a pulsatile pattern of GH secretion.

Corticotropin-releasing hormone

This hormone is a 41-amino acid polypeptide derived from a preprohormone of 192 amino acids. CRH is present in greatest abundance in parvicellular neurons in the paraventricular nuclei whose axons project to the median eminence.

About half of these cells in these nuclei are magnicellular neurons that express arginine vasopressin (AVP), which also acts as a corticotropin-releasing hormone. AVP has other important physiological functions and is transported to the posterior pituitary gland (see later and Chapter 9: Regulation of Salt and Water Balance) where it is released in response to axonal impulses as if it were a neurotransmitter. However, there is no second neuron. Instead, the released AVP diffuses into capillaries and is carried to the kidneys.

The wide distribution of CRH-containing neurons in the central nervous system suggests that it has other actions besides the regulation of ACTH secretion. CRH also is produced in the placenta and serves a critical role in pregnancy and parturition (see Chapter 14: Hormonal Control of Pregnancy and Lactation).

Dopamine and control of prolactin secretion

The simple monoamine neurotransmitter dopamine appears to satisfy most of the criteria for a PRL inhibitory factor whose existence was suggested by the persistent high rate of PRL secretion by pituitary glands transplanted outside the sella turcica. It is possible that there is also a PRL-releasing hormone, but although several candidates have been proposed, general agreement on its nature or even its existence is still lacking.

Secretion and actions of hypophysiotropic hormones

Although, in general, the hypophysiotropic hormones affect the secretion of one or another pituitary hormone specifically, TRH can increase the secretion of PRL at least as well as it increases the secretion of TSH. The physiological meaning of this experimental finding is not understood. Under normal physiological conditions, PRL and TSH appear to be secreted independently, and increased PRL secretion is not necessarily seen in circumstances that call for increased TSH secretion. However, in laboratory rats and possibly human beings as well, suckling at the breast increases both PRL and TSH secretion in a manner suggestive of increased TRH secretion. In the normal individual, somatostatin may inhibit the secretion of other pituitary hormones in addition to GH, but again the physiological significance of this action is not understood. With disease states, specificity of responses of various pituitary cells for their own hypophysiotropic hormones may break down, or cells might even begin to secrete their hormones autonomously.

The neurons that secrete the hypophysiotropic hormones are not autonomous. They receive input from many structures within the brain as well as from circulating hormones. Neurons that directly or indirectly are excited by actual or impending changes in the internal or external environment, from emotional changes, and from generators of rhythmic activity, signal to hypophysiotropic neurons by means of classical neurotransmitters as well as neuropeptides. In addition, their activity is modulated by hormonal changes in the general circulation. Integration of responses to all these signals may take place in the hypophysiotropic neurons themselves or information may be processed elsewhere in the brain and relayed to the hypophysiotropic neurons. Conversely, hypophysiotropic neurons or neurons that release hypophysiotropic peptides as their neurotransmitters communicate with other neurons dispersed throughout the central nervous system to produce responses that presumably are relevant to the physiological circumstances that call forth pituitary hormone secretion. Hypophysiotropic hormones increase both secretion and synthesis of pituitary hormones. All appear to act through stimulation of G-protein coupled receptors (see Chapter 1: Introduction) on the surfaces of anterior pituitary cells to increase the formation of cyclic AMP or inositol–trisphosphate–diacylglycerol second messenger systems. Release of hormone almost certainly is the result of an influx of calcium, which triggers and sustains the process of exocytosis. The actions of hypophysiotropic hormones on their target cells in the pituitary are considered further in the later chapters.

Feedback control of anterior pituitary function

We have already indicated that the primary drive for secretion of all the anterior pituitary hormones except PRL is provided by the hypothalamic-releasing hormones (Fig. 2.22).

In the absence of the hormones of their target glands, secretion of TSH (Fig. 2.23) and ACTH, GH, and the gonadotropins gradually increase manifold. Secretion of these pituitary hormones is subject to negative feedback inhibition by secretions of their target glands. Regulation of secretion of anterior pituitary hormones in the normal individual is achieved through the interplay of stimulatory effects of releasing hormones and inhibitory effects of target gland hormones (Fig. 2.24).

Regulation of the secretion of pituitary hormones by hormones of target glands could be achieved equally well if negative feedback signals acted at the level of (1) the hypothalamus to inhibit secretion of hypophysiotropic hormones or (2) the pituitary gland to blunt the response to hypophysiotropic stimulation. Some combination of the two mechanisms applies to all the anterior pituitary hormones except PRL.

In experimental animals it appears that secretion of GnRH is variable and highly sensitive to environmental influences; for example, day length, or even the act of mating. In humans and other primates, secretion of GnRH after puberty appears to be somewhat less influenced by changes in the internal and external environment, but there is ample evidence that GnRH secretion is modulated by factors in both the internal and external environment. It has been shown experimentally in rhesus monkeys and human subjects that all the complex changes in the rates of FSH and LH secretion characteristic of the normal menstrual cycle can occur when the pituitary gland is stimulated by pulses of GnRH delivered at an invariant frequency and amplitude. For such changes in pituitary secretion to occur, changes in secretion of target gland hormones that accompany ripening of the follicle, ovulation, and luteinization must modulate the responses of gonadotropes to GnRH (Chapter 13: Hormonal Control of Reproduction in the Female: The Menstrual). However, in normal humans, it is evident that target gland hormones also act at the level of the hypothalamus to regulate both the amplitude and frequency of GnRH secretory bursts (Fig. 2.25).

Adrenal cortical hormones exert a negative feedback effect both on pituitary corticotropes where they decrease transcription of POMC and on hypothalamic neurons where they decrease CRH synthesis and secretion (see Chapter 4: The Adrenal Glands) (Fig. 2.26).

The rate of CRH secretion is also profoundly affected by changes in both the internal and external environment. Physiologically, CRH is secreted in increased amounts in response to nonspecific stress. This effect is seen even in the absence of the adrenal glands, and the inhibitory effects of its hormones, indicating that CRH secretion must be controlled by positive inputs as well as the negative effects of adrenal hormones.

Control of GH secretion is more complex because it is under the influence of a releasing hormone, GHRH; a release-enhancing hormone, ghrelin; and a release-inhibiting hormone, somatostatin. In addition, GH secretion is under negative feedback to control byproducts of its actions in peripheral tissues. As is discussed in detail in Chapter 11, Hormonal Control of Growth, GH evokes the production of a peptide, called insulin-like growth factor I (IGF), which mediates the growth-promoting

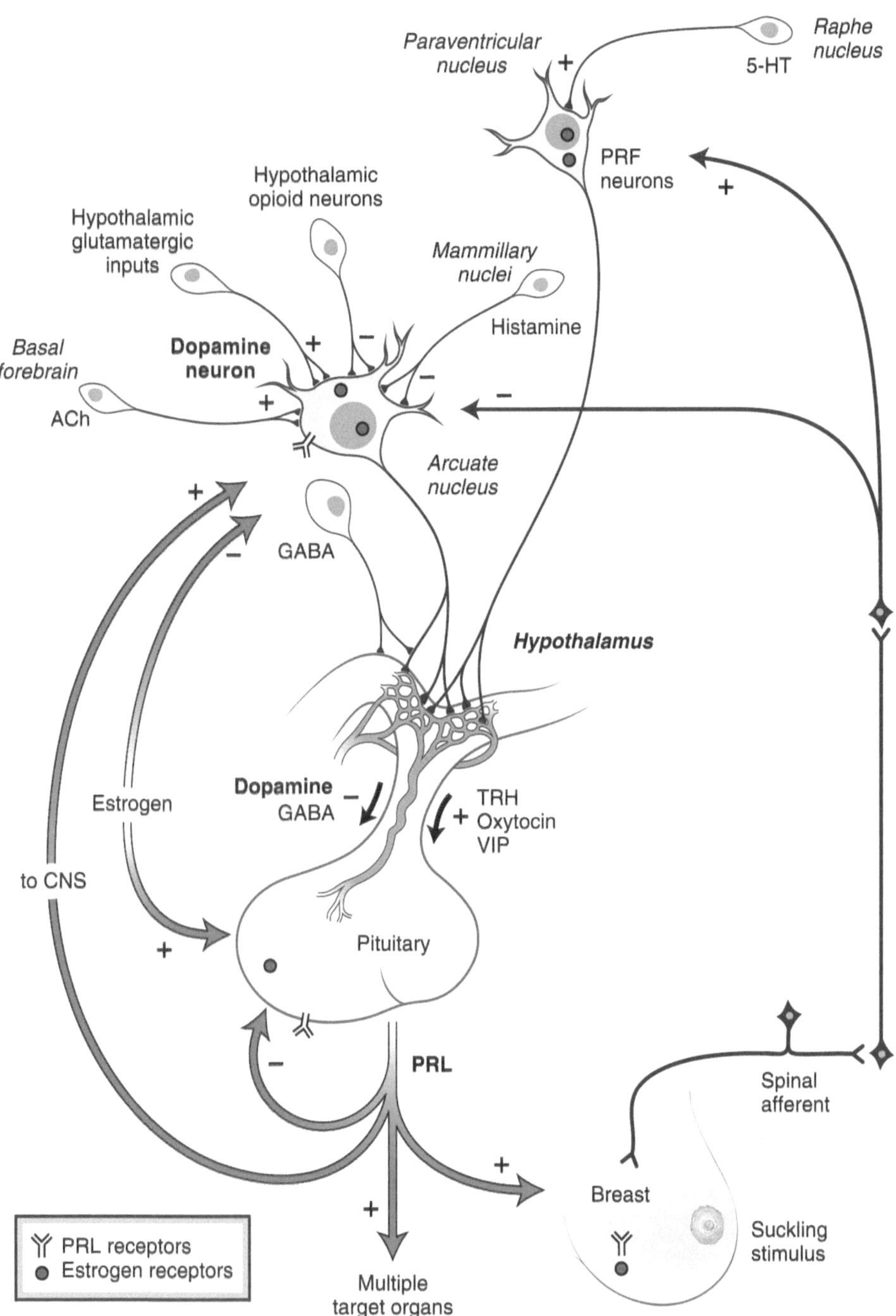

FIGURE 2.22 The hypothalamus–pituitary–prolactin axis. *5-HT*, 5-Hydroxytryptamine (serotonin); *ACh*, acetylcholine; *CNS*, central nervous system; *GABA*, gamma-aminobutyric acid; *PRF*, prolactin releasing factor; *PRL*, prolactin; *TRH*, thyrotropin-releasing hormone; *VIP*, vasoactive intestinal polypeptide. Source: *From Figure 7–27 in Low, M. J. (2016). Neuroendocrinology, Chapter 7. In S. Melmed, K. S. Polonsky, P. R. Larsen, H. M. Kronenberg. (Eds.),* Williams textbook of endocrinology *(13th ed., p. 149), Elsevier.*

actions of GH. IGF exerts powerful inhibitory effects on GH secretion by decreasing the sensitivity of somatotropes to GHRH. It also acts on the hypothalamic neurons to increase the release of somatostatin and to inhibit the release of GHRH. GH is also a metabolic regulator, and products of its metabolic activity such as increased glucose or free fatty acid concentrations in blood may inhibit its secretion. Modulating effects of target gland hormones on the pituitary gland are not limited to inhibiting secretion of their own provocative hormones. Target gland hormones may modulate pituitary function by increasing the sensitivity of other pituitary cells to their releasing factors or by increasing the synthesis of other pituitary hormones. Hormones of the thyroid and adrenal glands are required for normal responses of the somatotropes to GHRH. Similarly, estrogen secreted by the ovary in response to FSH and LH increases PRL synthesis and secretion. In addition to feedback inhibition exerted by target

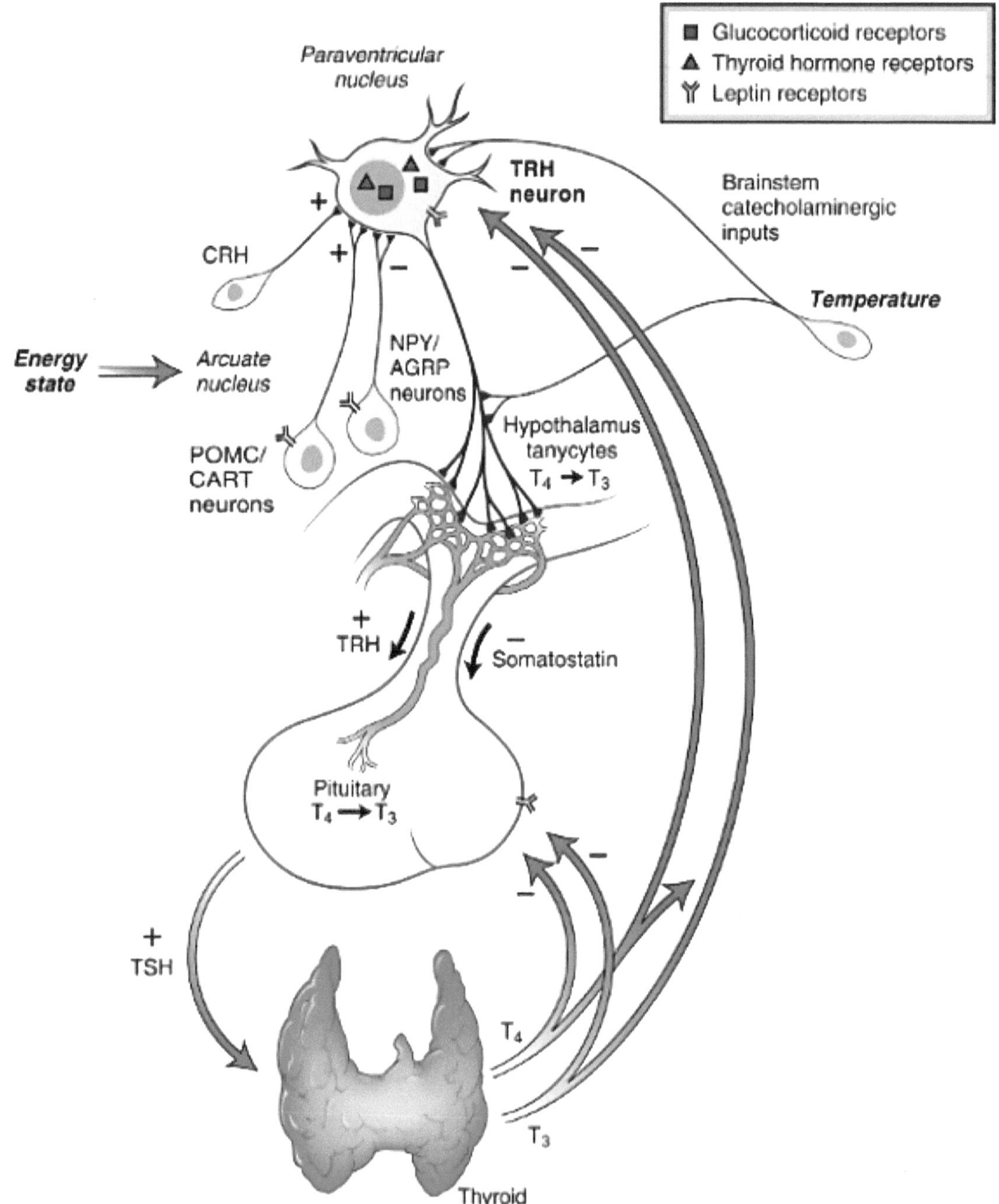

FIGURE 2.23 The hypothalamus–pituitary–thyroid axis. *AGRP*, Agouti-related peptide; *CART*, cocaine- and amphetamine-regulated transport; *CRH*, corticotropin-releasing hormone; *NPY*, neuropeptide Y; *POMC*, proopiomelanocortin; *T3*, triiodothyronine; *T4*, thyroxine; *TRH*, thyrotropin-releasing hormone.

gland hormones, there is evidence that pituitary hormones may inhibit their own secretion by actions on their cells of origin or by inhibiting secretion of their corresponding hypophysiotropic hormones. The physiological importance of such short-loop feedback systems has not been established, nor has that of the postulated ultrashort-loop feedback in which high concentrations of hypophysiotropic hormones may inhibit their own release.

Physiology of the posterior pituitary

The posterior pituitary gland is not a gland, but the axon endings of magnicellular neurons in the

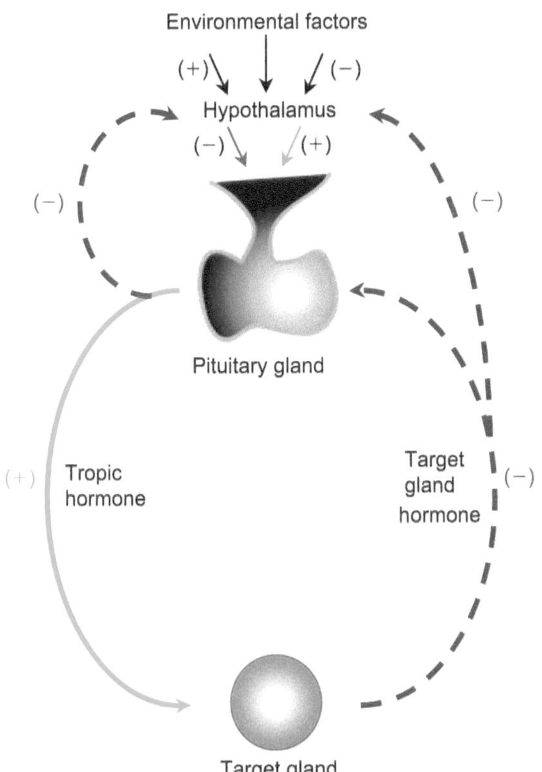

FIGURE 2.24 Regulation of anterior pituitary hormone secretion. Environmental factors may increase or decrease pituitary activity by increasing or decreasing hypophysiotropic hormone secretion. Pituitary secretions increase the secretion of target gland hormones, which may inhibit further secretion by acting at either the hypothalamus or the pituitary. Pituitary hormones may also inhibit their own secretion by a short feedback loop.

paraventricular nuclei and the supraoptic nuclei of the hypothalamus (Fig. 2.27).

These unmyelinated axons travel in the hypothalamic–hypophyseal tract to the posterior pituitary. There their axon endings store the hormones oxytocin and vasopressin. These are released a little at a time when an impulse travels down the axon from the hypothalamus. Oxytocin refers to *oxytocia* (Greek for rapid birth) in reference to its action to increase uterine contractions during parturition. Vasopressin contracts vascular smooth muscle and so raises blood pressure. Except for the pig, all mammals including humans have an arginine in position 8 of the protein hormone and are sometimes called AVP. The pig has a lysine in position 8 and so vasopressin from that source is called lysine vasopressin. Both oxytocin and vasopressin are nonapeptides and differ from each other by only two amino acids (Fig. 2.28).

A disulfide bond links cysteines at positions 1 and 6 to form a six-amino acid ring with a three amino acid side chain. Similarities in the structure and organization of their genes and in their posttranslational processing make it virtually certain that these hormones evolved from a single ancestral gene. The genes that encode them occupy adjacent loci on chromosome 20, but in opposite transcriptional orientation.

Each of the posterior pituitary hormones has other actions in addition to those for which it was named. Oxytocin also causes contraction of the myoepithelial cells that envelop the secretory alveoli of the mammary glands and thus enables the suckling infant to receive milk. Vasopressin is also called ADH for its action to promote reabsorption of "free water" by renal tubules (see Chapter 9: Regulation of Salt and Water Balance). These two effects are mediated by two different G-protein coupled receptors. The V1 receptors signal vascular muscle contraction by means of the inositol trisphosphate/diacylglycerol pathway (Chapter 1: Introduction), whereas V2 receptors utilize the cyclic AMP system to produce the antidiuretic effect in renal tubules. Oxytocin acts through a single class of G-protein receptors that signals through the inositol trisphosphate/diacylglycerol pathway. Physiological actions of these hormones are considered further in Chapter 9, Regulation of Salt and Water Balance and Chapter 14, Hormonal Control of Pregnancy and Lactation. Oxytocin and AVP are stored in and secreted by the neurohypophysis but are synthesized in magnicellular neurons whose cell bodies are present in both the supraoptic and paraventricular nuclei of the hypothalamus. Cells in the supraoptic nuclei appear to be the major source of vasopressin, while cells in the paraventricular nuclei may be the principal source of oxytocin. After transfer to the Golgi apparatus the oxytocin and AVP prohormones are packaged in secretory vesicles along with the enzymes that cleave them into the final secreted products. The secretory vesicles called Herring bodies are then transported down unmyelinated axons to the nerve terminals in the posterior pituitary where they are stored in relatively large amounts (Fig. 2.29).

It has been estimated that sufficient vasopressin is stored in the neurohypophysis to provide for 30–50 days of secretion at basal rates, or 5–7 days at maximal rates of secretion. Oxytocin and vasopressin are stored as 1:1 complexes with 93–95 residue peptides called neurophysins, which are adjacent segments of their prohormone molecules (Fig. 2.28). The neurophysins are cosecreted with vasopressin or oxytocin but have no known hormonal actions. The neurophysins, however, play an essential role in the posttranslational processing of the neurohypophysial hormones. The amino acid sequence of the central portion of the neurophysins is highly conserved across many vertebrate species, and mutations in this region of the preprohormone are responsible for hereditary deficiencies in

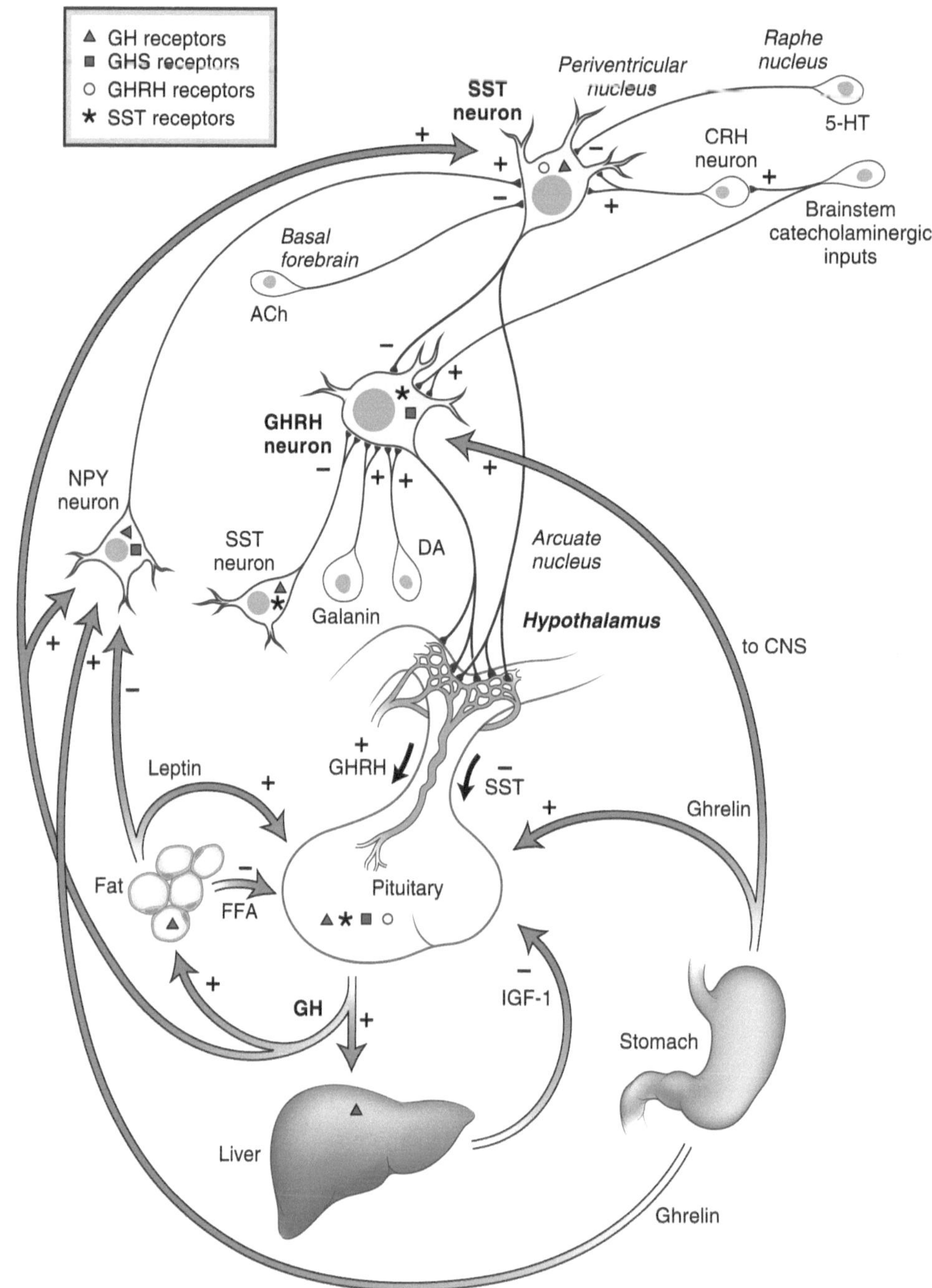

FIGURE 2.25 The hypothalamic–pituitary–growth hormone axis. *5-HT*, 5-Hydroxytryptamine (serotonin); *ACh*, acetylcholine; *CNS*, central nervous system; *CRH*, corticotropin-releasing hormone; *DA*, dopamine; *FFA*, free fatty acids (this is from fat); *GHRH*, growth hormone–releasing hormone; *IGF-1*, insulin-like growth factor 1 (older name is somatomedin C); *NPY*, neuropeptide Y (not covered in this text); *SST*, somatostatin. Source: *From Figure 7–22 in Low, M. J. (2016). Neuroendocrinology, Chapter 7. In S. Melmed, K. S. Polonsky, P. R. Larsen, H. M. Kronenberg. (Eds.),* Williams textbook of endocrinology *(13th ed., p. 141), Elsevier.*

vasopressin, which produce the disease diabetes insipidus (see Chapter 9: Regulation of Salt and Water Balance) even though expression of the vasopressin portion of the preprohormone is normal. It is likely that amino acid sequences in this region provide information directing folding and packaging of the posterior lobe hormones.

Vasopressin also serves as a neurotransmitter in neurons located elsewhere in the central nervous system. It is produced in considerably larger amounts in

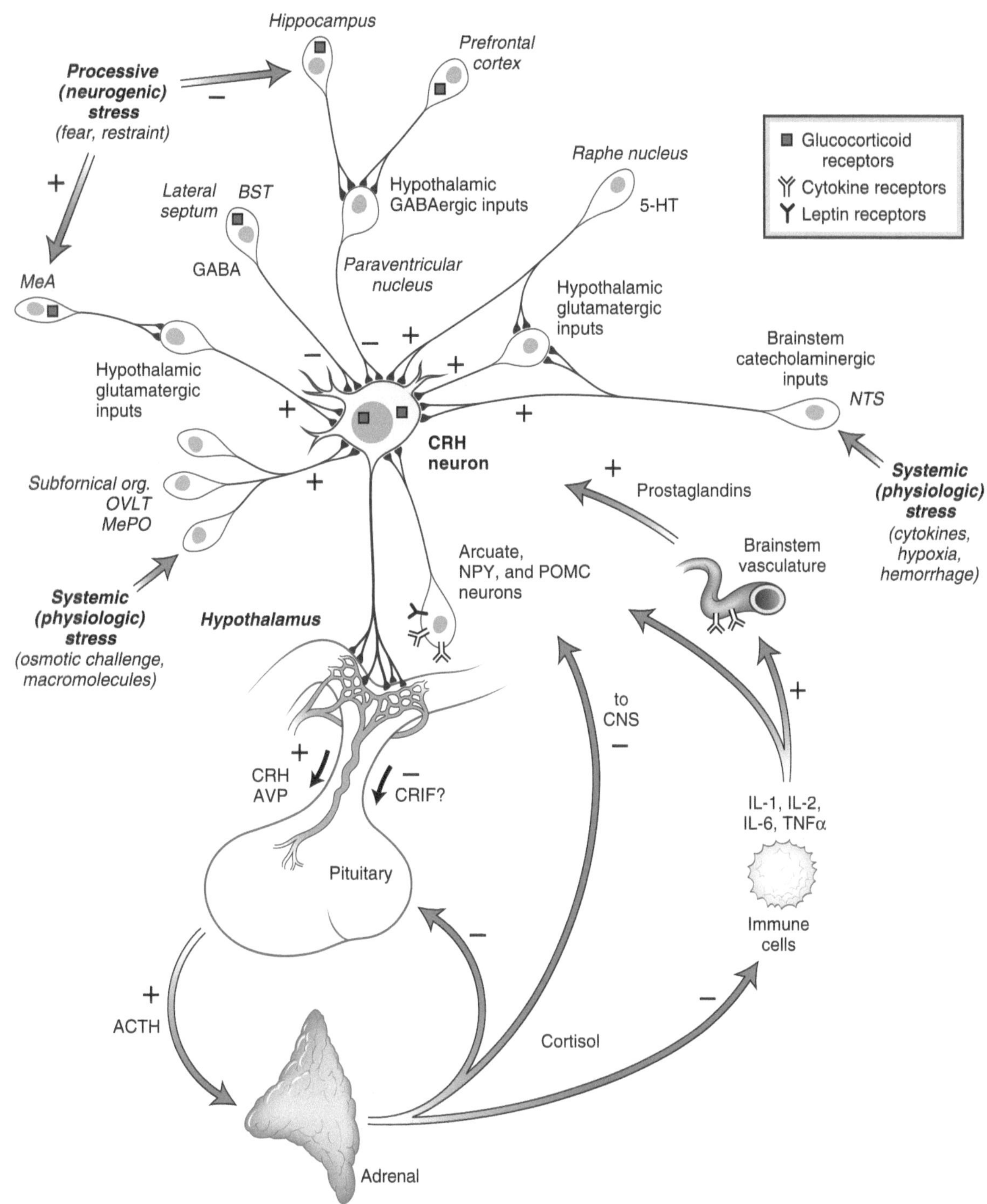

FIGURE 2.26 The hypothalamus–pituitary–adrenal axis. *5-HT*, 5-Hydroxytryptamine; *AVP*, arginine vasopressin; BST, bed nucleus of the stria terminalis; *CNS*, central nervous system; *CRH*, corticotropin-releasing hormone; *CRIF*, corticotropin release inhibitory factor; GABA, gamma-aminobutyric acid; *MeA*, medial amygdala; *MePO*, medial preoptic nucleus; *OVLT*, organum vasculosum of the lamina terminalis; *POMC*, proopiomelanocortin. Source: *From Figure 7–18 in Low, M. J. (2016). Neuroendocrinology, Chapter 7. In S. Melmed, K. S. Polonsky, P. R. Larsen, H. M. Kronenberg. (Eds.),* Williams textbook of endocrinology *(13th ed., p. 137), Elsevier.*

the magnicellular neurons that connect to the posterior lobe and is carried directly into the general circulation by veins that drain the posterior lobe. It is unlikely that AVP that originates in magnicellular neurons acts as a hypophysiotropic hormone, but it can reach the corticotropes and stimulate ACTH secretion when its concentration in the general circulation increases sufficiently. Oxytocin, like AVP, is

The hormones antidiuretic hormone (or arginine vasopressin) and oxytocin are synthesized in the neurons of the supraoptic and paraventricular nuclei, respectively

The hormones are transported along the axons forming the hypothalamic hypophyseal tract, together with the carrier protein neurophysin, and are released at the axon terminals. The hormones enter fenestrated capillaries derived from the inferior hypophyseal artery

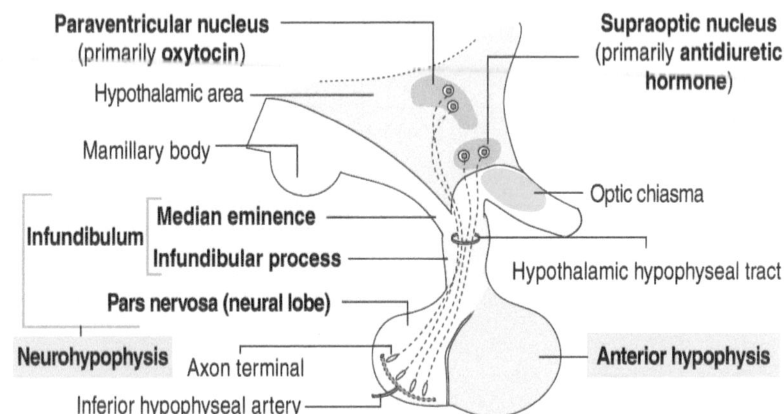

FIGURE 2.27 The posterior pituitary and its relationship to the hypothalamus. Source: *From Figure 18.12 in Kierszenbaum, A. L., Tres, L. L. (2016).* Histology and cell biology: An introduction to pathology *(4th ed., p. 569). Elsevier.*

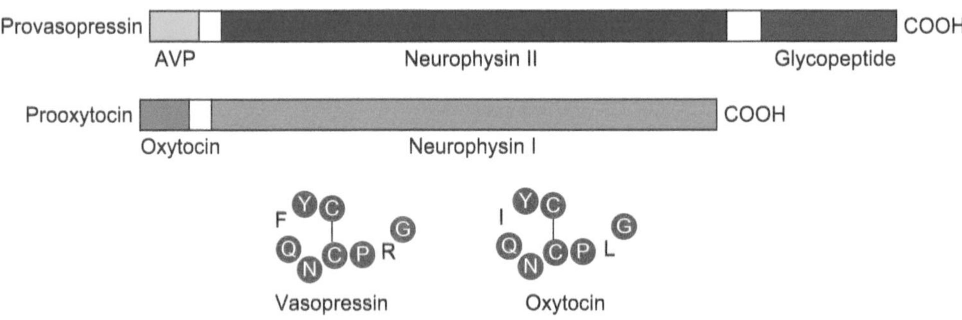

FIGURE 2.28 Structures of the hormones of the neurohypophysis and their prohormone precursors. Because final processing of the prohormones takes place in the secretory granules, the neurophysins and the glycopeptide fragment are cosecreted with oxytocin or vasopressin but have no known physiological actions. Amino acid sequences of oxytocin and vasopressin are shown in the single letter code: *C, Y, F, I, Q, N, P, R, L, G. C,* Cysteine; *F,* phenylalanine; *G,* glycine; *I,* isoleucine; *L,* leucine; *N,* asparagine; *P,* proline; *Q,* glutamine; *R,* arginine; *Y,* tyrosine.

also synthesized in parvicellular neurons at other sites in the nervous system and is released from axon terminals that project to a wide range of sites within the central nervous system.

Oxytocin also is produced in some reproductive tissues where it acts as a paracrine factor.

Regulation of posterior pituitary function

Because the hormones of the posterior pituitary gland are synthesized and stored in nerve cells, it should not be surprising that their secretion is controlled in the same way as that of conventional neurotransmitters. Action potentials that arise from synaptic input to the cell bodies within the hypothalamus course down the axons in the pituitary stalk, trigger an influx of calcium into nerve terminals, and release the contents of neurosecretory granules. Vasopressin or oxytocin is released along with their respective neurophysins and the processing enzymes. Tight binding of AVP or oxytocin to their respective neurophysins is favored by the acidic pH of the secretory granule, but upon secretion, the higher pH of the extracellular environment allows the hormones to dissociate from their neurophysins and circulate in an unbound form. Oxytocin and vasopressin are cleared rapidly from the blood with half-lives of about 2 minutes.

As is discussed in Chapter 1, Introduction, signals for the secretion of oxytocin originate in the periphery and are transmitted to the brain by sensory neurons. After appropriate processing in higher centers, cells in the supraoptic and paraventricular nuclei are signaled to release their hormone from nerve terminals in the posterior pituitary gland (Fig. 2.30).

The importance of neural input to oxytocin secretion is underscored by the observation that it may also be secreted in a conditioned reflex. A nursing mother sometimes releases oxytocin in response to the cries of her baby even before the infant begins to suckle.

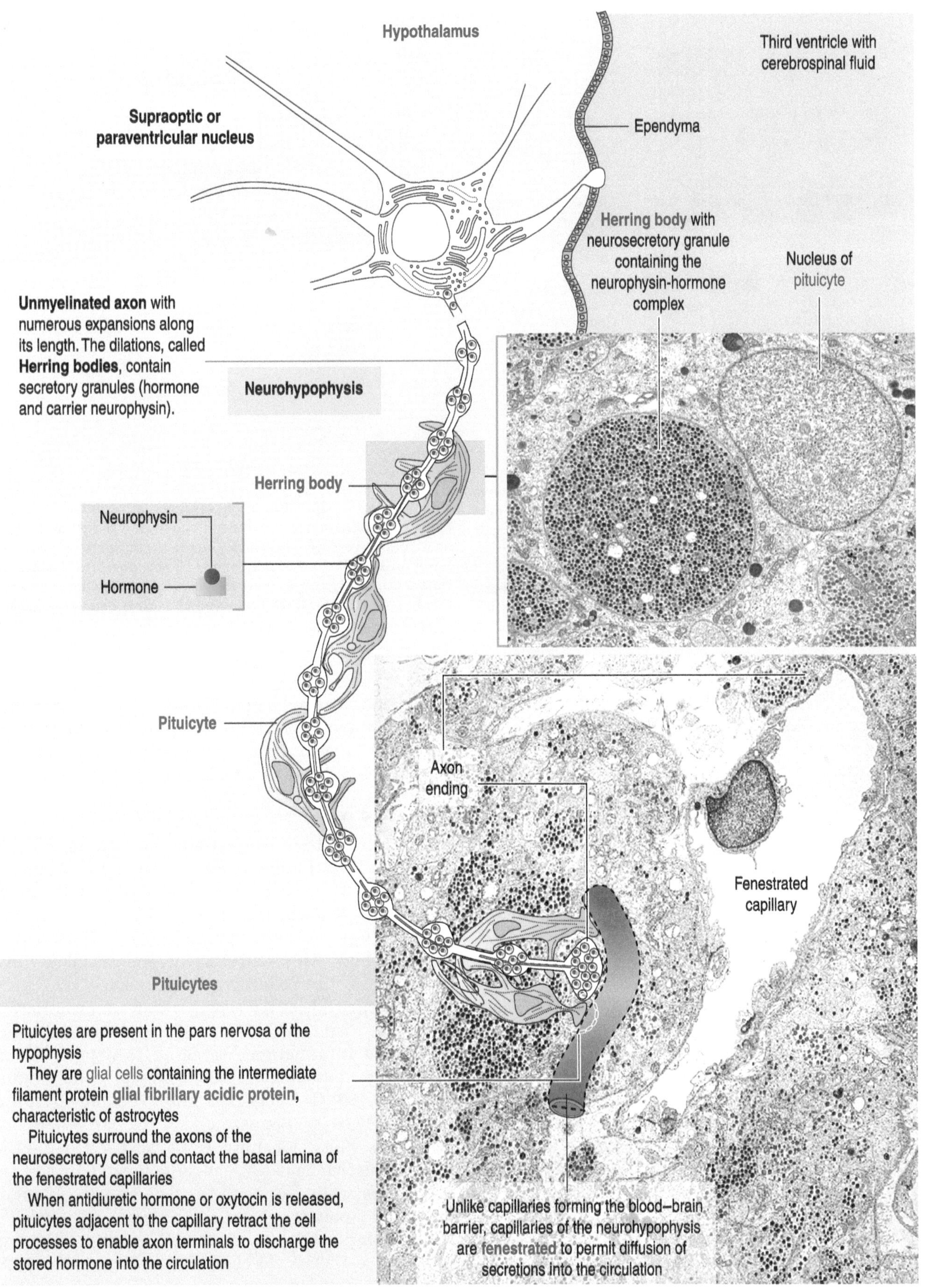

FIGURE 2.29 The secretion and transport of ADH and oxytocin from the hypothalamus to the neurohypophysis. *ADH*, Antidiuretic hormone. Source*: From Figure 18.13 in Kierszenbaum, A. L., Tres, L. L. (2016).* Histology and cell biology: An introduction to pathology *(4th ed., p. 570). Elsevier.*

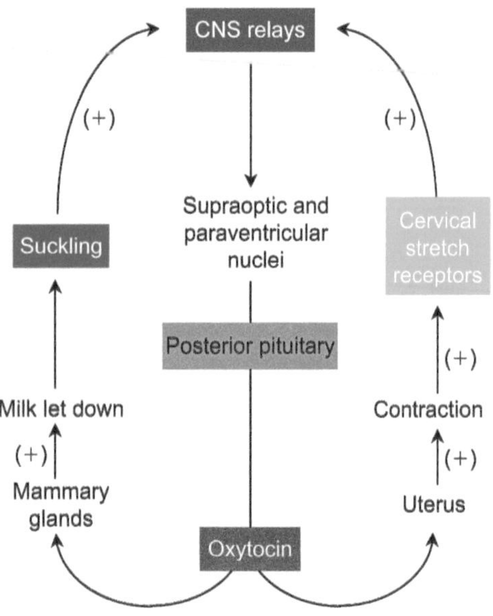

FIGURE 2.30 Regulation of oxytocin secretion showing a positive feedback arrangement. Oxytocin stimulates the uterus to contract and causes the cervix to stretch. Increased cervical stretch is sensed by neurons in the cervix and transmitted to the hypothalamus, which signals more oxytocin secretion. Oxytocin secreted in response to suckling forms an open-loop feedback system in which positive input is interrupted when the infant is satisfied and stops suckling. Further details are given in Chapter 14, Hormonal Control of Pregnancy and Lactation.

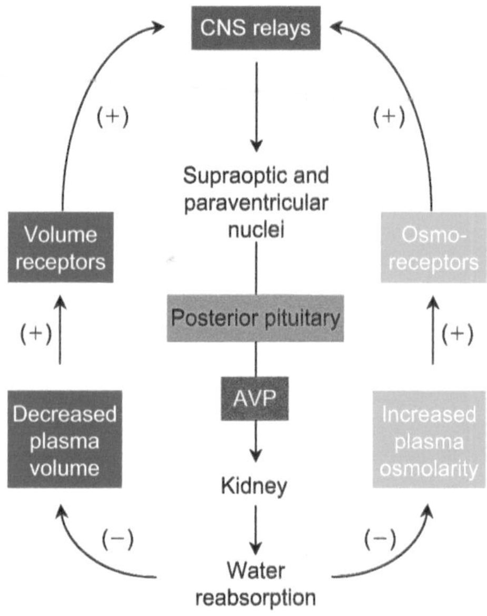

FIGURE 2.31 Regulation of vasopressin secretion. Increased blood osmolality or decreased blood volume are sensed in the brain or thorax, respectively, and increase vasopressin secretion. Vasopressin, acting principally on the kidney, produces changes that restore osmolality and volume, thereby shutting down further secretion in a negative feedback arrangement. Further details are given in Chapter 9, Regulation of Salt and Water Balance.

Oxytocin also is secreted at the same low basal rate in both men and women, but no physiological role has been established for basal oxytocin secretion. Recent findings that oxytocin is secreted during orgasm suggest a role in reproduction. Signals for vasopressin secretion in response to increased osmolality of the blood are thought to originate in hypothalamic neurons, and possibly in the AVP secretory cells themselves. Osmoreceptor cells are exquisitely sensitive to small increases in osmolality and signal cells in the paraventricular and supraoptic nuclei to secrete AVP. AVP is also secreted in response to decreased blood volume. Blood volume is monitored by pressure or stretch receptors in the thoracic vasculature. These receptors relay information to the central nervous system in afferent neurons in the vagus nerves. The control of AVP secretion is shown in Fig. 2.31 and is discussed more fully in Chapter 9, Regulation of Salt and Water Balance. Under basal conditions blood levels of AVP fluctuate in a diurnal rhythmic pattern that closely resembles that of ACTH.

Summary

Summary Long thought of as the master gland because its hormones affect diverse structures, many of which are hormone-producing structures in their own right, it is discovered in this chapter that it is really only a relay station between the hypothalamus of the brain and the rest of the body. The anterior and posterior divisions of the pituitary are explored embryologically, anatomically and physiologically.

Suggested readings

Chapter 2, **Basic Foundations** Kaiser, U., & Ho, K. K. Y. (2016). Pituitary Physiology and Diagnostic Evaluation. In S. Melmed, K. S. Polonsky, P. R. Larsen, & H. M. Kronenberg (Eds.), *Williams Textbook of Endocrinology* (13 ed., pp. 176–231). Philadelphia: Elsevier. Low, M. J. (2016). Neuroendocrinology. In S. Melmed, K. S. Polonsky, P. R. Larsen, & H. M. Kronenberg (Eds.), *Williams Textbook of Endocrinology* (13 ed., pp. 110–175). Philadelphia: Elsevier. **Advanced Information** Asa, S. L., & Mete, O. (2018). Endocrine pathology: past, present and future. *Pathology,* **50** (1), 111–118. http://doi.org/10.1016/j.pathol.2017.09.003 Boguszewski, C. L., Barbosa, E. J. L., Svensson, P.-A., Johannsson, G., & Glad, C. A. M. (2017). Mechanisms in endocrinology: Clinical and pharmacogenetic aspects of the growth hormone receptor polymorphism. *European Journal of Endocrinology,* **177** (6), R309–R321. http://doi.org/10.1530/eje-17-0549 Fischer, S., & Ehlert, U. (2018). Hypothalamic–pituitary–thyroid (HPT) axis functioning in anxiety disorders. A systematic review.

Depression and Anxiety, **35** (1), 98–110. http://doi.org/10.1002/da.22692 Kasuki, L., Wildemberg, L. E., & Gadelha, M. R. (2018). Management of endocrine disease: Personalized medicine in the treatment of acromegaly. *European Journal of Endocrinology*, **178** (3), R89–R100. http://doi.org/10.1530/eje-17-1006 Miyata, S. (2017). Advances in Understanding of Structural Reorganization in the Hypothalamic Neurosecretory System. *Frontiers in Endocrinology*, **8** (275). http://doi.org/10.3389/fendo.2017.00275 Rensen, N., Gemke, R. J. B. J., van Dalen, E. C., Rotteveel, J., & Kaspers, G. J. L. (2017). Hypothalamic-pituitary-adrenal (HPA) axis suppression after treatment with glucocorticoid therapy for childhood acute lymphoblastic leukaemia. *Cochrane Database of Systematic Reviews* (11). http://doi.org/10.1002/14651858.CD008727.pub4 Tsutsui, K., Son, Y. L., Kiyohara, M., & Miyata, I. (2018). Discovery of GnIH and Its Role in Hypothyroidism-Induced Delayed Puberty. *Endocrinology*, **159** (1), 62-68. http://doi.org/10.1210/en.2017-00300.

CHAPTER

3

Thyroid gland

Case study

Graves disease

A 32-year-old woman presents to her primary care physician reporting a variety of symptoms over the past 2 months. She has anxiety, a rapid heartbeat, difficulty sleeping, weight loss, and hand tremor. She feels too warm even when her officemates feel the room temperature is comfortable. On physical examination, she appears wide-eyed and has difficulty sitting still. Her vital signs are notable for a rapid but regular pulse. Her physical exam reveals damp, warm skin. She has a smooth, diffusely enlarged thyroid gland. Reflexes are abnormally brisk. Extension of her hands reveals a fine tremor.

Given this classic constellation of symptoms and physical findings, her physician orders a blood thyroid hormone panel. Thyroid-stimulating hormone (TSH) is undetectable, while T_3 and free T_4 are significantly elevated. A thyroid scan and uptake study is performed: an oral radioactive iodine dose is administered and its retention by the thyroid gland 24 h later is found to be elevated, with normal distribution of the tracer throughout the thyroid gland. A diagnosis of Graves disease is made.

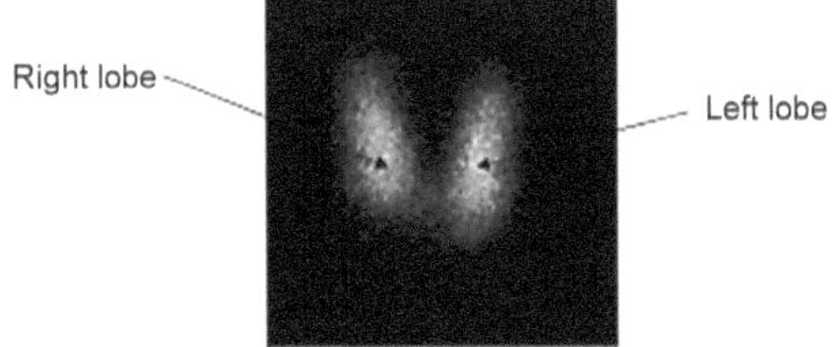

Figure: Radioactive iodine scan and uptake showing Graves disease. Retention of the I-123 radioisotope tracer by the disordered gland is above normal. I-123 distribution is uniform throughout the thyroid as is seen in a normal thyroid gland.

The diagnosis of Graves is confirmed by the presence of an antibody called thyroid-stimulating immunoglobulin (TSI) in the serum. The TSI acts by stimulating the thyroid follicular cells to make thyroid hormone in the absence of the normal regulation by TSH. This leads to higher than normal levels of thyroid hormone.

The patient is treated with a thionamide drug, the function of which is to inhibit the actions of the enzyme thyroid peroxidase, a catalyst for thyroid hormone synthesis. Over a few weeks, her thyroid levels return to normal and her symptoms resolve.

Goodman's Basic Medical Endocrinology.
DOI: https://doi.org/10.1016/B978-0-12-815844-9.00003-8

In the clinic

Hyperthyroidism

Introduction

Hyperthyroidism refers to the condition of a patient with abnormally elevated thyroid hormone levels. Thyroid hormone impacts the function of nearly every tissue in the body. Therefore the symptoms and signs of hyperthyroidism involve multiple organ systems. The task of the physician is to recognize the constellation of symptoms of hyperthyroidism. A complete physical exam will reveal the typical physical findings associated with hyperthyroidism. Laboratory studies to measure levels of thyroid hormones will confirm the suspicion of hyperthyroidism. Functional imaging of the thyroid gland may help in identifying the underlying cause of hyperthyroidism. Appropriate treatment of the condition varies, depending on the underlying cause. Rapid diagnosis and treatment of hyperthyroidism will help prevent complications of thyroid hormone excess.

Signs and symptoms

Thyroid hormone irregularities can vary in severity from mild (subclinical hyperthyroidism) to severe (thyroid storm). Because of the variation in thyroid hormone levels, the presentation of hyperthyroidism depends on the degree of hormonal abnormality. In milder cases, symptoms and physical findings may be absent and abnormalities may be discovered on routine laboratory screening. In the elderly, mild cases may be heralded by unexplained weight loss or a new diagnosis of irregular heartbeat (atrial fibrillation). As the severity of the hormonal abnormality increases, the number and severity of symptoms increase. Most of the symptoms reflect increased adrenergic tone seen in the setting of hyperthyroidism. These include a rapid heartbeat (tachycardia), anxiety, tremor, weight loss, heat sensitivity, increased sweating, and frequent bowel movements. In severe cases, known as thyroid storm, fever and delirium may be present.

On physical exam the patient's appearance will depend on the severity of the hormonal abnormality. In mild cases the appearance may be normal. In the setting of moderate hormone elevations, the individual may have difficulty sitting still and may appear anxious. Altered mental status can be evident in cases of thyroid storm. The vital signs will be notable for tachycardia. Skin will be warm and damp. A velvety texture to the skin may be noted, which is due to more rapid turnover in skin cells. Examination of the eyes will reveal a stare due to retraction of the upper eyelid. Examination of the thyroid gland will vary depending on the underlying cause of the hyperthyroidism. Possible findings on thyroid palpation include tenderness, diffuse enlargement, and a nodular texture. In some cases a venous hum or "bruit" may be audible over the gland with the aid of a stethoscope. Examination of the heart will confirm tachycardia and will reveal an irregular rhythm if atrial fibrillation is present. Extra heart sounds (gallops) may be audible in more severe cases if heart failure is present. On deep tendon reflex testing a more rapid than normal relaxation phase of the contraction will be observed. Extension of the hands will reveal a mild fine tremor.

Diagnosis

The physical exam, and the findings upon palpation of the thyroid, may provide some clues to the underlying cause of the hyperthyroidism. The thyroid is enlarged and smooth in Graves disease. It is firm and mildly enlarged, and occasionally tender, in thyroiditis. It is nodular or asymmetrically enlarged in the setting of a hyperfunctioning nodule. Simple blood tests will confirm the suspicion of hyperthyroidism and will provide information about the underlying cause. Typically the thyroid-stimulating hormone (TSH) is low, while thyroxine levels are elevated. An exception to this occurs with the rare entity of a TSH-secreting pituitary tumor, where TSH levels will be inappropriately normal or elevated in the setting of elevated thyroxine levels. Testing for the presence of a TSH receptor stimulating immunoglobulin or TSI will usually be positive in those with Graves disease.

Additional information about the underlying cause of the hyperthyroidism can be obtained by a thyroid scan and uptake. This is a two-part test where the patient swallows a capsule containing a small dose of a harmless isotope of radioactive iodine (I-123). This study takes the advantage of the natural tendency of the thyroid gland to take up iodine as it is needed for thyroid hormone synthesis. The thyroid gland is unable to distinguish between nonradioactive and radioactive iodine, so the radioactive compound is taken up in the same pattern as would be "cold" iodine. Twenty-four hours later the patient undergoes a scan to detect where the tracer has located within the thyroid gland. In addition, a calculation is also made of the percentage of the oral dose that is found in the thyroid at 24 h. Possible outcomes are shown in the figure below:

(cont'd)

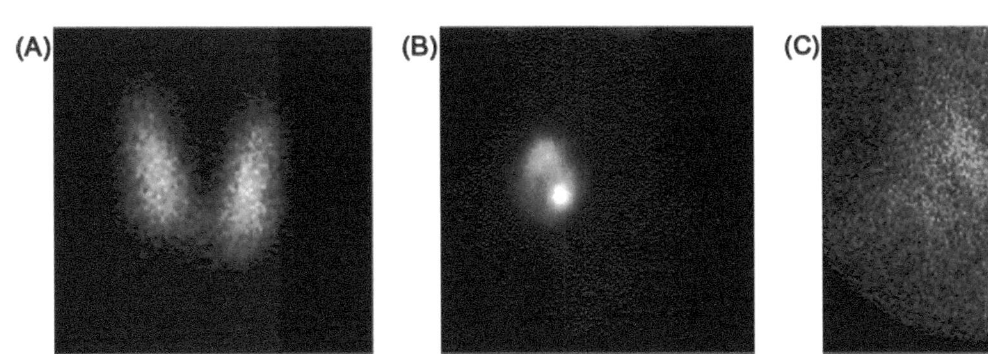

A. *Normal distribution of I-123 tracer throughout the thyroid gland, but elevated uptake of 78% at 24 h (normal, 10%–30%) as seen in Graves disease.*
B. *Distribution of I-123 tracer only in a nodule in the right thyroid lobe, with the absence of tracer in the left lobe. Percent uptake slightly elevated at 43%. This is consistent with a hyperfunctioning thyroid nodule in the right lobe.*
C. *Little-to-no distribution of tracer at 24 h, with low percent uptake of 1%. This is characteristic of thyroiditis.*

- In the normal thyroid, distribution of I-123 will be uniform throughout the gland and percent uptake at 24 h will be 10%–30% (the normal range will vary slightly from one hospital to the next).
- Graves disease is caused by abnormal production of an antibody that stimulates the TSH receptor on the surface of the thyroid follicular cells. This leads to overproduction of thyroid hormone. TSH will be appropriately low. Uptake of I-123 will be uniform throughout the thyroid gland as the antibody affects all parts of the thyroid. The percent uptake of iodine will be above normal, reflecting the excessive stimulation of the follicular cells by the TSI antibody. This is an autoimmune condition, the trigger of which is unknown. It is more common in women and may be present in multiple members of a family.
- A hyperfunctioning nodule develops when a mutation takes place for the gene encoding the TSH receptor in a follicular cell. This causes the TSH receptor to behave as if constantly being stimulated by TSH. Downstream effects include proliferation of the clone of mutated cells to produce a benign hyperfunctioning tumor or nodule in the thyroid, as well as unregulated excess production of thyroid hormone by the nodule. In this setting, thyroid hormone levels will be elevated, while TSH is low. The I-123 concentrates in the hyperfunctioning nodule where thyroid hormone is being made. The remaining normal parts of the thyroid gland will not take up tracer as the TSH level is low.
- Thyroiditis is usually caused by autoimmune destruction of the thyroid gland. This process usually involves the whole thyroid gland equally. Preformed thyroid hormone is released from the gland, resulting in high serum levels of thyroxine. The TSH will be appropriately suppressed. Due to the inflammatory injury to the thyroid tissue and the low TSH, the gland takes up little or no I-123. The scan will show absent tracer in thyroid gland and percent uptake of I-123 will be very low.

Management

Management of hyperthyroidism depends on its underlying cause.

For Graves disease the mainstay of treatment is the thionamide drugs (methimazole, carbamizole, and propylthiouracil or PTU). These medications interfere with function of thyroid peroxidase, the enzyme needed to catalyze key steps in thyroid hormone synthesis. In addition, PTU can decrease the activity of the deiodinase enzymes responsible for converting T4 into the more potent thyroid hormone, T_3, in peripheral tissues. In thyroid storm, additional agents are used along with thionamides. One such agent is a beta blocker, most commonly propranolol, which will slow the tachycardia and diminish anxiety and tremor. This agent can also reduce the conversion of T_4 to T_3. Glucocorticoids, such as prednisone, may be used to reduce the release of thyroid hormone from the gland and also interfere with the conversion of T_4 to T_3. Once thionamides are started, a brief treatment with iodine drops over several days can also block thyroid hormone release through the Wolff–Chaikoff effect. Beta blockers and steroids can be withdrawn when thyroid hormone levels normalize. In about one-third of Graves patients, the condition will remit over the course of months to years, and

(*cont'd*)

antithyroid medication can be discontinued. If it fails to remit, long-term stability can be achieved with thyroidectomy surgery, or more commonly with treatment with radioactive iodine I-131. Both of these interventions result in permanent hypothyroidism that is treated with T_4 supplementation.

In patients with hyperfunctioning thyroid nodules, hyperthyroidism is usually mild to moderate and can be managed with thionamide drugs in the short term. This condition is not expected to remit, so longer term control is achieved with surgery or more commonly with radioactive iodine therapy.

Thyroiditis is most commonly caused by an autoimmune condition that may be triggered by viral illness or childbirth. It is usually self-limited over a matter of several weeks, with thyroid hormone levels progressing from high to low and then back to normal. In some cases the resultant hypothyroidism is permanent and T4 supplementation is needed. During the hyperthyroid phase, beta blockers may help with symptom control. Nonsteroidal antiinflammatory medications or a brief course of glucocorticoids may help if there is tenderness of the thyroid gland.

Prognosis

Prognosis for hyperthyroidism is typically excellent, with the exception of thyroid storm where the condition is fatal in 10%–25%. More typical cases of hyperthyroidism can be successfully controlled with the interventions detailed previously.

Introduction

In the adult human, normal operation of a wide variety of physiological processes in virtually every organ requires appropriate amounts of thyroid hormone. Governing all of these processes, thyroid hormone acts as a modulator, rather than an all-or-none signal that turns the process on or off. In the immature individual, thyroid hormone plays an indispensable role in growth and development. Its presence in optimal amounts at a critical time is an absolute requirement for normal development of the nervous system. In its role in growth and development too, its presence seems to be required for the normal unfolding of processes, the course of which it modulates but does not initiate. Because thyroid hormone affects virtually every system in the body in this way, it is difficult to give a simple, concise answer to the naive but profound question: What does thyroid hormone do? The response of most endocrinologists would be couched in terms of consequences of hormone excess or deficiency. Indeed, deranged function of the thyroid gland is among the most prevalent of endocrine diseases and may affect as many as 12% of Americans during their lifetime. In regions of the world where the trace element iodine is scarce, the incidence of deranged thyroid function may be even higher.

Morphology

The human thyroid gland is located at the base of the neck and wraps around the trachea just below the cricoid cartilage (Figs. 3.1 and 3.2).

The two large lateral lobes that comprise the bulk of the gland lie on either side of the trachea and are connected by a thinner isthmus. A third structure, the pyramidal lobe, which is a remnant of the embryonic thyroglossal duct and its contents, is sometimes also seen as a finger-like projection extending superiorly from the isthmus. The thyroid gland in the normal human being weighs about 20 g but is capable of

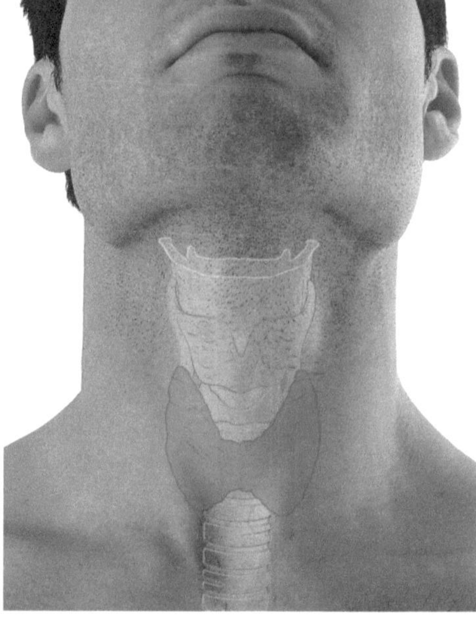

FIGURE 3.1 Location of the thyroid superimposed on a photographic image of the neck. Source: *From R. L. Drake, A. W. Vogl, A. W. M. Mitchell, R. M. Tibbitts, & P. E. Richardson. (2015).* Gray's atlas of anatomy *(2nd ed.) (p. 563). Elsevier.*

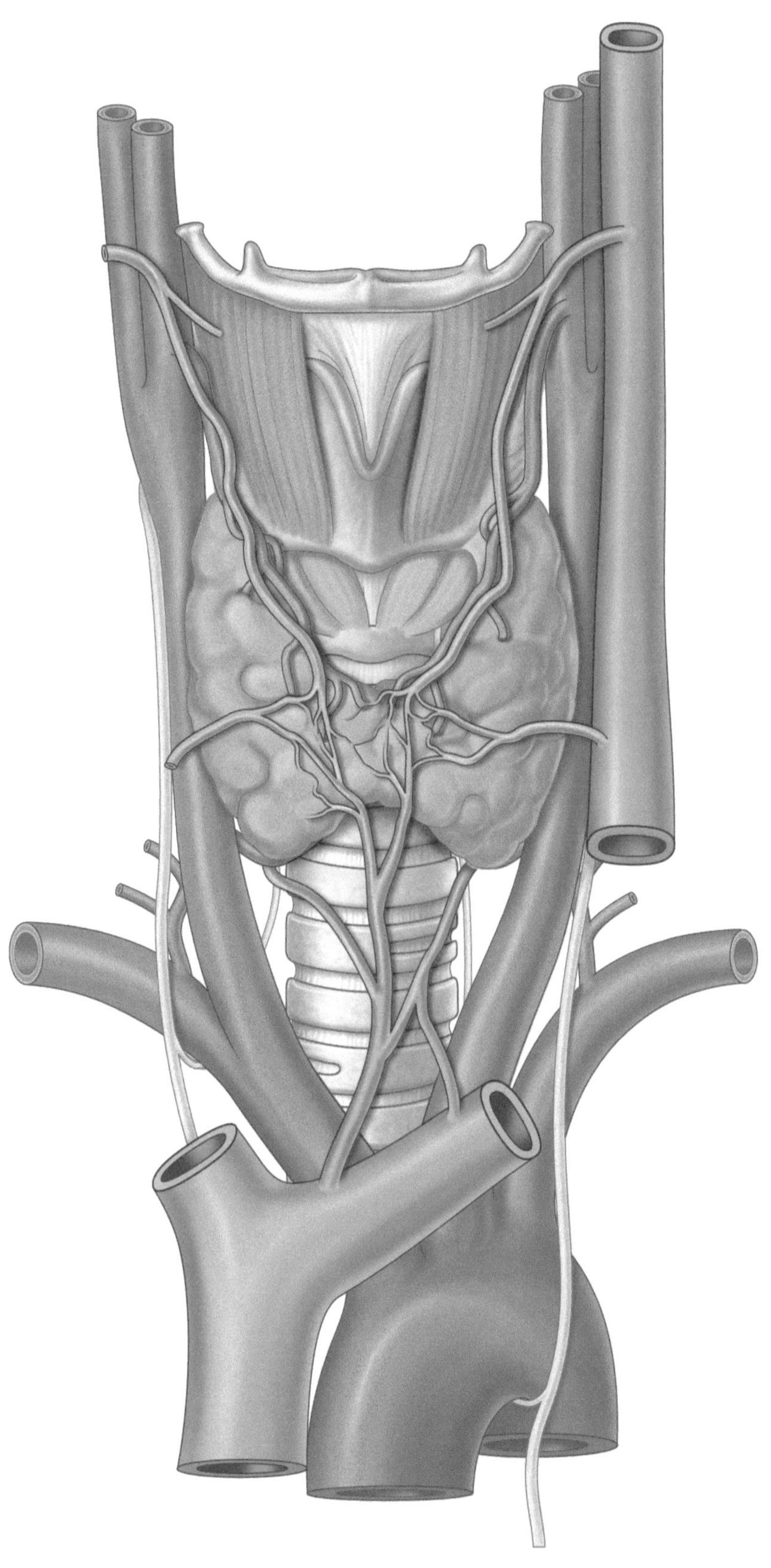

FIGURE 3.2 Blood supply to and from the thyroid gland. Source: *From R. L. Drake, A. W. Vogl, A. W. M. Mitchell, R. M. Tibbitts, & P. E. Richardson. (2015).* Gray's atlas of anatomy *(2nd ed.) (p. 564). Elsevier.*

enormous growth, sometimes achieving a weight of several hundred grams due to neoplasia or when stimulated intensely over a long period of time. Such enlargement of the thyroid gland, which may be grossly obvious, is called a goiter and is one of the most common manifestations of thyroid disease.

The thyroid gland receives its blood supply through the inferior and superior thyroid arteries, which arise from the external carotid and subclavian arteries. Relative to its weight, the thyroid gland receives a greater flow of blood than most other tissues of the body. Venous drainage is through the paired superior, middle, and inferior thyroid veins into the internal jugular and brachiocephalic veins. The gland is also endowed with a rich lymphatic system that may play an important role in delivery of hormone to the general circulation. The thyroid gland also has an abundant supply of sympathetic and parasympathetic nerves.

The functional unit of the thyroid gland is the follicle, which is composed of epithelial cells arranged as hollow vesicles of various shapes ranging in size from 0.02 to 0.3 mm in diameter; the follicle is filled with a glycoprotein colloid called thyroglobulin (Figs. 3.3–3.5).

There are about 3 million follicles in the adult human thyroid gland. Epithelial cells lining each follicle may be cuboidal or columnar, depending on their functional state, with the height of the epithelium being greatest when its activity is highest. Each follicle is surrounded by a dense capillary network separated from epithelial cells by a well-defined basement membrane. Groups of densely packed follicles are bound together by connective tissue septa to form lobules that receive their blood supply from a single small artery. Secretory cells of the thyroid gland are derived embryologically and phylogenetically from two sources. Follicular cells, which produce the thyroid hormones, thyroxine and triiodothyronine, arise from endoderm of the primitive pharynx. Parafollicular cells, or C cells, are scattered between the follicles and produce the polypeptide hormone calcitonin, which is discussed in Chapter 8, Hormonal Regulation of Fuel Metabolism. These neuroendocrine cells arise from the ultimobranchial body associated with the fifth branchial arch.

Thyroid hormones

The thyroid hormones are α-amino acid derivatives of tyrosine (Fig. 3.6).

Thyroxine was the first thyroid hormone to be isolated and characterized. Its name derives from thyroid oxyindole, which describes the chemical structure erroneously assigned to it when it was initially isolated in 1914 by Edward C. Kendall, who would later win the Nobel Prize for his work in isolating cortisol from the adrenal gland.

Triiodothyronine is considerably less abundant and was not discovered until 1953. It is considered the active form of thyroid hormone, whereas thyroxine is the storage form. Both hormone molecules are exceptionally rich in iodine, which comprises more than half of their molecular weight. Thyroxine contains four atoms of

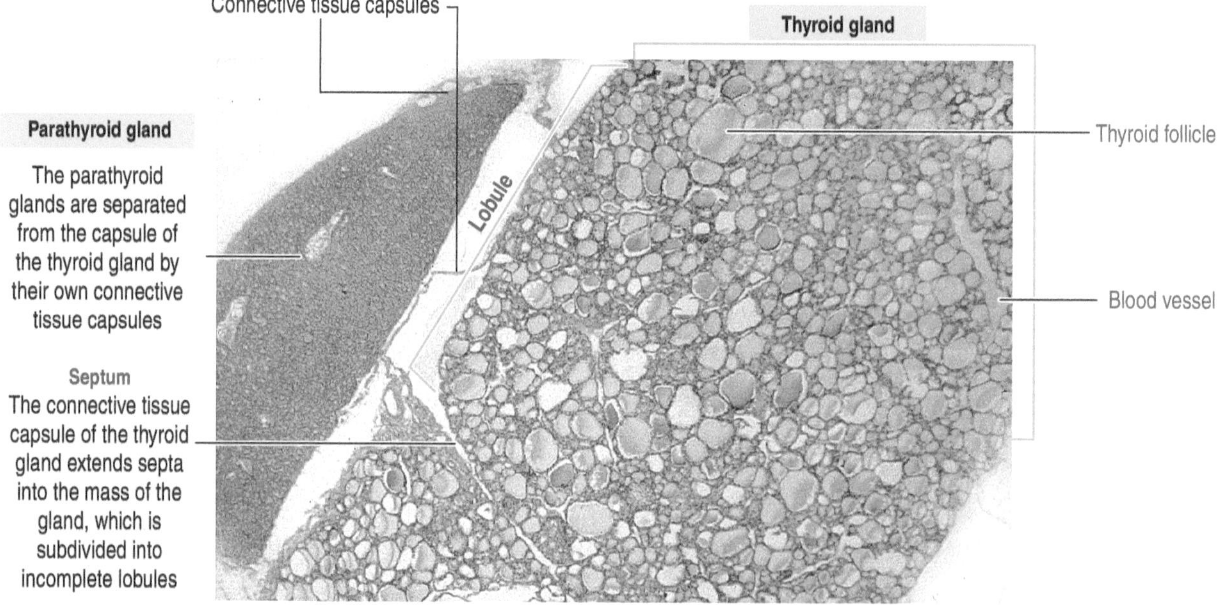

FIGURE 3.3 Low power magnification of part of the thyroid and parathyroid glands. The 2–4 parathyroid glands are on the posterior side of the thyroid. Source: *From Figure 19-1 in Kierszenbaum, A. L., & Tres, L. L. (2016).* Histology and cell biology: An introduction to pathology *(4th ed.) (p. 582). Elsevier.*

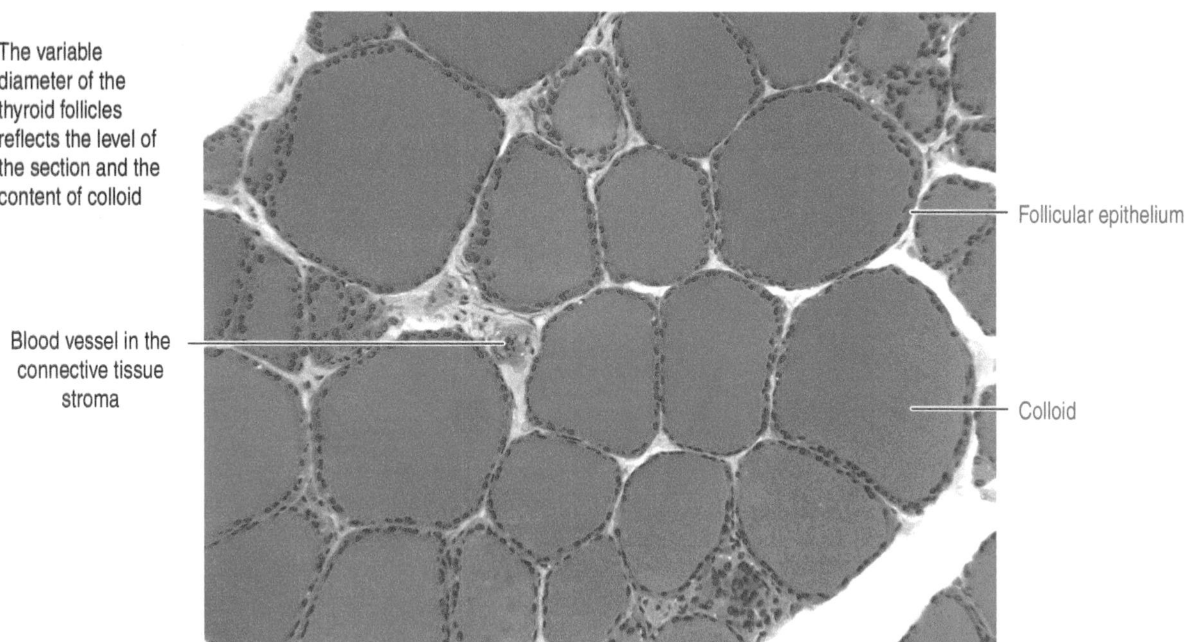

FIGURE 3.4 Higher magnification of the thyroid follicle. The epithelial cells surrounding the colloid are called the follicular cells or, collectively, follicular epithelium. Source: *From Figure 19-1 in Kierszenbaum, A. L., & Tres, L. L. (2016).* Histology and cell biology: An introduction to pathology *(4th ed.) (p. 582). Elsevier.*

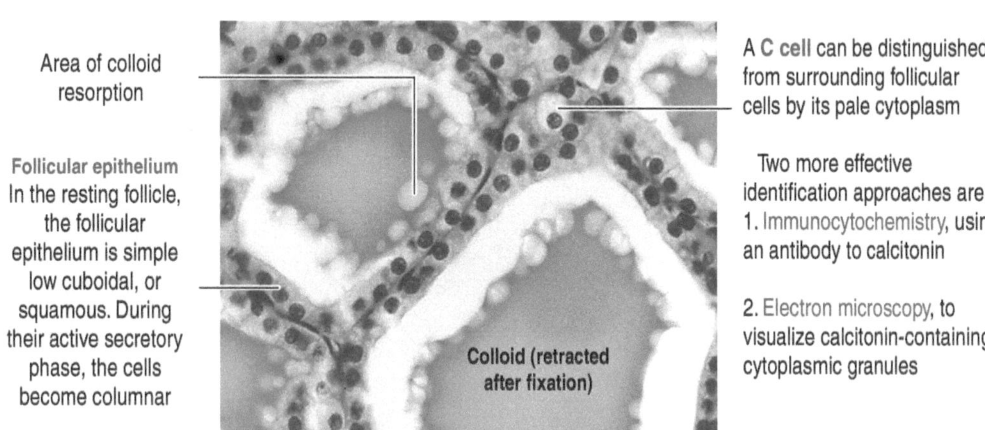

FIGURE 3.5 Higher power magnification showing the C cells (also called parafollicular cells) in between the follicles. C cells synthesize and secrete calcitonin. Source: *From Figure 19-1 in Kierszenbaum, A. L., & Tres, L. L. (2016).* Histology and cell biology: An introduction to pathology *(4th ed.) (p. 582). Elsevier.*

iodine and is abbreviated as T_4; triiodothyronine, which has three atoms of iodine and is abbreviated as T_3.

Biosynthesis

Several aspects of the production of thyroid hormone are unusual:

1. Thyroid hormones contain large amounts of iodine. Biosynthesis of active hormone requires adequate amounts of this element. This need is met by an efficient energy-dependent transport mechanism that allows thyroid cells to take up and concentrate iodide. The thyroid gland is also the principal site of storage of this rare dietary constituent.
2. Thyroid hormones are partially synthesized extracellularly at the luminal surface of follicular cells and stored in an extracellular compartment, the follicular lumen.

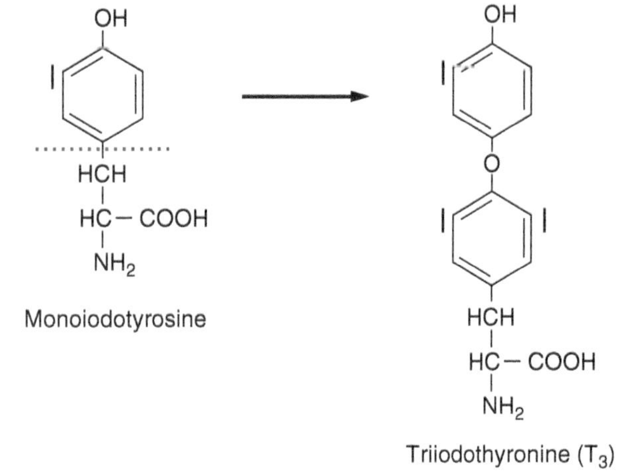

FIGURE 3.6 The first step is the conversion of phenylalanine to tyrosine in the liver. This is done with the enzyme phenylalanine hydroxylase that adds an OH to the ring. Tyrosine is taken up by the follicular cell and Iodine is added to the tyrosine. Either one iodine is added or two, to make monoiodotyrosine or diiodotyrosine, respectively. The iodinated ring can then be cleaved (leaving alanine) and added to a diiodotyrosine molecule. This will give either T_3 or T_4 depending on the number of iodine moities on the added ring.

3. The hormone therefore is doubly secreted, in that the precursor molecule, thyroglobulin, is released from apical surfaces of follicular cells into the follicular lumen, called colloid, only to be taken up again by follicular cells and degraded to release T_4 and T_3, which are then secreted into the blood from the basal surface of follicular cells.
4. Thyroxine, the major secretory product, is not the biologically active form of the hormone but must be transformed to T_3 by a deiodinase at extrathyroidal sites.

Biosynthesis of thyroid hormones can be considered as the sum of several discrete processes (Fig. 3.7), all of which depend upon the products of three genes that are expressed predominantly, if not exclusively, in thyroid follicle cells: the sodium iodide symporter (NIS), thyroglobulin, and thyroid peroxidase.

Iodine trapping

Under normal circumstances, iodide is about 25–50 times more concentrated in the cytosol of thyroid follicular cells than in blood plasma, and during periods of active stimulation, it may be as high as 250 times that of plasma. Iodine is accumulated against a steep concentration gradient by the action of an electrogenic "iodide pump" located in the basolateral membranes. The pump is a sodium iodide symporter that couples the transfer of two ions of sodium with each ion of iodide. Iodide is thus transported against its concentration driven by the favorable electrochemical gradient for sodium. Energy is expended by the sodium potassium ATPase (the sodium pump), which then extrudes three ions of sodium in exchange for two ions of potassium to maintain the electrochemical gradient for sodium. Outward diffusion of potassium maintains the membrane potential. Like other transporters, the sodium iodide symporter has a finite capacity and can be saturated. Consequently, other anions, such as perchlorate, pertechnetate, and thiocyanate, which compete for binding sites on the sodium iodide symporter, can block the uptake of iodide. This property can be exploited for diagnostic or therapeutic purposes.

Thyroglobulin synthesis

Thyroglobulin is the other major component needed for the synthesis of thyroxine and triiodothyronine. Thyroglobulin is the matrix for thyroid hormone synthesis and is the precursor form in which hormone is stored in the gland. It is a large glycoprotein composed of 300 carbohydrate and 5500 amino acid residues. Of these, only two to five modified amino acid residues will be thyroxine with an even smaller amount of triiodothyronine, the active hormone. Thyroglobulin is a stable dimer with a molecular mass of about 660 kD. Like other secretory proteins, thyroglobulin is synthesized on ribosomes, glycosylated in the cisternae of the endoplasmic reticulum, translocated to the Golgi apparatus, and packaged in secretory vesicles, which discharge it from the apical surface into the follicular lumen. Because thyroglobulin secretion into the lumen immediately follows its synthesis, follicular cells do not have the extensive accumulation of secretory granules characteristic of protein-secreting cells. Iodination to form mature thyroglobulin does not take place until after the thyroglobulin is discharged into the lumen of the colloid.

Incorporation of iodine

Iodide that enters at the basolateral surfaces of the follicular cell must be delivered to the follicular lumen where hormone biosynthesis takes place. Iodide diffuses throughout the follicular cell and exits from the apical membrane by way of a sodium-independent iodide transporter called pendrin, which is also expressed in brain and kidney. For iodide to be incorporated into tyrosine residues in thyroglobulin, it must first be converted to some higher oxidized state. This step is catalyzed by the thyroid-specific thyroperoxidase in the presence of hydrogen peroxide, the formation of which may be rate-limiting. Hydrogen peroxide

4 At the **apical plasma membrane, thyroid peroxidase** is activated and converts **iodide** into **iodine.** Two iodine atoms are linked to each tyrosyl residue. Iodination occurs within the lumen of the thyroid follicle.

After proteolytic processing, one monoiodotyrosine peptide combines with diiodotyrosine to form T_3 (triiodothyronine). Two diiodotyrosines combine to form T_4 (thyroxine). One iodinated thyroglobulin molecule yields four molecules of T_3 and T_4.

Clinical significance: Propylthiouracil and **methyl mercaptoimidazole** (MMI) inhibit thyroid peroxidase–mediated iodination of tyrosine in thyroglobulin.

5 A droplet in the colloid of the thyroid follicle, containing iodinated thyroglobulin, is endocytosed by a pseudopod extension of the apical domain of a follicular epithelial cell. The **intracellular colloid droplet**, guided by cytoskeletal components, fuses with a **lysosome.** T_3 and T_4 molecules are released by the proteolytic action of lysosomal enzymes.

Clinical significance: Propylthiouracil can block the conversion of T_4 to T_3 in peripheral tissues (liver).

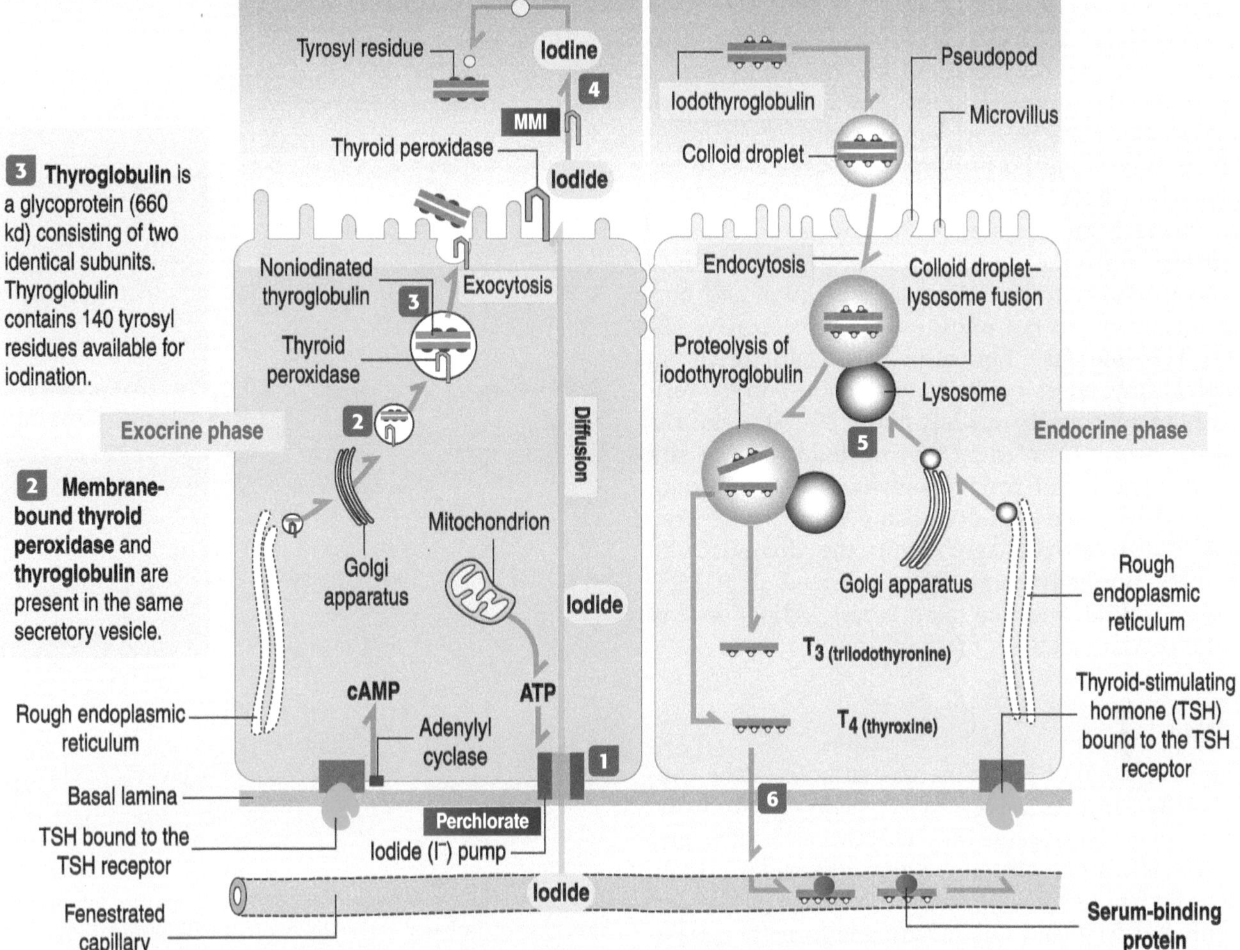

1 The **iodide** (I⁻) **pump** concentrates iodide within the thyroid follicular cell 20- to 100-fold above serum levels. An Na^+, K^+-dependent ATPase and adenosine triphosphate (ATP) provide the energy for iodide transport.

Clinical significance: Thyroid follicular cell activity can be determined by measuring **radioactive iodine uptake (RAIU).** Radiation thyroidectomy can be implemented by using larger amounts of radioactive iodine in cases of thyroid hyperfunction. Also, the iodide pump can be inhibited by **perchlorate,** a competitive anion.

6 T_3 **and** T_4 **are released from the cell across the basal lamina of the thyroid follicle into a fenestrated capillary** and bind to **serum-binding proteins.** Tissue-specific **deiodinases** expressed in peripheral tissues can increase local concentrations of T_3 from circulating T_4. T_3 has a shorter half-life (18 hours) than T_4 (5 to 7 days). T_3 is 2 to 10 times more active than T_4. Thyroid hormone action is predominantly mediated by **thyroid hormone receptors** (THRs), which are encoded by the thyroid hormone receptor α *(THRA)* and thyroid hormone receptor β *(THRB)* genes.

FIGURE 3.7 The synthesis and storage of thyroid hormone (left panel) and the secretion of T_3 and T_4 (right panel). Source: *Figure 19-3 in Kierszenbaum, A. L., & Tres, L. L. (2016).* Histology and cell biology: An introduction to pathology *(4th ed.) (p. 584). Elsevier.*

is generated by the catalytic activity of a calcium-dependent NADPH oxidase that is present in the brush border. Thyroperoxidase is the key enzyme in thyroid hormone formation and is thought to catalyze the iodination and coupling reactions described next in addition to the activation of iodide. Thyroperoxidase spans the brush border membrane on the apical surface of follicular cells and is oriented with its catalytic domain facing the follicular lumen.

Addition of iodine molecules to tyrosine residues in thyroglobulin is called organification. Thyroglobulin is iodinated at the apical surface of follicular cells as it is released into the follicular lumen. Iodide acceptor sites in thyroglobulin are in sufficient excess over the availability of iodide that no free iodide accumulates in the follicular lumen. Although posttranslational conformational changes orchestrated by endoplasmic reticular proteins organize the configuration of thyroglobulin to increase its ability to be iodinated, iodination and hormone formation do not appear to be particularly efficient. Tyrosine is not especially abundant in thyroglobulin and comprises only about 1 in 40 residues of the peptide chain. Only about 25–30 of the 134 tyrosine residues in each thyroglobulin dimer are iodinated. The initial products formed are monoiodotyrosine (MIT) and diiodotyrosine (DIT), and they remain in peptide linkage within the thyroglobulin molecules. Normally more DIT is formed than MIT, but when iodine is scarce there is less iodination and the ratio of MIT to DIT is reversed.

Coupling

The final stage of thyroxine biosynthesis is the coupling of two molecules of DIT to form T_4 within the peptide chain. This occurs only at residues 5, 1290, and 2553 and is also catalyzed by thyroperoxidase. Only three to four molecules become thyroxine with the rest remaining as MIT and DIT. Thyroxine formation takes place primarily nearer the amino end of thyroglobulin while triiodothyronine formation mostly occurs toward the carboxy terminus. There is only one site, residue 2746, where triiodothyronine is formed from one MIT and one DIT. T_3 may be formed either by deiodination of T_4 or by coupling one residue of DIT to one of MIT. Even so, there is usually only one T_3 formed for every five thyroglobulin molecules under iodine-sufficient conditions.

Exactly how coupling is achieved is not known. One possible mechanism involves joining two iodotyrosine residues that are near each other on either two separate strands of thyroglobulin or adjacent folds of the same strand. In lower animals the sequence Glu/AspTyr or Thr/SerTyrSer is needed before coupling.

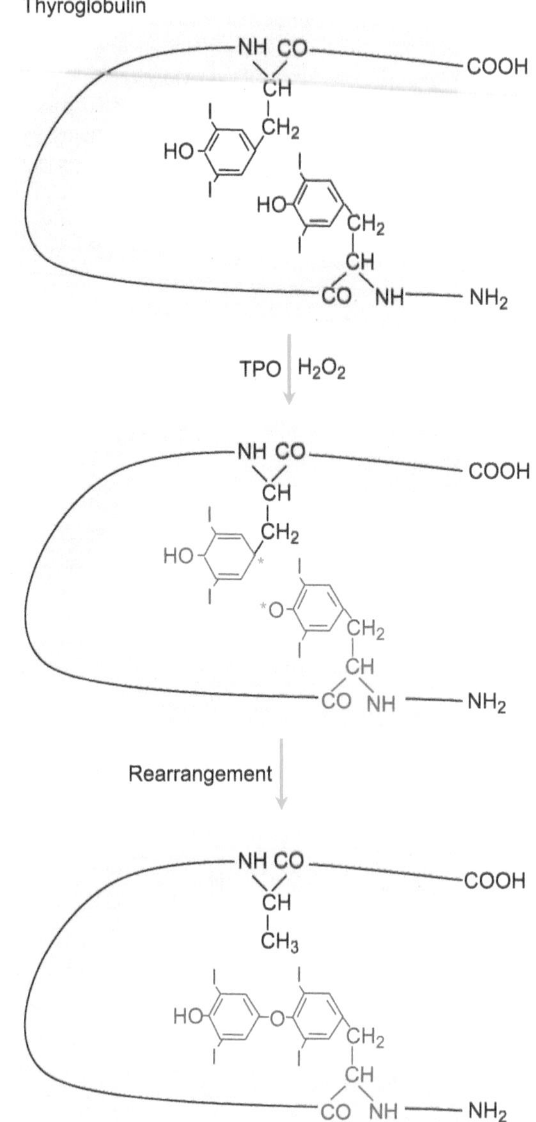

FIGURE 3.8 Hypothetical coupling scheme for intramolecular formation of T4 based on model reaction with purified thyroid peroxidase. Source: *Modified from Taurog, A. (2000). In L. E. Braverman & R. D. Utiger (Eds.).* Werner and Ingbar's The Thyroid *(8th ed.) (p. 71). Lippincott Williams and Wilkins, Philadelphia, PA.*

Free radicals formed by the action of thyroperoxidase react to form the ether linkage at the heart of the thyronine nucleus, leaving behind a dehydroalanine residue that was once attached to the phenyl group that now comprises the outer ring of T_4 (Fig. 3.8).

An alternative mechanism involves coupling a free diiodophenylpyruvate (deaminated DIT) with a molecule of DIT in peptide linkage within the thyroglobulin molecule by a similar reaction sequence. Regardless of which model proves correct, it is sufficient to recognize the central importance of thyroperoxidase for the formation of the thyronine nucleus as well as iodination of tyrosine residues. In addition, the mature hormone is formed while in peptide linkage within the thyroglobulin molecule and remains a part of that large storage molecule until thyroglobulin is endocytosed and lysosomal enzymes set thyroxine free during the secretory process.

Hormone storage

The thyroid is unique among endocrine glands in that it stores its hormone precursor called colloid extracellularly in follicular lumen (early histologists did not know its composition, so colloid is what they called it—and the name remains today). In the normal individual, approximately 30% of the mass of the thyroid gland is thyroglobulin, which corresponds to about 2–3 months' supply of hormone. Mature thyroglobulin is a high-molecular-weight molecule, a homodimer of the thyroglobulin precursor peptide, and contains about 10% carbohydrate and about 0.5% iodine. The iodine in thyroglobulin comprise an important reservoir for iodine and constitute about 90% of the total pool of iodine in the body.

Secretion

Thyroglobulin stored within the colloid is separated from extracellular fluid and the capillary endothelium by a virtually impenetrable layer of follicular cells. For secretion to occur, thyroglobulin must be brought back into follicular cells by a process of endocytosis. Upon acute stimulation with thyroid-stimulating hormone (TSH), long strands of protoplasm (pseudopodia) reach out from the apical surfaces of follicular cells to surround chunks of thyroglobulin, which are taken up in phagosomes (Fig. 3.9).

The phagosome fuses with lysosomes, which then migrates toward the basal membrane. During this migration, thyroglobulin is degraded to peptide fragments and free amino acids, including T_4, T_3, MIT, and DIT. Of these, only T_4 and T_3 are released into the bloodstream, in a ratio of about 20:1, by simple diffusion down a concentration gradient.

MIT and DIT cannot be utilized for the synthesis of thyroglobulin and are rapidly deiodinated by a specific microsomal deiodinase. Virtually all the iodide released from iodotyrosines is recycled into thyroglobulin. Deiodination of iodotyrosine provides about twice as much iodide for hormone synthesis as the iodide pump and is therefore of great significance in hormone biosynthesis. Patients who are genetically deficient in thyroidal tyrosine deiodinase readily suffer symptoms of iodine deficiency and excrete MIT and DIT in their urine. Normally, virtually no MIT or DIT escape from the gland.

Synthesis of thyroglobulin and its export in vesicles into the colloid is an ongoing process that takes place simultaneously with uptake of thyroglobulin in other vesicles moving in the opposite direction. These opposite processes, involving vesicles laden with thyroglobulin moving into and out of the cells, are somehow regulated so that under normal circumstances, thyroglobulin neither accumulates in follicular cells nor is the colloid depleted. The physiological mechanisms for such traffic control are not yet understood.

Control of thyroid function

Effects of thyroid-stimulating hormone

Although the thyroid gland can carry out all the steps of hormone biosynthesis, storage, and secretion in the absence of any external signals, autonomous function is far too sluggish to meet bodily needs for thyroid hormone. The principal regulator of thyroid function is the TSH, which is secreted by thyrotropes in the pituitary gland (see Chapter 2: Pituitary Gland). It may be recalled that TSH consists of two glycosylated peptide subunits, including the same α-subunit that is also found in follicle stimulating hormone and luteinizing hormone. The β-subunit is the part of the hormone that confers thyroid-specific stimulating activity, but free β-subunits are inactive and stimulate the thyroid only when linked to α-subunits in a complex three-dimensional configuration.

TSH binds to a single class of heptahelical G-protein-coupled receptors (see Chapter 1: Introduction and Fig. 3.10) in the basolateral surface membranes of thyroid follicular cells.

The TSH receptor is the product of a single gene, but it comprises two subunits held together by a disulfide bond. It appears that after the molecule has been properly folded and its disulfide bonds formed, a loop of about 50 amino acids is excised proteolytically from the extracellular portion of the receptor. The α-subunit includes about 300 residues at the amino terminus and contains most of the TSH-binding surfaces. The β-subunit contains the seven membrane-spanning alpha helices and the short carboxyl terminal tail in the cytoplasm. Reduction of the disulfide bond may lead to the release of the α-subunit into the extracellular fluid and may have important implications for the development of antibodies to the TSH receptor and thyroid disease.

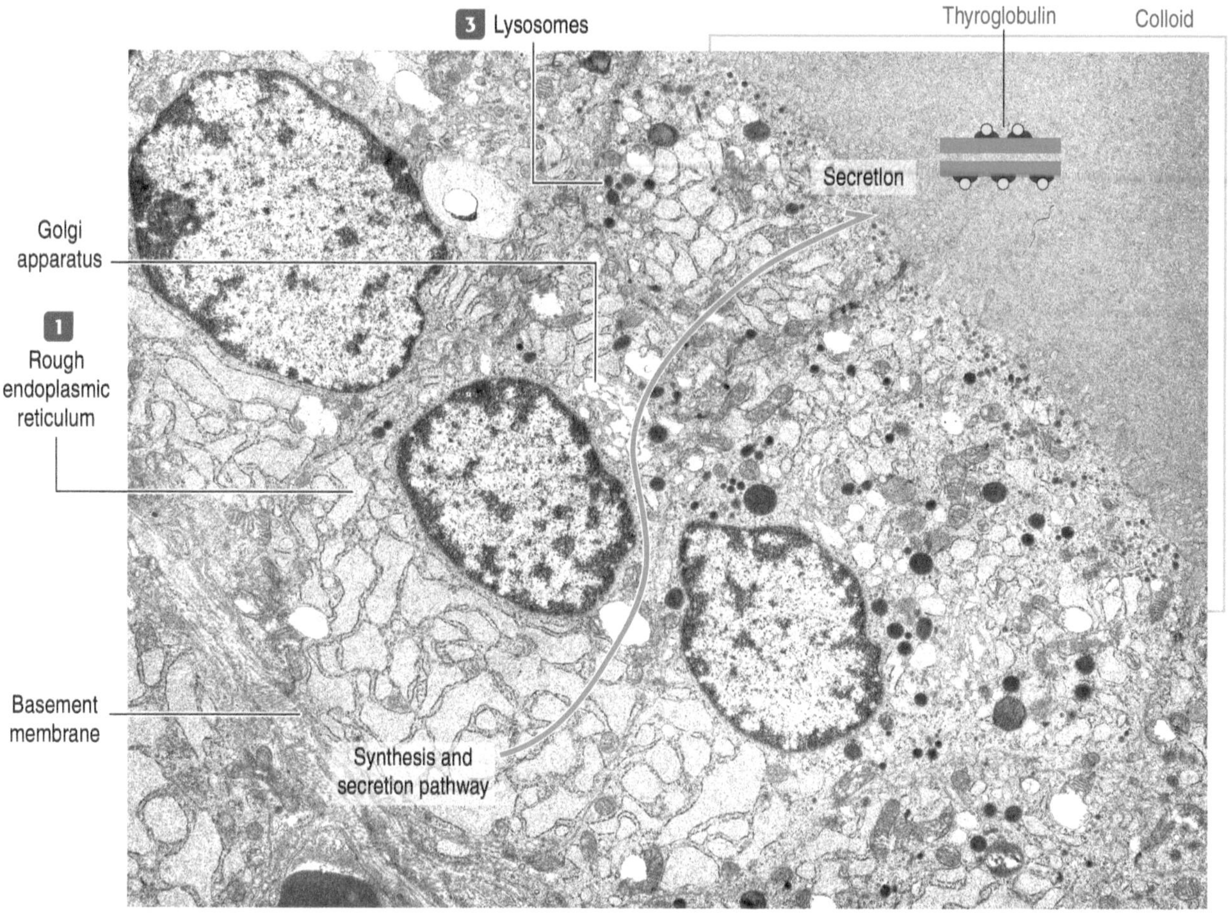

3 Lysosomes

Thyroglobulin

Colloid

Secretion

Golgi apparatus

1 Rough endoplasmic reticulum

Basement membrane

Synthesis and secretion pathway

1 The synthesis of thyroglobulin, the precursor of triiodothyronine (T_3) and thyroxine (T_4), starts in the rough endoplasmic reticulum (RER). The cisternae of the RER are distended by the newly synthesized precursor and the cytoplasmic regions are reduced to very narrow areas. Thyroglobulin molecules are glycosylated in the Golgi apparatus

2 Under the light microscope, thyroglobulin synthetic activity can be visualized in the cytoplasm of the follicular cells as optically clear vesicular spaces

3 The apical domain of the follicular cells displays abundant lysosomes involved in the processing of the prohormone thyroglobulin into thyroid hormones

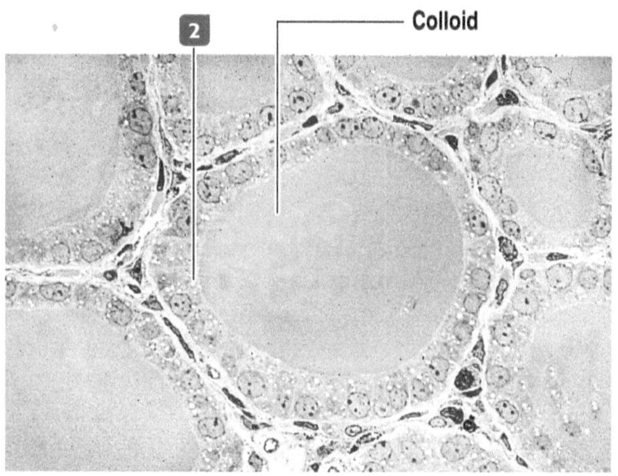

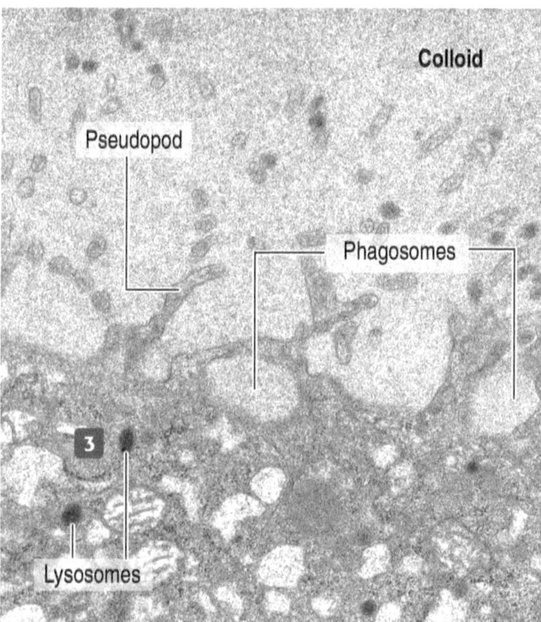

Pseudopods extend from the apical domain of the thyroid follicular cells and, after surrounding a portion of the colloid (thyroglobulin), organize an intracellular phagosome. Lysosomes fuse with the phagosome and initiate the proteolytic breakdown of thyroglobulin while moving toward the basal domain of the follicular cell

FIGURE 3.9 The formation and resorption of thyroglobulin. Note the long pseudopodia in the colloid and to reabsorb the thyroglobulin, pseudopodia extend into the colloid and surround a chunk of it. The arms fuse around the chunk creating a phagosome, a vesicle within the cell. Lysosomal enzymes then digest the thyroglobulin liberating T4 and a small amount of T3. Source: *From Figure 19-2 in Kierszenbaum, A. L., & Tres, L. L. (2020).* Histology and cell biology: An introduction to pathology *(5th ed.) (p. 634). Elsevier.*

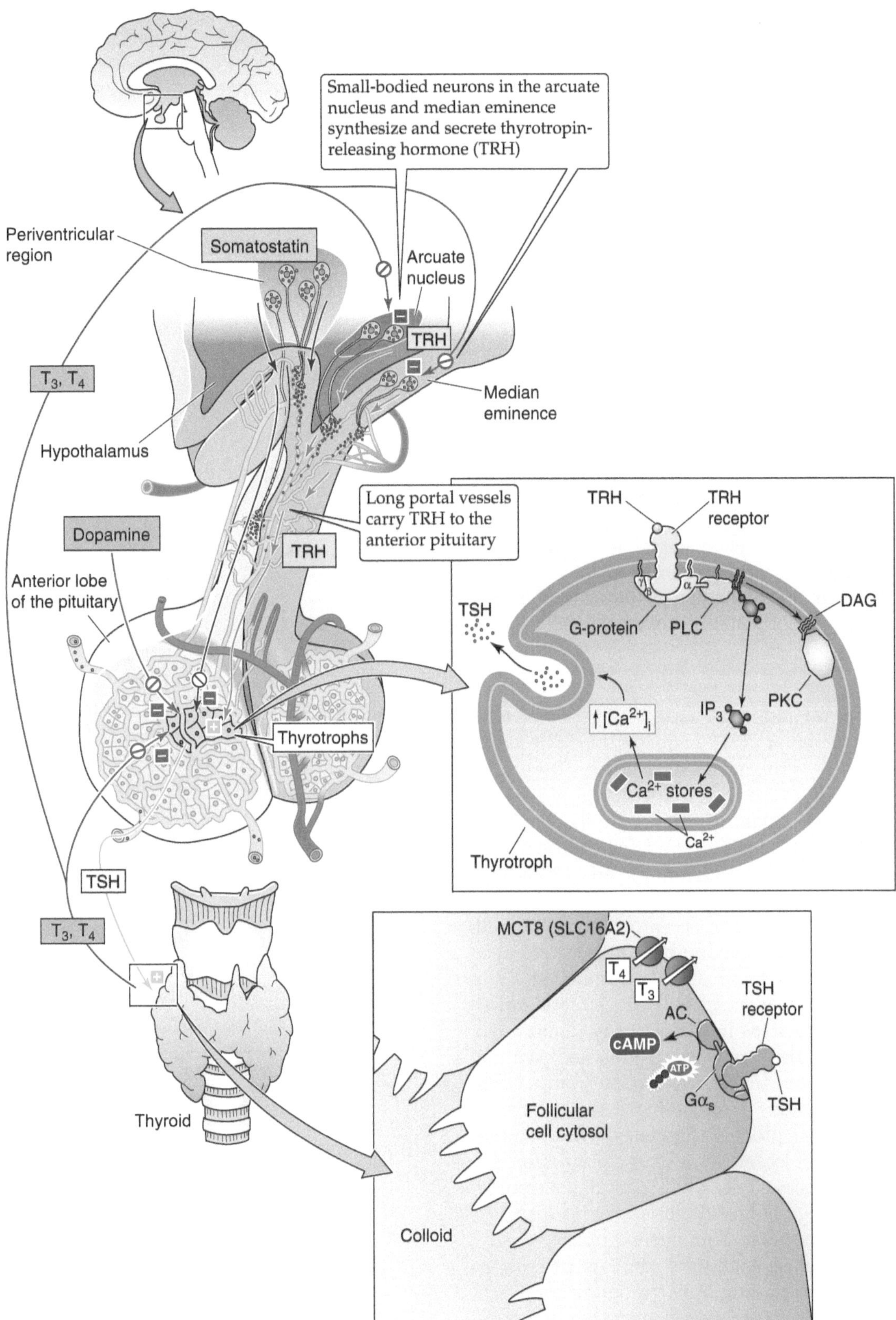

FIGURE 3.10 The hypothalamic–pituitary–thyroid axis. The effect of TSH on the receptor is also shown. *TSH*, Thyroid-stimulating hormone. Source: *From Figure 49-8 in Barrett, E. J. (2017). Chapter 49: The thyroid gland. In W. F. Boron & E. L. Boulpaep (Eds.),* Medical physiology *(3rd ed.) (p. 1015). Elsevier.*

Under the microscope—information in greater detail

Binding of thyroid-stimulating hormone (TSH) to the receptor results in the activation of both adenylyl cyclase through Gαs and phospholipase C through Gαq and leads to increases in both the cyclic adenosine monophosphate (AMP) and diacylglycerol (DAG)/inositol trisphosphate (IP3) second messenger pathways (see Chapter 1: Introduction). Activation of the cyclic AMP pathway appears to be the more important transduction mechanism, as all the known effects of TSH can be duplicated by cyclic AMP. Because TSH increases cyclic AMP production at much lower concentrations than are needed to increase phospholipid turnover, it is likely that IP3 and DAG are redundant mediators that reinforce the effects of cyclic AMP at times of intense stimulation, but it is also possible that these second messengers signal some unique responses. Increased turnover of phospholipid is associated with the release of arachidonic acid and the consequent increased the production of prostaglandins that also follows TSH stimulation of the thyroid.

In addition to regulating all aspects of hormone biosynthesis and secretion, TSH increases blood flow to the thyroid. With prolonged stimulation, TSH also increases the height of the follicular epithelium (hypertrophy) and can stimulate division of follicular cells (hyperplasia). Stimulation of thyroid follicular cells by TSH is a good example of a pleiotropic effect of a hormone in which there are multiple separate but complementary actions that collectively produce an overall response. Each step of hormone biosynthesis, storage, and secretion appears to be directly stimulated by a cyclic AMP–dependent process that is accelerated independently of the steps in the pathway. Thus, even when increased iodide transport is blocked with a drug that specifically affects the iodide pump, TSH nevertheless accelerates the remaining steps in the synthetic and secretory process. Similarly, when iodination of tyrosine is blocked by a drug specific for the organification process, TSH still stimulates iodide transport and thyroglobulin synthesis.

Most of the responses to TSH depend upon the activation of protein kinase A and the resultant phosphorylation of proteins, including transcription factors such as CREB (cyclic AMP response element-binding protein) (see Chapter 1: Introduction). TSH increases expression of genes for the sodium iodide symporter, thyroglobulin, thyroid oxidase, and thyroid peroxidase. These effects are exerted through cooperative interactions of TSH-activated nuclear proteins with thyroid-specific transcription factors, the expression of which is also enhanced by TSH. TSH appears to increase blood flow by activating the gene for the inducible form of nitric oxide synthase, which increases the production of the potent vasodilator, nitric oxide, and by inducing expression of paracrine factors that promote capillary growth (angiogenesis). Precisely how TSH increases thyroid growth is not understood, but it is apparent that synthesis and secretion of a variety of local growth factors is induced.

Autoregulation of thyroid hormone synthesis

Although production of thyroid hormones is severely impaired when too little iodide is available, iodide uptake and hormone biosynthesis are blocked temporarily when the concentration of iodide in blood plasma becomes too high. This effect of iodide is called the Wolff–Chaikoff effect and has been exploited clinically to produce short-term suppression of thyroid hormone secretion. This inhibitory effect of iodide apparently depends on its being incorporated into some organic molecule and is thought to represent an autoregulatory phenomenon that protects against overproduction of thyroxine. Blockade of thyroid hormone production is short-lived, and the gland eventually "escapes" from the inhibitory effects of iodide by mechanisms that include downregulation of the sodium iodide symporter. This is referred to as "escape" from the Wolff–Chaikoff effect.

Biosynthetic activity of the thyroid gland may also be regulated by thyroglobulin that accumulates in the follicular lumen. Acting through a receptor on the apical surface of follicular cells, thyroglobulin decreases expression of thyroid-specific transcription factors and thereby downregulates transcription of the genes for thyroglobulin, the thyroid peroxidase, the sodium iodide symporter, and the TSH receptor. Further effects of thyroglobulin include increased transcription of pendrin, which delivers iodide from the follicular cell to the lumen. Thus thyroglobulin may have significant effects in regulating its own synthesis and may temper the stimulatory effects of TSH, which remains the primary and most important regulator of thyroid function.

Thyroid hormones in blood

More than 99.8% of thyroid hormone circulating in blood is bound firmly to three plasma proteins,

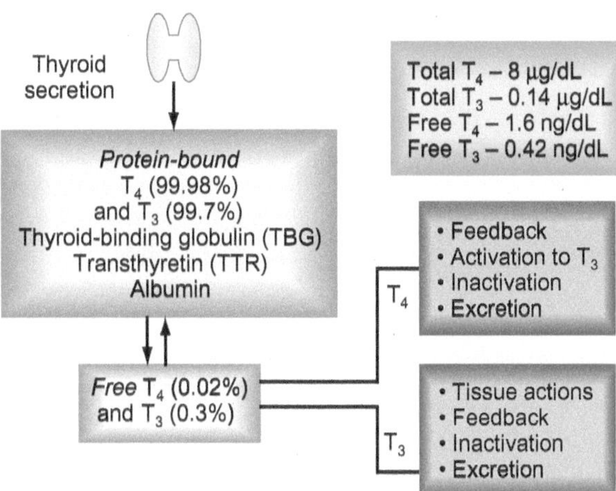

FIGURE 3.11 The transport of T_4 and T_3 in blood and the fate of each. Bound T4 and T3 are in equilibrium with free forms of T_4 and T_3, respectively. It is only the free forms of each that enter cells. It is only the T3 form that is the active thyroid hormone, although T4 does feedback to regulate the production of TRH and TSH by the hypothalamus and pituitary, respectively. *TRH*, Thyrotropin-releasing hormone; *TSH*, thyroid-stimulating hormone. Source: *From Figure 42-8 in Koeppen, B. M., & Stanton, B. A. (2018).* Berne and Levy physiology *(7th ed.) (p. 759). Elsevier.*

thyroxine-binding globulin (TBG), transthyretin (TTR), and albumin (Fig. 3.11).

Of these, TBG is quantitatively the most important and is the site for more than 70% of the total protein-bound hormone (both T_4 and T_3). About 10%–15% of circulating T_4 and 10% of circulating T_3 are bound to TTR and nearly equal amounts are bound to albumin. TBG carries the bulk of the hormone even though its concentration in plasma is only 6% that of TTR and less than 0.1% that of albumin because its affinity for both T_4 and T_3 is so much higher than that of the other proteins. All three thyroid hormone-binding proteins bind T_4 at least 10 times more avidly than T_3, so that the free, unbound concentrations of T_3 and T_4 are nearly equal. All three binding proteins are large enough to escape filtration by the kidney so that virtually no thyroid hormone appears in urine, and little crosses the capillary endothelium. The less than 1% of hormone present in free solution is in equilibrium with bound hormone and is the only hormone that can escape from capillaries to produce biological activity or be acted on by tissue deiodinase enzymes.

The total amount of thyroid hormone bound to plasma proteins represents about three times as much hormone as is secreted and degraded during a single day. Thus plasma proteins provide a substantial reservoir of extrathyroidal hormone. We therefore should not expect acute increases or decreases in the rate of secretion of thyroid hormones to bring about large or rapid changes in circulating concentrations of thyroid hormones. Thus changes in thyroid hormone secretion is an unlikely effector of minute-to-minute regulation of any homeostatic process. On the other hand, because so much of the circulating hormone is bound to plasma-binding proteins, we might expect that the total amount of T_4 and T_3 in the circulation would be affected significantly by chronic decreases in the concentration of plasma-binding proteins, as might occur with liver or kidney disease, or with increases in TBG as is seen in pregnancy.

Metabolism of thyroid hormones

Because T_4 is bound much more tightly by plasma proteins than T_3, a greater fraction of T_3 is free to diffuse out of the vascular compartment and into cells where it can produce its biological effects or be degraded. Consequently, it is not surprising that the halftime for disappearance of an administered dose of ^{125}I-labeled T_3 is only one-sixth of that for T_4, or that the lag time needed to observe effects of T_3 is considerably shorter than that needed for T_4. However, because of the binding proteins, both T_4 and T_3 have unusually long half-lives in plasma, measured in days rather than seconds or minutes (Fig. 3.12).

It is noteworthy that the half-lives of T_3 and T_4 are increased with thyroid deficiency and shortened with hyperthyroidism.

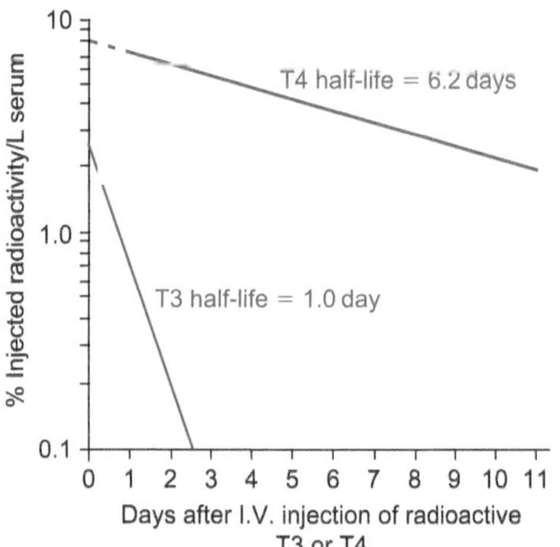

FIGURE 3.12 Rate of loss of serum radioactivity after injection of labeled thyroxine or triiodothyronine into human subjects. Source: *Plotted from data of Nicoloff, J. D., Low, J. C., Dussault, J. H., & Fisher, D. A. (1972). Simultaneous measurement of thyroxine and triiodothyronine peripheral turnover kinetics in man.* Journal of Clinical Investigation, 51, 473.

Although the main secretory product of the thyroid gland and the major form of thyroid hormone present in the circulating plasma reservoir is T_4, it is primarily T_3 and not T_4 that binds to thyroid hormone receptors (see later). T_4 could be considered to be a prohormone that serves as the precursor for extrathyroidal formation of T_3. Observations in human subjects confirm that most T_3 is formed outside the thyroid and can account for almost all the biological activity. Thyroidectomized subjects given pure T_4 in physiological amounts have normal amounts of T_3 in their circulation. Furthermore, the rate of metabolism of T_3 in normal subjects is such that about 30 μg of T_3 is replaced daily, even though the thyroid gland secretes only 5 μg each day. Thus nearly 85% of the T_3 that turns over each day must be formed by deiodination of T_4 in extrathyroidal tissues. This extrathyroidal formation of T_3 consumes about 35% of the T_4 secreted each day. The remainder is degraded to inactive metabolites.

Under the microscope—in depth information

Extrathyroidal metabolism of T4 centers around selective and sequential removal of iodine from the thyronine nucleus catalyzed by three different enzymes called iodothyronine deiodinases (Fig. 3.13).

These enzymes are selenoproteins and share the unusual feature of having the rare amino acid selenocysteine in their active sites. The type I deiodinase is expressed mainly in the liver and kidney but is also found in the

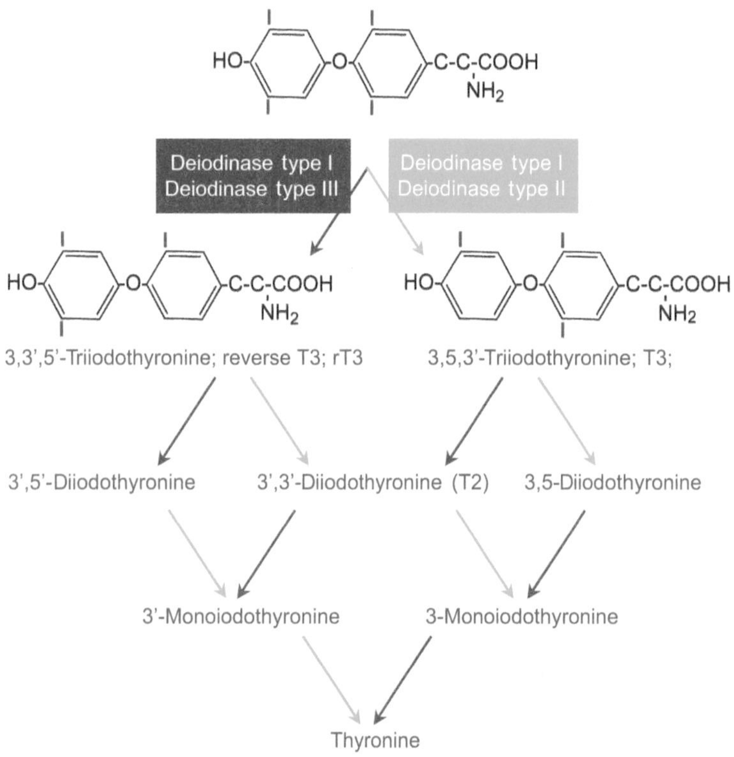

Deiodinase type I
Deiodinase type III

Deiodinase type I
Deiodinase type II

3,3',5'-Triiodothyronine; reverse T3; rT3

3,5,3'-Triiodothyronine; T3;

3',5'-Diiodothyronine

3',3'-Diiodothyronine (T2)

3,5-Diiodothyronine

3'-Monoiodothyronine

3-Monoiodothyronine

Thyronine

FIGURE 3.13 Metabolism of thyroxine. About 90% of thyroxine is metabolized by sequential deiodination catalyzed by deiodinases (types I, II, and III); the first step removes an iodine from either the phenolic or tyrosyl ring producing an active (T3) or an inactive (rT3) compound. Subsequent deiodinations continue until all the iodine is recovered from the thyronine nucleus. Green arrows designate deiodination of the phenolic ring and red arrows indicate deiodination of the tyrosyl ring. Less than 10% of thyroxine is metabolized by shortening the alanine side chain prior to deiodination.

(*cont'd*)

central nervous system, the anterior pituitary gland, and the thyroid gland itself. The type I deiodinase is a membrane-bound enzyme with its catalytic domain oriented to face the cytoplasm. T4 gains access to the enzyme after crossing the plasma membrane facilitated mainly by monocarboxylate transporter 8, which is present in most cells and also transports T3. After deiodination the newly produced T3 readily escapes into the circulation and accounts for about 80% of the T3 in blood. The type I deiodinase can remove an iodine molecule either from the outer (phenolic) ring of T4, or from the inner (tyrosyl) ring. Iodines in the phenolic ring are designated 3′ and 5′; iodines in the inner ring are designated simply 3 and 5. The 3 and 5 positions on either ring are chemically equivalent, but there are profound functional consequences of removing an iodine from the inner or outer rings of thyroxine. Removing an iodine from the outer ring produces 3′,3,5 triiodothyronine, usually designated as T3, and converts thyroxine to the form that binds to thyroid hormone receptors. Removal of an iodine from the inner ring produces 3′,5′,3 triiodothyronine, which is called reverse T3 (rT3). Reverse T3 cannot bind to thyroid hormone receptors. Hepatic expression of the type I deiodinase is under negative feedback control by T3 and is therefore most abundant when T3 levels are low. Whether the type I deiodinase produces predominately T3 or rT3 depends on the physiologic circumstances of the individual.

The type II deiodinase resides in the endoplasmic reticulum in many extrahepatic tissues but is absent from the liver. It accounts for most of the extrathyroidal production of T3 in normal humans. Its presence in the brain and pituitary gland is thought to account for about half of the T3 available to bind to receptors in these tissues. T3 and T4 are taken up by facilitated diffusion driven by blood levels of free hormone. However, circulating levels of T3 normally remain fairly constant, whereas tissue demands for hormone vary with changing physiological demands. The type II deiodinase provides an alternative means for satisfying needs for T3 through intracellular deiodination of T4, independently of the availability of the circulating hormone. As might be anticipated, the abundance of type II deiodinase is not constant; its expression is highest when blood concentrations of T4 are low. Both its synthesis and degradation are regulated. The enzyme turns over rapidly with a half-life of only about 20 min, compared to many hours for the type I enzyme. It is inactivated by ubiquitination and degraded in proteasomes. However, ubiquitination is reversible, and the type II enzyme can be rescued by the activation of deubiquitinating enzymes. Synthesis of the type II deiodinase also is regulated by other hormones and growth factors and by hormones that act through the cyclic AMP second messenger system (see Chapter 1: Introduction). These characteristics support the idea that this enzyme may provide T3 to meet local demands.

The type III deiodinase removes an iodine from the tyrosyl ring of T4 or T3; hence, its function is solely degradative. It is widely expressed by many tissues throughout the body. Reverse T3 is produced by both the type I and type III deiodinases and may be further deiodinated by the type III deiodinase by the inner ring (Fig. 3.13).

Reverse T3 (which is inactive) is also a favored substrate for the type I deiodinase, and although it is formed at a similar rate as T3, it is degraded much faster than T3. Some rT3 escapes into the bloodstream where it is avidly bound to thyroxine-binding globulin and transthyretin.

All three deiodinases can catalyze the oxidative removal of iodine from partially deiodinated hormone metabolites, and through their joint actions the thyronine nucleus can be completely stripped of iodine. The liberated iodide is then available for uptake by the thyroid and is recycled into hormone. A quantitatively less important route for degradation of thyroid hormones includes shortening of the alanine side chain to produce tetraiodothyroacetic acid (tetrac) and its subsequent deiodination products. Thyroid hormones also are conjugated with glucuronic acid and excreted intact in the bile. Bacteria in the intestine can split the glucuronide bond, and some of the thyroxine liberated can be taken up from the intestine and returned to the general circulation. This cycle of excretion in bile and absorption from the intestine is called the enterohepatic circulation and may be of importance in maintaining normal thyroid economy when thyroid function is marginal or dietary iodide is scarce. Thyroxine is one of the few naturally occurring hormones that is sufficiently resistant to intestinal and hepatic destruction that therapeutic doses can readily be given by mouth.

Physiological effects of thyroid hormones

Growth and maturation

Skeletal system

One of the most striking effects of thyroid hormones is its effects on bodily growth in the fetus and child (see Chapter 10: Hormonal Regulation of Calcium Balance). Growth of the fetus and neonate as well as attainment of normal adult stature require optimal amounts of thyroid hormone. Because stature or height is determined by the length of the skeleton, we might anticipate an effect of T_3 on growth of bones that elongate by expansion of cartilage in the epiphyseal plates followed by replacement of cartilage with bone (see Chapter 11: Hormonal Control of Growth). Cartilage cells at all stages of development express receptors for thyroid hormone and the type II deiodinase. Their progression from undifferentiated precursors, through mature and hypertrophic stages, is influenced by T_3, which also stimulates secretion of extracellular matrix proteins. In addition to these presumably direct actions, thyroid hormones appear to act permissively or synergistically with growth hormone, insulin-like growth factor I (see Chapter 11: Hormonal Control of Growth), and other growth factors that promote bone formation. They also promote bone growth indirectly by actions on the pituitary gland and hypothalamus. Thyroid hormone is required for normal growth hormone synthesis and secretion.

Skeletal maturation is distinct from skeletal growth. Maturation of bone results in the ossification and eventual fusion of the cartilaginous growth plates, which occurs with sufficient predictability in normal development that individuals can be assigned a specific "bone age" from radiological examination of ossification centers. Thyroid hormones profoundly affect skeletal maturation. Bone age is delayed relative to chronological age in children who are deficient in thyroid hormone and is advanced prematurely in hyperthyroid children. Uncorrected deficiency of thyroid hormone during childhood results in limitation of growth and malformation of facial bones' characteristic of juvenile hypothyroidism.

Central nervous system

The importance of the thyroid hormones for normal development of the nervous system is well established. Thyroid hormones and their receptors are present early in the development of the fetal brain, well before the fetal thyroid gland becomes functional. T_4 and T_3 present in the fetal brain at this time come from the mother and cross the placenta to the fetus, although the placenta is relatively impermeable to T_4 and T_3. Studies of children born to hypothyroid mothers show that maternal hypothyroidism may lead to deficiencies in postnatal neural development and reduced IQ. However, failure of thyroid gland development in babies born to mothers with normal thyroid function have normal brain development if properly treated with thyroid hormones immediately after birth. Maturation of the nervous system during the perinatal period has an absolute dependence on thyroid hormone. During this critical period, thyroid hormone must be present for normal development of the brain. In rats made hypothyroid at birth, cerebral and cerebellar growth and nerve myelination are severely delayed. Overall size of the brain is reduced along with its vascularity, particularly at the capillary level. The decrease in size may be partially accounted for by a decrease in axonal density and dendritic branching.

Thyroid hormone deficiency also leads to specific defects in cell migration and differentiation. In human infants the absence or deficiency of thyroid hormone during this period is catastrophic and results in permanent, irreversible mental retardation even if large doses of hormone are given later in childhood (Fig. 3.14).

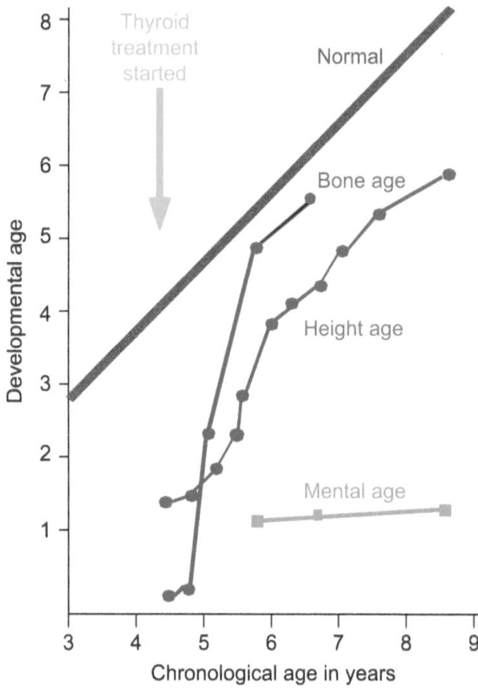

FIGURE 3.14 Effects of thyroid therapy on growth and development of a child with no functional thyroid tissue. Daily treatment with thyroid hormone began at 4.5 years of age (*green arrow*). Bone age rapidly returned toward normal, and the rate of growth (height age) paralleled the normal curve. Mental development, however, remained infantile. Source: *From Wilkins, L. (1965).* The diagnosis and treatment of endocrine disorders in childhood and adolescence. *Springfield, IL: Charles C Thomas.*

If replacement therapy is instituted early in postnatal life, however, the tragic consequences of neonatal hypothyroidism can be averted. Mandatory neonatal screening for hypothyroidism therefore has been instituted throughout the United States, Canada, and many other developed countries, but it is still performed in less than half of infants worldwide. Precisely what thyroid hormones do during the critical period, how they do it, and why the opportunity for intervention is so brief are the subjects of active research.

Effects of T_3 and T_4 on the central nervous system are not limited to the perinatal period of life. In the adult, hyperthyroidism produces irritability, restlessness, and exaggerated responses to environmental stimuli. Emotional instability that can lead to full-blown psychosis may also occur. Conversely, decreased thyroid hormone results in listlessness, lack of energy, slowness of speech, decreased sensory capacity, impaired memory, and somnolence. Mental capacity is dulled, and psychosis (myxedema madness) may occur. Conduction velocity in peripheral nerves is slowed and reflex relaxation time increased in hypothyroid individuals. The underlying mechanisms for these changes are not understood.

Autonomic nervous system

Interactions between thyroid hormones and the autonomic nervous system, particularly the sympathetic branch, are important throughout life. Increased secretion of thyroid hormone exaggerates many of the responses that are mediated by the neurotransmitters norepinephrine and epinephrine released from sympathetic neurons and the adrenal medulla (see Chapter 4: The Adrenal Glands). In fact, many symptoms of hyperthyroidism, including tachycardia (rapid heart rate) and increased cardiac output, resemble increased activity of the sympathetic nervous system. Thyroid hormones increase the abundance of receptors for epinephrine and norepinephrine (β-adrenergic receptors) in the myocardium and some other tissues. Thyroid hormones may also increase expression of the stimulatory G-protein ($G\alpha s$) associated with adrenergic receptors and downregulate the inhibitory G-protein ($G\alpha i$). Either of these effects results in greater production of cyclic AMP (see Chapter 1: Introduction). Furthermore, through the agency of cyclic AMP, sympathetic stimulation activates the type II deiodinase, which accelerates local conversion of T_4 to T_3. Because thyroid hormones exaggerate a variety of responses mediated by β-adrenergic receptors, pharmacological blockade of these receptors is useful for reducing some of the symptoms of hyperthyroidism. Conversely, the diverse functions of the sympathetic nervous system are compromised in hypothyroid states.

Cardiovascular system

In addition to the indirect effects produced through interaction with the sympathetic nervous system, thyroid hormones directly influence several aspects of cardiovascular function. Both the contraction and relaxation phases of the cardiac cycle are accelerated in the hyperthyroid heart because of increased rates of the release of calcium from the sarcoplasm reticulum and its reuptake. Opposite effects are seen in hypothyroidism. Thyroid hormones upregulate expression of the genes for the calcium channel (ryanodine receptor) through which calcium is released during contraction, and the sarcoplasmic reticular calcium ATPase (SERCa2) by which it is retrieved during relaxation. In addition, T_3 upregulates expression of the genes for the subunits of the sodium/potassium ATPase and the potassium channel proteins that restore the membrane potential.

Cardiac output is increased in hyperthyroidism and decreased in thyroid deficiency. Hyperthyroidism lowers peripheral resistance by promoting relaxation of arteriolar smooth muscle and by increasing venous tone. As a result, venous return is increased producing increased ventricular filling (preload). The decrease in peripheral resistance also decreases resistance to ventricular emptying (afterload). These effects may be indirect, but when combined with the direct effects on cardiac myocytes and enhanced sympathetic actions, they have profound implications for cardiovascular function.

Metabolism

Oxidative metabolism and thermogenesis

More than a century has passed since it was recognized that the thyroid gland exerts profound effects on oxidative metabolism in humans. The so-called basal metabolic rate (BMR), which is a measure of oxygen consumption under defined resting conditions, is highly sensitive to thyroid status. A decrease in oxygen consumption results from a deficiency of thyroid hormones, and excessive thyroid hormone increases BMR. Oxygen consumption in all tissues except brain, testis, and spleen is sensitive to the thyroid status and increases in response to thyroid hormone (Fig. 3.15).

Even though the dose of thyroid hormone given to hypothyroid animals in the experiment shown in Fig. 3.15 was large, there was a delay of many hours before effects were observable. In fact, the rate of oxygen consumption in the whole animal did not reach its maximum until 4 days after a single dose of hormone. The underlying mechanisms for increased oxygen consumption are incompletely understood.

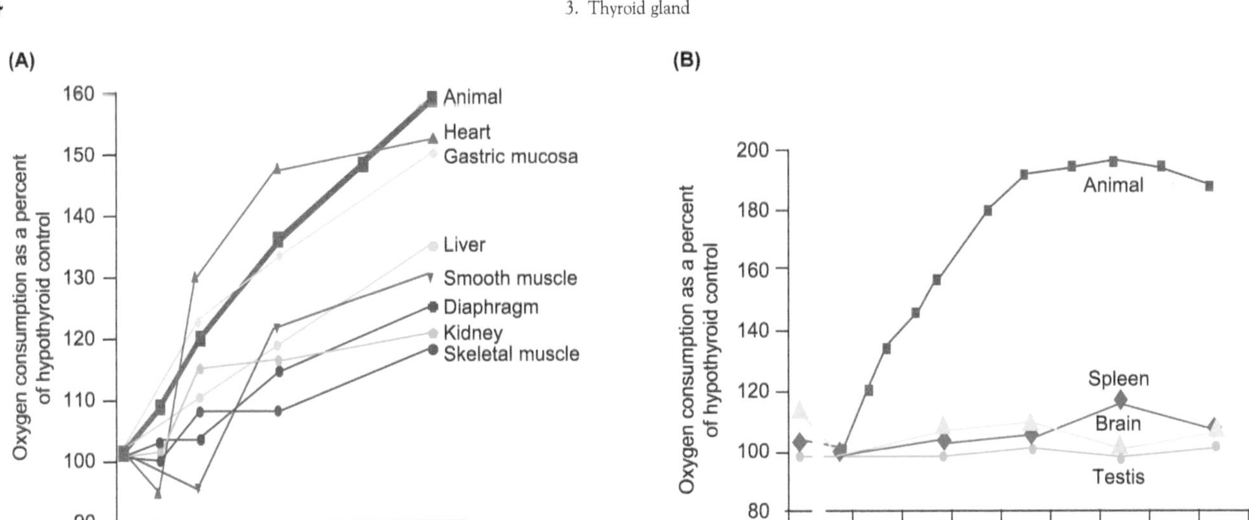

FIGURE 3.15 Effects of thyroxine on oxygen consumption by various tissues of thyroidectomized rats. Note that in (A) the abscissa is in units of hours and in (B) the units are days. Source: *Redrawn from Barker, S. B., & Klitgaard, H. M. (1952). Metabolism of tissues excised from thyroxine-injected rats.* American Journal of Physiology, 170, 81.

Oxygen consumption ultimately reflects the activity of mitochondria and is coupled with the formation of high-energy bonds in ATP. In general, oxygen consumption is proportional to energy utilization, but conversion of energy stored in metabolic fuels to the formation of ATP is not perfect, and some energy is lost as heat. Thus oxygen consumption and heat production are intimately related, and the effects of thyroid hormones on oxygen consumption seem to be byproducts of their essential role in calorigenesis. Although thyroid hormones have many functions in all vertebrates, their effects on oxygen consumption are seen only in those animals, birds, and mammals that maintain a constant body temperature (homeotherms). It is therefore not surprising that one of the classic signs of hypothyroidism is decreased tolerance to cold, whereas excessive heat production and sweating are seen in hyperthyroidism. Thyroid hormones increase oxygen consumption and heat production by increasing the rate of ATP breakdown and decreasing the efficiency of ATP synthesis.

Among the ATP-consuming processes that T_3 appears to accelerate are the maintenance of cellular ionic gradients. The sodium/potassium ATPase maintains ionic integrity of all cells and has been estimated to account for as much as 20% of total resting oxygen consumption, and the pumping of calcium from cytosol to the sarcoplasmic reticulum by calcium ATPases accounts for even more. Although most of the activity of the sodium/potassium ATPase resides in brain and kidney, the rates of metabolism of which are minimally increased by T_3, thyroid hormones are thought to promote entry of sodium into other cells and therefore increase the work of the sodium/potassium ATPase. Both the expression and activity of the sodium/potassium ATPase are decreased in hypothyroid and increased in hyperthyroid subjects. Similar changes are seen in calcium uptake and release from the sarcoplasmic reticulum in both resting and working skeletal muscle. These changes in calcium dynamics may account for the stiffness and delayed relaxation phase of reflexes seen in hypothyroid individuals. In addition, ATP-consuming cycles that are intrinsic components of carbohydrate, lipid, and protein metabolism are accelerated by thyroid hormones and contribute to the increase in oxygen consumption.

Thyroid hormones decrease the efficiency of ATP formation. Phosphorylation of ADP to form ATP is driven by the energy of the proton gradient that is generated across the inner mitochondrial membrane by the electron transport system. When ATP production is coupled optimally to oxygen consumption, 1.5–2.5 molecules of ATP are formed for each molecule of oxygen consumed. Leakage of protons across the inner mitochondrial membrane partially dissipates the gradient and results in fewer high-energy phosphate bonds formed for each atom of oxygen converted to water. Energy that would otherwise be stored in phosphate bonds is dissipated as heat. Leakage of protons is increased by uncoupling proteins (UCP) in the inner mitochondrial membrane. To date, three proteins thought to have uncoupling activity have been identified in mitochondrial membranes of various tissues. All three appear to be upregulated by T_3. Although the physiological importance of UCP-1 is firmly established (see later), the physiological roles of UCP-2 and UCP-3 remain uncertain.

The calorigenic effects of thyroid hormones are essential for maintaining constancy of body temperature. Upon exposure to a cold environment, heat production is increased through at least two mechanisms: (1) shivering, which is a rapid increase in involuntary activity of skeletal muscle and (2) the so-called nonshivering thermogenesis seen in cold acclimated individuals. As we have seen, the metabolic effects of T_3 have a long lag time and hence increased production of T_3 cannot be of much use for making rapid adjustments to cold temperatures. The role of T_3 in the shivering response is probably limited to maintenance of tissue sensitivity to sympathetic stimulation. In this context, the importance of T_3 derives from actions that were established before exposure to cold temperature. Maintenance of sensitivity to sympathetic stimulation permits efficient mobilization of stored carbohydrate and fat needed to fuel the shivering response and to make circulatory adjustments for increased activity of skeletal muscle. It may also be recalled that the sympathetic nervous system regulates heat conservation by decreasing blood flow through the skin. Piloerection in animals increases the thickness of the insulating layer of fur. These responses are important defenses in both acute and chronic exposure to cold.

Chronic nonshivering thermogenesis appears to require increased production of T_3, which acts in concert with the sympathetic nervous system to increase heat production and conservation. In humans and large animals, thyroid hormone dependency increases in the activity of ion pumps in muscle and provides the major source of increased heat production. Brown fat is an important source of heat in newborn humans and throughout life in small mammals. This form of adipose tissue is especially rich in mitochondria, which give it its unique brown color. Mitochondria in this tissue contain UCP-1, sometimes called thermogenin, which allows them to oxidize relatively large amounts of fatty acids and produce heat. Although both T_3 and the sympathetic neurotransmitter, norepinephrine, can upregulate expression of UCP-1, their cooperative interaction results in production of three to four times as much of this mitochondrial protein as the sum of their independent actions. In addition, T_3 increases the efficacy of norepinephrine to release fatty acids from stored triglycerides and thus provides fuel for heat production. Brown adipose tissue also upregulates type II deiodinase in response to sympathetic stimulation and produces abundant T_3 locally to meet its needs.

In rodents and other experimental animals, exposure to cold temperatures is an important stimulus for increased TSH secretion from the pituitary and the resultant increase in T_4 and T_3 secretion from the thyroid gland. Cold exposure does not increase TSH section in humans except in the newborn. In humans and experimental animals, however, exposure to cold temperatures increases the abundance of the type II deiodinase in skeletal muscle as well as brown fat. Consequently, the requirement for increased amounts of T_3 to satisfy demands imposed by the external environment is met by accelerated conversion of T_4 to T_3. Increased production of the type II deiodinase probably results from increased sympathetic nervous activity, which leads to increased cyclic AMP production in various tissues.

Carbohydrate metabolism

T_3 accelerates virtually all aspects of metabolism, including carbohydrate utilization. It increases glucose absorption from the digestive tract, glycogenolysis and gluconeogenesisin hepatocytes, and glucose oxidation in liver, fat, and muscle cells. No single or unique reaction in any pathway of carbohydrate metabolism has been identified as the rate-determining target of T_3 action. Rather, carbohydrate degradation appears to be driven by other factors, such as increased demand for ATP, the content of carbohydrate in the diet, or the nutritional state. Although T_3 may induce the synthesis of specific enzymes of carbohydrate and lipid metabolism (e.g., the malic enzyme, glucose 6-phosphate dehydrogenase, and 6-phosphogluconate dehydrogenase), it appears principally to behave as an amplifier working in conjunction with other signals (Fig. 3.16).

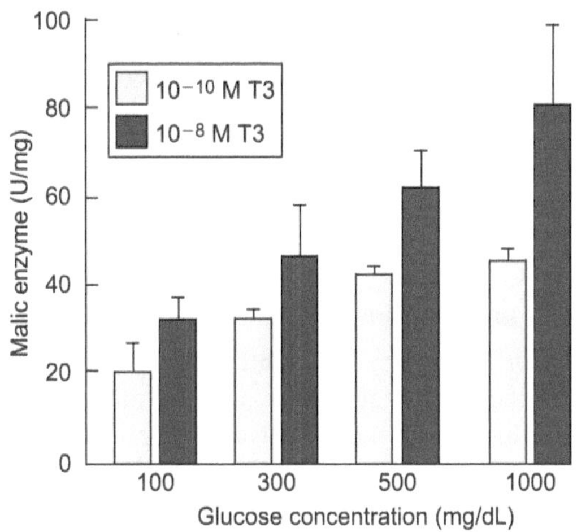

FIGURE 3.16 Effects of glucose and T3 on the induction of ME in isolated hepatocyte cultures. Note that the amount of enzyme present in tissues was increased by growing cells in higher and higher concentrations of glucose. Blue bars show effects of glucose in the presence of a low (10^{-10} M) concentration of T3. Red bars indicate that the effects of glucose that were exaggerated when cells were grown in a high concentration of T3 (10^{-8} M). *ME*, Malic enzyme. Source: *From Mariash, G. N., & Oppenheimer, J. H. (1982). Thyroid hormone-carbohydrate interaction at the hepatic nuclear level.* Federation Proceedings, 41, 2674.

In the example shown, induction of the malic enzyme in hepatocytes was dependent both on the concentration of glucose in the culture medium and on the concentration of T_3. T_3 had little effect on enzyme induction when there was no glucose but amplified the effectiveness of glucose as an inducer of genetic expression. This experiment provides a good example of how T_3 can amplify readout of genetic information.

Lipid metabolism

Because glucose is the major precursor for fatty acid synthesis in both liver and fat cells, it should not be surprising that optimal amounts of thyroid hormone are necessary for lipogenesis in these cells. Once again, the primary determinant of lipogenesis is not T_3, but rather, the amount of available carbohydrate or insulin (see Chapter 7: The Pancreatic Islets), with thyroid hormone acting as a gain control. Similarly, mobilization of fatty acids from storage depots in adipocytes is compromised in the thyroid-deficient subject and increased above normal when thyroid hormones are present in excess. Once again, T_3 amplifies physiological signals for fat mobilization without itself acting as such a signal.

Increased blood cholesterol (hypercholesterolemia), mainly in the form of low-density lipoproteins (LDL), typically is found in hypothyroidism. Thyroid hormones reduce cholesterol in the plasma of normal subjects and restore blood concentrations of cholesterol to normal in hypothyroid subjects. Hypercholesterolemia in hypothyroid subjects results from decreased ability to excrete cholesterol in bile rather than from overproduction of cholesterol. In fact, cholesterol synthesis is impaired in the hypothyroid individual. T_3 may facilitate hepatic excretion of cholesterol by increasing the abundance of LDL receptors in hepatocyte membranes, thereby enhancing uptake of cholesterol from the blood.

Nitrogen metabolism

Body proteins are constantly being degraded and resynthesized. Both synthesis and degradation of protein are slowed in the absence of thyroid hormones, and, conversely, both are accelerated by thyroid hormones. In the presence of excess T_4 or T_3 the effects of degradation predominate, and often there is severe catabolism of muscle. In hyperthyroid subjects, body protein mass decreases despite increased appetite and ingestion of dietary proteins. With thyroid deficiency, there is a characteristic accumulation of a mucus-like material consisting of protein complexed with hyaluronic acid and chondroitin sulfate in extracellular spaces, particularly in the skin. Because of its osmotic effect, this material causes water to accumulate in these spaces, giving rise to the edema typically seen in hypothyroid individuals and to the name myxedema for hypothyroidism.

Regulation of thyroid hormone secretion

As already indicated, secretion of thyroid hormones depends on the stimulation of thyroid follicular cells by TSH, which bears primary responsibility for integrating thyroid function with bodily needs (see Chapter 2: Pituitary Gland). In the absence of TSH, thyroid cells are quiescent and atrophy, and as we have seen, administration of TSH increases both synthesis and secretion of T_4 and T_3. Patients who lack functional TSH receptors present at birth with severe hypothyroidism accompanied by virtual absence of a functional thyroid gland, and high circulating levels of TSH. Secretion of TSH by the pituitary gland is governed by positive input from the hypothalamus by way of thyrotropin-releasing hormone (TRH) and negative input from the thyroid gland by way of T_3 and T_4. TRH increases expression of the genes for both the α- and β-subunits of TSH and also increases the posttranslational incorporation of carbohydrate that is required for normal potency of TSH. However, dependence of the thyrotropes on TRH in not complete, as these processes can go on at a reduced level in the absence of TRH. Disruption of the TRH gene reduces the TSH content of mouse pituitaries to less than half that of wild-type litter mate controls. Blood levels of thyroid hormones and TSH were just below the normal range in a rare case of a child with a genetic absence of TRH receptors. Growth was somewhat delayed, but hypothyroidism was otherwise mild. Similarly, blood levels of thyroid hormones are below normal in mice lacking a functional TRH gene, but they grow, develop, and reproduce almost normally.

Maintaining constant levels of thyroid hormones in blood depends upon negative feedback effects of T_4 and T_3, which inhibit the synthesis and secretion of TSH (Fig. 3.17).

The contribution of free T_4 in blood is quite significant in this regard. Because thyrotropes are rich in type II deiodinase, they can convert this more abundant form of thyroid hormone to T_3 and thereby monitor the overall amount of free hormone in blood. High concentrations of thyroid hormones may shut off TSH secretion completely and, when maintained over time, produce atrophy of the thyroid gland. Measurement of relative concentrations of TSH and thyroid hormones in the blood provides important information for diagnosing thyroid disease. For instance, low blood concentrations of free T_3 and T_4 in the presence of elevated levels of TSH signal a primary defect in the thyroid gland, while high concentrations of free T_3 and

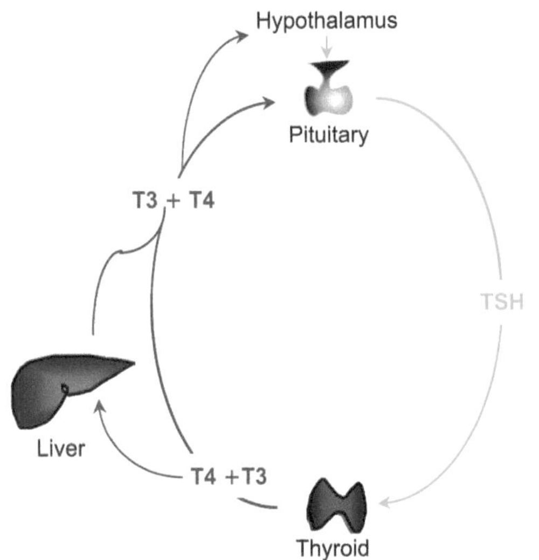

FIGURE 3.17 Feedback regulation of thyroid hormone secretion. Green arrow, stimulation; red arrow, inhibition.

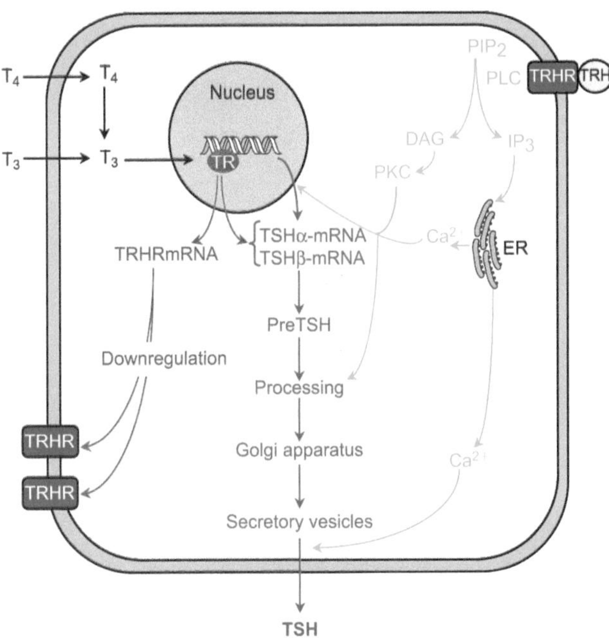

FIGURE 3.18 Effects of TRH, T3, and T4 on the thyrotrope. T3 downregulates expression of genes for TRHR and both subunits of TSH (*red arrows*). TRH effects (shown in green) include upregulation of TSH gene expression, enhanced TSH glycosylation, and accelerated secretion. *TR*, Thyroid hormone receptor; *TRH*, thyrotropin-releasing hormone; *TRHR*, TRH receptors; *TSH*, thyroid-stimulating hormone.

T_4 accompanied by high concentrations of TSH reflect a defect in the pituitary or hypothalamus. As already noted, the high concentrations of T_4 and T_3 seen in Graves disease are accompanied by very low concentrations of TSH in blood because of negative feedback inhibition of TSH secretion.

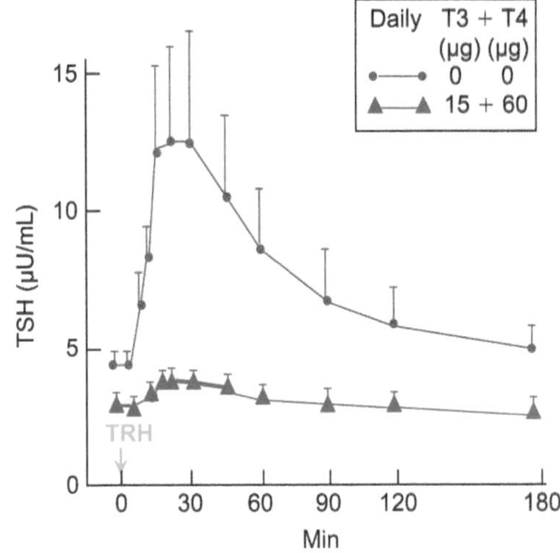

FIGURE 3.19 Effect of treatment of normal young men with thyroid hormones for 3–4 weeks on the response of the pituitary to TRH as measured by changes in plasma concentrations of TSH. The six subjects received 25 mg of TRH at time 0 as indicated by the green arrow. Values are expressed as means ± SEM. *TRH*, Thyrotropin-releasing hormone; *TSH*, thyroid-stimulating hormone. Source: *From Snyder, P. J., & Utiger, R. D. (1972). Inhibition of thyrotropin response to thyrotropin-releasing hormone by small quantities of thyroid hormones.* Journal of Clinical Investigation, 52, 2077.

Negative feedback inhibition of TSH secretion results from actions of thyroid hormones exerted both on TRH neurons in the paraventricular nuclei of the hypothalamus and on thyrotropes in the pituitary. Results of animal studies indicate that T_3 and T_4 inhibit TRH synthesis and secretion. Events thought to occur within the thyrotropes are illustrated in Fig. 3.18.

TRH binds its G-protein-coupled receptors (see Chapter 1: Introduction) on the surface of thyrotropes. The resulting activation of phospholipase C generates the second messengers inositol trisphosphate (IP3) and diacylglycerol (DAG). IP3 promotes calcium mobilization, and DAG activates protein kinase C, both of which rapidly stimulate the release of stored hormone. This effect is augmented by the influx of extracellular calcium following the activation of membrane calcium channels. In addition, transcription of genes for both subunits of TSH is increased. TRH also promotes processing of the carbohydrate components of TSH necessary for maximum biological activity. Meanwhile, both T_4 and T_3 are transported into thyrotropes at rates determined by their free concentrations in blood plasma. T_4 is deiodinated to T_3 in the cytoplasm by the abundant type II deiodinase. T_3 enters the nucleus, binds to its receptors, and downregulates transcription of the genes for both the α- and β-subunits of TSH and for TRH receptors. In addition, T_3 inhibits the release of stored hormone and accelerates TRH receptor degradation. The net consequence of these actions of T_3 is a reduction in the sensitivity of the thyrotropes to TRH (Fig. 3.19).

Mechanism of thyroid hormone action

As must already be obvious, virtually all cells appear to require optimal amounts of thyroid hormone for normal operation, even though different aspects of function may be affected in different cells. T_3 formed by deiodination of T_4 within target cells mixes freely with T_3 taken up from the plasma and enters the nucleus where it binds to its receptors (see Chapter 1: Introduction). Thyroid hormone receptors are members of the nuclear receptor superfamily of transcription factors and bind T_3 about 10 times more avidly than T_4. They contain about 400 amino acids arranged into regions or domains involved in ligand binding, dimerization with other receptors, DNA binding, and protein–protein interactions with coactivator or corepressor complexes (see Chapter 1: Introduction).

The biology of thyroid hormone receptors is complex and incompletely understood, and much of what is known has been learned from genetically manipulated mice. Thyroid hormone receptors are encoded in two genes, designated TRα and TRβ. The TRα gene resides on chromosome 17 in humans and gives rise to two isoforms, $TR\alpha_1$ and $TR\alpha_2$. Alternate RNA splicing deletes the T_3-binding site from the TRα2 isoform so that it cannot act as a hormone receptor but nevertheless plays a vital physiological role (see later).

Two additional truncated isoforms of the TRα gene, Δα1 and Δα2, arise by transcription from a downstream promoter and lack both DNA- and ligand-binding domains. Their physiological role is uncertain, but they may act as inhibitors of TRα1. The human TRβ gene maps to chromosome 3 and gives rise to two isoforms, TRβ1 and TRβ2, by alternate splicing, and both contain the hormone-binding site. TRα1 and TRβ1 are distributed widely throughout the body and are present in different ratios in the nuclei of all target tissues examined, but TRβ2 appears to be expressed primarily in the anterior pituitary gland and the brain.

Unlike most other nuclear receptors, thyroid hormone receptors bind to specific nucleotide sequences (thyroid response elements or TREs) in the genes they regulate whether or not the hormone is present. They may bind as monomers, but more typically as homodimers composed of two thyroid hormone receptors or as heterodimers formed with the receptor for an isomer of retinoic acid receptor or other nuclear receptor family members. In the absence of T_3, the unoccupied receptor, in conjunction with a corepressor protein complex, inhibits T_3-dependent gene expression by maintaining the DNA in a tightly coiled configuration that bars access of transcription activators or RNA polymerase. Upon binding T_3 the configuration of the receptor is modified in a way that causes it to release the corepressor and bind instead to a coactivator (Fig. 3.20).

Although T_3 acts in an analogous way to suppress expression of some genes, the underlying mechanism for negative control of gene expression is not understood.

The question of which T_3 responses are mediated by each form of the T_3 receptor has been addressed by examining the consequences of disrupting all or parts of the THRα or β genes in mouse embryos. Mice that lack both TRβ isoforms are fertile, exhibit no obvious behavioral abnormalities, and have minimal developmental deficiencies except for retinal and cochlear development. However, these animals have abnormally high concentrations of TSH, T_4, and T_3 in their blood presumably because TRβ2 mediates the negative feedback action of T_3. These symptoms are remarkably similar to those seen in a rare genetic disease that is characterized by resistance to thyroid hormone. Like

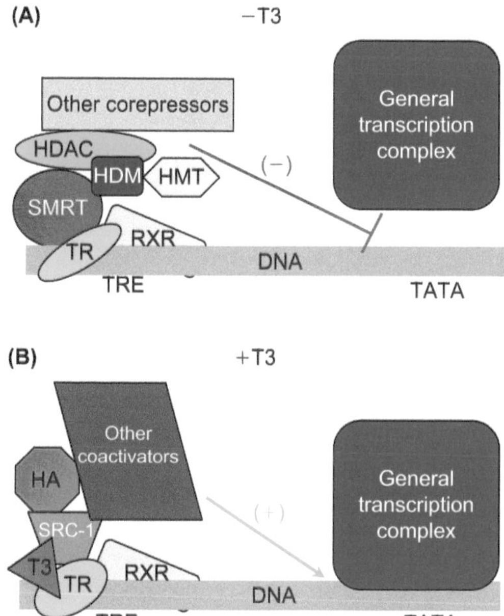

FIGURE 3.20 Models of the effects of *TR* on gene transcription. (A) In the absence of T3 the TR in heterodimeric union with the *RXR* binds to the thyroid hormone response element (*TRE*) in DNA. The unliganded TR also binds to a corepressor, in this case the *SMRT*, which recruits factors that remodel chromatin such as *HDAC*, *HDM*, *HMT*, and other factors that interfere with attachment of the RNA polymerase in the general transcription complex to the TATA box in the promoter of a thyroid hormone regulated gene. (B) Upon binding *T3* the *TR* changes its conformation, sheds the corepressor complex, and replaces it with a coactivator, in this case *SRC-1*, which recruits such chromatin remodeling factors as *HA* and other coactivators that make the gene accessible to the polymerase complex. *HA*, Histone acetylase; *HDAC*, histone deacetylase; *HDM*, histone demethylase; *HMT*, histone methyl transferase; *RXR*, retinoic acid receptor; *SMRT*, silencing mediator retinoic acid and TR; *SRC-1*, steroid receptor coactivator-1; *TR*, thyroid hormone receptor.

the knockout mice, patients with this disease exhibit few abnormalities but have increased circulating levels of TSH, T_4, and T_3. Their thyroid glands are enlarged (goiter) in response to the high TSH levels, but they typically suffer few of the consequences of T_4 hypersecretion, other than tachycardia. This disease typically results from mutations in the TRβ gene.

Manipulation of the gene for TRα so that only the α2 isoform can be expressed produced no deleterious effects on lifespan or fertility even though this isoform cannot bind T_3. However, lack of the TRα1 isoform in these mice resulted in low heart rate and low body temperature. When the TRα gene was knocked out so that neither the α1 nor the α2 isoform could be expressed, the animals stopped growing after about 2 weeks and died shortly after weaning with apparent failure of intestinal development. Although relatively few symptoms of hypothyroidism result from knockout of any of the three TR receptors that are capable of binding T_3, loss of the α2 isoform produced devastating effects, suggesting that products of the TRα gene play critical, though perhaps T_3-independent, roles in gene transcription and development.

It is possible that the α and β forms of the receptors regulate different complements of genes as suggested in the mouse studies, but the observed effects may simply reflect differences in distribution of the α and β thyroid hormone receptors in the various affected cell types. The combined absence of TRα1, TRβ1, and TRβ2 produces more pronounced symptoms of hypothyroidism than lack of either TRα1 or the TRβ isoforms, suggesting that these receptors have redundant or overlapping functions. However, the hypothyroid symptoms are mild compared to those seen when the complement of TRs is normal but thyroid hormones are absent. These and related observations in genetically manipulated cultured cells gave rise to the idea that unoccupied thyroid hormone receptors may repress gene expression and therefore produce harmful effects. Thus at least one of the physiological roles of T_3 may be to counteract the consequences of the silencing of some genes by unoccupied thyroid hormone receptors.

Although extensive evidence indicates that T_3 and T_4 produce most of their actions through nuclear receptors, it is likely that these receptors do not mediate all the actions of thyroid hormones. Extranuclear specific binding proteins for thyroid hormones have been found in the cytosol and mitochondria, although the functions, if any, of these proteins are not known. In addition, some rapid effects of T_3 and T_4 that may not involve the genome also have been described. It is highly likely that T_3 and T_4 have physiologically important actions that are not dependent on nuclear events, but detailed understanding will require further research. Thyroid hormones are critical factors in both prenatal and antenatal development and participate in a wide range of homeostatic processes, perhaps playing different roles at different stages of development. It should not be surprising therefore that multiple mechanisms are employed in expressing all the actions of these hormones or in the conclusion that much remains to be learned in this regard.

Summary

The butterfly-shaped gland lying just below the larynx is discussed from its embryological origins just below the tongue to its unique anatomical structure and physiological activity. Its secretory cells surround a cauldron of amorphous substance called colloid. Into this colloid the cells secrete a large protein from which ultimately will come the active hormone triiodothyronine and a storage form of this hormone, thyroxine. The transport and effect of triiodothyronine concludes this chapter.

Suggested readings

Advanced information

De la Vieja, A., & Santisteban, P. (2018). Role of iodide metabolism in physiology and cancer. *Endocrine-Related Cancer, 25*(4), R225–R245. Available from https://doi.org/10.1530/erc-17-0515.

Salvatore, D., Davies, T. F., Schlumberger, M.-J., Hay, I. D., & Larsen, P. R. (2016). Thyroid Physiology and Diagnostic Evaluation of Patients With Thyroid Disorders. In S. Melmed, K. S. Polonsky, P. R Larsen, & H. M. Kronenberg (Eds.), *Williams textbook of endocrinology* (pp. 334–368). Philadelphia, PA: Elsevier Inc.

Li, M., & Sirko, S. (2018). Traumatic brain injury: At the crossroads of neuropathology and common metabolic endocrinopathies. *Journal of Clinical Medicine, 7*(3), 59.

Mallya, M., & Ogilvy-Stuart, A. L. (2018). Thyrotropic hormones. *Best Practice & Research Clinical Endocrinology & Metabolism, 32*(1), 17–25. Available from https://doi.org/10.1016/j.beem.2017.10.006.

O'Kane, S. M., Mulhern, M. S., Pourshahidi, L. K., Strain, J. J., & Yeates, A. J. (2018). Micronutrients, iodine status and concentrations of thyroid hormones: A systematic review. *Nutrition Reviews*. Available from https://doi.org/10.1093/nutrit/nuy008, nuy008-nuy008.

Parmentier, T., & Sienaert, P. (2018). The use of triiodothyronine (T_3) in the treatment of bipolar depression: A review of the literature. *Journal of Affective Disorders, 229*, 410–414. Available from https://doi.org/10.1016/j.jad.2017.12.071.

Sinha, R. A., Singh, B. K., & Yen, P. M. (2018). Direct effects of thyroid hormones on hepatic lipid metabolism. *Nature Reviews Endocrinology, 14*, 259. Available from https://doi.org/10.1038/nrendo.2018.10.

Velasco, I., Bath, S., & Rayman, M. (2018). Iodine as essential nutrient during the first 1000 days of life. *Nutrients, 10*(3), 290.

CHAPTER

4

The adrenal glands

Case study

Cushing syndrome

He was referred to the endocrinology clinic. He was 55 and had truncal obesity, was hypertensive and hypokalemic and rather sleepy much of the time. His thyroid was normal so that was not the cause of his sleepiness. He had a round and flushed (florid) face. A presumptive diagnosis of Cushing syndrome had been made by his family physician.

In the clinic, a physical exam showed numerous large striae (up to 25 mm in width) on the abdomen similar to that seen in Fig. 4.1 as well as on the shoulder, back, and the back of his legs. He had a buffalo hump of fat on his neck. His arms and legs were thin when compared to his trunk. His bp was 180/95. He had a history of heavy smoking and did not drink excessively. He had a rasping voice and a smoker's dry cough.

A cortisol-to-creatinine ratio test on the first urine to be voided in the morning was done, this ratio confirmed that he had Cushing syndrome. An abdominal CT scan did not reveal any adrenal adenoma, but the adrenals were nodular and hyperplastic (Figs. 4.2–4.4).

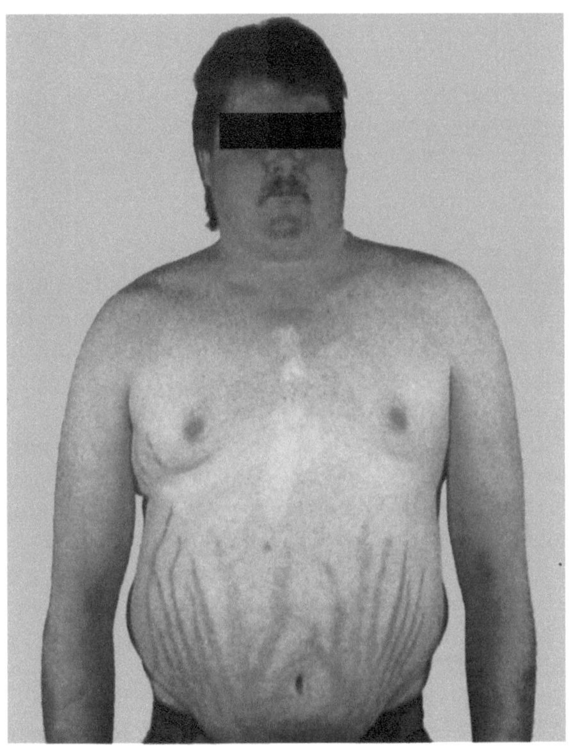

FIGURE 4.1 Cushing disease showing the florid moon face, truncal obesity but wasting away of the muscles of the arms. Note the large striae on the abdominal and chest. The old chest scar indicates previous cardiothoracic surgery (cause not stated in the caption). Source: *From Figure 24-44 in Maitra, A. (2015). The endocrine system, Chapter 24. In V. Kumar, A. K. Abbas, & J. C. Aster (Eds.),* Robbins and Cotran pathologic basis of disease *(9th ed., p. 1125). Elsevier.*

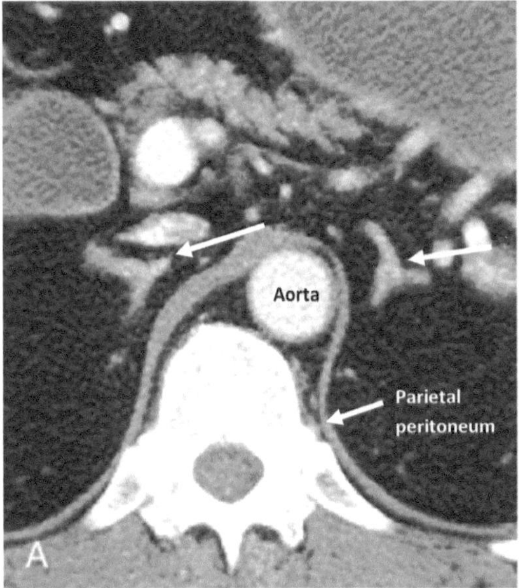

FIGURE 4.2 CT of normal adrenal glands (arrows) have the characteristic Y shape. Source: *From Figure 53-1 in Ho, L. M. (2017). Adrenal glands, Chapter 53. In J. R. Haaga & D. T. Boll (Eds.), CT and MRI of the whole body (6th ed., p. 1761). Elsevier.*

DOI: https://doi.org/10.1016/B978-0-12-815844-9.00004-X

(cont'd)

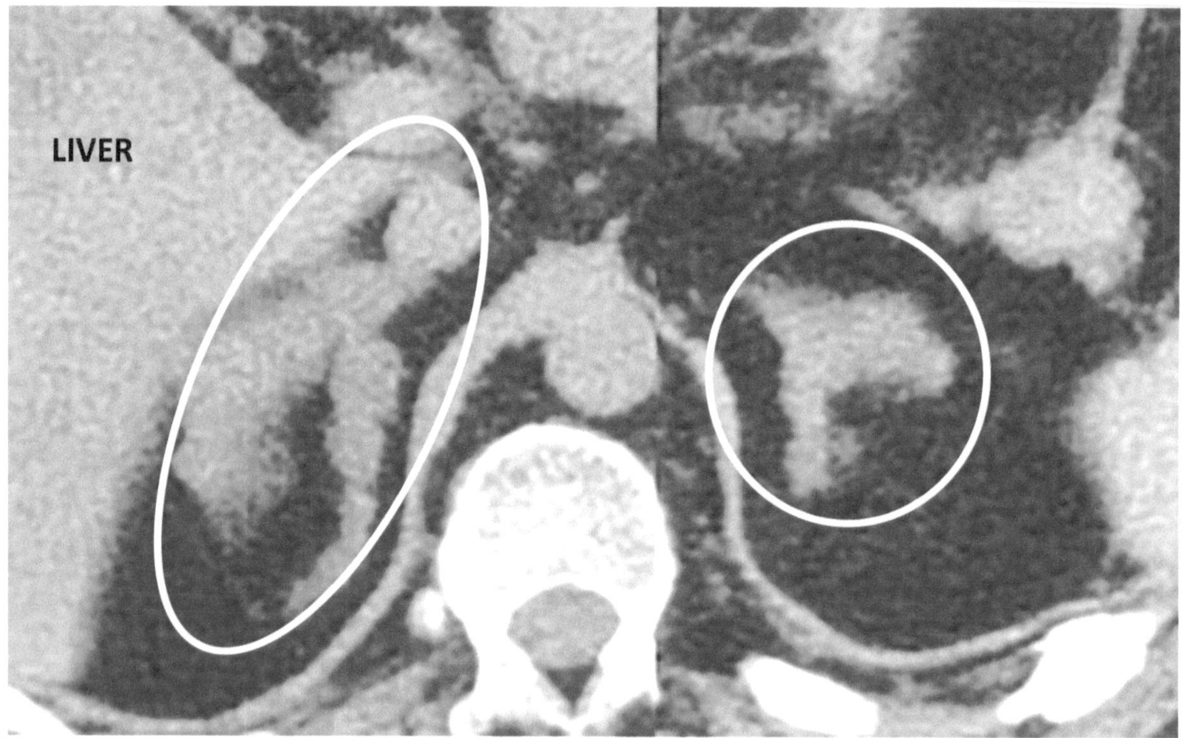

FIGURE 4.3 CT of nodular adrenal hyperplasia (circles) characteristic of that due to ACTH overstimulation. The "Y" shape is enlarged and distorted. The right is larger than the left. *ACTH*, Adrenocorticotropic hormone. Source: *From Figure 53-11 in Ho, L. M. (2017). Adrenal glands, Chapter 53. In J. R. Haaga & D. T. Boll (Eds.), CT and MRI of the whole body (6th ed., p. 1767). Elsevier.*

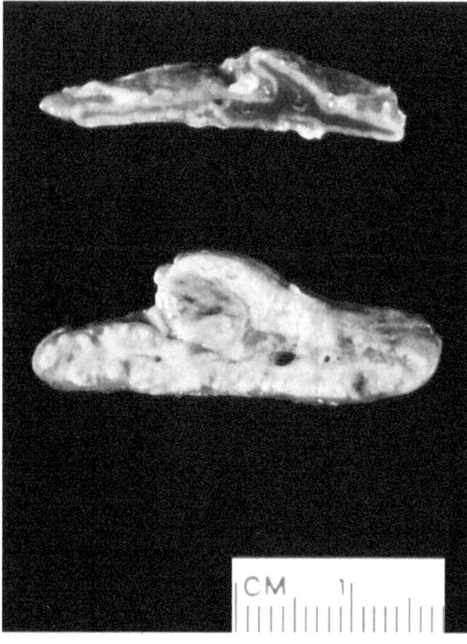

FIGURE 4.4 Adrenal nodular hyperplasia (bottom) compared to a normal adrenal (top). Source: *From Figure 24-42 in Maitra, A. (2015). The endocrine system, Chapter 24. In V. Kumar, A. K. Abbas, & J. C. Aster (Eds.),* Robbins and Cotran pathologic basis of disease *(9th ed., p. 1124). Elsevier.*

This usually implies that there is an external source that is stimulating the adrenal cortex, as tumors would show up as a mass. Blood levels of adrenocorticotropic hormone (ACTH) were very high which confirmed this hypothesis.

ACTH stimulates the adrenal cortex, and in most cases, this is due to a pituitary adenoma hypersecreting ACTH, so a head CT scan was done, but no tumor could be observed. A cannula was inserted by way of a cut down to the internal jugular and from there upstream to the hypophyseal veins (Fig. 2.7). The ACTH levels were below normal, so the pituitary was ruled out as the source of ACTH.

Since malignant neoplasms—especially small cell (oat cell) lung cancer—will produce hormones, and since he was a heavy smoker, a CT of his chest was done which revealed a tumor in the apex of the right lung similar to that seen in Figs. 4.5 and 4.6.

At surgery the superior lobe of the right lung was resected and chemotherapy initiated. A surgical biopsy was done on the resected tumor and immunohistochemistry revealed that the neoplasm was producing ACTH. Since he

(cont'd)

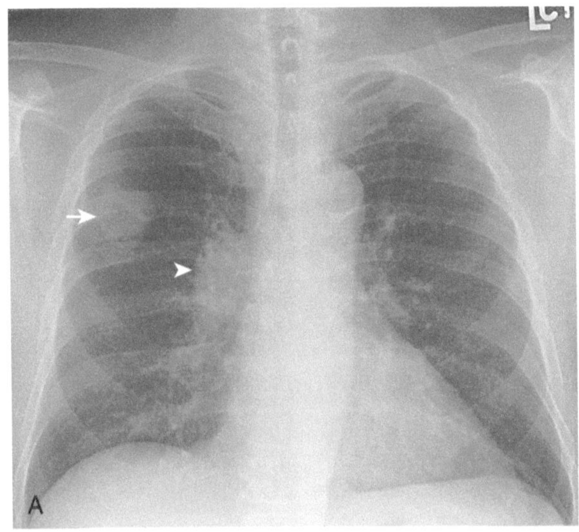

FIGURE 4.5 SCLC with disseminated metastases at presentation. Posteroanterior chest radiograph shows a lobular 3-cm right upper lobe nodule (arrow) and hilar adenopathy *(arrowhead)*. Source: *From Figure 37-31A in Erasmus, J. J., Rossi, S. E. (2017). Neoplastic disease of the lung, Chapter 37. In J. R. Haaga & D. T. Boll (Eds.),* CT and MRI of the whole body *(6th ed., p 1006). Elsevier.*

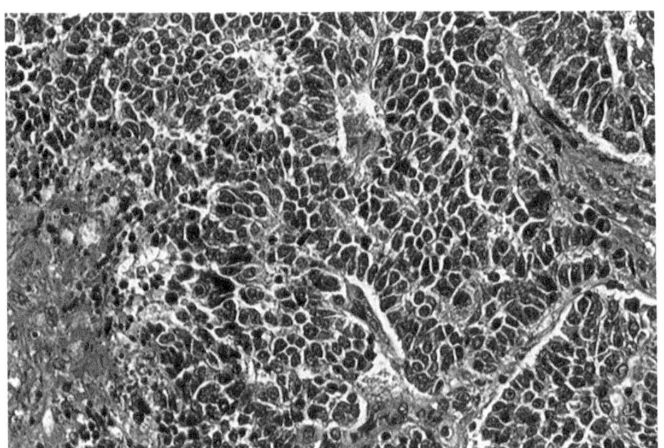

FIGURE 4.6 Small cell lung carcinoma under the microscope. The dark blue cells resemble rolled oats placed neatly in rows, hence the other name, oat cell carcinoma. Source: *From Figure 5-107 in Klatt, E. C. (Ed.) (2015).* Robbins and Cotran atlas of pathology *(3rd ed., p. 146). Elsevier.*

had little pituitary ACTH secretion, he was placed on glucocorticoid replacement therapy and weaned off gradually over the next several months to make certain he did not go into an adrenal crisis.

In the clinic

Cushing syndrome

Cushing syndrome is the most common adrenal disorder. In most cases, it is due to medications the patient is taking. Second to that, are pituitary adenomas as a cause. Third would be a malignancy in other parts of the body that are secreting ACTH. This is what happened to the patient in the case study.

Although all lung cancers can produce hormones, small cell lung carcinoma is most apt to do this, although usually the onset of the production of high levels of ACTH is sudden as small cell lung carcinomas are usually rapidly growing. Nonetheless, each malignancy is different and that was the case with the patient in the case study.

The effect of excessive ACTH production is an increase in glucocorticoid secretion from the zona fasciculata (Fig. 4.7), and not as many mineralocorticoids or androgens.

The secretion of ACTH by the pituitary is necessary for the secretion of cortisol by the adrenal cortex (Fig. 4.8).

The excessive glucocorticoid production has the effect on many different systems as shown in Fig. 4.9.

Signs and symptoms

Patients with Cushing syndrome may not complain until either headaches due to hypertension or some other symptoms bring them to a physician's office. There can also be a variety of other findings, including psychosis, peptic ulcers, muscular weakness, cardiac arrhythmias (due to hypokalemia), bone pain from osteoporosis, or it is due to a small cell lung carcinoma, metastasis to another organ causing secondary disturbances of function.

(cont'd)

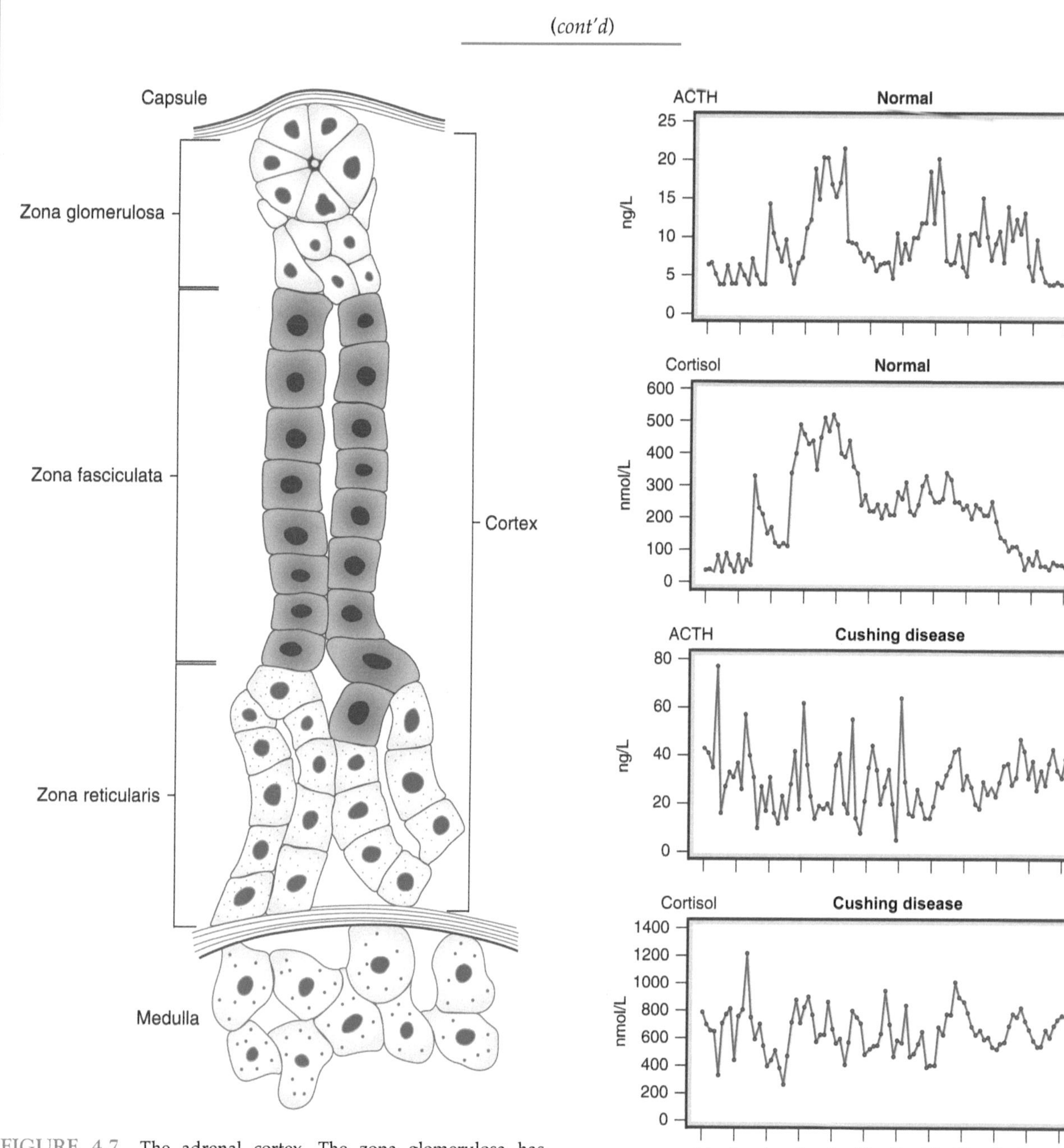

FIGURE 4.7 The adrenal cortex. The zona glomerulosa has many circular structures that reminded histologists of the glomerulus of the kidney, the zona fasciculata has many fascicles, or bundles, of rows of cells the zona reticularis refers to the network of cells. The zona glomerulosa secretes mineralocorticoids, the zona fasciculata secretes glucocorticoids, and the zona reticularis secretes androgens and a very small amount of estrogens. Source: *From Figure 15-2 in Stewart, P. M., & Newell-Price, J. C.C. (2016). The adrenal cortex, Chapter 15. In S. Melmed, K. S. Polonsky, P. R. Larsen, & H. M. Kronenberg (Eds.),* Williams textbook of endocrinology *(13th ed., p. 492). Elsevier.*

FIGURE 4.8 The normal secretion of ACTH is followed by an increase in secretion of cortisol. In Cushing disease, this diurnal pattern of ACTH secretion is not followed. *ACTH,* Adrenocorticotropic hormone. Source: *From Figure 15-8 in Stewart, P. M., & Newell-Price, J. C.C. (2016). The adrenal cortex, Chapter 15. In S. Melmed, K. S. Polonsky, P. R. Larsen, & H. M. Kronenberg (Eds.),* Williams textbook of endocrinology *(13th ed., p. 498). Elsevier.*

(cont'd)

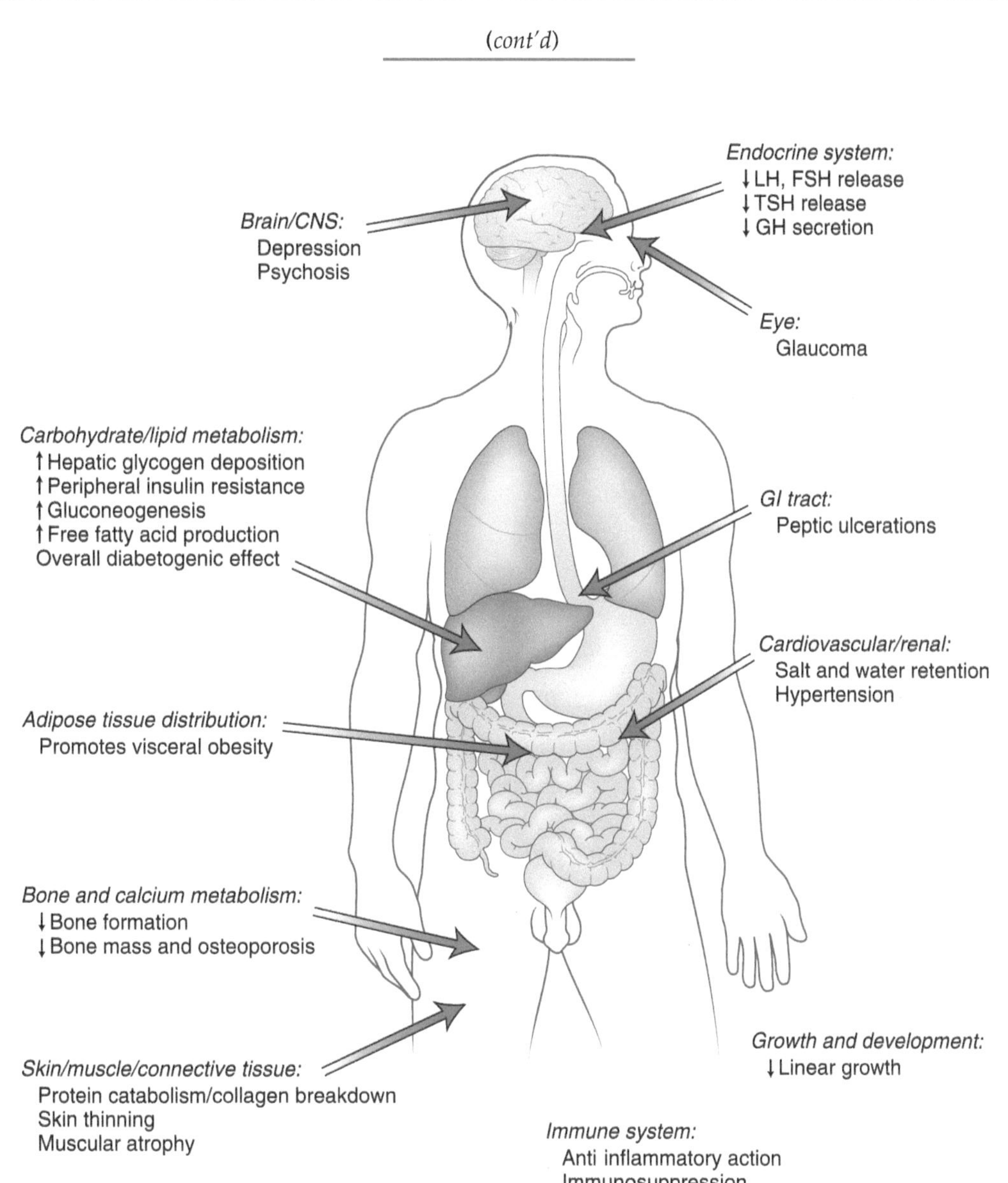

FIGURE 4.9 The effects of glucocorticoids on the major systems. The effects of excess cortisol are listed below each label. Source: *From Figure 15-13 in Stewart, P. M., & Newell-Price, J. C.C. (2016). The adrenal cortex, Chapter 15. In S. Melmed, K. S. Polonsky, P. R. Larsen, & H. M. Kronenberg (Eds.),* Williams textbook of endocrinology *(13th ed., p. 504). Elsevier.*

Diagnosis

Glucocorticoids are metabolized by the liver to more water-soluble compounds as shown in Fig. 4.10.

In addition, the kidney irreversibly metabolizes cortisol to cortisone. In past years, a 24-hour urine was collected to measure 17-hydroxycorticosteroids (17-OHCS) and 17-oxogenic (keto-) steroid excretion. But these tests are not very sensitive. Instead, they have been replaced with the urinary cortisol-to-creatinine ratio collected at the first voiding in the morning which can be done by the patient at home. In addition, a low dose of dexamethasone taken by the patient at home at 11 p.m. should suppress ACTH and, hence, cortisol production. This can be measured by collecting the urine at first voiding in the morning. In Cushing syndrome, there is no lowering of the cortisol and, if the cause is due to a tumor producing ACTH, neither will there be a drop in ACTH (Fig. 4.8). Another test that can be done by the patient is to collect saliva at midnight. Saliva contains cortisol that is not bound to cortisol-binding-globulin, on

(cont'd)

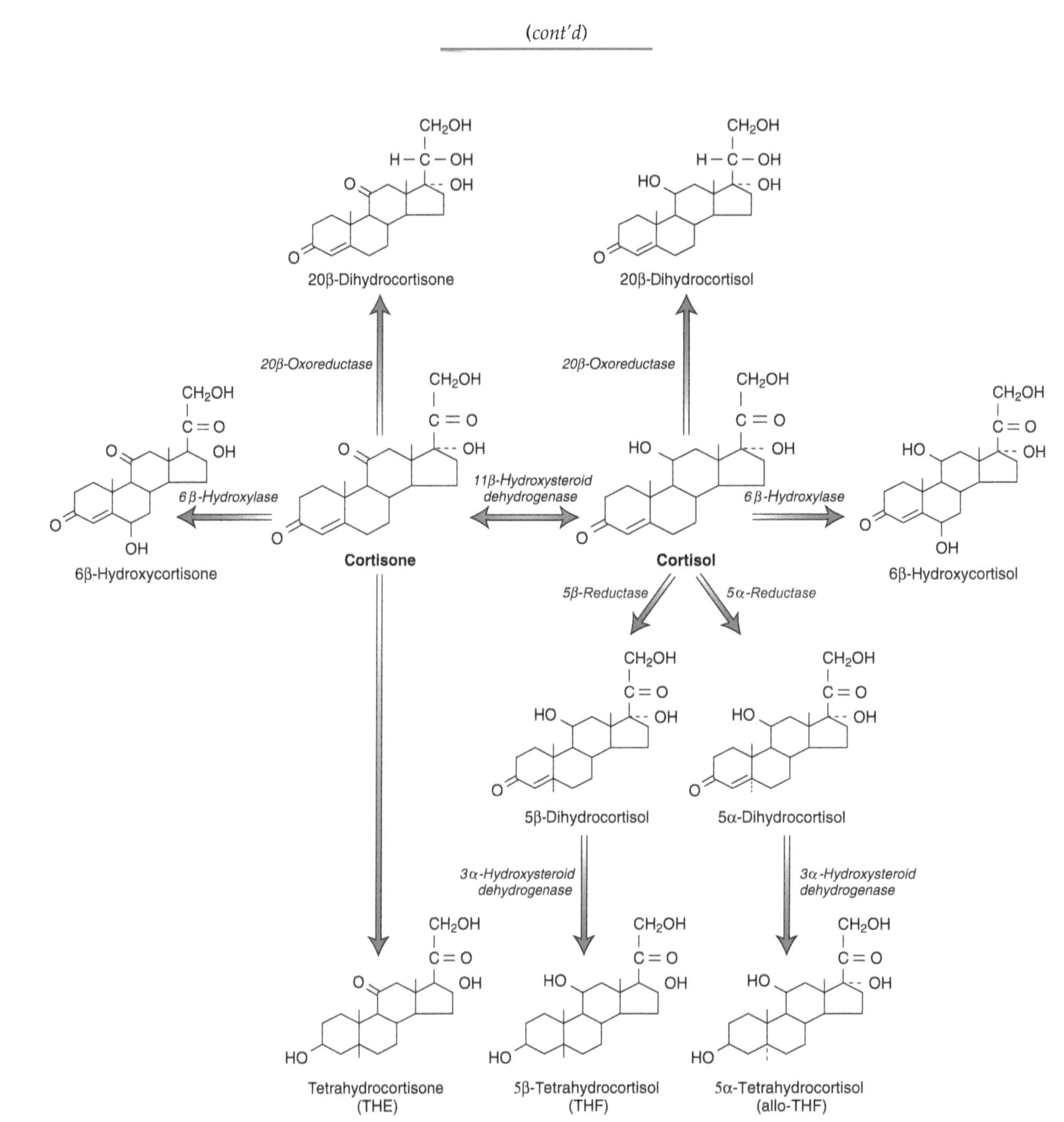

FIGURE 4.10 The metabolism of glucocorticoids by the liver. The kidney also metabolizes cortisol to cortisone in an irreversible process. Source: *From Figure 15-12 in Stewart, P. M., & Newell-Price, J. C.C. (2016). The adrenal cortex, Chapter 15. In S. Melmed, K. S. Polonsky, P. R. Larsen, & H. M. Kronenberg (Eds.),* Williams textbook of endocrinology *(13th ed., p. 502). Elsevier.*

Adrenal glands

(*cont'd*)

which cortisol is carried in the blood. Instead, salivary cortisol measures the free cortisol in plasma. This is the cortisol that gets into cells and is also excreted in saliva. The following algorithm can be used to determine Cushing syndrome (Fig. 4.11).

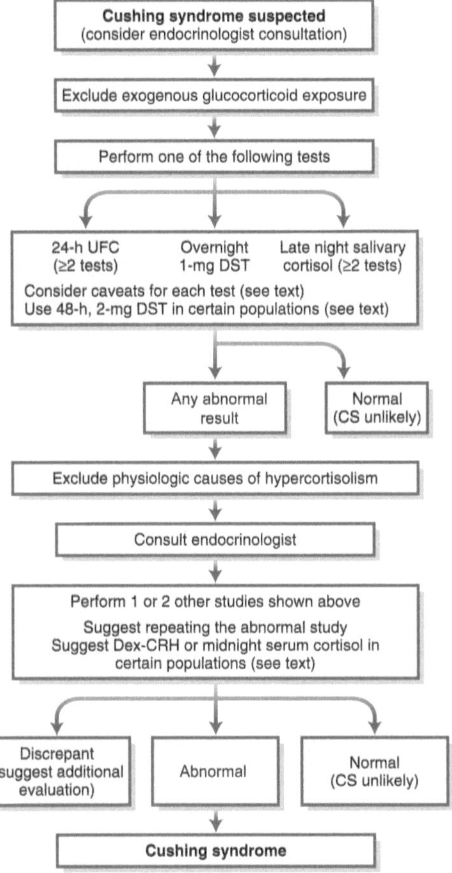

FIGURE 4.11 An algorithm for determining if a patient has CS. *CS*, Cushing syndrome. Source: *From Figure 15-20 in Stewart, P. M., & Newell-Price, J. C.C. (2016). The adrenal cortex, Chapter 15. In S. Melmed, K. S. Polonsky, P. R. Larsen, & H. M. Kronenberg (Eds.),* Williams textbook of endocrinology *(13th ed., p. 516). Elsevier.*

Management

The tumor that is secreting ACTH (or if it is a cortisol secreting tumor of the adrenal cortex) must be removed surgically or by chemotherapy. The following algorithm helps with the management (Fig. 4.12).

Prognosis

The prognosis depends on the nature of the tumor that caused Cushing syndrome. Small cell lung carcinoma has, overall, a very poor prognosis, whereas for pituitary or adrenal adenomas, once they are removed, the prognosis is very good for full recovery.

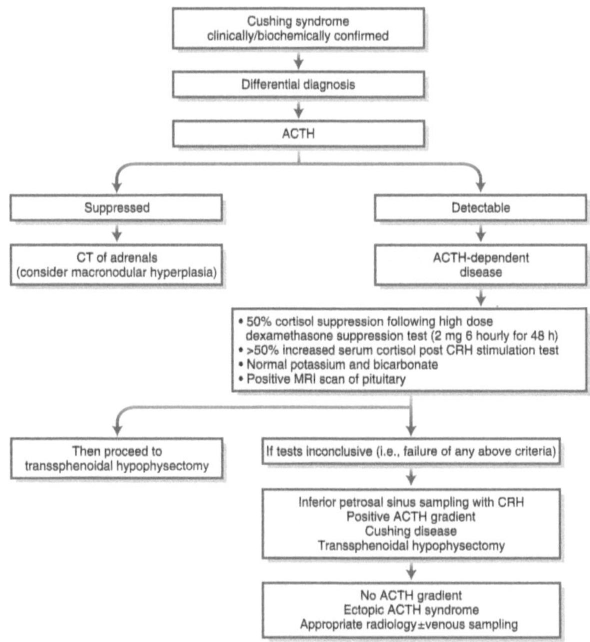

FIGURE 4.12 An algorithm for managing CS. *CS*, Cushing syndrome. Source: *From Figure 15-21 in Stewart, P. M., & Newell-Price, J. C.C. (2016). The adrenal cortex, Chapter 15. In S. Melmed, K. S. Polonsky, P. R. Larsen, & H. M. Kronenberg (Eds.),* Williams textbook of endocrinology *(13th ed., p. 517). Elsevier.*

The adrenal glands are complex polyfunctional structures whose secretions are required for maintenance of life. Without them, deranged electrolyte or carbohydrate metabolism leads to circulatory collapse or hypoglycemic coma and death. The hormones of the outer region, or cortex, are steroids and act at the level of the genome to regulate expression of genes that govern the operation of fundamental processes in virtually all cells. There are three major categories of adrenal steroid hormones: mineralocorticoids, whose actions regulate the body content of sodium and potassium; glucocorticoids, whose actions affect body fuel metabolism, responses to injury, and general cell function; and androgens, whose actions are similar to the hormone of the male gonad. We focus on actions of these hormones on those processes that are most thoroughly studied, but it should be kept in mind that adrenal cortical hormones directly or indirectly affect almost every physiological process and hence are central to the maintenance of homeostasis.

Secretion of mineralocorticoids is controlled primarily by the kidney through secretion of renin and the consequent production of angiotensin II. Secretion of glucocorticoids and androgens is controlled by the anterior pituitary gland through secretion of ACTH. The inner region, the adrenal medulla, is a component of the sympathetic nervous system and participates in the wide array of regulatory responses that are characteristic of that branch of the nervous system. The adrenal cortex and the medulla often behave as a functional unit and together confer a remarkable capacity to cope with changes in the internal or external environment. Fast-acting medullary hormones are signals for physiological adjustments, and slower-acting cortical hormones maintain or increase sensitivity of tissues to medullary hormones and other signals as well as maintain or enhance the capacity of tissues to respond to such signals. The cortical hormones thus tend to be modulators rather than initiators of responses.

Anatomy and histology

The adrenal (suprarenal) glands are bilateral structures situated above the kidneys (Fig. 4.13).

They comprised an outer region or cortex, which normally makes up more than three-quarters of the adrenal mass, and an inner region or medulla (Fig. 4.14).

The medulla is a modified sympathetic ganglion that, in response to signals reaching it through cholinergic, preganglionic fibers, releases either or both of its two hormones, epinephrine and norepinephrine, into adrenal venous blood. The cortex arises from mesodermal tissue and produces a class of lipid soluble hormones derived from cholesterol, called steroids. The cortex is subdivided histologically into three zones. Cells in the outer region, or zona glomerulosa, are arranged in clusters (glomeruli) and produce the hormone aldosterone. In the zona fasciculata, which comprises the bulk of the cortex, rows of lipid-laden cells are arranged radially in bundles of parallel cords (fasces). The inner region of the cortex consists of a tangled network of cells and is called the zona reticularis. The fasciculata and reticularis, which produce both cortisol and the adrenal androgens, are functionally separate from the zona glomerulosa.

The adrenal glands receive their blood supply from numerous small arteries that branch off the renal arteries or the lumbar portion of the aorta and its various major branches. These arteries penetrate the adrenal capsules and divide to form the subcapsular plexus from which small arterial branches pass centripetally toward the medulla. The subcapsular plexuses also give rise to long loops of capillaries that pass between the cords of fascicular cells and empty into sinusoids in the reticularis and medulla. Sinusoidal blood collects through venules into a single large central vein in each adrenal and drains into either the renal vein or the inferior vena cava.

Adrenal cortex

In all species studied thus far, the adrenal cortex is essential for maintenance of life. Insufficiency of adrenal cortical hormones (Addison's disease) produced by pathological destruction or surgical removal of the adrenal cortices results in death within 1–2 weeks unless replacement therapy is instituted. Virtually, every organ system goes awry with adrenal cortical insufficiency, but the most likely cause of death appears to be circulatory collapse secondary to sodium depletion. When food intake is inadequate, death may result instead of insufficient amounts of glucose in the blood (hypoglycemia).

Adrenal cortical hormones have been divided into two categories based on their ability to protect against these two causes of death. The mineralocorticoids are necessary for maintenance of sodium and potassium balance. Aldosterone is the physiologically most important mineralocorticoid, although some 11-deoxycorticosterone, another potent mineralocorticoid, is also produced by the normal adrenal gland (Fig. 4.15).

Cortisol and, to a lesser extent, corticosterone are the physiologically most important glucocorticoids and are so named for their ability to maintain carbohydrate reserves. Glucocorticoids have a variety of other effects as well. The adrenal cortex also produces androgens,

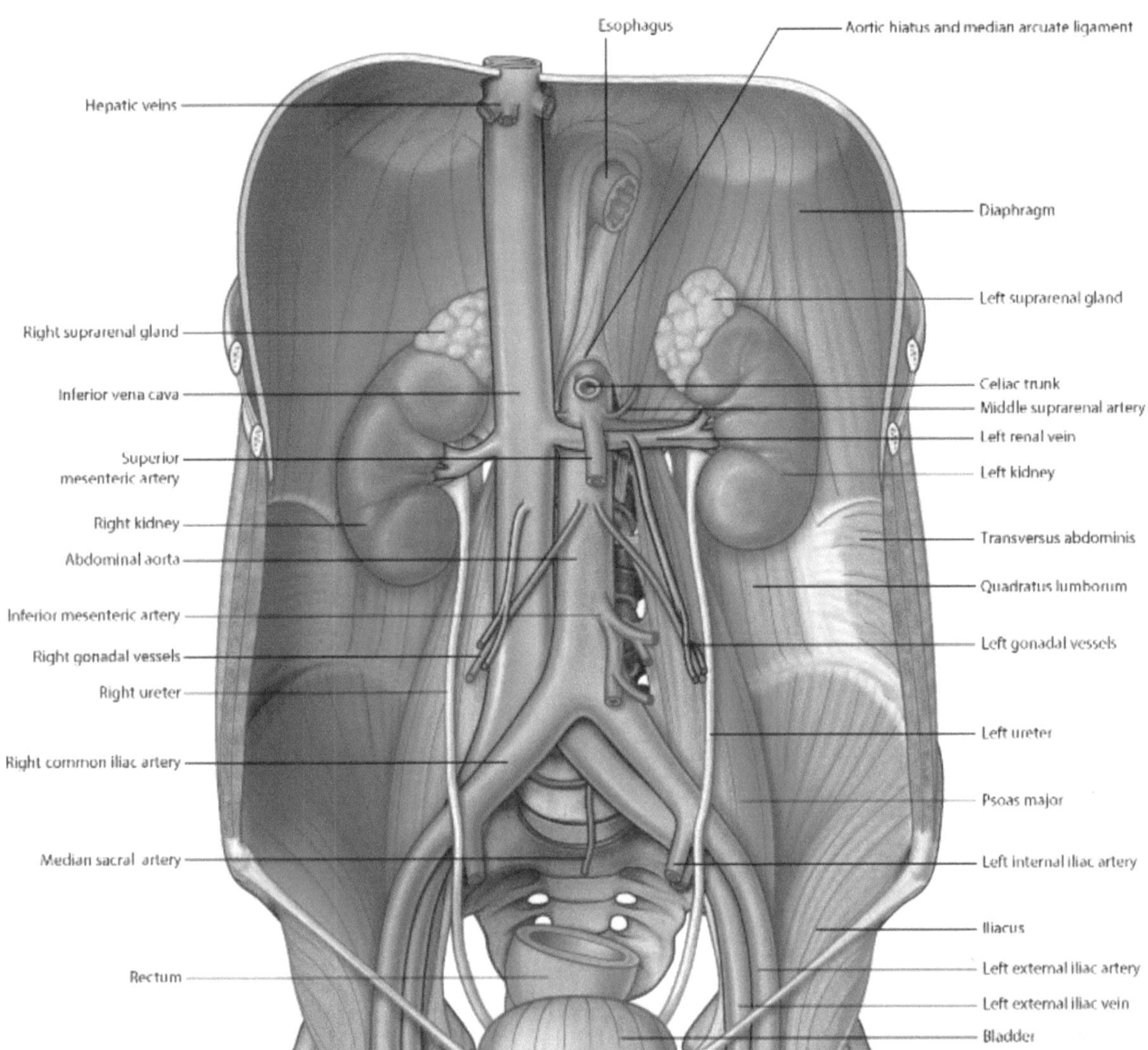

FIGURE 4.13 The location of the adrenal (suprarenal) glands behind the peritoneum (retroperitoneal). The liver and all other digestive structures have been removed. Source: *From R. L. Drake, A. W. Vogl, A. W. M. Mitchell, R. M. Tibbitts, & P. E. Richardson (Eds.) (2015).* Gray's atlas of anatomy *(2nd ed., p. 184). Elsevier.*

which, as their name implies, have biological effects similar to those of the male gonadal hormones (see Chapter 12: Hormonal Control of Reproduction in the Male). Adrenal androgens mediate some of the changes that occur at puberty and play an important role during fetal life (see Chapter 14: Hormonal Control of Pregnancy and Lactation). Adrenal steroid hormones are closely related to the steroid hormones produced by the testis and ovary and are synthesized from common precursors.

Adrenocortical hormones

All the adrenal steroids are derivatives of the polycyclic phenanthrene nucleus, present in cholesterol, which is the common molecular structure for ovarian and testicular steroids, bile acids, and precursors of vitamin D. Use of some of the standard conventions for naming the rings and the carbons facilitates discussion of the biosynthesis and metabolism of the steroid hormones. When drawing structures of steroid hormones, carbon atoms are indicated when reduced by carbon monoxide. The P450 enzymes utilize atmospheric oxygen and electrons donated from NADPH + to oxidize their substrates. Although they have only a single substrate-binding site, some of the P450 enzymes catalyze more than one oxidative step in steroid hormone synthesis.

The rate-limiting step in the biosynthesis of all the steroid hormones is the conversion of the 27-carbon cholesterol molecule to the 21-carbon pregnenolone molecule (Fig. 4.16).

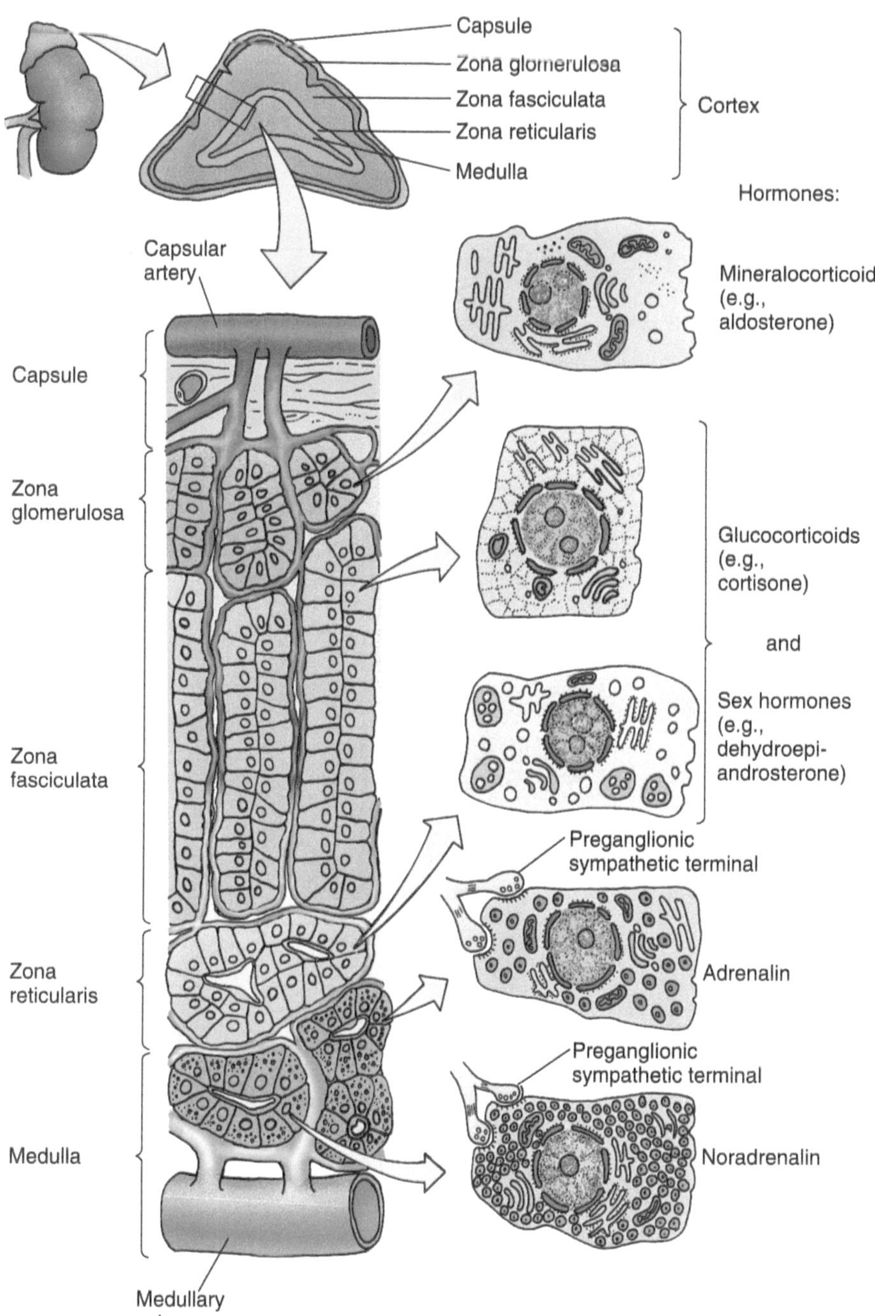

FIGURE 4.14 The layers of the adrenal gland from outside in. Note that the blood supply goes from the outside to the inside. Therefore sampling of the adrenal cortex can be made directly from the adrenal vein, into which the medullary vein goes. Source: *From Figure 13-10 in Gartner, L. P. (Ed.) (2017).* Textbook of histology *(4th ed., p. 362). Elsevier.*

This conversion is catalyzed by a unique enzyme, P450 side-chain cleavage enzyme (P450scc), which resides on the inner mitochondrial membrane. P450scc catalyzes three sequential oxidative reactions, the oxidation of carbons 20 and 22, and cleavage of the bond between them to shorten the side chain and reduce the number of carbons to 21. The rate of steroid hormone biosynthesis is determined by the rate at which cholesterol is presented to P450scc and converted to pregnenolone. To gain access to the enzyme, cholesterol must first be released from its esterified storage form in the cytosol by the action of an esterase. The free, but water-insoluble cholesterol must then be transferred to the mitochondrial surfaces through the agency of cholesterol-binding proteins with participation of cytoskeletal elements, and then must enter the mitochondria. Transit across the mitochondrial membrane bilayer requires synthesis and phosphorylation of the short-lived steroid acute regulatory (StAR) protein. Blockade of its synthesis blocks steroidogenesis. The StAR protein binds cholesterol and enters the mitochondria where it is inactivated, but it apparently does

Mineralocorticoids

Aldosterone 11-Deoxycorticosterone (DOC)

Glucocorticoids

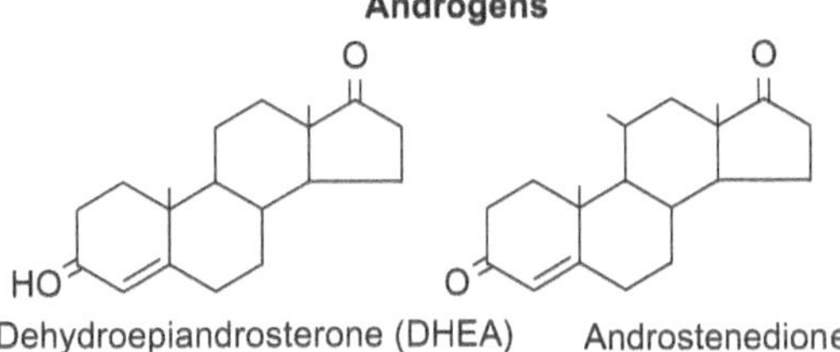

Androgens

Dehydroepiandrosterone (DHEA) Androstenedione

FIGURE 4.15 The principal adrenal steroid hormones.

not function simply as a membrane carrier protein. Precisely, how StAR facilitates delivery of cholesterol to the P450scc enzyme is not known, but constitutively expressed proteins in the outer mitochondrial membrane, particularly the benzodiazepine receptor, also play a role. StAR is present in all steroidogenic tissues except the placenta, and its synthesis is rapidly accelerated by agents that stimulate steroid hormone biosynthesis. Egress from mitochondria is independent of StAR protein, as 21 carbon steroids pass through the mitochondrial membranes rather freely.

Pregnenolone is the common precursor of all steroid hormones produced by the adrenals or the gonads. Early in the biosynthetic pathway the enzyme 3β-hydroxysteroid dehydrogenase (3β-HSD) catalyzes oxidation of the hydroxyl group at carbon 3 and causes a rearrangement that shifts the double bond from the B ring to the A ring. A ketone group at carbon 3 is found in all biologically important adrenal steroids and appears necessary for physiological activity. Biosynthesis of the various steroid hormones involves oxygenation of carbons 11, 17, 18, and 21, as depicted in Fig. 4.17.

The exact sequence of hydroxylations may vary, and some of the reactions may take place in a different order than that presented in the figure. The specific hormone that ultimately is secreted once the cholesterol–pregnenolone roadblock has been passed is determined by the enzymatic makeup of the particular cells involved. For example, there are two different P450 enzymes that catalyze the hydroxylation of carbon 11. They are encoded in separate genes that occupy adjacent loci on chromosome 8. The two enzymes are 93% identical in their amino acid sequence and appear to have arisen by gene duplication prior to the emergence of terrestrial vertebrates. One of the enzymes (P450c11AS) is expressed exclusively in cells of the zona glomerulosa and sequentially catalyzes the oxidation of both carbon 11 and carbon 18 to form aldosterone. The other enzyme (P450c11β) is found in cells of the zonae fasciculata and reticularis and can oxidize only carbon 11. Cells of the zonae fasciculata and reticularis, but not of the zona glomerulosa, express the enzyme P450c17, also called P450 17α-hydroxylase/lyase, which catalyzes the oxidation of the carbon at position 17. Hence, glomerulosa cells can produce corticosterone, aldosterone, and deoxycorticosterone, but not cortisol, whereas cells of the zonae fasciculata and reticularis can form cortisol and 17α-hydroxy-progesterone. When reducing equivalents are delivered to P450c17 rapidly enough, the reaction continues beyond the 17α-hydroxylation of progesterone to cleavage of the carbon 17–20 bond. Removal of carbons 20 and 21 produces the 19-carbon androgens. Hence, androgens may also be produced by these cells but not by glomerulosa cells.

As is probably already apparent, steroid chemistry is complex and can be bewildering; but because these compounds are so important physiologically and therapeutically, some familiarity with their structures is required. We can simplify the task somewhat by noting that steroid hormones can be placed into three major categories: those that contain 21 carbon atoms, those that contain 19 carbon atoms, and those that contain 18 carbon atoms. In addition, there are relatively few sites where modification of the steroid nucleus determines its physiological activity.

The physiologically important steroid hormones of the 21-carbon series are as follows:

- Progesterone has the simplest structure and can serve as a precursor molecule for all the other steroid hormones. Note that the only modifications to the basic carbon skeleton of the 21-carbon steroid nucleus are keto groups at positions 3 and 20. Normal adrenal cortical cells form little, if any, progesterone and none escapes into adrenal venous blood. Progesterone is a major secretory product of the ovaries and the placenta (Chapter 13: Hormonal Control of Reproduction in the Female: The Menstrual Cycle, and Chapter 14: Hormonal Control of Pregnancy and Lactation).

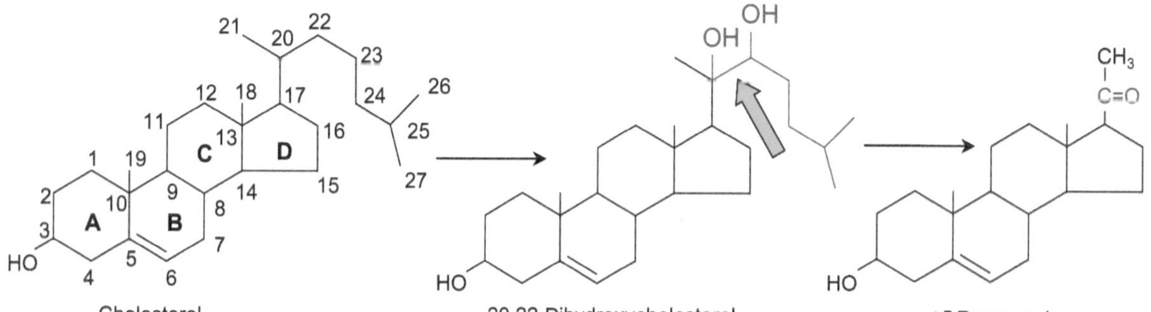

FIGURE 4.16 Conversion of cholesterol to pregnenolone, the rate determining reactions in steroid hormone biosynthesis. Carbons 20 and 22 are sequentially oxidized (in either order) followed by oxidative cleavage of the bond between them (*green arrow*). All three reactions are catalyzed by a single enzyme, cytochrome P450 side chain cleavage enzyme (P450scc).

- The presence of a hydroxyl group at carbon 21 of progesterone is the minimal change required for adrenal corticoid activity. This addition produces 11-deoxycorticosterone, a potent mineralocorticoid that is virtually devoid of glucocorticoid activity.
- Deoxycorticosterone is only a minor secretory product of the normal adrenal gland but may become important in some disease states.
- A hydroxyl group at carbon 11 is found in all glucocorticoids. Adding the hydroxyl group at carbon 11 confers glucocorticoid activity to deoxycorticosterone and reduces its mineralocorticoid activity 10-fold. This compound is corticosterone and can be produced in cells of all three zones of the adrenal cortex. Corticosterone is the major glucocorticoid in the rat but is of only secondary importance in humans.
- Corticosterone is a precursor of aldosterone, which is produced in cells of the zona glomerulosa by oxidation of carbon 18 to an aldehyde. The oxygen at carbon 18 increases the mineralocorticoid potency of corticosterone by a factor of 200 and only slightly decreases glucocorticoid activity.
- Cortisol differs from corticosterone only by the presence of a hydroxyl group at carbon 17. Cortisol is the most potent of the naturally occurring glucocorticoids. It has ten times as much glucocorticoid activity as aldosterone, but less than 0.25% of aldosterone's mineralocorticoid activity in normal human subjects. Synthetic glucocorticoids with even greater potency than cortisol are available for therapeutic use.

Steroids in the 19-carbon series usually have androgenic (male hormone) activity and are precursors of the estrogens (female hormones) (Figs. 4.18 and 4.19).

Hydroxylation of either pregnenolone or progesterone at carbon 17 is the critical prerequisite for cleavage of the C20,21 side chain to yield the adrenal androgens dehydroepiandrosterone or androstenedione (see Fig. 4.17). These compounds are also called 17-ketosteroids (17-KS). The principal testicular androgen is testosterone, which has a hydroxyl group rather than a keto group at carbon 17. Although the 19 carbon androgens are products of the same enzyme that catalyzes 17α-hydroxylation in the adrenals and the gonads, cleavage of the bond linking carbons 17 and 20 in the adrenals normally occurs to a significant extent only after puberty and then is confined an unsaturated A ring. Oxidation of the A ring (a process called aromatization) results in loss of the methyl carbon at position 19.

Control of adrenal cortical hormone synthesis

ACTH secreted by the anterior pituitary gland (see Chapter 2: Pituitary Gland) maintains normal secretory activity of the zonae fasciculata and reticularis of the adrenal cortex. After removal of the pituitary gland, little or no steroidogenesis occurs in the zona fasciculata or reticularis, but the zona glomerulosa continues to function. In cells of all three zones, ACTH interacts with a G protein–coupled membrane receptor, the melanocortin 2 receptor, and triggers production of cyclic AMP. Cyclic AMP activates protein kinase A, which catalyzes the phosphorylation of a variety of proteins and thereby modifies their activity. In the zonae fasciculata and reticularis, this results in accelerated deesterification of cholesterol esters, increased transport of cholesterol to the mitochondria, increased activity of preexisting StAR protein, and increased synthesis of StAR protein (Figs. 4.20 and 4.21).

The immediate actions of ACTH accelerate the delivery of cholesterol to the P450scc enzyme on the inner mitochondrial membrane to form pregnenolone.

Once pregnenolone is formed, remaining steps in hormone biosynthesis can proceed without further intervention from ACTH, although some evidence suggests that ACTH may also speed up some later reactions in the biosynthetic sequence. With continued

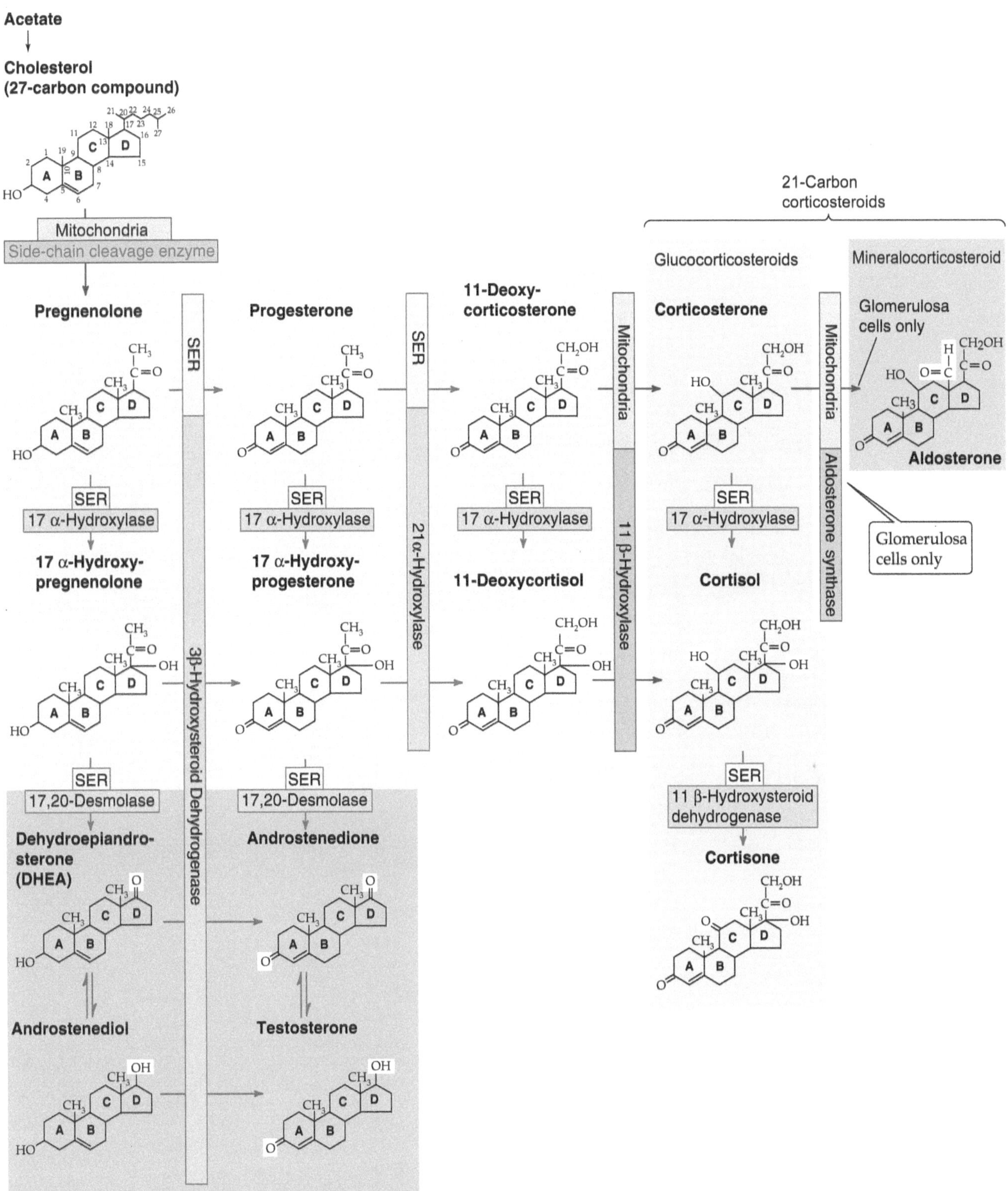

FIGURE 4.17 The enzymes 17a-hydroxylase is the same as 17, 20 desmolase. The enzymes are located in either the smooth endoplasmic reticulum or the mitochondria. Unless it says SER in the box, the reactions take place in the mitochondria. The image shows that reactions can go either horizontally or vertically. The group acted on by the enzyme is highlighted. *SER*, Smooth endoplasmic reticulum. Source: *From Figure 50-2 in Barrett, E. J. (2017). The adrenal gland, Chapter 50. In W. F. Boron & E. L. Boulpaep (Eds.),* Medical physiology *(3rd ed., p. 1020). Elsevier.*

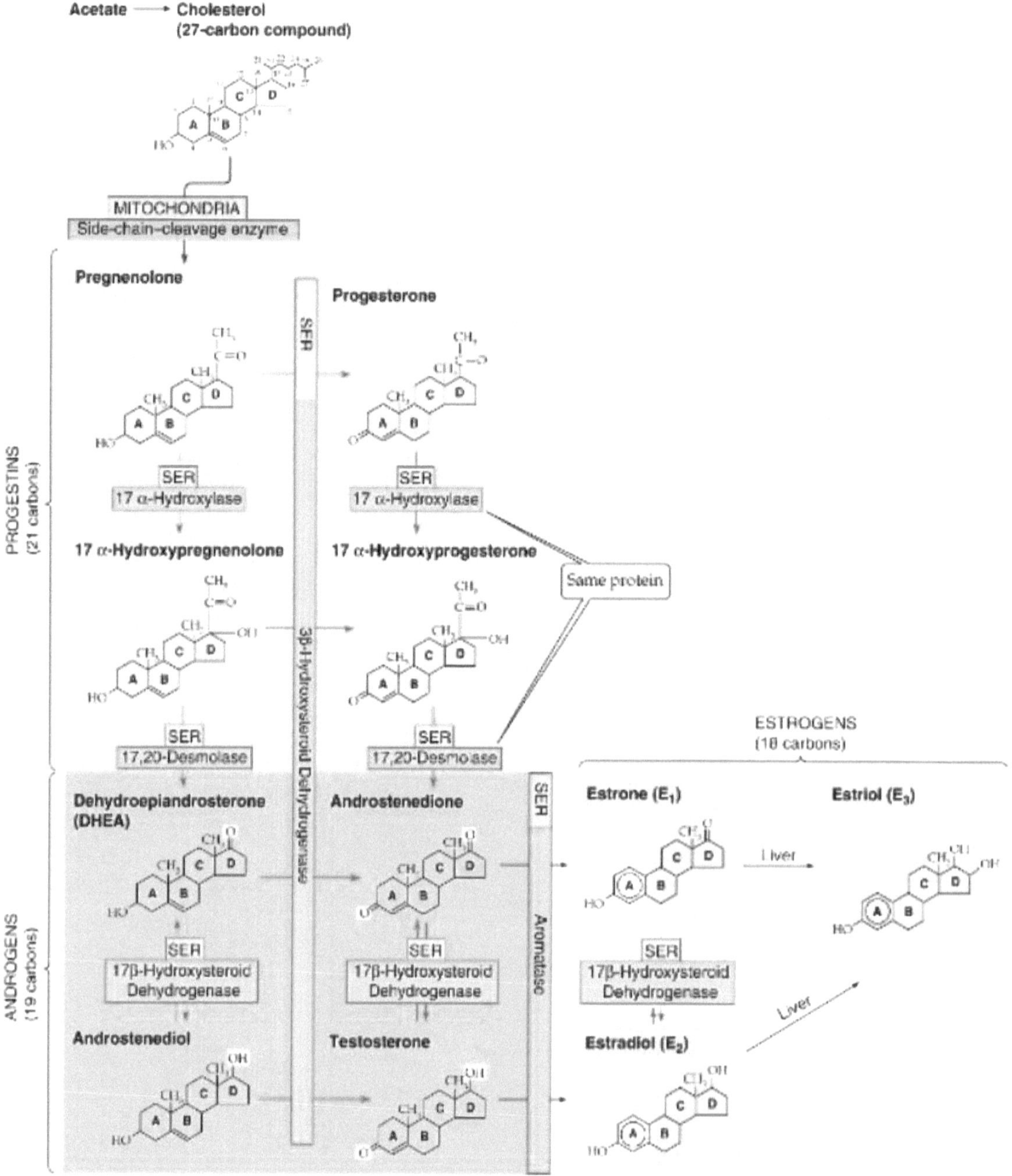

FIGURE 4.18 The synthesis of estrogens by the adrenal cortex is very limited. Most estrogen synthesis is done by the gonads. The adrenal cortex cannot synthesize estriol, which is only done in the liver. The highlighted areas are the group that the enzymes alter. The enzymatic reactions occur in either the SER or the mitochondria (no abbreviation). *SER*, Smooth endoplasmic reticulum. Source: *From Mesiano, S., & Jones, E, E. (2017). The female reproductive system, Chapter 55. In W. F. Boron & E. L. Boulpaep (Eds.),* Medical physiology *(3rd ed., p. 1118). Elsevier.*

stimulation, ACTH, acting through cyclic AMP and protein kinase A, also stimulates transcription of genes encoding the P450 enzymes (P450scc, P450c21, P450c17, and P450c11), the low-density lipoprotein receptor responsible for uptake of cholesterol, and the StAR protein.

ACTH is the only hormone known to control synthesis of the adrenal androgens. These 19-carbon steroids are produced primarily in the zona reticularis. Their production is limited first by the rate of conversion of cholesterol to pregnenolone and subsequently by the cleavage of the carbon 17–20 bond. As already mentioned, P450c17, the same enzyme that catalyzes α-hydroxylation of carbon 17 of cortisol, also catalyzes the second oxidative reaction at carbon 17 (17,20-lyase), which removes the C20,21 side chain. Some

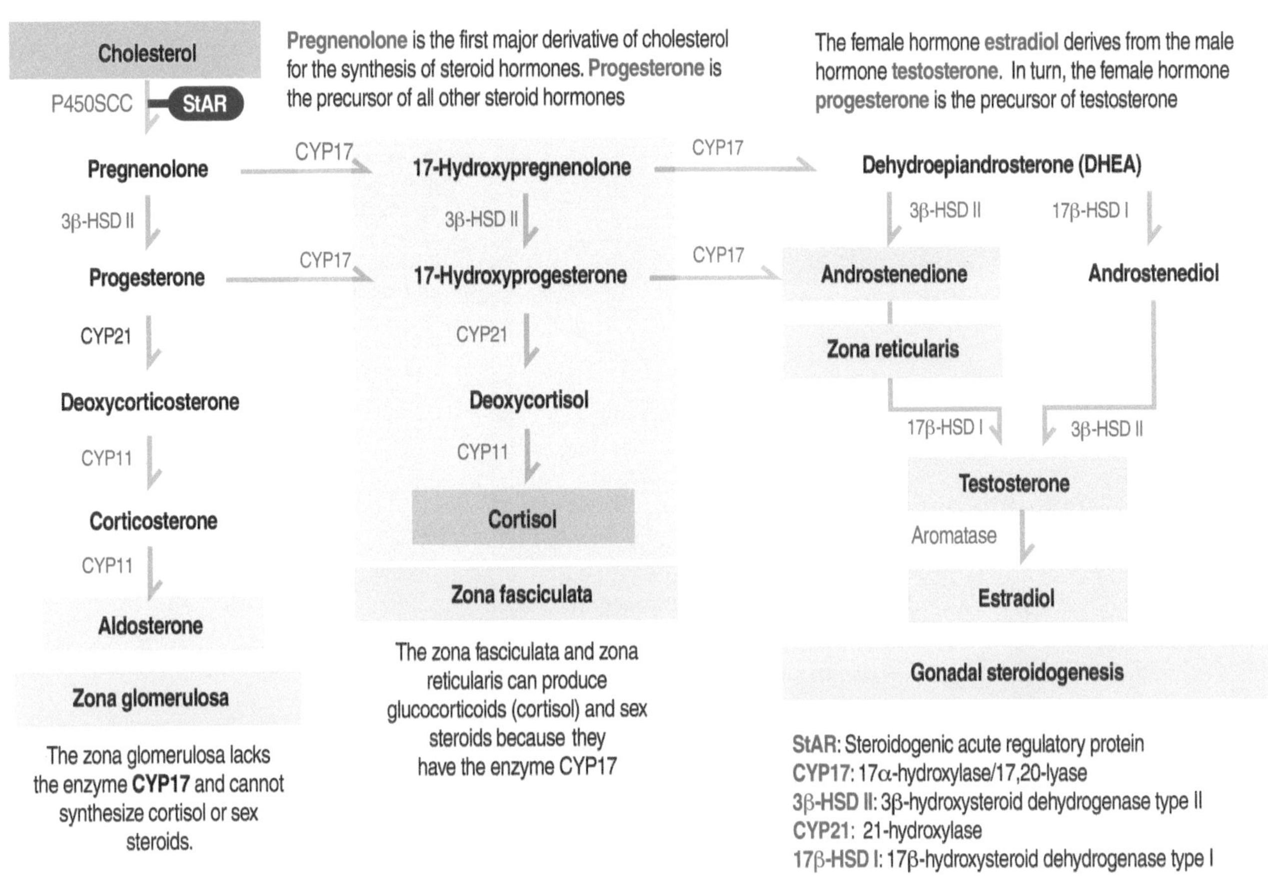

FIGURE 4.19 The synthesis of steroids by each zone in the adrenal cortex. Source: *From Figure 19.11 in Kierszenbaum, A. L., & Tres, L. L. (Eds.) (2020).* Histology and cell biology: An introduction to pathology *(5th ed., p. 648). Elsevier.*

evidence suggests that the lyase reaction is increased by phosphorylation of the P450c17, and other studies suggest that androgen production is driven by the capacity of reticularis cells to deliver reducing equivalents to the reaction. Little or no androgen is produced in young children whose adrenal glands contain only a rudimentary zona reticularis. The reticularis with its unique complement of enzymes develops shortly before puberty. The arrival of puberty is preceded by a dramatic increase in production of the adrenal androgens (adrenarche), principally dehydroepiandrosterone sulfate (DHEAS), which are responsible for growth of pubic and axillary hair. Secretion of DHEAS gradually rises to reach a maximum by age 20–25 and thereafter declines. This pattern of androgen secretion is quite different from the pattern of cortisol secretion and therefore appears to be governed by other factors than simply the ACTH-dependent rate of pregnenolone formation or the activity of the 17α-hydroxylase/lyase-enzyme (Fig. 4.22).

These findings have led some investigators to propose separate control of adrenal androgen production, possibly by another, as yet unidentified pituitary hormone, but to date no such hormone has been found. It is important to emphasize that increased stimulation of both the fasciculata and the reticularis by ACTH can profoundly increase adrenal androgen production.

Effects of ACTH on the adrenal cortex are not limited to accelerating the rate-determining step in steroid hormone production. ACTH either directly or indirectly also increases blood flow to the adrenal glands possibly by stimulating the release of arachidonic acid–derived vasodilators from cells of the zona glomerulosa. Increased blood flow provides not only needed oxygen and metabolic fuels but also increases the capacity to deliver newly secreted hormone to the general circulation. ACTH maintains the functional integrity of the inner zones of the adrenal cortex. Absence of ACTH leads to atrophy of these two zones, and chronic stimulation increases their mass. Stimulation with ACTH increases steroid hormone secretion within one to 2 minutes, and peak rates of secretion are achieved in about 15 minutes. Unlike other endocrine cells, steroid-producing cells do not store hormones, and hence,

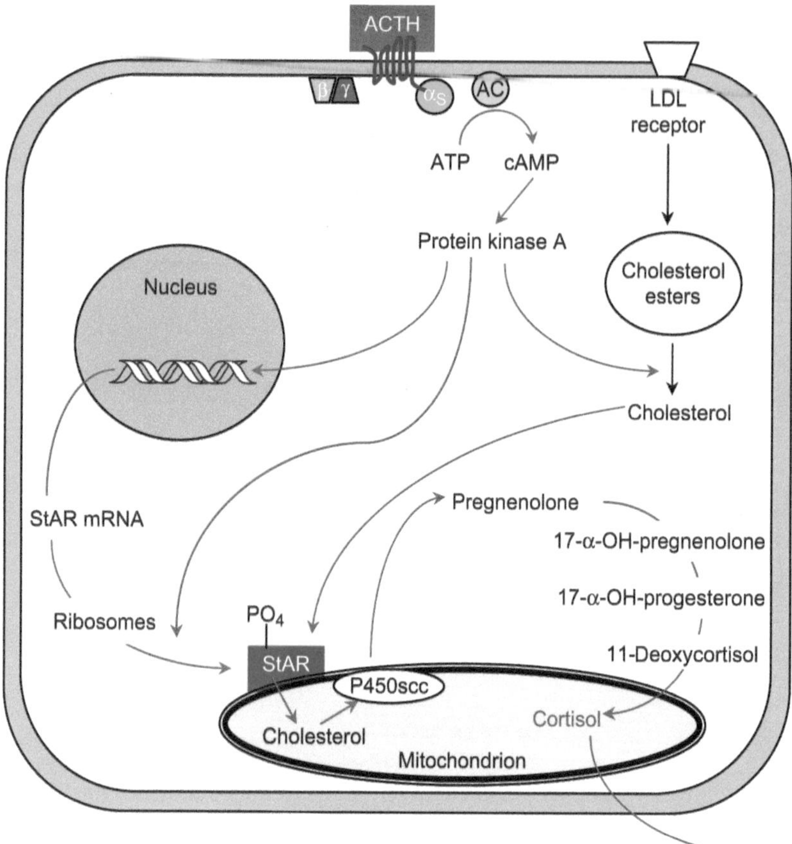

FIGURE 4.20 Stimulation of steroidogenesis by ACTH in zona fasciculata cells. Conversion of cholesterol to pregnenolone requires mobilization of cholesterol from its storage droplet and transfer to the P450scc (side-chain cleavage) enzyme on the inner mitochondrial membrane. See text for discussion. ACTH may also increase cholesterol uptake by increasing the number or affinity of LDL receptors. $\beta\gamma$, $\beta\gamma$ Subunits of the guanine nucleotide-binding protein; α_s, stimulatory α subunit of the guanine nucleotide–binding protein; *AC*, adenylyl cyclase; *ACTH*, adrenocorticotropic hormone; *LDL*, low-density lipoprotein; *StAR*, steroid acute regulatory protein.

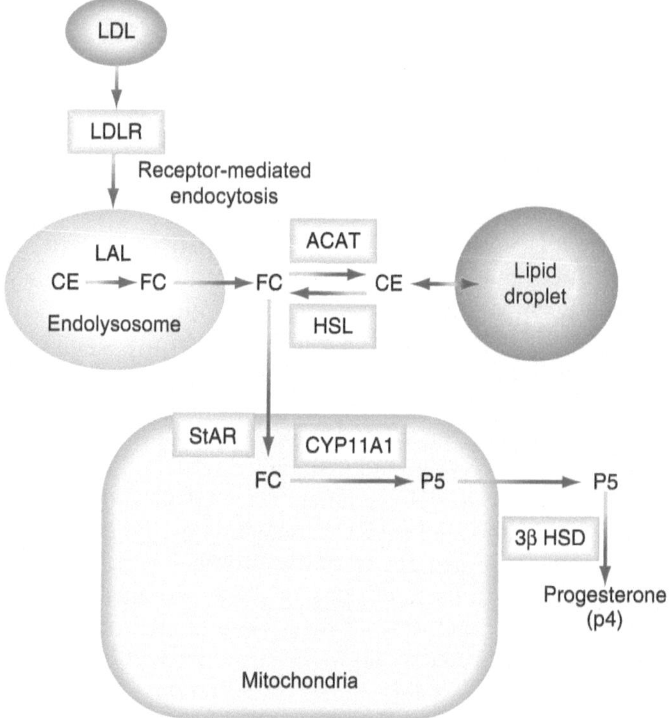

FIGURE 4.21 The pathway of cholesterol from LDL to lipid or endosome and thence to free cholesterol which can enter the mitochondria for conversion to pregnenolone then back outside the mitochondria in the smooth endoplasmic reticulum where it is converted to progesterone. CYP11A1 is also called P450 side-chain cleavage enzyme. *3β-HSD*, 3β-Hydroxysteroid dehydrogenase; *ACAT*, acyl CoA cholesterol; *CE*, cholesterol ester; *FC*, free cholesterol; *HSL*, hormone-sensitive lipase; *LAL*, lysosomal acid hydrolase; *LDL*, low-density lipoprotein; *LDLR*, low-density lipoprotein receptor; *P5*, pregnenolone; *StAR*, steroidogenic acute regulatory protein. Source: *From Figure 43.7 in Koeppen, B. M., & Stanton, B. M. (Eds.) (2018).* Berne and Levy physiology *(7th ed., p. 772). Elsevier.*

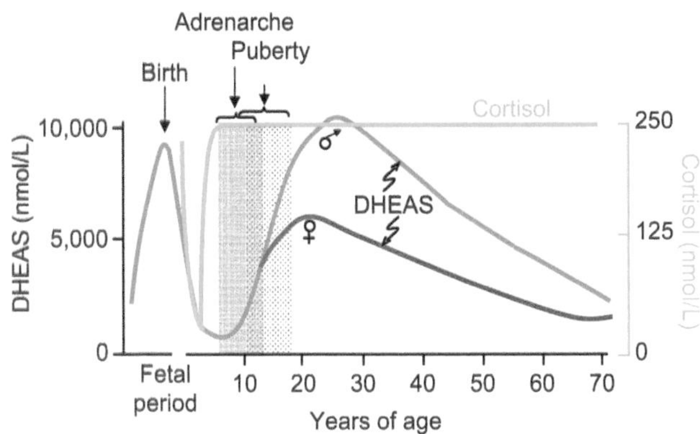

FIGURE 4.22 Average plasma concentrations of cortisol and DHEAS throughout life. DHEAS is abundant in fetal plasma (see Chapter 14: Hormonal Control of Pregnancy and Lactation) and declines precipitously after birth as the fetal zone of the adrenal involutes. DHEAS increases during adrenarche as the zona reticularis increases in mass. Although both the ovaries and testes contribute to circulating DHEAS, the difference in plasma levels between males and females reflects the greater contribution of the testes. Cortisol is secreted by the fetal adrenal cortex only in the latter part of pregnancy. Average adult levels are reached shortly after birth and remain within a constant range throughout life. *DHEAS*, Dehydroepiandrosterone sulfate. Source: *Adapted from Rainey, W. E., Carr, B. R., Sasano, H., Suzuki, T., & Mason, J. I. (2002). Dissecting human adrenal androgen production.* Trends in Endocrinology and Metabolism, *13, 234–239.*

biosynthesis and secretion are components of a single process regulated at the step of cholesterol conversion to pregnenolone. Because steroid hormones are lipid-soluble, they can diffuse through the plasma membrane and enter the circulation through simple diffusion down a concentration gradient. Even under basal conditions, cortisol concentrations are more than 100 times higher in fasciculata cells than in plasma. It is not surprising therefore that biosynthetic intermediates may escape into the circulation during intense stimulation. Adult human adrenal glands normally produce about 20 mg of cortisol, about 2 mg of corticosterone, 10–15 mg of androgens, and about 150 μg of aldosterone each day, but with sustained stimulation they can increase this output manyfold.

Control of aldosterone synthesis

The control of aldosterone synthesis is more complex than that of the glucocorticoids. Although cells of the zona glomerulosa express ACTH receptors and ACTH is required for optimal secretion, ACTH is not an important regulator of aldosterone production in most species. Angiotensin II, an octapeptide whose production is regulated by the kidney (see later and Chapter 7: The Pancreatic Islets), is the hormonal signal for increased production of aldosterone (Figs. 4.23 and 4.24).

Like ACTH, angiotensin II reacts with specific G protein–coupled membrane receptors, but angiotensin II does not activate adenyl cyclase or use cyclic AMP as its second messenger. Instead, it acts through IP3 and calcium to promote the formation of pregnenolone from cholesterol. The ligand-bound angiotensin receptor associates with Gαq and activates phospholipase C to release IP3 (see Chapter 1: Introduction) and diacylglycerol (DAG) from membrane phosphatidylinositol bisphosphate. Gαq may also interact directly with potassium channels and cause them to close. The resulting depolarization of the membrane opens voltage-gated calcium channels and allows calcium to enter. Simultaneously, the βγ subunits directly activate these calcium channels and further promote calcium entry.

Intracellular calcium concentrations are also increased by interaction of IP3 with its receptor in the endoplasmic reticulum to release stored calcium. Increased intracellular calcium activates a calmodulin-dependent protein kinase (CAM kinase II), which promotes transfer of cholesterol into the mitochondria by increasing the activity and synthesis of the StAR protein in the same manner as described for protein kinase A. Increase cytosolic calcium raises the intramitochondrial calcium concentration and stimulates P450c11AS, which catalyzes the critical final reactions in aldosterone synthesis. The DAG that is released by activation of phospholipase C activates protein kinase C, which may augment the phosphorylation and activity of StAR protein, and it may also contribute to opening calcium channels. In addition, protein kinase C may play an important role in mediating the hypertrophy of the zona glomerulosa seen after prolonged stimulation of the adrenal glands with angiotensin II.

Cells of the zona glomerulosa are exquisitely sensitive to changes in concentration of potassium in the extracellular fluid and adjust aldosterone synthesis and secretion accordingly. An increase of as little as 0.1 mM in the concentration of potassium, a change of only about 2%–3%, may increase aldosterone production by as much as 25%. This exquisite sensitivity is largely attributable to the abundance in the plasma membranes of two-pore potassium channels that allow outward "leak" of potassium. The especially high potassium conductance produces a highly negative membrane potential that becomes less negative as extracellular potassium increases. Voltage-sensitive calcium channels are activated by small decreases in membrane potential and allow calcium entry. Increasing intracellular calcium not only further depolarizes the membrane, but also activates calmodulin kinase II. Phosphorylation of these calcium channels increases their sensitivity to changes in membrane potential, producing further entry of calcium, and

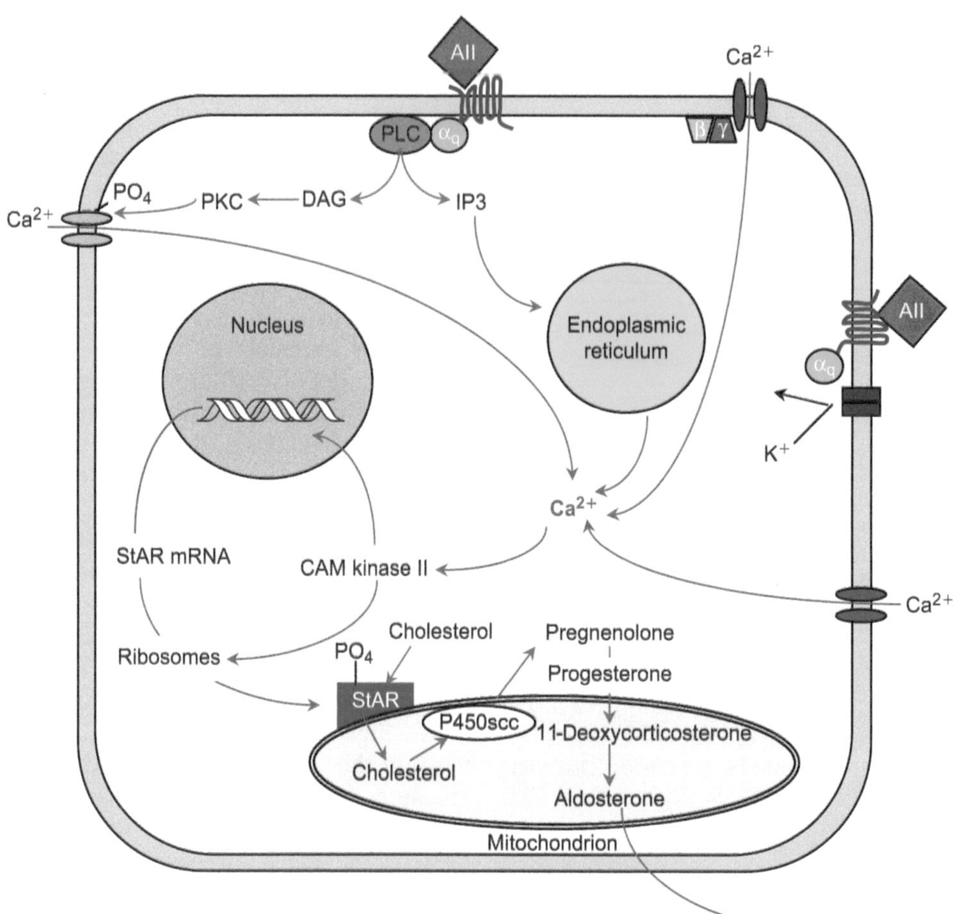

FIGURE 4.23 Stimulation of aldosterone synthesis by AII. AII accelerates the conversion of cholesterol to pregnenolone and 11-deoxycorticosterone to aldosterone. *AII*, Angiotensin II; *CAM kinase II*, calcium, calmodulin-dependent protein kinase II; *DAG*, diacylglycerol; *IP3*, inositol trisphosphate; *PKC*, protein kinase C; *PLC*, phospholipase C; *StAR*, steroid acute regulatory protein; αq, $\alpha\ \beta\ \gamma$, subunits of the guanine nucleotide-binding protein.

amplifies the response to increases in extracellular potassium. Intracellular calcium stimulates aldosterone synthesis as already described and heightens responsiveness to angiotensin II.

It is noteworthy that although aldosterone is the principal regulator of body sodium content, sodium has little if any direct effect on glomerulosa cells or the rate of aldosterone secretion. However, sodium profoundly affects aldosterone synthesis indirectly through its role as the major determinant of blood volume. Decreases in the effective plasma volume result in increased angiotensin II production, while increases in volume stimulate secretion of atrial natriuretic factor (ANF). Regulation of blood volume is discussed in Chapter 9, Regulation of Salt and Water Balance. Synthesis and secretion of aldosterone are negatively regulated by ANF, which activates potassium channels and thereby opposes opening of voltage-sensitive calcium channels. In addition, ANF reduces synthesis and phosphorylation of the StAR protein and inhibits transcription of its gene. ANF receptors have intrinsic guanylyl cyclase activity and, when bound to ANF, catalyze the conversion of guanosine triphosphate to cyclic guanosine monophosphate (cyclic GMP). Precisely, how an increase in cyclic GMP interferes with aldosterone synthesis has not been established. Cyclic GMP is known to activate the enzyme cyclic AMP phosphodiesterase and may thereby lower basal levels of cyclic AMP, or it may act through stimulating cyclic GMP-dependent protein kinase.

Adrenal steroid hormones in blood

Adrenal cortical hormones are transported in blood bound to a specific plasma protein, called transcortin or corticosteroid-binding globulin (CBG), and to a lesser extent to albumin. Like albumin, CBG is synthesized and secreted by the liver, but its concentration of $\sim 1\ \mu M$ in plasma is only about one-thousandth that of albumin. CBG is a glycoprotein with a molecular weight of about 58,000 and is a member of the

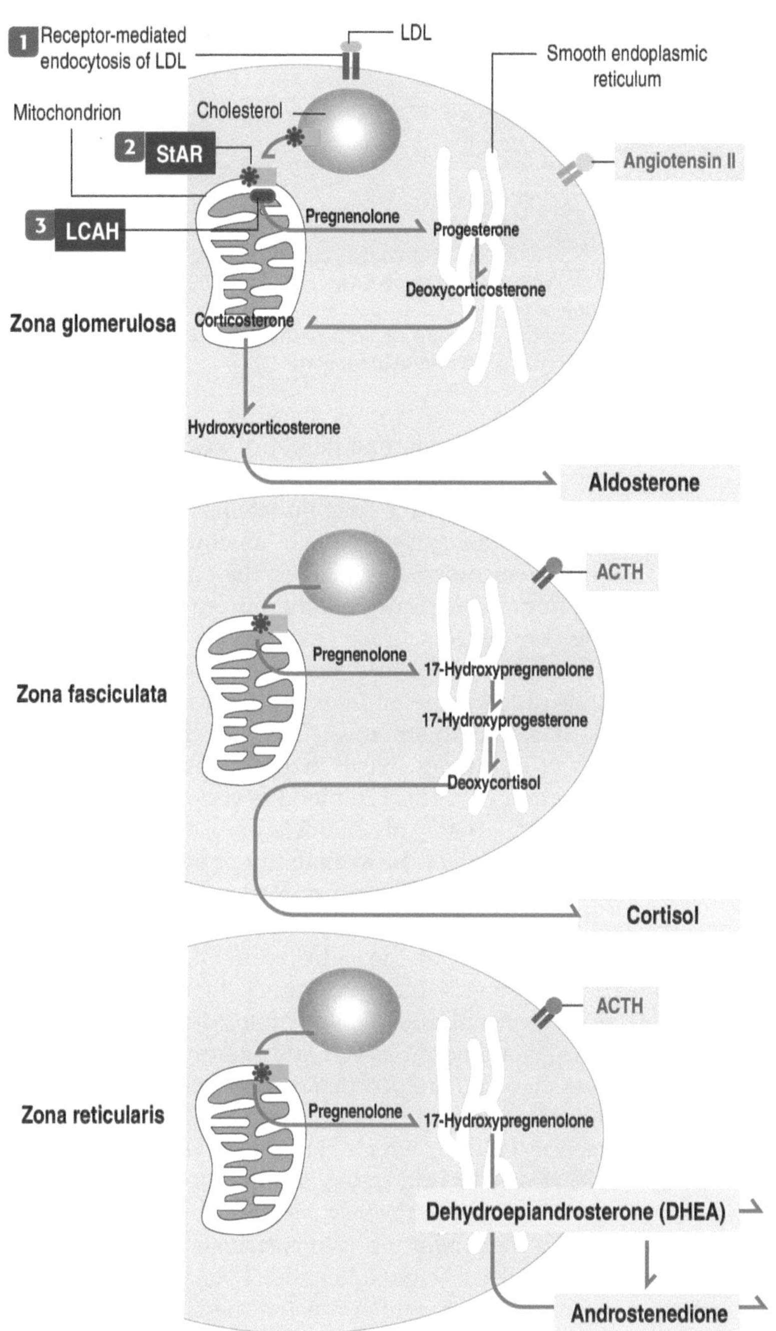

1 Most of the **cholesterol**, the precursor for the biosynthesis of all steroid hormones, derives from circulating **low-density lipoprotein (LDL)**. Cholesterol is esterified by acylCoA cholesterol acyltransferase to be stored in cytoplasmic lipid droplets

Cholesterol is modified by a series of hydroxylation reactions. Enzymes located in the mitochondria and smooth endoplasmic reticulum participate in the reactions. The substrates shuttle from mitochondria to smooth endoplasmic reticulum to mitochondria during steroidogenesis

Steroidogenic acute regulatory protein (StAR)

2 The **steroidogenic acute regulatory protein (StAR)** is a cholesterol transfer protein. StAR regulates the synthesis of steroids by **transporting cholesterol across the outer mitochondrial membrane to the inner mitochondrial membrane,** where cytochrome **P450SCC**, the rate-limiting enzyme of steroidogenesis is located

3 A mutation in the gene encoding StAR or P450SCC is detected in individuals with defective synthesis of adrenal and gonadal steroids (**lipoid congenital adrenal hyperplasia, LCAH**)

Congenital adrenal hyperplasia (CAH)

CAH results from genetic enzymatic defects in the synthesis of cortisol. However, the adrenal cortex is responsive to adrenocorticotropic hormone (ACTH) and, therefore, cortical hyperplasia develops

In a large number of patients (90%), CAH is caused by an inborn defect in 21-hydroxylase (CYP21), the enzyme that converts 17-hydroxyprogesterone to deoxycorticosterone. The precursor is instead converted to androgens. Aldosterone is lacking and hypoaldosteronism develops (with hypotension and low Na^+ in plasma). Circulating androgens are high and virilization is found in female infants

FIGURE 4.24 The formation of steroids in each of the zones of the adrenal cortex. Source: *From Figure 19.12 in Kierszenbaum, A. L., & Tres, L. L. (Eds.) (2020).* Histology and cell biology: An introduction to pathology *(5th ed., p. 649). Elsevier.*

serine proteinase inhibitor (SERPIN) super-family of proteins. It has a single steroid hormone binding site whose affinity for cortisol is nearly 20 times higher than for aldosterone. About 95% of the cortisol and about 60% of the aldosterone in blood are bound to protein. Under normal circumstances the concentration of free or unbound cortisol in plasma is about 100 times that of aldosterone. Probably because they circulate bound to plasma proteins, adrenal steroids have a relatively long half-life in blood: 1.5–2 hours for cortisol, and about 15 minutes for aldosterone (Table 4.1).

TABLE 4.1 Plasma concentrations and secretion rates of the principal adrenocortical hormones.

	8 a.m. Plasma concentration (μg/dL)	Secretion rate (mg/day)	Half-life (minutes)
Cortisol	15	15	100
Corticosterone	1	3	30
Deoxycorticosterone	0.07	0.6	40
Aldosterone	.012	0.15	15
DHEA	0.5	4[a]	20
DHEAS	150	15[a]	1200
Androstenedione	0.12	1.5[a]	20

[a]*About 30% originates in the gonads.*
DHEA, 5-Dehydroepiandrosterone; *DHEAS*, 5-dehydroepiandrosterone sulfate.

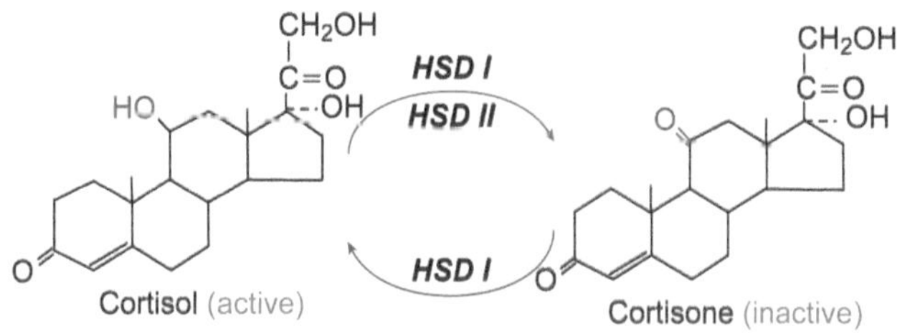

FIGURE 4.25 The cortisol-cortisone shuttle. Two enzymes, 11-hydroxysteroid dehydrogenase (HSD I and HSD II) catalyze the oxidation of cortisol to cortisone. HSD I can also catalyze the reaction in the reverse direction converting the inactive cortisone to cortisol. *HSD*, Hydroxysteroid dehydrogenase.

Postsecretory metabolism of adrenal cortical hormones

The cortisol/cortisone shuttle

Metabolic transformations of steroid hormones are not confined to the glands of origin but may continue after secretion, and may increase, decrease, or otherwise change biological activity. Several steroid metabolizing enzymes are expressed in steroid target tissues. Among these are two isoforms of the enzyme 11β-HSD (11β-HSD I and 11β-HSD II). The two enzymes are products of different genes and have different catalytic properties. 11β-HSD I catalyzes either the oxidation of the 11-hydroxyl group of cortisol to a ketone to form the inactive steroid cortisone (Fig. 4.25) or reduces the 11 keto-group of cortisone to form cortisol, depending upon the prevailing redox state. 11β-HSD II catalyzes only the oxidation of cortisol to the inactive cortisone. These reactions, which enable tissues to activate or inactivate glucocorticoid locally, are profoundly important for expression of both glucocorticoid and mineralocorticoid responses. Despite this potential cycle, not very much cortisone is produced by the adrenal cortex. However, HSD II is highly expressed in the renal distal tubule where it irreversibly converts cortisol to cortisone. By this means, aldosterone is able to regulate the mineralocorticoid receptor without competition from cortisol (see later).

Receptors for adrenal steroids originally were classified based upon their affinity and selectivity for mineralo- or glucocorticoids. The mineralocorticoid receptors, also called type I receptors, have a high and nearly equal affinity for aldosterone and cortisol. The type II, or glucocorticoid receptors, have a considerably greater affinity for cortisol than for aldosterone. Expression of mineralocorticoid receptors is confined largely to aldosterone target tissues and the brain, whereas glucocorticoid receptor expression is widely disseminated. In the unstimulated state, both receptors reside in the cytosol bound to other proteins. Upon binding hormone, they release their associated proteins and migrate as dimers to the nucleus where they activate or repress gene expression (see Chapter 1: Introduction). Because the mineralocorticoid receptor binds aldosterone and cortisol with nearly equal affinity, it cannot distinguish between the two classes of steroid hormones. Nevertheless, even though the concentration of cortisol in blood is about 1000 times higher than that of aldosterone, mineralocorticoid responses reflect the availability of aldosterone. This is due in part to differences in plasma protein binding; only 3% or 4% of cortisol is in free solution compared to nearly 40% of the aldosterone. Although hormone binding lowers the discrepancy in the available hormone concentrations by 10-fold, free cortisol is 100 times as abundant as free aldosterone and readily diffuses into mineralocorticoid target cells. Access to the mineralocorticoid receptor, however, is guarded by the enzyme HSD II, which colocalizes with mineralocorticoid receptors and defends mineralocorticoid specificity. The high efficiency of this enzyme inactivates cortisol by converting it to cortisone, which is released into the blood (Figs. 4.26 and 4.27).

The kidneys, which are the major targets for aldosterone, are a major source of circulating cortisone. Persons with a genetic defect in HSD II suffer from symptoms of mineralocorticoid excess (hypertension and hypokalemia) as a result of constant saturation of the mineralocorticoid receptor by cortisol. An acquired form of the same ailment is seen after ingestion of excessive amounts of natural black licorice. It contains glycyrrhizin which is an inhibitor of HSD-II.

A variety of glucocorticoid target tissues including adipose tissue and cells of the immune system express HSD I, which functions in the opposite direction in these tissues, converting cortisone to cortisol. Because of this ability, the effective concentrations of cortisol in

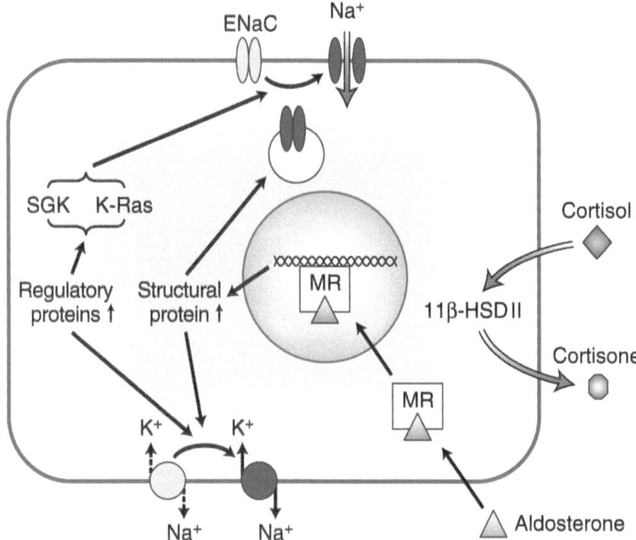

FIGURE 4.26 This can occur in the distal nephron or distal colon. The higher concentrations of cortisol are inactivated by 11β-HSD II which converts it to inactive cortisone. This permits aldosterone to combine with its MR which then translocates to the nucleus. In the nucleus, it stimulates the formation of structural proteins which, along with regulatory proteins, enhance the expulsion of Na into the extracellular space. The 11-hydroxyl group of aldosterone is protected from the enzyme because it forms a hemiacetal with the aldehyde group on carbon 18 (Fig. 4.13). SGK1, serum/glucocorticoid-regulated kinase; ENaC, epithelial sodium channel; MR, mineralocorticoid receptor. Source: *From Figure 15-11 in Stewart, P. M., & Newell-Price, J. C. C. (2016). The adrenal cortex, Chapter 15. In S. Melmed, K. S. Polonsky, P. R. Larsen, & H. M. Kronenberg (Eds.), Williams textbook of endocrinology (13th ed., p. 501). Elsevier.* HSD, *Hydroxysteroid dehydrogenase;* MR, *mineralocorticoid receptor.*

FIGURE 4.27 Formation of a hemiacetal with the aldehyde on carbon 18 protects the 11- hydroxyl group of aldosterone from oxidation by 11-HSD II. *HSD*, Hydroxysteroid dehydrogenase.

these tissues is considerably higher than in arterial blood, and glucocorticoid responses that might not otherwise occur can now take place. This phenomenon helps to resolve the long-standing question of how glucocorticoid responses that require hormone concentrations that are substantially higher than normal blood levels can nevertheless be produced under physiological circumstances.

Postsecretory transformations of androgens

DHEAS, the major product of the zona reticularis, is the most abundant steroid hormone in the circulation. Neither DHEAS nor its close relative androstenedione bind to the androgen receptor, but these 19 carbon steroids are converted to active male and female sex hormones within some peripheral target cells (Fig. 4.28).

For the most part these peripherally-formed hormones do not enter the circulation, and their biological actions are limited to the cells in which they are formed. The ability of peripheral target cells to carry out these transformations has profound consequences for progression of tumors in the prostate and breast, and also for the normal growth and maturation of bone (Chapter 11: Hormonal Control of Growth). The term intracrinology has been used to describe production of hormones by the cells in which they act without escaping into the extracellular fluid. Following removal of the sulfate ester at carbon 3, DHEAS is oxidized to androstenedione, which is the immediate precursor of testosterone or estrone.

Inactivation of adrenal cortical steroids

Mammals cannot degrade the ring structure of the steroid nucleus. Steroid hormones are inactivated by metabolic changes that make them unrecognizable to their receptors. Inactivation of glucocorticoids occurs mainly in liver and is achieved primarily by reduction of the A ring and its keto group at position 3. Conjugation of the resulting hydroxyl group on carbon 3 with glucuronic acid or sulfate increases water solubility and decreases binding to CBG so the steroid can now pass through renal glomerular capillaries and be excreted in the urine. The major products of adrenal steroid hormone degradation are glucuronide esters of 17-OHCS derived from cortisol, and 17-KS derived from glucocorticoids and androgens. Because recognizable hormonal derivatives are excreted in urine, it is possible to estimate daily secretory rates of steroid hormones by the noninvasive technique of measuring their abundance in urine.

Physiology of the mineralocorticoids

Although several naturally occurring adrenal cortical steroids, including glucocorticoids, can produce mineralocorticoid effects, aldosterone is by far the most important mineralocorticoid physiologically. In its absence, there is a progressive loss of sodium by the kidney, which results secondarily in a loss of extracellular fluid (see Chapter 9: Regulation of Salt and Water Balance). It may be recalled that the kidney adjusts the volume and composition of the

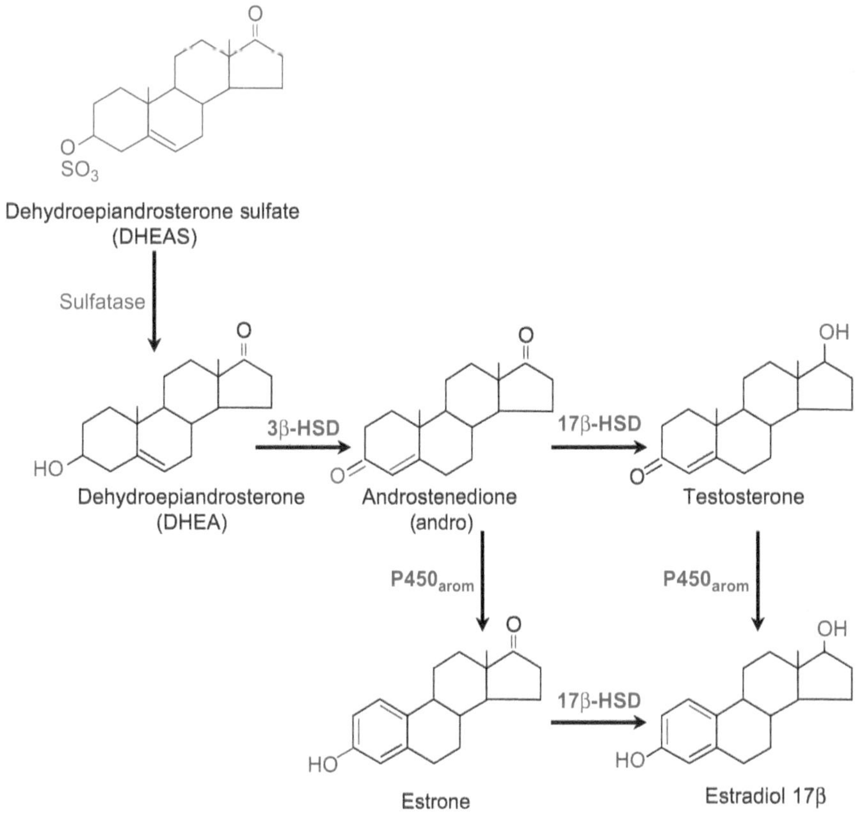

FIGURE 4.28 Pathways of extraadrenal synthesis of testosterone and estrogens from DHEAS. Enzyme-catalyzed changes are shown in red. *DHEAS*, Dehydroepiandrosterone sulfate.

extracellular fluid by processes that involve formation of an ultrafiltrate of plasma followed by secretion or selective reabsorption of solutes and water. Reabsorption of sodium is diminished in the absence of aldosterone, and with loss of sodium, there is an accompanying loss of water and a resulting decrease in blood volume. Decreased blood volume (hypovolemia) leads to a compensatory retention of "free" water (see Chapter 9: Regulation of Salt and Water Balance) with the result that the concentration of sodium in blood plasma may gradually fall (hyponatremia) from the normal value of 140– to 120 mEq/L or even lower in extreme cases.

With the decrease in concentration of sodium, the principal cation of extracellular fluid, there is a net transfer of water from extracellular to intracellular space, further aggravating hypovolemia. Diarrhea is frequently seen, and it too worsens hypovolemia. Loss of plasma volume increases the hematocrit (concentration of blood cells) and the viscosity of blood (hemoconcentration). Simultaneous with the loss of sodium, the ability to excrete potassium is impaired, and with continued dietary intake, plasma concentrations of potassium may increase from the normal value of 4 to 8–10 mEq/L (hyperkalemia). Increased concentrations of potassium in blood, and therefore in extracellular fluid, result in partial depolarization of plasma membranes of all cells, leading to cardiac arrhythmia and weakness of muscles including the heart. Blood pressure falls from the combined effects of decreased vascular volume, decreased cardiac contractility and decreased responsiveness of vascular smooth muscle to vasoconstrictor agents caused by hyponatremia. Mild acidosis is seen with mineralocorticoid deficiency, partly as a result of deranged potassium balance and partly from lack of the direct effects of aldosterone on hydrogen ion excretion.

All these life-threatening changes can be reversed by administration of aldosterone and can be traced to the ability of aldosterone to promote inward transport of sodium across epithelial cells of kidney tubules and the outward transport of potassium and hydrogen ions into the urine. It has been estimated that aldosterone is required for the reabsorption of only about 2% of the sodium filtered at the renal glomeruli; even in its absence, about 98% of the filtered sodium is reabsorbed. However, 2% of the sodium filtered each day corresponds to the amount present in about 3.5 L of extracellular fluid. Aldosterone also promotes sodium and potassium transport by the sweat glands, the colon, and the salivary glands. Of these target tissues the kidney is by far the most important.

Effects of aldosterone on the kidney

Initial insights into the action of aldosterone on the kidney were obtained from observations of the effects of hormone deprivation or administration on the composition of the urine. Mineralocorticoids decrease the ratio of sodium to potassium concentrations in urine; in the absence of mineralocorticoids, the ratio increases as sodium is lost from the body and potassium is retained. However, although aldosterone promotes both sodium conservation and potassium excretion, the two effects are not tightly coupled, and sodium is not simply exchanged for potassium. Indeed, when normal human subjects were given aldosterone for 25 days, the sodium-retaining effects lasted only for the first 15 days, but increased excretion of potassium persisted for as long as the hormone was given (Fig. 4.29).

Renal handling of sodium and potassium is complex, and compensatory mechanisms exerted at aldosterone insensitive loci within the kidney can offset sustained effects of aldosterone on sodium absorption in the otherwise normal subjects (see Chapter 9: Regulation of Salt and Water Balance).

The million or so tubules (nephrons) in each kidney reabsorb nearly all 180 L of plasma ultrafiltrate formed each day whether or not aldosterone is present. Aldosterone-sensitive cells, called principal cells, are found in a relatively short segment of the nephron comprised mainly of the connecting tubule and the cortical portion of the collecting duct (see Chapter 9: Regulation of Salt and Water Balance). Less than 10% of the filtrate remains by the time it reaches this distal segment, and hence aldosterone influences reabsorption of only a small fraction of the filtered sodium. Throughout the nephron reabsorption is driven by energy-dependent two-step transfer of sodium across the tubular epithelium. Sodium enters the tubular cells on transporters or through channels in the luminal membranes and is pumped out into the extracellular space by the action of the sodium–potassium-dependent ATPase (sodium pump) in the basolateral membranes. Each cycle of this enzyme extrudes three sodium ions and imports two potassium ions. Potassium, which would otherwise accumulate within the cells, diffuses out passively through channels located in the basolateral membranes. In aldosterone-sensitive principal cells, however, potassium channels called ROMK channels (for renal outer medullary K+) are also present in the luminal membranes. Aldosterone-driven movement of sodium from the lumen to the extracellular space in these cells may thus be accompanied by secretion of potassium into the tubular lumen. Although potassium secretion depends upon sodium reabsorption, the ratio of these ion movements is not constant. Rather, the amount of potassium

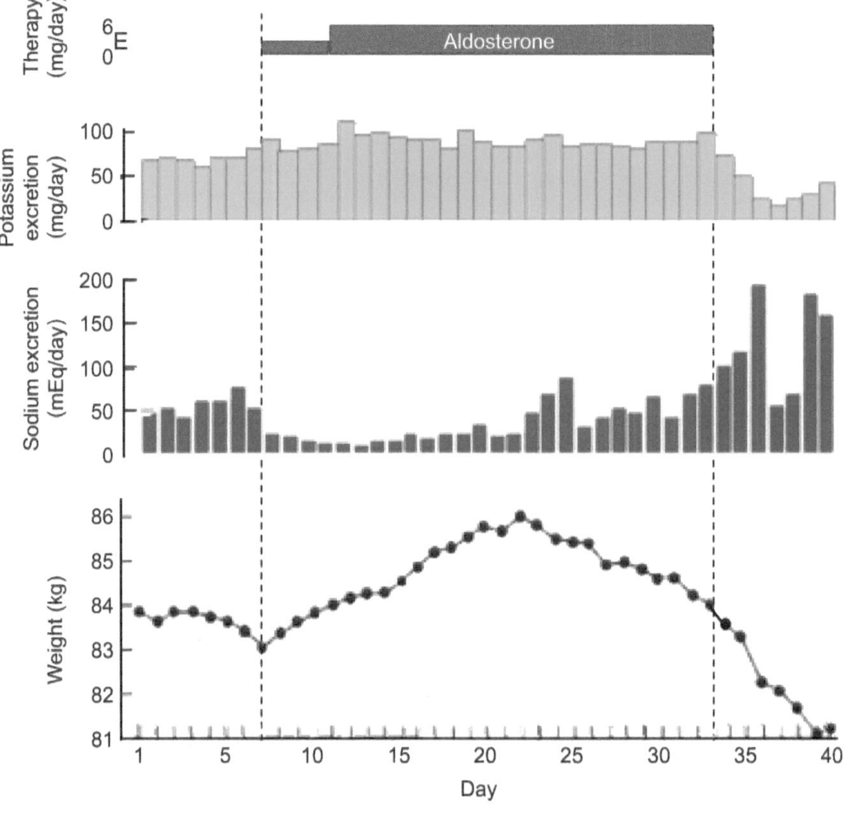

FIGURE 4.29 Effects of continuous administration of aldosterone to a normal man. Aldosterone (3–6 mg/day) increased potassium excretion and sodium retention represented here as a decrease in urinary sodium. The increased retention of sodium, which continued for 2 weeks, caused fluid retention and hence an increase in body weight. The subject "escaped" from the sodium-retaining effects but continued to excrete increased amounts of potassium for as long as aldosterone was given. Source: *From August, J.T., Nelson, D.H., & Thorn, G.W. (1958). Response of normal subjects to large amounts of aldosterone.* Journal of Clinical Investigation, 37, *1549–1559.*

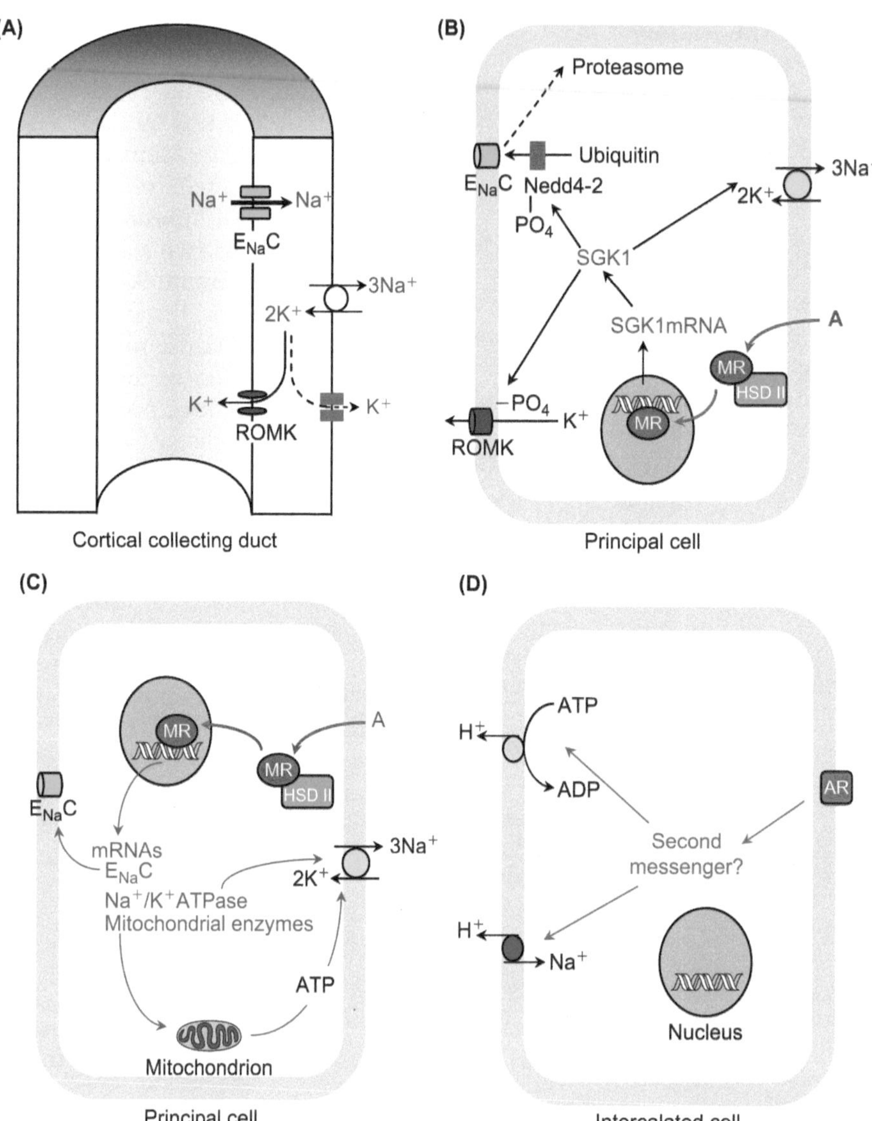

FIGURE 4.30 Proposed mechanisms of action of aldosterone in the kidney. (A) Sodium enters principal cells in the cortical collecting ducts through ENaC and is extruded into the interstitium by the sodium/potassium ATPase. Potassium exits through *ROMK* channels in the luminal surface or through basolateral potassium channels. (B) After a delay of ~30 min aldosterone increases expression of the serum/glucocorticoid-regulated kinase 1 (*SGK*). SGK1 increases ENaC in luminal membranes by phosphorylating and inactivating the ubiquitin ligase *Nedd4-2* that initiates ENaC retrieval. SGK1 also phosphorylates and increases the activity of ROMK channels. (C) Later effects of aldosterone include increased expression of proteins associated with increased sodium transport. (D) In intercalated cells, aldosterone promotes the secretion of protons by a mechanism that bypasses the nucleus and probably involves an aldosterone receptor on the cell surface (*AR*) acting through some second messenger. *AR*, Androgen receptor; *ENaC*, epithelial sodium channels; *HSD II*, 11-hydroxysteroid dehydrogenase II; *MR*, mineralocorticoid receptor; *ROMK*, renal outer medullary K.

that diffuses back into the extracellular space or that enters the tubular lumen is determined by the relative strengths of the electrochemical gradients across the luminal and basolateral membranes, and these in turn are determined by the potassium concentration of the interstitial fluid and the composition and rate of flow of tubular fluid (Fig. 4.30A).

Aldosterone increases the entry of sodium into the principal cells by increasing the abundance of functional epithelial sodium channels (ENaC) in the luminal membranes of the principal cells. This action of aldosterone requires a lag period of at least 30 minutes, is sensitive to inhibitors of RNA and protein synthesis, and is mediated by transcriptional events initiated by nuclear receptors (see Chapter 1: Introduction). That is, after binding to the mineralocorticoid receptor the aldosterone–receptor complex binds to hormone response elements that regulate transcription of certain genes. Surface expression of ENaC depends equally on the rates of insertion by exocytosis and retrieval by endocytosis. Aldosterone upregulates expression of genes whose products directly or indirectly enhance insertion and delay retrieval of ENaC. Epithelial sodium channels are composed of α, β, and γ subunits whose assembly in the endoplasmic reticulum is essential for transfer to the Golgi apparatus where the channels are proteolytically activated and dispatched to the luminal membrane. The channels are retrieved from the luminal membrane by endocytosis after a relatively short half-life. Retrieval of ENaC depends upon its ubiquitylation by the ubiquitin ligase Nedd4-2 and subsequent transfer to proteasomes for destruction.

One of the important proteins that is upregulated early in the response to aldosterone is the serum/glucocorticoid-regulated kinase 1 (SGK1). In the principal cells SGK1 phosphorylates and inactivates Nedd4-2, thereby prolonging the half-life of ENaC in the luminal membrane (Fig. 4.30B).

Aldosterone upregulates expression of the ENaC α subunit and therefore the abundance and availability of the channels. The rate of entry of sodium at the luminal surface of the principal cells is limited by the rate of extrusion at the basolateral surface. Aldosterone increases the expression and surface activity of the sodium/potassium ATPase in the basolateral membranes, and increases the capacity for ATP generation by promoting synthesis of some enzymes of the citric acid cycle in mitochondria, particularly isocitrate dehydrogenase (Fig. 4.30C).

In addition, aldosterone increases the activity of ROMK channels in the luminal membrane through phosphorylation by SGK1 and may also increase their surface abundance.

The intercalated cells in the distal nephron and collecting duct are also targets of aldosterone action. Aldosterone stimulates these cells to excrete hydrogen ions by increasing the activity and abundance of an electrogenic proton pump (H^+ATPase) in their luminal membranes and perhaps stimulating the activity of a sodium/hydrogen ion exchanger. At least some aspects of this effect are too rapid to be dependent on transcription and may be mediated by membrane-bound rather than nuclear receptors (Fig. 4.30D). This nongenomically mediated action of aldosterone appears to involve activation of protein kinase C, but the proteins phosphorylated by protein kinase C have not been identified. Transcriptional changes in the intercalated cells also contribute to these effects. Aldosterone-stimulated excretion of protons lowers the hydrogen ion concentration of the plasma, which indirectly lowers the potassium concentration, and thereby reinforces the kaliuretic (potassium losing) effect produced by the principal cells. Decreases in plasma hydrogen ion concentrations cause cells to release hydrogen ions into the extracellular fluid in exchange for potassium ions, which are taken up from the extracellular fluid. This effect may be augmented by the rapid nongenomic effect of aldosterone to decrease intracellular hydrogen ion concentrations by stimulating sodium hydrogen exchangers in the plasma membranes of cells throughout the body.

Aldosterone also regulates sodium and potassium movements in extrarenal tissues in the same manner as in renal principal cells. Aldosterone promotes the absorption of sodium and secretion of potassium in the colon and decreases the ratio of sodium to potassium concentrations in sweat and salivary secretions. The concentrations of sodium chloride and potassium in the initial secretions of sweat and saliva are similar to those of plasma. Epithelial cells of the secretory ducts modify the ionic composition of the fluid as it flows from its site of generation to the site of release. Aldosterone stimulates ductal epithelial cells and cells lining the colon to reabsorb sodium and secrete potassium by the same mechanisms as described for the renal cells. Because perspiration can be an important avenue for sodium loss, minimizing sodium loss in sweat is physiologically significant. Persons suffering from adrenal insufficiency are especially sensitive to extended exposure to a hot environment and may become severely dehydrated.

Regulation of aldosterone secretion

Angiotensin II is the primary stimulus for aldosterone secretion, although ACTH and high concentrations of potassium are also potent stimuli. Angiotensin II is formed in blood by a two-step process that depends upon proteolytic cleavage of the plasma protein, angiotensinogen, by the enzyme renin, to release the inactive decapeptide angiotensin I. Angiotensin I is then converted to angiotensin II by the ubiquitous angiotensin-converting enzyme. Control of angiotensin II production is achieved by regulating the secretion of renin from smooth muscle cells of the afferent glomerular arterioles. The principal stimulus for renin secretion is a decrease in the vascular volume. Although aldosterone secretion is regulated by negative feedback, its concentration in plasma is not the controlled variable that regulates renin secretion. Regulation of renin secretion is discussed further in Chapter 9, Regulation of Salt and Water Balance.

The principal physiological role of aldosterone is to defend the vascular volume. Reabsorption of sodium in the kidney is accompanied by a proportionate reabsorption of water, and because sodium remains extracellular, its retention expands the extracellular volume and hence blood volume. Conversely, loss of body sodium results in contraction of the vascular volume and signals increased renin and aldosterone secretion (Fig. 4.28).

Although preservation of body sodium is central to aldosterone action, the concentration of sodium in blood does not appear to be monitored directly, and fluctuations in plasma concentrations have little direct effect on the secretion of renin.

Unlike the plasma concentration of sodium, the concentration of potassium is directly monitored by the adrenal glomerulosa cells, which, as already mentioned, respond to increases with increased secretion of aldosterone. By stimulating potassium excretion, aldosterone lowers the plasma potassium concentration and thus decreases the stimulus for its secretion. The relationship between plasma potassium and aldosterone thus constitutes a second negative feedback loop that also regulates aldosterone secretion (Fig. 4.31).

Dual control mechanisms require mechanisms for integration of reinforcing or conflicting demands. Integration is achieved largely through the modulating effect of potassium on the response to angiotensin II. Reinforcement intensifies with increasing plasma potassium concentrations. Glomerulosa cells are most sensitive to angiotensin when vascular volume is decreased and potassium concentrations are high. When plasma volume is expanded, hyperkalemia-induced secretion of aldosterone promotes potassium excretion without causing further sodium retention as a result of renal compensatory mechanisms. When hypovolemia is accompanied by hypokalemia, maintenance of plasma volume takes precedence, and plasma concentrations of potassium may not be reduced further as low potassium concentrations in tubular and interstitial fluid favor potassium reabsorption. The roles of angiotensin II and aldosterone in the overall regulation of water and ionic balance are considered further in Chapter 9, Regulation of Salt and Water Balance.

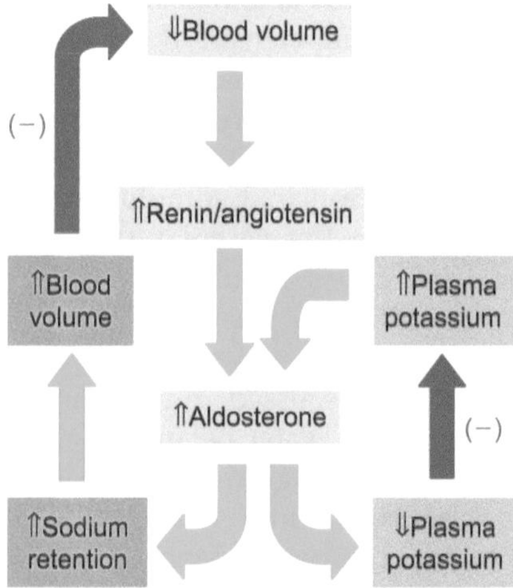

FIGURE 4.31 Dual negative feedback control of aldosterone secretion. One monitored variable is blood volume, and another is the plasma potassium concentration (see text for details).

Physiology of the glucocorticoids

Although named for their critical role in maintaining carbohydrate reserves, glucocorticoids produce diverse physiological actions, many of which are still not well understood and therefore can be considered only phenomenologically. Virtually, every tissue of the body is affected by an excess or deficiency of glucocorticoids (Fig. 4.9 and Table 4.2).

If any simple phrase could describe the role of glucocorticoids, it would be "coping with adversity." Even if sodium balance could be preserved and carbohydrate intake was adequate to meet energy needs, individuals suffering from adrenal insufficiency would still teeter on the brink of disaster when faced with a threatening environment. We shall consider here only the most thoroughly studied actions of glucocorticoids.

Effects on energy metabolism

Ability to maintain and draw on metabolic fuel reserves is ensured by actions and interactions of many hormones and is critically dependent on normal function of the adrenal cortex. Although we speak of maintaining carbohydrate reserves as the hallmark of glucocorticoid activity, it must be understood that metabolism of carbohydrate, protein, and in the absence of adrenal function, even relatively short periods of fasting may produce a catastrophic decrease in blood sugar (hypoglycemia) accompanied by depletion of muscle and liver glycogen. A drastically compromised ability to produce sugar from nonglucose precursors (gluconeogenesis) forces these individuals to rely almost exclusively on dietary sugars to meet their carbohydrate needs. Their metabolic problems are complicated further by decreased ability to access alternate substrates such as fatty acids and protein. Glucocorticoids promote hepatic gluconeogenesis and glycogen storage in liver and muscle by complementary mechanisms (Fig. 4.32).

1 Extrahepatic actions provide substrate. Glucocorticoids promote proteolysis and inhibit protein synthesis in muscle and lymphoid tissues, thereby causing amino acids to be released into the blood. In addition, they increase blood glycerol concentrations by acting with other hormones to increase breakdown of triglycerides in adipose tissue.

TABLE 4.2 Some effects of glucocorticoids.

Tissue	Effects
Central nervous system	Taste, hearing and smell: ↑in acuity with adrenal cortical insufficiency and ↓ in Cushing's disease
	↑CRH synthesis and secretion ↓ADH secretion
Cardiovascular system	Maintains sensitivity to epinephrine and norepinephrine
	↑Sensitivity to vasoconstrictor agents
	Maintains microcirculation
Gastrointestinal tract	↑Gastric acid secretion
	↓Gastric mucosal cell proliferation
Liver	↑Gluconeogenesis
Lungs	↑Maturation and surfactant production during fetal development
Pituitary	↓ ACTH secretion and synthesis
Kidney	↑GFR
	Required for excretion of dilute urine (free water clearance)
Bone	↑Resorption
	↓Formation
Muscle	↓Fatigue (probably secondary to cardiovascular actions)
	↑Protein catabolism
	↓Glucose oxidation
	↓Insulin sensitivity
	↓Protein synthesis
Immune system (see text)	↓Mass of thymus and lymph nodes
	↓Blood concentrations of eosinophils, basophils, and lymphocytes
	↓Cellular immunity
Connective tissue	↓Activity of fibroblasts
	↓Collagen synthesis

ACTH, Adrenocorticotropic hormone; *ADH*, antidiuretic hormone; *CRH*, Corticotropin-releasing hormone; *GFR*, Glomerular filtration rate.

2 Hepatic actions enhance the flow of glucose precursors through existing enzymatic machinery and induce the synthesis of additional gluconeogenic and glycogen-forming enzymes along with enzymes needed to convert amino acids to usable precursors of carbohydrate.

Nitrogen excretion during fasting is lower than normal with adrenal insufficiency, reflecting decreased conversion of amino acids to glucose. High concentrations of glucocorticoids, as seen in states of adrenal hyperfunction, inhibit protein synthesis and promote rapid breakdown of muscle and lymphoid tissues that serve as repositories for stored protein. These effects result in increased blood urea nitrogen (BUN) and enhanced nitrogen excretion. Individuals with hyperfunction of the adrenal cortex (Cushing's disease) characteristically have spindly arms and legs, reflecting increased breakdown of their muscle protein. Protein wasting in these patients may also extend to skin and connective tissue, and it contributes to their propensity to bruise easily.

Glucocorticoids defend against hypoglycemia in yet another way. In experimental animals, glucocorticoids decrease utilization of glucose by muscle and adipose tissue and lower the responsiveness of these tissues to insulin. Prolonged exposure to high levels of glucocorticoids often leads to diabetes mellitus (see Chapter 7: The Pancreatic Islets); about 20% of patients with Cushing disease are also diabetic, and virtually, all the remainders have some milder impairment of glucose metabolism. Decreased utilization of glucose coupled

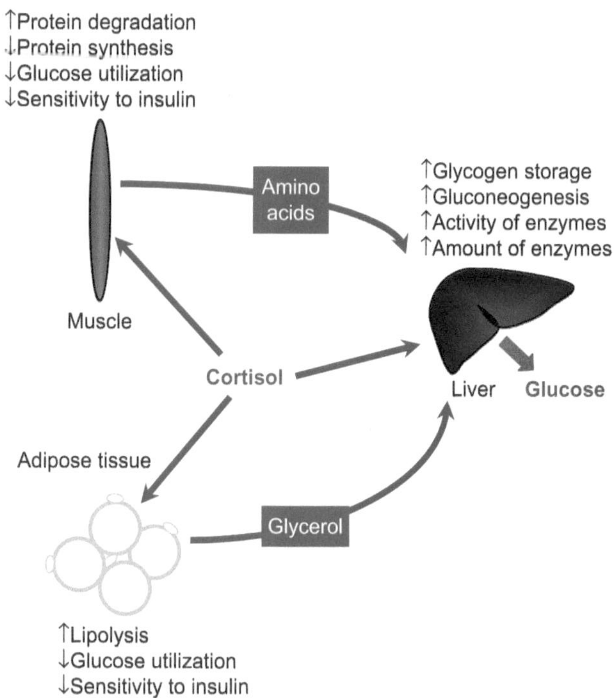

FIGURE 4.32 Principal effects of glucocorticoids on glucose production and the metabolism of body fuels.

with increased gluconeogenesis leads to increased storage of glucose as glycogen in muscles and liver. Despite the relative decrease in insulin sensitivity and increased tendency for fat mobilization seen in experimental animals, patients with Cushing's disease paradoxically accumulate fat in the face (moon face), between the shoulders (buffalo hump), and in the abdomen (truncal obesity). These tissues are particularly sensitive to the effects of glucocorticoids on fat cell differentiation (see Chapter 8: Hormonal Regulation of Fuel Metabolism).

Effects on water balance

In the absence of the adrenal glands, renal plasma flow and glomerular filtration are reduced and it is difficult to produce either concentrated or dilute urine. One of the diagnostic tests for adrenal cortical insufficiency is the rapidity with which a water load can be excreted. Glucocorticoids facilitate excretion of free water and are more important in this regard than mineralocorticoids. The mechanism for this effect is still debated. It has been suggested that glucocorticoids may maintain normal rates of glomerular filtration by acting directly on glomeruli or glomerular blood flow, or indirectly by facilitating the action or production of the atrial natriuretic hormone (see Chapter 9: Regulation of Salt and Water Balance). In addition, in the absence of glucocorticoids antidiuretic hormone (vasopressin) secretion is increased.

Effects on lung development

One of the dramatic physiological changes that must be accommodated in the newborn infant is the shift from the placenta to the lungs as site of oxygen and carbon dioxide exchange. Glucocorticoids play a crucial role in maturation of alveoli and production of surfactant, which facilitates expansion of the lungs. Surfactant, consisting largely of phospholipids and some protein, reduces alveolar surface tension, which increases lung compliance and allows even distribution of inspired air.

One of the major problems of preterm delivery is a condition known as respiratory distress syndrome caused by impaired pulmonary ventilation resulting from incomplete development of pulmonary alveoli and production of surfactant. Although the fetal adrenal gland is capable of secreting some glucocorticoids by about the 24th week of pregnancy, its major secretory products are androgens that serve as precursors for placental estrogen synthesis (see Chapter 14: Hormonal Control of Pregnancy and Lactation). Only in the final months of pregnancy does fetal production of glucocorticoids become sufficient to stimulate maturation of the lungs and other systems. Large doses of glucocorticoid given to women carrying fetuses at risk for premature delivery diminish the incidence of respiratory distress syndrome by promoting thinning of the alveolar walls and inducing transcription of genes that code for proteins found in surfactant. Steady-state levels of mRNA for surfactant proteins may be reached within about 15 hours after exposure of fetuses to glucocorticoids.

Glucocorticoids and responses to injury

One of the most remarkable effects of glucocorticoids was discovered almost by chance during the late 1940s when it was observed that glucocorticoids dramatically reduced the severity of disease in patients suffering from rheumatoid arthritis. This observation, in addition to leading to the award of a Nobel Prize, called attention to the antiinflammatory effects of glucocorticoids, which have been considered by some investigators to be pharmacological side effects because supraphysiological concentrations are needed to produce these effects therapeutically. As understanding of the antiinflammatory actions has increased, however, it has become clear that glucocorticoids are physiological modulators of the inflammatory response. It is likely that free cortisol concentrations are higher at local sites of tissue injury than in the general circulation. Partial degradation of CBG by the proteolytic enzyme, elastase, secreted by activated mononuclear leukocytes releases cortisol from its binding protein and increases its concentration locally at the site of inflammation. In addition, upregulation of 11β-HSD I by inflammatory mediators results in conversion of circulating cortisone to cortisol within the inflammatory cells in which it acts.

As might be anticipated, glucocorticoids and related compounds devised by the pharmaceutical industry are exceedingly important therapeutic agents for treating such diverse conditions as poison ivy, asthma, a host of inflammatory conditions, and various autoimmune diseases. The latter reflects their related ability to diminish the immune response.

Antiinflammatory effects

Inflammation is the term used to encompass the various responses of tissues to injury. It is characterized by redness, heat, swelling, pain, and loss of function (Fig. 4.33).

Redness and heat are manifestations of increased blood flow and result from vasodilation. Swelling is due to formation of a protein-rich exudate that collects because capillaries and venules become leaky to proteins. Pain is caused by chemical products of cellular injury and sometimes by mechanical injury to nerve endings. Loss of function may be a direct consequence of injury or secondary to the pain and swelling that injury evokes. An intimately related component of the early response to tissue injury is the recruitment of white blood cells to the injured area and the subsequent unfolding of the immune response.

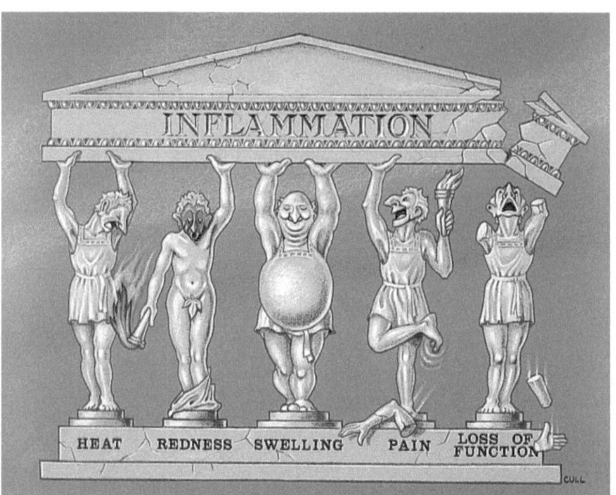

FIGURE 4.33 The five signs of inflammation. The first four were described in Roman times by Celsus, a Roman physician, who chose not to practice because it was considered beneath his aristocratic class to do so. The last one, disordered cellular function, was described in the 1800s by Dr. Rudolf Virchow, the founder of modern cellular pathology. Source: *From Figure 2-1 in Damjanov, I. (2017).* Pathology for the health professions *(5th ed., p. 24). Elsevier.*

The initial pattern of the inflammatory response is independent of the injurious agent or causal event. This response is presumably defensive and may be a necessary antecedent of the repair process. Increased blood flow accelerates delivery of the white blood cells that combat invading foreign substances or organisms and clean up the debris of injured and dead cells. Increased blood flow also facilitates dissemination of chemo-attractants to white blood cells and promotes their migration to the site of injury. In addition, increased blood flow provides more oxygen and nutrients to cells at the site of damage and facilitates removal of toxins and wastes. Increased permeability of the microvasculature allows fluid to accumulate in the extravascular space in the vicinity of the injury and thus dilute noxious agents.

Although we are accustomed to thinking of physiological responses as having beneficial effects, it is apparent that some aspects of inflammation may actually cause or magnify tissue damage. Lysosomal hydrolases released during phagocytosis of cellular debris or invading organisms may damage nearby cells that were not harmed by the initial insult. Loss of fluid from the microvasculature at the site of the injury may increase blood viscosity, slowing its flow, and even leaving some capillaries clogged with stagnant red blood cells. Decreased perfusion may cause further cell damage. In addition, massive disseminated fluid loss into the extravascular space sometimes compromises cardiovascular function. Consequently, long term survival demands that checks and balances be in place to prevent the defensive and positive aspects of the inflammatory response from becoming destructive. We may regard the physiological role of the glucocorticoids to modulate inflammatory responses as a major component of such checks and balances. Exaggeration of such physiological modulation with supraphysiological amounts of glucocorticoids upsets the balance in favor of suppression of inflammation and provides the therapeutic efficacy of pharmacological treatment.

Inflammation is initiated, sustained, and amplified by the release of a large number of chemical mediators derived from multiple sources. Cytokines are a diverse group of peptides that range in size from about 8 to about 40 kDa and are produced mainly by cells of the hematopoietic and immune systems, but they can be synthesized and secreted by virtually any cell. Cytokines may promote or antagonize development of inflammation or have a mixture of pro- and antiinflammatory effects depending upon the particular cells involved. Prostaglandins and leukotrienes are released principally from vascular endothelial cells and macrophages, but virtually all cell types can produce and release them. They may also produce either pro- or antiinflammatory effects depending upon the particular compound formed and the cells acted upon. Histamine and serotonin are released from mast cells and platelets. Enzymes and superoxides released from dead or dying cells or from cells that remove debris by phagocytosis contribute directly and indirectly to the spread of inflammation by activating other mediators (e.g., bradykinin) and leukocyte attractants that arise from humoral precursors associated with the immune and clotting systems. Glucocorticoids modulate virtually all aspects of the inflammatory response by multiple tissue-specific actions that modulate synthesis, secretion, and actions of inflammatory mediators.

Glucocorticoids and the metabolites of arachidonic acid prostaglandins and the closely related leukotrienes are derived from the polyunsaturated essential fatty acid arachidonic acid (Fig. 4.34).

Because of their 20-carbon backbone sometimes they are referred to collectively as eicosanoids. These compounds play a central role in the inflammatory response. They generally act locally on the cells that produced them and on cells in the immediate vicinity of their production, but some also survive in blood long enough to act on distant tissues. Prostaglandins act directly on blood vessels to cause vasodilation and indirectly increase vascular permeability by potentiating the actions of histamine and bradykinin. Prostaglandins sensitize nerve endings of pain fibers to other mediators of inflammation such as histamine, serotonin, bradykinin, and substance P, thereby increasing sensitivity to touch (hyperalgesia).

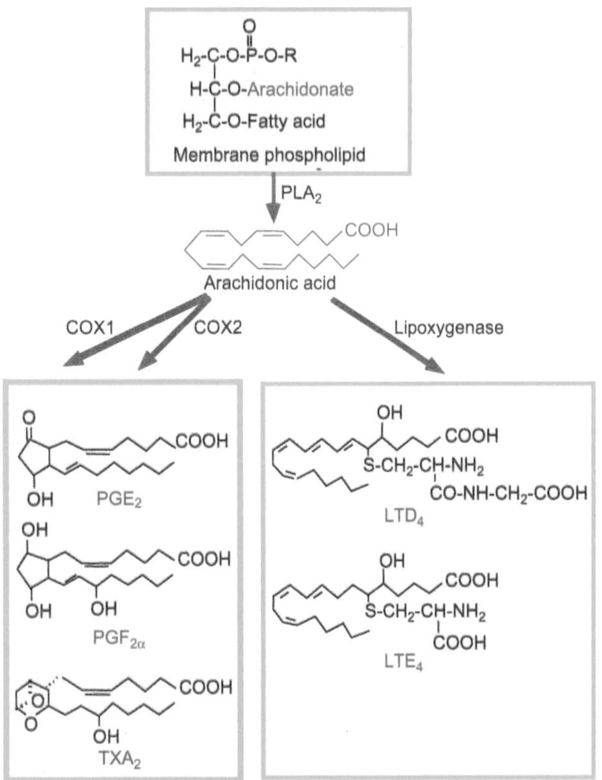

FIGURE 4.34 Synthesis and structures of some arachidonic acid metabolites. *R* may be choline, inositol, serine, or ethanolamine. The designations E_2 or $F_2\alpha$ refer to substituents on the ring structure of the PG. The designations *D4* and *E4* refer to glutathione derivatives in thioester linkage at carbon 6 of LT. *COX*, Cyclo-oxygenase; *LT*, leukotriene; *PG*, prostaglandin; PLA_2, phospholipase A_2; *TX*, thromboxane.

The leukotrienes stimulate production of cytokines and act directly on the microvasculature to increase permeability. Leukotrienes also attract white blood cells to sites of injury and increase their stickiness to vascular endothelium. The physiology of arachidonate metabolites is complex, and a thorough discussion is not possible here. There are a large number of these compounds with different biological activities. Although some eicosanoids have antiinflammatory actions that may limit the overall inflammatory response, arachidonic acid derivatives are major contributors to inflammation.

Arachidonic acid is released from membrane phospholipids by phospholipase A2 (PLA2; see Chapter 1: Introduction), which is activated by injury, phagocytosis, or a variety of other stimuli in responsive cells. Activation is mediated by a cytosolic PLA2 activating protein that closely resembles a protein in bee venom called melittin. In addition, PLA2 activity also increases as a result of increased enzyme synthesis. The first step in the conversion of arachidonate to prostaglandins is catalyzed by a cytosolic enzyme, cyclooxygenase. One isoform of this enzyme, called COX1, is constitutively expressed. A second form, COX2, is induced by cytokine mediators of the inflammatory response. Glucocorticoids suppress the formation of prostaglandins by inhibiting synthesis of COX2 and probably also by inducing expression of proteins that inhibit PLA2 and other enzymes in the prostaglandin synthetic pathway. Glucocorticoids stimulate expression of annexin I, which may mediate many of its effects on prostaglandin synthesis. Nonsteroidal antiinflammatory drugs such as indomethacin and aspirin also block the cyclooxygenase reaction catalyzed by both COX1 and COX2. Some of the newer antiinflammatory drugs specifically block COX2. Because prostaglandins produce varied and widespread effects, blockade of their production with cyclooxygenase inhibitors may produce undesirable long-term consequences.

Glucocorticoids and cytokines

The large number of compounds, perhaps 100 or more, designated as cytokines include one or more isoforms of the interleukins (IL-1−32), the tumor necrosis factor (TNF) family, the interferons (IFN-α, -β,-γ), colony stimulating factor (CSF), granulocyte-macrophage CSF, transforming growth factor family, leukemia inhibiting factor, oncostatin, and a variety of cell or tissue-specific growth factors. It is not clear just how many of these hormone-like molecules are produced. Not all have a role in inflammation, and a general discussion of cytokine biology is beyond the scope of this text. However, two cytokines, IL-1 and TNF-α, are particularly important in the development of inflammation and in the physiology of the glucocorticoids. The intracellular signaling pathways and biological actions of these two cytokines are remarkably similar. They enhance each other's actions in the inflammatory response, which differ only in the respect that TNF-α may promote cell death (apoptosis) whereas IL-1 does not.

IL-1 is produced primarily by macrophages and to a lesser extent by other connective tissue elements, skin, and endothelial cells. Its release from macrophages is stimulated by interaction with immune complexes, activated lymphocytes, and metabolites of arachidonic acid, especially leukotrienes. IL-1 is not stored in its cells of origin but is synthesized and secreted within hours of stimulation in a response mediated by increased intracellular calcium and protein kinase C (see Chapter 1: Introduction). IL-1 acts on many cells to produce a variety of responses, all of which are components of the inflammatory/immune response. They are illustrated in Fig. 4.35.

Many of the consequences of these actions can be recognized from personal experience as nonspecific symptoms of viral infection.

TNF-α also is produced in macrophages and other cells in response to injury and immune complexes and can act on many cells including those that secrete it. Secretion of both IL-1 and TNF-α and their receptors are increased by some of the cytokines and other mediators of inflammation whose production they increase, so that an amplifying positive feedback cascade is set in motion. Some products of these cytokines also feedback on their production in a negative way to modulate the inflammatory response. Glucocorticoids play an important role as negative modulators of IL-1 and TNF-α effect by inhibiting their production, by interfering with their signaling pathways, and by inhibiting the actions of their products. Glucocorticoids also interfere with the production and release of other proinflammatory cytokines as well, including IFN-γ, IL-2, IL-6, and IL-8, among others.

Production of IL-1 and TNF-α and many of their effects on target cells are mediated by activation of genes by the transcription factor, nuclear factor kappa B (NF-κB). In the inactivated state NF-κB resides in the cytoplasm bound to NF-κB inhibitor protein (I-κB). Stimulation of the signaling cascade by some tissue insult or the binding of IL-1 and TNF-α to their respective receptors is initiated by activation of a kinase that phosphorylates I-κB, which causes it to dissociate from NF-κB and to be degraded. Free NF-κB then is able to migrate to the nucleus where it binds to response elements in genes that it regulates, including genes for

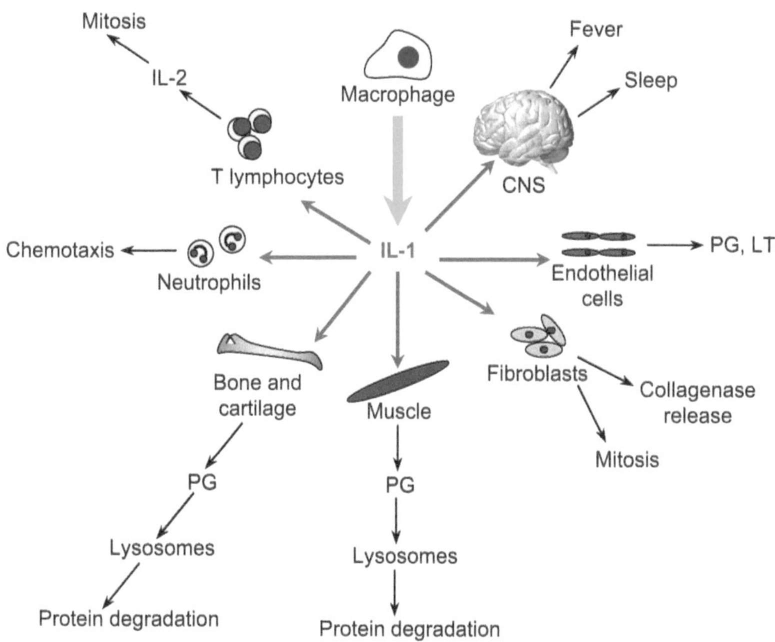

FIGURE 4.35 Effects of *IL-1*. *IL-1*, Interleukin-1; *LT*, leukotriene; *PG*, prostaglandin.

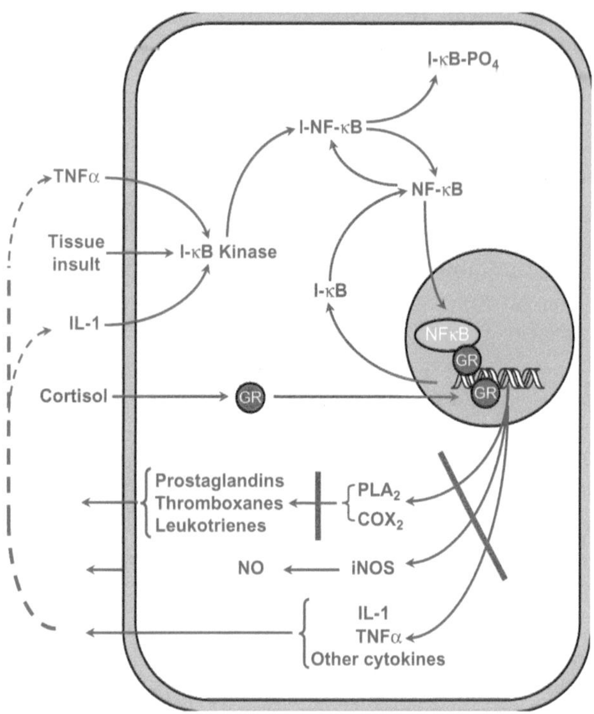

FIGURE 4.36 Antiinflammatory actions of cortisol. Cortisol induces the formation of the *I-κB*, which binds to *NF-κB* and prevents it from entering the nucleus and activating target genes. The activated *GR* also interferes with NF-κB binding to its response elements in DNA thus preventing the induction of *PLA2, COX2*, and the iNOS. By blocking further production of *TNF-α* and *IL-1* glucocorticoids disrupt the positive feedback cycle involving these cytokines. *COX2*, Cyclo-oxygenase 2; *GR*, glucocorticoid receptor; *IL-1*, interleukin-1; iNOS, inducible nitric oxide synthase; *I-κB*, inhibitor of nuclear factor κB; *NF-κB*, nuclear factor κB; *NO*, nitric oxide; *PLA2*, phospholipase A2; *TNF-α*, tumor necrosis factor-α.

the cytokines IL-1, TNF-α, IL-6, and IL-8 and for such enzymes as PLA2, COX2, and nitric oxide synthase (Fig. 4.36).

IL-6 is an important proinflammatory cytokine that acts on the hypothalamus, liver, and other tissues. IL-8 plays an important role as a leukocyte attractant. Nitric oxide is important as a vasodilator and may have other effects as well.

Glucocorticoids interfere with the NF-κB-dependent effects of IL-1 and TNF-α in two ways. They promote the synthesis of I-κB, which traps NF-κB in the cytosol, and they interfere with the ability of NF-κB that enters the nucleus to activate target genes. The mechanism for interference with gene activation is thought to invoke protein: protein interaction between the glucocorticoid receptor and NF-κB so that access of NF-κB, coactivators, or the RNA polymerase to the promoter regions of affected genes is blocked. Glucocorticoids also interfere in similar ways with IL-1 or TNF-α-dependent activation of other genes by the AP-1 (activator protein-1) transcription complex. In addition, cortisol induces expression of annexin 1, which decreases prostaglandin synthesis by inhibiting PLA2 and destabilizing the mRNA for COX2. It is noteworthy that many of the responses attributed to IL-1 may be mediated by prostaglandins or other arachidonate metabolites. For example, IL-1, which is identical with what once was called endogenous pyrogen, may cause fever by inducing the formation of prostaglandins in the thermoregulatory center of the hypothalamus. Glucocorticoids therefore might exert their antipyretic effect at two levels: at the level of the macrophage by inhibiting IL-1 production, and at the level of the hypothalamus by interfering with prostaglandin synthesis.

Glucocorticoids and the release of other inflammatory mediators

Granulocytes, mast cells, and macrophages contain vesicles filled with serotonin, histamine, or degradative enzymes, all of which contribute to the inflammatory response. These mediators and lysosomal enzymes are released in response to arachidonate metabolites, cellular injury, reaction with antibodies, or during phagocytosis of invading pathogens. Glucocorticoids protect against the release of all these compounds by inhibiting cellular degranulation. It has been suggested that glucocorticoids inhibit histamine formation and stabilize lysosomal membranes, but the molecular mechanisms for these effects are unknown.

Glucocorticoids and the immune response

The immune system, whose function is destruction and elimination of foreign substances or organisms, has two major components: The B lymphocytes are formed in bone marrow and develop in liver or spleen, and the thymus-derived T lymphocytes. Humoral immunity is the province of B lymphocytes, which, upon differentiation into plasma cells, are responsible for production of antibodies. Large numbers of B lymphocytes circulate in blood or reside in lymph nodes. Reaction with a foreign substance (antigen) stimulates B cells to divide and produce a clone of cells capable of recognizing the antigen and producing antibodies to it. Such proliferation depends on cytokines released from the macrophages and helper T cells. Antibodies, which are circulating immunoglobulins, bind to foreign substances and thus mark them for destruction. By inhibiting cytokine production by macrophages and T cells, glucocorticoids decrease normal proliferation of B cells and reduce circulating concentrations of immunoglobulins. They may also act directly on B cells to inhibit antibody synthesis and may even kill B cells by apoptosis.

T cells are responsible for cellular immunity and participate in destruction of invading pathogens or cells that express foreign surface antigens as might follow viral infection or transformation into tumor cells. IL-1 stimulates T lymphocytes to produce IL-2, which promotes proliferation of T lymphocytes that have been activated by contact with antigens. Antigenic stimulation triggers the transient expression of IL-2 receptors only in those T cells that recognize the antigen. Consequently, only certain clones of T cells are stimulated to divide because there are no receptors for IL-2 on the surface membranes of T lymphocytes until they interact with their specific antigens. Glucocorticoids block the production, but probably not the response, to IL-2 and thereby inhibit proliferation of T lymphocytes. IL-2 also stimulates T lymphocytes to produce INF-γ, which participates in destruction of virus-infected or tumor cells and, in addition, stimulates macrophages to produce IL-1. Macrophages, T lymphocytes, and secretory products are thus arranged in a positive feedback relationship and produce a self-amplifying cascade of responses. Glucocorticoids restrain the cycle by suppressing production of each of the mediators (Fig. 4.37).

Glucocorticoids also activate programed cell death in some T lymphocytes.

The physiological implications of the suppressive effects of glucocorticoids on humoral and cellular immunity are incompletely understood. It has been suggested that suppression of the immune response might prevent development of autoimmunity that might otherwise follow from the release of fragments of injured cells. However, it must be pointed out that much of the immunosuppression produced by therapeutic doses of glucocorticoids requires concentrations that may never be reached under physiological conditions. High doses of glucocorticoids can so impair immune responses that relatively innocuous infections with some organisms can become overwhelming and cause death. Thus excessive antiimmune or antiinflammatory influences are just as damaging as unchecked immune or inflammatory responses. Under normal physiological circumstances, these influences are balanced and protective. Nevertheless, the immunosuppressive property of glucocorticoids is immensely important therapeutically, and high doses of glucocorticoids often are administered to combat rejection of transplanted tissues and to suppress various immune and allergic responses.

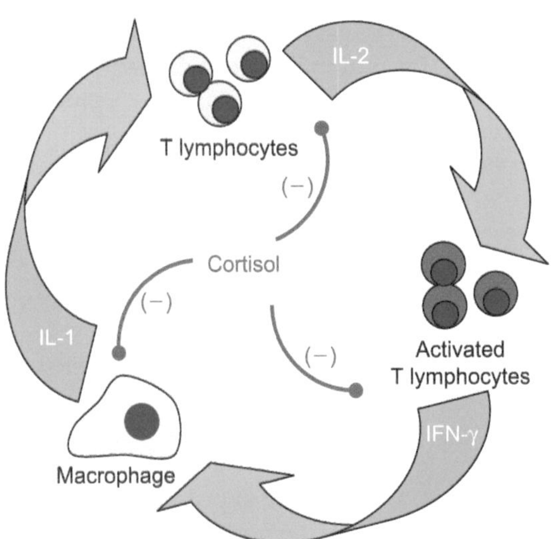

FIGURE 4.37 Cortisol inhibits proliferation of activated T cells by interfering with secretion of cytokines. *IFN-γ*, Interferon-γ; *IL-1*, interleukin-1; *IL-2*, interleukin-2.

Other effects of glucocorticoids on lymphoid tissues Sustained high concentrations of glucocorticoids produce a dramatic reduction in the mass of all lymphoid tissues including thymus, spleen, and lymph nodes. The thymus contains germinal centers for lymphocytes, and large numbers of T lymphocytes are formed and mature within it. Lymph nodes contain large numbers of both T and B lymphocytes. Immature lymphocytes of both lineages express glucocorticoid receptors and respond to hormonal stimulation by the same series of events as seen in other steroid-responsive cells except that the DNA transcribed contains the program for apoptosis. Although the physiological significance is not known, we have the unique situation of a hormone acting as a cytotoxic agent. Loss in mass of thymus and lymph nodes can be accounted for by the destruction of lymphocytes rather than the stromal or supporting elements. Mature lymphocytes and germinal centers are unresponsive to this action of glucocorticoids.

Glucocorticoids also decrease circulating levels of lymphocytes and particularly a class of white blood cells known as eosinophils (for their cytological staining properties). This decrease is partly due to the cytolytic effects described earlier and partly to sequestration in the spleen and lungs. Curiously, the total white blood cell count does not decrease because glucocorticoids also induce a substantial mobilization of neutrophils from bone marrow.

Maintenance of vascular responsiveness to catecholamines

A final action of glucocorticoids relevant to inflammation and the response to injury is maintenance of sensitivity of vascular smooth muscle to vasoconstrictor effects of norepinephrine released from autonomic nerve endings or the adrenal medulla. By counteracting local vasodilator effects of inflammatory mediators, norepinephrine decreases blood flow and limits the availability of fluid to form the inflammatory exudate. In addition, arteriolar constriction decreases capillary and venular pressure and favors reabsorption of extracellular fluid, thereby reducing swelling. The vasoconstrictor effect of norepinephrine is compromised in the absence of glucocorticoids. The mechanism for this action of glucocorticoids is not known, but at high concentrations, they may block inactivation of norepinephrine.

Adrenal cortical function during stress

During the mid-1930s the Canadian endocrinologist Hans Selye observed that animals respond to a variety of seemingly unrelated threatening or noxious circumstances with a characteristic pattern of changes that include an increase in size of the adrenal glands, involution of the thymus, and a decrease in the mass of all lymphoid tissues. He inferred that the adrenal glands are stimulated whenever an animal is exposed to any unfavorable circumstance, which he called "stress." Stress does not directly affect adrenal cortical function but, rather, increases the output of ACTH from the pituitary gland (see later). In fact, stress often is defined operationally by endocrinologists as any of the variety of conditions that increase ACTH secretion. Although it is clear that relatively benign changes in the internal or external environment may become lethal in the absence of the adrenal glands, we understand little more than Selye did about what cortisol might be doing to protect against stress. The favored experimental model used to investigate this problem was the adrenalectomized animal, which might have further complicated an already complex experimental question.

It is evident that many cellular functions require glucocorticoids either directly or indirectly for their maintenance. In addition, it has been found that glucocorticoids are required for normal responses to other hormones or to drugs, even though steroids themselves do not initiate similar responses in the absence of these agents. These findings suggest that these steroid hormones may govern some process that is fundamental to normal operation of most cells. Alternatively, emerging genomic data indicate that glucocorticoids directly or indirectly modulate expression of perhaps as many as 10,000 genes. Consequently, products of glucocorticoid-sensitive genes are likely to participate in a broad range of functions in virtually all cell types. Without glucocorticoids, many systems function only marginally even before the imposition of stress, and therefore any insult may prove overwhelming.

Treatment of adrenalectomized animals with a constant basal amount of glucocorticoid prior to and during a stressful incident prevents the devastating effects of stress and permits expression of expected responses to stimuli. This finding introduced the idea that glucocorticoids act in a normalizing, or permissive, way. That is, by maintaining normal operation of cells, glucocorticoids permit normal regulatory mechanisms to act. Because it was not necessary to increase the amounts of adrenal corticoids to ensure survival of stressed adrenalectomized animals, it was concluded that although their presence is essential, increased secretion of glucocorticoids was not required to combat stress. However, this conclusion is not consistent with clinical experience. Persons suffering from pituitary insufficiency or who have undergone hypophysectomy have severe difficulty withstanding stressful situations even though at other times they get along reasonably well on the small amounts of glucocorticoids produced by their adrenals in the absence of ACTH. Patients suffering from adrenal insufficiency are routinely given increased doses of glucocorticoids before undergoing surgery or other stressful procedures.

Mechanism of action of glucocorticoids

With few exceptions the physiological actions of the glucocorticoid hormones at the molecular level fit the general pattern of steroid hormone action described in Chapter 1, Introduction. The gene for the glucocorticoid receptor gives rise to two isoforms as a result of alternate splicing of RNA. The alpha isoform binds glucocorticoids, sheds its associated proteins, and migrates to the nucleus where it can form homodimers that bind to response elements in target genes. The beta isoform cannot bind hormone, is constitutively located in the nucleus, and apparently cannot bind to DNA. The beta isoform, however, can dimerize with the alpha isoform and diminish or block its ability to activate transcription or form protein:protein interactions with other transcription factors. Some evidence suggests that formation of the beta isoform may be a regulated process that modulates glucocorticoid responsiveness.

Glucocorticoids act on a great variety of cells and produce a wide range of effects that depend upon activating or suppressing transcription of specific genes. The ability to regulate different genes in different tissues presumably reflects differing accessibility of glucocorticoid-responsive genes to the activated glucocorticoid receptor in each differentiated cell type and presumably reflects the presence or absence of different coactivators and corepressors as well as differences in chromatin configuration. As described for NF-κB, glucocorticoids also inhibit expression of some genes that lack glucocorticoid response elements. Such inhibitory effects are thought to be the result of protein:protein interactions between the glucocorticoid receptor and other transcription factors to modify their ability to activate gene transcription. Through actions on histone acetylation, glucocorticoids may also modulate the accessibility of gene promoters to transcription regulators or to the RNA polymerase complex. The glucocorticoid receptor can be phosphorylated to various degrees on serine residues. Phosphorylation may modulate its affinity for hormone, or DNA, or for coactivators or repressors. Finally, glucocorticoids may also affect gene expression posttranscriptionally by restraining export of mRNA from nucleus to ribosomes, by destabilizing and shortening mRNA half-lives, and by interfering with mRNA translation.

Regulation of glucocorticoid secretion

Secretion of glucocorticoids is regulated by the anterior pituitary gland through the hormone ACTH, whose effects on the inner zones of the adrenal cortex were described earlier. In the absence of ACTH the concentration of cortisol in blood decreases to very low values, and the inner zones of the adrenal cortex atrophy. Regulation of ACTH secretion requires vascular contact between the hypothalamus and the anterior lobe of the pituitary gland and is driven primarily by corticotropin-releasing hormone (CRH). CRH containing neurons are distributed widely in the forebrain and brainstem but are concentrated heavily in the paraventricular nuclei in close association with vasopressin-secreting neurons. They stimulate the pituitary to secrete ACTH by releasing CRH into the hypophyseal portal system capillaries (see Chapter 2: Pituitary Gland). Vasopressin [arginine vasopressin (AVP)] also exerts an important influence on ACTH secretion by augmenting the response to CRH. AVP is cosecreted with CRH particularly in response to stress. It should be noted that the AVP that is secreted into the hypophyseal portal vessels along with CRH arises in a different population of paraventricular neurons from those that produce the AVP that is secreted by the posterior lobe of the pituitary in response to changes in blood osmolality or volume (see Chapter 2: Pituitary Gland).

Upon stimulation with ACTH, the adrenal cortex secretes cortisol, which inhibits further secretion of ACTH in a typical negative feedback arrangement (Fig. 4.38).

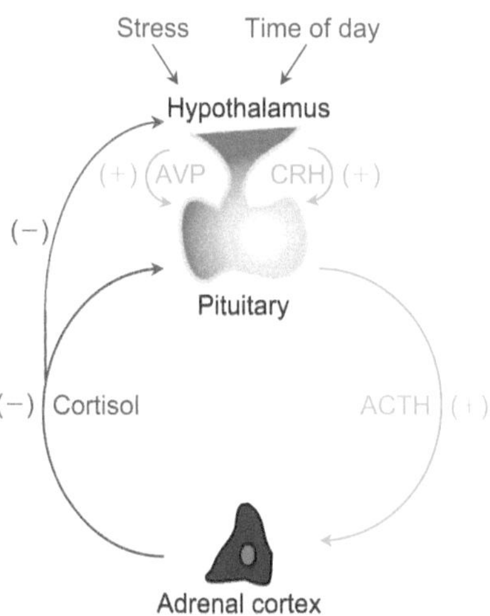

FIGURE 4.38 Negative feedback control of glucocorticoid secretion. (+), Stimulates; (−), inhibits; *AVP*, arginine vasopressin; *CRH*, corticotropin-releasing hormone.

Cortisol exerts its inhibitory effects both on CRH neurons in the hypothalamus and on corticotropes in the anterior pituitary. These effects are mediated by the glucocorticoid receptor. The negative feedback effects on secretion depend upon transcription of genes that code for proteins that either activate potassium channels or block the effects of PKA catalyzed phosphorylation on these channels and may also act at the level of secretory vesicle trafficking. Initial actions of glucocorticoids suppress secretion of CRH and ACTH from storage granules. Subsequent actions of glucocorticoids result from inhibition of transcription of the genes for CRH and POMC in hypothalamic neurons and corticotropes, perhaps by direct interaction of the glucocorticoid receptor with transcription factors that regulate CRH and POMC expression. This feedback system closely resembles the one described earlier for regulation of thyroid hormone secretion (see Chapter 3: Thyroid Gland) even though the adrenal–ACTH system is much more dynamic and subject to episodic changes.

CRH binds to G protein–coupled receptors in the corticotrope membrane and activates adenylyl cyclase. The resulting increase in cyclic AMP activates protein kinase A, which directly or indirectly inhibits potassium outflow through at least two classes of potassium channels. Buildup of positive charge within the corticotrope makes the membrane potential less negative and results in calcium influx through activated voltage-sensitive calcium channels. Protein kinase A–dependent phosphorylation of calcium channels may enhance calcium entry by lowering their threshold for activation. Increased intracellular calcium and perhaps additional effects of protein kinase A on secretory vesicle trafficking trigger ACTH secretion. Protein kinase A also phosphorylates CREB, which initiates production of the AP-1 complex that activates POMC transcription. AVP binds to its G protein–coupled receptor and activates phospholipase C to cause the release of DAG and IP3. This action of AVP has little effect on ACTH secretion in the absence of CRH but amplifies the effects of ACTH on ACTH secretion without affecting synthesis. As described in Chapter 1, Introduction, IP3 stimulates release of calcium from

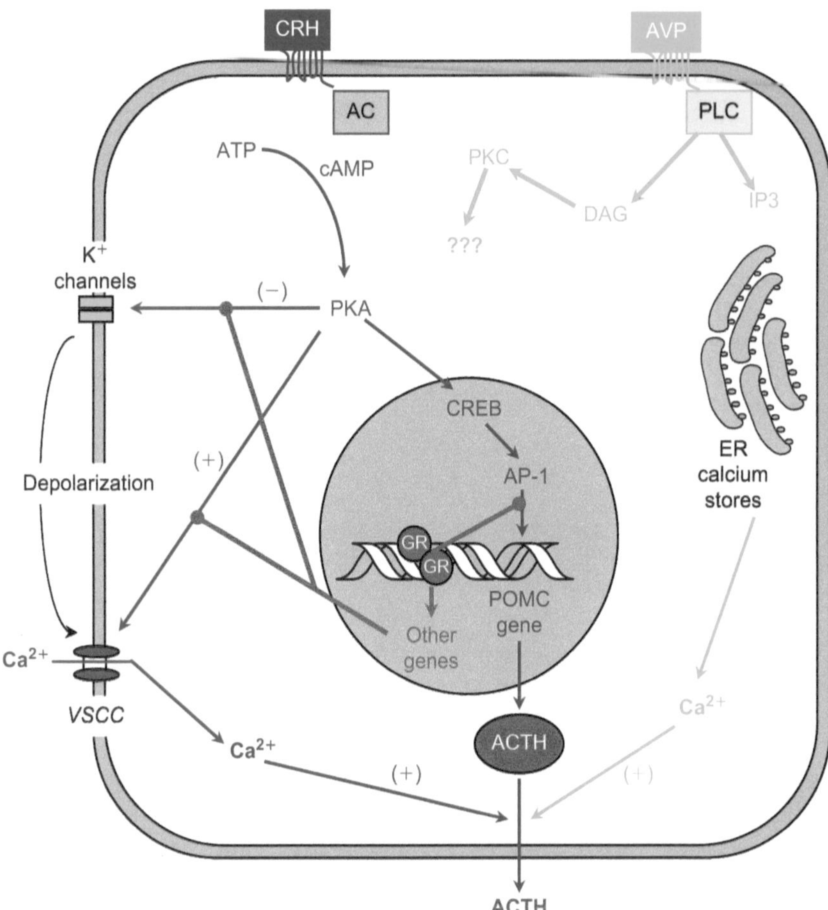

FIGURE 4.39 Hormonal interactions that regulate ACTH secretion by pituitary corticotrope. Glucocorticoids produce their negative feedback effects by interfering with POMC gene expression and membrane depolarization. *AC*, Adenylyl cyclase; *ACTH*, adrenocorticotropic hormone; *AP-1*, activator protein-1; *ATP*, adenosine triphosphate; *AVP*, arginine vasopressin; *cAMP*, cyclic adenosine monophosphate; *CREB*, cyclic AMP response element–binding protein; *CRH*, corticotropin-releasing hormone; *DAG*, diacylglycerol; *ER*, endoplasmic reticulum; *GR*, glucocorticoid receptor; *IP3*, inositol trisphosphate; *PKA*, protein kinase A; *PKC*, protein kinase C; *PLC*, phospholipase C; *POMC*, proopiomelanocortin; *VSCC*, voltage-sensitive calcium channels.

intracellular stores, and DAG activates protein kinase C, although the role of this enzyme in ACTH secretion is unknown. These effects are summarized in Fig. 4.39.

The relative importance of the pituitary and the CRH-producing neurons of the paraventricular nucleus for negative feedback regulation of ACTH secretion have been explored in mice that were made deficient in CRH by disruption of the CRH gene. These CRH knockout mice secrete normal amounts of ACTH and glucocorticoid under basal conditions, and their corticotropes express normal levels of mRNA for POMC. In normal mice, disruption of negative feedback by surgical removal of the adrenal glands results in a prompt increase both in POMC gene expression and ACTH secretion. Adrenalectomy of CRH knockout mice produced no increase in ACTH secretion, although POMC mRNA increased normally. These animals also suffer a severe impairment, but not total lack of ACTH secretion in response to stress. Thus it seems that basal function of the pituitary/adrenal negative feedback system does not require CRH, but that CRH is crucial for increasing ACTH secretion above basal levels. Further, it appears that transcription of the POMC gene is inhibited by glucocorticoids even under basal conditions. It was pointed out Chapter 1, Introduction, that negative feedback systems ensure constancy of the controlled variable. However, even in the absence of stress, ACTH and cortisol concentrations in blood plasma are not constant but oscillate within a 24-hour period. This so-called circadian rhythm is sensitive to the daily pattern of physical activity. For all but those who work the night shift, hormone levels are highest in the early morning hours just before arousal and lowest in the evening (Fig. 4.40).

This rhythmic pattern of ACTH secretion is consistent with the negative feedback model shown in Fig. 4.21 and is sensitive to glucocorticoid input throughout the day. In the negative feedback system the positive limb (CRH and ACTH secretion) is inhibited when the negative limb (cortisol concentration in blood) reaches some set point. For basal ACTH secretion the set point of the corticotropes and the CRH-secreting cells is thought to vary in its sensitivity to cortisol at different times of day.

Decreased sensitivity to inhibitory effects of cortisol in the early morning results in increased output of CRH, ACTH, and cortisol. As the day progresses

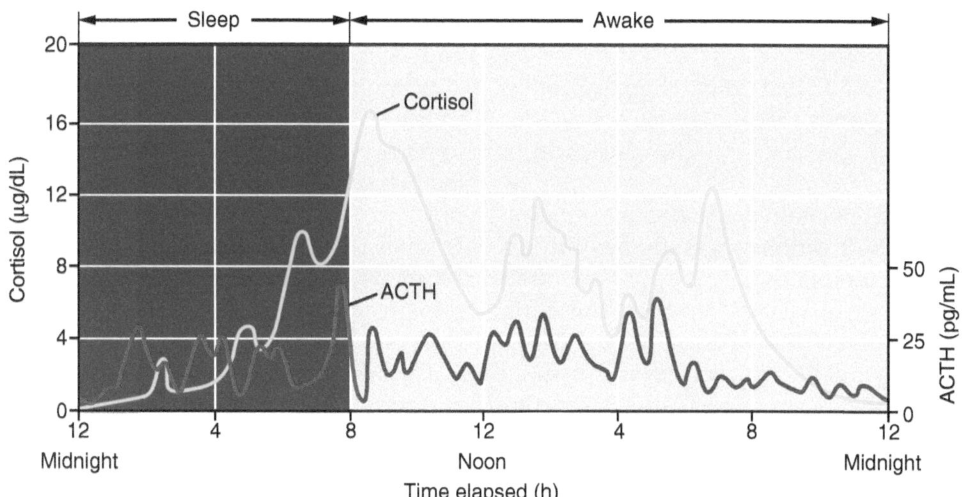

FIGURE 4.40 The correspondence between ACTH and cortisol production for a 24-hour period. *ACTH*, Adrenocorticotropic hormone. Source: *Redrawn from Figure 50-5 in Barrett, E. J. (2017). The adrenal gland, Chapter 50. In W. F. Boron & E. L. Boulpaep (Eds.),* Medical physiology *(3rd ed., p. 1026). Elsevier.*

sensitivity to cortisol increases, and there is a decrease in the output of CRH and consequently of ACTH and cortisol. The cellular mechanisms underlying the periodic changes in set point are not understood, but although they vary with time of day, cortisol concentrations in blood nevertheless are precisely controlled throughout the day.

Negative feedback also governs the response of the pituitary–adrenal axis to most stressful stimuli. Different mechanisms appear to apply at different stages of the stress response. With the imposition of a stressful stimulus, there is a sharp increase in ACTH secretion driven by CRH and AVP. The rate of ACTH secretion is determined by both the intensity of the stimulus to CRH-secreting neurons and the negative feedback influence of cortisol. In the initial moments of the stress response, pituitary corticotropes and CRH neurons monitor the rate of change rather than the absolute concentration of cortisol and restrain their output accordingly. After about 2 hours, negative feedback seems to be proportional to the total amount of cortisol secreted during the stressful episode. A new steady state is reached with chronic stress, and the negative feedback system again seems to monitor the concentration of cortisol in blood but with the set point readjusted at a higher level.

Each phase of negative feedback involves different cellular mechanisms. During the first few minutes the inhibitory effects of cortisol occur without a lag period and are expressed too rapidly to be mediated by altered genomic expression. Indeed, the rapid inhibitory action of cortisol is unaffected by inhibitors of protein synthesis. Its molecular basis is unknown, but receptors for steroids in neuronal membranes have been described. The negative feedback effect of cortisol in the subsequent interval occurs after a lag period and seems to require RNA and protein synthesis typical of the steroid actions discussed earlier. In this phase cortisol restrains secretion of CRH and ACTH but not their synthesis. At this time, corticotropes are less sensitive to CRH. With chronic administration of glucocorticoids or with chronic stress, negative feedback is also exerted at the level of POMC mRNA and ACTH synthesis.

Major features of the regulation of ACTH secretion include the following:

- Basal secretion of ACTH follows a diurnal rhythm driven by CRH.
- Stress increases CRH and AVP secretion through neural pathways.
- ACTH secretion is subject to negative feedback control under basal conditions and during the response to most stressful stimuli.
- Cortisol inhibits secretion of both CRH and ACTH.

Some observations suggest that cytokines produced by cells of the immune system may directly affect secretion by the hypothalamic–pituitary–adrenal axis. In particular, IL-1, IL-2, and IL-6 stimulate CRH secretion and may also act directly on the pituitary to increase ACTH secretion. IL-2 and IL-6 may also stimulate cortisol secretion by a direct action on the adrenal gland. In addition, lymphocytes express ACTH and related products of the POMC gene and are responsive to the stimulatory effects of CRH and the inhibitory effects of glucocorticoids. Because glucocorticoids inhibit cytokine production, there is another negative feedback relationship between the immune system and the adrenals (Fig. 4.41).

It has been suggested that this communication between the endocrine and immune systems provides a mechanism to alert the body to the presence of invading organisms or antigens.

Understanding the negative feedback relation between the adrenal and pituitary glands has important diagnostic and therapeutic applications. Normal adrenocortical function can be suppressed by injection of large doses of glucocorticoids. To test for deranged function a potent synthetic glucocorticoid, usually dexamethasone, is administered, and at a predetermined later time, the natural steroids or their metabolites are measured in blood or urine. If the hypothalamo-pituitary–adrenal system is intact, production of cortisol is suppressed and its concentration in blood is low. If on the other hand, cortisol concentrations remain high, an autonomous adrenal or ACTH-producing tumor may be present.

Another clinical application is treatment of the adrenogenital syndrome. As pointed out earlier, adrenal glands produce androgenic steroids by extension of the synthetic pathway for glucocorticoids (Figs. 4.18 and 4.28). Defects in production of glucocorticoids, particularly in enzymes responsible for hydroxylation of carbons 21 or 11, results in increased production of adrenal androgens. Overproduction of androgens in female patients leads to masculinization, which is manifest, for example, by enlargement of the clitoris, increased muscular development, and growth of facial hair. Severe defects may lead to masculinization of the genitalia of female infants and in male babies produce the supermasculinized "infant Hercules." Milder defects may show up simply as growth of excessive facial hair (hirsutism) in women. Overproduction of androgens occurs in the following way.

Stimulation of the adrenal cortex by ACTH increases pregnenolone production, most of which is normally converted to cortisol, which exerts negative feedback inhibition of ACTH secretion. With a partial block in cortisol production, much of the pregnenolone is diverted to androgens, which have no inhibitory effect on ACTH secretion. ACTH secretion therefore remains high and stimulates more pregnenolone production and causes adrenal hyperplasia (Fig. 4.42).

Eventually, the hyperactive adrenals produce enough cortisol for negative feedback to be operative, but at the expense of maintaining a high rate of androgen production. The whole system can be brought into proper balance by giving sufficient glucocorticoids to decrease ACTH secretion and therefore remove the stimulus for androgen production.

Adrenal medulla

The adrenal medulla accounts for about 10% of the mass of the adrenal gland and is embryologically and physiologically distinct from the cortex, although cortical and medullary hormones often act in a complementary manner. Cells of the adrenal medulla have an affinity for chromium salts in histological preparations and hence are called chromaffin cells. They arise from neuroectoderm and are innervated by neurons whose cell bodies lie in the intermediolateral cell column in the thoracolumbar portion of the spinal cord. Axons of

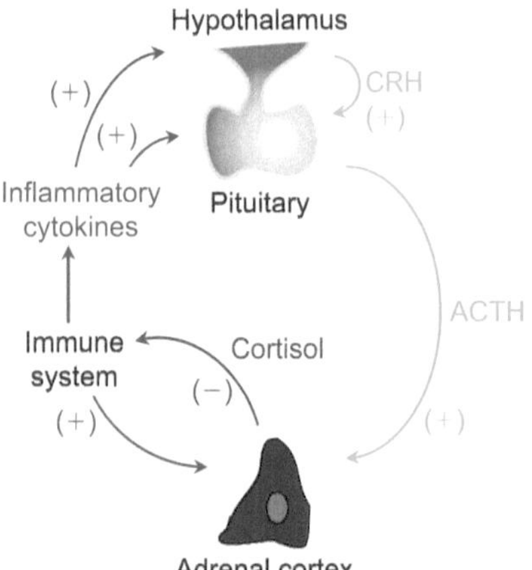

FIGURE 4.41 Negative feedback regulation of the hypothalamic–pituitary–adrenal axis by inflammatory cytokines. *CRH*, Corticotropin-releasing hormone.

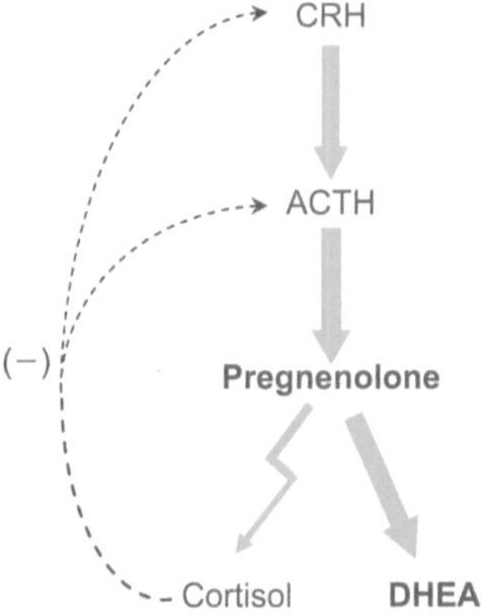

FIGURE 4.42 Consequences of a partial block of cortisol production by defects in either 11- or 21-hydroxylase. Pregnenolone is diverted to androgens, which exert no feedback activity on ACTH secretion. The thickness of the arrows connotes relative amounts. Broken arrows indicate impairment is in the inhibitory limb of the feedback system. Administration of glucocorticoids shuts down androgen production by inhibiting ACTH secretion. *ACTH*, Adrenocorticotropic hormone.

these cells pass through the paravertebral sympathetic ganglia to form the splanchnic nerves, which synapse with medullary chromaffin cells. Chromaffin cells are thus modified postganglionic neurons. Their principal secretory products, epinephrine and norepinephrine, are derivatives of the amino acid tyrosine and belong to a class of compounds called catecholamines. About 5–6 mg of catecholamines are stored in membrane-bound granules within chromaffin cells. Epinephrine is about nine times as abundant in the human adrenal medulla as norepinephrine, but only norepinephrine is found in postganglionic sympathetic neurons and extraadrenal chromaffin tissue. The adrenal medulla also produces and secretes at several neuropeptides including the vasodilator, adrenomedullin, and the opioid-like peptide, beta enkephalin, but the physiological role of medullary neuropeptides is incompletely understood. Although medullary hormones affect virtually every tissue of the body and play a crucial role in the acute response to stress, the adrenal medulla is not required for survival as long as the rest of the sympathetic nervous system is intact.

Biosynthesis of medullary catecholamines

The biosynthetic pathway for epinephrine and norepinephrine is shown in Fig. 4.43.

Hydroxylation of tyrosine to form dihydroxyphenylalanine (DOPA) is the rate-determining reaction and is catalyzed by the enzyme tyrosine hydroxylase. Activity of this enzyme is inhibited by catecholamines (product inhibition) and stimulated by phosphorylation. In this way, regulatory adjustments are made rapidly and are closely tied to bursts of secretion. A protracted increase in secretory activity induces synthesis of additional enzyme after a lag time of about 12 hours. Tyrosine hydroxylase and DOPA decarboxylase are cytosolic enzymes, but the enzyme that catalyzes the β-hydroxylation of dopamine to form norepinephrine resides within the secretory granule. Dopamine is pumped into the granule by an energy-dependent, stereospecific transport process. For sympathetic nerve endings and those adrenomedullary cells that produce norepinephrine, synthesis is complete with the formation of norepinephrine, and the hormone remains in the granule until it is secreted. Synthesis of epinephrine, however, requires that norepinephrine reenter the cytosol for the final methylation reaction. The enzyme required for this reaction, phenylethanolamine-*N*-methyltransferase, is at least partly inducible by glucocorticoids. Induction requires concentrations of cortisol that are considerably higher than those found in peripheral blood. The vascular arrangement in the adrenals is such that interstitial fluid surrounding cells of the medulla can equilibrate with venous blood that drains the cortex and therefore has a much higher content of glucocorticoids than arterial blood. Glucocorticoids may thus determine the ratio of epinephrine to norepinephrine production. Once methylated, epinephrine is pumped back into the storage granule, whose membrane protects stored catecholamines from oxidation by cytosolic enzymes.

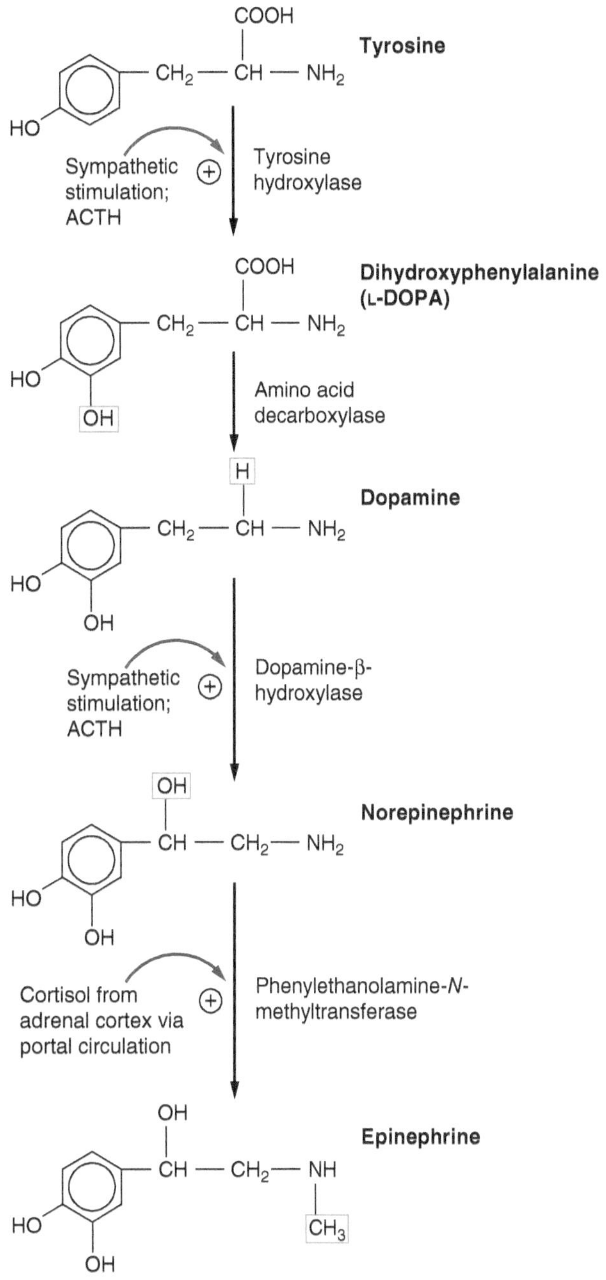

FIGURE 4.43 The synthesis of epinephrine from tyrosine. Source: *Redrawn from Figure 50-8A in Barrett, E. J. (2017). The adrenal gland, Chapter 50. In W. F. Boron & E. L. Boulpaep (Eds.),* Medical physiology *(3rd ed., p. 1031). Elsevier.*

Storage, release, and metabolism of medullary hormones

Catecholamines are stored in secretory granules in close association with ATP (Fig. 4.44) and at a molar ratio of 4:1, suggesting some hydrostatic interaction between the positively charged amines and the four negative charges on ATP. Some opioid peptides, including the enkephalins, β-endorphin, and their precursors, also are found in these granules and are cosecreted with catecholamines. Acetylcholine released during neuronal stimulation increases sodium conductance of the chromaffin cell membrane. The resulting influx of sodium ions depolarizes the plasma membrane, leading to an influx of calcium through voltage-sensitive channels. Secretion of catecholamines, like that of most other stored hormones, is triggered by increased cytosolic concentrations of calcium, which orchestrate the reactions of the regulated secretory pathway (see Chapter 1: Introduction). ATP, opioid peptides, and other contents of the granules are released along with epinephrine and norepinephrine. As yet, the physiological significance of opioid secretion by the adrenals is not known, but it has been suggested that the analgesic effects of these compounds may be of importance in the stress response.

All the epinephrine in blood originates in the adrenal glands. However, norepinephrine may reach the blood either by adrenal secretion or by diffusion from sympathetic synapses. The half-lives of medullary hormones in the peripheral circulation have been estimated to be less than 10 seconds for epinephrine and less than 15 seconds for norepinephrine. Up to 90% of the catecholamines are removed in a single passage through most capillary beds. Clearance from the blood requires uptake by both neuronal and nonneuronal tissues. Significant amounts of norepinephrine are taken up by sympathetic nerve endings and incorporated into secretory granules for release at a later time. Epinephrine and norepinephrine that is taken up in excess of storage capacity are degraded in neuronal cytosol principally by the enzyme monoamine oxidase. This enzyme catalyzes oxidative deamination of epinephrine, norepinephrine, and other biologically important amines (Fig. 4.45).

Catecholamines taken up by endothelium, heart, liver, and other tissues also are inactivated enzymatically, principally by catecholamine-*O*-methyl-transferase (COMT), which catalyzes transfer of a methyl group from *S*-adenosyl methionine to one of the hydroxyl groups. Both of these enzymes are widely distributed and can act sequentially in either order in

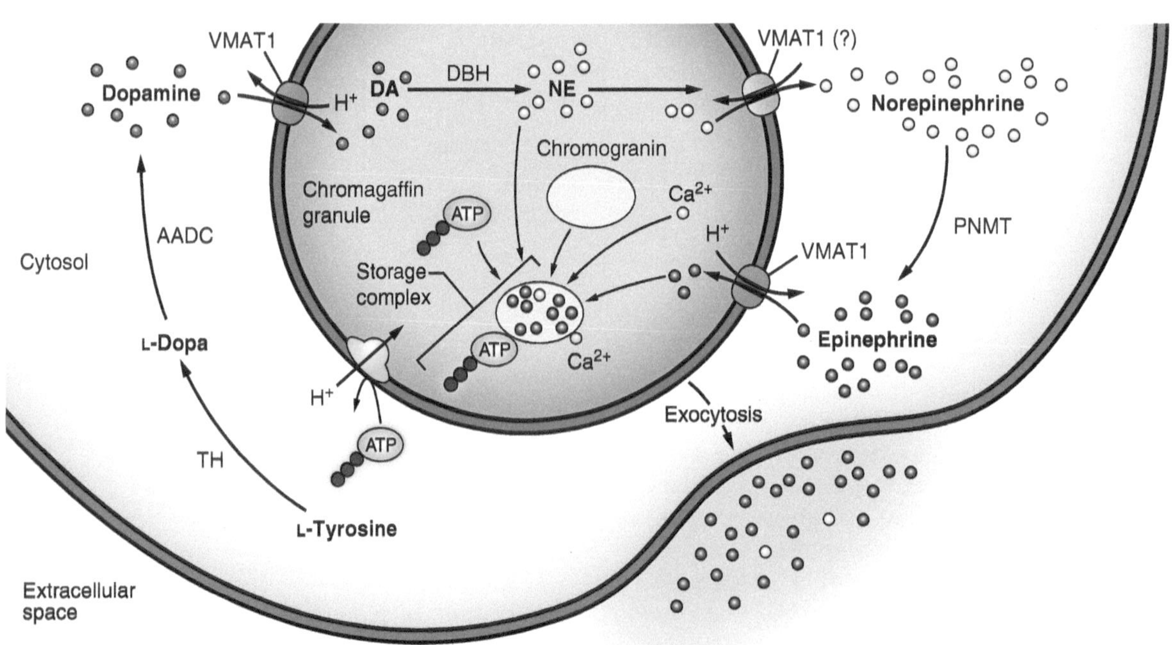

FIGURE 4.44 The synthesis and storage of catecholamines in the adrenal medulla cell. *AADC*, Amino-acid decarboxylase; *DA*, dopamine; *DBH*, dopamine β-hydroxylase; *Epi*, epinephrine; *NE*, norepinephrine; *TH*, tyrosine hydroxylase. Source: *Redrawn from Figure 50-9 in Barrett, E. J. (2017). The adrenal gland, Chapter 50. In W. F. Boron & E. L. Boulpaep (Eds.),* Medical physiology *(3rd ed., p. 1032). Elsevier.*

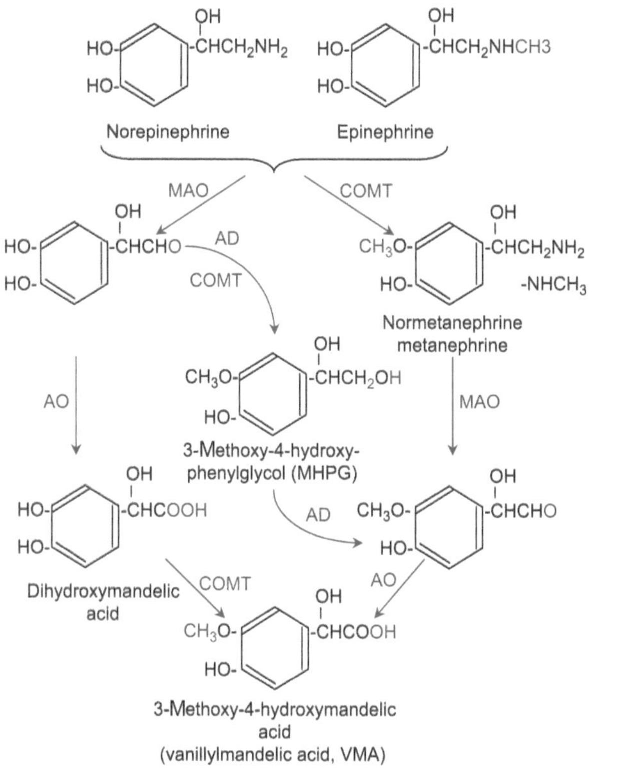

FIGURE 4.45 Catecholamine degradation. *AD*, Alcohol dehydrogenase; *AO*, aldehyde oxidase; *COMT*, catechol-*O*-methyl-transferase; *MAO*, monoamine oxidase. Source: *From Cryer (1987). In Philip Felig et al. (Eds.),* Endocrinology and metabolism *(2nd ed.). New York: McGraw Hill.*

metabolically inactivating epinephrine and norepinephrine. A number of pharmaceutical agents have been developed to modify the actions of these enzymes and thus modify sympathetic responses. Inactivated catecholamines, chiefly vanillylmandelic acid and 3-methoxy-4-hydroxyphenylglycol, are conjugated with sulfate or glucuronide and excreted in urine. As with steroid hormones, measurement of urinary metabolites of catecholamines is a useful, noninvasive source of diagnostic information.

Physiological actions of medullary hormones

The sympathetic nervous system and adrenal medullary hormones, like the cortical hormones, act on a wide variety of tissues to maintain the integrity of the internal environment both at rest and in the face of internal and external challenges. Catecholamines enable us to cope with emergencies and equip us for what Cannon called "fright, fight, or flight." Responsive tissues make no distinctions between blood-borne catecholamines and those released locally from nerve endings. In contrast to adrenal cortical hormones, effects of catecholamines are expressed within seconds and dissipate as rapidly when the hormone is removed. Medullary hormones are thus ideally suited for making the rapid short-term adjustments demanded by a changing environment, whereas cortical hormones, which act only after a lag period of at least 30 minutes, are of little use at the onset of stress. The cortex and medulla together, however, provide an effective "one–two punch," with cortical hormones maintaining and even amplifying the effectiveness of medullary hormones.

Cells in virtually all tissues of the body express G protein–coupled receptors for epinephrine and norepinephrine on their surface membranes (see Chapter 1: Introduction). These so-called adrenergic receptors originally were divided into two categories, α and β, based on their activation or inhibition by various drugs. Subsequently, the α and β receptors were further subdivided into α1, α2, β1, β2, and β3 receptors. All these receptors recognize both epinephrine and norepinephrine at least to some extent, and a given cell may have more than one class of adrenergic receptor. Biochemical mechanisms of signal transduction follow the pharmacological subdivisions of the adrenergic receptors. Stimulation of any of the β receptors activates adenylyl cyclase, but subtle differences distinguish them. Beta-adrenergic responses typically result from increased production of cyclic AMP, but β3 receptors may couple to both Gs and Gi heterotrimeric proteins and hence give a less robust response. From a physiological perspective, the only difference between β1 and β2 receptors is the low sensitivity of the β2 receptors to norepinephrine. Stimulation of α2 receptors inhibits adenylyl cyclase and may block the increase in cyclic AMP produced by other agents. For α2 effects, the receptor communicates with adenylyl cyclase through the inhibitory G protein (Gi). Responses initiated by the α1 receptor, which couples with Gq, are mediated by the inositol trisphosphate-DAG mechanism (see Chapter 1: Introduction). Glucocorticoids increase responses to catecholamines in some tissues by upregulating β adrenergic receptors or the αGs subunit.

Some of the physiological effects of catecholamines are listed in Table 4.3.

Although these actions may seem diverse, in actuality they constitute a magnificently coordinated set of responses that Cannon aptly called "the wisdom of the body." When producing their effects, catecholamines maximize the contributions of each of the various tissues to resolve challenges to survival. On the whole, cardiovascular effects maximize cardiac output and ensure perfusion of the brain and working muscles. Metabolic effects ensure an adequate supply of energy-rich

TABLE 4.3 Typical responses to stimulation of the adrenal medulla.

Target	Responses
Cardiovascular system	
Heart	↑Force and rate of contraction
	↑Conduction
	↑Blood flow (dilation of coronary arterioles)
	↑Glycogenolysis
Arterioles	
Skin	Constriction
Mucosae	Constriction
Skeletal muscle	Constriction
	Dilation
Metabolism	
Fat	↑Lipolysis
	↑Blood FFA and glycerol
Liver	↑Glycogenolysis and gluconeogenesis
	↑Blood sugar
Muscle	↑Glycogenolysis
	↑Lactate and pyruvate release
Respiratory system	Relaxation of bronchial muscle
Stomach and intestines	↑Motility
	↑Sphincter contraction
	↑Sphincter contraction
Urinary bladder	
Skin	↑Sweating
Eyes	Contraction of radial muscle of the iris
Salivary gland	↑Amylase secretion
	↑Watery secretion
Kidney	↑Renin secretion
	↑Sodium reabsorption
Skeletal muscle	↑Tension generation
	↑Neuromuscular transmission
	(defatiguing effect)

FFA, Free fatty acids.

substrate. Relaxation of bronchial muscles facilitates pulmonary ventilation. Ocular effects increase visual acuity. Effects on skeletal muscle and transmitter release from motor neurons increase muscular performance, and quiescence of the gut permits diversion of blood flow, oxygen, and fuel to reinforce these effects.

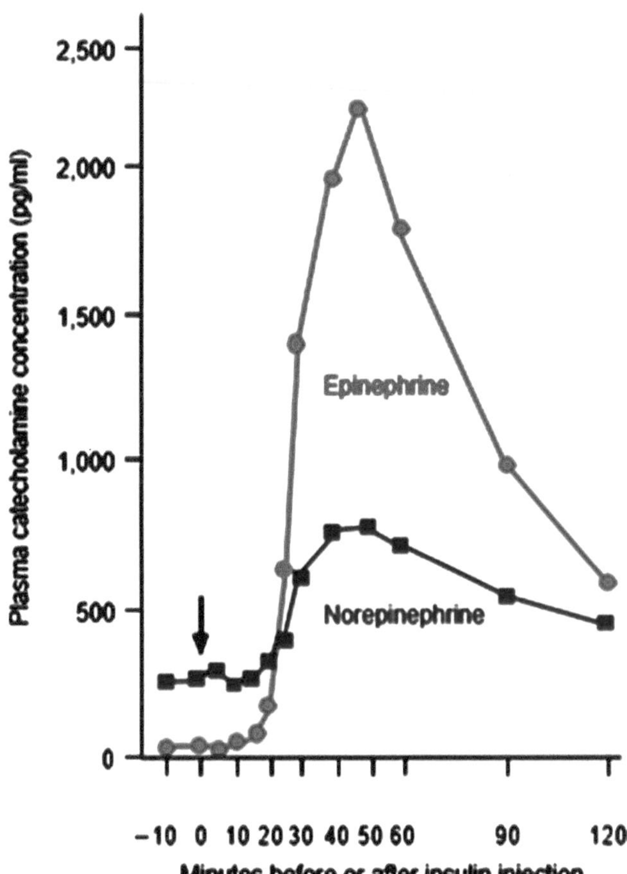

FIGURE 4.46 Changes in blood concentrations of epinephrine and norepinephrine in response to hypoglycemia. Insulin, which produces hypoglycemia, was injected at the time indicated by the arrow. Source: *From Garber, A. J., Bier, D. M., Cryer, P. E., & Pagliara, A. S. (1976). Hypoglycemia in compensated chronic renal insufficiency. Substrate limitation of gluconeogenesis.* Journal of Clinical Investigation, *58, 7–15.*

Regulation of adrenal medullary function

The sympathetic nervous system, including its adrenal medullary component, is activated by any actual or threatened change in the internal or external environment. It responds to physical changes, emotional inputs, and anticipation of increased physical activity. Input reaches the adrenal medulla through its sympathetic innervation. Signals arising in the hypothalamus and other integrating centers activate both the neural and hormonal components of the sympathetic nervous system but not necessarily in an all-or-none fashion. Activation may be general or selectively limited to discrete targets. Norepinephrine- or epinephrine-secreting cells can be preferentially and independently stimulated as shown in Fig. 4.46.

In response to hypoglycemia detected by glucose monitoring cells in the central nervous system, the concentration of norepinephrine in blood may increase threefold, whereas that of epinephrine, which tends to be a more effective hyperglycemic agent, may increase 50-fold. Metabolic actions of epinephrine are discussed further in Chapter 8, Hormonal Regulation of Fuel Metabolism.

Summary

The adrenal glands are perched atop each kidney and are embryologically divided into a central medulla and an outer cortex. The medulla is derived from the nervous system and is physiologically a ganglion in the sympathetic system. Unlike other ganglia, its postganglionic neurons have no axons and so secrete their neurotransmitters, epinephrine, and norepinephrine, directly into the extracellular space where they diffuse into the blood. The overlying cortex is divided into three zones each of which secretes a different hormone group that targets specific structures.

Suggested readings

Basic foundations

Stewart, P. M., & Newell-Price, J. D. C. (2016). The adrenal cortex. In S. Melmed, K. S. Polonsky, P. R. Larsen, & H. M. Kronenberg (Eds.), *Williams textbook of endocrinology* (pp. 490–555). Philadelphia, PA: Elsevier.

Advanced information

Angelousi, A., Kassi, E., Nasiri-Ansari, N., Weickert, M. O., Randeva, H., & Kaltsas, G. (2018). Clock genes alterations and endocrine disorders. *European Journal of Clinical Investigation, 48*(6), e12927. https://doi.org/10.1111/eci.12927. Epub 2018 Apr 16.

Gray, J. D., Kogan, J. F., Marrocco, J., & McEwen, B. S. (2017). Genomic and epigenomic mechanisms of glucocorticoids in the brain. *Nature Reviews Endocrinology, 13*, 661. Available from https://doi.org/10.1038/nrendo.2017.97.

Iacobucci, G. (2017). Consider corticosteroids for acute sore throat, says *BMJ* review. *BMJ*, 358. Available from https://doi.org/10.1136/bmj.j4333.

Kanczkowski, W., Sue, M., & Bornstein, S. R. (2017). The adrenal gland microenvironment in health disease and during regeneration. *Hormones, 16*(3), 251–265.

Kline, G., & Holmes, D. T. (2017). Adrenal venous sampling for primary aldosteronism: Laboratory medicine best practice. *Journal of Clinical Pathology, 70*(11), 911–916. Available from https://doi.org/10.1136/jclinpath-2017-204423.

Mifsud, K. R., & Reul, J. M. H. M. (2018). Mineralocorticoid and glucocorticoid receptor-mediated control of genomic responses to stress in the brain. *Stress*, 1–14. Available from https://doi.org/10.1080/10253890.2018.1456526.

Niu, M., Liu, A., Zhao, Y., & Feng, L. (2017). Malignant transformation of a mature teratoma of the adrenal gland: A rare case report and literature review. *Medicine, 96*(45), e8333. Available from https://doi.org/10.1097/md.0000000000008333.

Sadeghirad, B., Siemieniuk, R. A. C., Brignardello-Petersen, R., Papola, D., Lytvyn, L., Vandvik, P. O., ... Agoritsas, T. (2017). Corticosteroids for treatment of sore throat: Systematic review and meta-analysis of randomised trials. *BMJ, 358*. Available from https://doi.org/10.1136/bmj.j3887.

Seccia, T. M., Caroccia, B., Gomez-Sanchez, E. P., Vanderriele, P.-E., Gomez-Sanchez, C. E., & Rossi, G. P. (2017). Review of markers of zona glomerulosa and aldosterone-producing adenoma cells. *Hypertension, 70*(5), 867–874. Available from https://doi.org/10.1161/hypertensionaha.117.09991.

Stern, A., Skalsky, K., Avni, T., Carrara, E., Leibovici, L., & Paul, M. (2017). Corticosteroids for pneumonia. *Cochrane Database of Systematic Reviews* (12). Available from https://doi.org/10.1002/14651858.CD007720.pub3.

CHAPTER

5

Principles of hormone integration

Case study

Abraham Lincoln: did he have MEN3?

By all accounts, Abraham Lincoln was a very unusual-looking person—even ugly by some reports. He had had small pox, so there were lots of pits on his face; he had a large mole on his right cheek, his face was misshapen and not symmetrical, he had protruding lips, his ears were large, and his hair unruly (Fig. 5.1).

He stood 6 ft 4 in. and towered above men of the 1860s whose average height was 5 ft 7 in. (Fig. 5.2). Since then, historical clinicians have wondered what medical condition would cause such a habitus. In looking at the family history, his mother had the same stature and facial elements. She died of milk sickness at age 34 due to toxin (tremetol) from the white snakeroot plant which cows ate, and the toxin was subsequently secreted into the milk or stored in the meat before the animal had symptoms. His father, Thomas Lincoln, was of ordinary height and lived longer than Lincoln, dying in 1851 age 73. Only one of Lincolns four sons survived to maturity. The surviving son, Robert Todd Lincoln, was a successful lawyer and businessman and died age 82. He did not have his

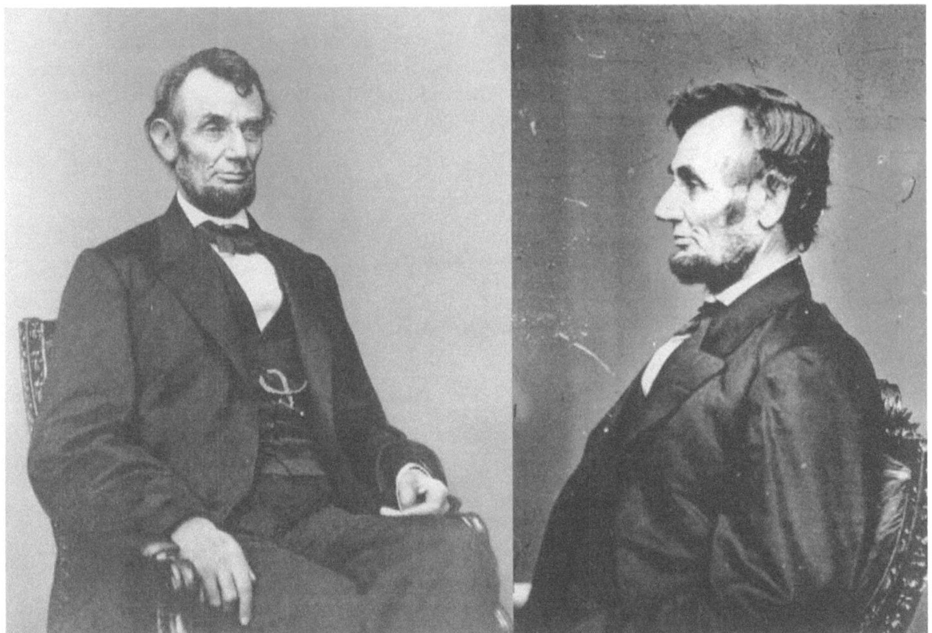

FIGURE 5.1 Two portraits of Lincoln by Matthew Brady. The one on the left is used for the $5 US bill and the one on the right is used for the US penny. Note the large ears and rugged facial features. Source: *Photographs from Sullivan, G. (1994).* Mathew Brady. *New York: Dutton.*

Goodman's Basic Medical Endocrinology.
DOI: https://doi.org/10.1016/B978-0-12-815844-9.00005-1

(*cont'd*)

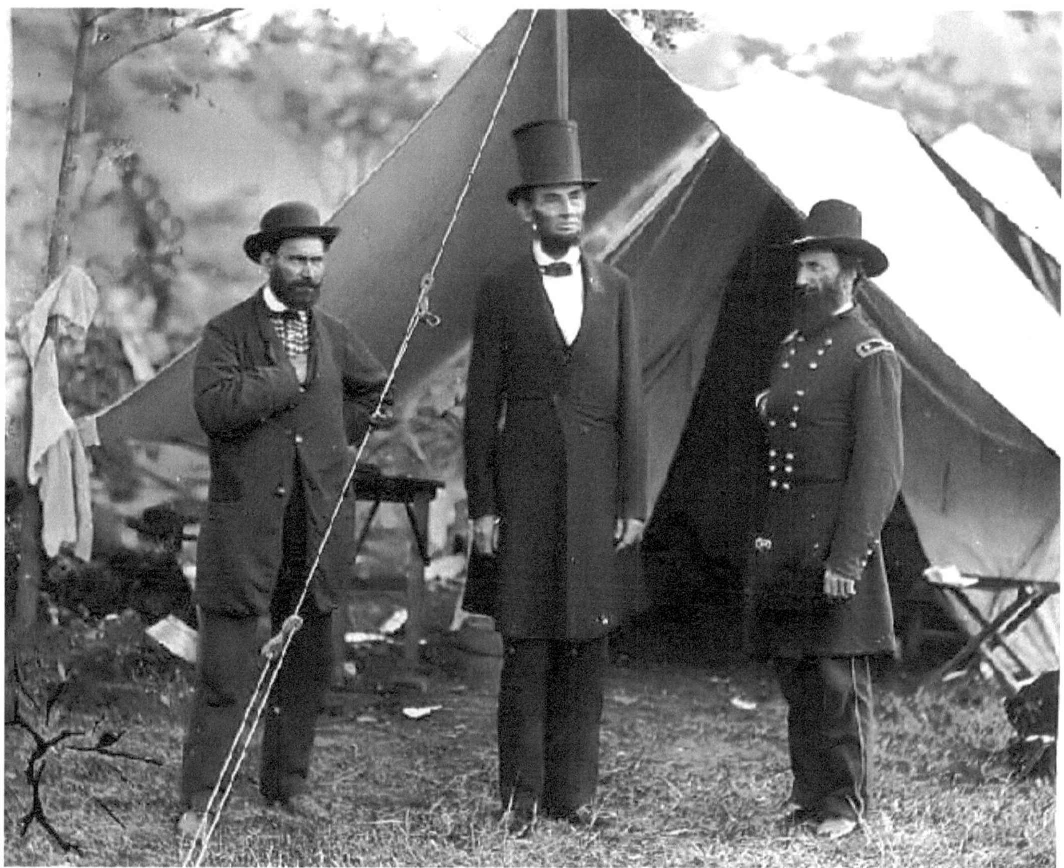

FIGURE 5.2 Lincoln at the Battle of Antietam, October 1862, with detective Allan Pinkerton (left) and Brigadier General McClernand (right). Lincoln's height at 6 ft 4 in. towered over that of Pinkerton and McClernand. The average height of men in the 1860s was 5 ft 7 in. His tall yet thin features are considered Marfanoid (like Marfan syndrome). Source*: (internet) and From Figure 50 in Sotos J. G. (2008).* The physical Lincoln *(pp. 50). Mt. Vernon Book Systems.*

father's features. His son and Abraham Lincoln's grandson, Abraham Lincoln II, died of septicemia at age 16.

Many clinicians think Lincoln had a variant of Marfan syndrome and there is a collateral Lincoln line with that disorder to reinforce this belief. However, in 2007 a clinician came up with a new diagnosis, multiple endocrine neoplasia (MEN 3). In his book *The Physical Lincoln*, Dr. John Sotos gives several arguments for Lincoln having this disorder.

MEN was described in the early 1900s and is now divided into four broad groups: MEN1, MEN2, MEN3, and MEN4. As the name implies, there are several endocrine systems that have formed tumors and produce too much hormone. In MEN1 the main neoplastic tumors are parathyroid, pancreaticoduodenal neuroendocrine, and carcinoid. A subset of MEN1, now renamed MEN4, is due to a *CDKN1B* mutation. In MEN2 the tumors are thyroid C-cell, adrenomedullary chromaffin, and parathyroid. MEN3 has, in addition, multiple neuromas, causing lumps—especially in the lips and oral cavity.

These are some of Dr. Soto's most salient arguments for Lincoln having MEN3:

1. Marfanoid appearance
2. facial characteristics (Fig. 5.3).
3. neuromas in lips (Fig. 5.4).
4. cancer (Fig. 5.5).

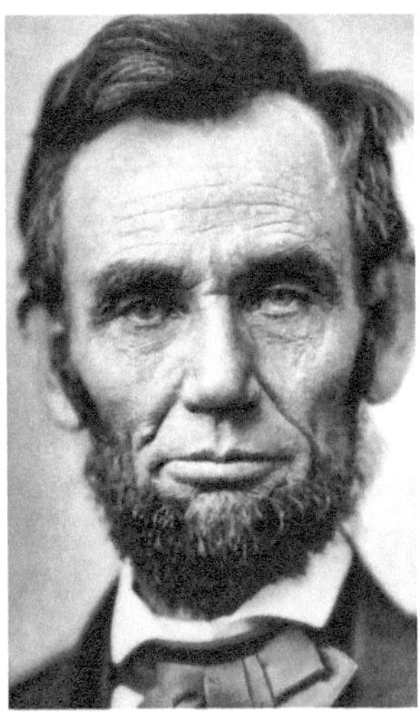

FIGURE 5.3 Lincoln in 1863 showing facial asymmetry noticeable on the left side where the face is indented and the eye is not moving correctly. Also notice the ptosis (drooping of the eyelid) and the large lips and ears. Source: *(internet) and From Figure 30 in Sotos J. G. (2008)*. The physical Lincoln *(pp. 30). Mt. Vernon Book Systems.*

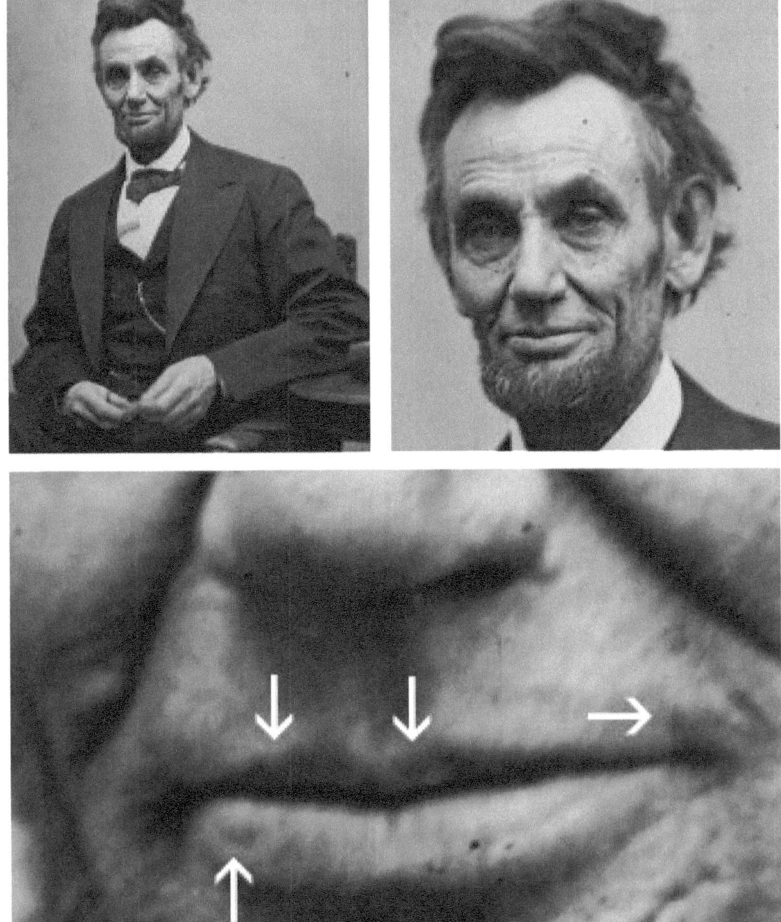

FIGURE 5.4 Dr. Sotos believes these lumps (his arrows) are neuromas. Source*: From Figure 128 in Sotos J. G. (2008)*. The physical Lincoln *(pp. 128). Mt. Vernon Book Systems.*

(cont'd)

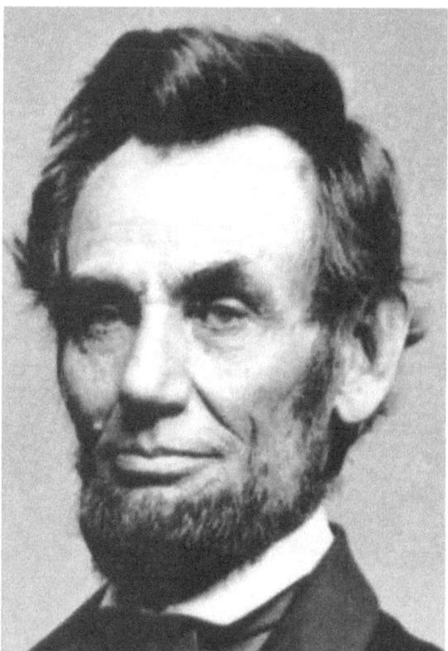
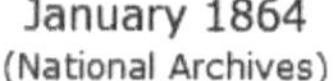

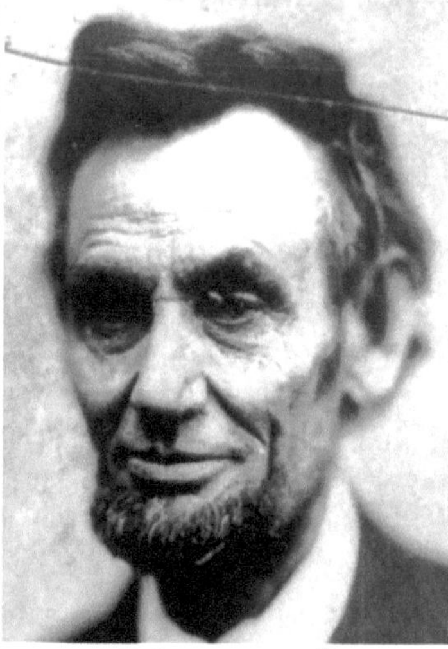

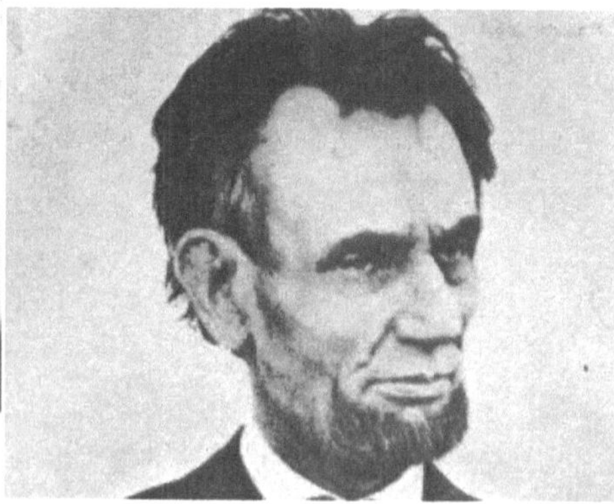

FIGURE 5.5 The loss of weight in 13 months is dramatic and led Dr. Sotos to believe that Lincoln was battling cancer. On the right a photograph also showing the weight loss and gaunt face taken by Warren in March 1865, a month before he was assassinated. Source: *From the Abraham Lincoln Research Site created by Roger Norton (internet). Internet and From Figure 146 in Sotos J. G. (2008).* The physical Lincoln *(pp. 146). Mt. Vernon Book Systems.*

In the clinic

Multiple endocrine neoplasia 3

MEN2 and MEN3 are rare disorders due to missense mutations resulting in medullary thyroid carcinoma (MTC) which is carcinoma of the calcitonin producing cells. Calcitonin is produced by C cells (also called parafollicular cells) in the superior half of each lateral lobe of the thyroid gland. In MEN3 the missense reading is most often (95%) at M918T in the RET protein which controls cell proliferation. In MEN3, there is the additional sign of neuromas in the lips and oral cavity (Fig. 5.6)—this is the major nonendocrine feature which further distinguishes MEN3 from MEN2. In 50% of MEN3 cases, there is also pheochromocytoma, a usually benign tumor of the chromaffin cells of the adrenal medulla. In MEN2, this percentage is increased to 100% a distinguishing endocrine feature.

Incidence

The incidence of MEN3 is 1.4–2.9 per million live births.

Signs and symptoms

Most cases are sporadic and arise de novo which have been attributed to an advanced age of the father (not the case with Lincoln, whose father was 31 when he was born), indicating a paternal preference for the inheritance of the *RET* gene. This gene is a proto-oncogene, so one mutation should suffice for it to initiate cancer. However, other factors not completely understood, slow the onset of cancer. Instead, the C cells undergo sequential hyperplasia before becoming malignant (Fig. 5.9). Because of its de novo origin and the slow progression

(cont'd)

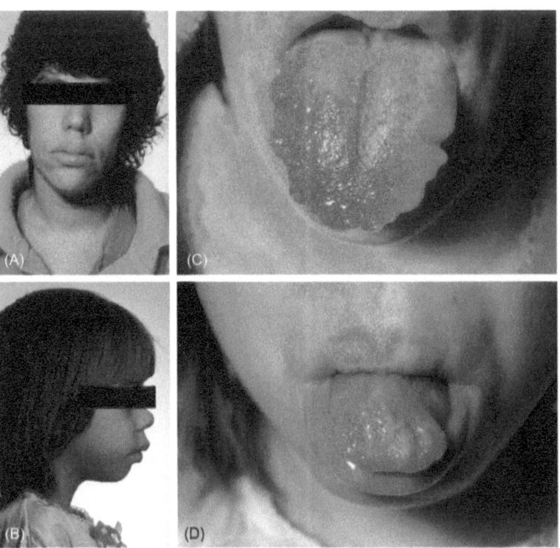

FIGURE 5.6 A mother (A and C) and daughter (B and D) with MEN3 syndrome showing the lumpy tongue and large lumpy lips. Notice the coarse facial features of the mother. Source: *From figure 39-11 in 9 in Melmed, S., Polonsky, K. S., Larsen, P. R., & Kronenberg, H. M. (2016).* Williams' textbook of endocrinology *(13th ed.) (pp. 1744). Elsevier.*

from normal C cells to carcinoma, it is the nonendocrine aspects of the disorder that usually first make their appearance. These aspects include a Marfanoid habitus (Fig. 5.7) asymmetrical face, large lips, the presence of neuromas on the lips, tongue and in the oral cavity; an everted eyelid (Fig. 5.8), alacrima, the failure to tear when crying, constipation with the potential for megacolon due to hyperplasia of ganglia (ganglioneuromatosis) within the intestinal wall.

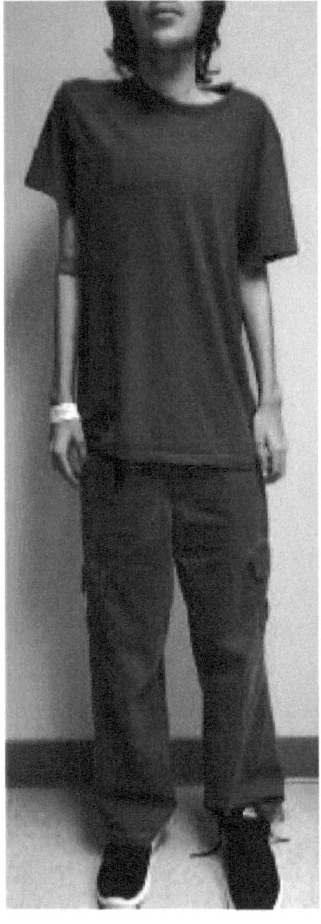

FIGURE 5.7 Marfanoid habitus in MEN3. Source: *From Figure 2 in Castinetti, F., Moley, J., Mulligan, L., & Waguespack, S. G. (2018). A comprehensive review of MEN2B.* Endocrine-Related Cancer, 25.

Diagnosis

Diagnosis is usually made in the second decade of life, with a range of 24–59 years, usually from the signs and symptoms. Calcitonin levels will be elevated.

Management

Complete thyroidectomy is the preferred method of treatment. Hopefully, the parathyroid glands can be spared, but these are hard to see in young children. Calcitonin and carcinoembryonic antigen levels are followed to make certain that there are no metastases. Most metastases will be in the cervical lymph nodes, with distant metastases to intrathoracic lymph nodes, lungs, liver, bones, and rarely the brain. Surgery is rarely curative and the approved tyrosine kinase inhibitor drugs, vandetanib and cabozantinib, will usually have to be employed.

Prognosis

The survival rate is 75%.

(cont'd)

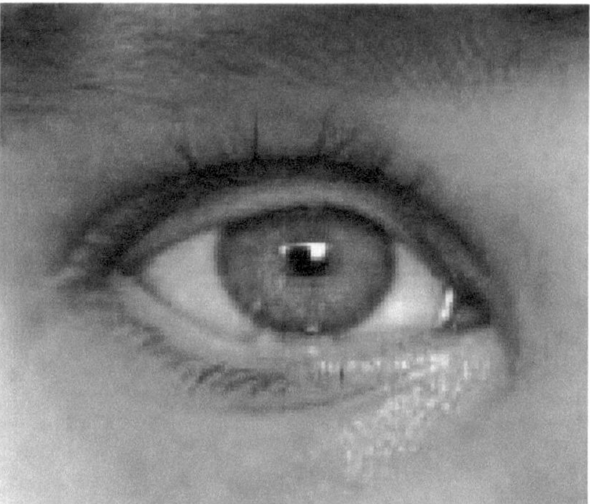

FIGURE 5.8 Everted eyelid with ptosis in MEN3. Source: *From Figure 2 in Castinetti, F., Moley, J., Mulligan, L., & Waguespack, S. G. (2018). A comprehensive review of MEN2B.* Endocrine-Related Cancer, 25.

Medullary thyroid carcinoma progression. Medullary thryoid carcinoma begins as a normal cell growth which undergoes successive stages of growth that evolves over time into carcinoma (Fig. 5.9).

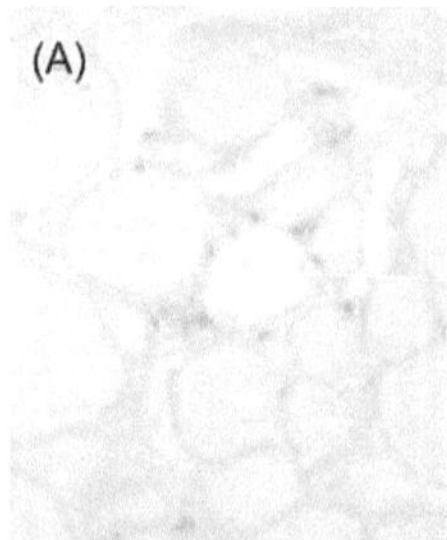

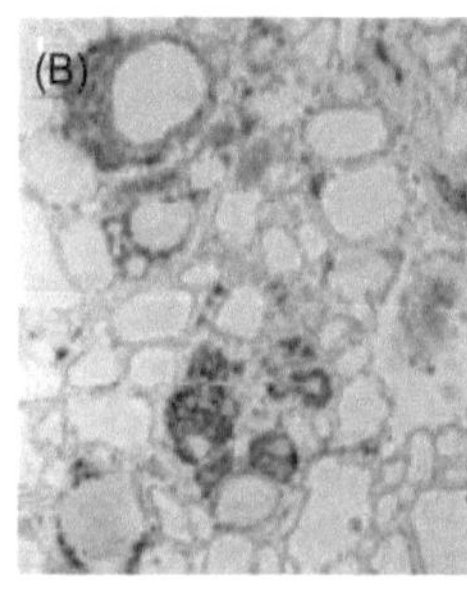

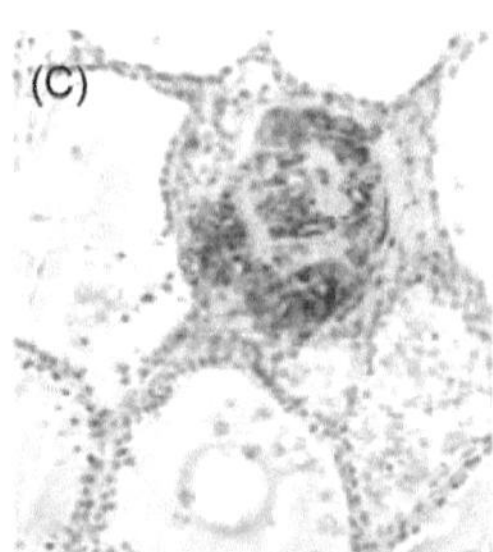

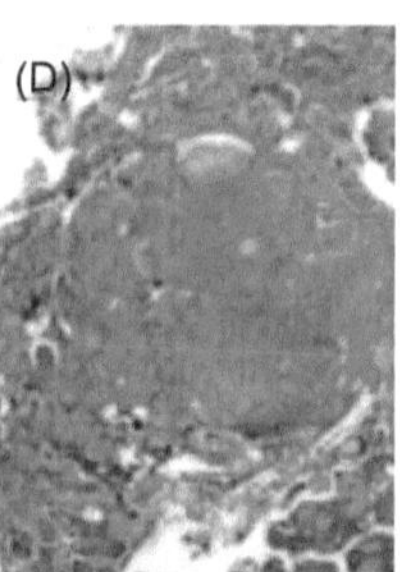

FIGURE 5.9 Microscopic progression of medullary thyroid carcinoma. The development of MTC. From normal C-cells (A), the tumor follows an asymptomatic hyperplasic state (B) before the development of micro-MTC (C, size ≤1 cm) and then macro-MTC (D, size >1 cm). *MTC*, Medullary thyroid carcinoma. Source: *From Figure 1 in Castinetti, F., Moley, J., Mulligan, L., Waguespack, S. G. (2018). A comprehensive review of MEN2B.* Endocrine-Related Cancer, 25.

At the molecular level (boxed material for additional information)

The genetic basis for MEN2

The genetic basis for MEN are mutations in specific genes. Those mutations for MEN1 involve the inactivation of a growth (tumor) suppressor genes, of which there are at least four: *MEN1*, *VHL*, *CNC*, and *NF1* with possible other genes involved. For MEN2, there are mutations in only one gene, *RET* (for ***RE***arranged during ***T***ransfection), which is a proto-oncogene that promotes cell growth. Mutations of *RET* are responsible for medullary thyroid tumors and MTC, both are tumors of the calcitonin secreting cells.

The normal RET protein has three domains: extracellular which combines with ligands and calcium, a transmembrane domain, and an intracellular domain. Once activated by several extracellular hormones, the intracellular tyrosine residues are autophosphorylated, enabling them to serve as docking sites for at least 18 different intracellular adaptor proteins (Fig. 5.10).

RET is found in all neural crest derived cells, including the autonomic nervous system (which includes the adrenal medulla—a modified sympathetic ganglion), enteric nervous system, thyroid parafollicular (C) cells, the branchial arch cells (parathyroid in particular), urogenital cells, including the kidneys.

Most of the mutations involving the RET protein are transcription point missense mutations resulting in defective extracellular or intracellular domains of RET. In about half of the cases of MTC—carcinoma of the C cells—the mutation is M918T (M = methionine, 918 is the number of the amino acid position in the protein, and T = threonine) where threonine is substituted for methionine.

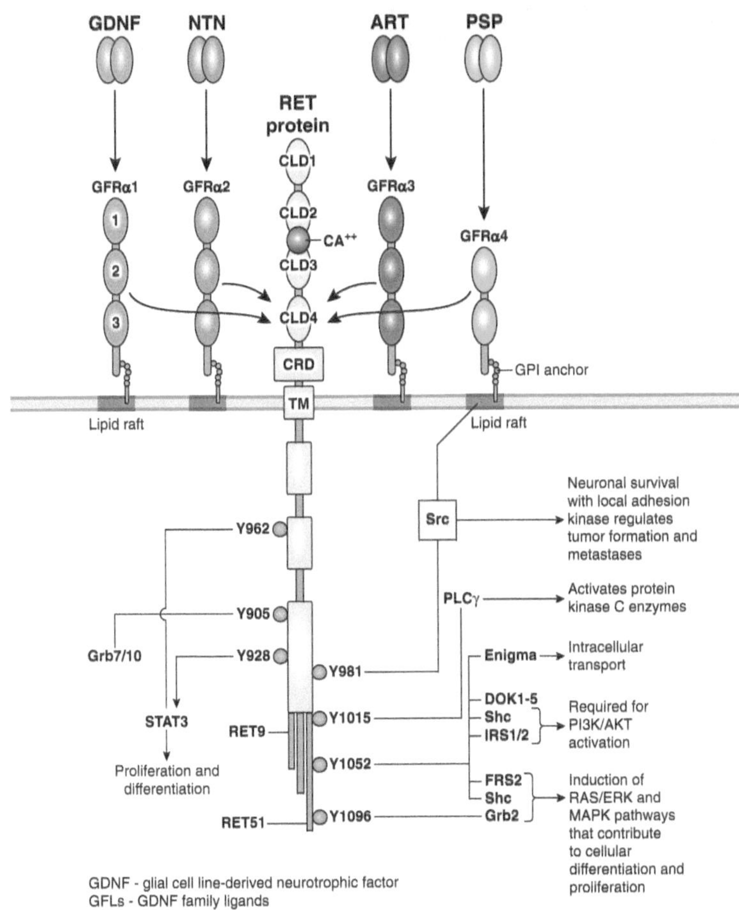

FIGURE 5.10 The RET protein and some of the intracellular phosphorylation sites on tyrosine residues. The adaptor proteins are to the right or left of the intracellular domain. Other acronyms are *ART*, artemin—a neurotropic ligand produced by glial cells; *CRD*, cysteine-rich domain; *DOK*, docking protein; *FRS2*, fibroblast growth factor receptor substrate; *GPI*, glycophosphatidylinositol—an anchor for ligands on the lipid raft (an area on the cell membrane high in cholesterol = lipid—where most receptors are located); *Grb*, granzyme B, which can have many different functions; *IRS* $^{1}/_{2}$, internal resolution sites $^{1}/_{2}$; *NTN*, neurturin—neurotropic ligand produced by glial cells; *PLC*γ, phospholipase C gamma; *PSP*, persephin—another neurotrophic ligand produced by glial cells; *Shc*, sarc homology; *Src*, sarc; *STAT*, signal transducer and activator of transcription; *TM*, transmembrane; Y1096, etc., docking sites. Source: *From figure 39-9 in Melmed, S., Polonsky, K. S., Larsen, P. R., & Kronenberg, H. M. (2016).* Williams' textbook of endocrinology *(13th ed.) (pp. 1741). Elsevier.*

Introduction

Introduction MEN involves more than one endocrine gland and several nonendocrine structures. Up to this chapter, individual endocrine glands have been considered along with some basic information about their physiological functions. Although it is helpful to first understand one hormone at a time or one gland at a time, it must be recognized that life is considerably more complex, and that endocrinological solutions to physiological problems require the integration of a large variety of simultaneous events. By integration is meant the coordination of reactions to separate physiological demands into a balanced overall response or group of responses. This chapter considers some of the general principles of endocrine integration at the cellular and whole-body level, and subsequent chapters consider integrated hormonal actions that govern homeostatic regulation, growth and development, and reproduction.

Integration of hormonal signals at the cellular and molecular level

Augmentation, antagonism, and synergy

Integration takes place at the level of individual cells as well as the whole body. Just as individual people must cope with a multiplicity of sensory inputs as each goes through a daily routine, so too must individual cells respond to the barrage of signals that reach them simultaneously. Most cells express receptors for multiple hormones and other signaling molecules and are simultaneously bombarded with excitatory, inhibitory, or a conflicting mixture of excitatory and inhibitory hormonal stimuli. Each hormone independently excites its receptors and initiates a cascade of transduction mechanisms, the immediate consequences of which contribute to determining the nature and magnitude of cellular responses. Therefore target cells must integrate the various inputs at both receptor and postreceptor levels and resolve them into productive responses. Detailed understanding of how cells accomplish this task is still emerging. A few examples and mechanisms are described to the given examples of the challenges that cells face in integrating hormone actions.

In the hypothetical example shown in Fig. 5.11, hormone B signals by stimulating the production of the second messenger cyclic 5′-adenosine monophosphate (AMP).

Its ability to increase cyclic AMP (cAMP) concentrations is mitigated by the hormones A and C whose actions lower cAMP concentrations by hastening its destruction (hormone A) and by diminishing its rate of production (hormone C). At the same time, hormone C may initiate other responses through activation of the diacylglycerol (DAG)/inositol trisphosphate (IP3) second messenger system. The net response of the cell is determined by the relative intensity of stimulation by hormones A, B, and C and hence will vary with the physiological circumstances that affect the degree to which each of these hormones is secreted. At times the

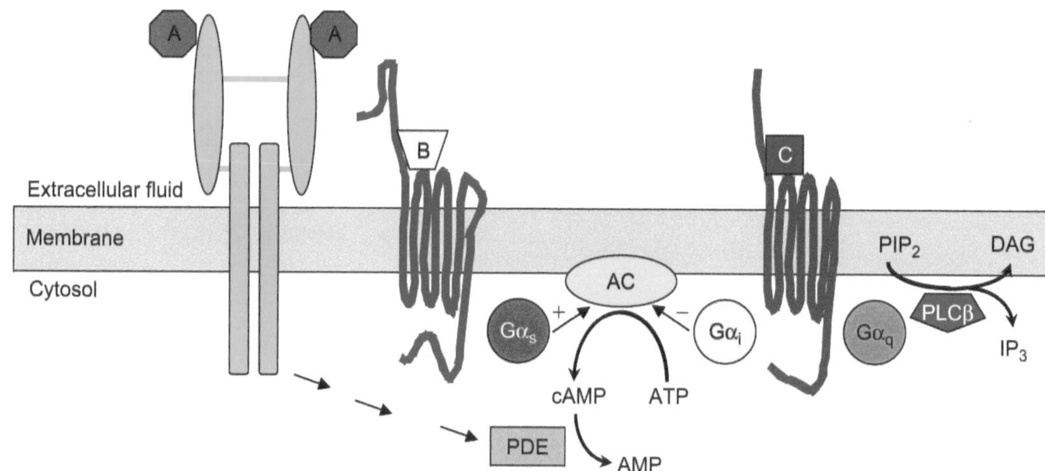

FIGURE 5.11 Integration at the cellular level. A cell may receive inputs from hormones A, B, and C simultaneously. Hormone B acting through a G-protein coupled receptor activates *AC* through the α stimulatory subunit $G\alpha_s$. Hormone C binds to its G-protein coupled receptor, which inhibits AC through the inhibitory subunit $G\alpha_i$ and activates phospholipase C through the $G\alpha_q$ subunit, resulting in cleavage of *PIP2* and the release of *DAG* and *IP3*. Hormone A, acting through a tyrosine kinase receptor, activates cAMP *PDE*, which degrades cAMP. The combined actions of the three hormones determines the concentration of cAMP. *AC*, Adenylyl cyclase; *AMP*, 5′-adenosine monophosphate; *cAMP*, cyclic adenosine monophosphate; *DAG*, diacylglycerol; *IP3*, inositol trisphosphate; *PDE*, phosphodiesterase; *PIP2*, phosphatidylinositol bis-phosphate.

action of hormone B will prevail; at other times, it will be overwhelmed by the combined actions of hormones A and C or by the dominant actions of either hormone A or hormone C.

One hormone may also influence responses to other hormones by regulating the expression of key components of transduction or signaling pathways. For example, responses to epinephrine depend on the availability of its receptors (called adrenergic receptors), G-proteins, and downstream mediators. Thyroid hormones increase the expression of adrenergic receptors in some tissues, and cortisol appears to increase the expression of adrenergic receptors, as well as $G\alpha_s$, and other components of G-protein signaling. Consequently, in the states of thyroid or adrenal insufficiency, responses to epinephrine are blunted or deficient, and conversely, after a period of increased secretion of thyroxine or cortisol, responses to epinephrine may be exaggerated. Interactions between hormones that occur downstream from the receptors may be seen in the final expression of the cellular response. Two or more hormones may produce overlapping effects in some target cells, and when present simultaneously may produce a final response that is of greater, equal, or lesser magnitude than the algebraic sum of their individual actions. If two hormones act through independent signaling pathways to achieve a response, the magnitude of their combined effects may simply summate. However, if they compete for some shared component of their signaling pathways of final effector molecules, the individual responses to each may be reduced, so that their combined response is of lesser magnitude than the sum of the responses each would have produced if acting alone. Conversely, if two hormones act through separate, but complementary pathways, they may enhance each other's actions, and the magnitude of the cellular response may be several-fold greater than the sum of the individual effects. This phenomenon is called synergism or potentiation. For example, both growth hormone and cortisol modestly increase lipolysis in adipocytes. When given simultaneously, however, lipolysis as measured by the rate of glycerol production (see Chapter 7: The Pancreatic Islets) was nearly twice as great as the sum of the effects of each (Fig. 5.12). Synergism is often seen, although the molecular mechanisms responsible are still not understood in most cases.

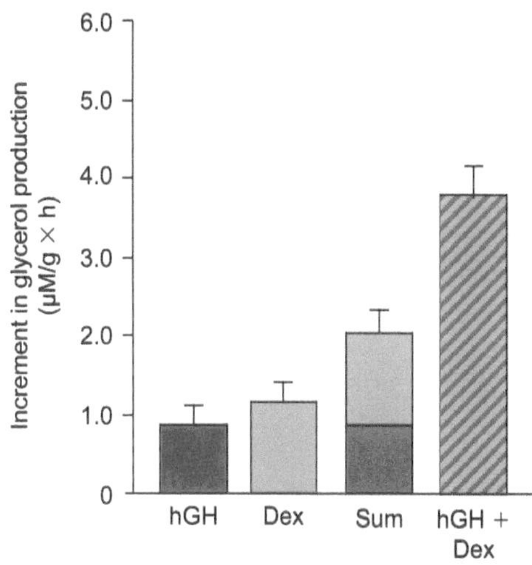

FIGURE 5.12 Synergistic effects of *hGH* and the synthetic glucocorticoid *DEX* on lipolysis as measured by the increase in glycerol release from rat adipocytes. Both hGH and Dex were somewhat effective when added individually, but when added together, the overall tissue response was greater than the sum of the responses produced by each hormone alone. *DEX*, Dexamethasone; *hGH*, human growth hormone. Source: *From Gorin, E., Tai, L. R, Honeyman, T. W, & Goodman, H. M. (1990). Evidence for a role of protein kinase C in the stimulation of lipolysis by growth hormone and isoproterenol.* Endocrinology, 126,2973.

Permissiveness

A related phenomenon is the permissive action of one hormone with respect to the actions of other hormones or other stimuli. A hormone acts permissively when its presence is necessary for, or permits, a response to occur, even though the hormone itself does not initiate the response. In this case, two hormones acting together may produce an effect that neither can produce alone. This phenomenon was mentioned in Chapter 4, The Adrenal Glands, with respect to the actions of the glucocorticoids, and originally was described in studies of glucocorticoid physiology, but permissive actions of other hormones are also seen. The underlying molecular mechanisms are not understood but probably relate to hormone effects on the expression of many genes that maintain normal cellular economy.

Maintaining signal fidelity

There are more hormones than there are signaling pathways, and virtually no signaling pathway is used exclusively by any one hormone. Many different hormones appear to signal by activating the same molecules or molecular complexes, and yet the final outcome produced by each is nearly always unique. While integrating or combining the actions of hormones in ways that increase or decrease the magnitude of a response, cells preserve the integrity of the actions of each hormone even when their transduction pathways appear to share common components. Even though the precise mechanisms that assure signal fidelity are not always understood, several factors appear to contribute to the specificity of hormone actions in cells that express receptors for different hormones that seemingly activate the same signaling pathways. Because most hormones do not simply activate a linear series of reactions, but rather signal through multiple parallel intracellular pathways, the particular combination of signaling pathways that are activated may determine the final outcome. It is now recognized that protein molecules involved in complex intracellular signal transmission do not float around freely in a cytoplasmic "soup" but are anchored at specific cellular loci by interactions with the cytoskeleton or the membranes of intracellular organelles, or in large signaling complexes. Protein kinase A, for example, may be localized to specific regions in the cell by specialized proteins called AKAPs (A kinase anchoring proteins), which may also act as scaffolds that anchor other participants in a signaling cascade. Although there are relatively few basic patterns of signal transduction, there is great versatility in their operation. Virtually all the intracellular signaling molecules discussed are represented in the human genome in multiple forms, often referred to as isoforms. In addition to being products of separate genes, different isoforms may arise by alternate splicing of mRNA from the same gene or by different posttranslational processing of the same gene product. A single cell often contains more than one isoform of various components of signaling pathways, each with unique regulatory properties and sometimes with discrete cellular loci. Many cells express more than one isoform of adenylyl cyclase, and although all nine isoforms of adenylyl cyclase are activated by any of the four different isoforms of $G\alpha_s$, some isoforms of adenyl cyclase are also activated or inhibited by different members of the protein kinase C family, or by calcium, or by some of the more than 50 possible combinations of G-protein $\beta\gamma$ subunit isoforms. There are also multiple uniquely regulated isoforms of cAMP phosphodiesterases, and of PI3 kinases. Similar statements can be made for the phospholipases C and the vast number of proteins that participate in tyrosine kinase and nuclear receptor signaling systems. Seven different proteins arise from alternate splicing of the CREB gene. In all, it has been estimated that more than 20% of the genome is devoted to signal transduction, and it is evident that there is ample complexity to account for all the regulated behaviors governed by hormones.

Modulation of responding systems

Biological systems are dynamic. Just as the amount of hormone secreted varies with changing circumstances, so too does the magnitude and duration of the response of target cells. Many factors in addition to the actions of other hormones influence how robust a response will be and for how long it may persist (Figs. 5.13 and 5.14).

Clearly, the most important determinants are the concentration of hormone present in the extracellular fluid surrounding target cells, the length of time that the concentration is maintained, and the competency of the target cells. For hormones that are secreted in a pulsatile fashion, both the amount secreted in each pulse and the frequency of secretory pulses are important determinants of the amount of hormone that reaches target cell receptors and how long effective concentrations (ECs) are maintained. In addition to the plasma concentration, the rate of delivery of a hormone to the extracellular fluid bathing its target cells also depends upon the rate of blood flow, capillary permeability, and the fraction of hormone that is bound to plasma proteins, all of which are sensitive to changing physiological circumstances and the actions

Determinants of the magnitude of hormonal responses

A. Concentration of hormone at the target cell surface
   1. Rate of secretion
   2. Rate of delivery by the circulation
   3. Rate of hormone degradation

B. Sensitivity of target cells
   1. Number of functional receptors per cell
   2. Receptor affinity for the hormone
   3. Post-receptor amplification capacity
   4. Abundance of available effector molecules

C. Number of functional target cells

FIGURE 5.13 Determinants of the magnitude of a hormonal response.

Determinants of the magnitude of hormonal responses

A. Concentration of hormone at the target cell surface
   1. Rate of secretion
   2. Rate of delivery by the circulation
   3. Rate of hormone degradation

B. Sensitivity of target cells
   1. Number of functional receptors per cell
   2. Receptor affinity for the hormone
   3. Post-receptor amplification capacity
   4. Abundance of available effector molecules

C. Number of functional target cells

FIGURE 5.14 Determinants of the duration of a hormonal response.

of hormones. Another critical determinant of the concentration of hormone available to target cells hormone is the rate of degradation either by target tissues or in blood and nontarget tissues. As we have seen regarding the rate of thyroxine metabolism, the rate of hormone degradation may also change with changing circumstances.

Sensitivity and capacity

Neither the sensitivity to hormonal stimulation nor the capacity of target tissues to respond is constant; they change with changing physiological or pathological circumstances. Sensitivity to stimulation and capacity to respond are two separate though related aspects of hormonal responses. Sensitivity describes the acuity of the ability of a cell or organ to recognize and respond to a signal in proportion to the intensity of that signal. The capacity to respond or the maximum response that a tissue or organ can achieve depends upon the number of target cells and their competence. Hormones regulate both the sensitivity and the capacity of target tissues to respond either to themselves or to other hormones.

The relationship between the magnitude of a hormonal response and the concentration of a hormone that produces the response can be described mathematically by a dose–response curve (Fig. 5.15). The typical dose–response curve usually is plotted with the magnitude of the response on the *Y* axis and the dose or concentration on the *X* axis. The lowest amount or concentration of hormone that produces a measurable response usually is called the threshold. The response is at a maximum when no further changes can be produced by further increases in hormone concentration. The slope of the linear portion of the curve describes the rate or degree of change in response per unit increase in hormone concentration. Each of these parameters may be modified by the actions of hormones or changes in physiological conditions. Because it is difficult to measure small responses with precision, the threshold is seldom used in describing sensitivity. Instead, sensitivity usually is described in terms of the concentration of hormone needed to produce a half-maximal response, which is sometimes abbreviated as EC50 (EC for 50% of the subjects).

When sensitivity is increased, a lower concentration of hormone is needed to achieve a half-maximal response, and when sensitivity is decreased, a higher concentration of hormone is needed to evoke the same response. In the example shown in Fig. 5.15, we may assume that curve B represents the basal or "normal" sensitivity with a half maximum response attained at a hormone concentration of 1 nmol/L.

Curve A reflects a 10-fold increase in sensitivity and Curve C represents a 10-fold decrease in sensitivity. In other words an increase in sensitivity shifts the dose response curve to the left, and a decrease shifts it to the right. We may consider the maximum response that can be elicited by a hormone as the capacity of the responding system.

Dose–response curves that reflect changes in capacity to respond are illustrated in Fig. 5.16.

Let us assume once again that Curve B represents the basal or "normal" condition. The maximum

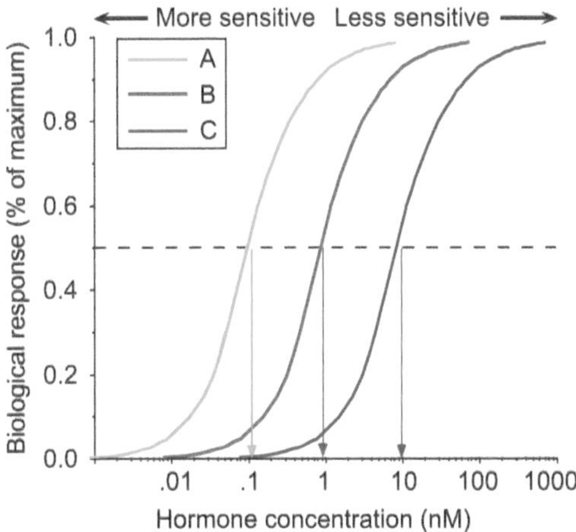

FIGURE 5.15 The relationship between concentration and response at three different levels of sensitivity. Arrows indicate the concentration of hormone that produces a half-maximal response for each level of sensitivity. Note that the abscissa is plotted on a logarithmic scale.

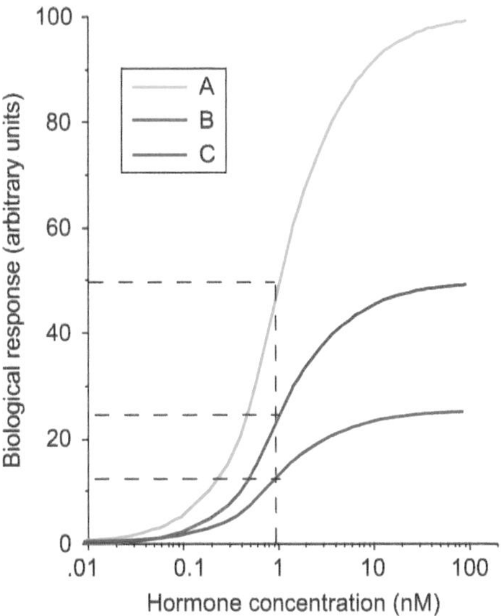

FIGURE 5.16 Concentration response relationships showing different capacities to respond. Note that the concentration needed to produce the half-maximal response is identical for all three response capacities. Note that the abscissa is plotted on a logarithmic scale.

response may be increased (Curve A) or decreased (Curve C), but the sensitivity (i.e., the concentration of hormone needed to produce the half-maximal response) remains unchanged at 1 ng/mL. Note that in this illustration the slope of the dose response curve also changes.

One mechanism by which the sensitivity of target tissues may be adjusted is by regulation of the availability of hormone receptors. The initial event in a hormonal response is the binding of the hormone to its receptor (see Chapter 1: Introduction). The higher the concentration of hormone, the more likely it is to interact with its receptors. If there are no hormone receptors, there can be no response, and the more receptors that are available to interact with any particular amount of hormone, the greater the likelihood of a response. In other words the probability that a molecule of hormone will encounter a molecule of receptor is related to the abundance of both the hormone and the receptor. The effects of changing receptor abundance on hormone sensitivity are shown in Fig. 5.17.

This relationship is not linear, and that doubling the receptor number lowers the hormone concentration needed to produce a half-maximal response by a factor of 2, while halving the number of receptors increases the needed concentration of hormone by a factor of 2.5.

Many hormones decrease the number of their own receptors in target tissues. This so-called downregulation originally was recognized as a real phenomenon in modern endocrinology when it was shown that the decreased sensitivity of some cells to insulin in hyperinsulinemic states resulted from a decrease in the number of receptors on the cell surface. However, a similar phenomenon was observed many years earlier by Cannon and Rosenblueth who described the "supersensitivity of denervated tissues." Cannon's original discovery of this phenomenon concerned the hypersensitivity of the denervated heart to circulating epinephrine and norepinephrine. The generality of this phenomenon for both endocrine and neural control systems is further indicated by the increase in acetylcholine receptors that occurs after a muscle is denervated and the restoration to normal after reinnervation. The phenomenon of tachyphylaxis, or loss of responsiveness to a pharmacological agent upon repeated or constant exposure, may be another example of downregulation of receptors. Downregulation may result from the inactivation of the receptors at the cell surface by covalent modifications or allosteric changes, from an increased rate of sequestration of internalized membrane receptors or a change in the rates of receptor degradation or synthesis.

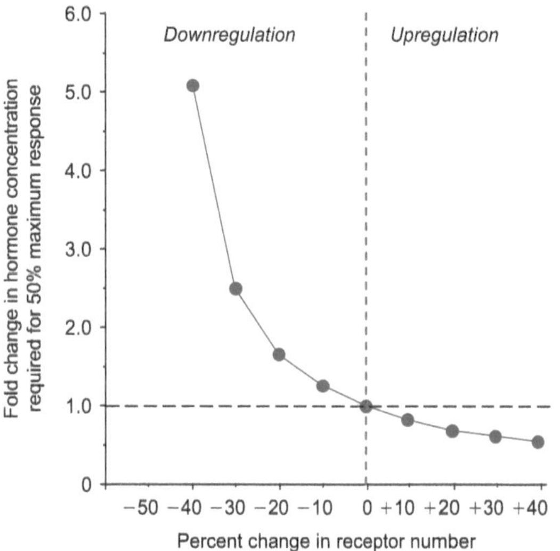

FIGURE 5.17 The effects of up- or downregulation of receptor number on sensitivity to hormonal stimulation. Note that the abscissa is plotted on a logarithmic scale.

Downregulation is not limited to the effects of a hormone on its own receptor or to the surface receptors for the water-soluble hormones. One hormone can downregulate receptors for another hormone. This appears to be the mechanism by which T3 decreases the sensitivity of the thyrotropes of the pituitary to thyrotropin releasing hormone (see Chapter 3: Thyroid Gland). Similarly, the ovarian hormone progesterone may downregulate both its own receptor and that of estrogen as well. Upregulation, or the increase in available receptors, also occurs. T3 and cortisol may increase adrenergic receptors in some tissues as already mentioned, and prolactin and growth hormone may upregulate their own receptors. Estrogen upregulates both its own receptors and those of luteinizing hormone in ovarian cells during the menstrual cycle and is essential for the expression of progesterone receptors (see Chapter 13: Hormonal Control of Reproduction in the Female: The Menstrual Cycle).

Spare receptors

Another determinant of sensitivity is the affinity of a receptor for its hormone. Hormones reversibly associate with their receptors according to the law of mass action. Affinity reflects the "tightness" of binding or the likelihood that an encounter between a hormone and its receptor will result in binding and usually is quantified in terms of the concentration of hormone at which half of the available receptors are occupied by hormone. Although the affinity of the receptor for its hormone may be increased or decreased by covalent modifications such as phosphorylation or dephosphorylation, more commonly, the number of receptors is modulated rather than their affinity.

Biological responses do not necessarily parallel hormone binding and, therefore, are not always limited by the affinity of the receptor for the hormone. Because they depend on many postreceptor events, responses to some hormones may be at a maximum at concentrations of hormone that do not saturate all the receptors (Fig. 5.18).

When fewer than 100% of the receptors need to be occupied to obtain a maximum response, cells are said to express "spare receptors." For example, glucose uptake by the fat cell is stimulated in a dose-dependent manner by insulin, but the response reaches a maximum when only a small percentage of available receptors are occupied by insulin. Consequently, the sensitivity of the cells to insulin is considerably greater than the affinity of the receptor for insulin. Recall that sensitivity is measured in terms of a biological response, which is the physiologically meaningful parameter, whereas affinity of the receptor is independent of the postreceptor events that produce the biological response. The magnitude of a cellular response to a hormone is determined by summation of the signals generated by each of the occupied receptors and, therefore, is related to the number of receptors that are activated rather than the fraction of the total receptor pool that is bound to hormone. However, because the fraction of available receptors that binds to hormone is determined by the hormone concentration, the number of activated receptors needed to produce a half-maximal response will represent a smaller and smaller fraction as the total number of receptors increases. In the example shown in Fig. 5.18, expression of five times more receptors than needed for a maximum response increases the sensitivity sevenfold.

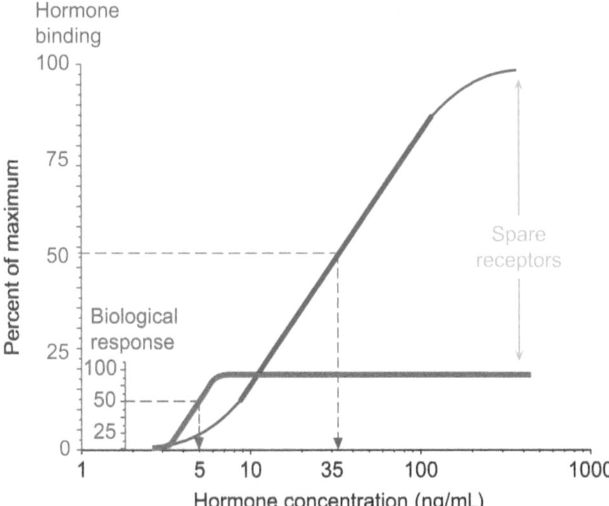

FIGURE 5.18 Spare receptors. Note that the concentration of hormone needed to produce a half-maximal response is considerably lower than that needed to occupy half of the receptors. Note that the abscissa is plotted on a logarithmic scale.

Another consequence of spare membrane receptors for peptide hormones relates to the rapidity with which a hormone can be cleared from the blood. It may be recalled that the degradation of peptide hormones depends, at least in part, upon receptor-mediated internalization of the hormone and hence access to proteolytic enzymes. It appears that cells have a greater capacity to degrade internalized hormone than to generate a hormone response. Receptors that may be spared with respect to producing a hormonal response may nevertheless play a physiologically important role in degrading their ligands. In fact, some membrane receptors such as the so-called clearance receptors for the atrial natriuretic factor (see Chapter 9: Regulation of Salt and Water Balance) lack the biochemical components needed for signal transduction, and function only in hormone degradation. Spare receptors thus may blunt potentially harmful overresponses to rapid changes in hormone concentrations and facilitate clearing hormone from blood.

Sensitivity to hormonal stimulation can also be modulated in ways that do not involve changes in receptor number or affinity. Postreceptor modulation may affect any of the steps in the biological pathway through which hormonal effects are produced. Up- or downregulation of effector molecules such as enzymes, ion channels, and contractile proteins may amplify or dampen responses and hence change the relationship between receptor occupancy and magnitude of response. For example, the activity of cAMP phosphodiesterase increases in adipocytes in the absence of pituitary hormones. It may be recalled (see Chapter 1: Introduction) that this enzyme catalyzes the degradation of cAMP. When its activity is increased, less cAMP can accumulate after the stimulation of adenylyl cyclase by a hormone such as epinephrine. Therefore if all other things were equal, a higher concentration of epinephrine would be needed to produce a given amount of lipolysis than might be necessary in the presence of normal amounts of pituitary hormones, and hence sensitivity to epinephrine would be reduced. Increased activity of phosphodiesterase is only one of several factors contributing to decreased responses to epinephrine in adipocytes of hypopituitary animals.

These tissues also express less hormone-sensitive lipase and changes in their content of G-proteins. Consequently, even when all their receptors are occupied, the maximum response that these cells can make is below normal. In this example, both the sensitivity and the capacity to respond are decreased.

At the tissue, organ, or whole-body level, the response to a hormone is the aggregate of the contributions of all the stimulated cells, so that the magnitude of the response is determined both by the number of responsive cells and their competence. For example, Adrenocorticotropic hormone (ACTH) produces a dose-related increase in blood cortisol concentration in normal individuals. However, immediately after the removal of one adrenal gland, changes in the concentration of cortisol in response to ACTH administration would be only half as large as seen when both glands are present. Therefore a much higher dose of ACTH will be needed to achieve the same change as was produced preoperatively. With time, however, as the adrenal cortical cells upregulate ACTH receptors and increase their enzymatic capacity for steroidogenesis, the concentration of ACTH needed to achieve a particular rate of cortisol secretion will decline. Another example of how changes in cell number and competence is reflected at the whole-body level is the gradual increase in estradiol secretion seen in the early part of the menstrual cycle despite an unchanging or even decreasing concentration of follicle stimulating hormone (FSH) (see Chapter 13: Hormonal Control of Reproduction in the Female: The Menstrual Cycle). This change in sensitivity to FSH reflects the activity of an increasing number of estradiol-producing cells.

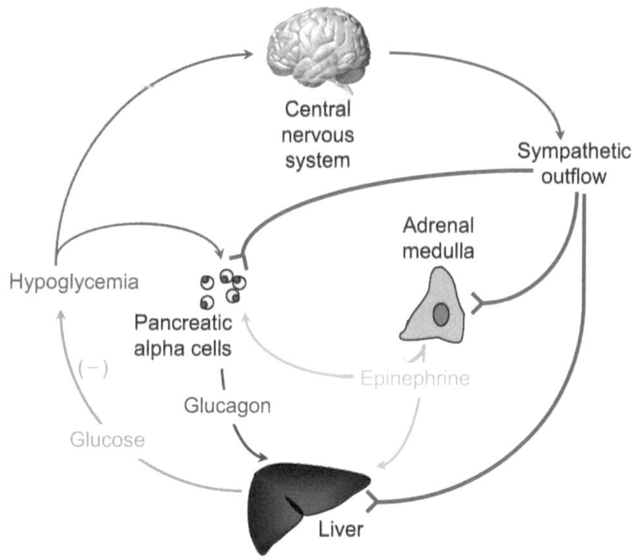

FIGURE 5.19 Redundant mechanisms to stimulate hepatic glucose production. Hormonal and neural mechanisms are marshaled to combat potentially life-threatening low blood glucose concentrations.

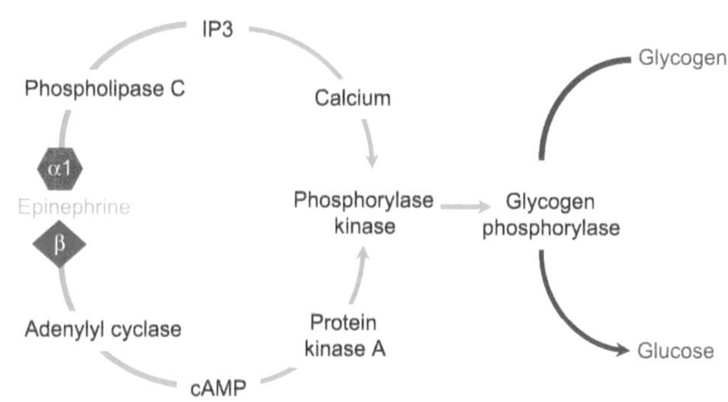

FIGURE 5.20 Redundant mechanisms to activate glycogen phosphorylase by a single hormone, epinephrine, acting through both α1 and β receptors.

Hormonal integration at the whole-body level

Redundancy

Survival in a hostile environment has been made possible by the evolution of fail-safe mechanisms to govern crucial functions. Just as each organ system has built in excess capacity giving it the potential to function at levels beyond the usual day-to-day demands, so too is there excess regulatory capacity provided in the form of seemingly duplicative or overlapping controls. Simply put, the body has more than one way to achieve a given end. For example, conversion of liver glycogen to blood glucose can be signaled by at least two hormones, glucagon from the alpha cells of the pancreas and epinephrine from the adrenal medulla (Fig. 5.19).

Both hormones increase cAMP production in the liver and thereby activate the enzyme, glycogen phosphorylase, which catalyzes glycogenolysis. Two hormones secreted from two different tissues, sometimes in response to different conditions, thus produce the same end result. When present simultaneously, their effects summate, so the overall response depends on both. When one is deficient or overproduced, greater or lesser secretion of the other may compensate, so that the overall response may remain unchanged.

Further redundancy can also be seen at the molecular level. Using the same example of conversion of liver glycogen to blood glucose, there are even two ways that epinephrine can activate phosphorylase. By stimulating beta adrenergic receptors, epinephrine increases cAMP formation as already mentioned. By stimulating α-1 adrenergic receptors, epinephrine activates phospholipase β and the resulting production of DAG and IP3. Calcium released from intracellular stores due to the effects of IP3 also activates phosphorylase (Fig. 5.20).

Redundant mechanisms not only assure that a critical process will take place, but they also offer opportunity for flexibility and subtle fine-tuning of a process.

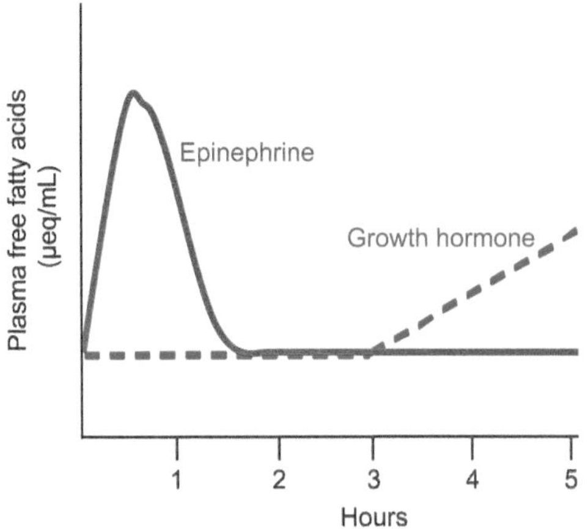

FIGURE 5.21 Idealized representation of the effects of epinephrine and growth hormone on plasma concentrations of free fatty acids.

Though redundant in the respect that two different hormones may have some overlapping effects, actions of the two hormones are usually not identical in all respects. Within the physiological range of its concentrations in blood, glucagon's action is restricted to the liver; epinephrine produces a variety of other responses in many extrahepatic tissues while increasing glycogenolysis in the liver. Variations in the relative input from both hormones allows for a wide spectrum of changes in blood glucose concentrations relative to such other effects of epinephrine as increased heart rate.

Two hormones that produce common effects may differ not only in their range of actions but also in their time constants (Fig. 5.21).

One may have a more rapid onset and short duration of action, whereas another may have a longer duration of action, but a slower onset. For example, epinephrine increases blood concentrations of free fatty acids (FFA) within seconds or minutes, and this effect dissipates as rapidly when epinephrine secretion is stopped. Growth hormone similarly increases the blood concentrations of FFA, but its effects are seen only after a lag period of 2 or 3 hours and persist for many hours. A hormone-like epinephrine may, therefore, be used to meet short-term needs, and another, like growth hormone, may satisfy sustained needs.

Redundancy also pertains to processes in which the same end may be achieved by more than one physiological means. For example, blood concentrations of calcium may be increased by an action of the parathyroid hormone to mobilize calcium stored in bone crystals (see Chapter 10: Hormonal Regulation of Calcium Balance), or by an action of vitamin D to promote calcium absorption from the gut. These processes, as might be expected, have different time constants as well.

One of the implications of redundancy for understanding both normal physiology and endocrine disease is that partial, or perhaps even complete, failure of one mechanism can be compensated by increased reliance on another mechanism. This point is particularly relevant to interpretation of results of gene knockout studies. In some cases, elimination of what was thought to be an essential protein resulted in no apparent functional changes, perhaps because of redundancy. Functional deficiencies may be masked by redundant mechanisms and be evident only in subtle ways. Some deficiencies may only show as overt disease after appropriate provocation or perturbation of the system. Conversely, strategies for therapeutic interventions designed to increase or decrease the rate of a process must consider the redundant inputs that regulate that process. Merely accelerating or blocking one regulatory input may not produce the desired effect since independent adjustments in redundant pathways may completely compensate for the intervention.

Reinforcement

It is an oversimplification to think of any hormone as simply having a single unique effect. In accomplishing any end, most hormones act at several locales either within a single cell or in different tissues or organs to produce separate but mutually reinforcing responses. In some cases a hormone may produce radically different responses at different locales, which nevertheless reinforce each other from the perspective of the whole organism. Let us consider, for example, some of the ways ACTH acts on the fasciculata cell of the adrenal cortex to promote the production of cortisol. It

- increases uptake of cholesterol, which serves as a substrate for hormone synthesis;
- activates the esterase enzyme needed for mobilization of cholesterol from storage droplets;
- increases the synthesis and activity of the STAR (steroid acute regulatory) protein needed for delivery of cholesterol to the intramitochondrial enzyme that converts it to pregnenolone; and
- increases adrenal blood flow, which facilitates the delivery not only of the cholesterol precursor to the adrenal cortex but also the newly synthesized hormone to the rest of the body.

Each of these effects contributes to the end of providing the body with cortisol, but, collectively, they make possible an enormously broader range of response in a shorter time frame.

Reinforcement can also take the form of a single hormone acting in different ways in different tissues to produce complementary effects. A good example of this is the action of glucocorticoid hormones to promote gluconeogenesis. As we have seen (see Chapter 4: The Adrenal Glands, Fig. 4.12), glucocorticoids promote protein breakdown in muscle and lymphoid tissues, and the consequent release of amino acids into the blood. In adipose tissue, glucocorticoids promote triglyceride lipolysis and the release of glycerol. In the liver, glucocorticoids induce the formation of the enzymes necessary to convert amino acids, glycerol, and other substrates into glucose. Either the extrahepatic action to provide substrate or the hepatic action to increase capacity to utilize that substrate would increase gluconeogenesis. Together, these complementary actions increase the overall magnitude and speed of the response.

Push–pull mechanisms

As discussed in Chapter 1, Introduction, many critical processes are under dual control by agents that act antagonistically either to stimulate or to inhibit. Such dual control allows for more precise regulation through negative feedback than would be possible with a single control system. The example cited was hepatic production of glucose, which is increased by glucagon and inhibited by insulin. In emergency situations or during exercise, epinephrine and norepinephrine released from the adrenal medulla and sympathetic nerve endings override both negative feedback systems by inhibiting insulin secretion and stimulating glucagon secretion (Fig. 5.22).

The effect of adding a stimulatory influence while simultaneously removing an inhibitory influence is a rapid and large response, more rapid and larger than could be achieved by simply affecting either hormone alone, or than could be accomplished by the direct glycogenolytic effect of epinephrine or norepinephrine.

Another type of push–pull mechanism can be seen at the molecular level. Net synthesis of glycogen from glucose depends upon the activities of two enzymes, glycogen synthase, which catalyzes the formation of glycogen from glucose, and glycogen phosphorylase, which catalyzes glycogen breakdown (Fig. 5.23).

The net reaction rate is determined by the balance of the activity of the two enzymes. The activity of both enzymes is subject to regulation by phosphorylation, but in opposite directions: addition of a phosphate group activates phosphorylase but inactivates synthase. In this case a single agent, cAMP, which activates protein kinase A, increases the activity of phosphorylase and simultaneously inhibits synthase.

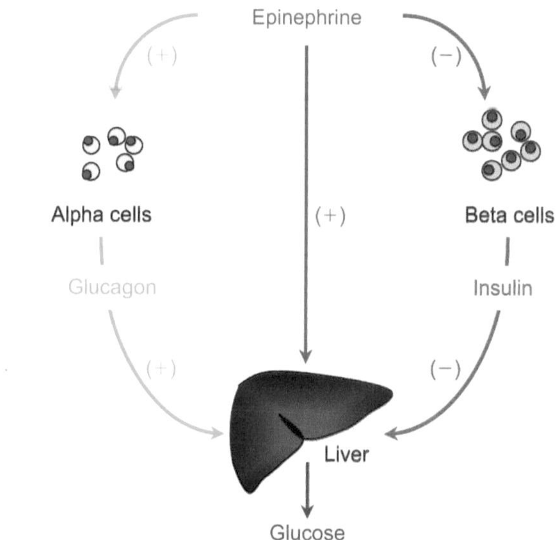

FIGURE 5.22 Push–pull mechanism. Epinephrine inhibits insulin secretion while promoting glucagon secretion. This combination of effects on the liver stimulates glucose production while simultaneously relieving an inhibitory influence. (+) = increases; (−) = decreases.

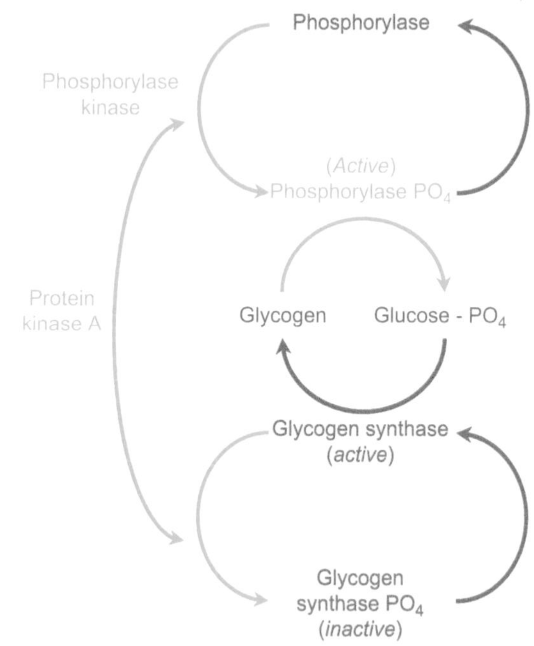

FIGURE 5.23 Push–pull mechanism to activate glycogen phosphorylase while simultaneously inhibiting glycogen synthase.

Numerous examples of the foregoing principles of hormonal integration can be seen in the succeeding chapters, which focus on the interactions of multiple hormones in addressing physiological problems.

Summary

Hormones rarely act alone and this chapter introduces the effect of integrated action of more than one hormone on target tissue. These actions include synergistic effect as a result of redundancy as well as additive responses as a result of opposite effects exerted by different hormones acting at different receptors.

Suggested readings

Basic foundations

Marx, S. J., & Wells, S. A. J. (2016). Multiple endocrine neoplasia. In S. Melmed, K. S. Polonsky, P. R. Larsen, & H. M. Kronenberg (Eds.), *Williams textbook of endocrinology* (pp. 1724–1761). Philadelphia, PA: Elsevier.

Sotos, J. G. (2008). *The physical Lincoln*. Mt. Vernon, VA: Mt. Vernon Book Systems.

Advanced information

Castinetti, F., Moley, J., Mulligan, L., & Waguespack, S. G. (2018). A comprehensive review of MEN2B. *Endocrine-Related Cancer, 25*.

Grey, J., & Winter, K. (2018). Patient quality of life and prognosis in multiple endocrine neoplasia type 2. *Endocrine-Related Cancer, 25* (2), T69–T77. Available from https://doi.org/10.1530/erc-17-0335.

Hughes, M., Feliberti, E., Perry, R. R., & Vinik, A. (2017). Multiple endocrine neoplasia type 2 A (including familial medullary carcinoma) and type 2B. In L. J. De Groot, G. Chrousos, & K. Dungan (Eds.), *Endotext*. South Dartmouth, MA: MD Text.com, Inc.

Hyde, S. M., Cote, G. J., & Grubbs, E. G. (2017). Genetics of multiple endocrine neoplasia type 1/multiple endocrine neoplasia type 2 syndromes. *Endocrinology and Metabolism Clinics of North America, 46*(2), 491–502. Available from https://doi.org/10.1016/j.ecl.2017.01.011.

Moramarco, J., Ghorayeb, N. E., Dumas, N., Nolet, S., Boulanger, L., Burnichon, N., ... Bourdeau, I. (2017). Pheochromocytomas are diagnosed incidentally and at older age in neurofibromatosis type 1. *Clinical Endocrinology, 86*(3), 332–339. Available from https://doi.org/10.1111/cen.13265.

Pacheco, M. C. (2016). Multiple endocrine neoplasia: A genetically diverse group of familial tumor syndromes. *Journal of Pediatric Genetics, 5*, 89–97.

Petr, E. J., & Else, T. (2016). Genetic predisposition to endocrine tumors: Diagnosis, surveillance and challenges in care. *Seminars in Oncology, 43*(2016), 582–590.

Plaza-Menacho, I. (2018). Structure and function of RET in multiple endocrine neoplasia type 2. *Endocrine-Related Cancer, 25*(2), T79–T90. Available from https://doi.org/10.1530/erc-17-0354.

Marx, S. J., & Wells, S. A., Jr. (2016). Multiple endocrine neoplasia, Chapter 39. In S. Melmed, K. S. Polonsky, P. R. Larsen, & H. M. Kronenberg (Eds.), *'Williams' textbook of endocrinology* (13th ed., pp. 1724–1761). Elsevier.

Pacheco, M. C. (2016). Multiple endocrine neoplasia: A genetically diverse group of familial tumor syndromes. *Journal of Pediatric Genetics, 5*, 89–97.

CHAPTER

6

Hormones of the gastrointestinal tract

Case study: Zollinger-Ellison syndrome (ZES)

"C.P., a 36-year-old married white female, was first admitted to the medical service of University Hospital, Columbus, Ohio, on July 22, 1952, with the chief complaints of abdominal pain and diarrhea of 8 years' duration. . ."

So begins gastric surgeons Robert Zollinger and Edwin Ellison's case history of the first patient to have the syndrome which bears their name. Their patient underwent repeated surgeries which removed successively more of her stomach and small intestine (Fig. 6.1).

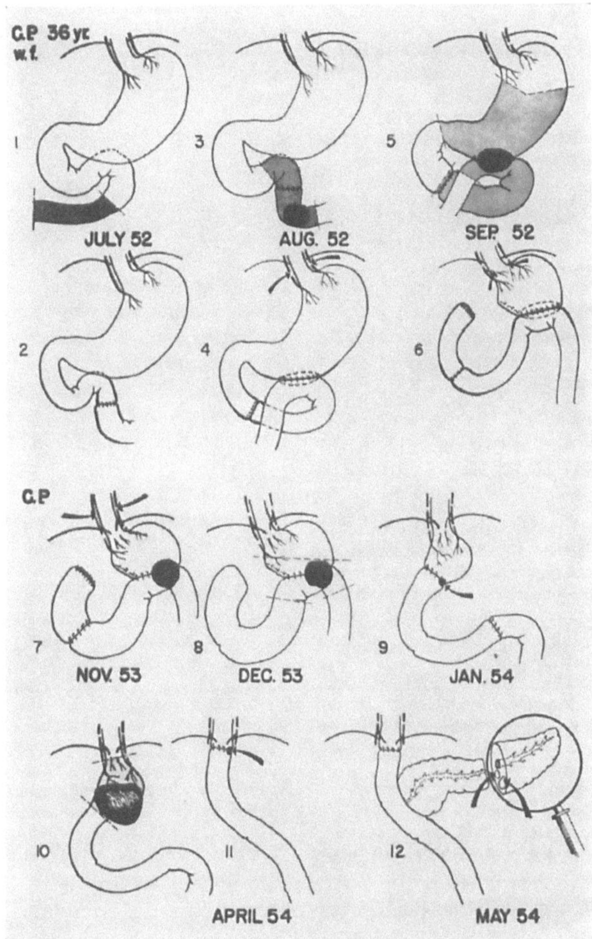

FIGURE 6.1 This shows the progressive surgeries performed in an attempt to stop the high production of hydrochloric acid and surgically treat the ulcers that were found. Source: *From Zollinger, R. M., & Ellison, E. H. (1955). Primary peptic ulcerations of the jejunum associated with islet cell tumors of the pancreas.* Annals of Surgery, 142*(4), 709–723.*

Goodman's Basic Medical Endocrinology.
DOI: https://doi.org/10.1016/B978-0-12-815844-9.00006-3

(*cont'd*)

In the first surgery (Diagram 1 in Fig. 6.1) a portion of the jejunum that was ulcerated (colored black) was removed and an end-to-end anastomosis between the duodenum and jejunum was done (Diagram 2). Within a month, multiple jejunal ulcers, further along the jejunum than the first one (Diagram 3), necessitated removal of another 22 cm (almost 10 in.) of jejunum (Diagram 4). At this time, both the right and left vagus nerves to the stomach were severed (arrows in Fig. 6.1, Diagram 4) in an effort to stop the high hydrochloric acid production (Fig. 6.2). It did not.

A month after the second surgery, signs and symptoms of another ulcer (Fig. 6.1, Diagram 5) necessitated another surgery in which 70% of the stomach was removed, along with more jejunum and the severing of additional potential vagal fibers (Fig. 6.1, Diagram 6). More ulcers occurred and more surgeries ensued (Fig. 6.1, Diagrams 7–11) so that by April of the next year, her stomach had been completely removed. Complications from her last surgery and her continued loss of weight (last reported weight was 72 lb) caused her demise 2 years after Zollinger and Ellison first saw her. At autopsy a pancreatic tumor was found. Only decades later would the picture become clearer: this tumor most likely secreted gastrin which stimulated the parietal cells of the stomach to produce large amounts of hydrochloric acid.

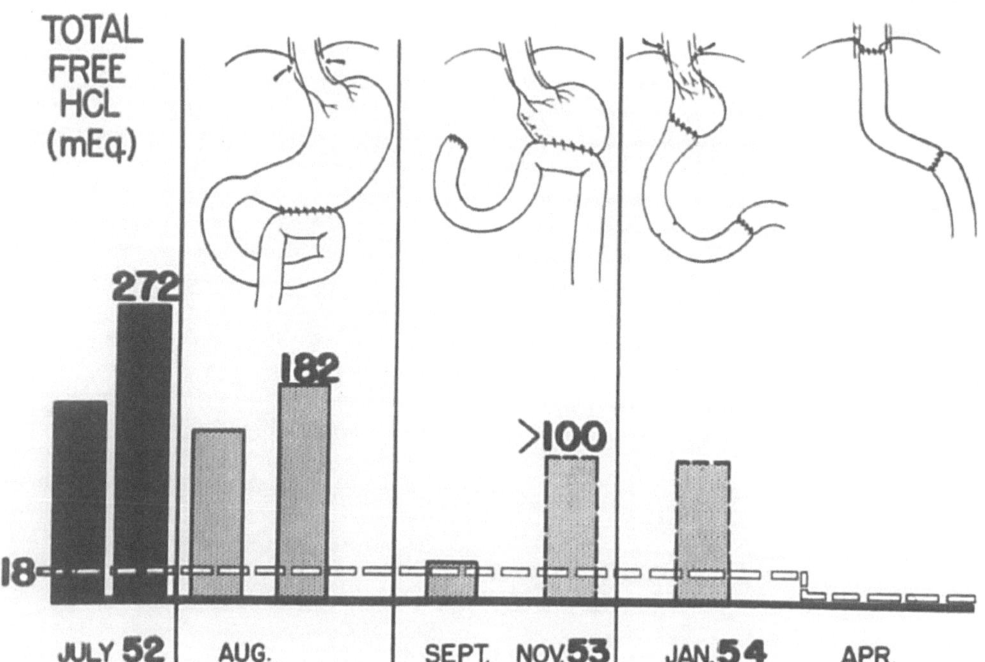

FIGURE 6.2 This shows the surgical attempt to reduce hydrochloric acid secretion. The dotted line is the normal level of hydrochloric acid secretion. Source: *From Zollinger, R. M., & Ellison, E. H. (1955). Primary peptic ulcerations of the jejunum associated with islet cell tumors of the pancreas.* Annals of Surgery, 142*(4), 709–723.*

In the clinic: Zollinger-Ellison syndrome

G cells produce gastrin. Normally, these cells predominate in the antrum of the stomach and duodenum of the small intestine, with lesser numbers in the central and peripheral nervous systems, other endocrine organs and tissues of the respiratory and reproductive tracts. While the gastrin gene is not normally present in pancreatic tissue, adenomas secreting gastrin (gastrinomas) are commonly found in that endocrine gland as well as in the duodenum. Gastrin is a hormone that stimulates the enterochromaffin-like (ECL) cells to produce

(cont'd)

histamine. In the presence of a lot of gastrin, the ECL cells will proliferate becoming hyperplastic (Fig. 6.3).

ECL cells are located throughout the stomach and small intestine as well as numerous other locations, but those near the gastric parietal cells secrete histamine into the extracellular space. The stimulation of H2 histamine receptors and gastrin receptors on the parietal cell membrane causes the production of hydrochloric acid (HCl). Production can be further enhanced by vagus nerve stimulation. Hydrochloric acid causes the activation of pepsinogen to the proteolytic enzyme, pepsin. Pepsinogen is secreted by the chief cells of the gastric glands. It is the pepsin that is primarily responsible for the ulcers seen in peptic ulcer disease (PUD) and Zollinger–Ellison syndrome. However, the excessive hydrochloric acid production itself will also be a major factor in ulcer formation.

Signs and symptoms

Because this syndrome is rare (Fig. 6.4), it is not usually accurately diagnosed for 4–6 years after the onset of symptoms.

The signs and symptoms of ZES include frequent diarrhea due to the irritation of the intestinal wall by high amounts of hydrochloric acid, pepsin, and the presence of undigested lipids; gastric ulcers and

(A)

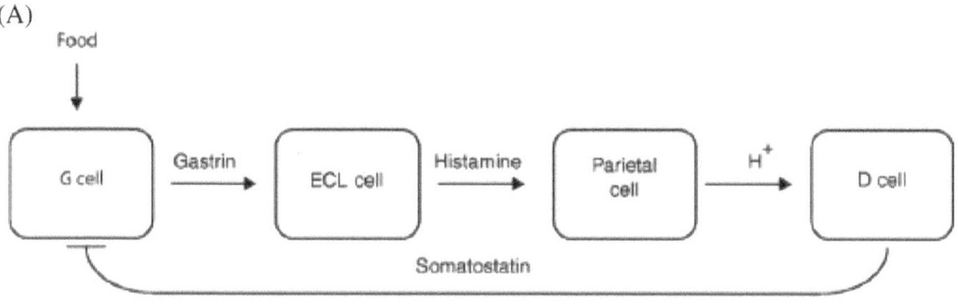

(B)

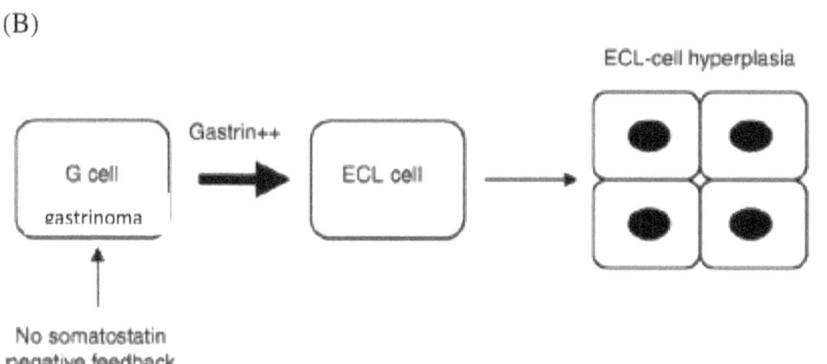

FIGURE 6.3 In (A), there is the normal sequence of secretion and regulation of that secretion by somatostatin negative feedback. In (B), there are no receptors on gastrinoma cells for somatostatin, so there is no negative feedback. The continued increase in gastrin causes histamine-secreting ECL hyperplasia with a resultant high increase in the parietal cell production of hydrochloric acid. Source: *Modified from Figure 3 of (A) Corey, B., & Chen, H. (2017). Neuroendocrine tumors of the stomach. Surgical Clinics of North America, 97, 333–343; (B) From Burkitt, M. D., & Pritchard, D. M. (2006). Review article: Pathogenesis and management of gastric carcinoid tumours.* Alimentary Pharmacology & Therapeutics, 24,*1306, with permission.*

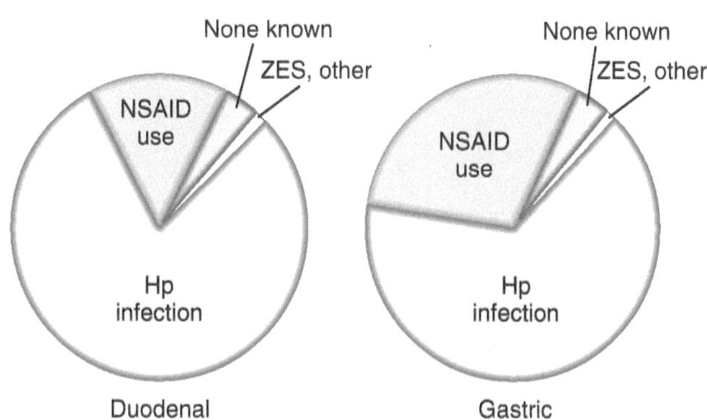

FIGURE 6.4 The most common causes of peptic ulcer disease are Hp infection, followed by NSAID overuse. ZES is only a small percentage of causes which explains why its diagnosis is often delayed for years. *Hp, Helicobacter pylori; NSAID,* nonsteroidal antiinflammatory drug; *ZES,* Zollinger–Ellison syndrome. Source: *Figure 53-1 in Chan, F. K. L., & Lau, J. Y. W. (2016). Peptic ulcer disease, Chapter 53. In M. Feldman, L. S. Friedman, & L. J. Brandt (Eds.),* Sleisenger and Fordtran's gastrointestinal and liver disease *(10th ed., p. 884). Elsevier.*

(*cont'd*)

associated pain, including heartburn, that do not respond well to drug therapy nor are caused by *Helicobacter pylori* infection; loss of weight due to duodenal destruction of pancreatic enzymes necessary to digest food; and gastric reflux into the esophagus (GERD—gastroesophageal reflux disease), a consequence of hypersecretion of HCl.

Diagnosis

Elevated serum levels of gastrin above 500 pg/mL. Secretin stimulation is often performed in patients whose gastrin levels are between 200 and 500 pg/mL to rule out other disorders. Secretin stimulates G cells. Normally, secretin also stimulates the release of somatostatin (SST) from D cells in the antrum, which has a negative effect on G cells so that gastrin production and hydrochloric acid production stops. However, there are no SST receptors on the G cells in gastrinomas, so secretin enhances hydrochloric acid production in ZES (Fig. 6.5), which is why it is used to test for this syndrome.

ZES should be considered with elevated gastric HCl levels above 15 mEq/h in an intact fasting stomach and above 5 mEq/h in a stomach that has had a gastric resection due to ulcers. Endoscopy can be used to detect the presence of gastric, duodenal, or jejunal ulcers. During the procedure, biopsies are taken of duodenal and upper jejunal tissue, especially around ulcers, to rule out malignancy (which can also cause ulcer formation). Finding the gastrinoma can be a challenge because it is not always visible by endoscopy if it is embedded in the intestinal wall or in the pancreas. Use of ultrasound in combination with endoscopy (endoscopic ultrasonography) has proven useful. Rare cases of ovarian or lymph node ectopic gastrin tumors have been reported. An algorithm for diagnosis is presented in Fig. 6.6 and for treatment in Fig. 6.7.

Management

Initially, the primary focus is to reduce the secretion of hydrochloric acid. This is best accomplished by hydrogen pump inhibitors [H^+/K^+-ATP (adenosine triphosphate) inhibitors] such as omeprazole. H2 receptor

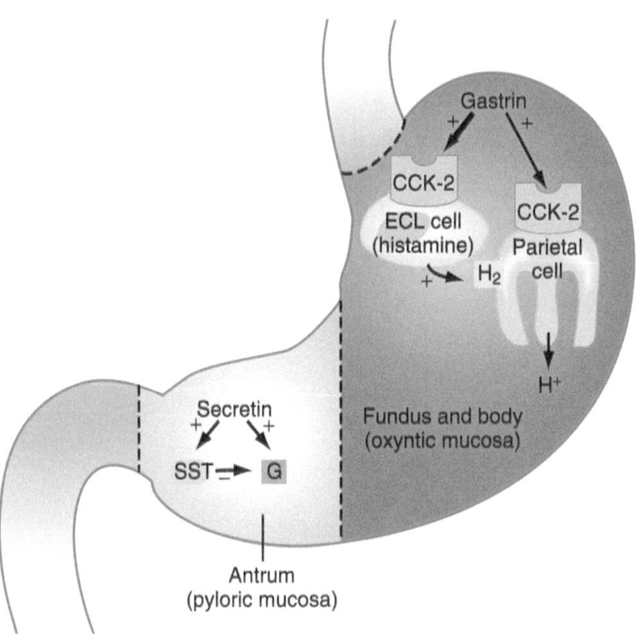

FIGURE 6.5 Secretin stimulates G cells and D cells, with the greater effect on D cells, resulting in SST release. Normally, the overall effect of secretin is to inhibit gastric acid secretion. However, in ZES, there are no receptors for somatostatin on the G cells in gastrinomas, so secretin in ZES stimulates the production of hydrochloric acid. *SST*, Somatostatin; *ZES*, Zollinger–Ellison syndrome. Source: *Figure 50-17 in Schubert, M. L., & Kaunitz, J. D. (2016). Gastric secretion, Chapter 50. In M. Feldman, L. S. Friedman, & L. J. Brandt (Eds.),* Sleisenger and Fordtran's gastrointestinal and liver disease *(10th ed., p. 851). Elsevier.*

(cont'd)

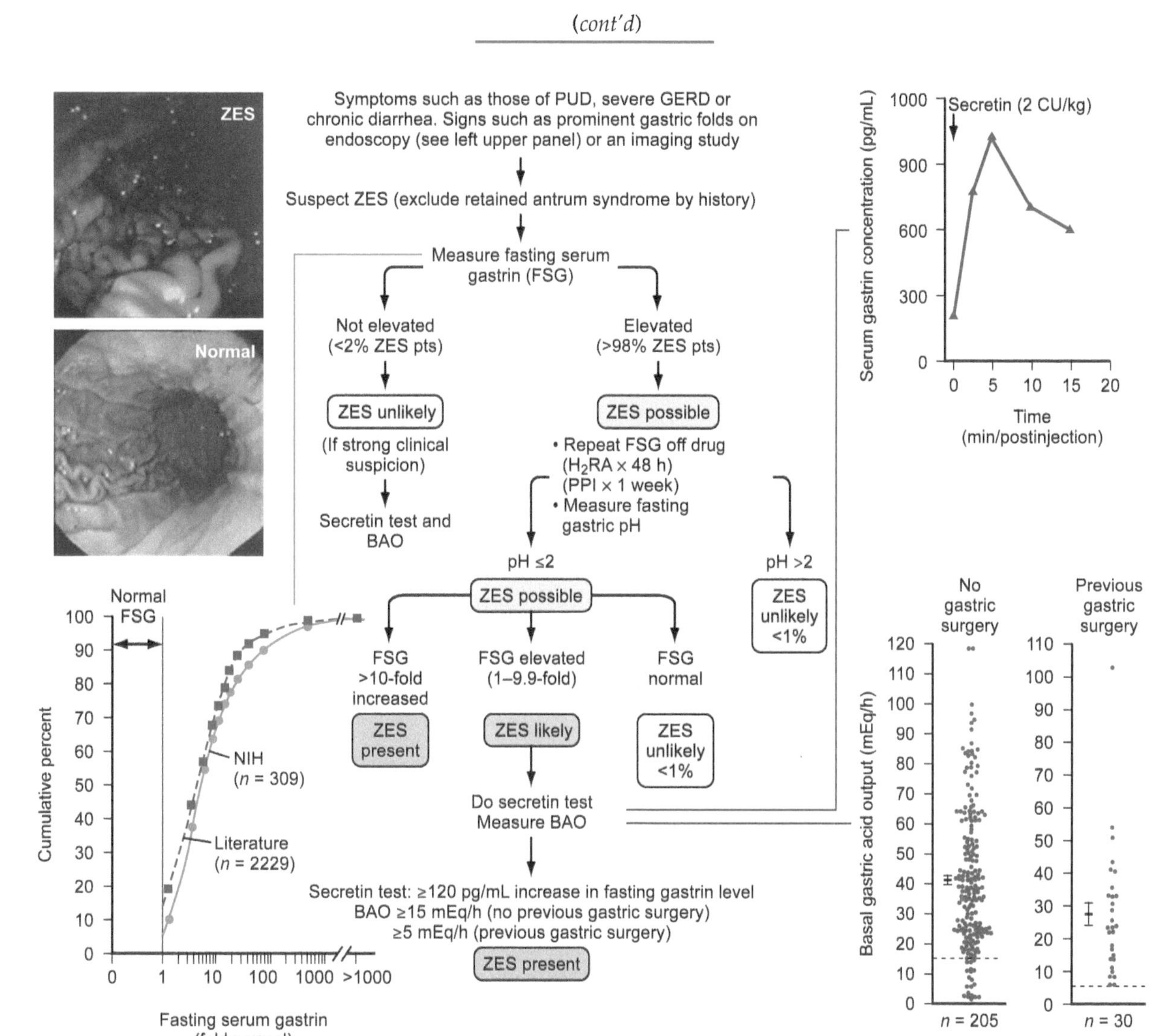

FIGURE 6.6 An algorithm for the detection of ZES. In the upper left are the enhanced gastric folds (rugae) seen by endoscopy in a patient with ZES compared to a normal patient. *BAO*, Basal acid (HCl) output; *CU*, clinical units; *FSG*, fasting serum gastrin; *GERD*, gastroesophageal reflux disease; *NIH*, National Institutes of Health (United States); *PUD*, peptic ulcer disease; *ZES*, Zollinger–Ellison syndrome. Source: *Figure 33-3 in Jensen, R. T., Norton, J. A., & Oberg, K. (2016). Neuroendocrine tumors, Chapter 33. In Feldman, M., Friedman, L. S., & Brandt, L. J. (Eds.),* Sleisenger and Fordtran's gastrointestinal and liver disease *(10th ed., Vol. 1, p. 512), Elsevier.*

blockers, such as cimetidine, have not worked as well. Once the acid secretion is under better control, an exploratory laparotomy can then be done to find the tumor. Usually, it is just a single tumor. Multiple tumors can indicate the presence of either metastases or other types of neuroendocrine tumors. Even with the most careful examination, the solitary tumor in ZES cannot be found in up to 20% of the cases. Only rarely is total gastrectomy performed and only then in cases where management by drug therapy is not effective (Fig. 6.7).

Prognosis

The prognosis depends on the natural history of the tumor, that is, its location and whether it metastasizes

(*cont'd*)

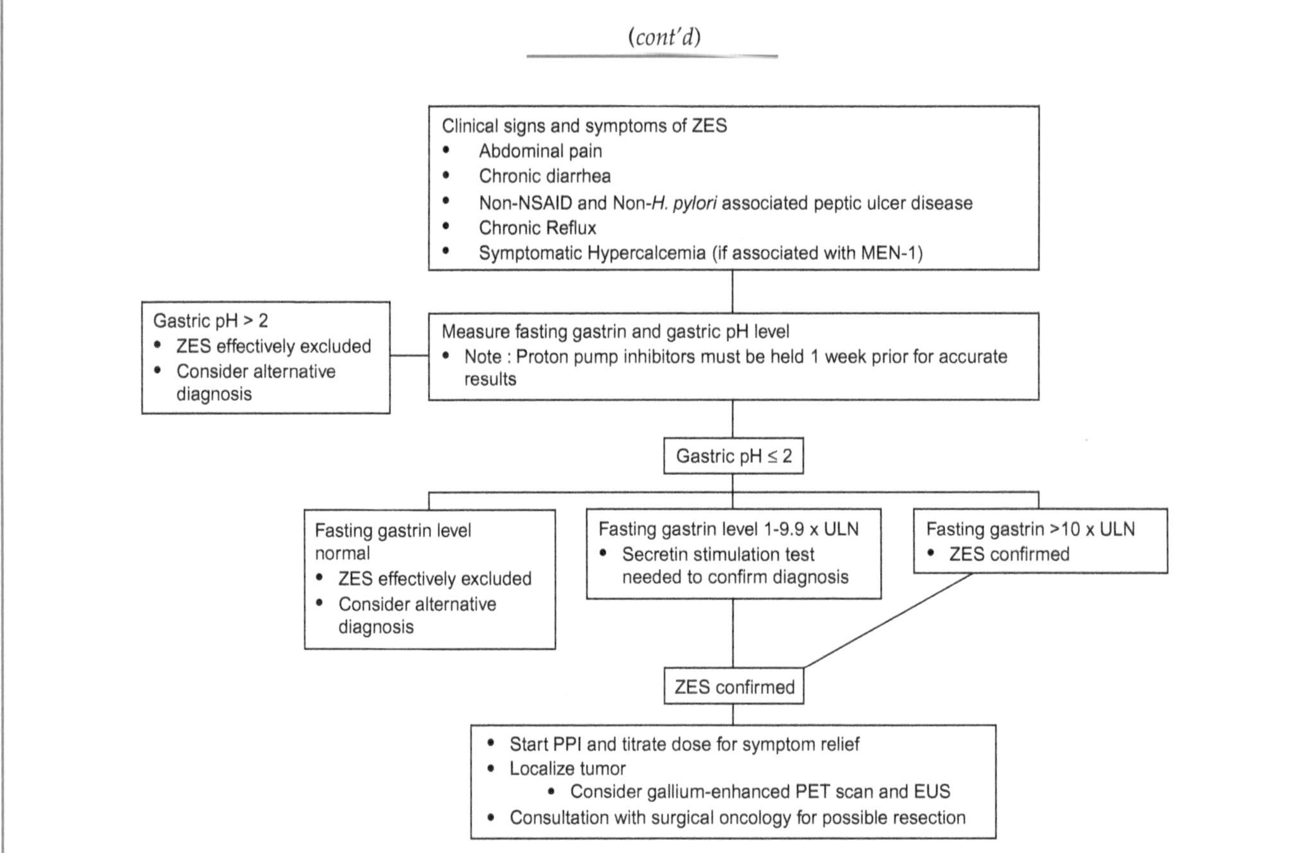

FIGURE 6.7 An algorithm for the detection and management of ZES. *EUS*, Endoscopic ultrasonography; *PI*, proton pump inhibitor; *ZES*, Zollinger–Ellison syndrome. Source: *Figure 1 from Mendelson, A. H., & Donowitz, M. (2017). Catching the zebra: Clinical pearls and pitfalls for the successful diagnosis of Zollinger–Ellison Syndrome.* Digestive Diseases and Sciences, 62, *2258–2265 (Springer Science and Business Media, LLC).*

and where that metastatic location will be. Pancreatic gastrinomas will metastasize to the liver in 50% of cases. Those from the duodenum have only an 8% probability of liver metastasis. Multiple metastases to the liver result in only a 10% survival rate after 10 years; those with a single liver metastasis have a 50% probability of surviving 20 years, while those with no liver metastases have a 90% survival rate after 20 years.

Additional note. 25% of patients with ZES have multiple endocrine neoplasia 1 (MEN1), a syndrome characterized by parathyroid neoplasia along with other endocrine neoplasms, including gastrinomas.

Gastrointestinal hormones

Introduction

Gastrinomas that cause Zollinger–Ellison syndrome are only 1 of over 20 different types of endocrine tumors found primarily in the gastrointestinal (GI) tract. Although only about 1% of the cells that line the GI tract secrete hormones, their total population is greater than that found in any other endocrine organ. Moreover, these cells secrete more than 30 peptides with endocrine functions. It is likely that other less understood peptides produced in the GI tract also function as hormones and as locally acting paracrine factors. More than 20 distinct enteroendocrine cell types containing characteristic secretory granules at their basolateral poles have been identified, and many of these are known to secrete more than one product. Unlike the cells of typical endocrine glands, hormone-secreting cells of the GI tract are not clustered together as discrete tissues but are widely scattered and interspersed among nonendocrine cells.

These cells interact extensively with both intrinsic and extrinsic neural elements in the GI tract and provide bidirectional communication with the brain as well as overlapping, redundant control of GI functions. This chapter focuses on the neuroendocrine regulation of the GI tract itself. The role of the GI hormones in nutrient assimilation is considered in Chapter 7, The Pancreatic Islets, and in the regulation of food intake in Chapter 8, Hormonal Regulation of Fuel Metabolism.

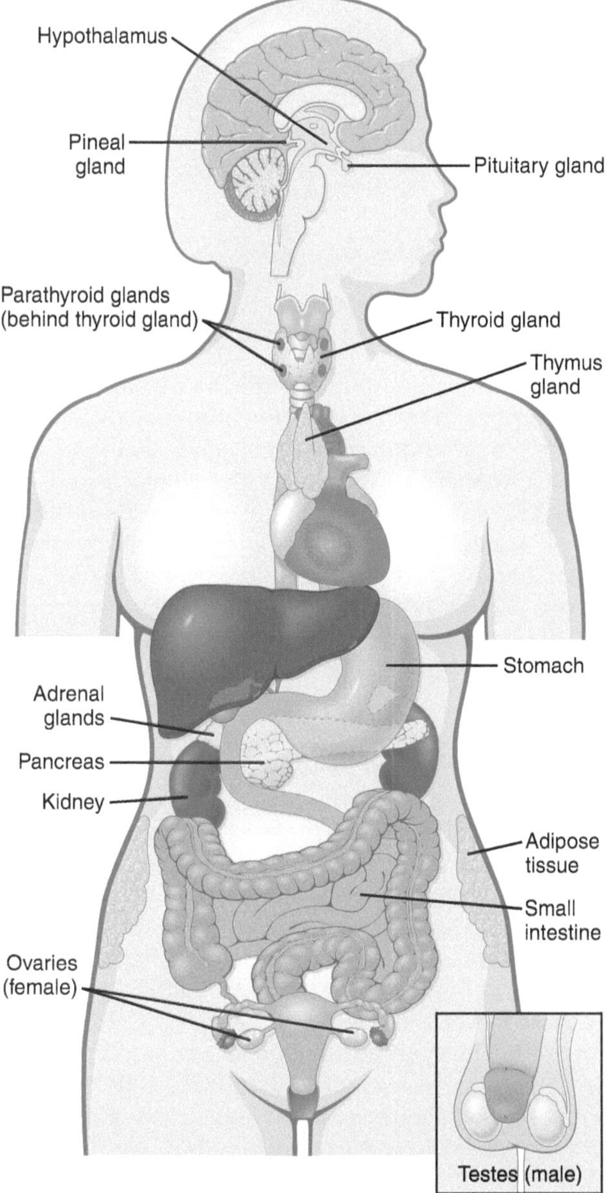

FIGURE 6.8 Anatomical loci of the principal endocrine glands and tissues of the body. Source: *From J.E. Hall, Guyton and Hall Textbook of Medical Physiology, 13th ed., Elsevier, 2016, p. 171, Figure 75.1.*

Functional anatomy of the gastrointestinal tract

From the mouth to the anus, the GI tract is a tube 16 ft long in the living person but 24–27 ft in the cadaver because the muscles are relaxed (Fig. 6.8).

The parotid, sublingual, and submandibular salivary glands as well as the pancreas and the liver are accessory digestive structures that deliver their secretions into the GI tract by way of ducts. The spleen, while not a GI structure, is connected to the liver via the splenic vein so that iron and bilirubin from old disintegrating erythrocytes within the spleen can be conveyed directly to the liver. The iron is stored in the liver, giving it its purple color, while the bilirubin is taken up and, after modification, is excreted as bile. The GI tract below the diaphragm is divided into a foregut, midgut, and hindgut each of which is supplied by a major arterial branch from the aorta, namely, the celiac trunk, superior mesenteric artery, and inferior mesenteric artery, respectively. Venous return from all structures from the lower esophagus to the upper rectum is by branches of the hepatic portal system. This system conveys oxygen, nutrients, drugs, bacteria (portal blood is not sterile), metabolic byproducts (such as ammonium ion), and cancer cells to the liver. In the liver the hepatic portal vein breaks down into capillaries, thus creating a portal system in which there are two capillary beds—one in the abdominal organ and the other in the liver. In the liver the oxygen is taken up by the approximately 2000 mitochondria per cell, bacteria are destroyed by Kupffer cells, the nutrients are assimilated, drugs and toxins are metabolized to more water-soluble compounds for excretion by the kidneys, and cancer cells invade and establish a secondary growth site called a metastasis. The liver becomes a major site of metastasis from all abdominal structures on the portal system.

Throughout its length, the wall of the GI tract is composed of concentric layers of tissue, which vary in thickness and complexity in the different segments. The mucosal surface is highly irregular and is thrown into deep folds and invaginations that amplify its surface area and house its secretory and absorptive cells. The mucosa consists of a single layer of epithelial cells supported by a lamina propria and is composed mainly of connective tissue. Contractions of the underlying thin layer of smooth muscle, the muscularis mucosae, alter the conformation of the ridges and folds of the mucosa, rearranging the exposed surfaces available for secretion or absorption. The submucosa that lies beneath the muscularis mucosa is a layer of dense connective tissue that contains arterioles, venules, and a network of lymphatics. Contractions of the circular and longitudinal smooth muscle layers that surround the mucosa promote mixing of the luminal contents and propel them along the length of the GI tract (Fig. 6.9).

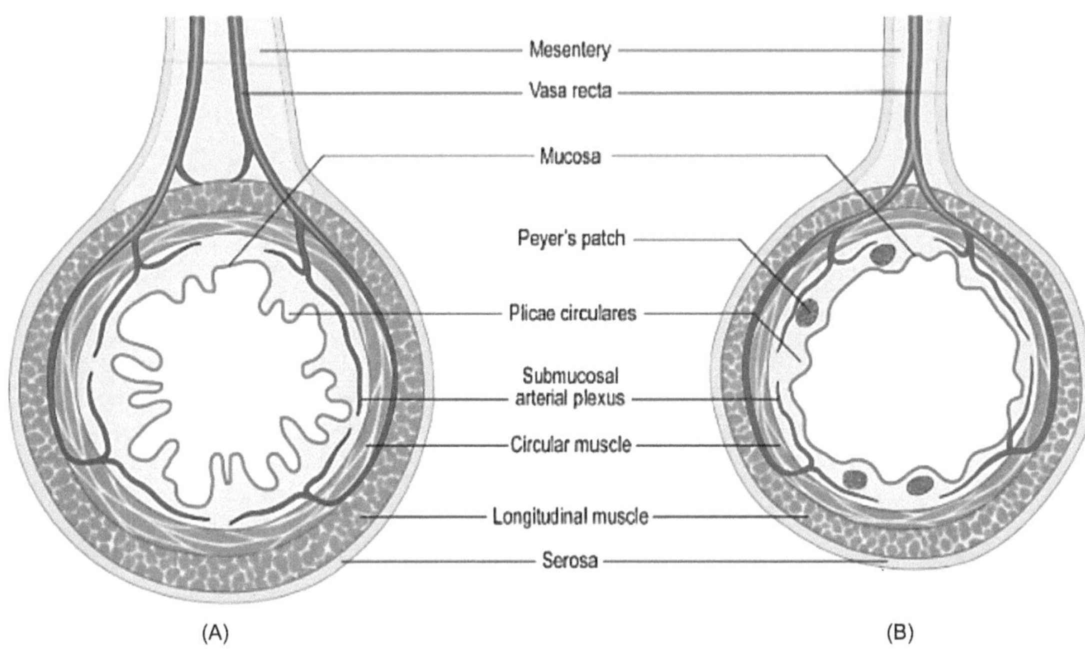

FIGURE 6.9 A representative diagram of the digestive tract wall, this taken from the duodenum. The serosa is visceral peritoneum and the single layer of squamous cells on its surface are called mesothelial cells. Cancer of these cells is called mesothelioma and is caused almost exclusively by asbestos. The mesentery is a double layer of visceral peritoneum through which arteries and hepatic portal veins go to and from the GI structures. *GI*, Gastrointestinal. Source: *Used with permission from Gray's Anatomy, 41st ed. p. 1127, Figure 65.5.*

The gastric and intestinal glands embedded in the mucosa are comprised of single layers of epithelial cells arranged to form deep invaginations of the mucosal surface called pits in the stomach and crypts in the intestines.

There are three types of influence on GI cells: endocrine, paracrine, and neural (Fig. 6.10). Endocrine and paracrine have already been discussed in Chapter 1, Introduction. Neural influence is by the autonomic nervous system, composed of parasympathetic, sympathetic, and enteric divisions. Parasympathetic fibers are 75%–80% sensory (afferent) and 20% motor, while sympathetic is the predominantly motor. Pain is carried on sympathetic fibers. Because these fibers synapse on or near cutaneous somatic sensory neurons, the brain cannot tell the location of origin and so records from the skin surface as referred pain, which is diffuse rather than localized.

Neural receptors are stimulated by parasympathetic and sympathetic nerves, the vagus nerve being the parasympathetic nerve for foregut and midgut structures (Fig. 6.8). Pelvic splanchnic parasympathetic nerves supply hindgut structures. Sympathetic nerves come only from the spinal cord, levels T5–8 for foregut structures, T9–12 for midgut structures, and L1–3 for hindgut structures. There is overlapping, so boundaries are not distinct.

Parasympathetic fibers synapse with other neurons within plexuses as part of the two layers within the wall of the GI tract. These other neurons are part of the enteric nervous system, which some classify as part of the autonomic nervous system (Figs. 6.11 and 6.12).

About three-quarters of the axons in the vagus nerve trunks transmit sensory impulses to the brainstem from abundant mechano- and chemo-receptors that are scattered throughout the stomach and intestines. In response, integrating centers in the brainstem signal secretory or contractile responses by way of motor nerve fibers that are also present in the vagus nerves. These reflexes are called *vago–vagal reflexes* because both afferent and efferent signals are carried by fibers in the vagus nerve trunks. Many of the responses that are governed by these reflexes also are produced by GI hormones. In addition, vagal afferent fibers express receptors for some of these hormones. Consequently, some effects of GI hormones are produced both indirectly by reflexes and directly by stimulation of receptors on target cells.

Cells that secrete hormones and locally acting chemical signals are called enteroendocrine cells. Some of these cells take up chromium salts in histological preparations and are called enterochromaffin (=affinity for chromium) cells and secrete serotonin. Cells that look like enterochromaffin cells but do not secrete serotonin are called enterochromaffin-like (ECL) cells. Most ECL in the stomach secrete histamine and are stimulated to do so by gastrin, produced by G cells (G for gastrin).

The stomach

The stomach regions are the fundus, body, and antrum, all containing gastric pits (Fig. 6.13). In the

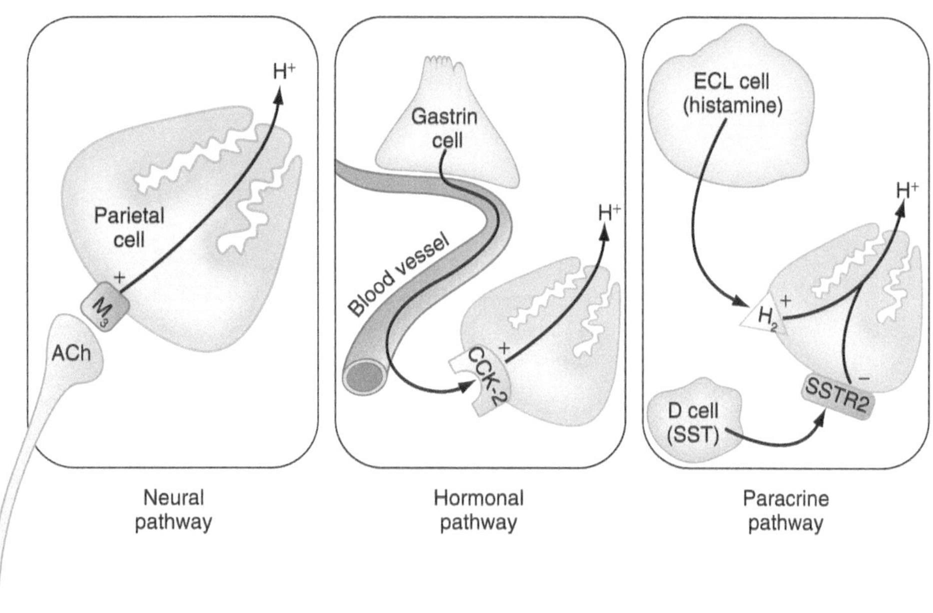

FIGURE 6.10 Endocrine, neural, and paracrine stimulation of the parietal cell. In this illustration the M3 receptor is muscarinic type 3 receptor, one of the receptor types for the neurotransmitter ACh released from the vagal fiber ending. CCK-2 is the receptor gastrin combines with on the parietal cell. ECL, enterochromaffin-like cell, which produces histamine; SST which is produced by D cells (so named from their sequence in pancreatic discovery—they were the fourth type of cell found in the pancreas [alpha, beta, gamma, and delta (D) cells]. Humans do not have gamma cells in their pancreas, but guinea pigs do!); SSTR2, the receptor for somatostatin on parietal cells. *Ach*, Acetylcholine; *CCK-2*, cholecystokinin type 2 receptor; *SST*, somatostatin. Source: *From Figure 50-1, Schubert, M. L., & Kaunitz, J. D. (2016). Gastric secretion, Chapter 50. In M. Feldman, L. S. Friedman, & L. J. Brandt (Eds.),* Sleisenger and Fordtran's gastrointestinal and liver disease *(10th ed., p. 840). Elsevier.*

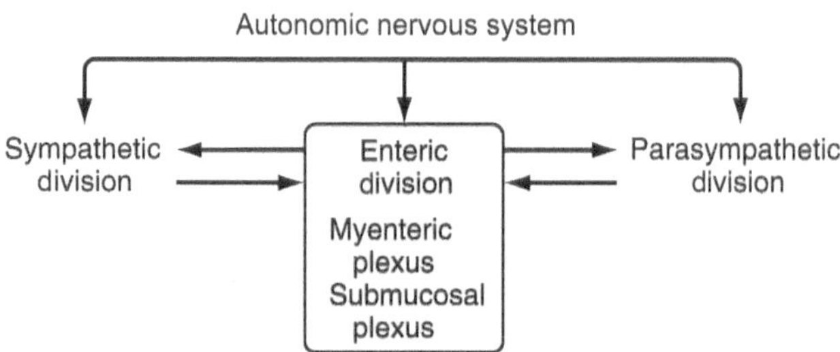

FIGURE 6.11 The enteric nervous system as part of the autonomic nervous system. It contains more neurons than are present in the spinal cord. Source: *Figure 50-6 Schubert, M. L., & Kaunitz, J. D. (2016). Gastric secretion, Chapter 50. In M. Feldman, L. S. Friedman, & L. J. Brandt (Eds.),* Sleisenger and Fordtran's gastrointestinal and liver disease *(10th ed., p. 842). Elsevier.*

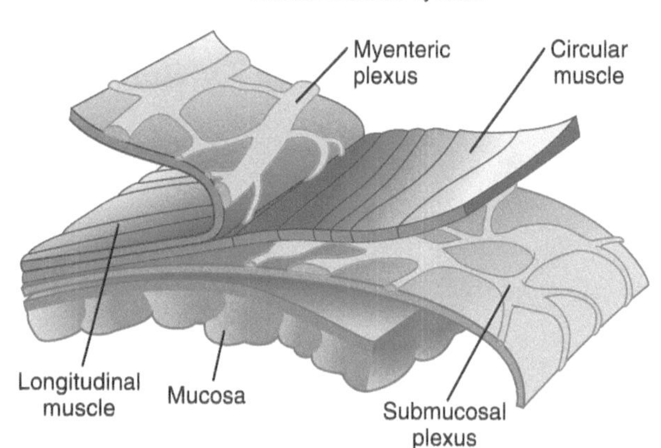

FIGURE 6.12 To facilitate gastrointestinal activity, there are two layers of enteric nerve plexuses, each one receiving input from the other branches of the autonomic nervous system. The myenteric plexus regulates motility while the submucosal plexus regulates secretion. Source: *Figure 50-7 in Schubert, M. L., & Kaunitz, J. D. (2016). Gastric secretion, Chapter 50. In M. Feldman, L. S. Friedman, & L. J. Brandt (Eds.),* Sleisenger and Fordtran's gastrointestinal and liver disease *(10th ed., p. 842). Elsevier.*

fundus and corpus (body) the pits are called gastric glands (Fig. 6.14) in which reside the chief cells, which produce pepsinogen (activated by HCl) and parietal (oxyntic) cells which secrete hydrochloric acid (HCl) and intrinsic factor, the latter essential for the absorption of extrinsic factor (later found to be vitamin B_{12}). In the antrum the pits are called pyloric glands and contain G cells that regulate the production of hydrochloric acid from parietal cells (Fig. 6.15).

Digestion of food begins in the mouth as the food is chewed and mixed with salivary enzymes. After swallowing the food passes from the esophagus into the stomach as a semisolid mixture. When ingested food reaches the antrum of the stomach, it stimulates the G cells to produce the hormone gastrin, which in

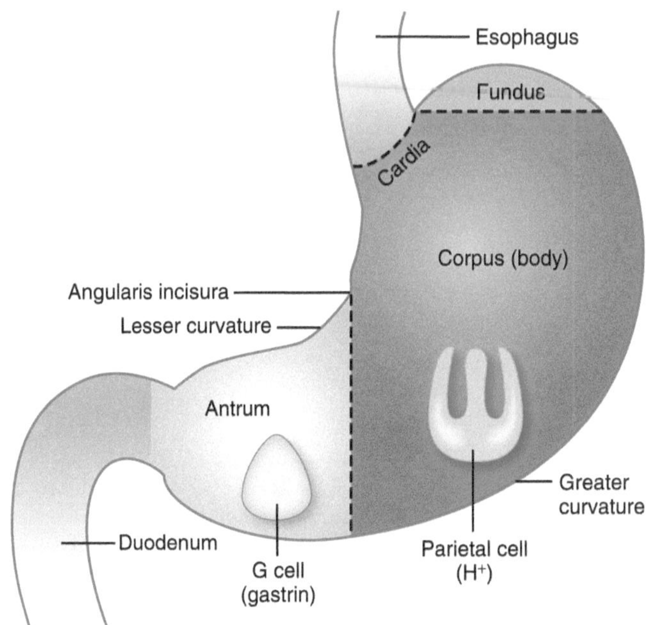

FIGURE 6.13 The functional regions of the stomach. The parietal cell is the dominant cell type in 80% of the stomach, while the G cell is the dominant cell type in the remaining 20%. There is debate as to whether the cardia is an actual anatomical region of the stomach or whether it develops in response to acid reflux. 50% of the population have no cardia. Source: *Figure 50-3 in Schubert, M. L., & Kaunitz, J. D. (2016). Gastric secretion, Chapter 50. In M. Feldman, L. S. Friedman, & L. J. Brandt (Eds.),* Sleisenger and Fordtran's gastrointestinal and liver disease *(10th ed., p. 841). Elsevier.*

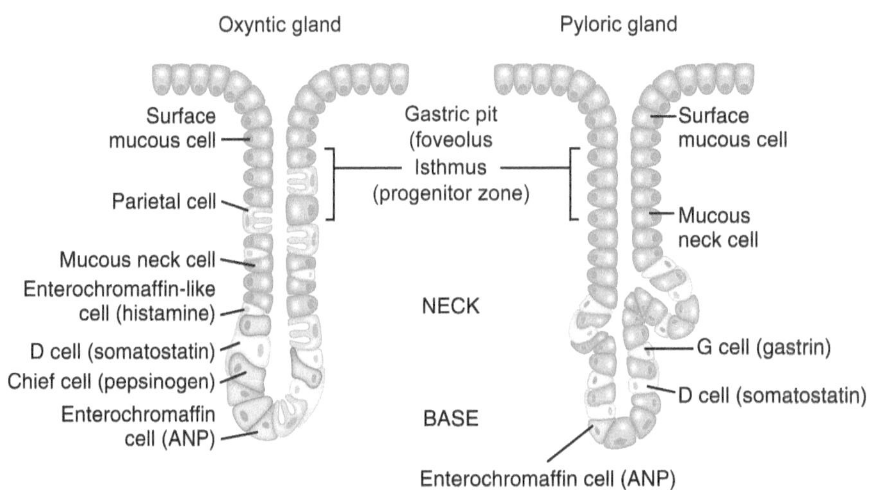

FIGURE 6.14 The oxyntic (Greek, acid) and pyloric glands and the cell types within each gland. Progenitor cells (not labeled) located in the isthmus give rise to all the other cell types. Mucus cells move upward, while parietal (oxyntic) and chief cells move downward in the oxyntic gland. Parietal cells will undergo senescence as they migrate down. Chief (zymogenic) cells migrate downward and are most numerous at the bottom of the gland. Enterochromaffin cells secrete atrial natriuretic peptide (first described in the heart). Source: *Figure 50-4 in Schubert, M. L., & Kaunitz, J. D. (2016). Gastric secretion, Chapter 50. In M. Feldman, L. S. Friedman, & L. J. Brandt (Eds.),* Sleisenger and Fordtran's gastrointestinal and liver disease *(10th ed., p. 841). Elsevier.*

turn stimulates the ECL cells to produce histamine. Histamine combines with H_2 histamine receptors (which are different from the H_1 receptors involved in allergic reactions) on the parietal cell. Gastrin also combines directly with its receptor on the parietal cell. Histamine and gastrin stimulate the parietal cell to produce hydrochloric acid (HCl). Parietal cell stimulation can be enhanced by the stimulation of the vagus nerve. When the pH in the stomach gets below 2, D cells in the gastric antrum produce somatostatin (SST) which

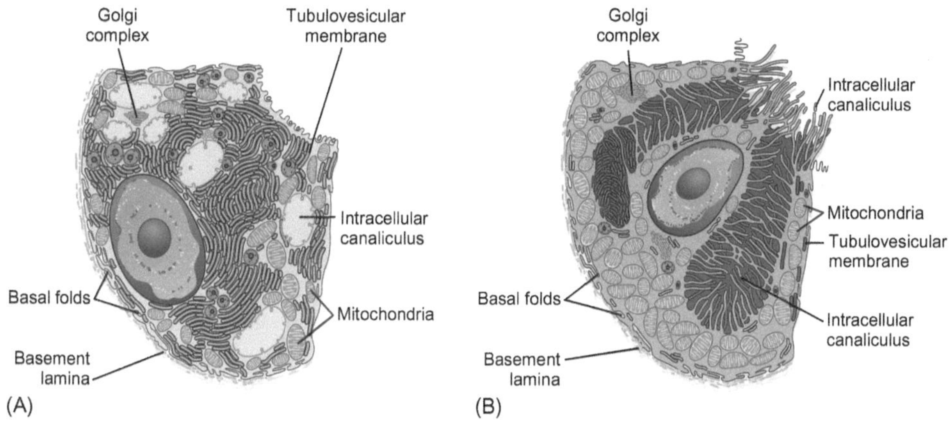

FIGURE 6.15 Parietal cell ultrastructure. (A) A resting parietal cell showing the tubulovesicular apparatus in the cytoplasm and the intracellular canaliculus. (B) An activated parietal cell that is secreting acid. The tubulovesicles have fused with the membranes of the intracellular canaliculus, which is now open to the lumen of the gland and lined with abundant long microvilli. Source: *From Figure 29.3 in Koeppen, B., Stanton, B., (2017). Berne & levy physiology (7th ed., p. 532), Chapter 29.*

inhibits both ECL cells and parietal cells (Fig. 6.16 summarized in Fig. 6.17).

Secretin, from S cells in the duodenum, is also a potent inhibitor of gastrin. It is secreted in response to fats and a low pH in the first part of the duodenal lumen and inhibits G cells indirectly by stimulating the D cells to secrete SST.

H. pylori infection may increase or decrease hydrochloric acid production by altering paracrine (histamine), endocrine (gastrin), and neural (vagal or enteric nervous system) activity depending on its location. If the infection is mainly in the antrum, there will be an increase in hydrochloric acid due to the inhibition of D-cell secretion of SST. This promotes the uninhibited secretion of gastrin with a subsequent increase in HCl by parietal cells. These patients have antral and gastric ulcers collectively called peptic ulcers. In contrast, acute infection or chronic infection involving the whole stomach will result in decreased acid production as these Gram-negative bacteria produce a number of exotoxins that inhibit the parietal cell directly through inhibition of the proton pump and indirectly by stimulating the release of SST (Fig. 6.18).

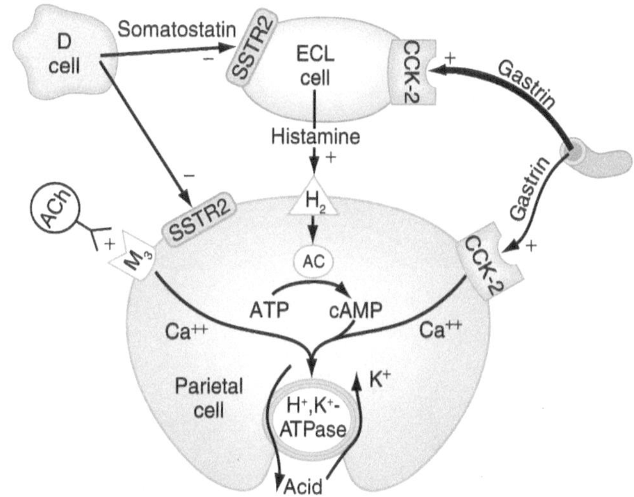

FIGURE 6.16 Major parietal cell activators and inhibitors. Histamine is a paracrine stimulus of the parietal cells via conversion of ATP to cyclic AMP and in the process the H^+, K^+ exchange pump is activated, expelling hydrogen out in exchange for potassium. Gastrin is an endocrine stimulus and the vagus nerve, releasing ACh, also helps to release acid. Inhibition is accomplished by somatostatin. *ACh*, Acetylcholine; *AMP*, 5′-adenosine monophosphate; *ATP*, adenosine triphosphate. Source: *Figure 50-9 in Schubert, M. L., & Kaunitz, J. D. (2016). Gastric secretion, Chapter 50. In M. Feldman, L. S. Friedman, & L. J. Brandt (Eds.),* Sleisenger and Fordtran's gastrointestinal and liver disease *(10th ed., p. 843). Elsevier.*

The duodenum and pancreas

When the pH of chyme (liquefied food) falls below 4.5 and enters the duodenum, S cells in the duodenal wall are stimulated to produce secretin. This hormone stimulates the production of SST by D cells in the antrum as well as causing the release of bicarbonate and fluid by the pancreatic ductal cells (Fig. 6.19).

Once the pH has risen, duodenal I cells downstream secrete cholecystokinin (CCK) which stimulates the pancreatic acinar cells to secrete digestive enzymes (Figs. 6.20 and 6.21). CCK also, as its name implies, stimulates the contraction of the gall bladder and the release of bile into the lumen of the duodenum. Bile is an emulsifying agent that makes fat water soluble so the lipases from the pancreas can digest it.

Phospholipids and bile salts emulsify fatty substances in the chyme, preparing them for further digestion by lipases secreted by the pancreas. Peptidases and amylase also present in pancreatic secretions continue the digestion of proteins and complex carbohydrates in concert with enzymes present on the apical surfaces of enterocytes. Absorption of nutrients and most pharmacological agents begins in the duodenum and continues as the

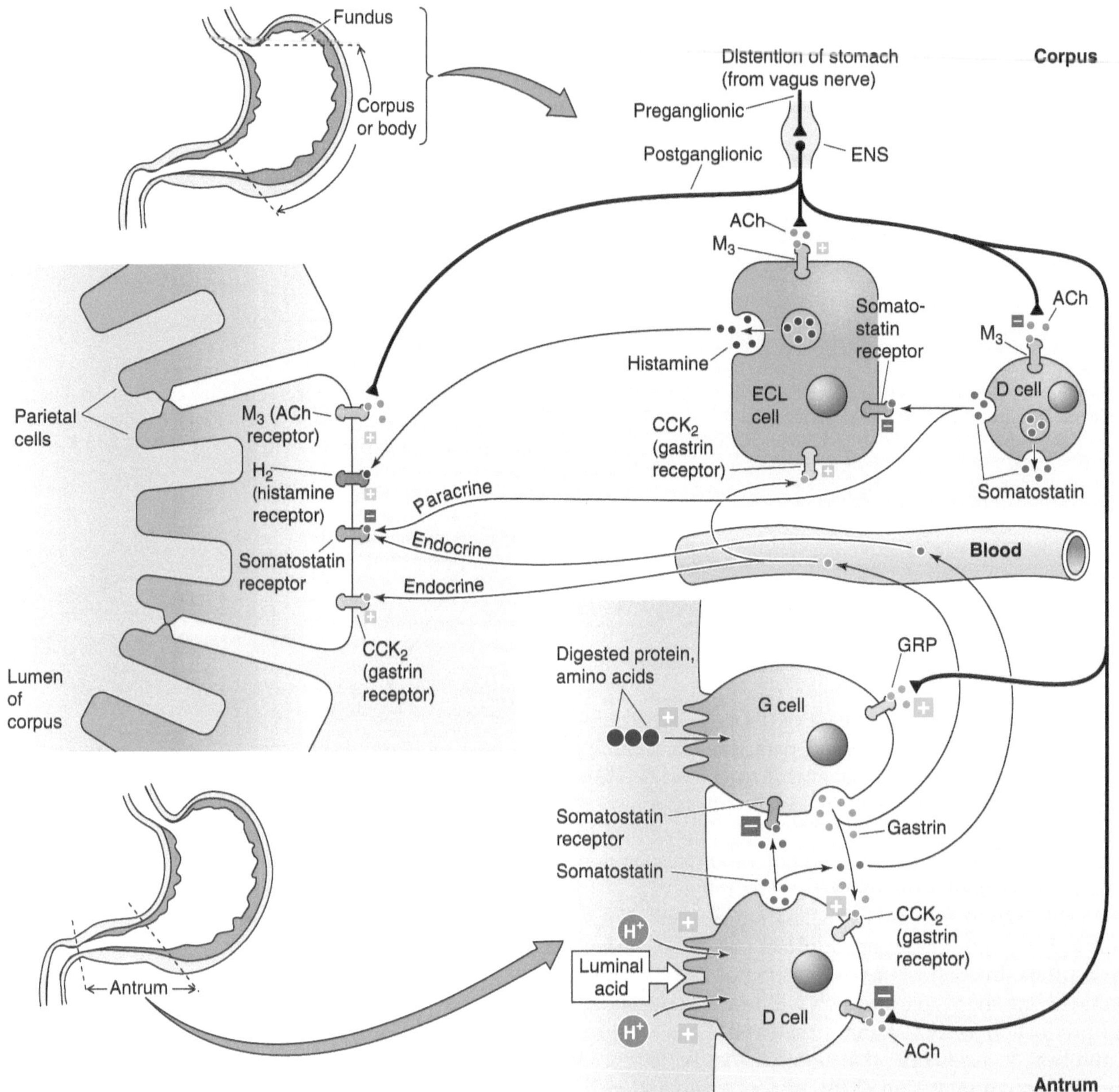

FIGURE 6.17 Actions of the hormones on the cells of the stomach. Histamine and gastrin as well as vagal innervation via the ENS, stimulate the production of hydrochloric acid. Somatostatin, from D cells in the antrum, inhibits the parietal cell directly and by inhibiting G cells and ECL cells. *ENS*, Enteric nervous system. Source: *Figure 42-8 in Binder, H. J. (2016). Gastric function, Chapter 42. In W. F. Boron, & E. L. Boulpaep (Eds.),* Medical physiology *(3rd ed., p. 869). Elsevier.*

chyme is propelled through the jejunum and ileum by peristaltic contractions. Peristaltic contractions are controlled mainly by the enteric nervous system with input from enteric hormones and both sympathetic and parasympathetic fibers. Most of the organic nutrients, water, salts, vitamins, and minerals are absorbed in the small intestine. The remaining chyme then passes into the colon, which carries out the final absorption of water and salts and stores the undigested dietary components and hepatic excretory products until defecation.

Additional hormones

Dozens of biologically active peptides and smaller molecules have been isolated from extracts of the GI tract. The precise physiological role of many of these remains to be established. Gastrointestinal peptides are produced and secreted by enteroendocrine cells and by both intrinsic and extrinsic nerve fibers. Those peptides that depend upon the general circulation to reach their target cells meet the classical definition of hormones presented in

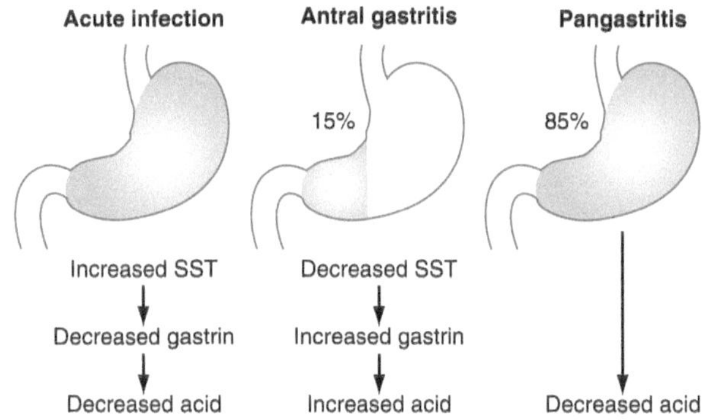

FIGURE 6.18 Infection by *Helicobacter pylori* can be acute (left) or chronic in which it is usually localized to the antrum (middle) in 15% of cases or involve the whole stomach (right) in 85% of cases. The effect of the bacteria on acid production is also shown. Source: *From Figure 50-16 in Schubert, M. L., & Kaunitz, J. D. (2016). Gastric secretion, Chapter 50. In M. Feldman, L. S. Friedman, & L. J. Brandt (Eds.),* Sleisenger and Fordtran's gastrointestinal and liver disease *(10th ed., p. 848). Elsevier.*

Chapter 1, Introduction. Others act locally in a paracrine manner, reaching their target cells by diffusion through interstitial fluid. However, particularly in the GI tract, the distinctions between endocrine, paracrine, and neural secretions are quite blurred, with many of these peptides reaching their targets by more than one route. Peptides that act locally may also enter the bloodstream to act systemically or they may excite receptors on afferent vagal neurons and initiate systemic responses through vaso–vagal reflexes. Some peptide secretions may diffuse through the interstitium to excite neurons of the enteric nervous system, which may respond by producing local effects or by transmitting signals to distant portions of the GI tract. A few may be secreted into the intestinal lumen and produce their effects on downstream targets in the intestinal mucosa. Many of the GI hormones have overlapping functions and their actions may be additive or synergistic (Chapter 5: Principles of Hormone Integration).

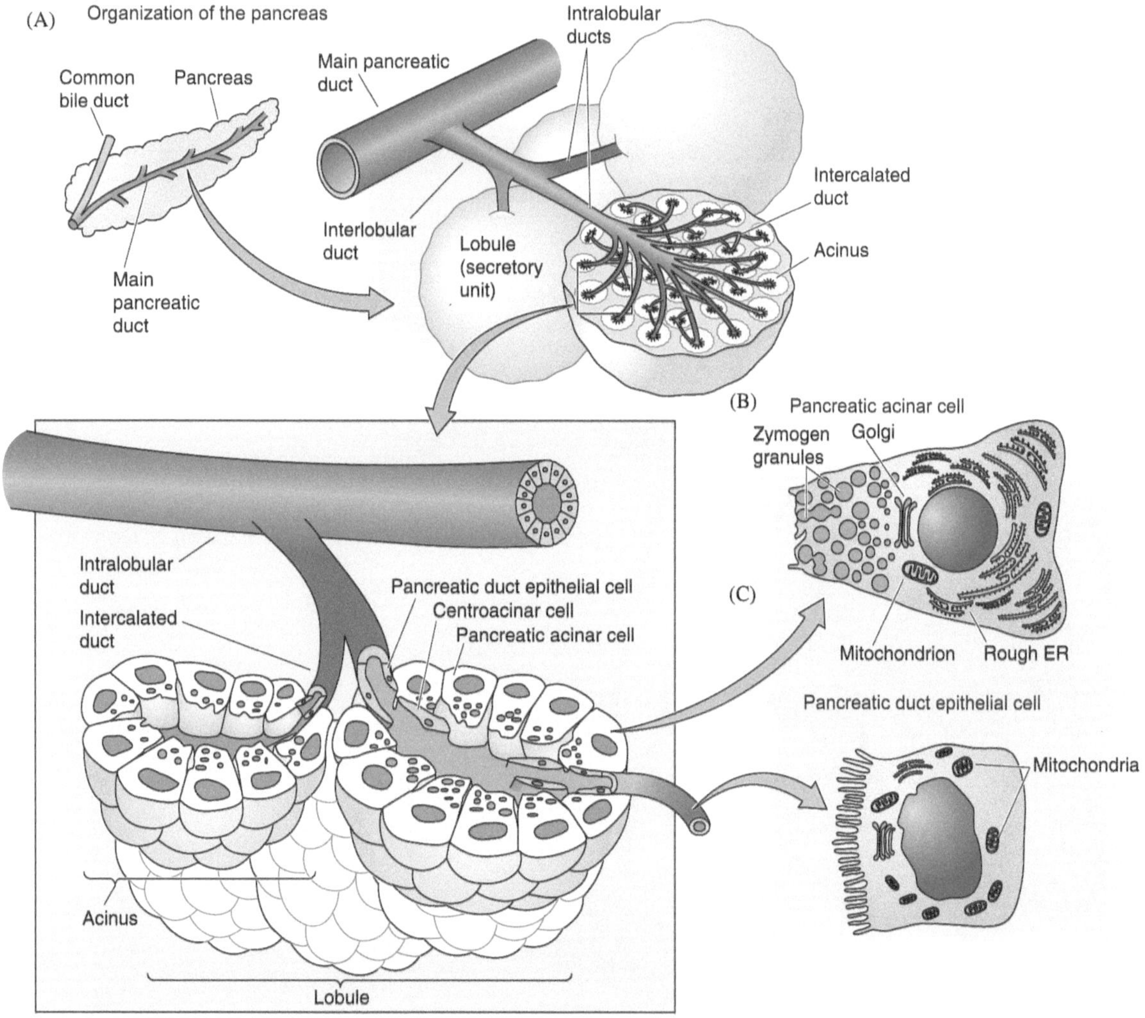

FIGURE 6.19 Pancreatic ductal cells secrete fluid and bicarbonate ion (usually as sodium bicarbonate) to dilute and neutralize the hydrochloric acid from the stomach. Once the optimum pH has occurred, cholecystokinin stimulates the secretion of digestive enzymes from the pancreatic acinar cells. Source: *Redrawn from Figure 43-1 in Marino, C. R., & Gorelick, F. S. (2016). Pancreatic and Salivary Glands, Chapter 43. In W. F. Boron & E. L. Boulpaep (Eds.),* Medical physiology *(3rd ed., p. 880). Elsevier.*

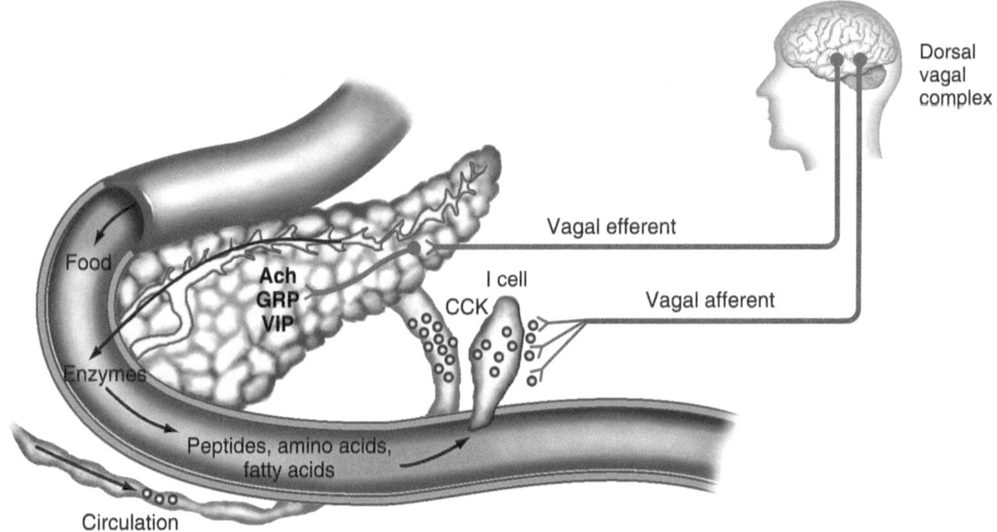

FIGURE 6.20 Once the pH is increased, CCK is released. This causes (1) direct activity on pancreatic acinar cells to release digestive enzymes and (2) stimulates vago–vagal reflex to cause the release of acetylcholine from vagal efferent endings. These stimulate the secretion of digestive enzymes as well as gastrin-releasing peptide and vasoactive intestinal peptide whose functions are not entirely clear. *CCK*, cholecystokinin. Source: *Figure 56-7 in Pandol, S. J. (2016). Pancreatic secretion, Chapter 56. In M. Feldman, L. S. Friedman, & L. J. Brandt (Eds.),* Sleisenger and Fordtran's gastrointestinal and liver disease *(10th ed., p. 934). Elsevier.*

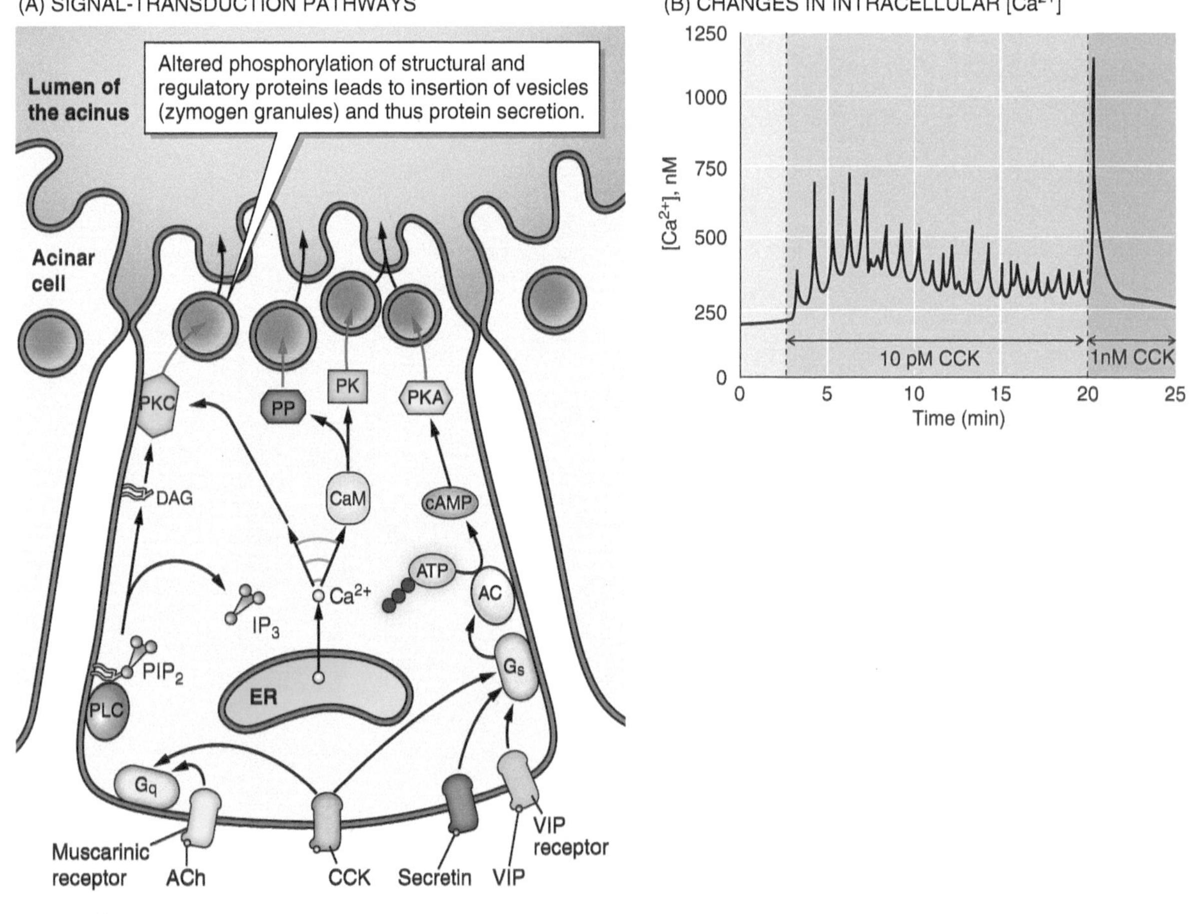

FIGURE 6.21 The actions of hormones, paracrines, and neurotransmitters on the pancreatic acinar cell. The effect of VIP is speculative. The product is inactive digestive enzymes which are activated in the lumen of the duodenum by either trypsin or enterokinase. *VIP*, Vasoactive intestinal peptide. Source: *Redrawn from Figure 43-4A in Marino, C. R., & Gorelick, F. S. (2016). Pancreatic and Salivary Glands, Chapter 43. In W. F. Boron & E. L. Boulpaep (Eds.),* Medical physiology *(3rd ed., p. 883). Elsevier.*

At the molecular level (boxed material for additional information)

Hormones of the gastrointestinal tract

The gastrin/cholecystokinin family

Because of the similarities in their structures, many of the GI hormones can be grouped into families. The following discussion focuses on those signaling molecules that have an established endocrine role. An ancestral gene appears to have duplicated in a primitive chordate about 500 million years ago, around the time of the emergence of the vertebrates, and gave rise to the genes that encode the hormones gastrin and CCK. The gastrin and CCK genes have retained similar organizational features, and are each comprised of three exons separated by two introns. Structural homologies are found in the 59 untranscribed regulatory region and in the coding region of exon 3. The preprohormone products have chain lengths of 101 and 115 amino acids for gastrin and CCK, respectively. An identical stretch of 12 amino acids is present near the carboxyl terminals of the precursors of both hormones (Fig. 6.22). Both prohormones undergo similar processing. Removal of the signal peptide occurs cotranslationally in the endoplasmic reticulum, and sulfation of tyrosine residues takes place as the hormones traverse the trans-Golgi apparatus. In the secretory granules, hormone convertases shorten the peptide chains and produce a mixture of peptides with identical C-termini. Cleavage of peptide bonds at the carboxyl terminals followed by amidation of phenylalanine completes the processing. The result of these posttranslational reactions is the production CCK and gastrin molecules of varying chain lengths but with identical amidated pentapeptide sequences at their C-terminals.

The four amino acid sequence at the carboxy terminus is required for biological activity of both hormones, and accounts for all the activity of gastrin. Pentagastrin consisting of the C-terminal five amino acids is not produced biologically but is used experimentally and clinically to reproduce all the effects of gastrin. The critical structural feature that distinguishes CCK from gastrin is the sulfate ester of the tyrosine located seven residues upstream from the carboxyl terminal (Fig. 6.22). CCK molecules that lack this sulfate ester behave like gastrin. Although the tyrosine located six residues upstream from the carboxyl terminal of gastrin may also be sulfated, the sulfate

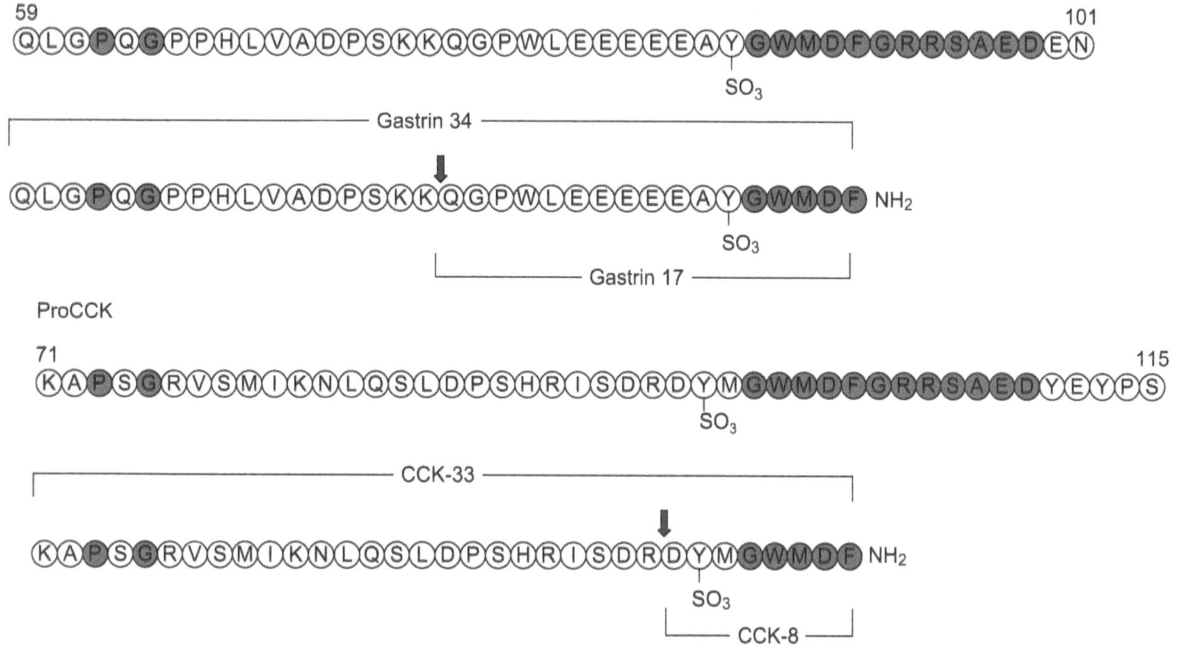

FIGURE 6.22 Progastrin, procholecystokinin (CCK), and their posttranslational processing. Amino acids are represented in the single-letter amino acid code. Identical amino acid residues in corresponding positions in both hormones are shown in red and are found largely in the carboxyl terminus. Posttranslational processing removes the 8 amino acids from the carboxyl terminal of progastrin and 11 amino acids from proCCK. The C-terminal glycine is then cleaved, leaving behind its amino group as an amide on the new C-terminal phenylalanine. Amidation is critical for bioactivity of both hormones. Subsequent cleavage by hormone convertases (*blue arrows*) produces the most prevalent forms of gastrin and CCK. *A*, alanine; *C*, cysteine; *CCK*, cholecystokinin; *D*, aspartic acid; *E*, glutamic acid; *F*, phenylalanine; *G*, glycine; *H*, histidine; *I*, isoleucine; *K*, lysine; *L*, leucine; *M*, methionine; *N*, asparagine; *P*, proline; *Q*, glutamine; *R*, arginine; *S*, serine; *T*, threonine; *V*, valine; *W*, tryptophan; *Y*, tyrosine.

(*cont'd*)

ester in this position has little influence on gastrin activity. About equal amounts of nonsulfated (gastrin-I) and sulfated (gastrin-II) normally are produced.

The close structural and evolutionary relationship between gastrin and CCK is also reflected in their receptors, which have about 50% sequence identity. These receptors originally were studied and characterized in CCK target tissues and are still called CCK receptors. The receptors that were found in rodent pancreatic acini-bind CCK with an affinity that is about 500–1000 times higher than for gastrin. They are called CCKA or CCK1 receptors (CCK1-R). Receptors of the type ubiquitously distributed throughout the brain bind CCK and gastrin with nearly equal affinity, and are called CCKB or CCK2 receptors (CCK2-R). The sulfated tyrosine 7 residues upstream from the carboxyl terminus are required for high-affinity binding to the CCK1-R, whereas the CCK2-R does not distinguish between sulfated and nonsulfated molecules. Under physiological circumstances, CCK1-R mediates the actions of CCK in the GI tract and its accessories, and CCK2-R mediates the actions of gastrin. Although the CCK2-R also is activated by CCK, gastrin is normally present in plasma at 5–10 times higher concentrations than CCK, and hence is the predominant ligand.

CCK1-R and CCK2-R are coupled to heterotrimeric G-proteins and signal through multiple transduction pathways that produce rapid protein phosphorylation-dependent changes and slower transcription-dependent changes. Both receptors are coupled to $G\alpha_{q/11}$ and phospholipase C and signal through the diacylglycerol (DAG)/inositol trisphosphate (IP_3) second messenger system and intracellular calcium. The CCK1-R, but not CCK2-R, is also coupled to $G\alpha_s$ and signals some responses by way of increased cyclic AMP (5′-adenosine monophosphate). The CCK2-R mediates some growth responses and appears to interact with several tyrosine kinases including src and the EGF receptor, and perhaps the JAK/STAT signaling pathway (see Chapter 1: Introduction).

Physiological actions of gastrin

Gastrin was discovered and named more than a century ago as the substance in extracts of stomach mucosa that stimulated gastric acid secretion when injected into anesthetized cats. However, its existence was soon cast in doubt by the discovery that histamine, which is abundant in the oxyntic mucosa, and hence in mucosal extracts, is a potent stimulator of gastric acid secretion. It was not until six decades later, after gastrin was isolated, purified, and chemically synthesized, that its status as a hormone and its role in gastric acid secretion finally was accepted.

Gastrin is secreted by G cells in the antrum of the stomach and to a lesser extent in the proximal portion of the duodenum. The predominant form secreted by antral G cells is the 17 amino acid peptide (G-17) called little gastrin. The longer, 34 amino acid peptide (G-34 or big gastrin), is the major form produced by the G cells in the duodenal mucosa. Because biological activity resides in the carboxyl end of the molecule, extension of the peptide chain toward the amino terminus has little effect on the ability of the hormone to interact with its receptor. Big and little forms of gastrin are equally able to elicit responses in target cells, but N-terminal extension increases the half-life in blood from about 7 minutes for little gastrin to about 38 minutes for big gastrin. CCK has the same last five amino acids as gastrin (Fig. 6.23).

Gastric acid secretion is stimulated by complex, redundant endocrine, paracrine, and neural mechanisms (Fig. 6.24).

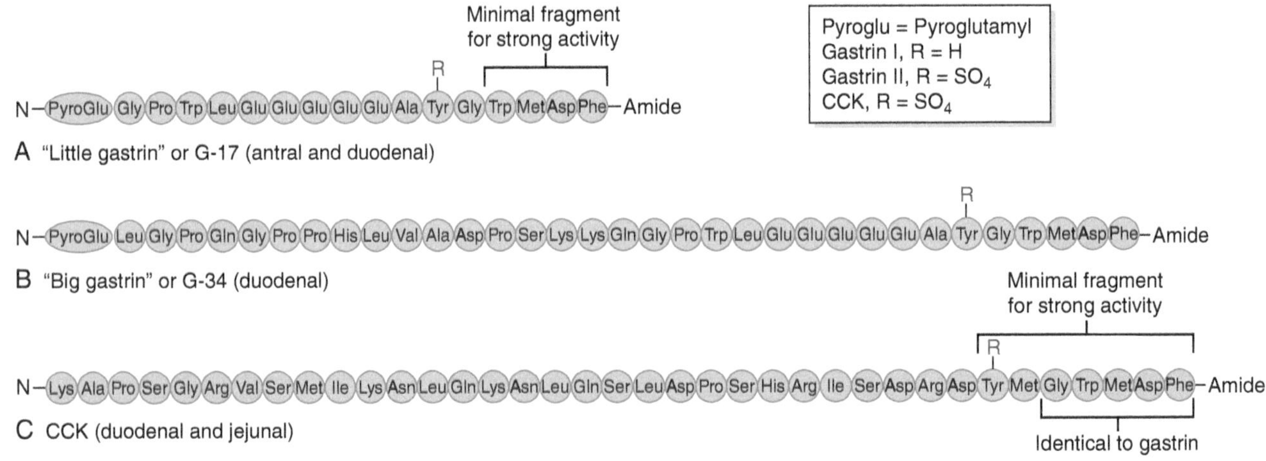

FIGURE 6.23 The structures of little and big gastrin compared to cholecystokinin. Source: *Redrawn from Figure 42-7 in Binder, H. J. (2016). Gastric function, Chapter 42. In W. F. Boron, & E. L. Boulpaep (Eds.),* Medical physiology *(3rd ed., p. 868). Elsevier.*

(cont'd)

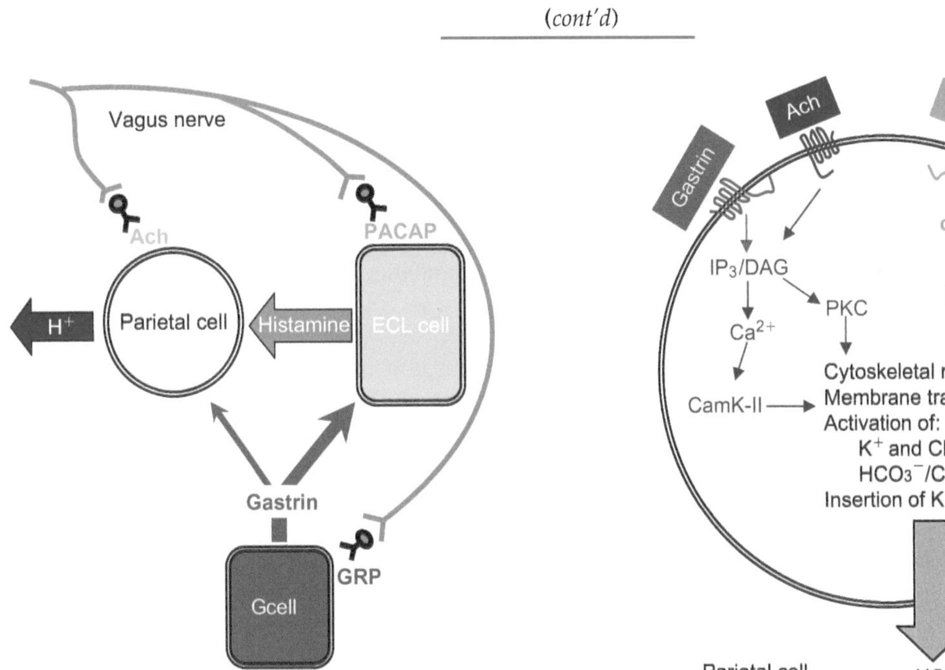

FIGURE 6.24 Stimulation of gastric acid secretion. Histamine secreted by enterochromaffin-like (ECL) cells is the principal stimulus for acid (H^+) secretion by parietal cells, which receive direct cholinergic (Ach) neural input and endocrine input from gastrin. The vagus provides stimulatory input to ECL cells with the postganglionic neurotransmitter PACAP (pituitary adenyl cyclase–activating peptide), and to the gastrin producing G cells with the postganglionic neurotransmitter GRP. G cells also secrete gastrin in response to direct stimulation by peptides and amino acids in the antral lumen. *ACh*, Acetylcholine; *GRP*, gastrin-releasing peptide.

FIGURE 6.25 Cellular actions of gastrin, acetylcholine, and histamine on the parietal cell. Convergence of signaling pathways results in synergistic stimulation of hydrochloride acid.

Parietal cells respond directly, but modestly to gastrin and acetylcholine, and both gastrin and vagal stimulation increase acid secretion indirectly by stimulating nearby ECL cells to release histamine, which is the primary driver of acid secretion. The postganglionic parasympathetic neurotransmitter that activates the ECL cell is probably the neuropeptide called pituitary adenyl cyclase–activating peptide (PACAP; see later). Blockade of histamine H_2 receptors nearly eliminates acid secretion evoked by gastrin and acetylcholine as well as by histamine. The interplay of histamine, gastrin, and acetylcholine in stimulating acid production is a good example of synergy in which the combined effects of agents that act through different signal transduction pathways exceeds the sum of their individual effects. Acting through its H_2 receptors, which are coupled to adenylyl cyclase through $G\alpha_s$, histamine increases cyclic AMP production and the activity of protein kinase A (see Chapter 1: Introduction). Receptors for both acetylcholine (muscarinic type 3 receptors) and gastrin (CCKR-2) are also coupled to G-proteins, but signal through the IP_3/DAG second messenger system and increased intracellular calcium. Activated protein kinase C isoforms and calmodulin-dependent kinase catalyze a series of protein phosphorylations. There is some overlap in the cellular substrates for these kinases. The patterns of protein phosphorylations produced by the different kinases presumably are complementary, with the result that histamine greatly amplifies responses to both acetylcholine and gastrin (Fig. 6.25).

An ATP-dependent "pump" that exchanges cytosolic hydrogen ions for luminal potassium ions (H^+/K^+ATPase) is the essential component of gastric acid secretion. In the inactive resting state, H^+/K^+ATPase pump molecules are sequestered in membranes of cytosolic tubulovesicles that lie beneath the apical membranes of parietal cells. Increased acid secretion requires translocation and insertion of the vesicles into the apical membranes, which greatly expands their surface area and throws it into tortuous folds. Activation of chloride and potassium channels allows passive ion rearrangements to maintain electrical neutrality and preserve the resting membrane potential. Exchange of bicarbonate for chloride at the basolateral membrane provides the needed chloride and disposes of the bicarbonate formed in the cell when hydrogen ions are generated. Potential substrates for activated protein kinases include cytoskeletal and enzymatic components of the

(cont'd)

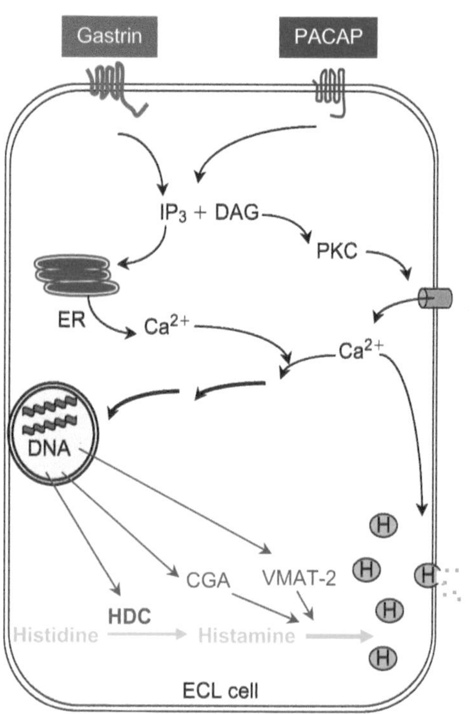

FIGURE 6.26 Actions of gastrin and PACAP in ECL cells. Both gastrin and PACAP stimulate G protein–coupled receptors to activate the IP_3/DAG pathway and increase intracellular Ca^{2+}. IP_3 stimulates the release of Ca^{2+} from the ER, and DAG-dependent activation of PKC results in phosphorylation and activation of membrane calcium channels. Increased Ca^{2+} triggers release of preformed histamine from storage granules and induces expression of HDC, the enzyme that catalyzes histamine formation, and expression of at least two proteins, CGA and VMAT-2. *CGA*, Chromagranin; *DAG*, diacylglycerol phosphate; *ER*, endoplasmic reticulum; *HDC*, histidine decarboxylase; *IP_3*, inositol trisphosphate; *PKC*, protein kinase C; *VMAT-2*, vesicular monoamine transporter type 2.

machinery of the translocation and insertion processes, ion channels, and the H1/K1ATPase itself. However, the precise molecular sites of action and interaction of the gastrin and histamine signaling pathways are not known.

Gastrin stimulates ECL cells to secrete preformed histamine and to transcribe genes that are critical for histamine synthesis and storage (Fig. 6.26).

It increases expression and activity of histidine decarboxylase, the enzyme that catalyzes histamine formation from its amino acid precursor. Gastrin also increases expression of vesicular monoamine transporter type 2 and chromogranin A, which are essential for transport, concentration, and storage of the newly synthesized histamine in secretory granules. Chromogranin A is cosecreted with histamine and may be partially cleaved to release a fragment called pancreastatin, which in some experimental systems inhibits pancreatic endocrine and exocrine secretion. A physiological role for pancreastatin has not been established.

Gastrin contributes to gastric acid secretion in yet another way. It is a trophic hormone that supports proliferation and maintenance of the oxyntic mucosa. Chronic inhibition of gastrin secretion or loss of G cells results in a severe reduction in the abundance and activity of ECL cells and atrophy of the oxyntic mucosa. Overproduction of gastrin results in hypertrophy and hyperplasia of the oxyntic mucosa and excessive acid production that can result in gastric and duodenal ulcers. Overproduction of gastrin is seen in Zollinger–Ellison syndrome, which is characterized by gastrin-secreting tumors located principally in the pancreas. All the cells of the mucosa are derived from the same pluripotential stem cells, but these cells lack gastrin receptors and must proliferate in response to some other growth factor(s). ECL cells are capable of self-replication and increase disproportionately in the presence of excess gastrin. They, or perhaps the parietal cells, may be the source of growth factors that control stem cell proliferation and differentiation.

Regulation of gastrin secretion

Gastrin concentrations in blood increase about two- to threefold with food intake and decline during interdigestive (between meal) periods. In the initial cephalic phase, gastrin secretion is triggered by sensations of smell and taste, or even just thoughts of food, and results from parasympathetic stimulation of the oxyntic mucosa. Vagal input to secretomotor fibers in the antral mucosa stimulates the release of a 27-amino acid neurotransmitter called gastrin-releasing peptide (GRP). GRP belongs to a large family of neuropeptides that are widely expressed in peripheral and central neurons in mammals and in the skin of amphibia. The sequence of 13 out of the 14 amino acids at the C terminus is identical to the amino acid sequence of the peptide bombesin, found in the skin of the frog *Bombina bombina*.

In the gastric phase, food entering the stomach neutralizes the acid in the previously empty stomach. The resulting increase in pH and distention of the stomach are detected by chemo- and mechanoreceptors that signal G cells to release gastrin through vago–vagal reflexes. Partially degraded proteins, small peptides, and amino acids, particularly phenylalanine and tryptophan, in the antral lumen directly stimulate G cells to secrete gastrin. Calcium ions are also potent stimulants of gastrin secretion. There is little direct information concerning how G cells detect these metabolites. The G

(*cont'd*)

protein–coupled calcium-sensing receptor expressed by parathyroid and other cells (see Chapter 10: Hormonal Regulation of Calcium Balance) is also expressed in G cells and may be involved. Amino acids and peptides bind to the calcium receptor and increase its sensitivity to calcium, which in turn activates the intracellular signaling pathways that may culminate in gastrin secretion.

Passage of chyme into the duodenum begins the intestinal phase. Although the duodenal mucosa contains some G cells, their contribution to gastrin secretion is normally very small. Inhibition of gastrin secretion is more characteristic of the intestinal phase. The acidic pH, lipid content, and high osmolarity of the chyme that enters the duodenum trigger hormonal and neural responses that directly and indirectly decrease secretion of both gastrin and gastric acid. Intestinal secretions that inhibit acid secretion and stomach motility are called enterogastrones. Several intestinal hormones (see later) behave as enterogastrones and produce their inhibitory effects indirectly by stimulating D cells in the gastric mucosa to secrete SST. In addition, vago–vagal reflexes triggered by the same stimuli shut down GRP release in the antral mucosa, and relieve vagal inhibition of SST secretion in the oxyntic mucosa (Fig. 6.27).

Somatostatin

SST is the most important negative feedback inhibitor of both gastrin and gastric acid secretion. It was discovered as the hypothalamic peptide that inhibits growth hormone secretion (see Chapter 2: Pituitary Gland, and Chapter 11: Hormonal Control of Growth), but subsequent studies revealed that its production and actions are not limited to the hypothalamus. SST is synthesized and secreted by enteric neurons and by D cells that are widely distributed throughout the mucosa of the stomach and intestines, and by delta cells in the pancreatic islets (see Chapter 7: The Pancreatic Islets). SST secreted by enteroendocrine cells acts both as a local paracrine factor and a circulating hormone. Two biologically active forms consisting of 14 (SST-14) or 28 (SST-28) amino acids are produced in the normal processing of the 116 amino acid preprosomatostatin gene product. Both contain the same 14 amino acid sequence at the carboxyl terminus. A disulfide bond links the carboxyl terminal cysteine with the cysteine residue 11 amino acids upstream to produce a cyclized molecule. For most responses SST-14 and SST-28 have similar potencies, although SST-28 has a longer half-life in blood (15 vs 2 minutes). Consistent with its widespread distribution, SST serves a variety of functions mediated by five distinct receptor isoforms, all of which are G protein–coupled and activate multiple signaling pathways including inhibition of adenylyl cyclase and activation or inhibition of specific ion channels.

The D cells that are present in the oxyntic and antral mucosae differ somewhat in their anatomical and physiological characteristics. The D cells of the oxyntic mucosa have long cytoplasmic processes that extend from the perikaryal regions to end in close proximity to parietal cells, chief cells, and ECL cells. SST secreted by these cells is thought to act in a purely paracrine manner to inhibit histamine release from ECL cells and acid secretion by parietal cells, but has little impact on gastrin secretion by G cells in the antrum. D cells in the oxyntic mucosa have no direct contact with the stomach contents and cannot monitor luminal pH. Secretion of SST by these cells is inhibited by vagal cholinergic input that is coordinated with stimulation of ECL and parietal cells. SST secretion is stimulated by catecholamines released from sympathetic nerves and by intestinal hormones as discussed later.

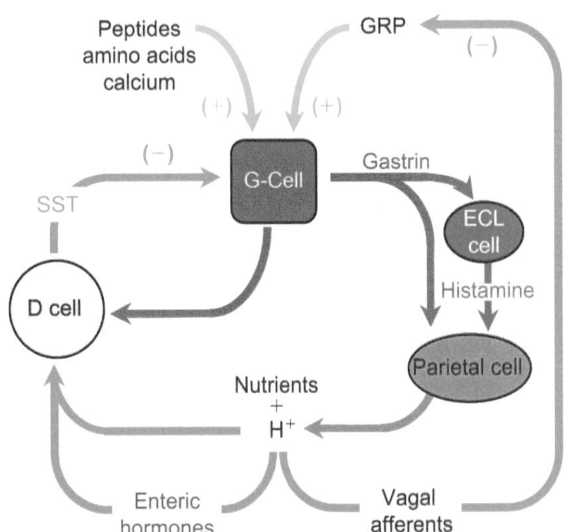

FIGURE 6.27 Direct and indirect feedback regulation of gastrin secretion. Gastrin secretion is positively regulated by luminal nutrients and GRP and is negatively regulated by SST. Gastrin reaches D cells in both the antral and oxyntic mucosae by paracrine or endocrine pathways and stimulates them to secrete SST. Increased luminal H^+ concentrations stimulate antral and duodenal D cells to secrete SST. Increased H^+ concentrations in the duodenum and luminal nutrients in the intestine increase the secretion of enteric hormones, which stimulate D cells in the gastric and duodenal mucosae to secrete SST. Increased luminal H^+ concentrations are sensed by neuronal chemoreceptors and initiate vago–vagal reflexes, which result in decreased release of GRP and decreased cholinergic inhibition of D cells. *GRP*, Gastrin-releasing peptide; *SST*, somatostatin.

(cont'd)

D cells in the antral mucosa are in contact with chyme in the antral lumen and secrete SST in response to low pH. SST acts as a paracrine inhibitor of gastrin secretion from nearby G cells and travels through the blood to reach distant cells in the antral and oxyntic mucosae. Blood concentrations of SST may increase 6- to 10-fold after eating a mixed meal, but the relative contributions of intestinal, oxyntic, and antral D cells to the circulating pool of SST have not been determined. It is likely that increased hydrogen ion concentration directly stimulates antral D cells. Peptides, amino acids, and fat in the intestinal lumen may require neural or humoral intervention to stimulate antral, oxyntic mucosal, and intestinal D cells (Fig. 6.28).

Cholecystokinin

In 1928 Ivy and Oldberg discovered a substance in extracts of duodenal mucosa that causes the gall bladder to contract and empty. They named it cholecystokinin (CCK), meaning "that which excites or moves the gall bladder." About 15 years later it was found that injections of crude extracts of the duodenal mucosa caused the pancreas to secrete digestive enzymes, which are stored as zymogen granules. The active substance in the extract was named pancreozymin (PZ). Only after purification of CCK-33 to homogeneity more than two decades later was it recognized that both the gall bladder contraction and the enzyme secreting activities reside in the same molecule, which for a while was called CCK/PZ, and now is simply CCK. In addition to its role as a GI hormone, CCK also functions as a neurotransmitter in peripheral nerves, particularly in relation to GI function, and CCK-8 appears to be the most abundant neuropeptides produced in the human brain.

CCK is produced by I cells in the duodenal and jejunal mucosae. The principal form of CCK in human plasma is the 33 amino acid peptide, but CCK molecules with peptide chain lengths of 58, 22, and 8 amino acids also are secreted by these cells. All active forms of CCK have the same amidated carboxyl terminals and tyrosine-sulfated octapeptide required for recognition by the CCK-1 receptor. CCK peptides circulating in blood have half-lives that range from less than 1 minute for CCK-8 to about 5 minutes for CCK-58. The kidney is the major site of CCK clearance.

Physiological actions of cholecystokinin

Pancreatic enzyme secretion Efficient breakdown and absorption of ingested proteins, fats, and starches require the catalytic activities of enzymes that are synthesized in abundance in pancreatic acinar cells and stored in membrane-bound secretory vesicles. The pancreas maintains the highest rates of protein synthesis in the body and

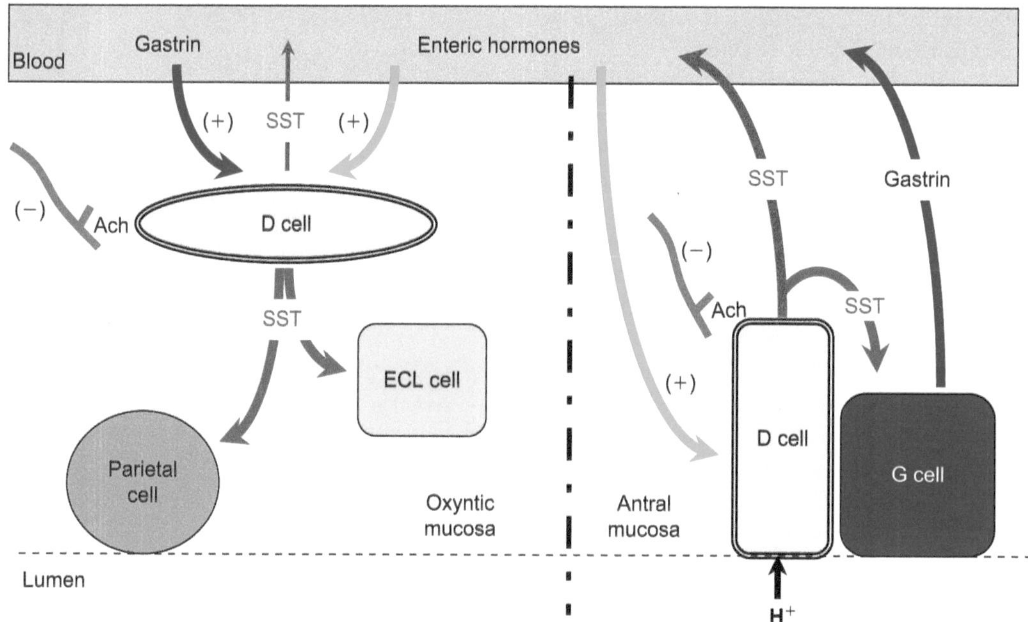

FIGURE 6.28 Effects of SST and control of its secretion in the gastric mucosa. D cells in the oxyntic mucosa have no access to the luminal contents and are stimulated to secrete SST by hormones secreted by endocrine cells downstream in the GI tract and inhibited by vagal cholinergic nerves. SST secreted by these cells acts mainly as a paracrine factor. D cells in the antral mucosa are stimulated by increases in H^+ concentrations and circulating enteric hormones and are inhibited by vagal cholinergic neurons. *SST*, Somatostatin.

(*cont'd*)

in a normal day may release as much as 15 g of protein into the duodenum. Pancreatic enzymes are released into the pancreatic exocrine ducts by a calcium-dependent process that is activated both by acetylcholine and by CCK. Proteolytic enzymes secreted as inactive proenzymes called zymogens are activated by proteases in the duodenal lumen. Lipases and amylase are secreted as active enzymes. In response to stimulation, acinar cells secrete enough watery fluid to carry the secreted enzymes through the pancreatic duct system. The pancreatic duct joins the common bile duct at the sphincter of Oddi, and its contents enter the duodenum along with bile.

Plasma concentrations of CCK increase about 5- to 10-fold within 30 minutes after eating a typical meal containing protein and fat (Fig.6.29).

The appearance of pancreatic enzymes in the intestinal lumen coincides with increased blood concentrations of CCK, and administration of CCK in amounts that produce comparable increases in plasma concentrations increase pancreatic enzyme secretion. Receptors for CCK (CCKR-1) originally were isolated and characterized in preparations of rodent pancreatic acinar tissue, consistent with the classical view that these cells are targets of CCK. Indeed, addition of CCK to isolated rodent acinar cells causes intracellular calcium to increase, and zymogen granules to fuse with the apical membranes and discharge their contents. However, human pancreatic acinar cells express very few CCK-1 receptors, and accordingly, CCK has little effect on enzyme secretion when added directly to isolated human pancreatic acini. In humans, acetylcholine released from parasympathetic neurons provides most of the direct input for pancreatic exocrine secretion. Cholinergic stimulation operates through the same intracellular signaling pathway as described for CCK in rodent acini. Vagal afferent neurons express CCK-1 receptors, which, upon binding CCK, initiate the reflex that activates cholinergic secretomotor efferent neurons in the pancreas (Fig. 6.30). Although it is clear that acetylcholine released from parasympathetic nerve endings accounts for most of the classical pancreatic response to CCK, the question of whether or not CCK has any direct input to pancreatic enzyme secretion in humans is still unresolved.

Gall bladder contractions Bile provides the phospholipids, cholesterol, and bile salts needed to emulsify fats and facilitate their digestion and absorption by the small intestine. Bile is also a vehicle for excreting detoxified metabolites. Hepatocytes secrete bile into bile canaliculi, which converge to form interlobular ductules, and ultimately the common hepatic bile duct. The cystic duct, which carries bile to and from the gall bladder, branches

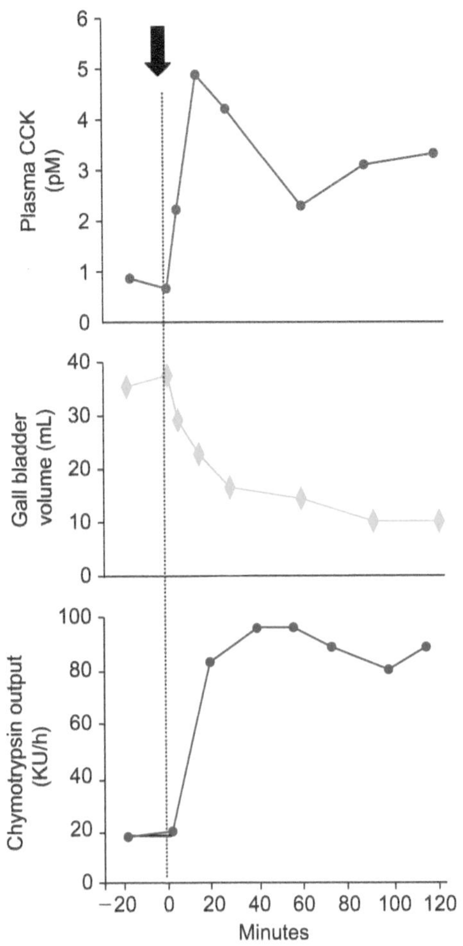

FIGURE 6.29 Effects of ingestion of a standardized liquid meal (*arrow*) on plasma concentrations of cholecystokinin, gall bladder contraction, and pancreatic chymotrypsin secretion in normal subjects. Source: *Redrawn from data of Liddle, R. A., Goldfine, I. D., Rosen, M. S., Taplitz, R. A., & Williams, J. A. (1985). Cholecystokinin activity in human plasma. Molecular forms, responses to feeding and relationship to gall bladder contraction.* Journal of Clinical Investigation, 75, 1144–1152; *Owyang, C., Louie, D. S., & Tatum, D. (1986). Feedback regulation of pancreatic enzyme secretion. Suppression of cholecyctokinin release by trypsin.* Journal of Clinical Investigation, *77*, *2042–2047.*

off the common bile duct after it emerges from the liver (Fig. 6.8). Epithelial cells (cholangiocytes) that line the walls of the ducts actively secrete a watery fluid that is rich in bicarbonate. Nearly a liter of dilute bile is produced each day, about half of which enters the duodenum directly through the common bile duct. Flow of bile into the duodenum is controlled by the sphincter of Oddi, which surrounds the insertion of the common bile duct through the duodenal wall. The sphincter is formed by longitudinal and circular muscles in the duodenal

(cont'd)

wall. Phasic contractions of these muscles during interdigestive periods occlude the opening of the common bile duct and divert the flow of bile into the gall bladder where the organic constituents are concentrated as much as 20-fold by selective reabsorption of water and electrolytes. The gall bladder is a hollow sac with a capacity of about 50 mL. Its walls are comprised of a single layer of epithelial cells overlying a network of transverse, longitudinal and oblique smooth muscle fibers. The gall bladder, bile ducts, and sphincter of Oddi are richly innervated with both sympathetic and parasympathetic nerves.

As its name implies, CCK stimulates the gall bladder to contract and expel its content of bile. For bile to enter the duodenum, however, CCK must also relax the sphincter of Oddi. Vagal efferent nerves also stimulate the gall bladder to contract and cause the sphincter to relax. Smooth muscle cells of the human gall bladder have receptors for both CCK (CCKR-1) and acetylcholine (M3) and isolated strips of gall bladder wall contract in response to physiologically relevant amounts of both these agents. CCKR-1 are also present in vagal and enteric afferent neurons, and their stimulation by CCK initiates a reflex that duplicates and reinforces the direct action of CCK on the gall bladder. Thus CCK acts both directly and indirectly to contract the gall bladder (Fig. 6.29).

Although CCKR-1 are present in the sphincter of Oddi, relaxation is produced primarily through neural mechanisms (Fig. 6.30) and is severely impaired by pharmacologic blockade of axonal transmission. Activation of CCKR-1 increases intracellular calcium, which is associated with contraction rather than relaxation of smooth muscle, consistent with the response of the gall bladder, but not the sphincter. It is likely that vasoactive intestinal peptide (VIP, see later), which acts through the cyclic AMP second messenger system, rather than acetylcholine is the neurotransmitter that signals relaxation.

Other effects of cholecystokinin

Although CCK can bind to the same receptors as gastrin (CCKR-2) on ECL and parietal cells, its net effect in the stomach is to inhibit rather than stimulate acid secretion. The inhibitory effect is best explained as a consequence of stimulating gastric D cells to secrete SST. CCK also inhibits the release of pepsinogens and gastric lipase by chief cells, again perhaps by way of increased secretion of SST. Delayed gastric emptying results from complex effects on the smooth muscle layers of the stomach.

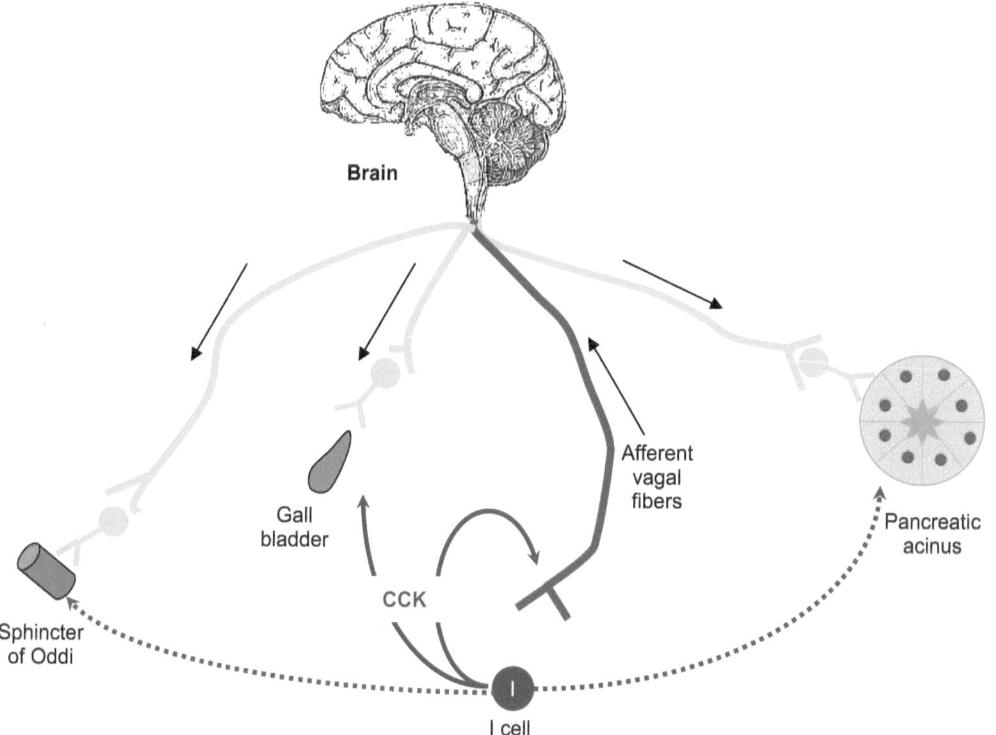

FIGURE 6.30 Actions of CCK on pancreatic secretion and bile flow. Major direct actions are indicated by solid blue arrows. Effects of questionable physiological significance are indicated by the dotted blue arrows. *CCK*, Cholecystokinin.

(cont'd)

At the same time that it stimulates phasic contractions of pyloric, antral, and duodenal smooth muscles, CCK causes smooth muscles in the fundus to relax. To at least some extent these actions are mediated by CCKR-1 on smooth muscle cells, but it is likely that vaso–vagal reflexes initiated by CCK acting on vagal afferent neurons play an important role. Stimulation of vagal afferents by CCK is also likely to contribute to the inhibitory effect of CCK on food intake and its role in limiting meal size. The delay in gastric emptying may contribute to the feeling of fullness that is a component of satiety. Factors involved in the control of food intake are discussed further in Chapter 8, Hormonal Regulation of Fuel Metabolism. CCK also accelerates the passage of chyme along the intestine by stimulating rhythmic contractions of circular and longitudinal smooth muscle. Whether these effects of CCK are direct or are mediated by vaso–vagal reflexes remains to be established. It is noteworthy that CCK-8 is present in neurons that innervate intestinal smooth muscle. It is possible that some of the effects of CCK noted earlier result from its role as a neurotransmitter rather than as a hormone.

Regulation of cholecystokinin secretion As already mentioned, plasma concentrations of CCK increase dramatically after eating (Fig. 6.29). The apical surfaces of CCK-secreting I cells are exposed to the luminal contents of the duodenum and upper jejunum. In rodents, and probably humans as well, the intestinal mucosa constitutively secretes peptides called luminal CCK–releasing factors (LCRF), which, as their name implies, stimulate secretion of CCK. Degradation of LCRF by pancreatic proteases that are intermittently released into the duodenum in interdigestive periods maintains secretion of CCK at low basal levels. After eating, LCRF are protected from degradation by ingested proteins that compete for access to proteolytic enzymes, and CCK secretion increases. CCK secretion is also increased by components in the chyme, the most important of which are fatty acids with chain lengths of at least 12 carbons. Through mechanisms that are incompletely understood, exposure of I cells to fatty acids causes intracellular calcium concentrations to increase sufficiently to trigger CCK secretion. Some evidence suggests that fatty acids may produce this effect by entering the cytosol and stimulating the endoplasmic reticulum to release its calcium stores. Other evidence supports the idea that fatty acids activate a G protein–coupled receptor at the I cell surface. Amino acids and small peptides also stimulate I cells to secrete CCK possibly by stimulating the G protein–coupled calcium receptor, as described earlier. Carbohydrates have little, if any, effect on CCK secretion.

Feedback control of CCK secretion is achieved through direct inhibition of I cells and through reduction or elimination of positive stimuli (Fig. 6.31).

Bile salts that enter the duodenum in response to CCK act directly on I cells to inhibit further secretion of CCK. In addition, bile salts facilitate the absorption and disposition of luminal fats, and thus decrease the drive for CCK secretion. Similarly, pancreatic proteases accelerate

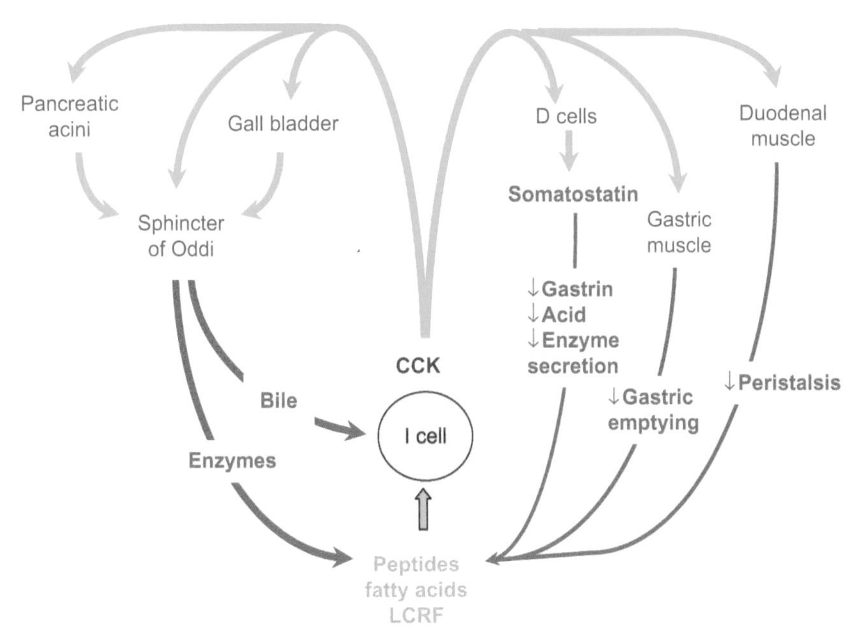

FIGURE 6.31 Regulation of CCK secretion. Red arrows indicate inhibitory influences. *CCK*, Cholecystokinin; *LCRF*, luminal cholecystokinin–releasing factors.

(cont'd)

the degradation of LCRF and peptide secretagogues in the chyme. CCK stimulates D cells in the gastric mucosa to secrete SST, which inhibits the secretion of enzymes from chief cells, histamine from ECL cells, gastrin from G cells, and acid from parietal cells. This effect and the slowing of stomach emptying decrease the presentation of fatty acids, peptides, and amino acids to the I cells and thus further diminish the drive for CCK secretion. SST may also directly inhibit the I cells. Finally, by inducing feelings of satiety, CCK reduces food intake and hence the abundance of luminal factors that increase its secretion.

The secretin/glucagon superfamily

The secretin/glucagon superfamily (Fig. 6.32) includes nine highly homologous hormones, paracrine factors, or neuropeptides encoded in six single-copy genes. It is likely that this superfamily of peptides evolved from an ancient DNA sequence by both exon and gene duplication. In addition to secretin and glucagon, the superfamily includes glucose-dependent insulinotropic polypeptide (GIP), glucagon-like peptides 1 and 2 (GLP-1, GLP-2), VIP, peptide histidine methionine (PHM), pituitary adenylate cyclase–activating peptide (PACAP), and growth hormone–releasing hormone (GHRH). Glucagon, GLP-1, and GLP-2 are all encoded in separate exons of the same gene, and the VIP gene also encodes PHM. The PACAP gene product contains an additional homologous peptide called PACAP-related peptide, but this peptide appears to be biologically inactive. Curiously, in birds the PACAP gene also encodes GHRH. Two other genes in this superfamily are found only in lizards and encode four peptides (exendins 1–4) that closely resemble GLP-1 and PACAP. These peptides are components of the venom secreted by the salivary glands of the Gila monster and related lizards.

Secretin, GLP-1, GLP-2, and GIP, are produced in endocrine cells in the intestinal mucosa, whereas VIP, PHM, and PACAP are present in enteric and vagal neurons. Traces of GHRH and of glucagon also are found in the GI tract, but they are produced in much greater abundance in the hypothalamus (see Chapter 2: Pituitary Gland, and Chapter 8: Hormonal Regulation of Fuel Metabolism) and pancreatic islets (see Chapter 7: The Pancreatic Islets) and are discussed elsewhere. All these peptides are also produced by neurons in the brain where they function as neurotransmitters and neuromodulators. Receptors for these peptides are closely related structurally and belong to the branch of the G protein–coupled receptor superfamily that includes the visual receptor, rhodopsin. They appear to have coevolved with their ligands by duplications of the gene for

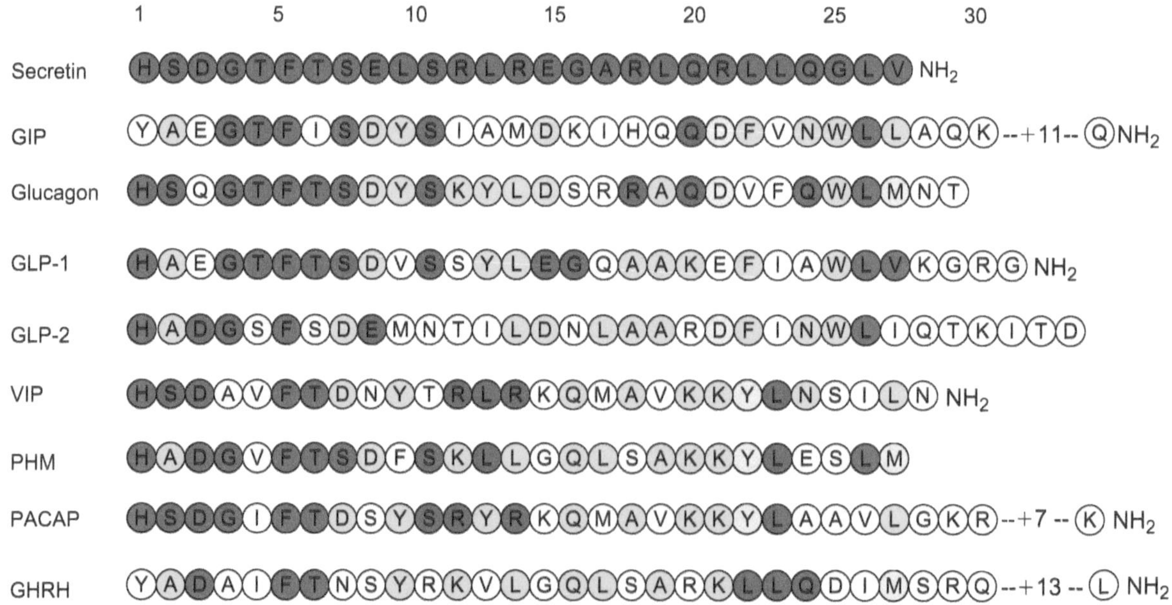

FIGURE 6.32 The secretin/glucagon family of peptides. Amino acids are represented by the single-letter amino acid code. Residues colored red are identical with those in corresponding positions in secretin. Residues colored cyan or green are identical with those in corresponding positions in at least three family members. Beyond residue 30, in the C terminal region, sequence divergence is almost complete. In most of these peptides the carboxyl terminal amino acid is amidated. *A*, alanine; *C*, cysteine; *D*, aspartic acid; *E*, glutamic acid; *F*, phenylalanine; *G*, glycine; *H*, histidine; *I*, isoleucine; *K*, lysine; *L*, leucine; *M*, methionine; *N*, asparagine; *P*, proline; *Q*, glutamine; *R*, arginine; *S*, serine; *T*, threonine; *V*, valine; *W*, tryptophan; *Y*, tyrosine.

(cont'd)

an ancient receptor progenitor, and produce their effects through activating G protein–coupled receptors that signal through the cyclic AMP second messenger system.

Secretin The discovery of secretin in 1902 by Bayliss and Starling laid the foundation for the science of endocrinology by establishing the concept that a chemical substance released into the blood by one organ in response to a particular stimulus can signal another organ to respond. These investigators found that instilling acid into an isolated loop of dog jejunum resulted in the secretion of pancreatic fluid even though all nervous connections were severed. They subsequently obtained the same results by injecting dogs with an extract of duodenal mucosa. They called the active substance secretin and coined the name "hormone" from the Greek word meaning to urge on, to initiate, or to stimulate. Before the discovery of secretin, communication between organs was thought to occur only through neural mechanisms.

Secretin is produced in S in the duodenal and proximal jejunal mucosae. Its secretion increases sharply when the pH of intestinal contents falls below 4.5. The major physiological role of secretin is to stimulate secretion of bicarbonate and water by the epithelial cells that line the secretory ducts of the pancreas and the cholangiocytes of the bile ducts. Increased delivery of bicarbonate to the duodenum buffers the hydrogen ions in the chyme and raises the pH to near neutrality. Both pancreatic juice and bile contribute to neutralization of the duodenal contents, but the contribution of the pancreas is considerably greater.

Cellular effects of secretin Secretin stimulates secretion of water and bicarbonate by regulating ion movements across the plasma membranes of epithelial cells that form the pancreatic and intrahepatic biliary ducts (Fig. 6.33).

As in other polarized epithelia, different complements of ion channels, exchangers, and transporters are present in the membranes that face the duct lumen (apical surface) and those that face the interstitium (basolateral surfaces). These cells are linked by junctional complexes that are permeable to water and selectively permeable to ions. The driving force for electrolyte transfer is the steep electrochemical sodium gradient between the cytosol and extracellular fluids. The driving force for movement of water into the lumen is the osmotic gradient established by these ion movements. Sodium ions are carried across the basolateral membranes on carrier molecules that cotransport two ions of bicarbonate with each ion of sodium. Bicarbonate ions are discharged across the apical membrane into the lumen in exchange for chloride ions. Accumulation of excess negatively charged chloride ions in the cytosol is prevented by extrusion through apical chloride channels, which allows the chloride molecules to recycle as bicarbonate accumulates in luminal fluid. The negatively charged bicarbonate creates an electrical gradient that provides the driving force for sodium to diffuse through intercellular junctions. The resulting increase in sodium bicarbonate concentration creates the osmotic force that drives water through and between the epithelial cells. The sodium gradient that is required for the system to operate is preserved by continuous extrusion of sodium by the sodium/potassium ATPase (the sodium pump) in the basolateral membranes. Continued operation of this system may produce as much as a liter of bicarbonate-rich pancreatic fluid in a day.

According to the current model, in the unstimulated, basal state, membranes embedded with chloride/bicarbonate exchangers, chloride channels, and water channels called aquaporin 1 are sequestered as vesicles in the cytoplasm beneath the apical membranes. Stimulation

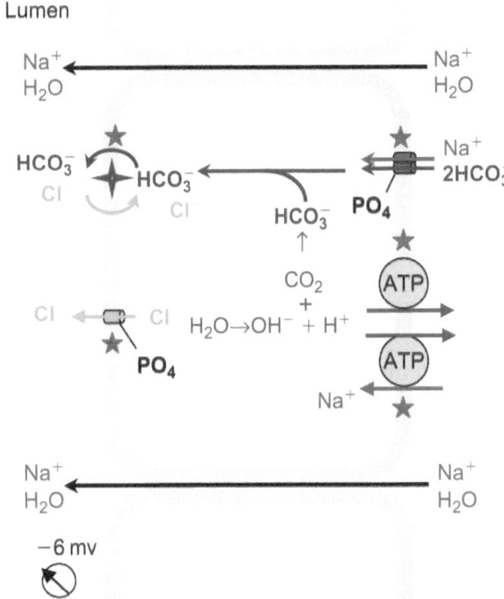

FIGURE 6.33 Actions of secretin on bicarbonate secretion by pancreatic and bile duct epithelial cells. Stars indicate processes that are stimulated by secretin through increased cyclic AMP formation and protein kinase A-dependent phosphorylation (see text for explanation). *AMP*, 5′-Adenosine monophosphate.

(*cont'd*)

by secretin results in cyclic AMP–dependent phosphorylation of critical proteins associated with the cytoskeleton and causes these vesicles to fuse with the apical membrane. In addition, the newly inserted luminal chloride channel, known as the cystic fibrosis transmembrane regulator (CFTR), is activated by protein kinase A–catalyzed phosphorylation. Activation of this channel is a critical component of fluid secretion. Genetic defects in the CFTR chloride channel severely impair secretory processes not only in the pancreas but also in the bronchiolar mucosa and elsewhere and are the cause of the devastating disease, cystic fibrosis.

On the basolateral side of the epithelial cells, protein kinase A catalyzed phosphorylation activates the sodium/bicarbonate cotransporter, increasing the rate of bicarbonate entry. Most of the bicarbonate that is added to bile and pancreatic juice is derived from interstitial fluid and plasma, but some are generated from carbon dioxide and water in the epithelial cells through the action of carbonic anhydrase, which catalyze the formation of carbonic acid from carbon dioxide and water. The alkaline intracellular environment favors dissociation of carbonic acid to bicarbonate and hydrogen ions. The hydrogen ions are eliminated by exchange for sodium and by an ATP-dependent hydrogen ion pump in the basolateral membrane. The sodium/hydrogen ion exchanger and the hydrogen ion pump may be sequestered in submembranous vesicles and inserted in the basolateral membrane by cyclic AMP–dependent processes. The net effect of stimulation by secretin is production of pancreatic juice and bile with a sodium concentration that is about equal to that of extracellular fluid, a bicarbonate concentration that is as much as fivefold higher than that of plasma, and a reciprocal reduction in chloride.

Secretin/cholecystokinin/acetylcholine interactions Secretin, CCK, and acetylcholine are the major stimulants of pancreatic secretion. Acetylcholine released from parasympathetic neurons, and perhaps CCK stimulates acinar cells to secrete proteins accompanied by small amounts of fluid. These agents alone have little effect on secretion of water and bicarbonate by the duct epithelia. However, CCK, probably by way of vagally released acetylcholine, strongly potentiates the actions of secretin on water and bicarbonate secretion (Fig. 6.34).

The potentiated response probably results from the complementary phosphorylation of key proteins, catalyzed by kinases activated by cyclic AMP, and the IP_3/diacyl glycerol second messenger systems (see Chapter 1: Introduction). Although the individual actions of CCK, acetylcholine, and secretin are described separately to provide insight into the actions of each, it cannot be overemphasized that these agents are present simultaneously and operate together in normal physiology along with still undetermined other factors whose effects are more subtle.

Other effects of secretin The principal outcome of stimulating bicarbonate production by pancreatic and bile ducts is neutralization of chyme in the duodenum. This effect of secretin is complemented by actions on the stomach to decrease the delivery of hydrogen ions to the duodenum (Fig. 6.17). Secretin indirectly inhibits gastric acid production and gastrin secretion by stimulating D cells in both the oxyntic and antral mucosae to secrete SST. SST inhibits acid secretion by its effects on G cells, ECL cells, and parietal cells as already described. Some evidence indicates that secretin and CCK may have synergistic effects on SST secretion. In addition, by activating receptors on vagal afferent neurons, secretin and CCK signal a reduction in the tonic inhibition of D cells, slow gastric emptying, and cause smooth muscle in the proximal stomach to relax. Other effects on the stomach include stimulation of mucus, pepsinogen, and gastric lipase secretion. Along with CCK, secretin is a trophic hormone that stimulates the growth of the exocrine pancreas. Secretin receptors are found in a variety of cells in the brain and

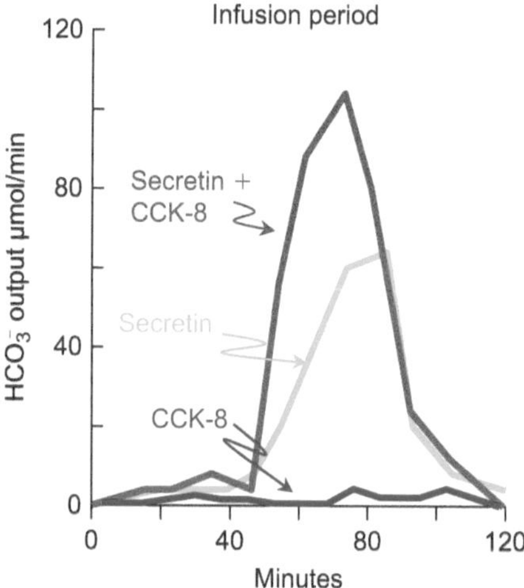

FIGURE 6.34 Synergistic effects of secretin and CCK on bicarbonate secretion. Secretin alone, CCK alone or secretin and CCK in combination were infused intravenously in six normal human subjects. Bicarbonate output was assessed in samples of duodenal fluids collected through a nasogastric tube. *CCK*, Cholecystokinin. Source: *Redrawn from data of Refeld, J. F. (2004).* Best Practice and Research in Clinical Endocrinology and Metabolism, 18, *569–586.*

(cont'd)

other organs, but its physiological role outside of the digestive remains to be established.

Regulation of secretin secretion A decrease in luminal pH is the principal stimulus for the release of secretin from duodenal S cells. Fatty acids in the chyme provide a secondary stimulus. Although S cells are in direct contact with the luminal contents, it appears that they do not respond directly to luminal pH, but rather respond to a "secretin-releasing factor" secreted into the duodenal lumen by some other, uncharacterized chemoreceptive cells probably associated with the enteric nervous system. The secretin releasing factor in rodents is a small peptide, but the human counterpart has not been identified. Destruction of the secretin releasing factor by proteolytic enzymes in pancreatic juice serves a negative feedback function. Similarly, the decreased delivery of acid to the duodenum also reduces the drive for secretion. Finally, SST secreted by D cells in the duodenal mucosa as well as in the gastric mucosa inhibits secretin output (Figs. 6.35 and 6.36).

GIP (glucose-dependent insulinotropic polypeptide/gastric inhibitory peptide) A 42-amino acid peptide that was devoid of CCK and secretin activities was isolated from extracts of intestinal mucosa based upon its ability to inhibit gastric acid secretion and gastric motility in dogs. It was given the descriptive name gastric inhibitory polypeptide (GIP). Despite its potency in dogs, rats, and other experimental animals, GIP is virtually devoid of gastric inhibitory activities in humans. When subsequent studies revealed that GIP produced a glucose-dependent stimulation of insulin secretion in humans and experimental animals, the GIP acronym came to stand for glucose-dependent insulinotropic polypeptide. GIP and GLP-1 (see later) are called incretins, intestinal hormones that increase the secretion of insulin. Their function is to prepare the body for an impending influx of nutrients and to facilitate the disposition of those nutrients through accelerating and amplifying the availability of insulin. The original demonstration of the incretin effect is shown in Fig. 6.36

Plasma insulin concentrations increased more rapidly and to a far greater extent when glucose was infused intrajejunally rather than intravenously, even though the intravenous infusion produced a much greater increase in plasma glucose concentration. Incretin actions are discussed further in Chapter 7, The Pancreatic Islets.

GIP is synthesized and secreted by K cells, which reside mainly in the proximal duodenum and to a lesser extent in the jejunum. The concentration of GIP in peripheral blood increases abruptly after a meal rich in carbohydrates and fat (Fig. 6.37).

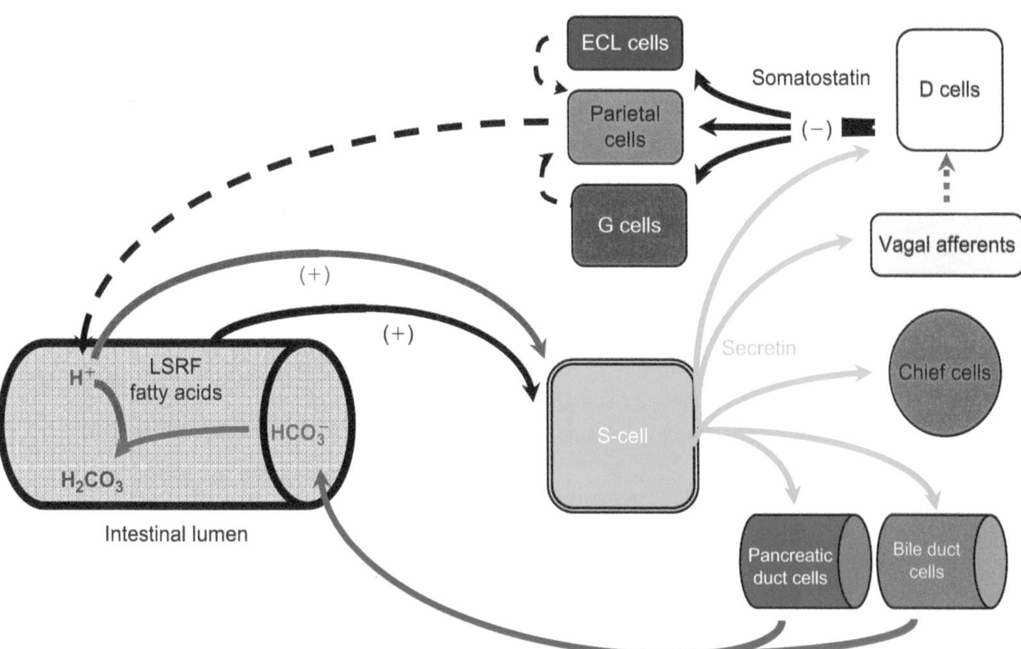

FIGURE 6.35 Schematic representation of the actions of secretin and feedback regulation of its secretion. Solid arrows indicate stimulation; dashed arrows indicate inhibition. *LSRF*, Luminal secretin releasing factors.

(cont'd)

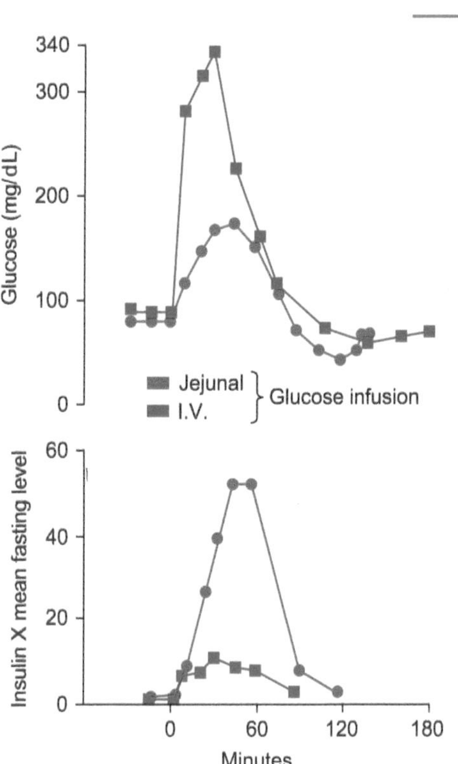

FIGURE 6.36 The incretin effect. Infusion of a solution of 500 mg of glucose intrajejunally produces a smaller increase in plasma glucose concentration than infusion of the same amount of glucose intravenously (upper panel), but the jejunal infusion elicits a much greater increase (55- vs 12-fold) in insulin secretion. Source: *Reproduced from McIntyre, N., Holdsworth, C. D., & Turner, D. S. (1965). Intestinal factors in the control of insulin secretion.* Journal of Clinical Endocrinology and Metabolism, *25, 1317.*

Peak concentrations are seen within 20–30 minutes, when only about 10% of the ingested nutrients have entered the duodenum. A similarly rapid increase is seen following infusion of a mixture of nutrients or only glucose directly into the duodenum of human subjects. The presence of glucose in the intestinal lumen is the primary stimulus for secretion. Apical surfaces of K cells directly contact luminal contents and appear to sense ingested nutrients. Detection of glucose results in a series of cyclic AMP and calcium-dependent reactions that culminate in GIP secretion into the mucosal interstitium. GRP secreted by neurons of the enteric nervous system during the cephalic phase also stimulates GIP secretion through a similar cascade of reactions.

Although glucose in the duodenum produces a robust increase in GIP secretion, no increase is seen after infusion of glucose into the blood, indicating that only the apical surfaces of K cells are sensitive to glucose. Just how glucose is detected by K cells remains a matter of speculation. To be effective stimuli of GIP secretion, sugars must be transported across apical cellular membranes by the sodium-coupled glucose transporter (SGLT). Glucose, galactose, and even glucose analogs that are transported, but not metabolized, stimulate GIP secretion, whereas fructose, which enters enteric cells by facilitated diffusion, is not an effective stimulant. Partial depolarization of apical membranes by the positively charged sodium ions that accompany sugars into cells may activate voltage-sensitive calcium channels and initiate the cascade of reactions that culminate in GIP release. In addition, G protein–coupled receptors, akin to the sweet taste receptors of the tongue, are present in intestinal mucosa and may reside in K cells and enteric nerves. Stimulation of these "taste receptors" by glucose engages the cyclic AMP signaling pathway and may lead to GIP secretion.

Unlike CCK and gastrin, in which only a small C-terminal fragment is needed for biological activity, both the amino and carboxyl terminals of GIP and other peptides in the secretin/glucagon family are required for receptor activation. GIP is rapidly inactivated by the enzyme, dipeptidyl peptidase (DPP-IV), which cleaves a dipeptide from the amino terminus. Dipeptidyl peptidase is found in soluble form in blood plasma and is present as an ectoenzyme bound to the surface of capillary endothelial cells throughout the body. GIP has a half-life in plasma of about 5–7 minutes. Other members of the glucagon/secretin family, particularly those with an alanine residue in position 2, are also rapidly inactivated by DPP-IV, but glucagon and secretin, which have a serine residue in position 2, are poor substrates.

The principal physiological targets for GIP are the insulin-secreting beta cells of the pancreatic islets. GIP enhances the secretion of insulin only when plasma glucose concentrations are above fasting levels (Fig. 6.36). The magnitude of this enhancement increases with increasing glucose concentrations. It has been estimated that stimulation by GIP may account for as much as 30% of the insulin secreted by the pancreas in normal individuals. Beta cells express GIP receptors and respond to it with increased production of cyclic AMP, which, through activation of protein kinase A, augments both the secretory process and transcription of the insulin gene. GIP also stimulates beta-cell proliferation and decreases apoptosis. These actions are considered further in Chapter 7, The Pancreatic Islets.

(cont'd)

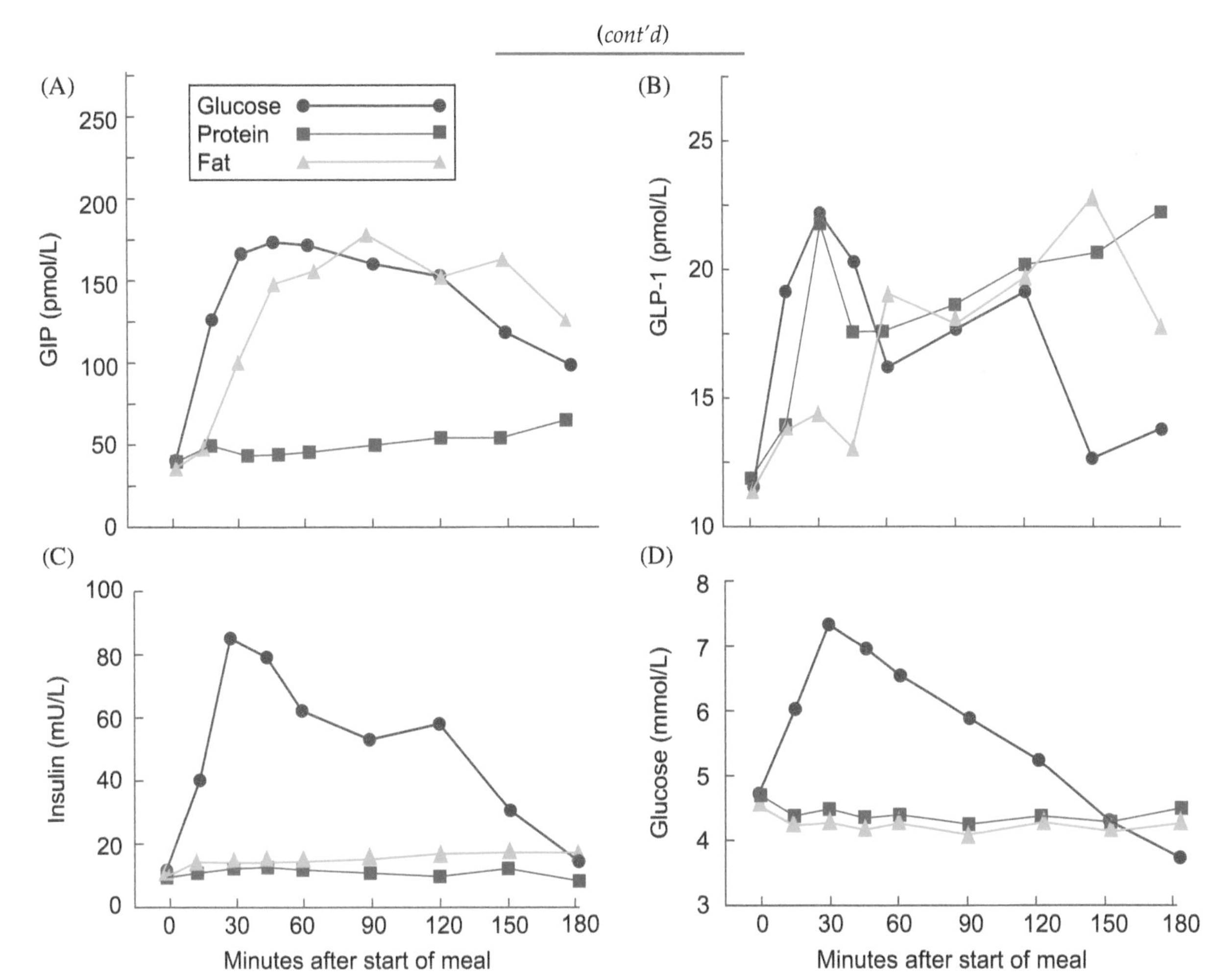

FIGURE 6.37 Effects of different dietary nutrients in the secretion of incretin hormones. Eight healthy volunteers were fed 375-calorie meals consisting of only glucose, protein, or fat. Venous blood was sampled at the indicated times. (A) Glucose and fat promptly increased plasma concentrations of GIP (glucose-dependent insulinotropic peptide), but proteins had no effect on GIP secretion. (B) Glucose and protein promptly increased plasma levels of GLP-1, but the response to the fatty meal was delayed. Note the difference in the scales for plasma concentrations of GIP and GLP in panels A and B, and note also that peak-plasma concentrations of both hormones were achieved in 30 min after the glucose meal. (C) Plasma concentrations of insulin were increased only after the glucose meal, which also increased plasma insulin concentrations [panel (D)]. Plasma glucose and insulin concentrations were unchanged after ingesting protein or fat, despite increased secretion of GIP and GLP-1, illustrating the glucose dependence of the incretin effect. *GLP-1*, Glucagon-like peptide 1. Source: *Redrawn from the data of Elliot, R. M., Morgan, L. M., Tredger, L. A., Deacon, S., Wright, J., & Marks, V. (1993). Glucagon-like peptide-1 (7-36) amide and glucose-dependent insulinotropic polypeptide secretion in response to nutrient ingestion in man: Acute post-prandial and 24-h secretion patterns.* Journal of Endocrinology, *138, 162.*

Regulation of GIP secretion Secretion of GIP is stimulated by eating, but unlike other hormones we have considered, the major consequence of its actions, increased secretion of insulin, does not produce a negative feedback signal. Insulin does not inhibit GIP secretion. GIP may increase SST secretion somewhat, and although SST may restrain GIP secretion, plasma levels of GIP remain elevated as long as glucose is present in the intestinal lumen. Clearance of nutrients from the duodenal lumen is the major event that terminates secretion of GIP.

Glucagon-like peptides 1 and 2 The glucagon gene encodes three biologically important peptides—glucagon, GLP-1, and GLP-2—each in a separate exon. The gene is expressed in L cells in the intestinal mucosa, alpha cells in the endocrine portion of the pancreas, and neurons in several locations in the brain. The proglucagon gene product is a 160-amino acid polypeptide that contains six pairs of basic amino acids that are primary sites for cleavage by processing enzymes (convertases), and at least one monobasic cleavage site. The nature and

(cont'd)

length of the final products secreted by these cells are determined by the complement of processing enzymes present in each cell type in which the gene is expressed. Cleavages of specific peptide bonds proceed at different rates, creating a potential for about 15 different peptides. Because these processing enzymes are present and act within the secretory granules, incompletely processed products enter the bloodstream along with mature hormones.

Proglucagon processing in both pancreatic and intestinal cells begins with cleavage into two large fragments (Fig. 6.38).

The N-terminal fragment, which contains glucagon, was isolated from pig ileal mucosa and was erroneously thought to consist of 100 amino acids. It was named glicentin for glucagon-like immunoactive peptide of 100 ('cent') amino acids. In pancreatic alpha cells, glicentin is cleaved to release a 30 amino acid peptide called glicentin-related pancreatic peptide (GRPP), authentic glucagon, and a small peptide fragment. The carboxyl terminal peptide, which is not further processed in pancreatic alpha cells, was aptly named the major proglucagon fragment. Of these products of alpha cells, only glucagon is biologically active (see Chapter 7: The Pancreatic Islets). In L cells, glicentin is cleaved to release GRPP, and a larger peptide, called oxyntomodulin, which consists of glucagon extended by eight amino acids at its carboxyl terminus. Oxyntomodulin inhibits gastric acid secretion when present in blood in high enough concentrations.

The physiologically important products of proglucagon in the intestine are GLP-1 and GLP-2, which are derived from the major proglucagon fragment. Based on the location of the paired basic amino acids, it was predicted that GLP-1 would consist of the 37 amino acids encompassing amino acids 72–108 of proglucagon. However, when this 37 amino acid peptide was synthesized, it was found to be biologically inactive. L cells produce enzymes that process this peptide further, removing six amino acids from the N terminus and converting the glycine at the C terminus to an amide. The product of these reactions is sometimes called GLP-1 (7–36) amide and is the biologically active hormone we call GLP-1. Small amounts of the 37 amino acid peptide along with other partially processed fragments of proglucagon are found in blood along with partially degraded GLP-1 and GLP-2.

L cells are the most abundant peptide producing endocrine cells in the GI tract. They are found throughout the small intestine and colon with the highest abundance in the distal ileum and colon. Contact of their apical surfaces with luminal contents enables them to monitor nutrients in chyme. L cells respond to glucose, amino acids, or fatty acids, with an increase in intracellular calcium concentrations and the release of GLP-1 and GLP-2 (Fig. 6.37). In addition to the glucose-sensing mechanisms proposed for K cells, L cells may sense glucose by the same mechanisms as described for pancreatic beta cells in Chapter 7, The Pancreatic Islets. Amino acids and long-chain fatty acids probably signal their presence by activating G protein–coupled receptors in the apical membrane. Chemoreceptors of the enteric nervous system also contribute to nutrient sensing and probably signal to L cells with small molecule neurotransmitters.

The observation that L cells are present in greatest abundance in the distal regions of the intestine, beyond where most of the ingested nutrients have been absorbed, appears inconsistent with their ability to monitor nutrients and signal insulin secretion. Yet GLP-1

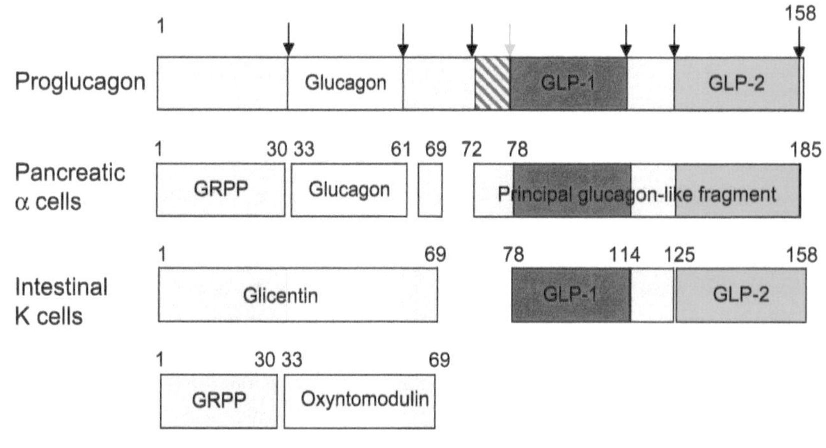

FIGURE 6.38 Posttranslational processing of proglucagon. Black arrows indicate dibasic sites of cleavage by hormone convertases. The green arrow points to a monobasic cleavage site. The cross-hatched area represents the hexapeptide N-terminal extension found in the immature GLP-1. The final products of pancreatic alpha cells and intestinal L cells are determined by the presence of different convertases in the two cell types. *GLP-1*, Glucagon-like peptide 1; *GLP-2*, glucagon-like peptide 2; *GRPP*, glicentin-related pancreatic peptide.

(cont'd)

secretion increases as rapidly after food intake as GIP (Fig. 6.37), whose origin is in K cells of the duodenum and proximal jejunum. It is likely that enteric neurons sense nutrients in the duodenum and communicate with distally located L cells. In addition, although only a minority of the total L cell population is present in the upper intestine, L cells in the duodenum and jejunum are as numerous as K cells. Furthermore, some cells in the jejunal and duodenal mucosae secrete both GLP-1 and GIP.

Physiological actions of glucagon-like peptide 1 The principal role of GLP-1 is to facilitate nutrient disposition and minimize changes in plasma glucose and amino acid concentrations after meals. Coordinated actions in the pancreas, the stomach, and the brain contribute to this role.

Effects on the pancreas As already mentioned, GLP-1 is an incretin, and like GIP, stimulates insulin secretion in a glucose-dependent manner. Mole for mole GLP-1 is considerably more potent than GIP, but because plasma concentrations of GIP are so much higher than those of GLP-1, the two incretins probably contribute about equally to insulin secretion, and their effects on pancreatic beta cells are additive. The glucagon-secreting pancreatic alpha cells also respond to both GLP-1 and GIP. Insulin lowers plasma glucose concentrations, and glucagon has the opposite effect. GLP-1 inhibits glucagon secretion and thereby increases the effectiveness of insulin. In contrast, GIP is a mild stimulator of glucagon secretion. In experimental animals and isolated tissues, GLP-1 increases insulin synthesis, promotes the differentiation of new insulin-producing beta cells, and reduces beta-cell apoptosis. These actions and their implications are discussed further in Chapter 7, The Pancreatic Islets.

Effects on the stomach GLP-1 contributes further to minimizing postprandial hyperglycemia by slowing gastric emptying and hence the rate of delivery of ingested nutrients to intestinal sites of absorption (Fig. 6.39).

GLP-1 lowers intragastric pressure by relaxing smooth muscle in proximal portions of the stomach and stimulates tonic and phasic contractions of smooth muscle in the pylorus and adjacent antral duodenal regions. These effects require intact vagal innervation. GLP-1 may retard gastric emptying by stimulating vagal afferent neurons to initiate vago–vagal reflexes, or perhaps by acting directly at the level of vagal motor centers in the brain. GLP-1 also decreases gastric acid secretion both by direct inhibitory actions on parietal cells, which express receptors for GLP-1, and by stimulating D cells to secrete SST.

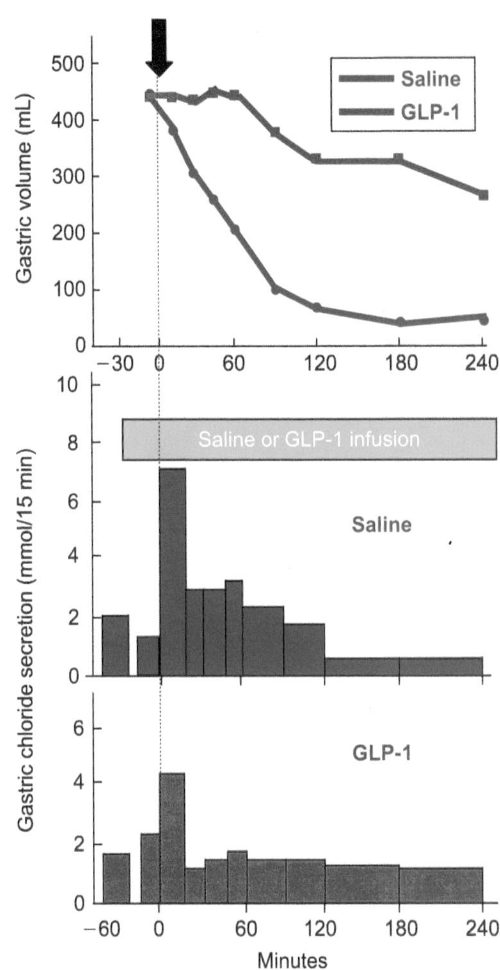

FIGURE 6.39 Effects of GLP-1 infusion on gastric emptying and acid secretion following the ingestion of a standardized liquid meal in nine healthy male volunteers. Subjects were given a constant infusion of either saline or 1.2 pmol of GLP-1/kg/min beginning 30 min before eating and continuing through the subsequent 4 h (*green bar*). The arrow indicates the time of meal ingestion. *GLP-1*, Glucagon-like peptide 1. Source: *Redrawn from the data of Nauck, M. A., Niedereichholz, U., Ettler, R., Holst, J. J., Orskov, C., Ritzel, R., & Schmiegel, W. H. (1997). Glucagon-like peptide 1 inhibition of gastric emptying outweighs its insulinotropic effects in healthy humans.* American Journal of Physiology: Endocrinology and Metabolism, 273, *E981–E988.*

Effects on the brain Studies in experimental animals and human subjects indicate that GLP-1 inhibits food intake. GLP-1 receptors are present in regions of the hypothalamus and brainstem that are associated with appetite control. These receptors may be stimulated by GLP-1 that arises in the intestines and crosses the blood–brain barrier and also by GLP-1 that is synthesized in the brain.

(cont'd)

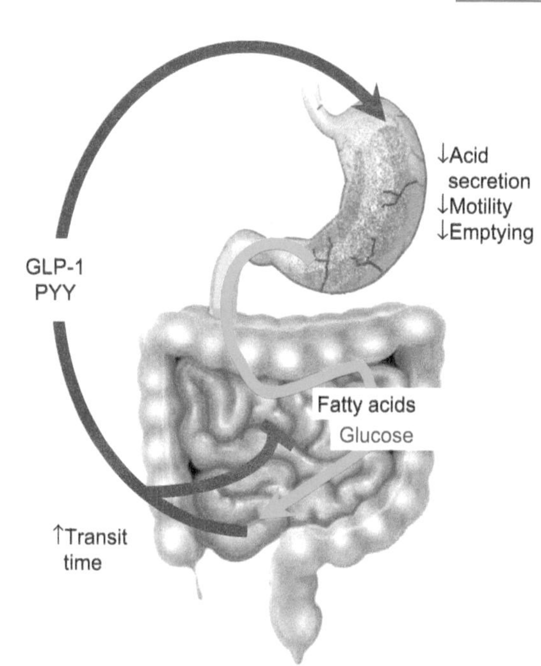

FIGURE 6.40 The ileal brake. *GLP-1*, Glucagon-like peptide 1.

In addition, GLP-1 may signal to appetite centers in the brain through activating receptors on afferent vagal neurons. By slowing gastric emptying, GLP-1 contributes to a feeling of fullness that also limits meal size. Control of appetite is complex and subject to regulation by multiple redundant signaling mechanisms, only one of which involves GLP-1. Detailed consideration of this topic is found in Chapter 8, Hormonal Regulation of Fuel Metabolism.

Ileal brake mechanism Another related physiological role for GLP-1 is in the so-called ileal brake mechanism (Fig. 6.40).

The ileal brake refers to the slowing of gastric and pancreatic exocrine secretion, stomach emptying, and intestinal motility in response to the presence of unabsorbed nutrients in the distal ileum. The abundant presence of L cells in the distal ileum and colon positions them well to gauge the efficiency of nutrient absorption in more proximal sections of the small intestine. Fatty acids rather than glucose may be more important for this response since little or no carbohydrate remains in the chyme that reaches these distal portions of the intestinal tract. Secretion of GLP-1 provides a feedback signal to the stomach to slow the delivery of nutrients into the intestine. GLP-1, presumably via vagal reflexes, also slows contractions of intestinal smooth muscles, which prolongs intestinal transit time and permits greater fractional absorption of nutrients.

Regulation of glucagon-like peptide 1 secretion Luminal nutrients are the most important stimuli for GLP-1 secretion, but stimulation of L cells by enteric neurons may also contribute to the rapid rise in GLP-1 concentrations in plasma after eating. L cells are unresponsive to changes in plasma levels of glucose, fatty acids, or insulin. GLP-1 may stimulate secretion of SST from D cells in the stomach, intestines, and pancreatic islets, and thereby restrain secretory activity of L cells. However, GLP-1 largely regulates its own secretion through its action of decreasing the delivery of glucose and fat to L cells.

Physiological actions of glucagon-like peptide 2 GLP-2 is co-secreted with GLP-1 in equimolar amounts. It produces similar but less pronounced effects on gastric motility and acid production as GLP-1 but has little or no effect on insulin secretion. Its principal biological target is the intestinal mucosa, where it has a trophic effect to stimulate cell proliferation and inhibit apoptosis. The resulting increase in depth of mucosal folds expands the surface area for nutrient absorption. In addition, GLP-2 stimulates amino acid and glucose transport by enterocytes and increases expression of SGLTs in their apical membranes. GLP-2 also promotes mucosal repair, reduces inflammatory responses to bowel injury, and maintains the mucosal permeability barrier to bacteria and enterotoxins. Although changes in enterocyte abundance and activity are the end result of GLP-2 action, GLP-2 receptors are expressed only in enteroendocrine cells of unknown function, myofibroblasts, and enteric neurons. The absence of GLP-2 receptors in enterocytes and stem cells in the mucosal crypts indicates these effects are produced indirectly and mediated by unknown growth factors. Promising results of clinical trials suggest that GLP-2 may have important therapeutic effects in the treatment of patients with inflammatory bowel diseases or following intestinal resection (short bowel syndrome).

The pancreatic polypeptide family

Pancreatic polypeptide (PPP) originally was isolated from pancreatic extracts in the course of purifying avian insulin. Two structurally related peptides, peptide YY (PYY) and neuropeptide Y (NPY), subsequently were isolated from intestinal mucosa and brain extracts. The name PYY was given to the peptide isolated from intestinal mucosa because one of its distinguishing features is the presence of tyrosine residues at both the carboxyl and amino terminals (Fig. 6.41).

In the single-letter amino acid code Y designates tyrosine. NPY is found predominantly, and perhaps exclusively,

(*cont'd*)

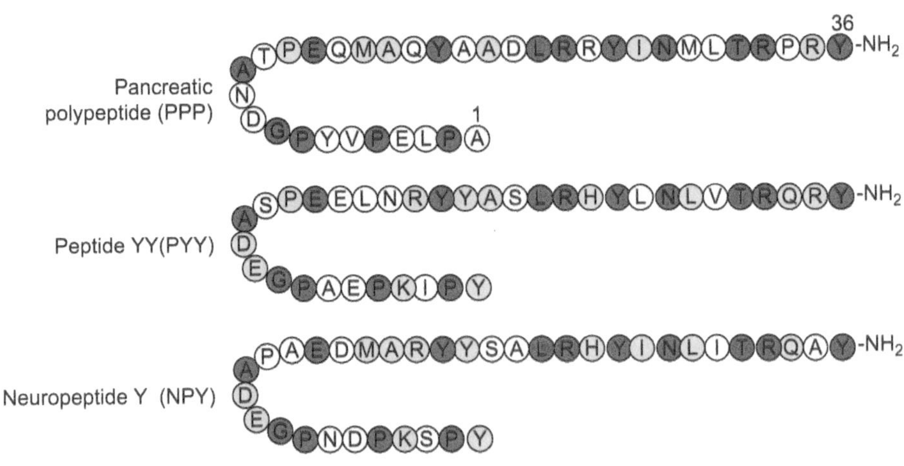

FIGURE 6.41 Amino acid sequences of the PPY family of peptides using the single-letter amino acid code. Residues shown in red are identical in corresponding positions in all three peptides. Residues shown in cyan or green are identical with those in corresponding positions in two family members. *A*, alanine; *C*, cysteine; *D*, aspartic acid; *E*, glutamic acid; *F*, phenylalanine; *G*, glycine; *H*, histidine; *I*, isoleucine; *K*, lysine; *L*, leucine; *M*, methionine; *N*, asparagine; *P*, proline; *PPY*, PP-fold; *Q*, glutamine; *R*, arginine; *S*, serine; *T*, threonine; *V*, valine; *W*, tryptophan; *Y*, tyrosine.

in central and peripheral nerves. It is one of the most abundant neuropeptides in the brain where it plays an important role in regulating food intake (see Chapter 8: Hormonal Regulation of Fuel Metabolism). The N in its name designates its neuronal abundance, although it, too, has tyrosine residues at both ends. All three peptides have 36 amino acids and are amidated at their carboxyl ends. Their U-shaped tertiary structure gives rise to the alternate name of PP-fold peptide family.

PPP is produced in F cells located in the periphery of pancreatic islets and in small clumps scattered among the acini. PYY is coproduced with the glucagon-like peptides in L cells predominantly in distal regions of the ileum and in the colon. Most of the PYY stored in these cells and about 40% of the circulating hormone is the so-called 3–36PYY in which the N-terminal dipeptide has been removed through the action of dipeptidylpeptidase IV. Both forms of PYY are biologically active. PYY also is produced in peripheral and central neurons where it might function in regulating metabolism. The similarity of the tertiary structures of the PP-fold peptides allows them to bind to the same subfamily of receptors, but with different affinities. Five distinct G protein–coupled receptor isoforms distributed widely in the brain and intestinal tract mediate the actions of these peptides.

Physiological effects of the pancreatic polypeptide hormone family Plasma concentrations of both PPP and PYY increase within moments after eating a mixed meal and may remain elevated for several hours. Secretion of PPP increases even in the absence of nutrients when the stomach is distended with water or when subjects are given a sample meal to smell, taste, and chew without swallowing (sham feeding). This response is elicited by vagal stimulation of pancreatic F cells. It is possible that enteric or vagal nerves also stimulate secretion of PYY by L cells in the distal ileum and colon, but the major stimulus for its secretion appears to be long-chain fatty acids in the ileum. Plasma concentrations of PYY usually increase in parallel with those of GLP-1.

PYY not only is co-secreted with GLP-1 but also functions along with GLP-1 as another component of the ileal brake mechanism described earlier (Fig. 6.39). When infused into experimental subjects in physiologically relevant amounts, PYY and PPP inhibit gastric acid secretion, gastric motility, and gastric emptying. Both PPP and PYY antagonize the effects of CCK and secretin on pancreatic enzyme secretion and gall bladder contraction. In addition, PYY slows the movement of chyme along the intestine. These effects on the GI tract and the inhibitory effects on delivery of pancreatic and hepatic secretions to the intestine are produced mainly through vagal reflexes. Finally, PYY, especially the 3–36 truncated form, may act as a satiety signal to the brain to limit meal size. Such an effect, like those exerted in the proximal GI tract, also would decrease the delivery of nutrients to the distal ileum and colon. Most of the actions of PYY are quite similar to those of GLP-1 and presumably reinforce those of GLP-1. Unlike GLP-1, however, PYY does not affect insulin or glucagon secretion.

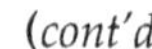

(cont'd)

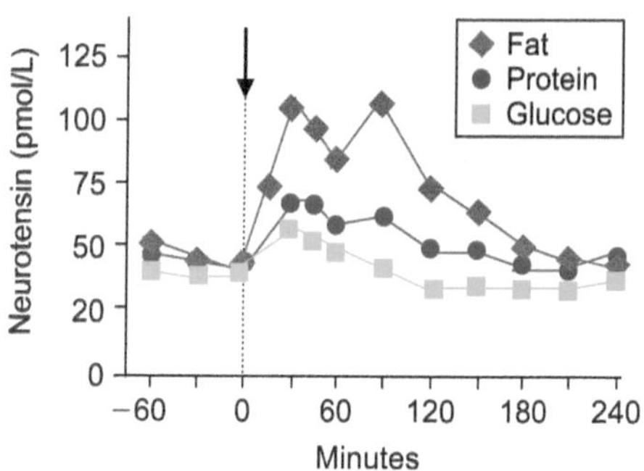

FIGURE 6.42 The effects of isocaloric test meals of carbohydrate, protein, and fat on plasma concentrations of neurotensin in healthy young adult subjects. Source: *Redrawn from Rosell, S., & Rökaeus, Ä. (1979). The effect of ingestion of amino acids, glucose and fat on circulating neurotensin-like immunoreactivity (NTLI) in man.* Acta Physiologica, *107, 263–267.*

Neurotensin

The tridecapeptide neurotensin, secreted by N cells in the distal jejunum throughout the ileum and in the colon, may be a third contributor to the ileal break mechanism. Like PYY and GLP-1, it is secreted mainly in response to fatty acids in the intestinal lumen, although carbohydrates and amino acids are also somewhat effective (Fig. 6.42).

It is likely that N cells respond directly to long-chain fatty acids and other nutrients sensed at their apical surfaces, but a neurally mediated stimulus for secretion is also possible. Just as already described for GLP-1 and PYY, neurotensin inhibits gastric acid secretion, slows gastric emptying, and decreases motility of the small intestine. In contrast, it may increase contractile activity in the colon. Neurotensin may also have a general trophic effect on the intestinal mucosa, stimulating mucosal proliferation and repair. Although neurotensin receptors have been identified in intestinal smooth muscle and in the gastric mucosa, it is likely that at least some of its actions are indirect and mediated by vago–vagal reflexes and SST.

In addition to the foregoing enterogastrone-like actions, neurotensin acts as a facilitator of fat digestion and absorption. Not only does it increase secretion of pancreatic lipase and bile acids, which play essential and cooperative roles in fat digestion, but it also increases the hepatic supply of bile acids. Bile acids are secreted into the bile by hepatocytes and recycled back to the liver in an enterohepatic circulation. Neurotensin stimulates the uptake of bile acids by ileal enterocytes, facilitating their return to the liver for resecretion into the bile. In addition, neurotensin stimulates bile secretion and may increase the contraction of the gall bladder, thereby hastening delivery of the bile acids to the intestinal lumen. Finally, by slowing the movement of chyme through the small intestine, it increases the time for digestion and absorption of fat.

Neurotensin originally was isolated from bovine hypothalamus, but soon was found to be expressed at 10-fold higher levels in the GI tract. Neurotensin is synthesized as a large 148-residue prohormone that also contains a biologically active hexapeptide called neuromedin N just downstream from the 13 amino acids of neurotensin. Intestinal N cells secrete neurotensin in greater abundance than neuromedin N, which is incompletely cleaved from the prohormone precursor in these cells. Both neurotensin and neuromedin N are produced by brain neurons and serve as neurotransmitters and neuromodulators. The two peptides have the same four amino acid sequence at their carboxyl terminals and bind to the same receptors. Consequently, they produce the same effects on the intestine, but neuromedin is considerably less effective due to its lower affinity for the receptor. The GI receptor for neurotensin (NTR1) belongs to the G protein–coupled superfamily and signals by way of the IP_3/DAG second messenger system. A closely related receptor (NTR2) is expressed largely in brain. A third receptor is a single membrane-spanning protein, which forms a heterodimer with NTR1.

The motilin/ghrelin family

The intestinal hormones discussed to this point are all secreted in response to eating, and govern GI functions associated with digestion and assimilation of ingested nutrients. Only two GI hormones are secreted in increased amounts in the interdigestive periods, and both belong to the motilin/ghrelin family. The two single copy genes of this family encode the precursors of a 22 amino acid peptide called motilin, and a 28 amino acid peptide called ghrelin at their amino terminals. The amino acid sequences of ghrelin and motilin are about 30% identical. The ghrelin precursor (Fig. 6.43) contains an additional peptide called obestatin, which may also have biological activity, but no activity has yet been found for the larger C-terminal peptide released from promotilin. A unique structural feature of ghrelin is the octanoic acid moiety bound in ester linkage to the serine in position three. Octanoate is added during posttranslational processing of the molecule and is required for binding to the ghrelin receptor and for transport across the blood–brain barrier. However, less than a quarter of the ghrelin stored in secretory granules is octanoylated,

(cont'd)

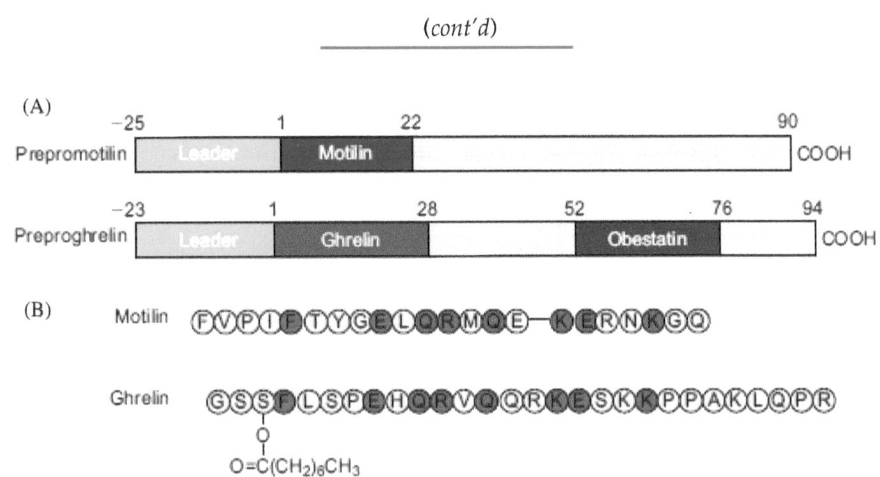

FIGURE 6.43 The motilin ghrelin family. (A) Posttranslational processing of prepromotilin and preproghrelin. Cleavage of proghrelin releases ghrelin from the N terminus and a second peptide called obestatin, which may have biological activity. (B) Amino acid sequences of motilin and ghrelin represented with the single amino acid code. Insertion of a gap between residues 15 and 16 in motilin optimizes the correspondence to the sequence of ghrelin and probably represents the loss of a codon. The octanoate held in ester linkage with the serine at position 3 of ghrelin is essential for activity.

and only about 5% of the circulating hormone contains octanoate, probably because the deacylated form of ghrelin has a half-life in plasma of about 30 minutes compared to only about 10 minutes for the active hormone. Both motilin and ghrelin are expressed in the brain and peripheral neurons as well as mucosal cells in the GI tract. Like their ligands, receptors for motilin and ghrelin are closely related and have about half of their amino acid sequences in common. These receptors and a possible receptor for obestatin are coupled to heterotrimeric G-proteins and signal through the IP3/DAG second messenger system.

Physiological actions of motilin The stomach is quiescent between emptying and the onset of the next meal, except for brief episodes of contractions spaced about 90 minutes apart. These contractions, which begin at about the midpoint of the stomach and continue distally toward the pylorus, are called the migrating motility complex and propel any remaining food particles and accumulated mucus into the duodenum. The waves of contractions continue through the duodenum and jejunum with diminishing intensity. These contractions coincide with, and are probably initiated by, motilin secreted by enteroendocrine cells in the duodenum and upper jejunum (Fig. 6.44).

Other effects of motilin include stimulation of enzyme secretion by the stomach and pancreas, and contractions of the gall bladder. This constellation of effects is consistent with a housekeeping role for motilin in clearing the stomach and intestine in preparation for the next episode of feeding.

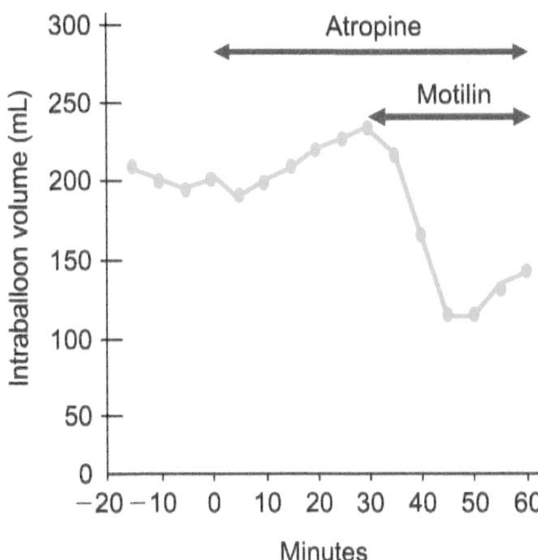

FIGURE 6.44 Effects of motilin on gastric muscle tone. An intragastric balloon was placed in the stomachs of normal fasted volunteers and filled with air. Changes in gastric muscle tone were detected as changes in balloon volume: Increased muscle tone decreases balloon volume. Infusion of atropine, which blocks acetylcholine receptors, resulted in expansion of the balloon, indicating a decrease in tone. Infusion of motilin alone (not shown) or during the continued infusion of atropine increased gastric tone as indicated by the decreased volume of the balloon. This effect of motilin is not mediated by parasympathetic stimulation of gastric muscle. Source: *Redrawn from the data of Cuomo, R., Vandaele, P., Coulie, B., Peeters, T., Depoortere, I., Janssens, J., et al. (2006). Influence of motilin on gastric fundus tone and on meal-induced satiety in man: Role of cholinergic pathways.* American Journal of Gastroenterology, 101, *804–811.*

(cont'd)

Detailed understanding of the regulation of motilin secretion is still lacking.

Motilin secreting cells in the duodenal mucosa receive cholinergic neural input from the enteric nerves, but the physiological mechanism for the intermittent activity of these neurons is not understood. Motilin secretion is inhibited both by sham feeding and by the presence of fatty acids in the duodenum. Motilin receptors are found in the greatest abundance in smooth muscle of the stomach and to a lesser extent in the duodenum, the small intestine, and colon. They are found on afferent vagal neurons and neurons of the myenteric plexus. Curiously, in addition to motilin, these receptors are activated by the antibiotic erythromycin, which can produce strong contractions of the stomach and intestine. This finding has led to the development of orally effective agents for the treatment of delayed gastric emptying encountered in some disease states.

Discovery of ghrelin The route to the discovery of ghrelin followed an unusual and circuitous path that began decades earlier with attempts to prepare analogs of the neuropeptide, enkephalin, that might greatly enhance its ability to stimulate growth hormone secretion. The success in producing potent growth hormone–releasing peptides fueled efforts to identify the receptor that mediates this activity in the pituitary and hypothalamus. The search uncovered a G protein–coupled receptor that is highly conserved among vertebrate animals and is closely related to the motilin family. Like motilin, it stimulates gastric contraction and emptying. Efforts to find the natural ligand for this receptor resulted in the isolation of a peptide from extracts of the rat stomach. The peptide was named ghrelin from the Proto-Indo-European word for "grow." Ghrelin is secreted by relatively abundant P/D1 endocrine cells that are located primarily in the oxyntic mucosa and are of two types. The open type has its surface on the gastric lumen whereas the closed type has no luminal surface. Both types secrete ghrelin into the blood. Ghrelin cells are also present to a lesser extent in the antrum and in the mucosae of the small and large intestines. Some ghrelin-producing cells are found in the endocrine portion of the pancreas. Ghrelin-producing cells are particularly prominent in the pancreas during fetal development. Hypothalamic neurons in the arcuate nucleus also produce ghrelin, but most of the ghrelin circulating in blood originates in the oxyntic mucosa.

Physiological actions of ghrelin As already stated, discovery of ghrelin was the outcome of efforts to enhance secretion of growth hormone. This effect is due mainly to ghrelin released from hypothalamic neurons, but some crosstalk may also take place between the growth hormone–producing cells of the pituitary and the P/D1 cells of the GI tract. The role of ghrelin in regulating growth hormone secretion is discussed in Chapter 11, Hormonal Control of Growth.

The physiological actions of ghrelin on the GI tract are quite similar to motilin. Ghrelin receptors are found in smooth muscle and neurons in the stomach and intestines. Ghrelin increases gastric acid secretion, gastric motility, and gastric emptying. In addition, it accelerates the propulsion of chyme through the small and large intestines. These actions are at least partly indirect and depend upon stimulation of smooth muscles by acetylcholine and neuropeptides released from vagal and enteric motor neurons. Excitation of ghrelin receptors on afferent neurons in the GI wall initiates vago–vagal reflexes and local reflexes of the enteric nervous system. Analogous actions on colonic contractions involve reflexive release of acetylcholine from pelvic nerves. However, no GI abnormalities were reported for mice lacking ghrelin, suggesting that its effects are not essential, or that redundant mechanisms compensate for its absence.

Ghrelin concentrations in plasma increase during interdigestive periods. They rise just before eating and are suppressed by ingestion of fat and carbohydrates (Fig. 6.45).

This pattern suggested that ghrelin might have a role in regulating food intake. Experiments in humans and rodents indicate that ghrelin increases feelings of hunger

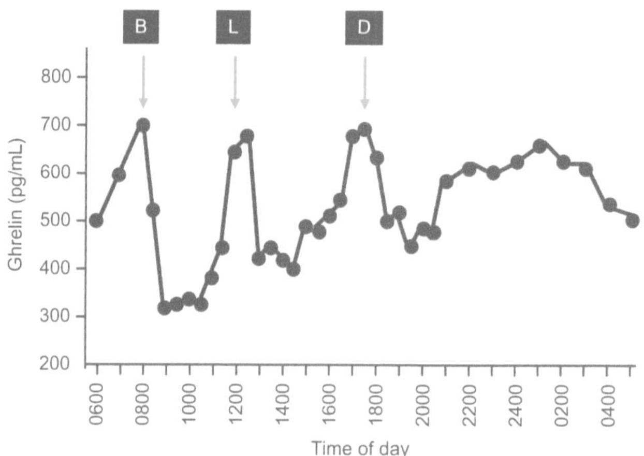

FIGURE 6.45 Average plasma ghrelin concentrations during a 24-h period in 10 human subjects consuming breakfast (B), lunch (L), and dinner (D) at the times indicated (0800, 1200, and 1730, respectively). Source: *From Cummings, D. E., Purnell, J. Q., Frayo, R. S., Schmidova, K., Wisse, B. E., & Weigle, D. S. (2001). A preprandial rise in plasma ghrelin levels suggests a role in meal initiation in humans.* Diabetes, *50, 1714–1719.*

(cont'd)

and stimulates hypothalamic neurons in appetite control centers. Treatment of experimental animals with ghrelin increases food intake and causes weight gain. Regulation of ghrelin secretion is clearly related to energy balance, but understanding of the mechanisms involved is incomplete. The possible role of ghrelin in appetite control and its relation to insulin secretion are discussed in Chapter 8, Hormonal Regulation of Fuel Metabolism.

TABLE 6.1 Hormones and neuropeptides that regulate gastric functions.

Peptide	Source	Targets	Actions
Gastrin	Antral G cells	ECL cells	↑ Histamine synthesis and secretion
		Parietal cells	↑ Acid secretionGrowth and maintenance of oxyntic mucosa
GRP	Vagal and enteric efferent neurons	Antral G cells	↑ Gastrin secretion
SST	Oxyntic and antral D cells	G cells, ECL cells	↓ Secretion of gastrin, histamine, and acid
		Parietal cells	
Ghrelin	Oxyntic P/D1 cells	Vagal and enteric	↑ Gastric motility
		Afferent neurons	↑ Gastric emptying
		Smooth muscle cells	
Motilin	Duodenal and jejunal endocrine cells	Vagal and enteric	↑ Gastric motility; initiates migrating motility complex
		Afferent neurons	
		Smooth muscle cells	
GLP-1	L cells in intestinal mucosa	Gastric D cells	↑ SST secretion
		Parietal cells	↓ Acid secretion
		Afferent neurons	↓ Gastric motility; delays gastric emptying
GLP-2	L cells in intestinal mucosa	Gastric D cells	↑ SST secretion
		Parietal cells	↓ Acid secretion
		Afferent neurons	↓ Gastric motility; delays gastric emptying
Oxyntomodulin	L cells in intestinal mucosa	Gastric D cells	↑ SST secretion
	Alpha cells in pancreatic islets	Parietal cells	↓ Acid secretion
		Afferent neurons	↓ Gastric motility; delays gastric emptying (activates GLP-1 receptors)
PPP	F cells in pancreas	Vagal afferent and enteric neurons?	Delays gastric emptying
PYY	L cells is distal ileum and colon	Gastric D cells	↑ SST secretion
		Afferent neurons?	↓ Acid secretion
			↓ Gastric motility; delays gastric emptying

(Continued)

TABLE 6.1 (Continued)

Peptide	Source	Targets	Actions
Secretin	Duodenal S cells	Oxyntic and antral D cells	↑ SST secretion
		Chief Cells	↓ Acid secretion
			↑ Pepsinogen and lipase secretion
Cholecystokinin	Duodenal I cells	Oxyntic and Antral D cells	↑ SST secretion
		Chief cells	↓ Acid, pepsinogen, and lipase secretion
		Afferent neurons	Contracts antral-pyloric area and relaxes fundic area; delays gastric emptying
		Smooth muscle cells	
Neurotensin	Jejunal and ileal N cells	? Oxyntic and antral D cells, chief cells?	↓ Acid secretion
		Afferent neurons?	↓ Gastric motility; delays gastric emptying
		Smooth muscle cells?	
Pituitary adenyl cyclase activating peptide (PACAP)	Vagal and enteric efferent neurons	ECL cellsSmooth muscle cells	↑ Histamine secretion
			↑ Relaxation of smooth muscle
VIP	Vagal and enteric efferent neurons	Smooth muscle cells	↑ Relaxation

GLP-1, Glucagon-like peptide 1; *GLP-2*, glucagon-like peptide 2; *GRP*, gastrin-releasing peptide; *PPP*, pancreatic polypeptide; *PYY*, peptide YY; *SST*, somatostatin; *VIP*, vasoactive intestinal peptide.

TABLE 6.2 Hormones and neuropeptides that regulate pancreatic and hepatic function.

Peptide	Source	Targets	Actions
CCK	Duodenal I cells	Gall bladder smooth muscle	↑ Gall bladder contraction
		Pancreatic acinar cells	↑ Bile secretion
		Vagal afferent neurons	↑ Pancreatic enzyme secretion
			Growth and maintenance of pancreatic acini
Secretin	Duodenal S cells	Bile duct cells	↑ Water and bicarbonate secretion
		Pancreatic duct cells	
Glucose-dependent insulinotropic	Duodenal K cells	Pancreatic beta cells	↑ Insulin secretion
		Pancreatic alpha cells	↓ Glucagon secretion
Peptide (GIP)			Growth and maintenance of beta cells
GLP-1	Intestinal L cells	Pancreatic beta cells	↑ Insulin secretion
		Pancreatic alpha cells	↓ Glucagon secretion
			Growth and maintenance of beta cells
PPP	Pancreatic F cells	Pancreatic acinar and islet cells	↓ Enzyme and hormone secretion
PYY	Intestinal L cells	Pancreatic acinar and ductal cells, hepatocytes	↓Enzyme, bicarbonate, water, and bile secretion
Neurotensin	Intestinal N cells	Hepatocytes	↑ Bile production
		Gall bladder smooth muscle	↑ Contraction

(*Continued*)

TABLE 6.2 (Continued)

Peptide	Source	Targets	Actions
		Pancreatic acinar cells	↑ Enzyme secretion
GRP	Vagal efferent neurons	Vagal afferent neurons	Pancreatic acinar cells
↑ Enzyme secretion			
VIP	Vagal efferent neurons	Smooth muscles of the sphincter of Oddi	↑ Relaxation
Somatostatin	D cells of the GI tract, pancreatic delta cells	Pancreatic acinar and islet cells	↓ Hormone, enzyme, bicarbonate, water, and bile secretion
		Biliary duct cells	

CCK, Cholecystokinin; *GI*, gastrointestinal; *GLP-1*, glucagon-like peptide 1; *GRP*, gastrin-releasing peptide; *PPP*, pancreatic polypeptide; *PYY*, peptide YY; *VIP*, vasoactive intestinal peptide.

TABLE 6.3 Hormones and neuropeptides that regulate intestinal function.

Peptide	Source	Target	Actions
Motilin	Intestinal endocrine cells	Smooth muscle	↑ Contraction
Ghrelin	Oxyntic mucosal P/D1 cells	Smooth muscle	↑ Contraction
GLP-1	L cells	Smooth muscle?	↓ Contraction
		Enteric neurons?	
GLP-2	L cells	Enterocytes?	↑ Nutrient absorption
		unknown	↓ Growth, repair and maintenance of mucosa
Luminal secretin–releasing peptides	? Gastric or duodenal mucosa?	Duodenal S cells	↑ Secretion
Luminal CCK–releasing peptides	? Gastric or duodenal mucosa?	Duodenal I cells	↑ Secretion
PYY	Ileal and colonic L cells	Smooth muscle?	↓ Contraction
		Enteric neurons?	
SST	Stomach and intestinal D cells and pancreatic ∂ cells	Endocrine cells	↓ Secretion
		Smooth muscle cells	↓ Contraction
Neurotensin	Jejunal and duodenal N cells	Enterocytes?	↑ Nutrient absorption
		Unknown	↑ Growth, repair, and maintenance of mucosa

CCK, Cholecystokinin; *GLP-1*, glucagon-like peptide 1; *GLP-2*, glucagon-like peptide 2; *PYY*, peptide YY; *SST*, somatostatin.

Concluding comments

Neuroendocrine regulation of the GI tract is exceedingly complex and still incompletely understood. Redundancy of control mechanisms, the absence of discrete aggregates of endocrine cells that can be excised and studied or eliminated, and wide species differences make studying human GI endocrinology enormously challenging. Yet impressive progress is being made with respect to understanding GI regulation and its relationship to overall energy balance. We have focused the discussion of GI endocrinology hormone by hormone. Tables 6.1–6.3 aim to highlight the convergence and redundancy of hormonal actions on their principal targets. Much is left to learn about the endocrine control of the GI tract and the relative importance of these hormones for expression of the effects listed.

Summary

Digestion is a multiorgan task, beginning with the stomach. In this chapter the relevant structures and their endocrine-responsive cells are described in the normal sequence of digestion starting with the fundus and body of the stomach. From the stomach, food moves into the duodenum and from there through the jejunum and ileum to the colon. At each step along the way, hormonal regulation ensures maximum efficiency in obtaining nutrients from food.

Suggested readings

Basic foundations

Binder, H. J. (2017). Gastric function. In W. F. Boron, & E. L. Boulpaep (Eds.), *Medical physiology* (3rd ed., pp. 863–878). Philadelphia, PA: Elsevier.

Corey, B., & Chen, H. (2017). Neuroendocrine tumors of the stomach. *Surgical Clinics of North America*, *97*(2), 333–343. Available from https://doi.org/10.1016/j.suc.2016.11.008.

Marino, C. R., & Gorelick, F. S. (2017). Pancreatic and salivary glands. In W. F. Boron, & E. L. Boulpaep (Eds.), *Medical physiology* (3rd ed., pp. 879–898). Philadelphia, PA: Elsevier.

Advanced information

Jensen, R. T., Norton, J. A., & Oberg, K. (2016). Neuroendocrine tumors. In (10th ed.M. Feldman, L. S. Friedman, & L. J. Brandt (Eds.), *Sleisenger and Fordtran's gastrointestinal and liver disease* (Vol. 1Philadelphia, PA: Elsevier.

Mendelson, A. H., & Donowitz, M. (2017). Catching the zebra: Clinical pearls and pitfalls for the successful diagnosis of Zollinger–Ellison syndrome. *Digestive Diseases and Sciences*, *62*(9), 2258–2265. Available from https://doi.org/10.1007/s10620-017-4695-7.

Metz, D. C., Cadiot, G., Poitras, P., Ito, T., & Jensen, R. T. (2017). Diagnosis of Zollinger–Ellison syndrome in the era of PPIs, faulty gastrin assays, sensitive imaging and limited access to acid secretory testing. *International Journal of Endocrine Oncology*, *4*(4), 167–185. Available from https://doi.org/10.2217/ije-2017-0018.

Norton, J. A., Krampitz, G. W., Poultsides, G. A., Visser, B. C., Fraker, D. L., Alexander, H. R., & Jensen, R. T. (2018). Prospective evaluation of results of reoperation in Zollinger-Ellison syndrome. *Annals of Surgery*, *267*(4), 782–788. Available from https://doi.org/10.1097/sla.0000000000002122.

Öberg, K. (2018). Management of functional neuroendocrine tumors of the pancreas. *Gland Surgery*, *7*(1), 20–27. Available from https://doi.org/10.21037/gs.2017.10.08.

Tariq, H., Kamal, M. U., Vootla, V., ElZaeedi, M., Niazi, M., Gilchrist, B., ... Chilimuri, S. (2018). A rare cause of abdominal pain and mass in an 18-year-old patient: A diagnostic dilemma. *Gastroenterology Research*, *11*(1), 75–78. Available from https://doi.org/10.14740/gr955w.

Historical information

Zollinger, R. M., & Ellison, E. H. (1955). Primary peptic ulcerations of the jejunum associated with islet cell tumors of the pancreas. *Annals of Surgery*, *142*(4), 709–723.

CHAPTER

7

The pancreatic islets

Case study: type 1 diabetes mellitus

Patient is a 25-year-old female without significant past medical history who presented to the emergency room with 7 days of polyuria, polydipsia, dry mouth, polyphagia, 10 lb weight loss, blurry vision, and diffuse abdominal pain. On physical examination, her body mass index was normal at 20. She was afebrile but tachycardic (heart rate 120) and blood pressure was 100/65. She had a fruity odor to her breath and had a tender but nonsurgical abdomen. Laboratory evaluation revealed a serum glucose of 550, anion gap was elevated at 25 (normal <12), arterial pH was low at 7.1 (normal arterial pH 7.35–7.45), and positive serum and urine ketones. Her hemoglobin A1c was elevated at 9.5%. Based on her clinical presentation and biochemical evaluation, she was diagnosed with diabetic ketoacidosis and was started on intravenous fluids and insulin. After 12 h, her hyperglycemia and metabolic acidosis were corrected. She was able to eat and was transitioned to subcutaneous long acting and mealtime insulin. Once her blood sugars were well controlled on the insulin regimen, she was discharged home. Outpatient laboratory evaluation revealed low C-peptide of 0.3 ng/mL (normal range 0.8–3.85 ng/mL) and elevated titers of glutamic acid decarboxylase 65 antibodies (2.7 U/mL, normal <1 U/mL), IA-2 antibodies (1.8 U/mL, normal <0.8 U/mL), and antiinsulin antibodies (2.3 U/mL, normal <0.4 U/mL) confirming a diagnosis of type 1 diabetes mellitus.

Type 1 diabetes mellitus, once known as juvenile diabetes or insulin-dependent diabetes, is a chronic condition in which the pancreas produces little or no insulin. Insulin is a hormone needed to allow glucose to enter cells to produce energy. The exact cause of type 1 diabetes is unknown. Usually, the body's own immune system mistakenly destroys the insulin-producing islets of Langerhans in the pancreas. Type 1 diabetes has no cure. Treatment focuses on managing blood sugar levels with insulin, diet, and lifestyle to prevent complications. Until the discovery of insulin, type 1 diabetes was a lethal disease. In 1869 Paul Langerhans, a medical student in Berlin, Germany, discovered the later known islets of Langerhans but their role became evident only in 1901 when Eugene Lindsay Opie established the link between the islets of Langerhans and diabetes. Over the following two decades, several attempts were made to isolate insulin from the pancreatic tissue. In 1916 Nicolae Paulescu, a Professor of Physiology at the University of Medicine and Pharmacy in Bucharest, Romania, developed an aqueous pancreatic extract that normalized hyperglycemia when was administered to a diabetic dog. In 1921 Frederick Banting in collaboration with J.J.R. Macleod, Charles H. Best and James B. Collip at the University of Toronto, Canada, were able to isolate an extract from the pancreatic islets. A year later, Leonard Thompson, a 14-year-old very sick Canadian diabetic patient, was given the first injection of insulin. Banting and MacLeod were awarded the Nobel Prize in Physiology or Medicine in 1923 for the discovery of insulin (Fig. 7.1). Banting and MacLeod shared the award money with Best and Collip.

Goodman's Basic Medical Endocrinology.
DOI: https://doi.org/10.1016/B978-0-12-815844-9.00007-5

(cont'd)

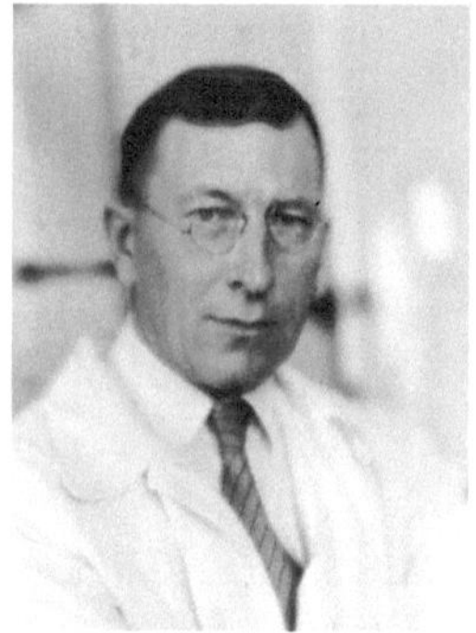
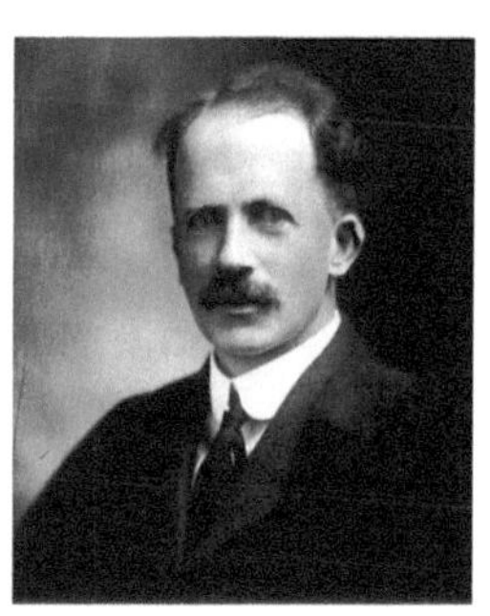
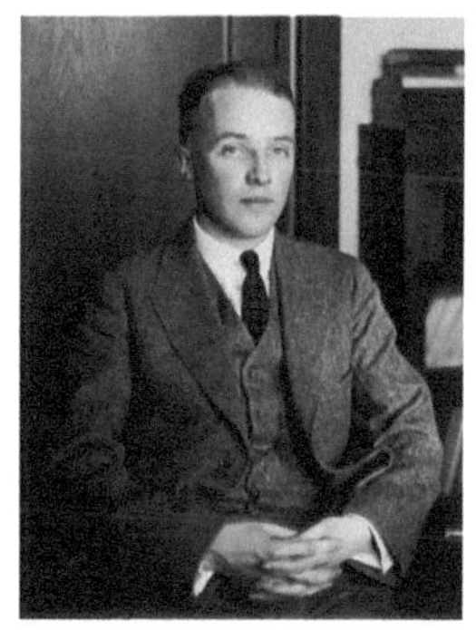
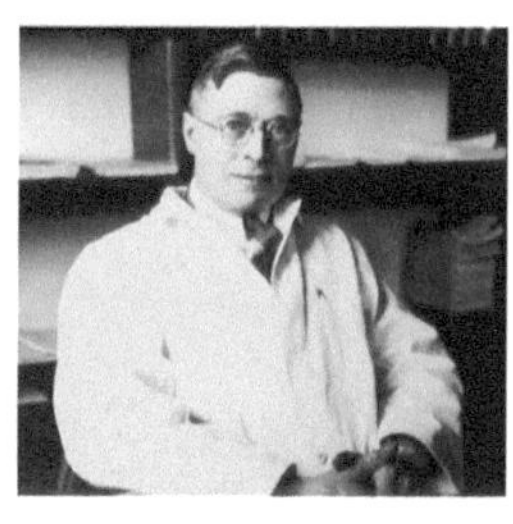

FIGURE 7.1 The four people who made insulin possible. *From left: Frederick Banting, J.J. R. MacLeod, Charles H. Best and James B. Collip.*

In the clinic: diabetes mellitus

Introduction

Diabetes mellitus is a disease that occurs when the blood glucose is elevated. In diabetes the pancreas does not make insulin or the body does not use the insulin well (insulin resistance). The two most common types of diabetes are type 1 and type 2 diabetes. In type 1 diabetes the body does not make insulin because the immune system destroyed the pancreatic beta cells that secreted insulin. Type 1 diabetes is usually diagnosed in children and young adults, although it can appear at any age. People with type 1 diabetes need to take insulin every day to stay alive. Type 2 is the most common type of diabetes. In this type the body does not make enough insulin or there is resistance to it. Type 2 diabetes can develop at any age but is most common in middle-aged and older people. Usually, type 2 diabetes is being associated with being overweight or obese, which causes insulin resistance.

Signs and symptoms

The most common presentation of new onset diabetes is with hyperglycemia without acidosis. Patients present with polyuria, polydipsia, weight loss, fatigue, and blurry vision. Less commonly patients present with diabetic ketoacidosis, which is more frequently seen in type 1 rather than type 2 diabetes. Symptoms are similar but usually more severe than those of patients without acidosis. In addition to polyuria, polydipsia, and weight loss, patients with ketoacidosis may present symptoms caused by the acidosis such as fruity-smelling breath, abdominal pain, and change in mental status, including drowsiness and lethargy. On clinical exam, patient with diabetic ketoacidosis appears sick and dehydrated. Signs include hypotension, tachycardia and tachypnea, hypothermia, Kussmaul breathing, ileus, acetone breath, and altered sensorium. Type 2 diabetes patients can present with extreme hyperglycemia and hyperosmolality but without or with minimum ketosis. This condition is called hyperglycemic hyperosmolar state. Patients presenting with hyperglycemic hyperosmolar state are very dehydrated and present with more significant changes in mental status than patients with diabetic ketoacidosis.

Diagnosis

Diabetes mellitus is diagnosed based on one of the following criteria:

1. fasting plasma glucose ≥126 mg/dL (7 mmol/L) on more than one occasion;
2. random plasma glucose ≥200 mg/dL (11.1 mmol/L) in a patient with classic symptoms of hyperglycemia;
3. plasma glucose ≥200 mg/dL (11.1 mmol/L) measured 2 h after an oral glucose tolerance test; and

(*cont'd*)

4. hemoglobin A1c ≥ 6.5% (using an assay that is certified by the National Glycohemoglobin Standardization Program)

Unless patient has unequivocal symptoms of hyperglycemia, the diagnosis of diabetes mellitus should be confirmed by repeat testing.

Management

The goal of treatment in diabetes is to control hyperglycemia and prevent micro- and macrovascular diabetes complications. As type 1 diabetes is caused by lack of insulin production due to the destruction of pancreatic beta cells, all patients with type 1 diabetes should receive insulin. Insulin is a hormone administered by injection or via insulin pump into subcutaneous fat tissue. Different types of insulin are available, including long acting, intermediate acting, short/rapid acting, and premixed preparations. As in type 2 diabetes, there is often time some residual insulin production; these patients can be treated with oral agents, insulin, or a combination of these agents. There are several classes of noninsulin antidiabetic medications which work through different mechanisms, including biguanides, sulfonylureas, glinides, thiazolidinedione, glucagon-like protein-1 (GLP-1) agonists, dipeptidyl peptidase-4 inhibitors, sodium–glucose cotransporter 2 inhibitors, and alpha-glucosidase inhibitors.

Prognosis

Diabetes mellitus is a chronic disease. Diabetes-related complications include microvascular complications (retinopathy, nephropathy, and neuropathy) and macrovascular complications (heart attack, stroke, and peripheral artery disease). As good glycemic control has been shown to decrease the risk of diabetes-related complications, in particular, microvascular disease, the goal of treatment is to control hyperglycemia while not exposing patients to severe hypoglycemia. A reasonable treatment goal for most patients is a hemoglobin A1c 6%–7%; however, the target should be individualized especially for older patients who in general should have a higher hemoglobin A1c target.

The pancreatic islets

The pancreas (Fig. 7.2) has both an exocrine and an endocrine function. Exocrine secretions of the pancreas are digestive enzymes and will not be covered further. The endocrine portion secretes hormones (Table 7.1).

The principal pancreatic hormones are insulin and glucagon, whose opposing effects on the liver regulate hepatic storage, production, and release of energy-rich fuels. Insulin is an anabolic hormone that promotes sequestration of carbohydrate, fat, and protein in storage depots throughout the body. Its powerful actions are

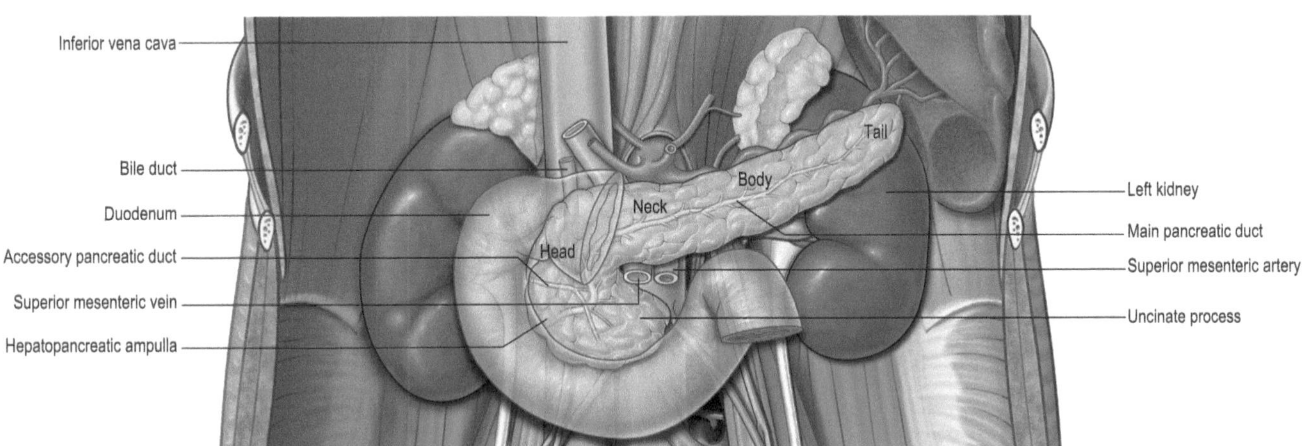

FIGURE 7.2 The pancreas in the abdominal cavity lies behind the stomach. In this illustration the liver is not shown. It would lie above the right kidney. The regions of the pancreas are also shown. The pancreas gets some of its arterial blood from the splenic artery which is unlabeled but is visible as a series of curves just above the neck, body, and tail of the pancreas and from branches of the superior mesenteric artery. Source: *From Figure 69.1 in S. Standring. (2016),* Gray's anatomy *(41st ed.) (p. 1179). Elsevier.*

TABLE 7.1 The endocrine hormones produced by the islet cells in the pancreas.

Cell	Percentage of total	Location	Fine structure of granules	Hormone and molecular weight	Function
β Cell	70	Scattered throughout islet (but concentrated in center)	300 nm in diameter; dense core granule surrounded by a wide electron-lucent halo	Insulin 6000 Da	Decreases blood glucose levels
				Amylin, ~3200 Da	Inhibits gastric emptying and glucagon release from α cells
α Cell	20	Islet periphery	250 nm in diameter; dense core granule with a narrow electron-lucent halo	Glucagon, 3500 Da	Increases blood glucose levels
δ Cell D D_1	5	Scattered throughout islet	350 nm in diameter; electron-lucent homogeneous granule	Somatostatin, 1640 Da	*Paracrine:* inhibits hormone release from endocrine pancreas and enzymes from exocrine pancreas
					Endocrine: reduces contractions of alimentary tract and gallbladder smooth muscles
				Vasoactive intestinal peptide, 3800 Da	Induces glycogenolysis; regulates smooth muscle tonus and motility of gut; controls ion and water secretion by intestinal epithelial cells
G cell	1	Scattered throughout islet	300 nm in diameter	Gastrin, 2000 Da	Stimulates production of hydrochloric acid by parietal cells of stomach
PP cell (F cell)	1	Scattered throughout islet	180 nm in diameter	Pancreatic polypeptide 4200 Da	Inhibits exocrine secretions of pancreas
ε Cell (Epsilon cell)	1	Scattered throughout islet	?	Ghrelin	Induces the sensation of hunger and modulates receptive relaxation of the smooth muscle fibers of the muscularis externa of the gastrointestinal tract

From Table 18.1 from Histology *(4th ed.), by Leslie P. Gartner. Elsevier, 2017, p. 480.*

exerted principally on skeletal muscle, liver, and adipose tissue, whereas the effects of glucagon are restricted to the liver, which responds by forming and secreting energy-rich water-soluble fuels: glucose, acetoacetic acid, and β-hydroxybutyric acid. Interplay of these two hormones contributes to constancy in the availability of metabolic fuels to all cells. Somatostatin is also an islet hormone and was discussed in Chapter 6, Hormones of the Gastrointestinal Tract, as was pancreatic polypeptide. Ghrelin, produced by epsilon cells, is discussed in Chapter 8, Hormonal Regulation of Fuel Metabolism.

Glucagon acts in concert with other fuel-mobilizing hormones to counterbalance the fuel-storing effects of insulin. Insulin, on the other hand, acts alone, and prolonged survival is not possible in its absence. Inadequacy of insulin due to insufficient production results in the disease called diabetes mellitus type 1; a second disease, diabetes mellitus type 2, results primarily from decreased end organ sensitivity to insulin (insulin resistance).

Morphology of the endocrine pancreas

The 1–2 million islets of the human pancreas range in size from about 50 to about 500 mm in diameter and contain from 50 to 300 endocrine cells (Fig. 7.3).

Collectively, the islets make up only 1%–2% of the pancreatic mass. They are highly vascular, with each cell seemingly, in direct contact with a capillary. Blood is supplied by the pancreatic artery and eventually drains into the portal vein, which thus delivers the entire output of pancreatic hormones to the liver. Blood entering each islet through one or more arterioles flows through an anastomosing network of capillaries before forming a vein and exiting at the opposite pole. The blood then flows through the acini. The transition from arterioles to capillaries in the islets and acini and then back to a venule forms the insuloacinar portal system. The islets then have some control over the digestive enzyme secretions of the acini (Figs. 7.4 and 7.5).

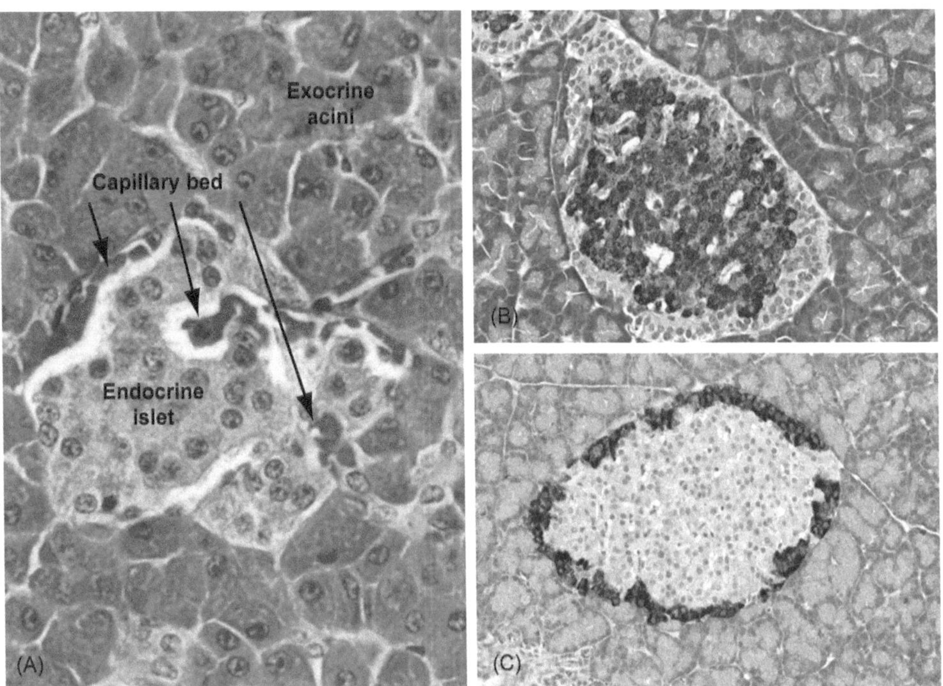

FIGURE 7.3 Rat islets of Langerhans. The islets are surrounded by acini that secrete digestive enzymes. Note the extensive blood vessel network in (A). In (B) the beta cells have been stained for insulin and in (C) the alpha cells have been stained for glucagon. Note that the alpha cells are organized around the periphery of each islet, while the beta cells are centrally located. In humans the alpha and beta cells are randomly scattered throughout each islet. Source: *From Figure 39.5 in Koeppen B. M., & Stanton B. A. (2018).* Berne and levy physiology *(7th ed.) (p. 704). Elsevier.*

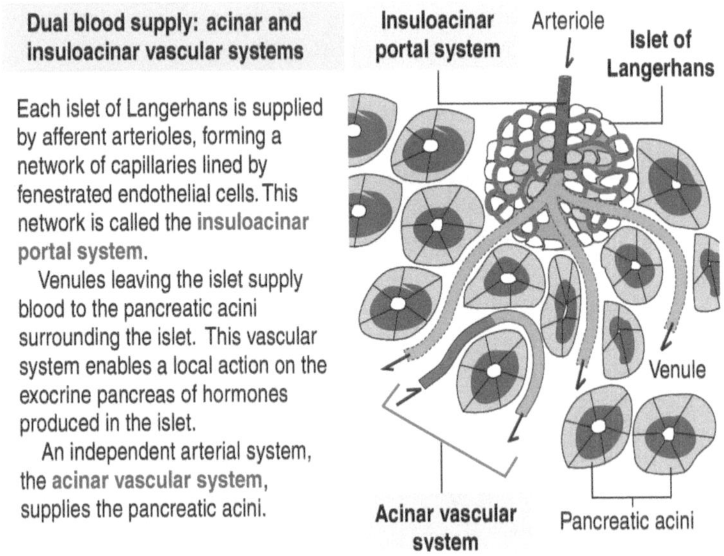

Dual blood supply: acinar and insuloacinar vascular systems

Each islet of Langerhans is supplied by afferent arterioles, forming a network of capillaries lined by fenestrated endothelial cells. This network is called the **insuloacinar portal system.**

Venules leaving the islet supply blood to the pancreatic acini surrounding the islet. This vascular system enables a local action on the exocrine pancreas of hormones produced in the islet.

An independent arterial system, the **acinar vascular system**, supplies the pancreatic acini.

Insuloacinar portal system
Arteriole
Islet of Langerhans
Venule
Acinar vascular system
Pancreatic acini

FIGURE 7.4 Blood flow through the islets and acini and demonstrating the insuloacinar portal system. By this system the islets may exert some control over nearby acini. More distal acini are supplied with blood from branches of the splenic artery. Source: *From Figure 19-15 from Kierszenbaum A. L., & Tres L. L. (2020).* Histology and cell biology: An introduction to pathology *(5th ed.) (p. 653). Elsevier.*

This pattern of blood flow in human islets differs from the classic description of islet blood flow derived from studies in rodents. The same is true of the location of alpha and beta cells. In rodents the alpha cells are on the periphery of the islet, while the beta cells are in the center (Fig. 7.3), but in humans, the alpha and beta cells are distributed randomly throughout the islet (Fig. 7.6).

The islets are richly innervated with both sympathetic and parasympathetic fibers that terminate on or near the secretory cells. Parasympathetic preganglionic fibers arise from cell bodies in the dorsal motor

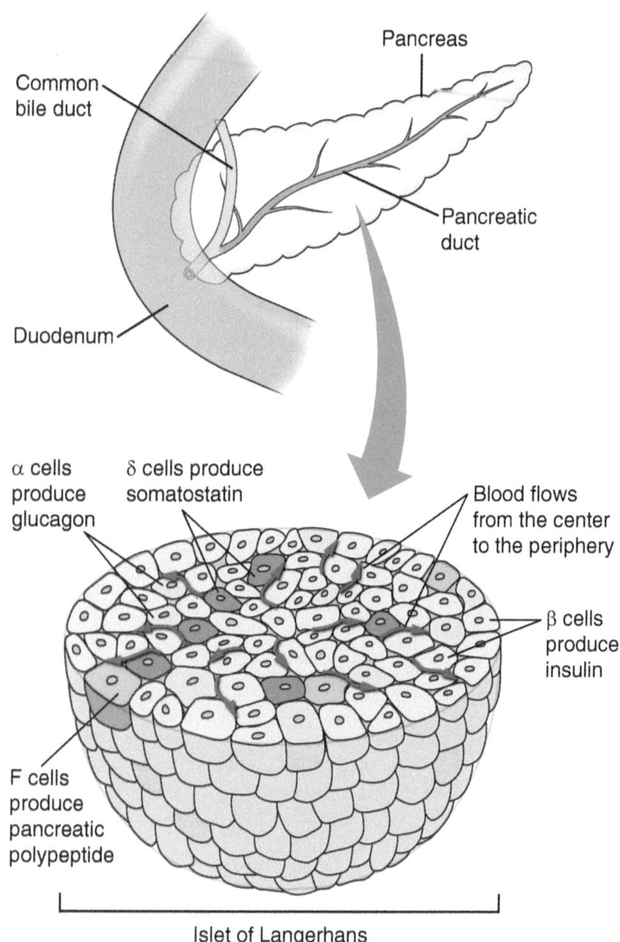

FIGURE 7.5 The blood flow within an islet and the different cell types. The blood flows from the center of the islet toward the periphery. Epsilon cells are not illustrated. Source: *Redrawn from Figure 51.1 from Barrett E. J. (2017). Chapter 51: The endocrine pancreas. In W. F. Boron, & E. L. Boulpaep (Eds.)* Medical physiology *(3rd ed.) (p. 1036). Elsevier.*

nucleus of the vagus and synapse with postganglionic cholinergic and peptidergic neurons in pancreatic ganglia buried within the pancreas. Sympathetic fibers originate in the hypothalamus and terminate on cell bodies in the intermediolateral column of the spinal cord. The preganglionic fibers to the pancreas pass through the sympathetic chain and without synapsing and travel in the greater splanchnic nerve to synapse in the celiac or superior mesenteric ganglia. The postganglionic fibers from these ganglia end in the pancreas but it has not been determined if they synapse directly on individual cells (Fig. 7.7).

These neurons release norepinephrine and several neuropeptides. The islets also contain a rich complement of sensory fibers. Pain fibers return to the spinal cord via the sympathetic fibers in the greater splanchnic nerve.

Histologically, the islets consist of three major and at least two minor cell types. Beta cells, which synthesize and secrete insulin, make up about 60% of a typical islet. Alpha cells are the source of glucagon and comprise perhaps as much as 30% of islet tissue. Delta cells, which are considerably less abundant, produce somatostatin.

F cells, which secrete pancreatic polypeptide, may also appear in the exocrine part of the pancreas. A fifth cell type, epsilon cells, that secretes ghrelin has been identified in both fetal and adult islets. In humans, these cells and the F cells occupy the perimeters of islets, with alpha cells, whereas beta cells are more centrally located (Figs. 7.3 and 7.4) and are situated along the lengths of capillaries. In humans as well as rodents the close contacts between the different cell types is thought to favor paracrine communication and may have a role in regulating islet cell function.

Glucagon

Biosynthesis, secretion, and metabolism

Glucagon is a simple unbranched peptide chain that consists of 29 amino acids and has a molecular weight of about 3500 Da. Its amino acid sequence has been remarkably preserved throughout evolution of the vertebrates. The glucagon gene, which is located on chromosome 2, is expressed primarily in alpha cells, L-cells of the intestinal epithelium, and discrete brain areas. It is secreted from a preproglucagon peptide (Fig. 7.8).

Glucagon formation and its relation to other products of the same gene and to other hormones and neuropeptides are discussed in Chapter 6, Hormones of the Gastrointestinal Tract. Glucagon is packaged, stored in membrane-bound granules, and secreted by exocytosis like other peptide hormones. It circulates without binding to carrier proteins and has a half-life in blood of about 5 minutes. Glucagon concentrations in peripheral blood are considerably lower than in portal venous blood. This difference reflects not only greater dilution in the general circulation but also the fact that about 25% of the secreted glucagon is destroyed during passage through the liver. The kidney is another important site of degradation, and a considerable fraction of circulating glucagon is destroyed by plasma peptidases.

Physiological actions of glucagon

The physiological role of glucagon is to stimulate hepatic production and secretion of glucose and to a lesser extent, ketone bodies, which are derived from fatty acids (Fig. 7.9).

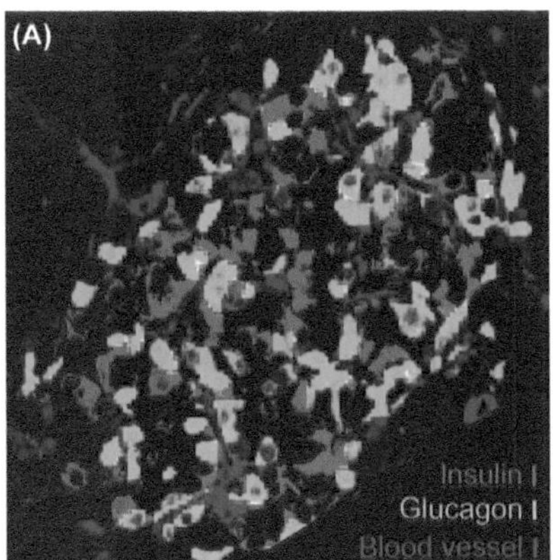

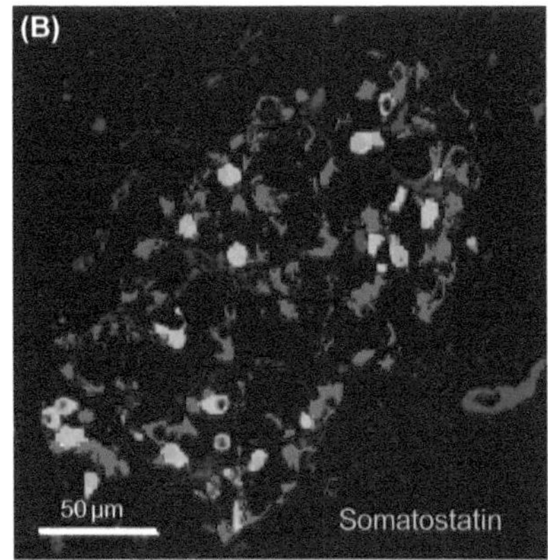

FIGURE 7.6 Cytoarchitecture of a typical human pancreatic islet as revealed in immunostained confocal scanning microscopic images. Endocrine cells are closely but randomly associated with vascular cells. Most (A) insulin- (red) and glucagon- (green), and (B) somatostatin- (cyan) immunoreactive cells are in close proximity to vascular cells immunoreactive for smooth muscle cell actin (blue). Endocrine cells are aligned along the blood vessels in a random order. Source: *From Cabrera, O., Berman, D. M., Kenyon, N. S., Ricordi, C., Berggren, P. O., & Caicedo, A. (2006). The unique cytoarchitecture of human pancreatic islets has implications for islet cell function.* Proceedings of the National Academy of Sciences of the United States of America, 103, *2334–2339, with permission.*

Under normal circumstances, liver and possibly pancreatic beta cells are the only targets of glucagon action (Fig. 7.10).

A number of other tissues, including fat, and heart express glucagon receptors and can respond to glucagon experimentally, but considerably higher concentrations of glucagon are needed than are normally found in peripheral blood. Glucagon stimulates the liver to release glucose and produces a prompt increase in blood glucose concentration. Glucose that is released from the liver is obtained from breakdown of stored glycogen (glycogenolysis) and new synthesis (gluconeogenesis). Because the principal precursors for gluconeogenesis are amino acids, especially alanine, glucagon also increases hepatic production of urea (ureagenesis) from the amino groups taken off the amino acids (two amine groups are combined with CO_2 to form urea). Glucagon also increases production of ketone bodies (ketogenesis) by directing metabolism of long-chain fatty acids toward oxidation and away from esterification and export as lipoproteins. Concomitantly, glucagon may also promote breakdown of hepatic triacylglycerols to yield long-chain fatty acids, which, along with fatty acids that reach the liver from peripheral fat depots, provide the substrate for ketogenesis.

All the effects of glucagon appear to be mediated by cyclic adenosine monophosphate (cAMP) (see Chapter 1: Introduction). In fact, it was studies of the glycogenolytic action of glucagon that led to the discovery of cAMP and its role as a second messenger. Activation of protein kinase A by cAMP results in phosphorylation of enzymes, which increases or decreases their activity, or phosphorylation of the transcription factor cAMP response element-binding protein, which usually increases transcription of target genes. Glucagon may also increase intracellular concentrations of calcium by a mechanism that depends upon activation of protein kinase A. Increased intracellular calcium may reinforce some cAMP–mediated actions of glucagon, particularly on glycogenolysis.

Glucose production

To understand how glucagon stimulates the hepatocyte to release glucose, we must first consider some of the biochemical reactions that govern glucose metabolism in the liver. Biochemical pathways that link these reactions are illustrated in Fig. 7.11.

It is important to recognize that not all enzymatic reactions are freely reversible under conditions that prevail in living cells. Phosphorylation and dephosphorylation of substrates usually require separate enzymes. This arrangement sets up substrate cycles that would spin futilely in the absence of some regulatory influence exerted on either or both opposing reactions. These reactions are often strategically situated at or near branch points in metabolic pathways and can therefore direct flow of substrates toward one fate or another.

Regulation is achieved both by modulating the activity of enzymes already present in cells and by increasing or decreasing rates of enzyme synthesis and therefore the amounts of enzyme molecules. Enzyme activity can be regulated allosterically by changes in conformation produced by interactions with substrates or cofactors, or covalently by phosphorylation and dephosphorylation of regulatory sites in the enzymes themselves. Changing the activity of an enzyme requires only seconds, whereas many

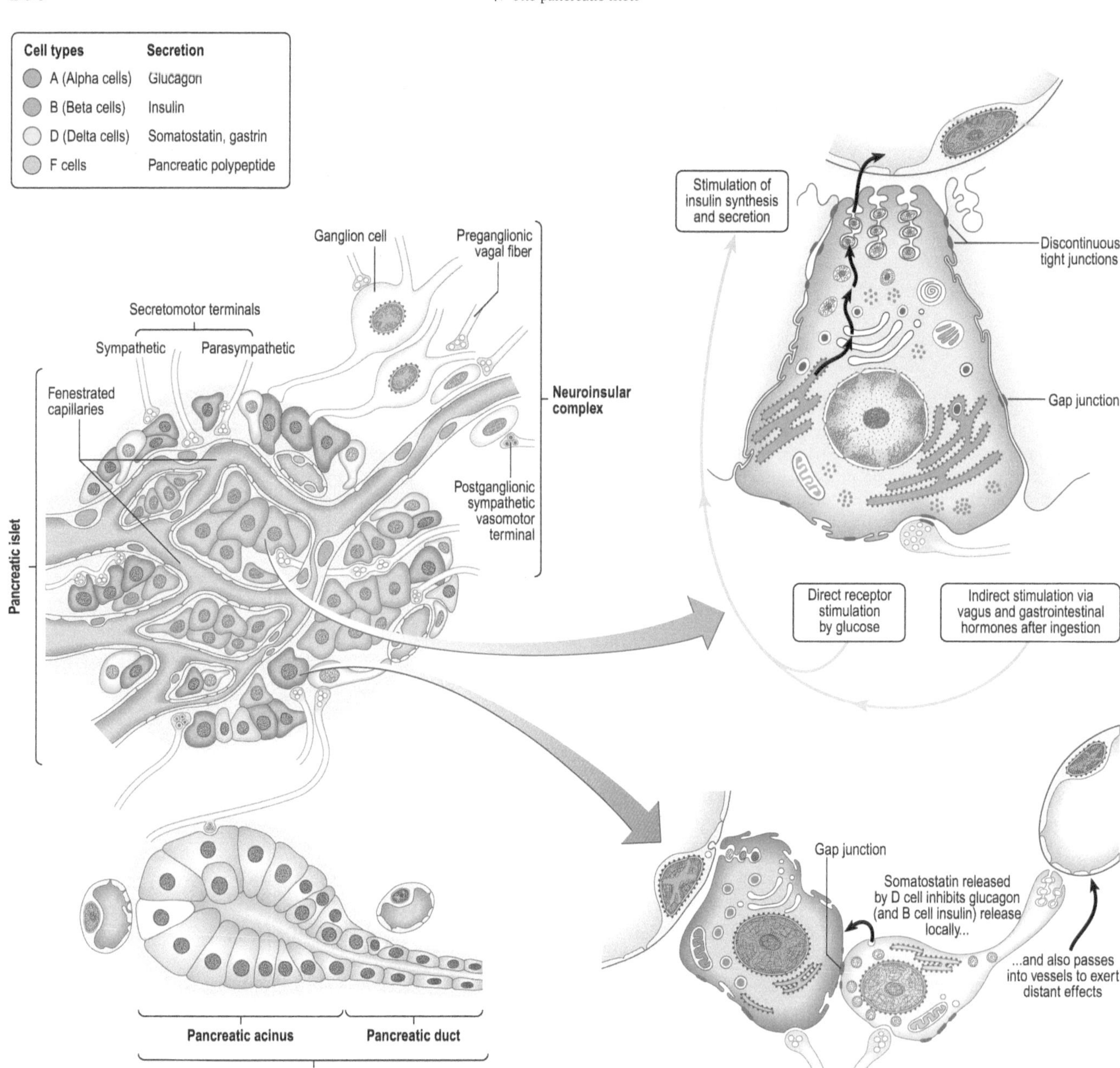

FIGURE 7.7 (A) The structure of one of the more than one million islets in the human pancreas. Blue cells are beta cells, red are alpha cells, green are somatostatin-forming cells, and orange are F cells. Not shown are epsilon cells. This image depicts the beta cells as being in the center with the alpha cells in the periphery. As was indicated, in humans, the alpha and beta cells are distributed randomly throughout the islet; (B) (boxed inset) a beta cell showing direct vagal stimulation. Black arrows show the direction of insulin synthesis; (C) (boxed inset) the relationship between an alpha cell (red) and a delta cell (green). The neural modulation is via the vagus nerve. Source: *From Figure 60.10 from S. Standring (2016).* Gray's anatomy *(41st ed.) (p. 1186). Elsevier.*

minutes or even hours are needed to change the amount of an enzyme.

Glycogenolysis

cAMP formed in response to the interaction of glucagon with its G protein–coupled receptors on the surfaces of hepatocyte (see Chapter 1: Introduction) activates protein kinase A, which catalyzes phosphorylation, and hence activation, of an enzyme called phosphorylase kinase (Fig. 7.12).

This enzyme, in turn, catalyzes phosphorylation of another enzyme, glycogen phosphorylase, that cleaves glycogen stepwise to release glucose-1-

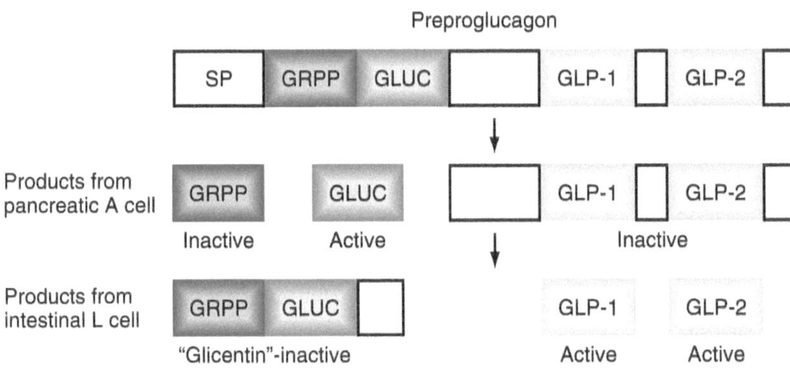

FIGURE 7.8 The synthesis of different molecules from the preproglucagon molecule and whether they are active or inactive. *GLUC*, Glucagon; *GLP*, glucagon-like peptide, *GRPP*, glucagon-related polypeptide. Source: *From Figure 39.10 in Koeppen B. M., & Stanton B. A. (2018).* Berne and levy physiology *(7th ed.) (p. 708). Elsevier.*

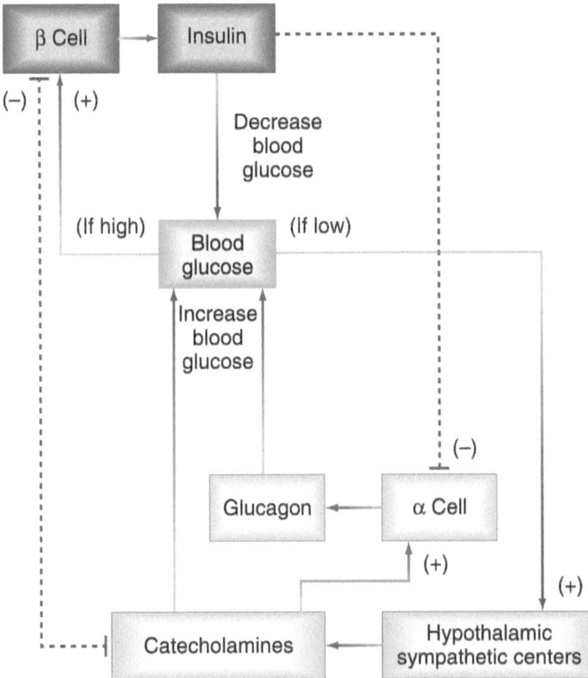

FIGURE 7.9 Integrated regulation of blood glucose showing the effect of glucagon, insulin, and catecholamines (norepinephrine and epinephrine) on blood glucose. Source: *From Figure 39.11 in Koeppen B. M., & Stanton B. A. (2018).* Berne and levy physiology *(7th ed.) (p. 709). Elsevier.*

phosphate. Glucose-1-phosphate is the substrate for glycogen synthase which catalyzes the incorporation of glucose into glycogen. Glycogen synthase is also a substrate for protein kinase A and is inactivated when phosphorylated. Thus by increasing the formation of cAMP, glucagon simultaneously promotes glycogen breakdown and prevents recycling of glucose to glycogen. cAMP–dependent phosphorylation of enzymes that regulate the glycolytic pathway at the level of phosphofructokinase and acetyl coenzyme A (CoA) carboxylase (see later) minimizes consumption of glucose-6-phosphate by the hepatocyte itself, leaving dephosphorylation and delivery into the blood as the major pathway open to newly depolymerized glucose.

Gluconeogenesis

Precursors of glucose enter the gluconeogenic pathway as 3- or 4-carbon compounds. Glucagon directs their conversion to glucose by accelerating their condensation to fructose phosphate while simultaneously blocking their escape from the gluconeogenic pathway (cycles III and IV in Fig. 7.7). cAMP controls production of a potent allosteric regulator of metabolism called fructose-2,6-bisphosphate. This compound, when present even in tiny amounts, activates phosphofructokinase and inhibits fructose-1,6-bisphosphatase, thereby directing flow of substrate toward glucose breakdown rather than glucose formation (Fig. 7.13).

Fructose-2,6-bisphosphate, which should not be confused with fructose-1,6-bisphosphate, is formed from fructose-6-phosphate by the action of an unusual bifunctional enzyme that catalyzes either phosphorylation of fructose-6-phosphate to fructose-2,6-bisphosphate or dephosphorylation of fructose-2,6-bisphosphate to fructose-6-phosphate, depending on its own state of phosphorylation. This enzyme is a substrate for protein kinase A and behaves as a phosphatase when it is phosphorylated. Its activity in the presence of cAMP rapidly depletes the hepatocyte of fructose-2,6-bisphosphate, and substrate therefore flows toward glucose production.

The other important regulatory step in gluconeogenesis is phosphorylation and dephosphorylation of pyruvate (cycle IV in Fig. 7.7). It is here that 3- and 4-carbon fragments enter or escape from the gluconeogenic pathway. The cytosolic enzyme that catalyzes dephosphorylation of phosphoenol pyruvate (PEP) was inappropriately named pyruvate kinase before it was recognized that direct phosphorylation of pyruvate does not occur under physiological conditions, and that this enzyme acts only in the direction of dephosphorylation (Fig. 7.14).

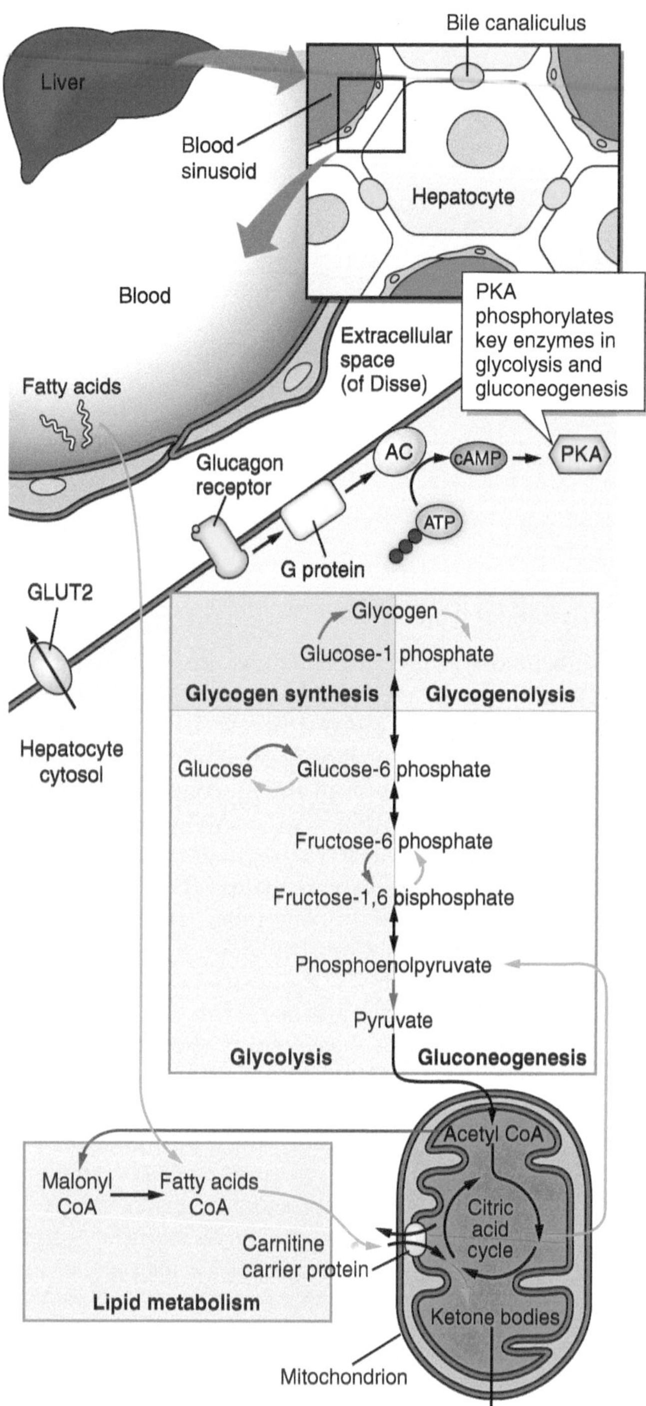

FIGURE 7.10 The effect of glucagon on the liver cell (hepatocyte). The liver is the main target for glucagon. Source: *Redrawn from Figure 51-12 from Barrett E. J. (2017). Chapter 51: The endocrine pancreas. In W. F. Boron, & E. L. Boulpaep (Eds.),* Medical physiology *(3rd ed.) (p. 1052). Elsevier.*

Pyruvate kinase is another substrate for protein kinase A and is powerfully inhibited when phosphorylated, but the inhibition can be overcome allosterically by fructose-6-bisphosphate. Thus activation of protein kinase A has the duel effect of decreasing pyruvate kinase activity directly and of decreasing the abundance of its activator, fructose-1,6-bisphosphate, by reactions shown in Fig. 7.9. Inhibiting pyruvate kinase may be the single most important effect of glucagon on the gluconeogenic pathway. On a longer time scale, glucagon inhibits the synthesis of pyruvate kinase. Phosphorylation of pyruvate requires a complex series of reactions in which pyruvate must first enter mitochondria where it is carboxylated to form oxaloacetate.

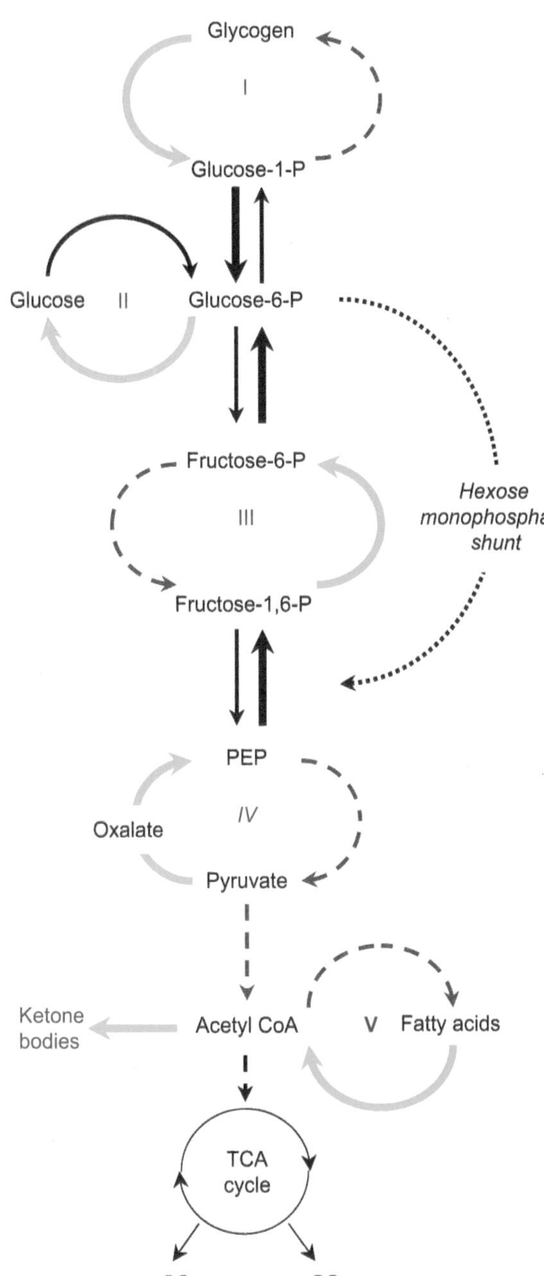

FIGURE 7.11 Biochemical pathways of glucose metabolism in hepatocytes. Reactions that are accelerated in the presence of glucagon are shown in green. Broken red arrows indicate reactions that are inhibited by protein kinase A catalyzed phosphorylation. The hexose-monophosphate shunt is indirectly inhibited. Roman numerals indicate substrate cycles.

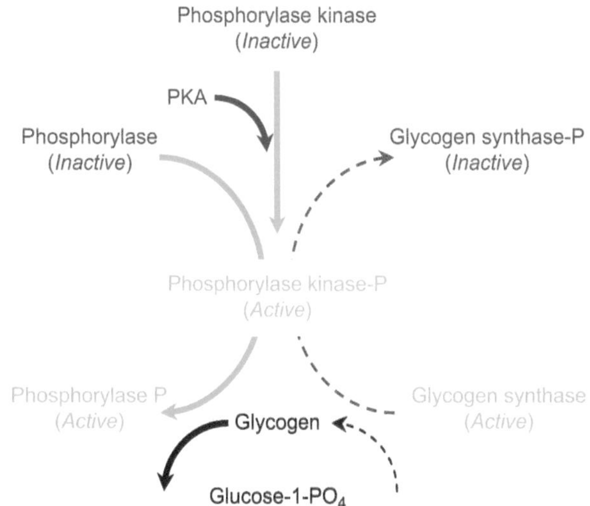

FIGURE 7.12 Role of protein kinase A (cyclic AMP-dependent protein kinase) in glycogen metabolism.

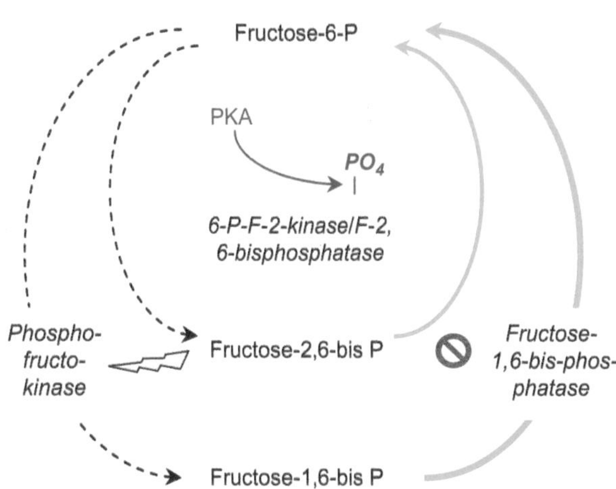

FIGURE 7.13 Regulation of fructose-1,6-bisphosphate metabolism by protein kinase A (cyclic AMP–dependent protein kinase). Formation of fructose-1,6-bis phosphate is accelerated by the metabolite fructose-2,6-bisphosphate, which stimulates phosphofructokinase and inhibits fructose-1,6-phosphatase. Protein kinase A lowers the concentration of fructose-2,6-bisphosphate by catalyzing phosphorylation of the bifunctional enzyme 6 phosphofructose-2 kinase/fructose-2,6-bisphosphatase, which promotes its phosphatase activity. The resulting decrease in fructose-2,6-bisphosphate concentration removes the stimulation of phosphofructokinase, and the inhibition of fructose-1,6-phosphatase, and drives substrate flow from fructose-1,6-bisphosphate to fructose-1-phosphate.

Entry of pyruvate across the mitochondrial membrane is accelerated by glucagon, but the mechanism for this effect is not known. Oxaloacetate is converted to cytosolic PEP by the catalytic activity of PEP carboxykinase. Synthesis of this enzyme is accelerated by increased cAMP.

Lipogenesis and ketogenesis

The alternate fate of pyruvate in mitochondria is decarboxylation to form acetyl CoA (Fig. 7.15).

This 2-carbon acetyl unit is the building block of fatty acids and eventually finds its way back to the cytosol where fatty acid synthesis (lipogenesis) takes place.

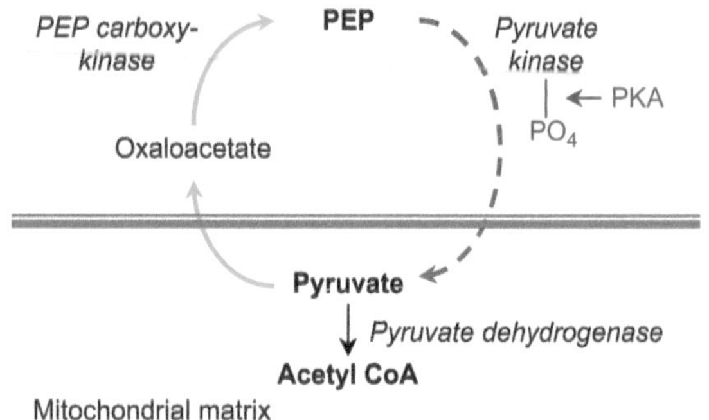

FIGURE 7.14 Regulation of *PEP* formation by PKA (cyclic AMP–dependent protein kinase). PKA catalyzes the phosphorylation and, hence, inactivation of *pyruvate kinase* whose activity limits the conversion of PEP to pyruvate. *PEP*, Phosphoenol pyruvate; *PKA*, protein kinase A.

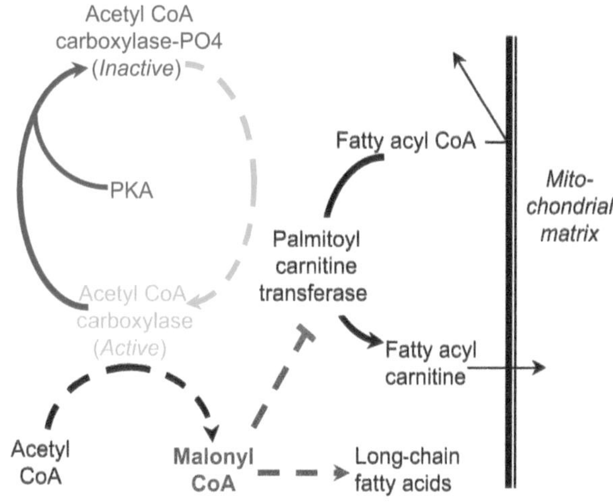

FIGURE 7.15 *Protein kinase A* (cyclic AMP–dependent protein kinase) indirectly stimulates ketogenesis by decreasing the formation of *malonyl CoA*, thus removing a restriction on accessibility of fatty acids to intramitochondrial oxidative enzymes. *CoA*, Coenzyme A.

Lipogenesis is the principal competitor of gluconeogenesis for 3-carbon precursors. The first committed step in fatty acid synthesis is the carboxylation of acetyl CoA to form malonyl CoA. Acetyl CoA carboxylase, the enzyme that catalyzes this reaction, is yet another substrate for protein kinase A and is powerfully inhibited when phosphorylated. Inhibition of fatty acid synthesis not only preserves substrate for gluconeogenesis but also prevents oxidation of glucose by the hexose monophosphate shunt pathway (Fig. 7.11). NADP, which is required for shunt activity, is reduced in the initial reactions of this pathway and can be regenerated only by transferring protons to the elongating fatty acid chain.

Fatty acid synthesis and oxidation constitute another substrate cycle and another regulatory site for cAMP action. The same reaction that inhibits fatty acid synthesis promotes fatty acid oxidation and consequently ketogenesis (ketone body formation) (Fig. 7.11). Long-chain fatty acid molecules that reach the liver can be either oxidized or esterified and exported to adipose tissue as the triacylglycerol. To be esterified, fatty acids must remain in the cytosol, and to be oxidized they must enter the mitochondria. Long-chain fatty acids can cross the mitochondrial membrane only when linked to carnitine. Carnitine acyltransferase, the enzyme that catalyzes this linkage, is powerfully inhibited by malonyl CoA.

Malonyl CoA thus has two distinct and crucial roles: it is both an indispensable metabolite for fatty acid synthesis and an allosteric regulator of the enzyme that permits fatty acids to be oxidized. When hepatic concentrations of malonyl CoA are high, coincident with fatty acid synthesis, fatty acid oxidation is inhibited. Conversely, when its concentration is low, fatty acids readily enter mitochondria and are oxidized to acetyl CoA. Because long-chain fatty acids typically contain 16 and 18 carbons, each molecule that is oxidized yields eight or nine molecules of acetyl CoA. The ketone bodies, β-hydroxybutyrate and acetoacetate, are formed from condensation of two molecules of acetyl CoA and the subsequent removal of the CoA moiety.

By blocking the formation of malonyl CoA, glucagon sets the stage for ketogenesis, but the actual rate of ketone production is determined by the abundance of long-chain fatty acids that are available for oxidation. Most fatty acids oxidized in liver are derived from the plasma free fatty acids (FFA) released from adipose tissue. In addition, glucagon, through its stimulation of cAMP production, may also activate a lipase in liver and thereby make fatty acids available from the breakdown of hepatic triacylglycerols. The metabolic effects of glucagon are summarized in Table 7.2.

Ureagenesis

Whenever carbon chains of amino acids are used as substrate for gluconeogenesis, amino groups must be disposed of in the form of urea, which thus becomes a by-product of gluconeogenesis. By promoting gluconeogenesis, therefore, glucagon also increases the formation of urea (ureagenesis). Carbon skeletons of most amino acids can be converted to glucose, but because of peculiarities of peripheral metabolism alanine is quantitatively the most important glucogenic amino acid. By accelerating conversion of pyruvate to glucose (see earlier), glucagon indirectly accelerates transamination of alanine to pyruvate. Glucagon also accelerates ureagenesis by increasing transport of amino acids across hepatocyte plasma membranes by an action that requires synthesis of new RNA and protein. In

TABLE 7.2 The effect of glucagon on glucose, fat, ketone, and protein metabolism.

Glucagon effect on glucose metabolism
Stimulation of liver glycogenolysis
Increase of gluconeogenesis
Glucagon effect on fat metabolism
Stimulation of lipolysis
Enhancement of hepatic oxidation of fatty acids
Glucagon effect on ketone body metabolism
Stimulation of ketone body formation
Glucagon effect on protein metabolism
Stimulation of amino acid uptake by the liver providing substrate for gluconeogenesis (ureagenesis)

addition, glucagon also promotes the synthesis of some urea cycle enzymes. The metabolic effects of glucagon are summarized in Table 7.2.

Regulation of glucagon secretion

The concentration of glucose in blood is the most important determinant of glucagon secretion in normal individuals. When the plasma glucose concentration exceeds 200 mg/dL, glucagon secretion is maximally inhibited. Inhibitory effects of glucose are proportionately less at lower concentrations and disappear when its concentration falls below 50 mg/dL. Except immediately after a meal rich in carbohydrate, the blood glucose concentration remains constant at around 90 mg/dL. This set point for glucose concentration thus falls well within the range over which glucagon secretion is regulated, so alpha cells can respond to fluctuations in blood glucose with either an increase or a decrease in glucagon output. It is possible that alpha cells directly sense glucose concentrations, but molecular mechanisms conferring such monitoring ability await discovery. Alternatively, changes in glucagon secretion may be controlled by insulin released from adjacent beta cells, whose well-documented capacity to monitor blood glucose concentrations is discussed later. Insulin inhibits glucagon secretion and is required for expression of inhibitory effects of glucose. A precipitous decline in insulin secretion in response to hypoglycemia may trigger glucagon release. In persons suffering from insulin deficiency (see later), glucagon secretion is deranged and may be brisk despite high blood glucose concentrations or may fail to increase in response to hypoglycemia. Somatostatin, GLP-1 (see Chapter 6: Hormones of the Gastrointestinal

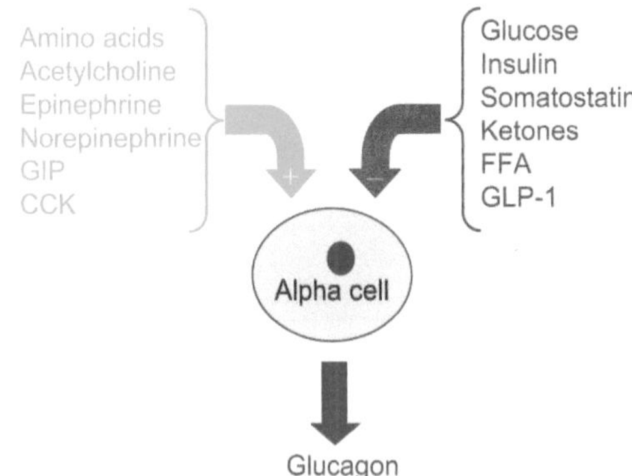

FIGURE 7.16 Stimulatory and inhibitory signals for glucagon secretion.

Tract), and FFA also exert inhibitory influences on glucagon secretion (Fig. 7.16).

Hypoglycemia is detected not only at the level of the islet, but this life-threatening circumstance also is detected by glucose-sensing neurons in the hypothalamus, which alert autonomic centers to activate both sympathetic and parasympathetic responses. Parasympathetic nerve endings within the islets release their neurotransmitters, acetylcholine and VIP (vasoactive intestinal peptide) and perhaps PACAP (pituitary adenylate cyclase activating peptide), and norepinephrine and NPY (neuropeptide Y) are released from sympathetic nerve fibers. These peptides are described in Chapter 6, Hormones of the Gastrointestinal Tract. Alpha cells express receptors for all these neurotransmitters and increase their secretion of glucagon in response to both parasympathetic and sympathetic stimulation. The sympathetic response to hypoglycemia also stimulates the adrenal medulla to secrete epinephrine and norepinephrine (see Chapter 4: The Adrenal Glands). These adrenomedullary hormones not only reinforce the glycogenolytic actions of glucagon on the liver but also further stimulate alpha cells to secrete glucagon.

Glucagon secretion also is evoked by a meal rich in amino acids. Alpha cells may respond directly to increased blood levels of certain amino acids, particularly arginine, which also increases insulin secretion. In addition, digestion of protein-rich foods triggers the release of cholecystokinin (CCK) and GIP (glucose-dependent insulinotropic peptide) from cells in the duodenal mucosa (see Chapter 6: Hormones of the Gastrointestinal Tract). CCK is a secretagogue for islet hormones as well as pancreatic enzymes and GIP may stimulate secretion of glucagon as well as insulin. Both of these gastrointestinal hormones alert alpha cells to an impending influx of amino acids. The resulting increased secretion of glucagon not only prepares the liver to dispose of excess amino acids by gluconeogenesis but also signals the liver to release glucose and thus counteracts the potentially hypoglycemic effects of insulin, whose secretion is simultaneously increased by amino acids (see later).

Insulin

Biosynthesis, secretion, and metabolism

Insulin is composed of two unbranched peptide chains joined together by two disulfide bridges (Fig. 7.17).

The single gene that encodes the 110-amino acid preproinsulin molecule consists of three exons and two introns and is located on chromosome 11. After removal of the leader sequence in the endoplasmic reticulum, the proinsulin molecule undergoes folding and disulfide bond formation before it is transferred to the Golgi apparatus where it is packaged in secretory granules and stored complexed with zinc. Processing of the single-chain proinsulin molecule to form the two-chained mature insulin takes place in the secretory granules where a 31-residue peptide, called the connecting peptide (C peptide), is excised by stepwise actions of two endopeptidase enzymes called prohormone convertases 2 and 3. The C peptide therefore accumulates within granules in equimolar amounts with insulin. When insulin is secreted, the entire contents of secretory vesicles are disgorged into extracellular fluid (Fig. 7.18).

Consequently, the C peptide and any remaining proinsulin and processing intermediates enter the circulation along with insulin. When secretion is rapid, proinsulin may comprise as much as 20% of the circulating peptides detected by insulin antibodies, but it contributes little biological activity. Although several biological actions of the C peptide have been described, no physiological role for the C peptide has yet been established.

The insulin storage granule contains a variety of proteins that are also released whenever insulin is secreted. Most of these proteins are thought to maintain optimal conditions for storage and processing of insulin, but some may also have biological activity. One such protein, called amylin, has a synergistic effect to the action of insulin in various tissues. In addition, the amylin causes decreased gastric emptying, inhibits the digestive secretions, and, as a result, reduces the food intake. The precursor molecule proamylin may contribute to the amyloid that accumulates in and around beta cells in states of insulin hypersecretion and may contribute to islet pathology.

Insulin is cleared rapidly from the circulation with a half-life of 4–6 minutes. The first step in insulin degradation is receptor-mediated internalization by an endosomic mechanism. Degradation may take place following fusion of endosomes with lysosomes. The liver is the principal site of insulin degradation and inactivates from 30% to 70% of the insulin that reaches it in hepatic portal blood. Insulin degradation in the

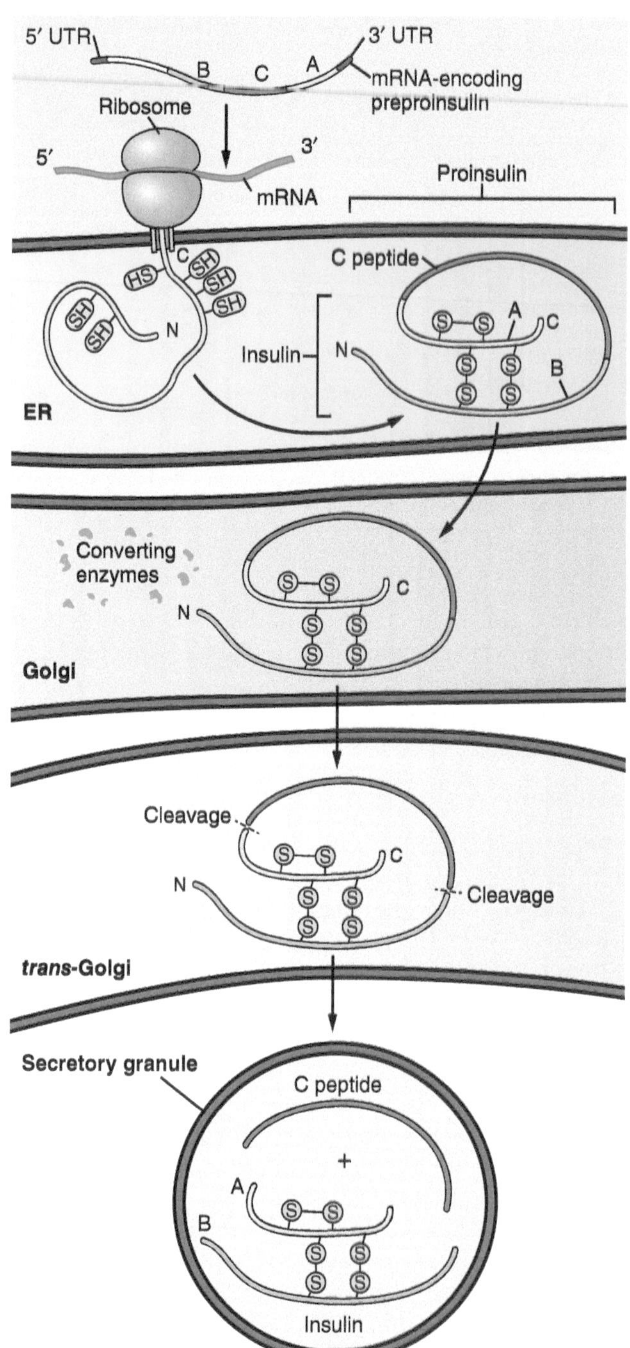

FIGURE 7.17 Synthesis and processing of the insulin molecule. UTR, 5′untranslated region which refers to the gray area. Source: *Redrawn from Figure 51-2 from Barrett E. J. (2017). Chapter 51: The endocrine pancreas. In W. F. Boron, & E. L. Boulpaep (Eds.).* Medical physiology *(3rd ed.) (p. 1037). Elsevier, 2017.*

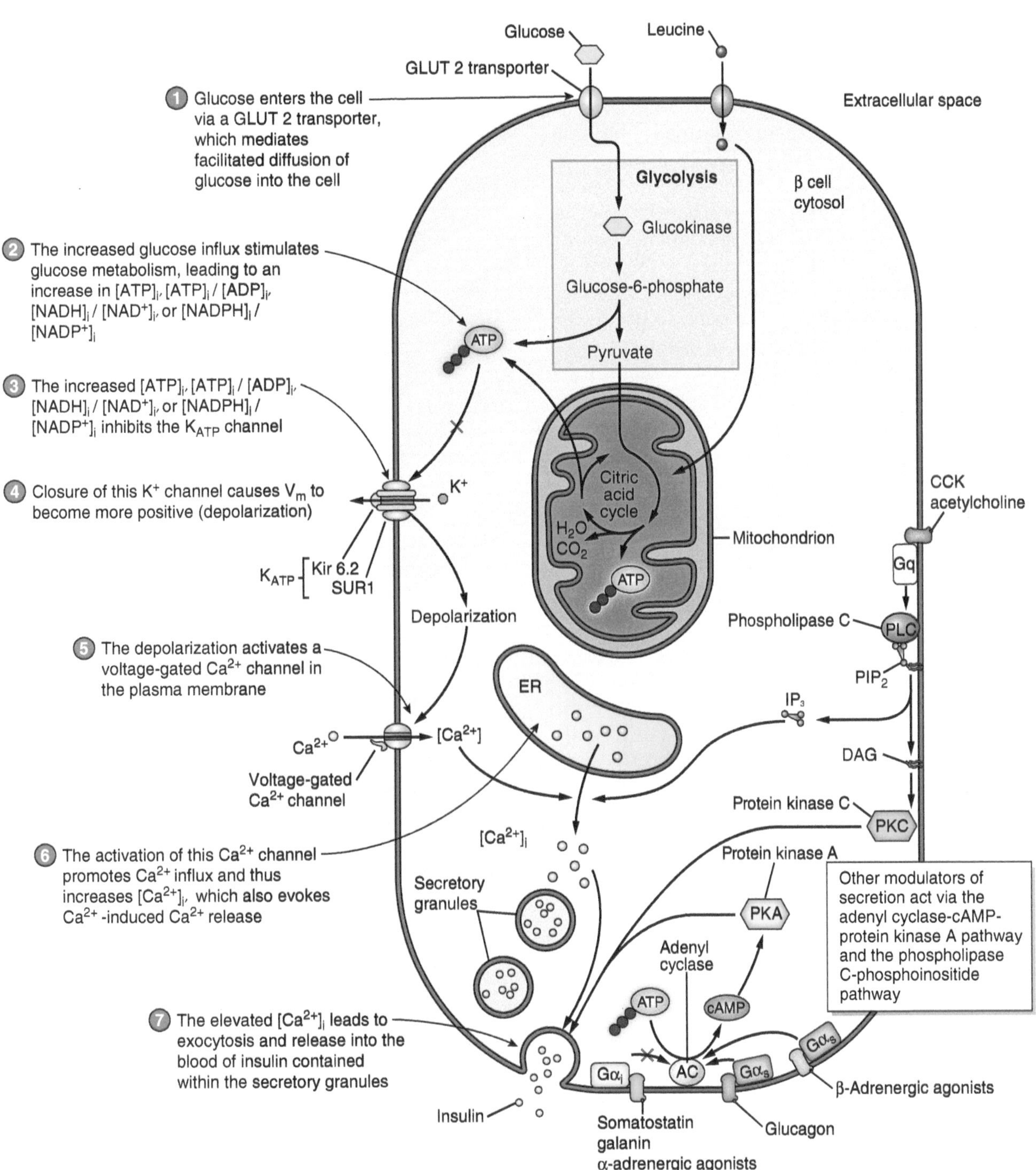

FIGURE 7.18 A detailed summary of the synthesis of insulin. Source: *Redrawn from Figure 51.4 from Barrett E. J. (2017). Chapter 51: The endocrine pancreas. In* Medical Physiology *(3rd ed.) by Walter F. Boron and Emile L. Boulpaep. Elsevier, 2017, p. 1040.*

liver appears to be a regulated process governed by changes in availability of metabolic fuels and changing physiological circumstances. The liver may thus regulate the amount of insulin that enters the systemic circulation. The kidneys account for destruction of about half the circulating insulin following receptor-mediated uptake both from the glomerular filtrate and from postglomerular blood plasma. Normally, little or no insulin is found in urine. The remainder is degraded in muscle and other insulin-sensitive tissues throughout the body. Proinsulin has a half-life that is at least twice as long as insulin and is not converted to insulin outside the pancreas. The kidney is the principal site of degradation of proinsulin and the C peptide. Because little degradation of the C peptide occurs in the liver, its concentration in blood is useful for estimating the rate of insulin secretion and evaluation of beta cell function.

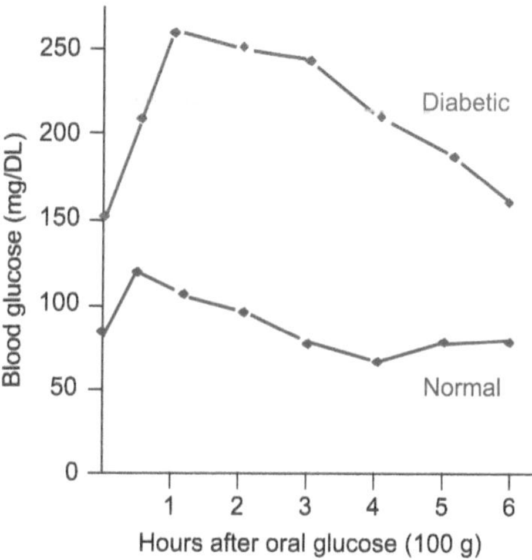

FIGURE 7.19 Idealized glucose tolerance tests in normal and diabetic subjects. Subjects are given a standardized solution of glucose to drink and blood samples are taken at the indicated times thereafter. An impairment of glucose disposition results in a greater than normal and prolonged increase in blood glucose concentration.

Physiological actions of Insulin

Effects of insulin deficiency

In many areas of endocrinology, basic insights into the physiological role of a hormone can be gained from examining the consequences of its absence. In such studies, secondary or tertiary effects may overshadow the primary cellular lesion but nevertheless ultimately broaden our understanding of cellular responses in the context of the whole organism. Insights into the physiology of insulin and the physiological processes it affects directly and indirectly were gained originally from clinical observations. Consideration of some of the classic signs of this disease therefore provides a good starting point for discussing the physiology of insulin.

Hyperglycemia

In the normal individual the concentration of glucose in blood is maintained at around 90 mg/dL of plasma (5 mM). Blood glucose in diabetics is higher, sometimes reaching levels of more than 1000 mg/dL. Diabetics have particular difficulty removing excess glucose from their blood. Normally, after ingestion of a meal rich in carbohydrate, excess glucose disappears rapidly from plasma, and there is only a small and transient increase in blood glucose. The diabetic, however, is intolerant of glucose, and the ability to remove it from plasma is severely impaired. Oral glucose tolerance tests, which assess the ability to dispose of a glucose load, are used diagnostically to evaluate existing or impending diabetic conditions. A standard load of glucose is given by mouth and the blood glucose concentrations are measured periodically over several hours. In normal subjects, blood glucose peak values do not rise above 180 mg/dL. In the diabetic or "prediabetic," blood glucose levels rise much higher and take a longer time to return to basal levels (Fig. 7.19).

Glycosuria

Normally, renal tubules have adequate capacity to transport and reabsorb all the glucose filtered at the glomeruli so that little or none escapes in the urine. When the serum glucose concentration rises above 180 mg/dL (10 mmol/L), the renal threshold for glucose is exceeded, which leads to increased urinary glucose excretion (glycosuria).

Polyuria

Polyuria is defined as excessive production of urine. Because more glucose is present in the glomerular filtrate than can be reabsorbed by proximal tubules, some remains in the tubular lumen and exerts an osmotic hindrance to water and salt reabsorption in this portion of the nephron, which normally reabsorbs about two-thirds of the glomerular filtrate. The abnormally high volume of fluid that remains cannot be reabsorbed by more distal portions of the nephrons, with the result that water excretion is increased (osmotic diuresis). Increased flow through the nephron increases urinary loss of sodium and potassium as well.

Polydipsia

Dehydration results from the copious flow of urine and stimulates thirst, a condition called polydipsia, or excessive drinking. The untreated diabetic is characteristically thirsty and consumes large volumes of water to compensate for water lost in urine. Polydipsia is often the first symptom that is noticed by the patient or parents of a diabetic child.

Polyphagia

By mechanisms that likely stem from insulin's role in regulating food intake (see Chapter 8: Hormonal Regulation of Fuel Metabolism), appetite is increased in what seems to be an effort to compensate for urinary loss of glucose. The condition is called polyphagia (excessive food consumption).

Weight loss

Despite increased appetite and food intake, however, insulin deficiency reduces all anabolic processes and accelerates catabolic processes. Accelerated protein degradation, particularly in muscle, provides substrate for gluconeogenesis. Insulin is the most potent antilipolytic hormone. Insulin deficiency increases the activity of hormone sensitive lipase (HSL), which causes lipolysis of the fat stores. FFA and glycerol are released into the circulation causing hyperlipidemia. The fatty acids are transported to the liver where they are oxidized. After oxidation, they can enter the ketogenic metabolic pathway to form ketone bodies (acetoacetate, β-hydroxybutyrate, and acetone). Ketones can be used as source of energy when glucose is not available. Acetoacetate and β-hydroxybutyrate are true acids and their accumulation in diabetic ketoacidosis leads to an anion gap metabolic acidosis.

Effects of insulin excess

The effect of insulin excess on glucose metabolism is hypoglycemia. Insulin lowers blood glucose in two ways: it increases uptake of glucose by muscle and adipose tissue and decreases the glucose output by the liver. There is no absolute blood glucose cutoff that should be used to define hypoglycemia. In patients with diabetes, hypoglycemia is defined as an episode of low blood sugar with or without symptoms that exposes the patient to harm (usually blood glucose <60–70 mg/dL). In individuals without diabetes, it is best to use Whipple's triad to define hypoglycemia: (1) symptoms consistent with hypoglycemia; (2) documented low plasma glucose when symptoms are present; and (3) alleviation of symptoms by administering glucose or glucagon. Hypoglycemia causes neurogenic and neuroglycopenic symptoms. The neurogenic symptoms include tremor, palpitations, anxiety (adrenergic symptoms), sweating, hunger, and paresthesias (cholinergic symptoms). The neuroglycopenic symptoms are cognitive impairment, behavioral and motor abnormalities, loss of consciousness, seizure, and coma.

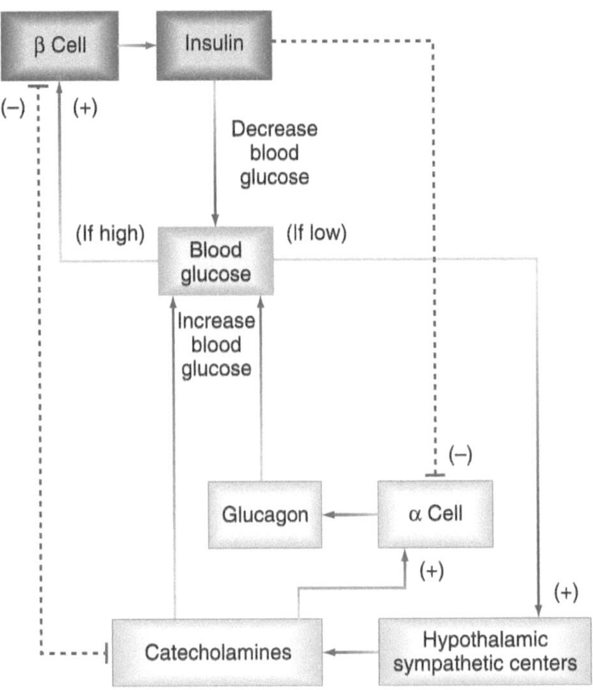

FIGURE 7.20 The effect of insulin on blood glucose and the counterregulatory factors glucagon and catecholamines (norepinephrine and epinephrine) that increase blood glucose. Source: *From Figure 39.11 from Koeppen B. M., & Stanton B. A. (2018).* Berne and levy physiology *(7th ed.) (p. 709). Elsevier.*

Effects on glucose metabolism

Insulin affects glucose production and glucose utilization (Fig. 7.20).

Insulin acts directly to limit hepatic glucose output by inhibiting the glycogenolytic enzyme glycogen phosphorylase. Insulin also acts indirectly to suppress hepatic gluconeogenesis through several mechanisms, including decrease in the flow of gluconeogenic precursors and FFA to the liver (Fig. 7.21), inhibition of glucagon secretion, in part by direct inhibition of the glucagon gene in the pancreatic alpha cells, and change in neural input to the liver.

Insulin stimulates glucose uptake by skeletal muscle and fat. In these tissues, glucose transport across cell membranes is mediated by glucose transporter 4 (GLUT 4) which is located in the cytoplasm. Insulin signal causes translocation of GLUT 4 to the cell membrane, where it facilitates glucose entry into these tissues. When blood glucose is normal, most insulin-mediated glucose uptake occurs in muscle and less in the adipose tissue. But adipose tissue can indirectly promote glucose utilization via insulin-mediated inhibition of lipolysis. This occurs through the mechanism of competing substrates. When the availability of FFA as a fuel source is low, glucose uptake and metabolism

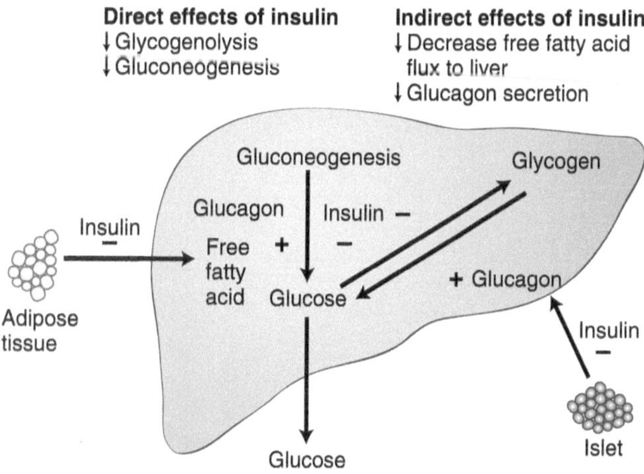

FIGURE 7.21 Effect of insulin on hepatic glucose production. Insulin suppresses hepatic glucose production directly by inhibiting gluconeogenesis and the breakdown of glycogen to glucose and indirectly by inhibiting lipolysis by adipose tissue and inhibiting the production of glucagon by the islet alpha cells. Source: *From Figure 31-5 in Polonsky K. S., & Burant C. F. (2016). Chapter 31: Type 2 diabetes mellitus. In S. Melmed, K. S. Polonsky, P. R. Larsen, & H. M. Kronenberg (Eds.),* Williams textbook of endocrinology *(13th ed.) (p. 1396). Elsevier.*

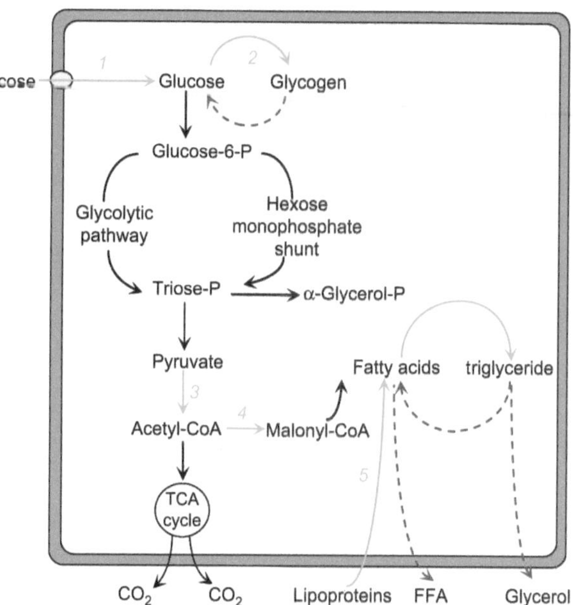

FIGURE 7.22 Carbohydrate and lipid metabolism in adipose tissue. Reactions enhanced by insulin (*green arrows*) are as follows: (1) transport of glucose into adipose cell; (2) conversion of excess glucose to glycogen; (3) decarboxylation of pyruvate; (4) initiation of fatty acid synthesis; and (5) uptake of fatty acids from circulating lipoproteins. Breakdown of triacylglycerols is inhibited by insulin (*dashed red arrows*). Esterification of fatty acids to triacylglycerols follows from availability of α-glycerol phosphate.

in the muscle is increased. Insulin also promotes glucose disposal within cells through its effects on glycogen synthesis and glucose breakdown (glycolysis). Insulin increases the activity of glycogen synthase in several tissues, including adipose tissue, muscle, and liver. This action of insulin does not result in net glycogen synthesis unless glycogen phosphorylase is strongly inhibited. Insulin stimulates the rate of glycolysis in skeletal muscle and adipose tissue by increasing the activity of two key enzymes in the glycolytic pathway, hexokinase, and 6-phosphofructokinase.

Effects on adipose tissue

Storage of fat in adipose tissue depends on multiple insulin-sensitive reactions, including: (1) synthesis of long-chain fatty acids from glucose; (2) synthesis of triacylglycerols from fatty acids and glycerol (esterification); (3) breakdown of triacylglycerols to release glycerol and long-chain fatty acids (lipolysis); and (4) uptake of fatty acids from the lipoproteins of blood. The relevant biochemical pathways are shown in Fig. 7.22.

Lipolysis and esterification are central events in the physiology of the adipocyte. Fat, in the form of triacylglycerols, is stored in a single large droplet coated by a protein called perilipin. The rate of lipolysis depends largely, but not exclusively, on the activity of an enzyme called HSL that catalyzes the breakdown of triacylglycerols into fatty acids and glycerol. In the absence of stimulation, lipolysis proceeds at a low basal rate, while HSL resides in the cytoplasm and is denied access to the lipid droplet by its coating of perilipin. In response to stimulation, cAMP is formed and activates protein kinase A, which catalyzes phosphorylation of both HSL and perilipin. The resulting association of activated HSL with the lipid droplet dramatically increases the breakdown of triacylglycerols to fatty acids that can either escape from the adipocyte and become the FFA of blood or be reesterified to triacylglycerol.

Fatty acid esterification requires a source of glycerol that is phosphorylated in its α-carbon; free glycerol cannot be used. Because adipose tissue lacks the enzyme α-glycerol kinase, all of the free glycerol that is produced by lipolysis escapes into the blood. The α-glycerol phosphate used for esterification of fatty acids is derived primarily from phosphorylated 3-carbon intermediates formed from oxidation of glucose. However, when glucose is in short supply, as in fasting, some α-glycerol phosphates can also be formed from plasma lactate or alanine in a process of glyceroneogenesis that depends on the availability of the enzyme PEP carboxykinase.

As its name implies, HSL is activated by lipolytic hormones that stimulate the formation of cAMP and thereby promote its phosphorylation and the phosphorylation of perilipin by protein kinase A. Insulin accelerates the degradation of cAMP by activating the enzyme cAMP phosphodiesterase and thus interferes with activation of lipolysis. Simultaneously, insulin increases the rate of fatty acid esterification by accelerating glucose oxidation, which increases the availability of α-glycerol phosphate. The net result of these actions is preservation of triacylglycerol stores at the expense of plasma FFA, whose concentration in blood plasma promptly falls. Decreases in FFA concentrations are seen with doses of insulin that are too low to affect blood glucose and appear to be the most sensitive response to insulin.

Because glucose does not readily diffuse across the plasma membrane, its entry into adipocytes and most other cells depends on carrier-mediated transport. Insulin increases cellular uptake and metabolism of glucose by accelerating transmembrane transport of glucose and structurally related sugars. This process starts with the insulin receptor that has a cytosolic tyrosine kinase domain (Fig. 7.23).

This action depends upon the availability of glucose transporters in the plasma membrane. Glucose transporters (abbreviated GLUT) are large proteins that weave in and out of the membrane 12 times to form stereospecific channels through which glucose can diffuse down its concentration gradient Fig. 7.24).

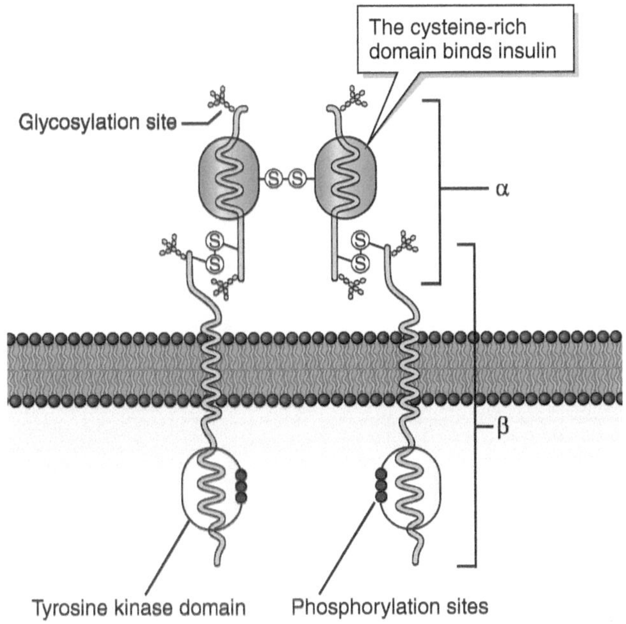

FIGURE 7.23 Insulin combines with its receptor on the cell membrane of a typical cell. This activates tyrosine kinase which sets off a series of reactions (see Fig. 7.24) which ends up inserting one of the GLUT transporters into the cell membrane. Glucose is transported on the GLUT into the cell. Source: *Redrawn from Figure 51.5 from Barrett E. J. (2017). Chapter 51: The endocrine pancreas. In W. F. Boron, & E. L. Boulpaep (Eds.)* Medical physiology *(3rd ed.) (p. 1042). Elsevier.*

There are at least five isoforms of GLUT expressed in various cell types. The liver has GLUT 2 (Fig. 7.25).

In addition to GLUT 1, which is present in the plasma membrane of most cells, insulin-sensitive cells such as adipocytes contain pools of intracellular membranous vesicles that are rich in GLUT 4 (Fig. 7.26).

Insulin increases the number of glucose transporters on the adipocyte surface by stimulating the translocation of GLUT 4–containing vesicles toward the cell surface and fusion of their membranes with the adipocyte plasma membrane (Fig. 7.26).

Insulin accelerates synthesis of fatty acids by increasing the uptake of glucose and by activating at least two enzymes that direct the flow of glucose carbons into fatty acids. Insulin increases conversion of pyruvate to acetyl CoA, which provides the building blocks for long-chain fatty acid synthesis and stimulates carboxylation of acetyl CoA to malonyl CoA, which is the initial and rate-determining reaction in fatty acid synthesis. In humans, adipose tissue is not an important site of fatty acid synthesis, particularly in Western cultures where the diet is rich in fat. Fat stored in adipose tissue is derived mainly from dietary fat and tri-glycerides synthesized in the liver. Fat destined for storage reaches adipose tissue in the form of low density lipoproteins and chylomicrons. Uptake of fat from lipoproteins depends on cleavage of ester bonds in triacylglycerols by the enzyme lipoprotein lipase to release fatty acids. Lipoprotein lipase is synthesized and secreted by adipocytes and adheres to the endothelium of adjacent capillaries. Insulin promotes synthesis of lipoprotein lipase and thus facilitates the transfer of fatty acids from lipoproteins to triacylglycerol storage droplets in adipocytes.

Effects on muscle

Insulin increases uptake of glucose by muscle and directs its intracellular metabolism toward the formation of glycogen (Fig. 7.27).

Because muscle comprises nearly 50% of body mass, uptake by muscle accounts for the majority of the glucose that disappears from blood after injection of insulin. As in adipocytes, glucose utilization in muscle is limited by permeability of the plasma membrane. Insulin accelerates entry of glucose into muscle by mobilizing GLUT 4–containing vesicles by the same mechanism that is operative in adipocytes. Metabolism of glucose begins with conversion to glucose-6-phosphate catalyzed by either of the two isoforms of the enzyme hexokinase that are present in muscle. Insulin not only increases the synthesis of hexokinase II, but it also appears to enhance the efficiency of hexokinase II activity by promoting its association with the outer membrane of mitochondria, which optimizes its access to ATP. In the basal state, glucose is

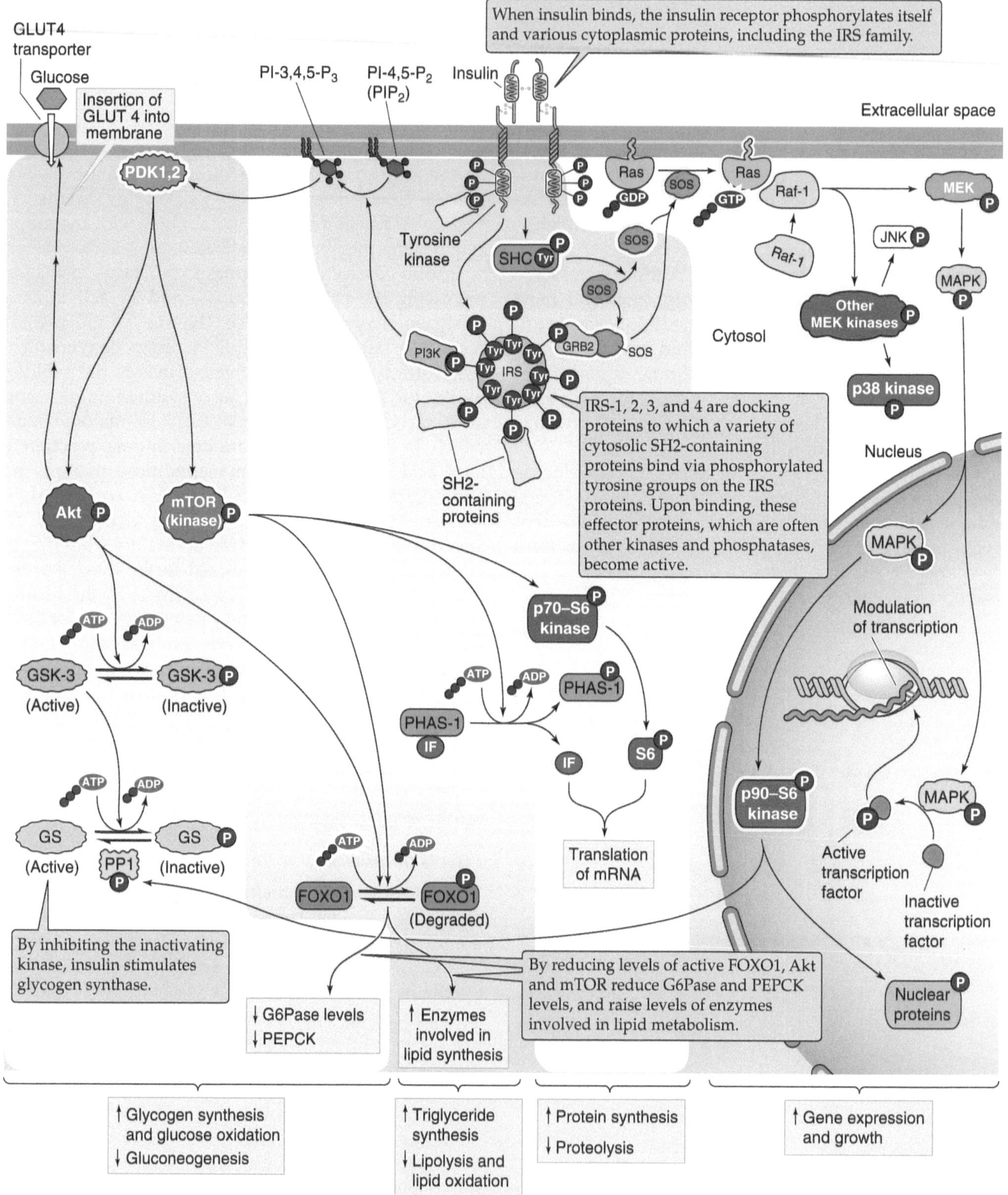

FIGURE 7.24 Glucose uptake by a cell that has been activated by insulin. The tyrosine kinase in the insulin receptor sets off a chain reaction that results in GLUT 4 being incorporated into the cell membrane. Glucose can then slide down the concentration gradient into the cell via GLUT 4 (upper left). *GS*, Glycogen synthetase; *GSK-3*, glycogen synthetase kinase 3; *IF*, initiation factor; *PDK*, phosphatidylinositol-dependent kinase; *IRS*, insulin-receptor substrates; *SHC*, Src homology C terminus. Source: *From Figure 51.6 from Barrett E. J. (2017). Chapter 51: The endocrine pancreas. In W. F. Boron, & E. L. Boulpaep (Eds.)* Medical physiology *(3rd ed.) (p. 1043). Elsevier.*

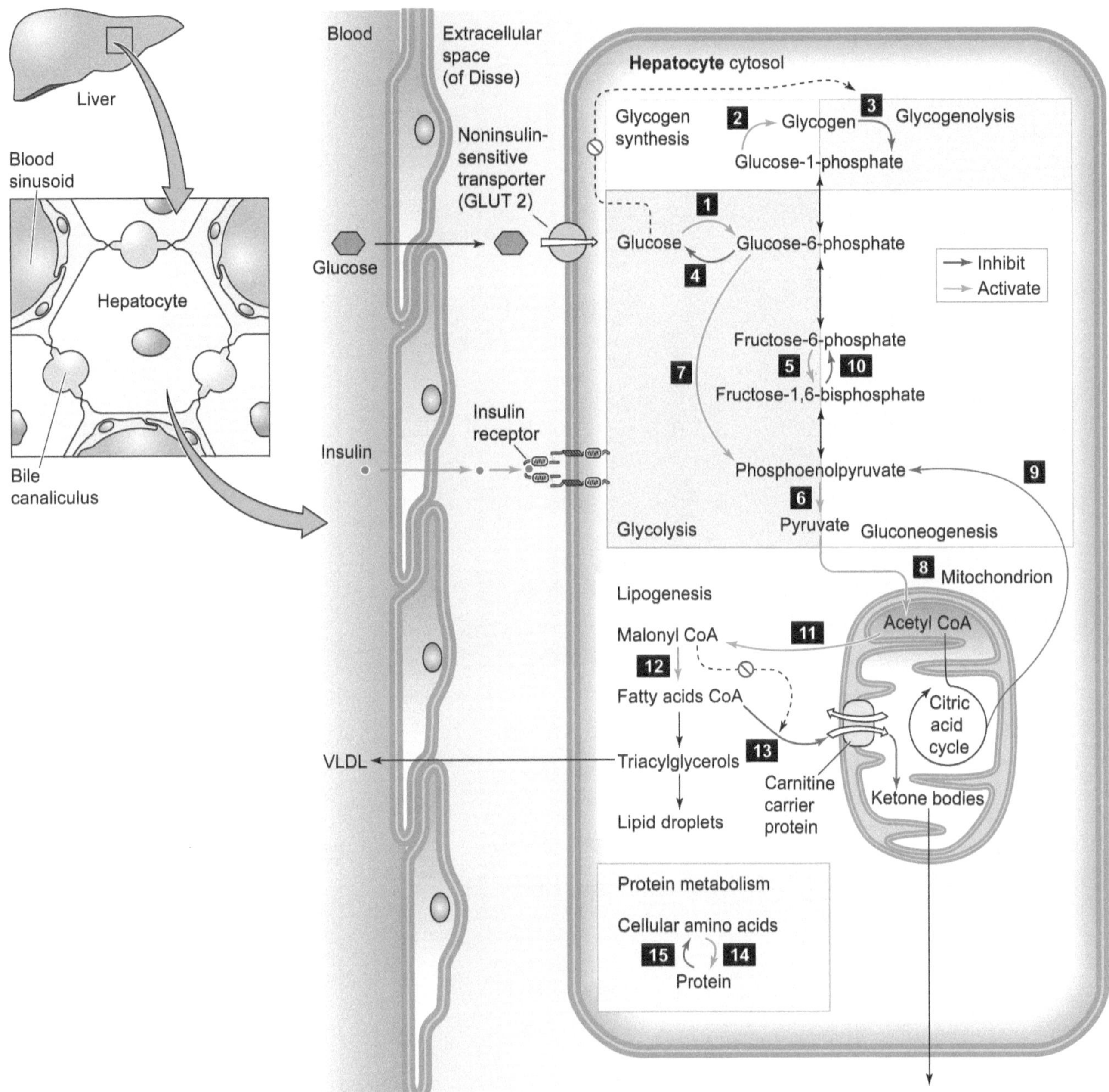

FIGURE 7.25 The effect of insulin on a liver cell. Note that GLUT 2 is the transporter in liver. Insulin has a direct effect on the liver as it receives blood directly from the pancreas via the hepatic portal system. Source: *From Figure 51-8 Barrett E. J. (2017). Chapter 51: The endocrine pancreas. In W. F. Boron, & E. L. Boulpaep (Eds.)* Medical physiology *(3rd ed.) (p. 1046). Elsevier.*

phosphorylated almost as rapidly as it enters the cell, and hence the intracellular concentration of free glucose is only about one-tenth to one-third that of extracellular fluid. Glucose-6-P is an allosteric inhibitor of hexokinase and an allosteric activator of glycogen synthase. Stimulation of glycogen synthesis by insulin and glucose-6-phosphate protects hexokinase from the inhibitory effect of glucose-6-phosphate when entry of glucose into the muscle cell is rapid. Glycogen synthase activity is low when the enzyme is phosphorylated and increased when it is dephosphorylated. The degree of phosphorylation of glycogen synthase is determined by the balance of kinase and phosphatase activities. Insulin shifts the balance in favor of dephosphorylation in part by inhibiting the enzyme, glycogen synthase kinase 3 (GSK-3), and in part by activating a phosphatase. Dephosphorylation of glycogen synthase not only increases its activity directly but also increases its responsiveness to stimulation by its substrate, glucose-6-P. Hence, the powerful effects of insulin on muscle

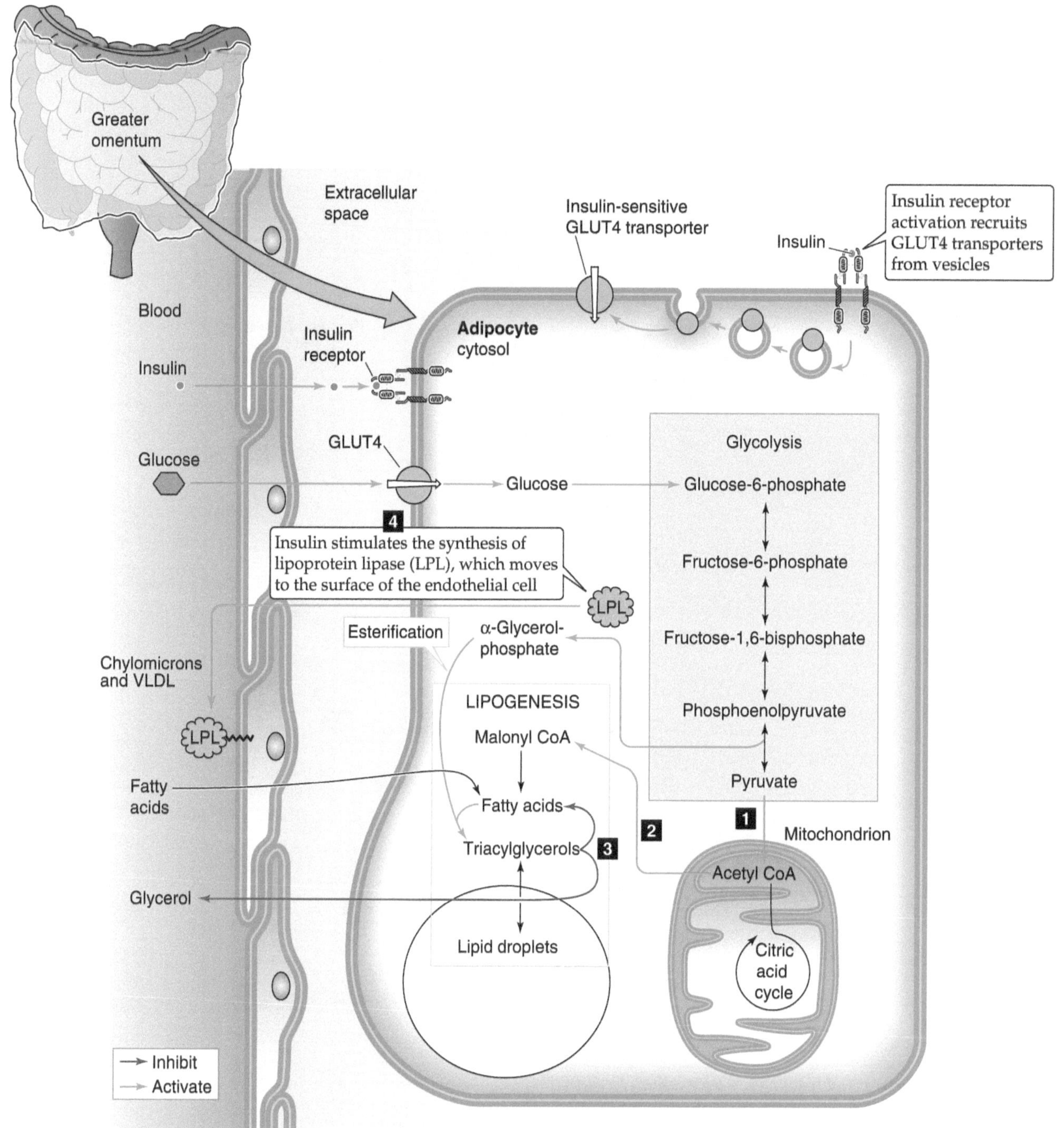

FIGURE 7.26 Effect of insulin on adipocytes, here being shown located in the greater omentum, the apron-like structure that covers the abdominal surface. Source: *From Figure 51-10 Barrett E. J. (2017). Chapter 51: The endocrine pancreas. In W. F. Boron, & E. L. Boulpaep (Eds.)* Medical physiology *(3rd ed.) (p. 1049). Elsevier.*

glycogen synthesis are achieved by the complementary effects of increased glucose transport, increased glucose phosphorylation, and increased glycogen synthase activity.

The alternative fate of glucose-6-P, metabolism to pyruvate in the glycolytic pathway, is also increased by insulin. Access to the glycolytic pathway is guarded by phosphofructokinase, whose activity is precisely regulated by a combination of allosteric effectors, including ATP, ADP, and fructose-2,6-bisphosphate. This complex enzyme behaves differently in intact cells and in the broken cell preparations typically used by biochemists to study enzyme regulation. Because conflicting findings have been obtained under a variety of

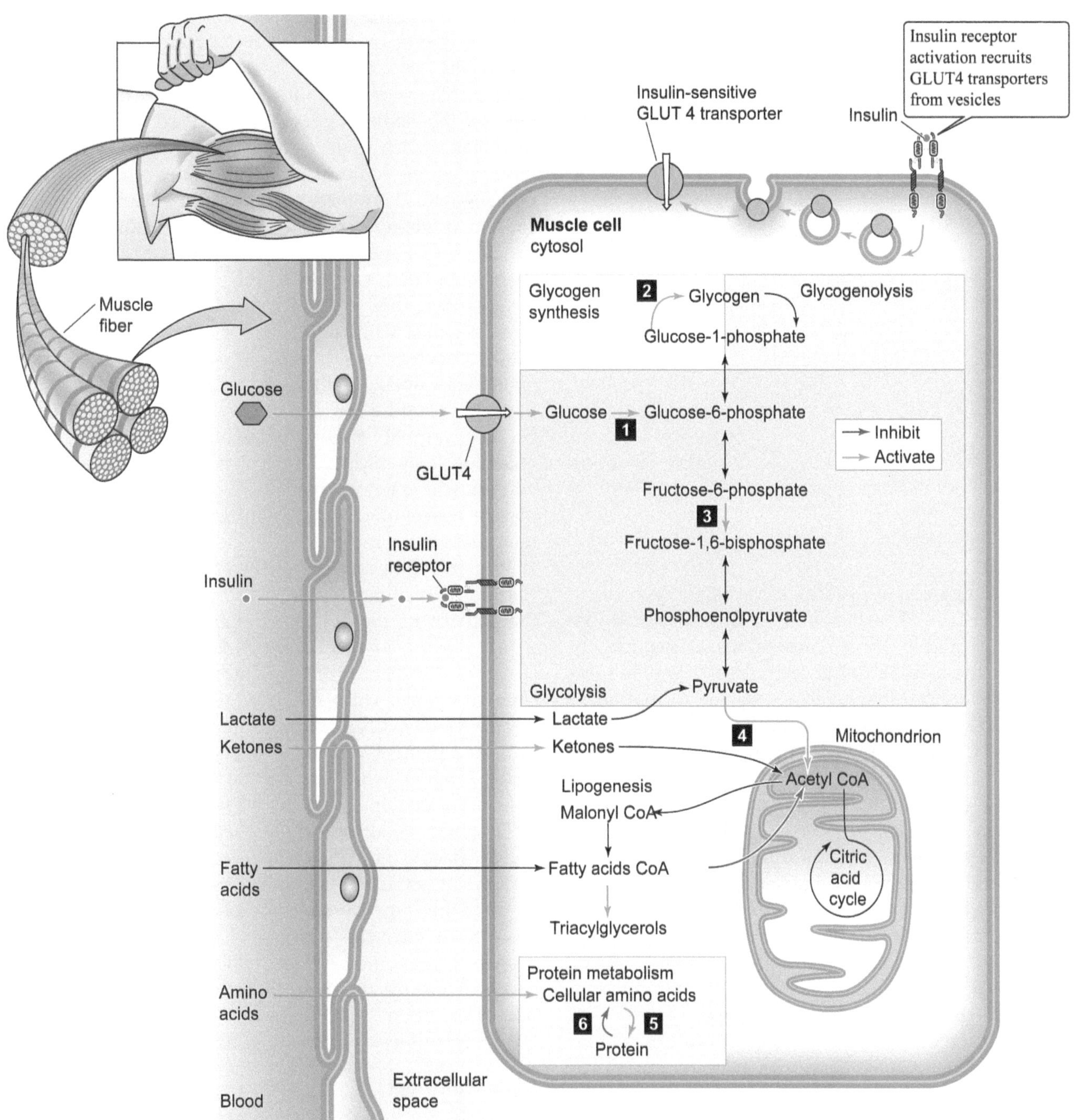

FIGURE 7.27 Effect of insulin on muscle cells. Source: *From Figure 51-9 Barrett E. J. (2017). Chapter 51: The endocrine pancreas. In W. F. Boron, & E. L. Boulpaep (Eds.)* Medical physiology *(3rd ed.) (p. 1048). Elsevier.*

experimental circumstances, no general agreement has been reached on how insulin increases phosphofructokinase activity. In contrast to the liver the isoform of the enzyme that forms fructose-2,6-bisphosphate in muscle is not regulated by cAMP. The effects of insulin are likely to be indirect.

It should be noted that oxidation of fat profoundly affects the metabolism of glucose in muscle and that insulin also increases all aspects of glucose metabolism in muscle as an indirect consequence of its action on adipose tissue to decrease FFA production. When insulin concentrations are low, increased oxidation of fatty acids decreases oxidation of glucose by inhibiting the decarboxylation of pyruvate and the transport of glucose across the muscle cell membrane. In addition, products of fatty acid oxidation appear also to inhibit

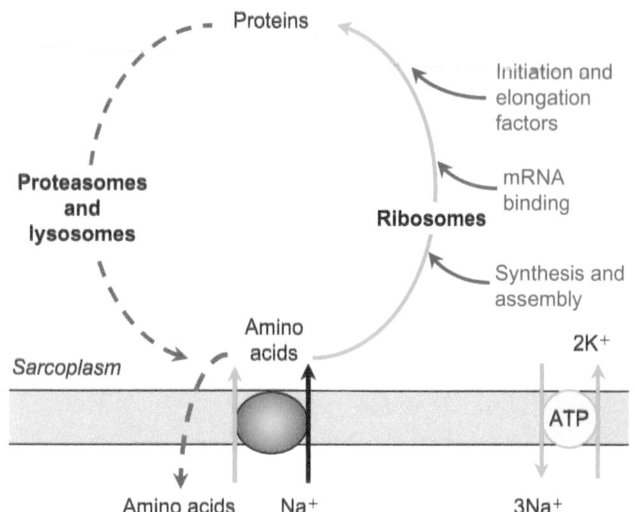

FIGURE 7.28 Effects of insulin on protein turnover in muscle. Reactions stimulated by insulin are shown in green. The dashed red arrows indicate reactions inhibited by insulin.

hexokinase, but recent studies have called into question the relevance of earlier findings that fatty acid oxidation may inhibit phosphofructokinase. Insulin not only limits the availability of fatty acids but also inhibits their oxidation. Insulin increases the formation of malonyl CoA, which blocks entry of long-chain fatty acids into the mitochondria as described for liver (Fig. 7.23). These effects are discussed further in Chapter 8, Hormonal Regulation of Fuel Metabolism.

Protein synthesis and degradation are ongoing processes in all tissues and in the nongrowing individual are completely balanced so that on average there is no net increase or decrease in body protein (Fig. 7.28).

Insulin intercedes in protein turnover at several levels and has both rapid and delayed effects. One of the hallmarks of insulin deficiency is the massive breakdown of muscle protein. Protein degradation begins with the attachment of ubiquitin to the protein molecules destined for breakdown. Ubiquitinated proteins enter the proteasomes and are cleaved to small fragments that subsequently are hydrolyzed to their amino acid constituents in the lysosomes. Insulin reduces the protein degrading activity of the ubiquitin–proteasomal system by decreasing expression of ubiquitin conjugating enzymes and by modulating the protease activity of its components.

Protein synthesis is a complex process that begins with adequate supplies of amino acids to charge the transfer RNA molecules that deliver them to the protein synthetic apparatus. Insulin stimulates the transport of amino acids from blood into muscle cells by recruiting carrier molecules to the plasma membrane in a manner analogous to the recruitment of GLUT 4. Amino acids are transported across the plasma membrane accompanied by sodium ions by a process of secondary active transport that is driven by the favorable electrochemical gradient for sodium. The sodium gradient is preserved by the operation of the sodium/potassium ATPase in the plasma membrane. Each cycle of this "sodium pump" extrudes three ions of sodium into the extracellular space in exchange for two ions of potassium. Insulin increases sodium pumping activity by recruiting pump molecules to the plasma membrane and by promoting their phosphorylation. Because more positively charged ions (Na +) are extruded than enter (K +), the cell interior becomes more negative with respect to the extracellular fluid, and the electrochemical driving force for sodium-coupled amino acid uptake is increased. The effects of insulin on the sodium pump are of considerable clinical importance. Because normal plasma potassium concentrations are quite low (~4 mM/L), transfer of even small amounts into muscle may produce relatively large decreases in plasma concentrations and may lead to cardiac arrhythmias and other problems.

Protein synthesis requires the attachment of mRNA to ribosomes. Insulin stimulates phosphorylation and hence the activity of the eukaryotic initiation factor 4 (eIF4), which plays a pivotal role in the binding of mRNA to ribosomes. Initiation of the synthesis of any particular protein begins with the engagement of methionine-loaded transfer RNA with the start codon in its mRNA. This engagement depends on the eukaryotic initiation factor 2 (eIF2), which is inactive when phosphorylated. One of the enzymes that catalyzes its phosphorylation is GSK, which, as already mentioned, is inhibited by insulin. By inactivating GSK, insulin accelerates dephosphorylation of eIF2. Elongation of the nascent protein requires the stepwise translocation of the ribosome along the mRNA after the addition of each amino acid. This process is governed by elongation factors that insulin also activates by inhibiting the kinase that catalyzes their phosphorylation. On a longer time scale, insulin increases synthesis of ribosomal RNA.

Effects on liver

Insulin reduces outflow of glucose from the liver and promotes its storage as glycogen. It inhibits glycogenolysis, gluconeogenesis, ureagenesis, and ketogenesis, and it stimulates the synthesis of fatty acids and proteins. These effects are accomplished by a combination of actions that change the activity of some hepatic enzymes and rates of synthesis of other enzymes. Hence, not all the effects of insulin occur on the same timescale. Although we use the terms "block" and "inhibit" to describe the actions of insulin, it is important to remember that these verbs are used in the relative and not the absolute sense. Rarely would inhibition of an enzymatic transformation be absolute.

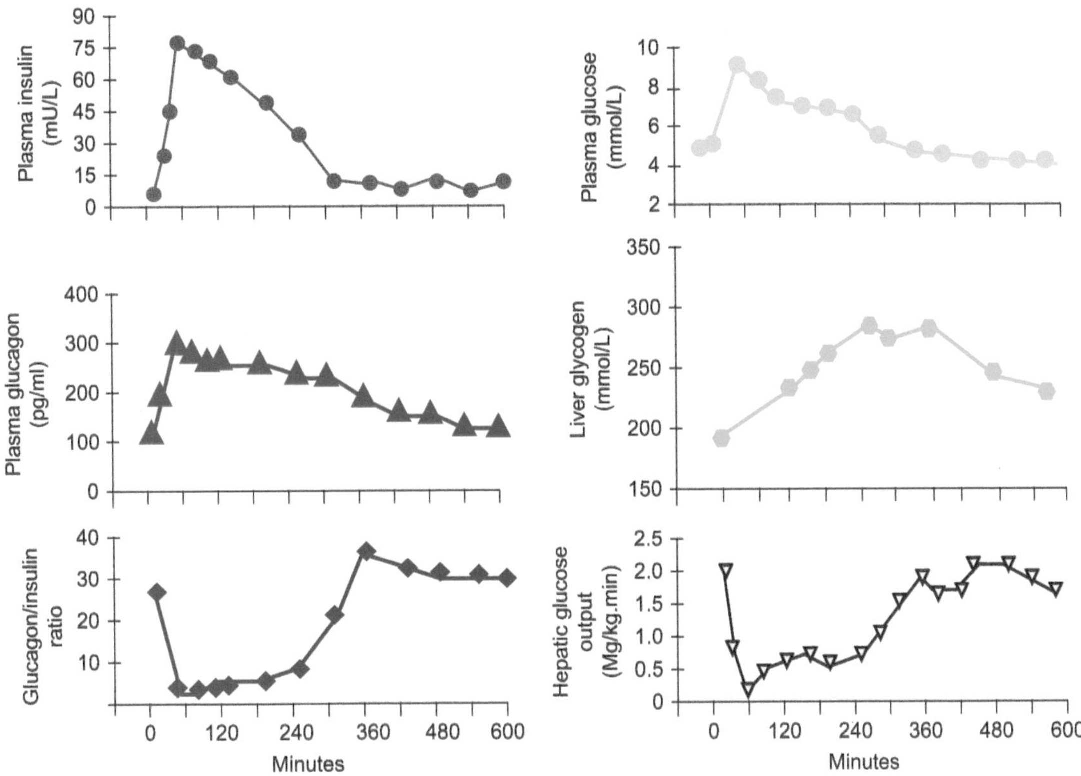

FIGURE 7.29 Changes in insulin and glucagon in plasma and carbohydrate metabolism in normal subjects following ingestion of a liquid meal rich in carbohydrate. Although secretion of both insulin and glucagon was stimulated, insulin increased about 25-fold, while glucagon increased only 3-fold so that the ratio of glucagon to insulin fell dramatically. Plasma glucose increased transiently, but release of glucose from the liver fell precipitously, and liver glycogen increased. Source: *From Taylor, R., Magnusson, I., Rothman, D. L., Cline, D.W., Caumo, A., Cobelli, C., & Shulman, G. L. (1996). Direct assessment of liver glycogen storage by* ^{13}*C nuclear magnetic resonance spectroscopy and regulation of glucose homeostasis after a mixed meal in normal subjects.* Journal of Clinical Investigation *97, 126–132, with permission.*

In addition, all the hepatic effects of insulin are reinforced indirectly by actions of insulin on muscle and fat to reduce the influx of substrates for gluconeogenesis and ketogenesis (Figs. 7.25 and 7.29).

The actions of insulin on hepatic metabolism are always superimposed on a background of other regulatory influences exerted by metabolites, glucagon, and a variety of other regulatory agents. The magnitude of any change produced by insulin thus is determined not only by the concentration of insulin but also by the strength of the opposing or cooperative actions of these other influences. Rates of secretion of both insulin and glucagon are dictated by physiological demand. Because of their antagonistic influences on hepatic function, however, it is the ratio rather than the absolute concentrations of these two hormones that determines the overall hepatic response (Fig. 7.30).

Glucose production

In general, liver takes up glucose when the circulating concentration is high and releases it when the blood level is low. Glucose transport into or out of hepatocytes depends upon the high-capacity insulin-insensitive glucose transporter, GLUT 2. Because the movement of glucose is passive, net uptake or release depends upon whether the concentration of free glucose is higher in extracellular or intracellular fluid. The intracellular concentration of free glucose depends on the balance between phosphorylation and dephosphorylation of glucose (Fig. 7.30, cycle II). The two enzymes that catalyze phosphorylation are hexokinase, which has a high affinity for glucose and other 6-carbon sugars, and glucokinase, which is specific for glucose. The kinetic properties of glucokinase are such that phosphorylation increases proportionately with glucose concentration over the entire physiological range. In addition, glucokinase activity is regulated by glucose. When glucose concentrations are low, much of the glucokinase is bound to an inhibitory protein that sequesters it within the nucleus. An increase in glucose concentration releases glucokinase from its inhibitor and allows it to move into the cytosol where glucose phosphorylation can take place.

Phosphorylated glucose cannot pass across the hepatocyte membrane. Dephosphorylation of glucose

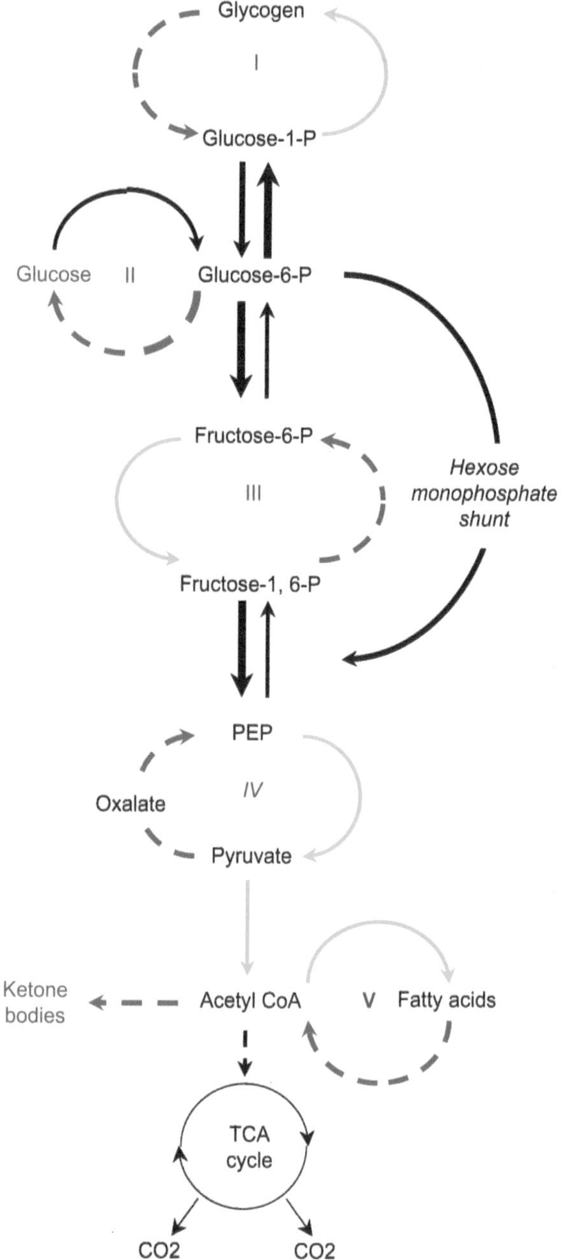

FIGURE 7.30 Effects of insulin on glucose metabolism in hepatocytes. Green arrows indicate reactions that are increased, and dashed red arrows indicate reactions that are decreased.

requires the activity of glucose-6-phosphatase. Insulin suppresses synthesis of glucose-6-phosphatase and increases synthesis of glucokinase, thereby decreasing net output of glucose while promoting net uptake. This response to insulin is relatively sluggish and contributes to long-term adaptation rather than to minute-to-minute regulation. The rapid effects of insulin to suppress glucose release are exerted indirectly through decreasing the availability of glucose-6-phosphate, hence starving the phosphatase of substrate. Uptake and phosphorylation by glucokinase is only one source of glucose-6-P. Glucose-6-P is also produced by glycogenolysis and gluconeogenesis. Insulin not only inhibits these processes, but it also drives them in the opposite direction. Most of the hepatic actions of insulin are opposite to those of glucagon, discussed earlier, and can be traced to inhibition of cAMP accumulation. Rapid actions of insulin largely depend on changes in the phosphorylation state of enzymes already present in hepatocytes. Insulin decreases hepatic concentrations of cAMP by accelerating its degradation by cAMP phosphodiesterase and may also interfere with cAMP formation and perhaps, activation protein kinase A. The immediate consequences can be seen in Fig. 7.28 and are in sharp contrast to the changes in glucose metabolism produced by glucagon shown in Fig. 7.11. Insulin promotes glycogen synthesis and inhibits glycogen breakdown. These effects are accomplished by the combination of interference with cAMP–dependent processes that drive these reactions in the opposite direction (Fig. 7.12); inhibition of glycogen synthase kinase, which, like protein kinase A, inactivates glycogen synthase; and by activation of the phosphatase that dephosphorylates both glycogen synthase and phosphorylase. The net effect is that glucose-6-P is incorporated into glycogen.

By lowering cAMP concentrations, insulin decreases the breakdown and increases the formation of fructose-2,6-phosphate, which potently stimulates phosphofructokinase and promotes the conversion of glucose to pyruvate. Insulin affects several enzymes in the PEP substrate cycle (Fig. 7.30, cycle IV) and in so doing directs substrate flow away from gluconeogenesis and toward lipogenesis (Fig. 7.31).

With relief of inhibition of pyruvate kinase, PEP can be converted to pyruvate, which then enters mitochondria. Insulin activates the mitochondrial pyruvate dehydrogenase enzyme complex that catalyzes decarboxylation of pyruvate to acetyl CoA. Insulin also indirectly accelerates this reaction by decreasing the inhibition imposed on it by fatty acid oxidation. Decarboxylation of pyruvate to acetyl CoA irreversibly removes these carbons from the gluconeogenic pathway and makes them available for fatty acid synthesis. The roundabout process that transfers acetyl carbons across the mitochondrial membrane to the cytoplasm, where lipogenesis occurs, requires condensation with oxaloacetate to form citrate. Citrate is transported to the cytosol and cleaved to release acetyl CoA and oxaloacetate. It might be recalled from earlier discussion that oxaloacetate is a crucial intermediate in gluconeogenesis and is converted to PEP by PEP carboxykinase. Insulin bars the flow of this lipogenic substrate into the gluconeogenic pool by inhibiting synthesis of PEP carboxykinase. The only

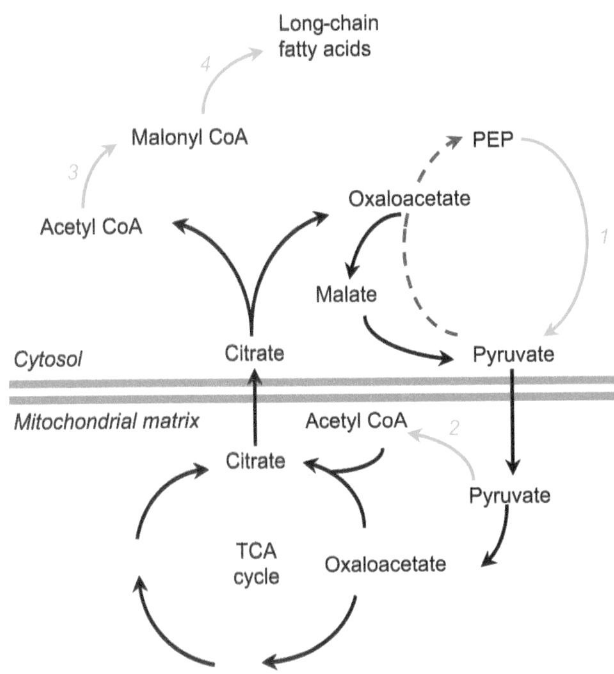

FIGURE 7.31 Effects of insulin on lipogenesis in hepatocytes. Green arrows indicate reactions that are increased, and the dashed red arrow indicates a reaction that is decreased. (1) Pyruvate kinase, (2) pyruvate dehydrogenase, (3) acetyl CoA carboxylase, and (4) fatty acid synthase.

fate left to cytosolic oxaloacetate is decarboxylation to pyruvate.

Finally, insulin increases the activity of acetyl CoA carboxylase, which catalyzes the rate determining reaction in fatty acid synthesis. Activation is accomplished in part by relieving cAMP–dependent inhibition and in part by promoting the polymerization of inactive subunits of the enzyme into an active complex. The resulting malonyl CoA not only condenses with acetyl CoA to form long-chain fatty acids but also prevents oxidation of newly formed fatty acids by blocking their entry into mitochondria (Fig. 7.27). On a longer timescale, insulin increases the synthesis of acetyl CoA carboxylase.

It may be noted that hepatic oxidation of either glucose or fatty acids increases delivery of acetyl CoA to the cytosol, but ketogenesis results only from oxidation of fatty acids. The primary reason is that lipogenesis usually accompanies glucose utilization and provides an alternate pathway for disposal of acetyl CoA. There is also a quantitative difference in the rate of acetyl CoA production from the two substrates: 1 mol of glucose yields only 2 mol of acetyl CoA compared to 8 or 9 mol for each mole of fatty acids. The effects of insulin on glucose, fat, ketone, and protein metabolism are summarized in Table 7.3 and a comparison of the metabolic effects of insulin and glucagon is outlined in Table 7.4.

TABLE 7.3 The effects of insulin on glucose, fat, ketone, and protein metabolism.

Insulin effects on glucose metabolism
Inhibition of glycogenolysis
Inhibition of gluconeogenesis
Stimulation of glucose transport into fat and muscle
Increase of glycolysis in fat and muscle
Stimulation of glycogen synthesis
Insulin effects on fat metabolism
Increase clearance from circulation of triglyceride-rich chylomicrons via lipoprotein lipase
Stimulation of reesterification of free fatty acids into triglycerides within fat cells
Inhibition of lipolysis of triglyceride stores by inhibiting hormone-sensitive lipase
Insulin effects on ketone body metabolism
Reduction of circulating ketone bodies by decreasing the supply of free fatty acids to the liver (decrease of lipolysis)
Inhibition of ketogenesis in the liver
Enhancement of peripheral clearance of ketone bodies
Insulin effects on protein metabolism
Stimulation of protein synthesis
Inhibition of protein breakdown (proteolysis)
Inhibition of urea formation

TABLE 7.4 Comparison of the metabolic effects of insulin and glucagon.

	Insulin	Glucagon
Glycogen synthesis	↑	↓
Glycolysis	↑	↓
Glycogenolysis	↓	↑
Gluconeogenesis	↓	↑
Lipogenesis	↑	↓
Lipolysis	↓	↑
Ketogenesis	↓	↑
Protein synthesis	↑	↓

Mechanism of insulin action

The many changes that insulin produces at the molecular level—membrane transport, enzyme activation, gene transcription, and protein synthesis—have been described. The molecular events that link these changes to the interaction of insulin and its receptor are still incompletely understood, although much progress has been made in recent years. More than a hundred different molecules have already been identified as participants in the complex panoply of events entrained by the activated insulin receptor. Transduction of the insulin signal is not accomplished by a linear series of biochemical changes, but rather multiple intracellular signaling pathways are activated simultaneously and may intersect at one or more points before the final result is expressed.

The insulin receptor is a tetramer composed of two α- and two β-glycoprotein subunits that are held together by disulfide bonds that link the α subunits to each other and to the β subunits (Fig. 7.23). The α and β subunits of insulin are encoded in a single gene that contains 22 exons. The α subunits are completely extracellular and contain the insulin-binding domain. The β subunits span the plasma membrane and contain tyrosine kinase activity in the cytosolic domain. Binding to insulin is thought to produce a conformational change that relieves each β subunit from the inhibitory effects of the α subunit, allowing it to phosphorylate itself and other proteins at tyrosine residues. Autophosphorylation of the kinase domain is required for full activation. Tyrosine phosphorylation of the receptor also provides docking sites for other proteins that participate in transducing the hormonal signal. Docking on the phosphorylated receptor may position proteins optimally for phosphorylation by the receptor kinase.

Among the proteins that are phosphorylated on tyrosine residues by the insulin receptor kinase are four cytosolic proteins called insulin receptor substrates (IRS-1, IRS-2, IRS-3, and IRS-4). These relatively large proteins contain multiple tyrosine phosphorylation sites and act as scaffolds upon which other proteins are assembled to form large signaling complexes. IRS-1 and IRS-2 appear to be present in all insulin target cells, whereas IRS-3 and IRS-4 have more limited distributions. Despite their names the IRS proteins are not functionally limited to transduction of the insulin signal but participate in expression of the effects of other hormones and growth factors. Moreover, they are not the only substrates for the insulin receptor kinase.

Two other scaffold proteins called Shc and Cbl serve a similar function. A variety of other proteins that are tyrosine phosphorylated by the insulin receptor kinase have also been identified. Proteins recruited to the insulin receptor and IRS proteins may have enzymatic activity or they may have a coupling function by providing binding sites for recruiting other proteins. The assemblage of proteins initiates signaling cascades that ultimately express the various actions of insulin described earlier.

One of the most important of the proteins that is activated is phosphatidylinositol-3 (PI3) kinase. PI3 kinase plays a critical role in activating many downstream effector molecules, including protein kinase B (also called AKT), which mediates the effects of insulin on glycogen synthesis and GLUT 4 translocation. Like the IRS proteins, PI3 kinase also is activated by a variety of other hormones, cytokines, and growth factors whose actions do not necessarily mimic those of insulin. The uniqueness of the response to insulin probably reflects the unique combination of biochemical consequences produced by the simultaneous activity of multiple signaling pathways and the particular set of effector molecules expressed in insulin target cells. Insulin is known to regulate expression of more than 150 genes, but the functions of many of the proteins encoded by these genes and how the receptor communicates with these regulatory proteins is under extensive study. Fig. 7.32 presents a simplified map of some of the signaling pathways that produce the cellular responses to insulin.

Regulation of insulin secretion

As might be expected of a hormone whose physiological role is promotion of fuel storage, insulin secretion is greatest immediately after eating and decreases during between-meal periods (Fig. 7.33).

Coordination of insulin secretion with nutritional state as well as with fluctuating demands for energy production is achieved through stimulation of beta cells by metabolites, hormones, and neural signals. Because insulin plays the primary role in regulating storage and

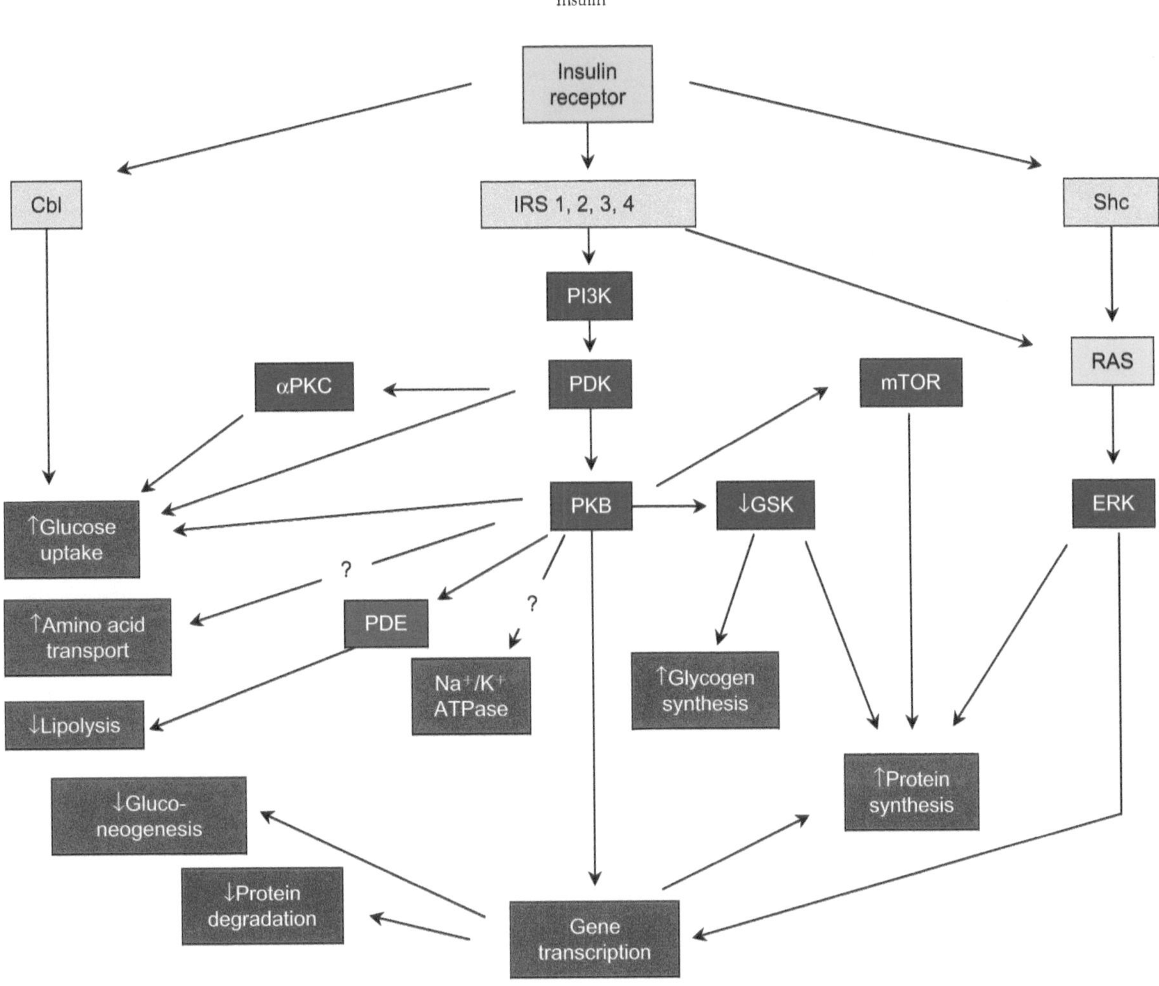

FIGURE 7.32 Simplified model of insulin signaling pathways. The insulin receptor proteins *(IRS 1,2,3,4)*, *Cbl*, *Shc*, and the β subunits of the insulin receptor are phosphorylated on tyrosine residues by the insulin receptor kinase and serve as anchoring sites for cytosolic proteins that form signaling cascades. Proteins shown in blue boxes are serine/threonine kinases. Specific isoforms and/or subunits are not shown nor are the relevant phosphatases. *Cbl*, Cacitas B lineage lymphoma protein; *ERK*, extracellular receptor kinase; *GSK*, glycogen synthase kinase; *mTOR*, mammalian target of rapamycin; *PDE*, phosphodiesterase; *PDK*, phosphoinositide-dependent kinase; *PI3K*, phosphoinositol-3-kinase; *PKB*, protein kinase B; *RAS*, Ras oncogene, a small G-protein; *Shc*, Src homology containing protein; *α PKC*, α isoform of protein kinase C.

mobilization of metabolic fuels, the beta cells must be constantly apprised of bodily needs, not only with regard to feeding and fasting, but also to the changing demands of the environment. Energy needs differ widely when an individual is at peace with the surroundings and when (s)he is fighting for survival. Maintaining constancy of the internal environment is achieved through direct monitoring of circulating metabolites by beta cells themselves. This input can be overridden or enhanced by hormonal or neural signals that prepare the individual for rapid storage of an influx of food or for massive mobilization of fuel reserves to permit a suitable response to environmental demands.

Glucose

Glucose is the most important regulator of insulin secretion (Fig. 7.34).

In the normal individual, its concentration in blood is maintained within the narrow range of about 70 or 80 mg/dL after an overnight fast to about 150 mg/dL immediately after a glucose-rich meal. When blood glucose increases, insulin secretion increases proportionately. At low concentrations of glucose, adjustments in insulin secretion are influenced most heavily by other stimuli (see next) that act as amplifiers or inhibitors of the effects of glucose. The effectiveness of these agents therefore decreases as glucose concentration decreases.

Other circulating metabolites

Amino acids are important stimuli for insulin secretion. The transient increase in plasma amino acids after a protein-rich meal is accompanied by increased secretion of insulin. Arginine, lysine, and leucine are the

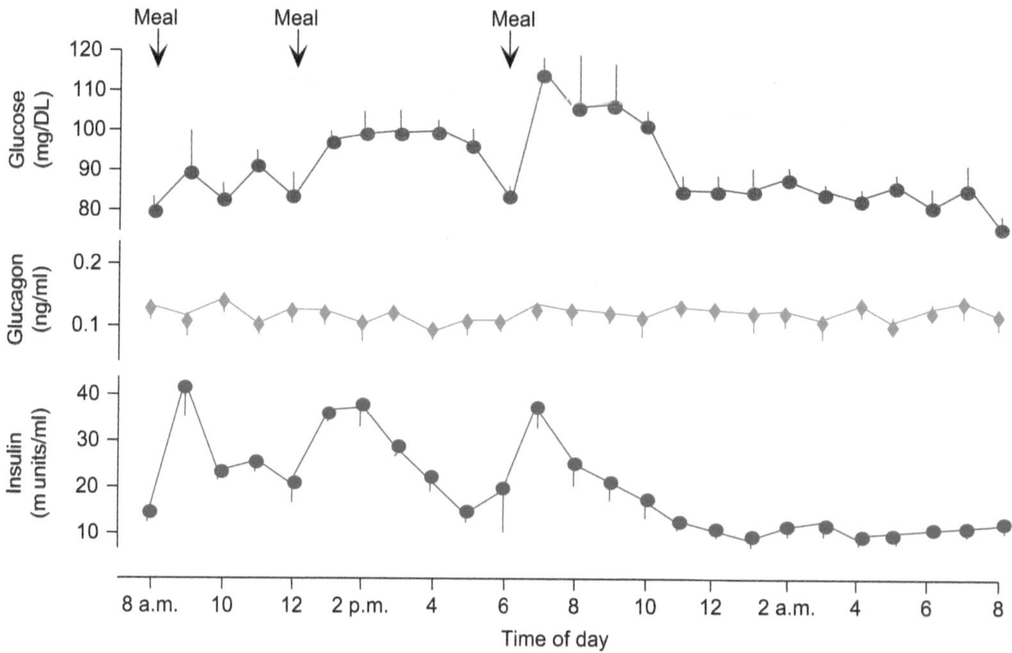

FIGURE 7.33 Changes in the concentrations of plasma glucose, *IRG*, and *IRI* throughout the day. Values are the mean ± SEM ($n = 4$). *IRG*, immunoreactive glucagon; *IRI*, immunoreactive insulin. Source: *From Tasaka, Y., Sekine, M., Wakatsuki, M., Ohgawara, H., & Shizume, K. (1975). Levels of pancreatic glucagon, insulin and glucose during twenty-four hours of the day in normal subjects.* Hormone and Metabolic Research 7, *205–206.*

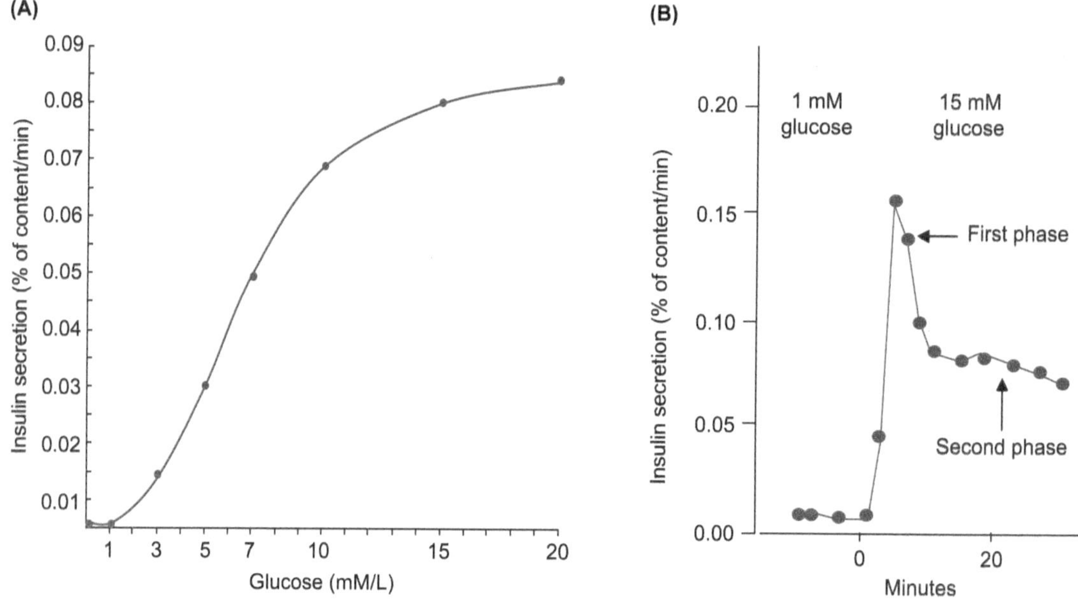

FIGURE 7.34 Insulin secretion by isolated human pancreatic islets in response to increasing concentrations of glucose. (A) Stimulus:response curve. The threshold for increased secretion in vivo may be somewhat higher than between 1 and 3 mM/L shown here. (B) Insulin secretion in response to a sudden rise in glucose concentration has two phases: an early transient spike followed by a sustained plateau. Source: *Drawn from the data of Henquin, J. C., Dufrane, D., & Nenquin, M. (2006). Nutrient control of insulin secretion in isolated normal human islets.* Diabetes, 55, *3470–3477.*

most potent amino acid stimulators of insulin secretion. Insulin secreted at this time may facilitate storage of dietary amino acids as protein and prevents their diversion to gluconeogenesis. Amino acids are effective signals for insulin release only when blood glucose concentrations are adequate. Failure to increase insulin secretion when glucose is in short supply prevents hypoglycemia that might otherwise occur after a protein meal that contains little carbohydrate. Fatty acids and ketone bodies may also increase insulin secretion, but only when they are present at rather high concentrations. Because fatty acid mobilization and ketogenesis are inhibited by insulin, their ability to stimulate insulin secretion provides a feedback mechanism to protect against excessive mobilization of fatty acids and ketosis.

Hormonal and neural control

In response to carbohydrate in the lumen, the intestinal mucosa secretes at least two hormones, called incretins, that reach the pancreas through the general circulation and stimulate the beta cells to release insulin even though the increase in blood glucose is still quite small (see Fig. 6.35). Incretins are thought to act by amplifying the stimulatory effects of glucose. This anticipatory secretion of insulin prepares tissues to cope with the coming influx of glucose and dampens what might otherwise be a large increase in blood sugar. Various gastrointestinal hormones, including gastrin, secretin, CCK, glucagon-like peptide (GLP-1), and glucose-dependent insulinotropic peptide (GIP), can evoke insulin secretion when tested experimentally, but of these hormones, only GLP-1 and GIP appear to be physiologically important incretins.

Secretion of insulin in response to food intake is also mediated by a neural pathway. The taste or smell of food or the expectation of eating may increase insulin secretion during this cephalic phase of feeding. Parasympathetic fibers in the vagus nerve stimulate beta cells by releasing acetylcholine or the neuropeptide VIP. Activation of this pathway is initiated at integrative centers in the brain and involves input from sensory endings in the mouth, stomach, small intestine, and portal vein. An increase in the concentration of glucose in portal blood is detected by glucose sensors in the wall of the portal vein and the information is relayed to the brain via vagal afferent nerves. In response, vagal efferent nerves stimulate the pancreas to secrete insulin and the liver to take up glucose.

Insulin secretion is virtually shut off by epinephrine or norepinephrine delivered to beta cells by either the circulation or sympathetic neurons. This inhibitory effect is seen not only as a response to low blood glucose but may occur even when the blood glucose level is high. It is mediated through α2-adrenergic receptors on the surface of beta cells. Physiological circumstances that activate the sympathetic nervous system thus can shut down insulin secretion and thereby remove the major restraint on mobilization of metabolic fuels needed to cope with an emergency.

Secretory activity of beta cells is also enhanced by growth hormone and prolactin by mechanisms that are not yet understood. During pregnancy and lactation the capacity for insulin secretion is greatly enhanced (see Chapter 14: Hormonal Control of Pregnancy and Lactation). Although growth hormone does not directly evoke a secretory response, basal insulin secretion is increased when it is present in excess, and beta cells become hyperresponsive to signals for insulin secretion. Excessive secretion of growth hormone or cortisol decreases tissue sensitivity to insulin and provokes compensatory increases in both basal and stimulated secretion. These hormones can produce transient or even permanent diabetes when beta cells are overtaxed (see Chapter 8: Hormonal Regulation of Fuel Metabolism). In high concentrations, glucocorticoids may directly inhibit insulin synthesis and secretion and may even cause beta cell apoptosis, but paradoxically, perhaps, insulin secretion is reduced when cortisol or growth hormone are deficient. The adipose hormone leptin (see Chapter 8: Hormonal Regulation of Fuel Metabolism) also inhibits insulin gene expression. Factors that regulate insulin secretion are shown in Fig. 7.35.

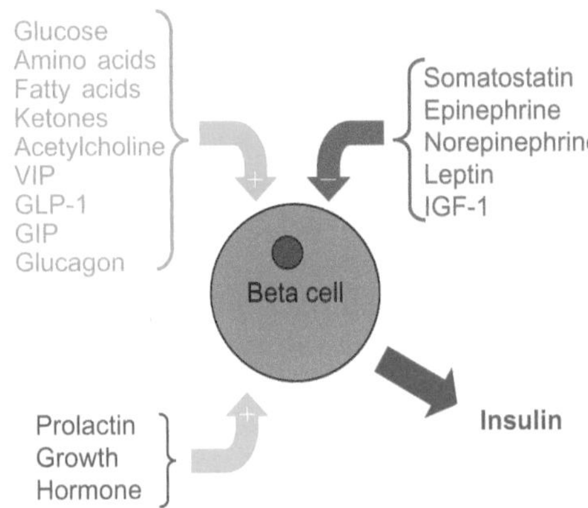

FIGURE 7.35 Metabolic, hormonal, and neural influences on insulin secretion.

Cellular events

Beta cells increase their rates of insulin secretion within a few seconds of exposure to increased concentrations of glucose and can shut down secretion as rapidly. Secretion in response to a sudden increase in glucose takes place in two distinct phases (Fig. 7.32B): an initial short-lived burst followed by a lower, but sustained rate that lasts as long as the glucose concentration is elevated. Insulin secreted in the first phase is released from storage granules that are already primed and docked at fusion sites on the plasma membrane (see Chapter 1: Introduction). These granules are part of the "readily releasable pool" that may account for about 5% of the granules stored in the beta cell. The second phase of secretion represents the rate of replenishment of the readily releasable pool by storage granules from the larger "reserve pool" located deeper in the cytosol and the requisite docking at specific sites on the membrane, priming, and ultimately fusion and hormone release. In normal beta cells the reserve pool is large enough to sustain maximal rates of secretion for prolonged periods without a need for de novo synthesis, but signals that increase secretion also activate insulin gene expression and ensure that the reserve pool is replenished.

The event that triggers insulin secretion is an influx of extracellular calcium through voltage-sensitive channels. Secretion of insulin in both phases depends upon increased intracellular calcium and is amplified by processes that are sensitive to the availability of extracellular glucose, hormonally induced cAMP and other second messengers, and to both intracellular and extracellular lipids and other metabolites. Normal beta cells secrete insulin in a pulsatile manner with each pulse coinciding with a transient increase in cytosolic calcium. The cellular mechanisms that govern these complex events are the subject of intense investigation motivated by the growing need to develop therapeutic approaches to correct beta cell dysfunction in type 2 diabetes.

The question of how the concentration of glucose is monitored and translated into rates of insulin secretion has not been answered completely, but many of the important steps are known. The beta cell has specific receptors for hormones and neurotransmitters that augment or inhibit secretion, but it does not have specific receptors for glucose. To stimulate insulin secretion, glucose must be metabolized by the beta cell, indicating that some consequence of glucose oxidation, rather than glucose itself, is the critical determinant. Glucose enters the cells on two transporters, GLUT 1 and GLUT 2, which have a high capacity, but relatively low affinity for glucose. At plasma concentrations at or above about 100 mg/dL, glucose enters the beta cell primarily on GLUT 2 at a rate that is determined by its concentration and not by the capacity of transporters. Glucose can potentially cross the cell membrane 100 times faster than it can be phosphorylated. Glucokinase, which catalyzes the rate determining reaction for glucose metabolism, has the requisite kinetic characteristics to behave as a glucose sensor. Mutations that affect its function result in decreased insulin secretion in response to glucose and may be severe enough to cause a form of diabetes. Increased metabolism of glucose results in increased phosphorylation of adenosine diphosphate (ADP) to form adenosine triphosphate (ATP).

Glucose metabolism and calcium influx are linked by their mutual relationship to cellular concentrations of ATP and ADP. In resting beta cells, efflux of potassium through open ATP-sensitive potassium channels (KATP) offsets the slow influx of positive charge and maintains the membrane potential at about −70 mV. KATP channels are octamers composed of four pore-forming subunits bound to four regulatory subunits called sulfonylurea receptors (SUR). The SUR subunits are so named for their role in the action of a class of drugs, the sulfonylureas, that stimulate insulin secretion. These channels are activated (opened) by MgADP, which binds to the regulatory subunits, and inhibited (closed) by ATP, which binds to the pore-forming subunits. When blood glucose concentrations are low, the effects of ADP predominate even though its concentration in beta cell cytoplasm is less than a third that of ATP. When glucose concentrations increase, accelerated oxidation of glucose increases the rate of phosphorylation of ADP to ATP. As a result, the inhibitory effects of ATP become dominant (Fig. 7.36).

Closure of the KATP channels results in accumulation of positive charge in the cells and causes the membrane to depolarize. Voltage-sensitive calcium channels open when the depolarizing membrane potential reaches about −50 mV. Influx of positively charged calcium produces a transient reversal of the membrane potential. This increase in cytosolic calcium inhibits voltage-sensitive calcium channels and activates calcium-sensitive and voltage-sensitive potassium channels allowing potassium to exit and the cell to repolarize briefly. Calcium may exit the cells via the action of calcium ATPases (calcium pumps) in the plasma membrane. Electrical recording of these events reveals a pattern of voltage changes that resembles an action potential. Oscillations in membrane potential thus produced are accompanied by oscillations in cytosolic calcium concentrations and bursts of insulin secretion. The frequency and duration of electrical discharges in beta cells increase as glucose concentrations increase.

The role of calcium is not limited to triggering insulin release from storage granules that are poised to fuse with the plasma membrane. The increase in cytosolic calcium also stimulates further release of calcium from endoplasmic reticulum stores by a process known as calcium-induced calcium release. Calcium has multiple roles in mobilizing and priming storage granules to replenish the readily releasable pool. Acting in conjunction with calmodulin, calcium also activates adenylyl cyclase and cAMP formation. cAMP stimulates insulin secretion at multiple steps in the exocytotic pathway by activating both protein kinase A and a guanine nucleotide exchange factor (EPAC, see Chapter 1: Introduction) that, in turn, activates small G-protein regulators of granule translocation and fusion with the plasma membrane.

The increase in cytosolic calcium is mirrored by an increase in calcium within mitochondria whose role in amplifying insulin secretion extends beyond supplying

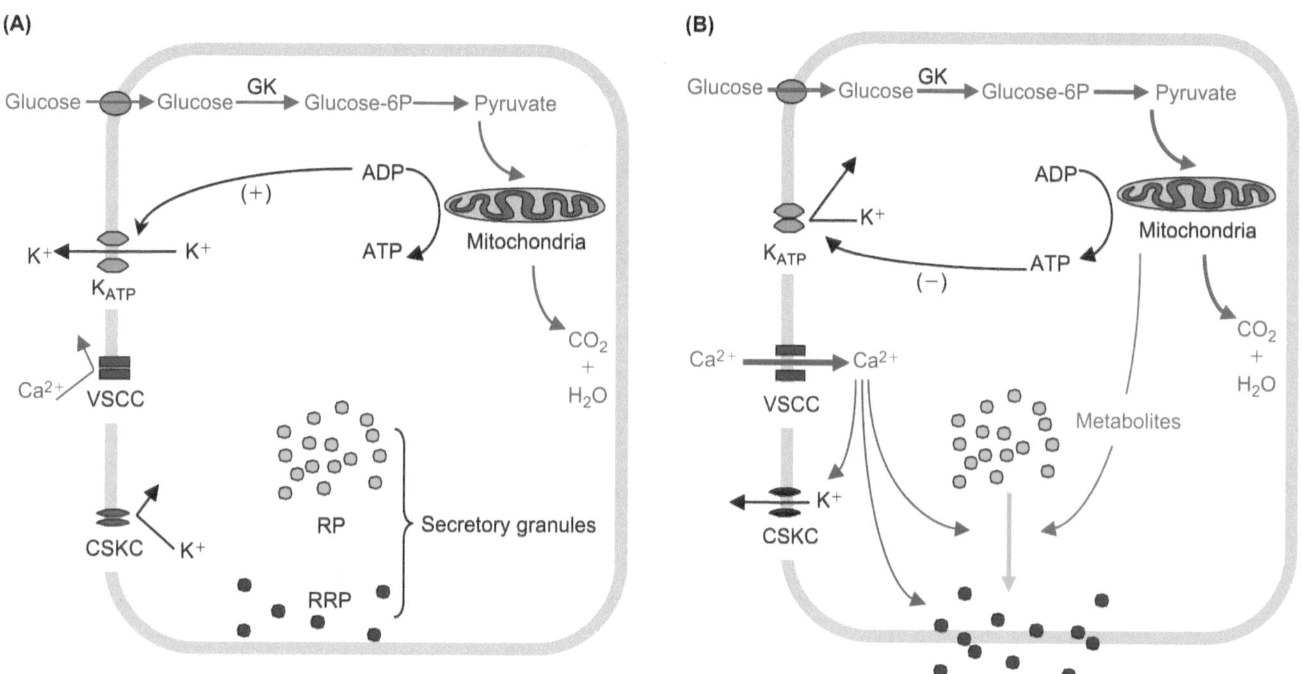

FIGURE 7.36 Triggering of insulin secretion by glucose. (A) "Resting" beta cell (blood glucose <100 mg/dL). ADP/ATP ratio is high enough so that ATP-sensitive potassium channels (K_{ATP}) are open, and the membrane potential is about −70 mV. *VSCC* and *CSKC* are closed. (B) Beta cell response to increased blood glucose. Increased entry and metabolism of glucose decreases the ratio of ADP/ATP, and K_{ATP} channels close. VSCC are activated; calcium enters and stimulates insulin secretion. Mitochondrial metabolites formed in response to glucose and calcium amplify secretion. Influx of calcium inhibits VSCC and activates calcium-sensitive and voltage-sensitive potassium channels, thereby allowing the cell membrane to repolarize and calcium channels to close. Calcium is extruded by membrane calcium ATPase. Persistence of high glucose results in repeated spiking of electrical discharges and oscillation of intracellular calcium concentrations. *CSKC*, Calcium-sensitive potassium channels; *VSCC*, voltage-sensitive calcium channels.

the requisite ATP. Increased intramitochondrial calcium increases the activity of pyruvate dehydrogenase and other dehydrogenases that are critical for generating metabolites that modulate insulin secretion. Pyruvate is the major product of glycolysis and may be decarboxylated by the pyruvate dehydrogenase complex to form acetyl CoA or carboxylated to form oxaloacetate within the mitochondria. These two products can then combine to form citrate, which, upon transfer to the cytosol, serves as a precursor of malonyl CoA and other metabolic regulators of islet cell metabolism.

Unstimulated beta cells derive the bulk of their energy from the oxidation of long-chain fatty acids, but malonyl CoA blocks access of fatty acid CoA to intramitochondrial sites of oxidation and switches beta cells to use glucose as their primary fuel. Long-chain fatty acids that accumulate in the cytosol amplify insulin secretion through their effects on secretory granule trafficking and the activities of enzymes and ion channels. Fatty acids are also converted to more complex lipids that appear to have additional signaling functions. Other metabolites derived from citrate and amino acids or arising from mitochondrial transformations that contribute to both the triggering and amplifying aspects of insulin secretion remain subjects of active investigation.

In addition to stimulating insulin secretion, glucose is the most important stimulator of insulin synthesis. Both glucose and cAMP increase transcription of the insulin gene, and glucose stabilizes the mRNA transcript. The mRNA template for insulin turns over slowly and has a half-life of about 30 hours. Hyperglycemia prolongs its half-life more than twofold, while hypoglycemia accelerates its degradation. In addition, glucose increases translation of the proinsulin mRNA by stimulating both the initiation and elongation reactions. Concurrently, glucose also upregulates production of the convertase enzymes that process proinsulin to insulin.

Effects of incretins

GIP and GLP-1 (see Chapter 6: Hormones of the Gastrointestinal Tract) are secreted by K and L cells of the intestinal mucosa in response to luminal nutrients. They activate specific G protein–coupled receptors on beta cells to accelerate glucose-dependent insulin secretion in a manner that blunts the increase in

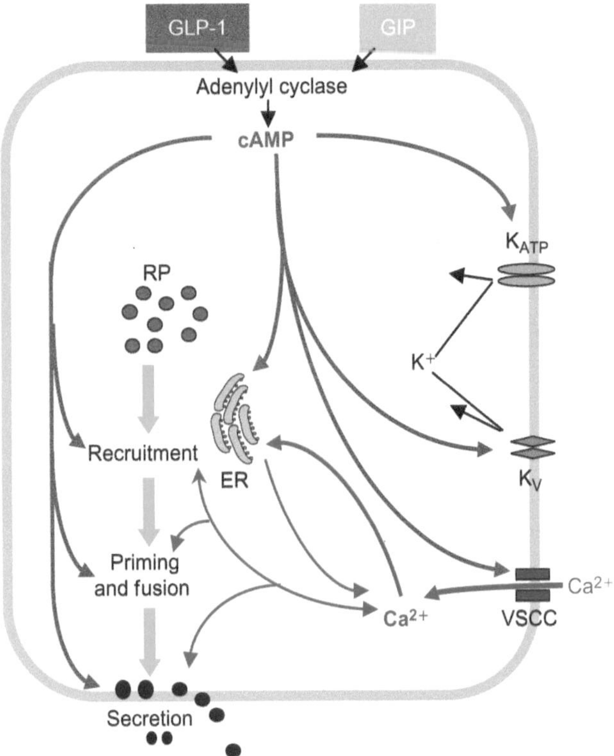

FIGURE 7.37 Major acute cellular actions of incretins. *GLP-1* and *GIP* acting through G peptide–coupled receptors activate adenylyl cyclase to increase intracellular concentrations of *cAMP*. cAMP increases the activity of protein kinase A or binds to a GTP exchange factor to increase cytosolic calcium and enhance the effects of calcium of insulin secretion. *cAMP*, Cyclic AMP; *ER*, endoplasmic reticulum; *GIP*, glucose-dependent insulinotropic peptide; *GLP-1*, glucagon-like peptide 1; *GTP*, guanosine triphosphate; K_{ATP}, ATP-sensitive potassium channels; K_V, voltage-sensitive potassium channels; *RP*, reserve pool of secretory granules; *VSCC*, voltage-sensitive calcium channels. See text for details.

plasma glucose concentration produced by intestinal absorption. Stimulation of beta cells by these agents may account for as much as 60% of the insulin secreted each day. Activation of GLP-1 and GIP receptors and the subsequent production of cAMP enhance glucose-dependent insulin secretion at multiple sites in the stimulation–secretion pathway (Fig. 7.37).

At the level of the plasma membrane, cAMP–dependent phosphorylation of channel proteins facilitates closure KATP in response to ATP and impedes opening of the voltage-sensitive K channels that contribute to repolarization. At the same time, cAMP–dependent phosphorylation partially activates the voltage sensitive calcium channels and prolongs their open state. Together these effects magnify the influx of calcium produced by increases in plasma glucose. cAMP–dependent release of calcium from intracellular stores further augments the increase in cytosolic calcium. In addition to increasing cytosolic calcium, the incretins sensitize the secretory apparatus to the effects of calcium and promote both secretion of insulin from the readily releasable pool and its replenishment from the reserve pool.

On a longer timescale, GLP-1 in conjunction with glucose increases transcription of the insulin gene and stabilizes its mRNA transcript. Prolonged stimulation with GLP-1 increases islet cell mass by stimulating proliferation of beta cells and by inhibiting apoptosis. Some data indicate that GLP-1 may also stimulate beta cell development from precursor stem cells. GLP-1 receptor agonists are a novel class of antihyperglycemic medications used in management of type 2 diabetes. All the actions of GLP-1 are shared by GIP, but receptors for GIP tend to be downregulated by hyperglycemia.

Effects of other hormones and neurotransmitters

Acetylcholine and CCK, whose receptors are coupled through Gαq to phospholipase C, stimulate insulin secretion by way of the IP3/DAG second messenger system. IP3 stimulates release of calcium from intracellular storage sites and thus augments the influx of extracellular calcium triggered by metabolism of glucose. In addition, activated protein kinase C enhances aspects of the secretory process that are both dependent and independent of calcium. Receptors for norepinephrine and somatostatin are coupled to the inhibitory guanine nucleotide-binding protein Gi and block insulin secretion primarily by inhibiting adenylyl cyclase and lowering cAMP. Through the effects on ion channels, the βγ subunits of the somatostatin receptor may also cause the plasma membrane to hyperpolarize and hence prevent activation of voltage-sensitive calcium channels.

Somatostatin

Although somatostatin produced in delta cells is the third most abundant of the pancreatic islet hormones, the physiological importance of pancreatic somatostatin is not understood. Its major role may be as a paracrine regulator of insulin and glucagon secretion. Somatostatin originally was isolated from hypothalamic extracts that inhibited the secretion of growth hormone. It is found in many secretory cells (delta cells) outside of the pancreatic islets, particularly in the lining of the gastrointestinal tract (see Chapter 6: Hormones of the Gastrointestinal Tract), and is widely distributed in many neural tissues where it presumably functions as a neurotransmitter. Measurable increases in somatostatin concentration can be found in peripheral blood after ingestion of a meal rich in fat or protein, with the vast majority secreted by intestinal cells rather than islet cells. It is cleared rapidly from the blood and has a half-life of only about 3 minutes. Further discussion of somatostatin is found in

Chapter 2, Pituitary Gland, Chapter 6, Hormones of the Gastrointestinal Tract, and Chapter 11, Hormonal Control of Growth.

Summary

The pancreas is divided into two parts: an exocrine part for the digestion of food and an endocrine part for the regulation of blood glucose and potassium, the results of digestion. The interaction of pancreatic hormones with other hormones and the imbalance when this interaction is not good is discussed in the last part of this chapter.

Suggested readings

Basic foundations

Atkinson, M. A. (2017). Type 1 diabetes mellitus. In S. Melmed, K. S. Polonsky, P. R. Larson, & H. M. Kronenberg (Eds.), *Williams textbook of endocrinology* (13th ed., pp. 1451–1483). Philadelphia, PA: Elsevier.

Brownlee, M., Aiello, L. P., Cooper, M. E., Vinik, A. I., Plutzky, J., & Boulton, A. J. M. (2017). Complications of diabetes mellitus. In S. Melmed, K. S. Polonsky, P. R. Larson, & H. M. Kronenberg (Eds.), *Williams textbook of endocrinology* (13th ed., pp. 1484–1581). Philadelphia, PA: Elsevier.

Marino, C. R., & Gorelick, F. S. (2017). Pancreatic and salivary glands. In W. F. Boron, & E. L. Boulpaep (Eds.), *Medical physiology* (3rd ed., pp. 879–898). Philadelphia, PA: Elsevier.

Polonsky, K. S., & Burant, C. F. (2017). Type 2 diabetes mellitus. In S. Melmed, K. S. Polonsky, P. R. Larson, & H. M. Kronenberg (Eds.), *Williams textbook of endocrinology* (13th ed., pp. 1386–1450). Philadelphia, PA: Elsevier.

Advanced information

Downie, M. L., Ulrich, E. H., & Noone, D. G. (2018). An update on hypertension in children with type 1 diabetes. *Canadian Journal of Diabetes, 42*(2), 199–204. Available from https://doi.org/10.1016/j.jcjd.2018.02.008.

Nambam, B., & Haller, M. J. (2016). Updates on immune therapies in type 1 diabetes. *European Endocrinology, 12*(2), 89–95. Available from https://doi.org/10.17925/EE.2016.12.02.89.

Shibao, C. A., Celedonio, J. E., Tamboli, R., Sidani, R., Love-Gregory, L., Pietka, T., ... Flynn, C. R. (2018). CD36 modulates fasting and preabsorptive hormone and bile acid levels. *The Journal of Clinical Endocrinology & Metabolism*. Available from https://doi.org/10.1210/jc.2017-01982, jc.2017-01982-jc.02017-01982.

Turton, J. L., Raab, R., & Rooney, K. B. (2018). Low-carbohydrate diets for type 1 diabetes mellitus: A systematic review. *PLoS One, 13*(3), e0194987. Available from https://doi.org/10.1371/journal.pone.0194987.

Vella, A. (2016). Gastrointestinal hormones and gut endocrine tumors. In S. Melmed, K. S. Polonsky, P. R. Larson, & H. M. Kronenberg (Eds.), *Williams textbook of endocrinology* (13th ed., pp. 1701–1723). Philadelphia, PA: Elsevier.

You, C.-j, Liu, D., Liu, L.-l, & Li, G.-z (2018). Correlation between acute stroke-induced white matter lesions and insulin resistance. *Medicine, 97*(11), e9860. Available from https://doi.org/10.1097/md.0000000000009860.

CHAPTER

8

Hormonal regulation of fuel metabolism

Case study: lipodystrophy

Patient is a 35-year-old woman who was noticed since childhood to have increased muscle mass in her arms and legs, which was attributed to being athletic. Menarche was around the age of 11 and her periods were irregular occurring every 4–6 months. Her parents also noticed an increased appetite. Her father had the same phenotype. At the age of 32 the patient was diagnosed with type II diabetes mellitus, insulin resistance, hypertriglyceridemia, and fatty liver. She was 1.7 m tall and weighed 86 kg (body mass index, 28). On physical examination, she had markedly decreased subcutaneous adipose tissue sparing her face and neck. Her arms and legs were muscular with prominent veins. She had acanthosis nigricans around her neck, in the axilla and inguinal area and mild hepatomegaly. On laboratory evaluation, her fasting blood sugar was 129 mg/dL (normal <100 mg/dL), insulin level was 33 μU/mL (normal range 2.6–24 μU/mL), hemoglobin A1c was 7.6% (normal <5.6%), aspartate aminotransferase 94 U/L (normal range 0–32 U/L), alanine aminotransferase 88 U/L (normal 0–33 U/L), low-density lipoproteins was 64 mg/dL (optimal level <100–160 mg/dL depending on the cardiovascular risk), high-density lipoprotein was 34 mg/dL (optimal level >40 mg/dL), and triacylglycerols were 301 mg/dL (optimal level <150 mg/dL). Leptin level was low at 4.6 ng/mL (normal leptin level for her body mass index, 8.0–38.9 ng/mL). Abdominal ultrasound revealed hepatic steatosis. She was diagnosed with familial partial lipodystrophy of the Dunnigan variety caused by a mutation in the LMNA gene. To control her metabolic abnormalities, she was started on metformin and fenofibrate.

Leptin was discovered when the gene mutation in the *ob/ob* mouse, an animal model of obesity, was identified. Leptin is a polypeptide of 167 amino acids that is encoded by the obese (*ob*) gene. Leptin is produced primarily by the adipose cells and helps regulate the energy balance by inhibiting hunger. *Ob/ob* mice make a defective leptin protein and are extremely obese and hyperphagic. Since leptin administration causes a significant reduction in weight and food intake in these mice, it was hoped that leptin could be used to treat obesity in humans. However, leptin levels are proportional to fat tissue mass and are high in obese humans, suggesting that obese humans have leptin resistance. Administration of exogenous leptin in obese individuals had limited effect in inducing weight loss. But exogenous recombinant leptin has been successfully used to treat conditions characterized by low leptin levels such as lipodystrophy.

Lipodystrophies are a group of acquired or inherited disorders characterized by the selective loss of subcutaneous adipose tissue and low leptin levels. Individuals with lipodystrophy present with various degrees of subcutaneous fat tissue loss. Some lack fatty tissue in the face, neck, or extremities and some lack fat tissue altogether. While lipodystrophy is characterized by the loss of subcutaneous adipose tissue in certain areas of the body, organs such as liver and muscle have significant abnormal accumulation of fat, which impairs their metabolic activity. These patients have insulin resistance and are at risk for diabetes. They may also have lipid abnormalities, fatty infiltration of the liver, and polycystic ovarian syndrome. Typically, lipodystrophy patients have voracious appetite. Treatment of lipodystrophy includes the administration of insulin, oral hypoglycemic agents, and lipid-lowering drugs. Patients with generalized lipodystrophy who remain uncontrolled despite conventional treatment are candidates for injectable recombinant human leptin analog (metreleptin) treatment.

Goodman's Basic Medical Endocrinology.
DOI: https://doi.org/10.1016/B978-0-12-815844-9.00008-7

In the clinic: lipodystrophy

Introduction

Lipodystrophy is characterized by the loss of adipose tissue and low leptin levels. The etiology may be congenital or acquired and the involvement may be generalized or partial (Fig. 8.1).

Patients with lipodystrophy have extreme insulin resistance, diabetes, dyslipidemia, and hepatic steatosis.

Generalized lipodystrophies are rare disorders that can be congenital (Seip–Berardinelli syndrome) or acquired (Lawrence syndrome). These conditions are characterized by complete loss of subcutaneous fat. Congenital generalized lipodystrophy is an autosomal recessive disorder caused by mutations in the *AGPAT2*, *BSCL2*, *CAV1*, or *PTRF* genes. Acquired generalized lipodystrophy develops in previously healthy individuals. It is sometimes preceded by an episode of panniculitis. It may be associated with other autoimmune conditions, particularly juvenile dermatomyositis.

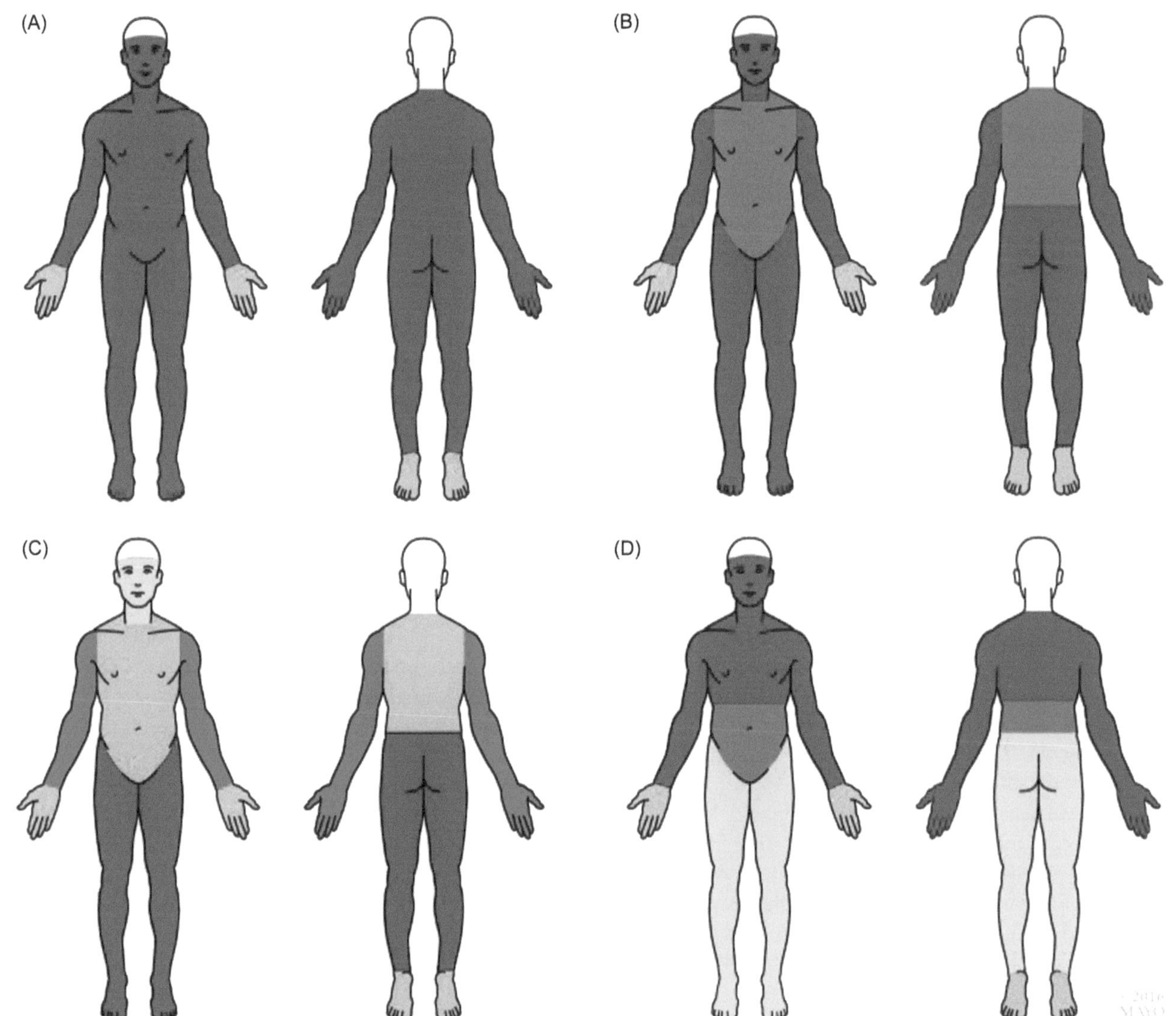

FIGURE 8.1 Distribution of adipose tissue in four major lipodystrophies [(A) congenital generalized lipodystrophy, (B) acquired generalized lipodystrophy, (C) familial partial lipodystrophy, and (D) acquired partial lipodystrophy]. Red, fat loss in >72% patients; brown, fat loss in 57%–72% patients; blue, fat loss in <57% patients; and green, fat sparing. For the purposes of uniformity in the pictorial representation, frequency cutoffs of >72%, 57%–72%, and <57% were used. Source: *Figure 2 from Gupta, N., Asi, N., Farah, W., Almasri, J., Barrionuevo, P., Alsawas, M., et al. Clinical features and management of non-HIV-related lipodystrophy in children: A systematic review.* The Journal of Clinical Endocrinology and Metabolism, 102*(2), 363–374.*

(*cont'd*)

Partial lipodystrophy is characterized by regional loss of subcutaneous fat with concurrent excess fat accumulation in nonatrophic areas. Congenital partial lipodystrophy includes familial partial lipodystrophy (most commonly caused by mutations in the *LMNA* or *PPARG* gene with autosomal dominant transmission, although other affected genes have been recently identified), partial lipodystrophy is due to *CAV1* mutation, mandibuloacral dysplasia, and a few other conditions that are extremely rare. In acquired partial lipodystrophy (Barraquer–Simons syndrome) the fat loss occurs during childhood or adolescence. This disease is thought to be caused by accelerated complement activation and a serum immunoglobulin G called C3 nephritic factor, which can cause lysis of adipose tissue. It is sometimes seen in association with other autoimmune conditions such as systemic lupus erythematosus and juvenile dermatomyositis, Patients with human immunodeficiency virus infection treated with antiretroviral therapy, especially HIV-1 protease inhibitors, can develop acquired partial lipodystrophy.

Signs and symptoms

Individuals with lipodystrophy present with generalized or localized loss of subcutaneous fat. This is evident at birth or in childhood in cases of congenital lipodystrophy or later in life in cases of acquired lipodystrophy. Patients with generalized lipodystrophy have complete or near complete lack of subcutaneous adipose tissue while patients with partial lipodystrophy lack subcutaneous fat tissue in certain areas such as face, neck, or extremities. Some patients with partial lipodystrophy have increased fat deposition in other parts of their body. As these patients have low leptin level, and leptin regulates satiety, individuals with lipodystrophy tend to have excessive appetite. On physical exams, lipodystrophy patients can have acanthosis nigricans (marker of insulin resistance), eruptive xanthomas (caused by hypertriacylglycerolemia), and signs of hyperandrogenism (associated with polycystic ovarian syndrome) such as hirsutism, acne, hair loss, and irregular periods. Fatty infiltration of the liver can cause hepatomegaly.

Diagnosis

Diagnosis of lipodystrophy is made based on clinical features (generalized or localized loss of subcutaneous fat tissue, increased appetite) and biochemical evaluation (low serum leptin levels, elevated blood sugar, dyslipidemia, in particular high triacylglycerol levels and elevated liver function tests if fatty liver is present). A positive family history of lipodystrophy can be present in congenital cases.

Management

The initial treatment of metabolic disturbances associated with lipodystrophy (diabetes, hypertriglyceridemia) consists in lifestyle modification (diet and exercise). If needed, insulin-sensitizing agents such as metformin and pioglitazone, insulin- and cholesterol-lowering medications such as statins or fibrates can be used. If metabolic disturbances persist, generalized lipodystrophy patients who have low leptin levels can be treated with injectable recombinant human leptin analog (metreleptin).

Hormonal regulation of fuel metabolism

Mammalian survival in a cold, hostile environment demands an uninterrupted supply of metabolic fuels to maintain body temperature, to escape from danger, and to grow and reproduce. Glucose and other energy-rich metabolic fuels must be absorbed and be available (Fig. 8.2).

It then must be available to the brain and other vital organs at all times despite wide fluctuations in food intake and energy expenditure. Constant availability of metabolic fuel is achieved by storing excess carbohydrate, fat, and protein principally in liver, adipose tissue, and muscle, and drawing on those reserves when needed. We consider here how fuel homeostasis is maintained minute-to-minute, day-to-day, and year-to-year by regulating fuel storage and mobilization, the mixture of fuels consumed in different physiological circumstances, and food intake.

Homeostatic regulation is provided by the endocrine system and the autonomic nervous system. The strategy of hormonal regulation of metabolism during starvation or exercise is to provide sufficient substrate to working muscles while maintaining an adequate concentration of glucose in blood to satisfy the needs of brain and other glucose-dependent cells. When dietary or stored carbohydrate is inadequate, availability of glucose is ensured by (1) gluconeogenesis from lactate, glycerol, and alanine and (2) inhibition of glucose utilization by those tissues that can satisfy their energy needs with other substrates, notably fatty acids and ketone bodies. The principal hormones that govern fuel homeostasis are insulin, glucagon, epinephrine, cortisol, growth hormone (GH), thyroid hormones, and leptin. The principal target organs for these hormones are adipose tissue, liver, and skeletal muscle.

General features of energy metabolism

In discussing how hormones regulate fuel metabolism, we consider first the characteristics of metabolic fuels and the intrinsic biochemical regulatory mechanisms upon which hormonal control is superimposed. This is summarized in Fig. 8.3.

Body fuels

Glucose

Glucose is readily oxidized by all cells. One gram yields about 4 cal. The average 70-kg man requires approximately 2000 cal/day and therefore would require a reserve supply of approximately 500 g of glucose to ensure sufficient substrate to survive 1 day of food deprivation (Fig. 8.4).

If glucose were stored as an isosmolar solution, approximately 10 L of water (10 kg) would be needed to accommodate a single day's energy needs, and the 70-kg man would have to carry around a storage depot equal to his own weight if he were to survive only 1 week of starvation. Actually, only about 20 g of free glucose are dissolved in extracellular fluids, or enough to provide energy for about 1 hour.

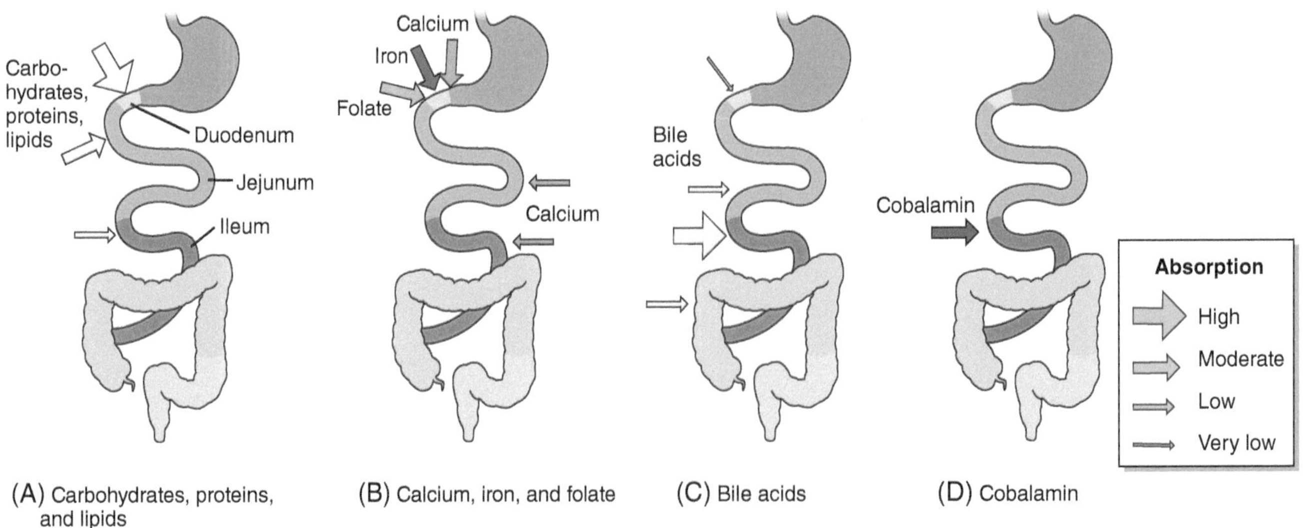

FIGURE 8.2 The absorption areas of the intestinal tract. Of interest for this chapter is the absorption of carbohydrates, proteins, and lipids that are absorbed best in the duodenum. Source: *Redrawn from Figure 45-2 in Binder, H. J., & Mansbach, C. M., II. (2017). Chapter 45: Nutrient digestion and absorption. In W. F. Boron, & E. Boulpaep (Eds.),* Medical physiology *(3rd ed.) (p. 914). Elsevier.*

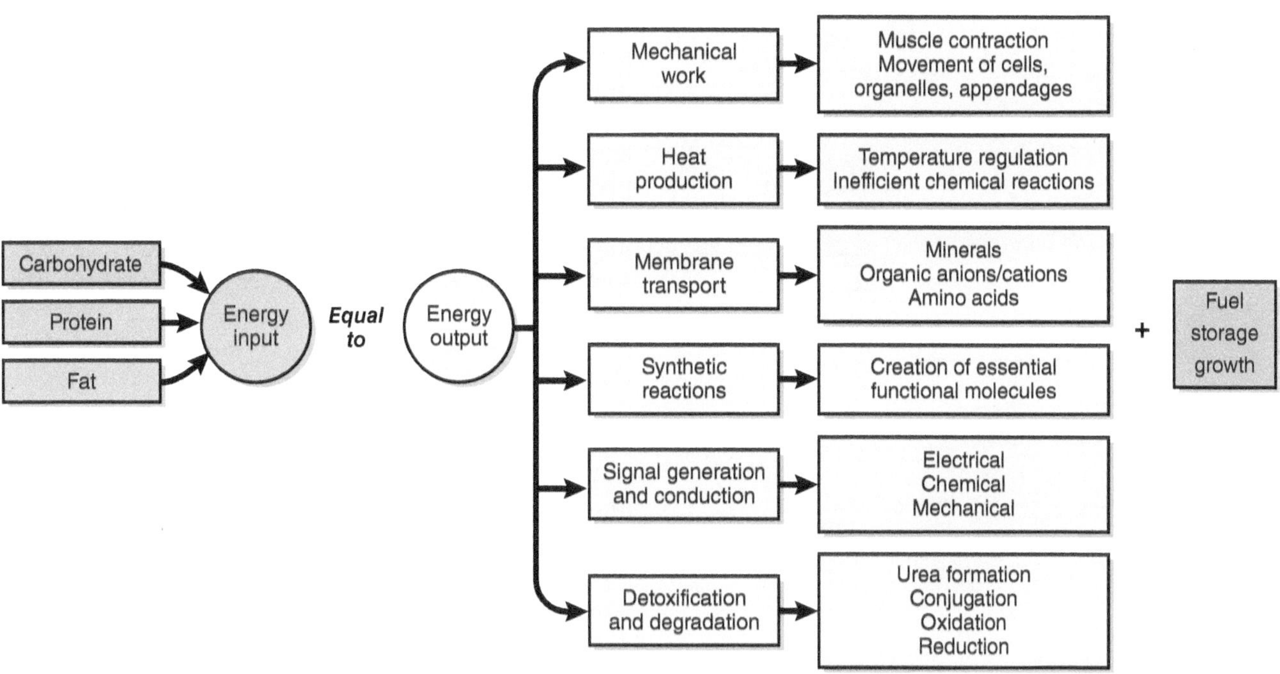

FIGURE 8.3 Energy balance: where the energy goes when food is ingested. Source: *Redrawn from Figure 58.4 from Shulman, G. I., & Peterson, K. F. (2017). Chapter 58: Metabolism. In W. F. Boron, & E. Boulpaep (Eds.),* Medical physiology *(3rd ed.) (p. 1173). Elsevier.*

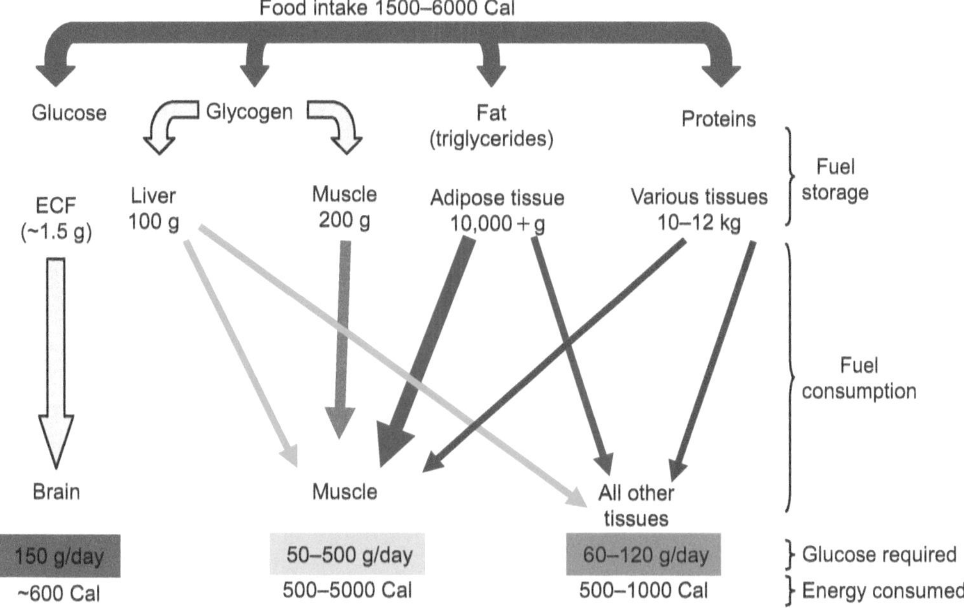

FIGURE 8.4 Storage and utilization of biological fuels.

Glycogen

Polymerizing glucose to glycogen eliminates the osmotic requirement for large volumes of water (Fig. 8.5).

To meet a single day's energy needs, only about 1.8 kg of "wet" glycogen is required; that is, 500 g of glycogen requires only about 1.3 L of water. Glycogen stores in the well-fed 70-kg man are enough to meet only part of a day's energy needs—about 100 g of glycogen in the liver and about 200 g in muscle.

Protein

Calories can also be stored in somewhat more concentrated form as protein. Storage of protein, however,

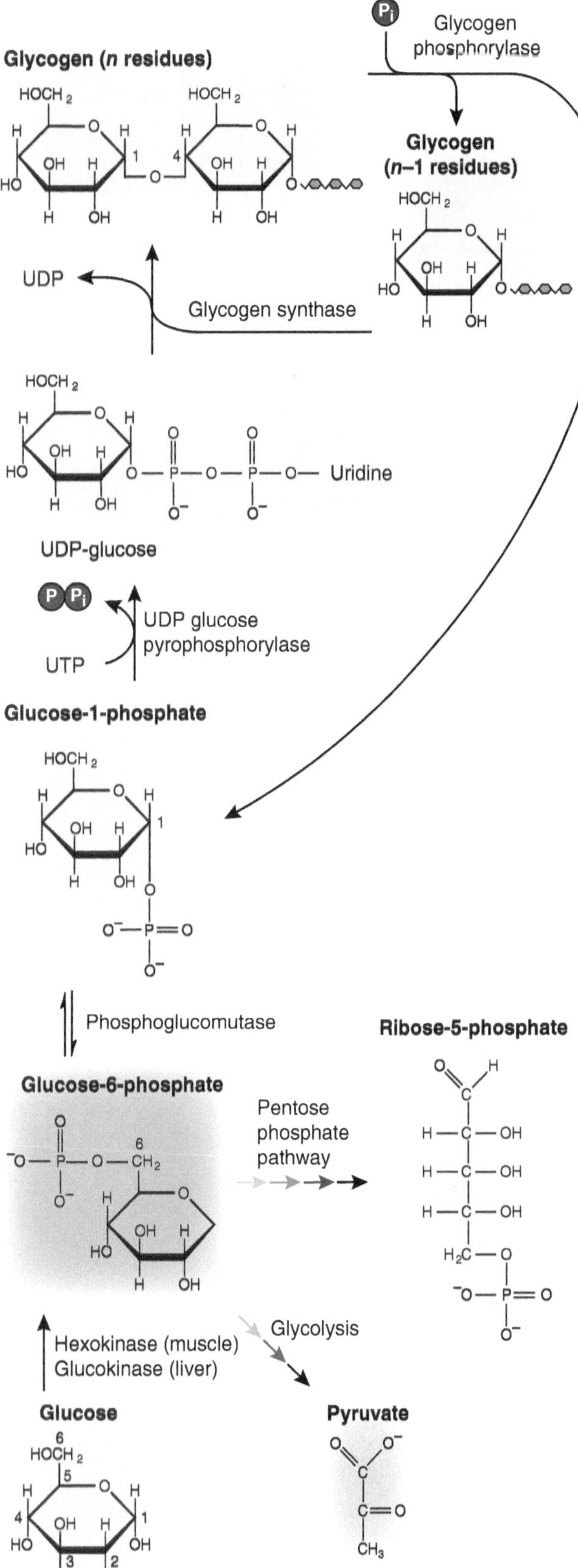

FIGURE 8.5 The formation of glycogen from glucose. Glucose (bottom) is phosphorylated and then joined to other glucose molecules in either a straight chain (1–4 linkage) or branched chain (1–6 linkage). Glycogen (animals) and starch (plants) are both formed the same way but glycogen is more branched. Source: *Redrawn from Figure 58-1 in Shulman, G. I., & Peterson, K. F. (2017). Chapter 58: Metabolism. In W. F. Boron, & E. Boulpaep (Eds.),* Medical physiology *(3rd ed.) (p. 1171). Elsevier.*

also obligates storage of some water, and oxidation of protein creates unique by-products: ammonia, which must be detoxified to form urea at metabolic expense, and sulfur-containing acids. The body of a normal 70-kg man in nitrogen balance contains about 10–12 kg of protein, most of which is in skeletal muscle. Little or no protein is stored as an inert fuel depot, so that mobilization of protein for energy necessarily produces some functional deficits. Under conditions of prolonged starvation, as much as one-half of the body protein may be consumed for energy before death ensues, usually from failure of respiratory muscles.

Fat

Triacylglycerols (TAGs, formerly called triglycerides) are by far the most concentrated storage form of high-energy fuel (9 cal/g), and they can be stored essentially without water. They are formed from glycerol and three free fatty acids (FFAs) (Fig. 8.6).

One day's energy needs can be met by less than 250 g of TAG. Thus a 70-kg man carrying 10 kg of fat maintains an adequate depot of fuel to meet energy needs for more than 40 days. Most fat is stored in adipose tissue, but other tissues such as muscle and bone marrow also contain small reserves of TAGs.

Problems inherent in the use of glucose and fat as metabolic fuels

Fat is the most abundant and efficient energy reserve, but efficiency has its price. When converting dietary carbohydrate to fat, about 25% of the energy is dissipated as heat. More importantly, the synthesis of fatty acids from glucose is an irreversible process. Once the carbons of glucose are converted to fatty acids, virtually none can be reconverted to glucose. The glycerol portion of TAGs remains convertible to glucose, but glycerol represents only about 10% of the mass of TAG.

Limited water solubility of fat complicates transport between tissues. TAGs are "packaged" as very low-density lipoproteins or as chylomicrons for transport in blood to storage sites. Uptake by cells follows breakdown to fatty acids by lipoprotein lipase at the external surface or within capillaries of muscle or fat cells. Mobilization of stored TAGs also requires breakdown

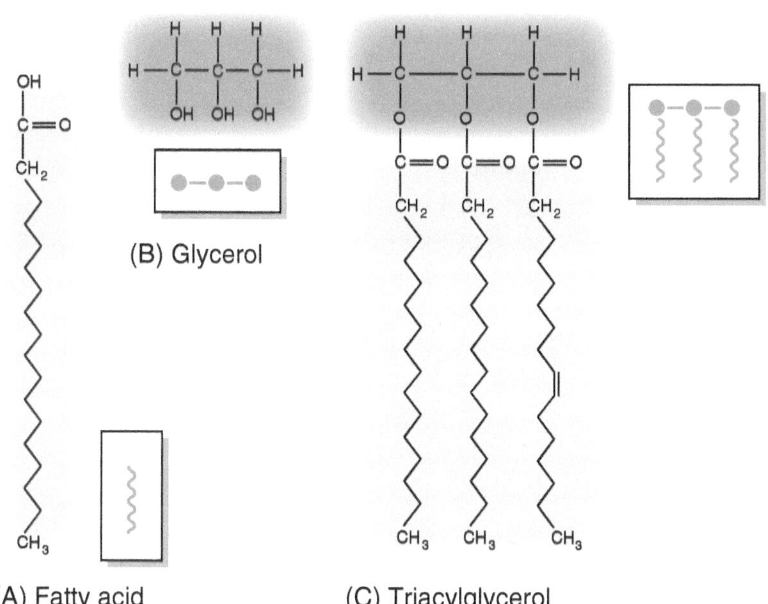

FIGURE 8.6 The formation of a TAG from glycerol and three fatty acids, in this case two palmitic and one palmitoleic (it has one double bond) acid. Glycerol is a trihydroxy alcohol derived from glucose. *TAG*, Triacylglycerol. Source: *Redrawn from Figure 45-11 in Binder, H. J., & Mansbach, C. M., II. (2017). Chapter 45: Nutrient digestion and absorption. In W. F. Boron, & E. Boulpaep (Eds.),* Medical physiology *(3rd ed.) (p. 926). Elsevier.*

to fatty acids, which leave adipocytes in the form of FFAs. FFAs are not very soluble in water and are transported in blood firmly bound to albumin. Because they are bound to albumin, FFAs have limited access to tissues such as brain; they can be processed to water-soluble forms in the liver, however, which converts them to 4-carbon ketone bodies, which can cross the blood–brain barrier.

Energy can be derived from glucose without simultaneous consumption of oxygen, but oxygen is required for degradation of fat. Therefore glucose must be constantly available in the blood to satisfy the needs of red blood cells, which lack mitochondria, and cells in the renal medullae, which function under low oxygen tension. Under basal conditions, these cells consume about 50 g of glucose each day and release an equivalent amount of lactate into the blood. Because lactate is readily reconverted to glucose in the liver, however, these tissues do not act as a drain on carbohydrate reserves.

In a well-nourished person the brain relies almost exclusively on glucose to meet its energy needs and consumes nearly 150 g/day. The brain does not derive energy from oxidation of FFA or amino acids. Ketone bodies are the only alternative substrates to glucose, but studies in experimental animals indicate that only certain regions of the brain can substitute ketone bodies for glucose. Total fasting for 4–5 days is required before the concentrations of ketone bodies in blood are high enough to provide a significant fraction of the brain's energy needs. Even after several weeks of total starvation, the brain continues to satisfy about one-third of its energy needs with glucose. The brain stores little glycogen and hence must depend on the circulation to meet its minute-to-minute fuel requirements. The rate of glucose delivery depends on its concentration in arterial blood, the rate of blood flow, and the efficiency of extraction. Although an increased flow rate might compensate for decreased glucose concentrations, the mechanisms that regulate blood flow in brain are responsive to oxygen and carbon dioxide, rather than glucose. Under basal conditions the concentration of glucose in arterial blood is about 5 mM (90 mg/dL), of which the brain extracts about 10%. The fraction extracted can double, or perhaps even triple, when the concentration of glucose is low, but when the blood glucose concentration falls below about 30 mg/dL, metabolism and function are compromised. Thus the brain is exceedingly vulnerable to hypoglycemia, which can quickly produce coma or death.

Fuel consumption

The amount of metabolic fuel consumed in a day varies widely and normally is balanced by variations in food intake, but the adipose tissue reservoir of TAGs can shrink or expand to accommodate imbalance in fuel intake and expenditure. Muscle comprises about 50% of body mass and is by far the major consumer of metabolic fuels. Even at rest muscle metabolism accounts for about 30% of the oxygen consumed. Although normally a 56-kg woman or a 70-kg man consumes about 1600 or 2000 cal in a typical day, daily caloric requirements may range from about 1000 with complete bed rest to as much as 6000 with prolonged physical activity. For example, marathon running may consume 3000 cal in only 3 hours.

Under basal conditions an individual on a typical mixed diet derives about half of the daily energy needs from the oxidation of glucose, a small fraction from consumption of protein, and the remainder from fat. With starvation or with prolonged exercise, limited carbohydrate reserves are quickly exhausted unless some restriction is placed on carbohydrate consumption by muscle, the fuel needs of which far exceed those of any other tissue and can be met by increased utilization of fat. In fact, simply providing muscle with fat restricts its ability to consume carbohydrate. Hormonal regulation of energy balance is accomplished largely through adjusting the flux of energy-rich fatty acids and their derivatives to muscle, and the consequent sparing of carbohydrate and protein.

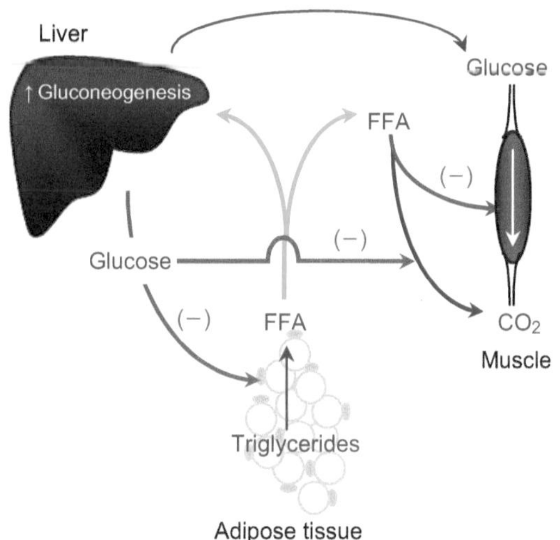

FIGURE 8.7 Intraorgan flow of substrate and the competitive regulatory effects of glucose and fatty acids that comprise the glucose–fatty acid cycle. See text for details.

The glucose fatty acid cycle

The reciprocal relationship in which availability of fatty acids to muscle limits glucose utilization while abundance of glucose limits fat utilization has been called the glucose fatty acid cycle (Figs. 8.7 and 8.8).

The biochemical mechanisms originally proposed to account for this relationship were based on studies of rodent muscle and have since been challenged by more recent studies in human subjects. Nevertheless, the fact that fatty acids can curtail the metabolism of glucose by muscle and that glucose can curtail the availability and hence the oxidation of fatty acids remains a cornerstone of metabolic regulation. Fatty acids are released from their TAG storage form in adipose tissue in an ongoing cycle of lipolysis and reesterification. The fatty acids that escape reesterification diffuse out of adipocytes and become the plasma FFAs.

Reesterification or uptake of FFA from circulating lipids depends on the availability of α-glycerol phosphate in adipocytes. In the fed individual the only source of α-glycerol phosphate is the pool of triose phosphates derived from glucose oxidation, as adipose tissue is deficient in the enzyme required to phosphorylate and hence reuse the glycerol that is released from TAGs. Consequently, when glucose and insulin are abundant, α-glycerol phosphate is readily available, the rate of reesterification is high relative to lipolysis, and the rate of release of FFA is low. Conversely, when glucose is scarce or insulin concentrations are low, more fatty acids escape and plasma concentrations of FFA increase.

FFAs are taken up by muscle in proportion to their plasma concentration. Exposure of muscle to elevated levels of FFA for several hours decreases transport of glucose across the plasma membrane and phosphorylation to glucose-6-phosphate. The mechanism for this effect is incompletely understood, but it is likely that accumulation of some fatty acid–derived metabolite interferes with elements of the insulin signaling pathway that lead to recruitment and retention of glucose transporters to the plasma membrane. The decrease in glucose transport decreases glucose-6-phosphate, which is both a substrate and an allosteric activator of glycogen synthase, and results in decreased glycogen formation and glucose oxidation by glycolysis. Downstream effects on carbohydrate oxidation may also occur. Oxidation of fatty acids or ketone bodies limits the oxidation of pyruvate to acetyl coenzyme A (CoA).

It may be recalled (see Chapter 7: The Pancreatic Islets) that long-chain fatty acids must be linked to carnitine to gain entry into mitochondria where they are oxidized (Fig. 8.9).

Accumulating long-chain fatty acid CoA molecules allosterically increase the activity of acylcarnitine transferase, which is required for their entry into mitochondria. In the mitochondria, long-chain fatty acids or ketone bodies compete with pyruvate for limited amounts of CoA and the oxidized form of the cofactor nicotinamide adenine dinucleotide (NAD). The resulting scarcity of NAD and CoA limits the breakdown of pyruvate. It should be noted that oxidation of pyruvate to acetyl CoA is the reaction that irreversibly removes carbons from the pool of metabolites that are convertible to glucose.

Influx of fatty acids to the liver promotes ketogenesis (Fig. 8.10) and gluconeogenesis (Fig. 8.11).

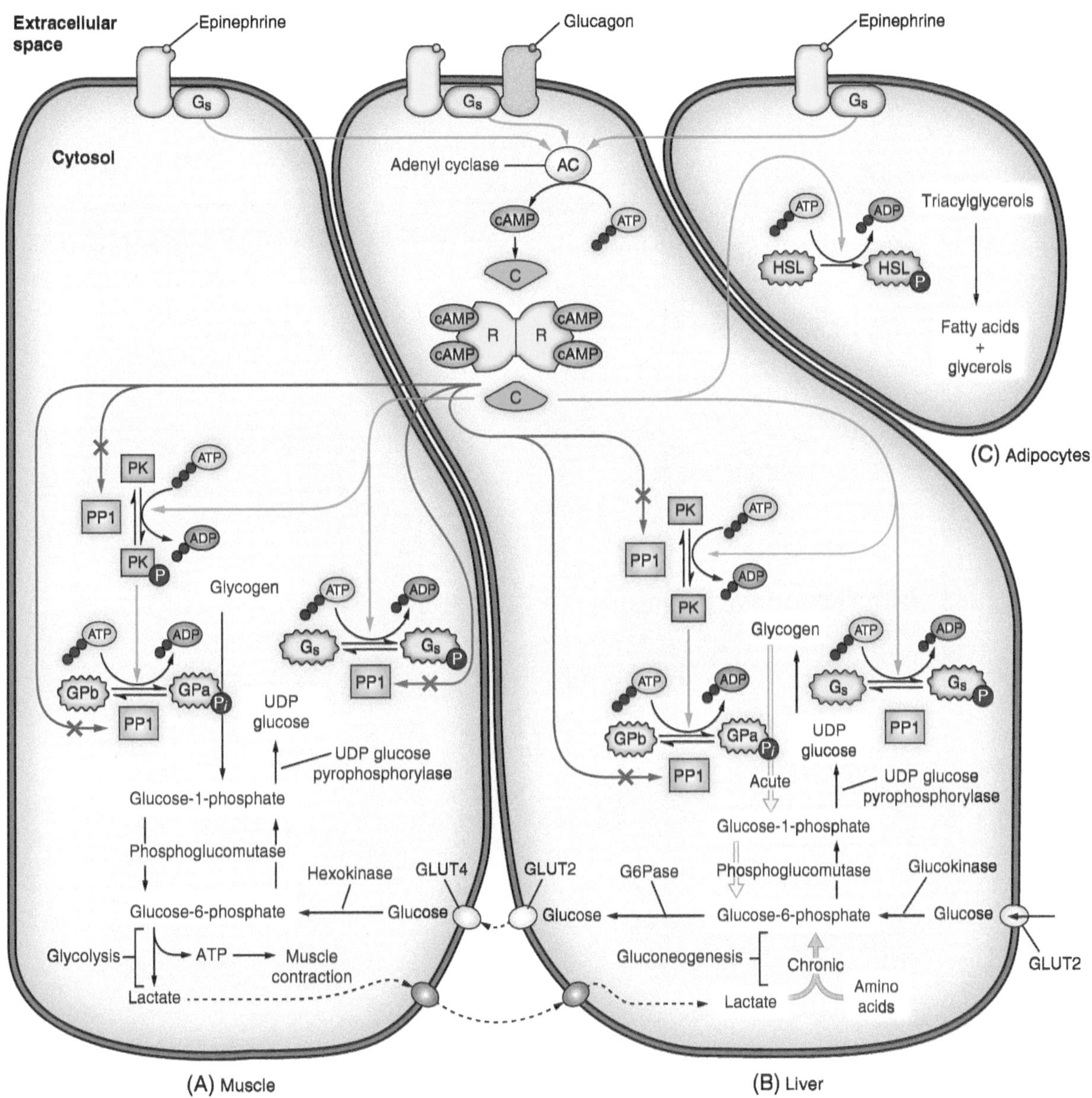

FIGURE 8.8 A more detailed illustration of the relationship between (A) muscle, (B) liver, and (C) adipocytes. Source: *Redrawn from Figure 58-9 in Shulman, G. I., & Peterson, K. F. (2017). Chapter 58: Metabolism. In W. F. Boron, & E. Boulpaep (Eds.),* Medical physiology *(3rd ed.) (p. 1183). Elsevier.*

Metabolism of long-chain fatty acids inhibits the intramitochondrial oxidation of pyruvate to acetyl CoA. Gluconeogenic precursors arriving at the liver in the form of pyruvate, lactate, alanine, or glycerol are thus spared oxidation in the tricarboxylic acid cycle and instead are converted to phosphoenol pyruvate and thence to glucose. Conversely, when glucose is abundant, the concentration of glucose-6-phosphate increases, and gluconeogenesis is inhibited both at the level of fructose-1,6-bisphosphate formation and at the level of pyruvate kinase (Chapter 7: The Pancreatic Islets, Fig. 7.3). Under these circumstances, malonyl CoA formation is increased and fatty acids are restrained from entering the mitochondria and subsequent degradation.

Through the reciprocal effects of glucose and fatty acids, glucose indirectly regulates its own rate of utilization and production by a negative feedback process that depends on intrinsic allosteric regulatory properties of metabolites and enzymes of the glucose fatty acid cycle. Hormones regulate fuel metabolism by altering the activities or amounts of enzymes, and by influencing the flow of metabolites. The glucose fatty

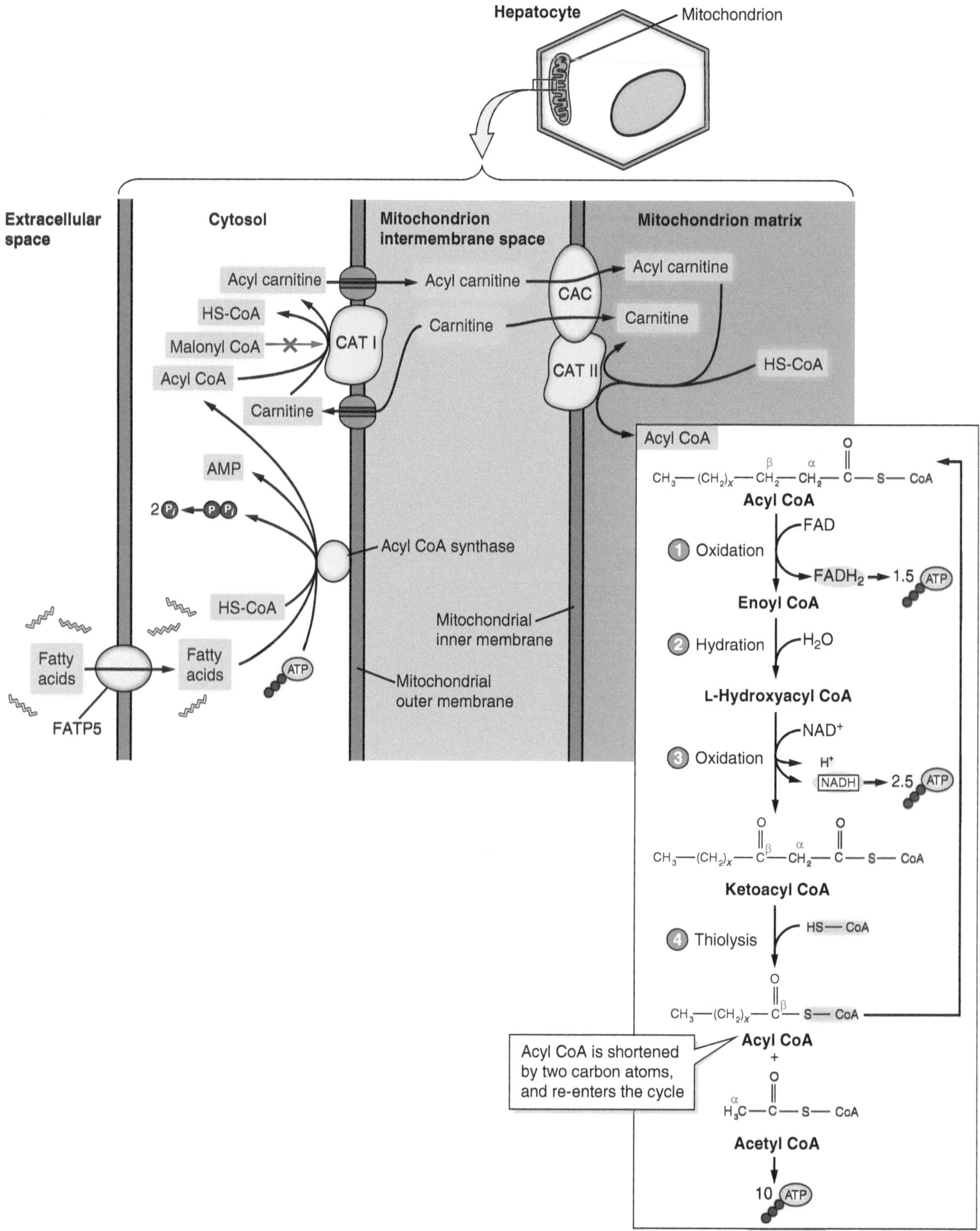

FIGURE 8.9 The transport of fatty acids into the mitochondrion and beta oxidation within the mitochondria. Source: *Redrawn from Figure 58-10 in Shulman, G. I., & Peterson, K. F. (2017). Chapter 58: Metabolism. In W. F. Boron, & E. Boulpaep (Eds.),* Medical physiology *(3rd ed.) (p. 1184). Elsevier.*

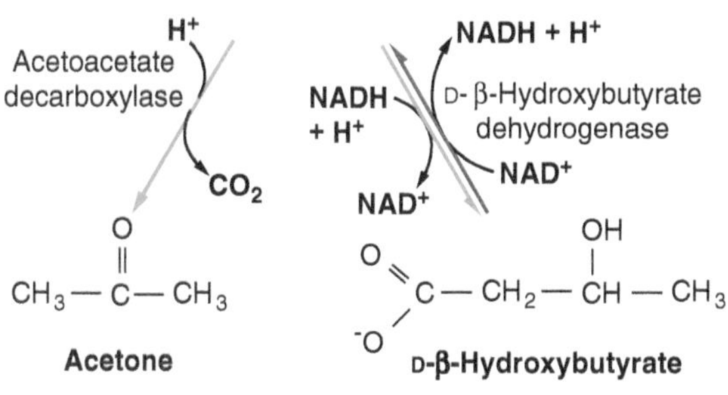

FIGURE 8.10 Ketogenesis in the liver. Source: *Redrawn from Figure 58.12 in Shulman, G. I., & Peterson, K. F. (2017). Chapter 58: Metabolism. In W. F. Boron, & E. Boulpaep (Eds.),* Medical physiology *(3rd ed.) (p. 1187). Elsevier.*

acid cycle operates in normal physiology even though the concentration of glucose in blood remains nearly constant. In fact, the contribution of some hormones, notably glucocorticoids and GH, to the maintenance of blood glucose and muscle glycogen stores depends in part on the glucose fatty acid cycle. Conversely, in addition to stimulating glucose entry into muscle, insulin indirectly increases glucose metabolism by decreasing FFA mobilization from adipose tissue, thereby reducing the inhibitory influence of the glucose fatty acid cycle. This effect is accelerated by a further effect of insulin to increase the formation of malonyl CoA in liver and muscle, thereby diminishing access of fatty acids to the mitochondrial oxidative apparatus and redirecting their disposition to formation of TAGs.

Adenosine monophosphate–activated kinase (AMPK)

All cells require adequate amounts of adenosine triphosphate (ATP) to survive and have the capacity to adjust their metabolism to maximize energy production and minimize energy utilization. Depletion of cellular energy is monitored as accumulation of 5′-adenosine monophosphate (AMP) relative to ATP. It may be recalled that energy-consuming processes are fueled by the conversion of ATP to adenosine diphosphate (ADP). ATP is regenerated by oxidative phosphorylation in mitochondria when adequate amounts of metabolic fuels are available, and by the transfer of a high-energy phosphate from one ADP to another according to the reaction: ADP + ADP → ATP + AMP. Cellular concentrations of AMP therefore increase dramatically and ATP concentrations fall when ATP consumption exceeds mitochondrial production. Increases in the ratio of AMP concentrations to ATP allosterically activate the ubiquitously expressed enzyme AMP-activated kinase (AMPK). The activity of AMPK also is increased by phosphorylation. AMPK catalyzes reactions that amplify availability of metabolic fuels and dampen ATP-consuming processes.

In muscle (Fig. 8.12), AMPK increases glucose availability by stimulating the translocation of the glucose transporter GLUT4 to plasma membranes in a manner similar to that described for insulin in Chapter 7, The Pancreatic Islets. AMPK also stimulates glycolysis and inhibits glycogen synthesis. Activated AMPK increases fatty acid oxidation. It catalyzes the phosphorylation and hence inactivation of acetyl CoA carboxylase, the enzyme that forms malonyl CoA. It also catalyzes the phosphorylation, and hence activation, of the enzyme malonyl CoA decarboxylase and thus depletes malonyl CoA, which impedes the access of fatty acids to intramitochondrial oxidative machinery. Accelerated oxidation of intramuscular lipids has the additional effect of relieving inhibition of glucose transport discussed earlier.

In liver, as in muscle, AMPK decreases malonyl CoA and channels long-chain fatty acid CoA molecules toward oxidation in mitochondria and away from the

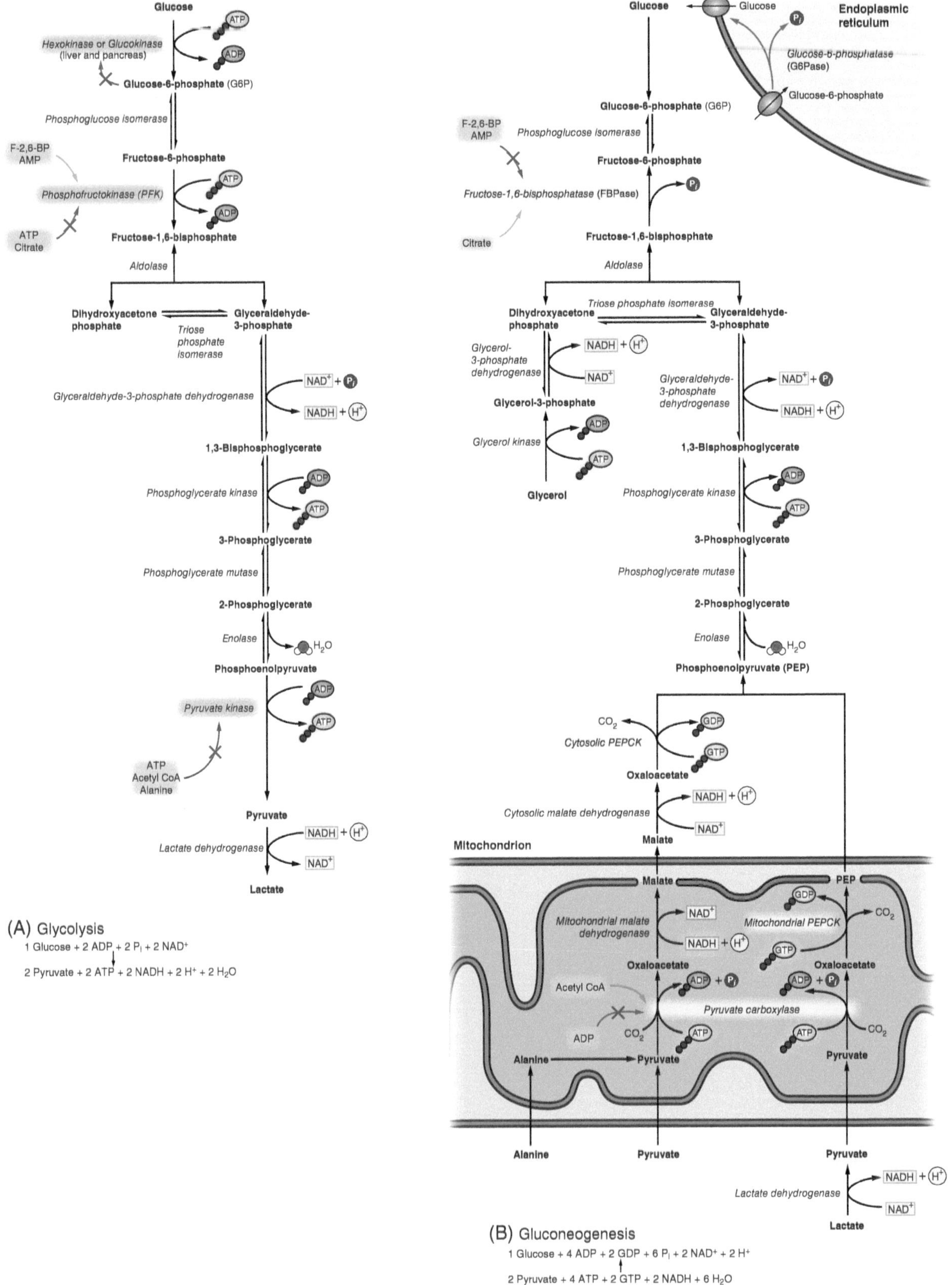

FIGURE 8.11 Gluconeogenesis from alanine, pyruvate, and lactate. Highlighted in blue are the three cytosolic and two mitochondrial enzymes that bypass the irreversible enzymes of glycolysis and allows the formation of glucose from alanine, pyruvate, and lactate. Source: *Redrawn from Figure 58-6 B in Shulman, G. I., & Peterson, K. F. (2017). Chapter 58: Metabolism. In W. F. Boron, & E. Boulpaep (Eds.),* Medical physiology *(3rd ed.) (p. 1175). Elsevier.*

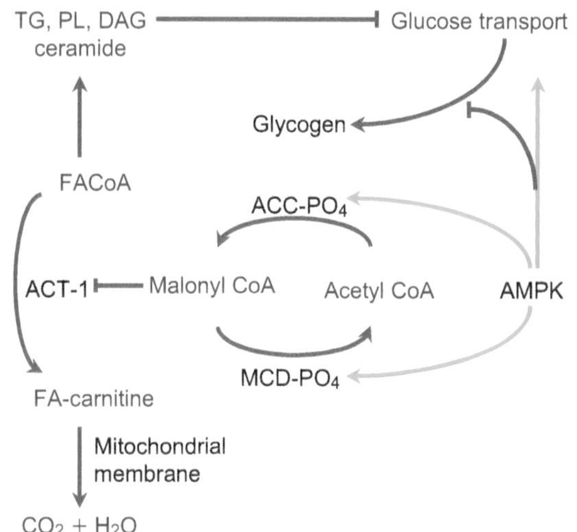

FIGURE 8.12 Actions of AMP-activated protein kinase (*AMPK*) in muscle increase oxidation of fatty acids and glucose. Phosphorylation inactivates *ACC* and activates *MCD*. (See text for details). *ACC*, Acetyl CoA carboxylase; *ACT-1*, acyl carnitine transferase-1; *AMP*, adenosine monophosphate; *DAG*, diacylglycerol; *FA-carnitine*, fatty acyl carnitine; *FACoA*, fatty acyl coenzyme A; *MCD*, malonyl CoA decarboxylase; *PL*, phospholipids; *TG*, triglyceride.

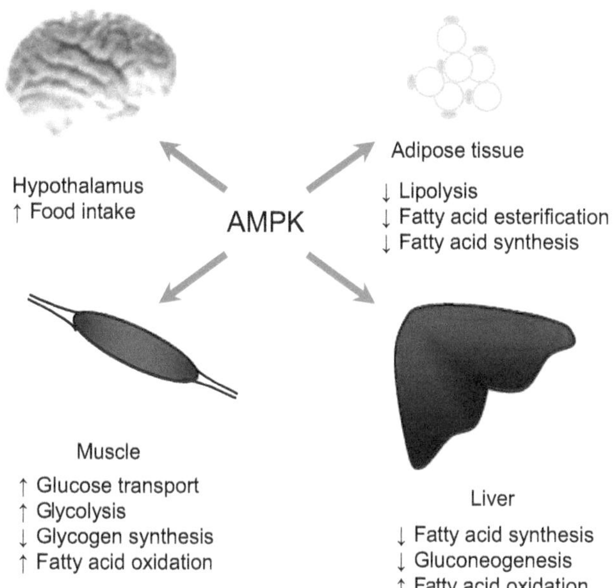

FIGURE 8.13 Multiple effects of AMP-activated kinase (*AMPK*) that summate to increase energy-producing reactions and inhibit energy-consuming reactions.

energy-consuming processes of formation of TAGs and lipoproteins (Fig. 8.4). Because malonyl CoA formation is the rate-determining step in fatty acid synthesis, a decrease in its production decreases the ATP-consuming process of fatty acid synthesis. AMPK also inhibits a key enzyme in the conversion of acetyl CoA to cholesterol.

In adipose tissue, AMPK slows the costly cycle of lipolysis and reesterification by inhibiting both hormone-sensitive lipase and glucose transport. Because only a small fraction of the fatty acids that participate in this process escape as FFA, this apparently paradoxical effect actually conserves ATP without significantly cutting off the supply of plasma FFA. AMPK also inhibits fatty acid synthesis, uptake of fatty acids from circulating lipids, and their esterification to TAGs.

Because its actions accelerate the metabolism of both glucose and fatty acids in ATP-deficient states, activation of AMPK overrides competition between glucose and fatty acids. In addition to responding to local conditions in individual cells, AMPK is also responsive to hormonal and neural regulation and thus participates in coordinated actions at the whole-body level. As discussed later in this chapter, such coordination is reflected in regulation of food intake and preserving sensitivity to insulin stimulation of carbohydrate metabolism in states of excessive fat storage. The effects of AMPK in regulating malonyl CoA levels in key areas of the brain complement the overall actions of this metabolite as the body's "fuel gauge" as reflected in its importance in controlling food intake and energy expenditure (Fig. 8.13)

Overall regulation of blood glucose concentration

Despite vagaries in dietary input and large fluctuations in food consumption, the concentration of glucose in blood remains remarkably constant. Its concentration at any time is determined by the rate of input and the rate of removal by the various body tissues (Fig. 8.14).

The rate of glucose removal from the blood varies over a wide range depending on physical activity and environmental temperature. Even immediately after eating, the rate of input largely reflects activity of the liver because glucose and other metabolites absorbed from the intestine must pass through the liver before entering the circulation.

Liver glycogen is the immediate source of blood glucose under most circumstances. Hepatic gluconeogenesis contributes to blood glucose directly and is important for replenishing glycogen stores. The kidneys are also capable of gluconeogenesis, but their contribution to blood glucose has not been studied as thoroughly as that of the liver. However, some recent estimates credit the kidneys with the production of as much as 20%–40% of the glucose released during fasting. In acidosis, renal glucose production from glutamate accompanies production and excretion of ammonium.

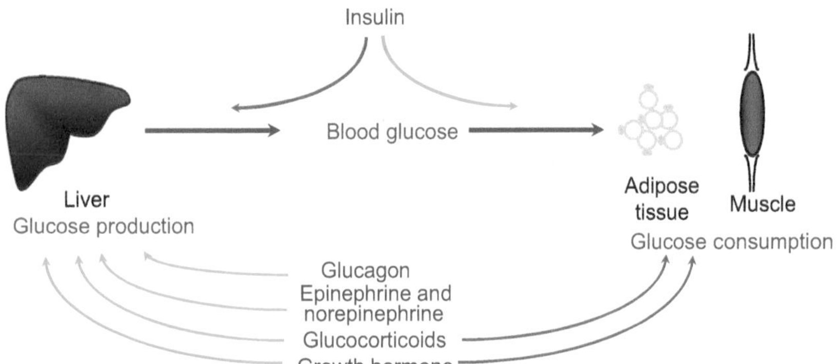

FIGURE 8.14 Interaction of hormones to maintain the blood glucose concentration. Green arrows denote increase and red arrows denote decrease.

Short-term regulation

Minute-to-minute regulation of blood glucose depends on (1) insulin, which, in promoting fuel storage, drives glucose concentrations down and (2) glucagon, and to a lesser extent catecholamines, which, in mobilizing fuel reserves, drive glucose concentrations up. Effects of these hormones are evident within seconds or minutes and dissipate as quickly. Insulin acts at the level of the liver to inhibit glucose output, and on muscle and fat to increase glucose uptake.

Liver is more responsive to insulin than muscle and fat, and because of its anatomical location, is exposed to higher hormone concentrations. Smaller increments in insulin concentration are needed to inhibit glucose production than to promote glucose uptake. Glucagon and catecholamines act on hepatocytes to promote glycogenolysis and gluconeogenesis. They have no direct effects on glucose uptake by peripheral tissues, but epinephrine and norepinephrine may decrease the demand for blood glucose by mobilizing alternative fuels, glycogen and fat, within muscle and adipose tissue. Increased blood glucose is perceived directly by pancreatic beta cells, which respond by secreting insulin.

Hypoglycemia is perceived not only by the glucagon-secreting alpha cells of pancreatic islets but also by glucose-sensing neurons in the hypothalamus and the hindbrain. These neurons communicate with neurons in autonomic centers and activate sympathetic outflow to the islets of Langerhans, the liver, and the adrenal medullae. Sympathetic stimulation of pancreatic islets increases the secretion of glucagon and inhibits the secretion of insulin. In addition, hypoglycemia evokes the secretion of the hypothalamic-releasing hormones that stimulate adrenocorticotropic hormone (ACTH) and GH secretion from the pituitary gland. Cortisol, secreted in response to ACTH, and GH act only after a substantial delay and hence are unlikely to contribute to rapid restoration of blood glucose. However, they are important for withstanding a sustained hypoglycemic challenge. Collectively, hormones that oppose the actions of insulin on blood glucose are referred to as counterregulatory hormones (Fig. 8.15).

Long-term regulation

Operative on a time scale of hours or perhaps days, long-term regulation depends on direct and indirect actions of many hormones and ultimately ensures (1) that the peripheral drain on glucose reserves is minimized and (2) that liver contains an adequate reservoir of glycogen to satisfy minute-to-minute needs of glucose-dependent cells. To achieve these ends, peripheral tissues, mainly muscle, must be provided with alternate substrate and must limit their consumption of glucose. At the same time, gluconeogenesis must be stimulated and supplied with adequate precursors to provide the 150–200 g of glucose needed each day by the brain and other glucose-dependent tissues. Long-term regulation includes all the responses that govern glucose utilization as well as all those reactions that govern storage of fuel as glycogen, protein, or TAGs.

Integrated actions of metabolic hormones

Metabolic fuels absorbed from the intestine are converted largely to storage forms in liver, adipocytes, and muscle. It is fair to state that storage is virtually the exclusive province of insulin, which stimulates biochemical reactions that convert simple compounds to more complex storage forms and inhibits fuel mobilization. Counterregulatory hormones that mobilize fuel and defend the glucose concentration include glucagon, epinephrine, whenever there is increased demand for energy. These hormones act synergistically and together produce effects that are greater than the sum of their individual actions. In the example shown in Fig. 8.16, glucagon and epinephrine raised the blood glucose level primarily by increasing hepatic production. When cortisol was given simultaneously, these effects were magnified, even though cortisol had little effect when given alone. Triiodothyronine (T3) must also be considered in this context, as its actions increase the rate of fuel consumption and the sensitivity of target cells to insulin and counterregulatory

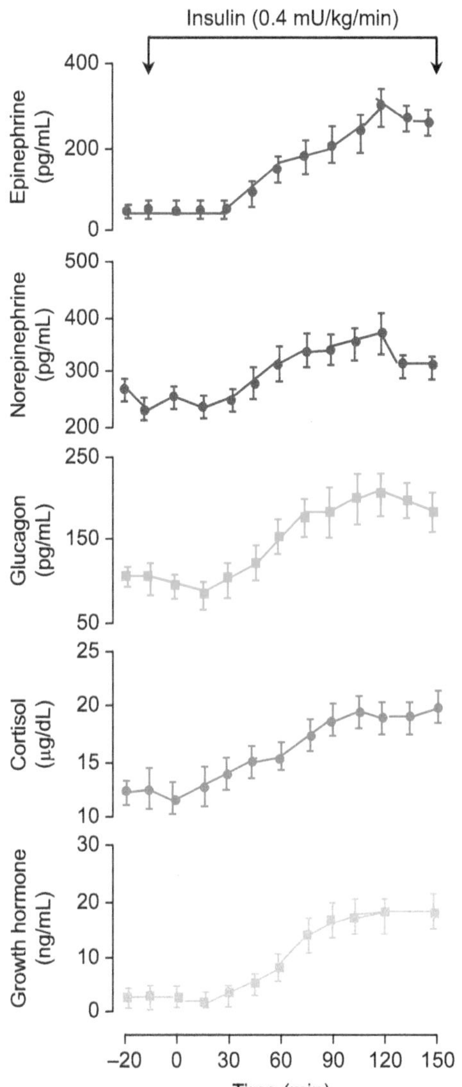

FIGURE 8.15 Counterregulatory hormonal responses to insulin-induced hypoglycemia. The infusion of insulin reduced plasma glucose concentration to 50–55 mg/dL. Source: *From Sacca, L., Sherwin, R., Hendler, R., & Felig, P. (1979). Influence of continuous physiologic hyperinsulinemia on glucose kinetics and counterregulatory hormones in normal and diabetic humans.* Journal of Clinical Investigation, 63, *849–857.*

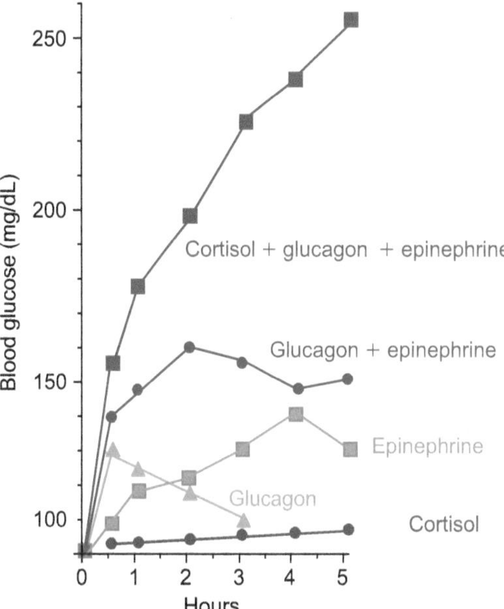

FIGURE 8.16 Synergistic effects of cortisol, glucagon, and epinephrine on increasing plasma glucose concentration. Note that the hyperglycemic response to the triple hormone infusion is far greater than the additive response of all three hormones given singly. Source: *Redrawn from data of Eigler, N., Sacca, L., & Sherwin, R. S. (1979). Synergistic interactions of physiologic increments of glucagon, epinephrine, and cortisol in the dog.* Journal of Clinical Investigation, 63, *114–123.*

hormones. Before examining the interactions of these hormones in the whole body, it is useful to summarize their effects on individual tissues.

Adipose tissue

The central event in adipose tissue metabolism is the cycle of fatty acid esterification and TAG lipolysis (Fig. 8.17).

Although reesterification of fatty acids can regulate FFA output from fat cells, regulation of lipolysis and hence the rate at which the cycle spins provides a wider range of control. It has been estimated that under basal conditions 20% of the fatty acids released in lipolysis are reesterified to TAGs, and that reesterification may decrease to 9% or 10% during active fuel consumption. Under the same conditions, lipolysis may be varied over a 10-fold range. Catecholamines and insulin, through their antagonistic effects on cyclic AMP metabolism, increase or decrease the activity of hormone-sensitive lipase. Human adipocytes express β-adrenergic receptors that signal through increased cyclic AMP and hence increase lipolysis. Responses to catecholamines and insulin are expressed within minutes. Other hormones, especially cortisol, T3, and GH, modulate the sensitivity of adipocytes to insulin and catecholamines. Modulation is not a reflection of abrupt changes in hormone concentrations but, rather, stems from long-term tuning of metabolic machinery. Finally, GH produces a sustained increase in lipolysis after a delay of about 2 hours. GH and cortisol also decrease fatty acid esterification by inhibiting glucose metabolism in adipose tissue both directly and by decreasing responsiveness to insulin. These hormonal effects on adipose tissue are summarized in Fig. 8.18.

Muscle

By inhibiting FFA mobilization, insulin promptly decreases plasma FFA concentrations and thus

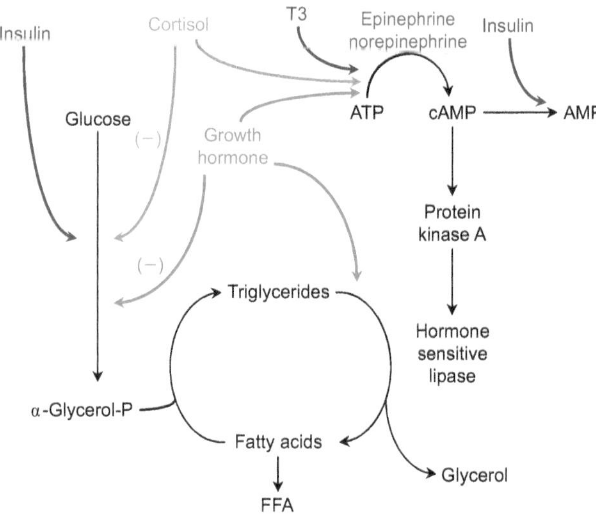

FIGURE 8.17 Hormonal effects on FFA production. Epinephrine and norepinephrine stimulate hormone-sensitive lipase through a cyclic AMP-mediated process. Insulin antagonizes this effect by stimulating cyclic AMP degradation. T3, cortisol, and growth hormone increase the response of adipocytes to epinephrine and norepinephrine. Growth hormone also directly stimulates lipolysis. Insulin indirectly antagonizes the release of FFA by increasing reesterifi cation. Growth hormone and cortisol increase FFA release by inhibiting reesterification. *AMP*, Adenosine monophosphate; *FFA*, free fatty acid.

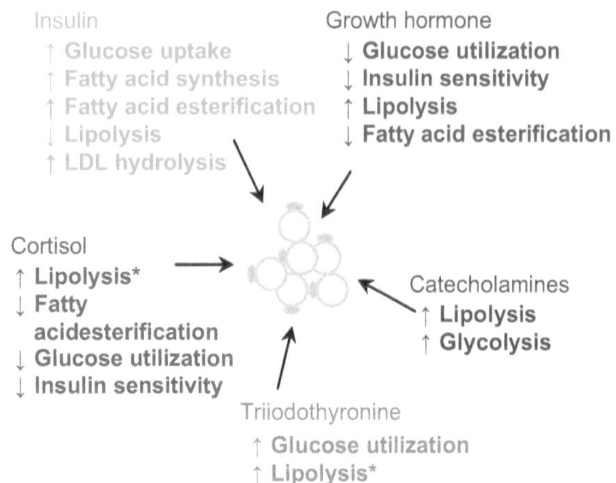

FIGURE 8.18 Effects of metabolic hormones on adipose tissue. * Lipolytic effects of cortisol are permissive.

removes a deterrent of glucose utilization in muscle while it promotes transport of glucose into myocytes. The response to insulin can be divided into two components. Stimulation of glucose transport and glycogen synthesis are direct effects and are seen within minutes. Increased oxidation of glucose that results from release of fat-induced inhibition requires several hours. Epinephrine and norepinephrine promptly increase cyclic AMP production and glycogenolysis.

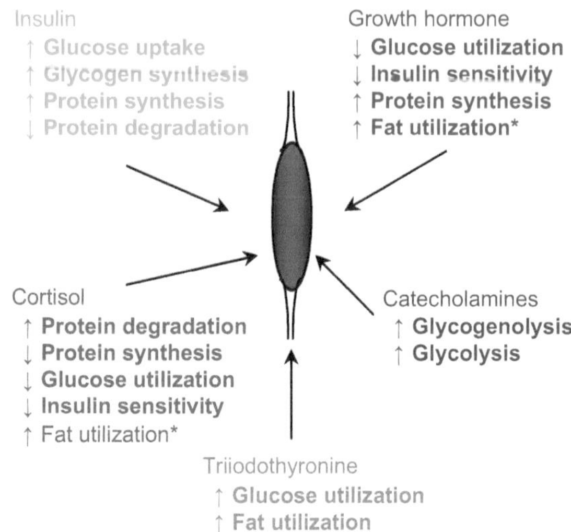

FIGURE 8.19 Effects of metabolic hormones on skeletal muscle. * The stimulations of fatty acid oxidation by GH and cortisol are indirect and result from increased fatty acid mobilization.

When the rate of glucose production from glycogen exceeds the need for ATP production, muscle cells release pyruvate and lactate, which can be reconverted to glucose in liver. GH and cortisol directly inhibit glucose uptake by muscle and indirectly decrease glucose metabolism in myocytes through their actions on FFA mobilization. By indirectly inhibiting glucose metabolism, GH and cortisol decrease glycogen breakdown. The resulting preservation of muscle glycogen has been called the glycostatic effect of GH and is part of the overall effect of cortisol that gives rise to the term glucocorticoid.

Cortisol also inhibits the uptake of amino acids and their incorporation into proteins and simultaneously promotes degradation of muscle protein. As a result, muscle becomes a net exporter of amino acids, which provide substrate for gluconeogenesis in liver. These events are summarized in Fig. 8.19. Insulin and GH antagonize the effects of cortisol on muscle protein metabolism.

Liver

The antagonistic effects of insulin and glucagon on gluconeogenesis, ketogenesis, and glycogen metabolism in hepatocytes are described in Chapter 7, The Pancreatic Islets. Epinephrine and norepinephrine, by virtue of their effects on cyclic AMP metabolism, share all the actions of glucagon. In addition, these medullary hormones also activate α1-adrenergic receptors and reinforce these effects through the agency of the diacylglycerol/inositol trisphosphate–calcium system (see Chapter 1: Introduction). Cortisol is indispensable as a permissive agent for the actions of glucagon and catecholamines on gluconeogenesis and

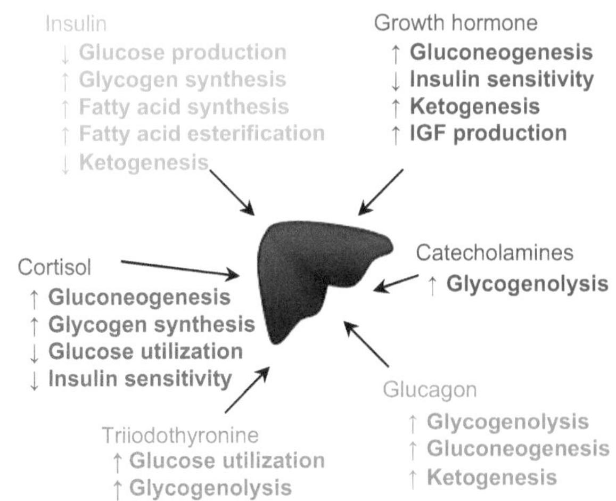

FIGURE 8.20 Effects of metabolic hormones on the liver.

glycogenolysis. In addition, cortisol induces the synthesis of a variety of enzymes responsible for gluconeogenesis and glycogen storage. By virtue of its actions on protein degradation in muscle, cortisol is also indispensable for providing substrate for gluconeogenesis. T3 promotes glucose utilization in liver by promoting the synthesis of enzymes required for glucose metabolism and lipid formation. GH is thought to increase hepatic glucose production, probably because of increased FFA mobilization, and it also increases ketogenesis largely by increasing mobilization of FFA. These hormonal influences on hepatic metabolism are summarized in Fig. 8.20.

Pancreatic islets

Alpha and beta cells of pancreatic islets are targets for metabolic hormones as well as producers of glucagon and insulin. Glucagon can stimulate insulin secretion but the physiological significance of such an action is not understood. Insulin inhibits glucagon secretion, and in its absence, responsiveness of alpha cells to glucose is severely impaired. Conversely, insulin apparently also exerts autocrine effects on the beta cells and is required to maintain the normal secretory response to increased glucose concentrations. Epinephrine and norepinephrine inhibit insulin secretion and stimulate glucagon secretion. GH, cortisol, and T3 are required for normal secretory activity of beta cells, the capacity of which for insulin secretion is reduced in their absence.

The effects of GH and cortisol on insulin secretion are somewhat paradoxical. Although their effects in adipose tissue, muscle, and liver are opposite to those of insulin, GH and cortisol nevertheless increase the sensitivity of beta cells to signals for insulin secretion and exaggerate responses to hyperglycemia. When cortisol or GH is present in excess, higher than normal concentrations of insulin are required to maintain blood glucose in the normal range. Higher concentrations of insulin itself may contribute to decreased sensitivity by downregulating insulin receptors in fat and muscle. When either GH or glucocorticoids is present in excess for prolonged periods, diabetes mellitus often results. Approximately 30% of patients suffering from excess GH (acromegaly) and a similar percentage of persons suffering from Cushing's disease (excess glucocorticoids) develop type II diabetes mellitus as a complication of their disease. In the early stages, diabetes is reversible and disappears when excess pituitary or adrenal secretion is corrected. Later, however, diabetes may become irreversible, and islet cells may be affected. This so-called diabetogenic effect is an important consideration with chronic glucocorticoid therapy and argues against the use of large amounts of GH to build muscle mass in athletes.

Regulation of metabolism during feeding and fasting

Postprandial period

Immediately after eating, metabolic activity is directed toward the processing and sequestration of energy-rich substrates that are absorbed by the intestines. This phase is dominated by insulin, which is secreted in response to three inputs to the beta cells. The cephalic, or psychological, aspect of eating stimulates insulin secretion though acetylcholine and vasoactive inhibitory peptide released from vagal fibers that innervate the islets. Food in the small intestine stimulates the secretion of the incretins, glucagon-like peptide-1 (GLP-1) and glucose-dependent insulinotropic peptide. Finally, the beta cells respond directly to increased glucose and amino acids in arterial blood (see Chapter 7: The Pancreatic Islets).

During the postprandial period the concentration of insulin in peripheral blood may rise from a resting value of about 10 μU/mL to perhaps as much as 50 μU/mL. Glucagon secretion may also increase at this time in response to amino acids in arterial blood. Dietary amino acids may also stimulate GH secretion.

Characteristically, the sympathetic nervous system is relatively quiet during the postprandial period, and there is little secretory activity of the adrenal medulla or cortex at this time. Under the dominant influence of insulin, dietary carbohydrates and lipids are transferred to storage depots in liver, adipose tissue, and muscle, and amino acids are converted to proteins in various tissues. Extrahepatic tissues use dietary glucose and fat to meet their needs instead of glucose derived from hepatic glycogen or fatty acids mobilized from adipose tissue. Hepatic glycogen increases by an amount equivalent to about half of the ingested carbohydrate. Fatty acid mobilization is inhibited by the high concentrations of insulin and glucose in blood. Of course, the composition of the diet profoundly affects postprandial responses. Obviously, a diet rich in carbohydrate elicits quantitatively different responses from one that is mainly composed of fat.

Postabsorptive period

Several hours after eating, when metabolic fuels largely have been absorbed from the intestine, the body begins to draw on fuels that were stored during the postprandial period. During this period, insulin secretion returns to relatively low basal rates and is governed principally by the concentration of glucose in blood, which has returned to about 5 mM (90 mg/dL). About 75% of the glucose secreted by the liver derives from glycogen, and the remainder comes from gluconeogenesis, driven principally by glucagon. Although the rate of glucagon secretion is relatively low at this time, the decline in insulin enables the actions of glucagon to prevail. GH and cortisol are also secreted at relatively low basal rates in the postabsorptive period. About 75% of the glucose consumed by extrahepatic tissues during this period is taken up by brain, blood cells, and other tissues, the consumption of fuels of which is independent of insulin. Muscle and adipose tissue, which are highly dependent on insulin, account for the remaining 25%.

Blood levels of FFA gradually increase as adipose tissue is progressively relieved of the restraint imposed by high levels of insulin during the postprandial period. Blood glucose remains constant during this period, but glucose metabolism in muscle decreases as the restrictive effects of the glucose–fatty acid cycle become operative. Liver gradually depletes its glycogen stores and begins to rely more heavily on gluconeogenesis from amino acids and glycerol to replace glucose consumed by extrahepatic tissues as would occur in an overnight fast (Fig. 8.21).

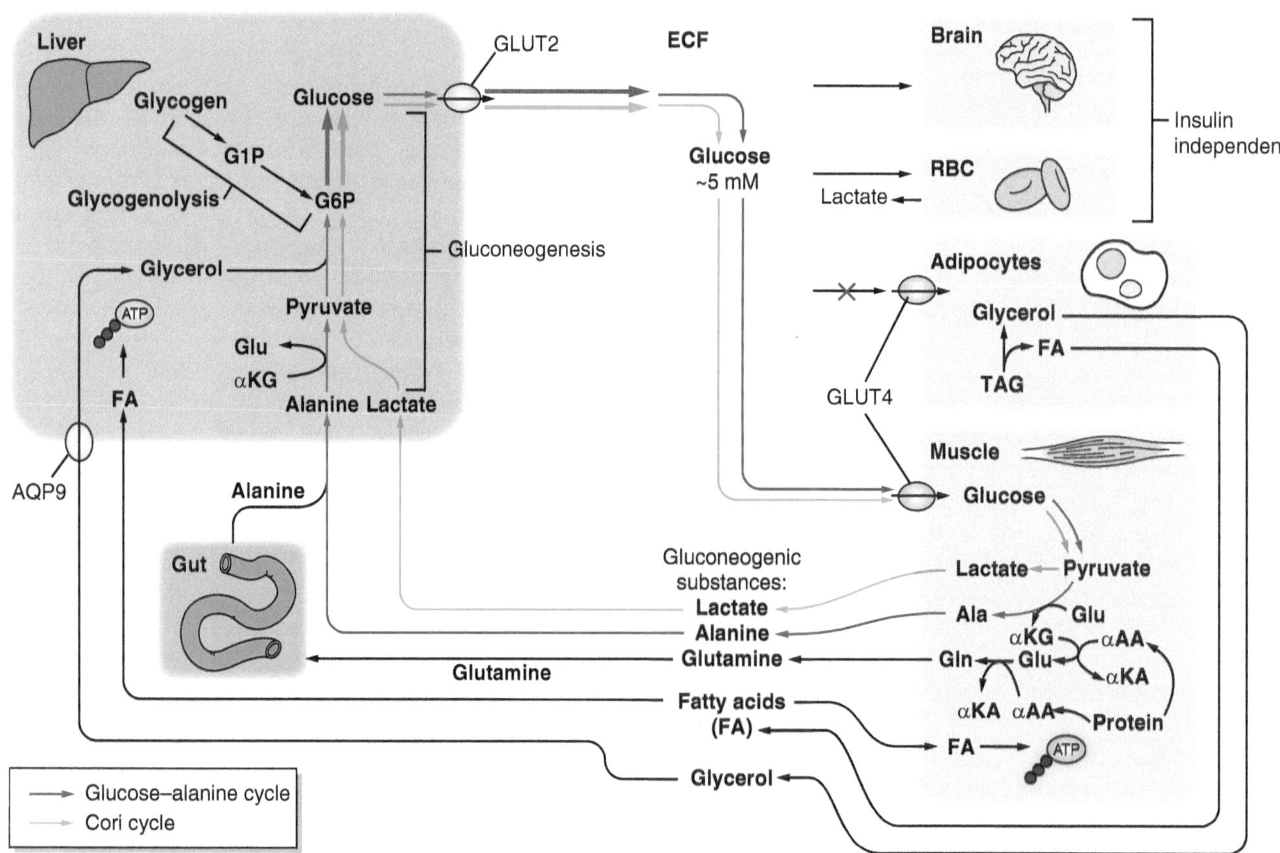

FIGURE 8.21 An overnight fast showing the metabolic interactions. *αAA*, Alpha amino acid; *αKA*, alpha keto acid; *αKG*, alpha ketoglutarate; *AQP9*, aquaporin 9; *ECF*, extracellular fluid, *RBC*, red blood cell. Source: *Redrawn from Figure 58.13 in Shulman, G. I., & Peterson, K. F. (2017). Chapter 58: Metabolism. In W. F. Boron, & E. Boulpaep (Eds.),* Medical physiology *(3rd ed.) (p. 1190). Elsevier.*

Fasting

More than 24 hours after the last meal, the individual is in a fasting state. At this time, circulating insulin concentrations decrease further, and glucagon and GH increase. Cortisol secretion follows its basal diurnal rhythmic pattern (see Chapter 4: The Adrenal Glands) unaffected by fasting at this early stage, but basal concentrations of cortisol play their essential permissive role in allowing gluconeogenesis and lipolysis to proceed (Fig. 8.22).

Glucocorticoids and GH also exert a restraining influence on glucose metabolism in muscle and adipose tissue. With the further decrease in insulin concentration, there is a further decrease in restraint of lipolysis. The lipolytic cycle speeds up, fatty acid esterification decreases, and FFA mobilization is accelerated. This effect is supported and accelerated by GH and cortisol. Decreased insulin permits a net breakdown of muscle protein; and the amino acids that consequently leave muscle, mainly as alanine, provide the substrate for gluconeogenesis. Fuel consumption after 24 hours of fasting is summarized in Fig. 8.23.

With prolonged fasting of 3 days or more, increased GH and decreased insulin result in even greater mobilization of FFA. Ketogenesis becomes significant, driven by the almost unopposed action of glucagon. By about the third day of starvation, ketone bodies in blood reach concentrations of 2–3 mM and begin to provide for an appreciable fraction of the brain's metabolic needs. Urinary nitrogen excretion decreases to the postabsorptive level or below as the pool of rapidly turning over proteins diminishes. During subsequent weeks of total starvation, nitrogen excretion continues at a low but steady rate with carbon skeletons from amino acids providing substrate for gluconeogenesis and the intermediates needed to maintain the tricarboxylic acid cycle.

Glycerol liberated from TAGs provides the other major substrate for gluconeogenesis. Renal gluconeogenesis from glutamate accompanies the production of

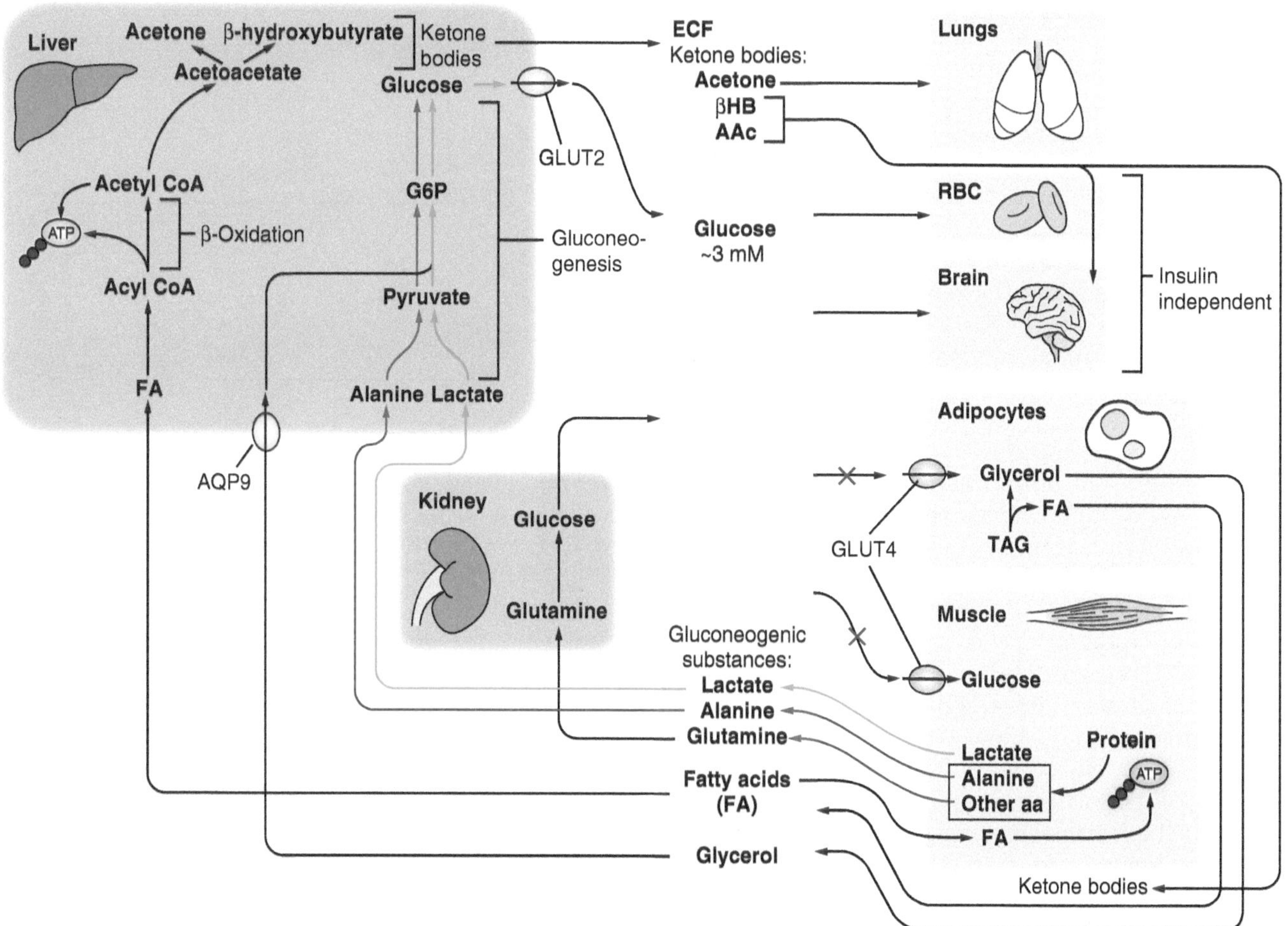

FIGURE 8.22 Fasting for longer than 24 h. *αAA*, Alpha amino acid; *αKA*, alpha keto acid; *αKG*, alpha ketoglutarate; *AQP9*, aquaporin 9; *ECF*, extracellular fluid; *RBC*, red blood cell. Source: *Redrawn from Figure 58.14 in Shulman, G. I., & Peterson, K. F. (2017). Chapter 58: Metabolism. In W. F. Boron, & E. Boulpaep (Eds.),* Medical physiology *(3rd ed.) (p. 1192). Elsevier.*

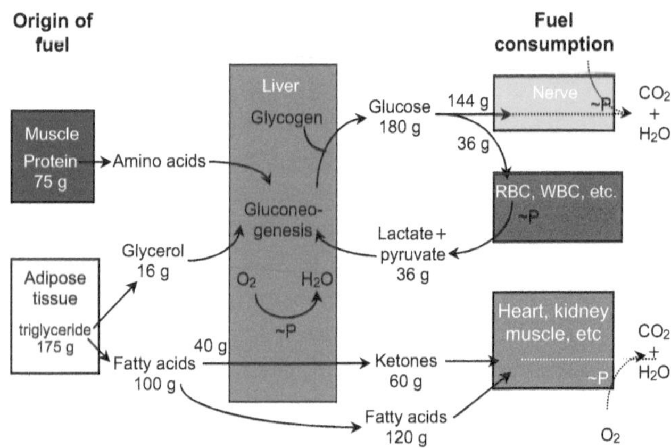

FIGURE 8.23 Quantitative turnover of substrates in a hypothetical person in the basal state after fasting for 24 h (−1800 cal). Source: *From Cahill, G. F., Jr. (1970). Starvation in man.* The New England Journal of Medicine, 282, *668–675.*

ammonium stimulated by ketoacidosis. Virtually, all other energy needs are met by oxidation of fatty acids and ketones until TAG reserves are depleted. In the terminal stages of starvation, proteins may become the only remaining substrate and are rapidly broken down to amino acids. Gluconeogenesis briefly increases once again until cumulative protein loss precludes continued survival. Curiously, continued slow loss of protein during starvation of the extremely obese individual may result in death from protein depletion even before fat depots are depleted.

Fig. 8.24 shows some of the changes in plasma hormone concentrations in the transition from the fed to the fasting state.

Values for cortisol remain unchanged or might even decrease somewhat until late in starvation reflecting, perhaps, a decrease in cortisol-binding globulin. Concentrations of cortisol shown in Fig. 8.24 represent morning values and change with the time of day in a diurnal rhythmic pattern that is not altered by fasting (see Chapter 4: The Adrenal Glands). Even though its concentration does not increase during fasting, cortisol nevertheless is an essential component of the survival mechanism. In its absence, mechanisms for producing and sparing carbohydrates are virtually inoperative, and death from hypoglycemia is inevitable.

The role of glucocorticoids in fasting is a good example of permissive action, in which a hormone maintains the instruments of metabolic adjustments so that other agents can manipulate those instruments effectively. Hypoglycemia or perhaps nonspecific stress may account for increased cortisol in the terminal stages of starvation.

The decrease in plasma concentrations of T3 reflect decreased conversion of plasma T4 to T3. At least

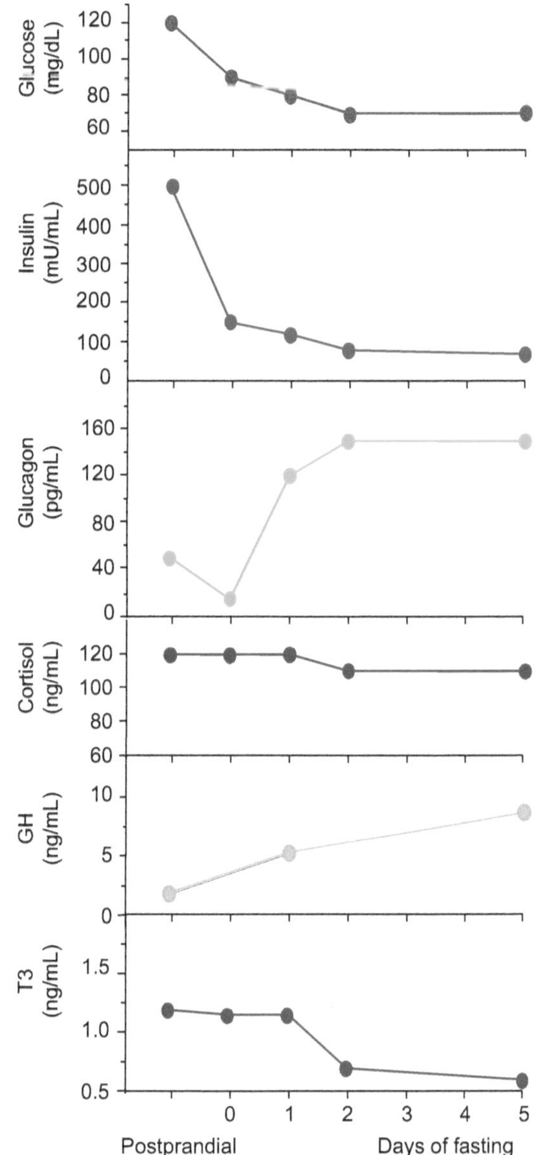

FIGURE 8.24 Representative values for plasma glucose and metabolic hormones during fasting. Values for growth hormone are averaged over 24 hours. The small decline in cortisol may reflect a decrease in cortisol-binding globulin.

during the first few days of fasting, T4 concentrations in plasma remain constant. The slight decline in T4 seen with more prolonged fasting probably reflects a decrease in plasma-binding proteins. Recall that T3, which is formed mostly in extrathyroidal tissue, is the biologically active form of the hormone (see Chapter 3: Thyroid Gland). Deiodination of T4 can lead to the formation of T3 or the inactive metabolite rT3. With starvation the concentration of rT3 in plasma increases, suggesting that metabolism of T4 shifted from the formation of the active to the inactive metabolite. Some of this increase may also be accounted for by a somewhat slower rate of degradation of rT3. Decreased

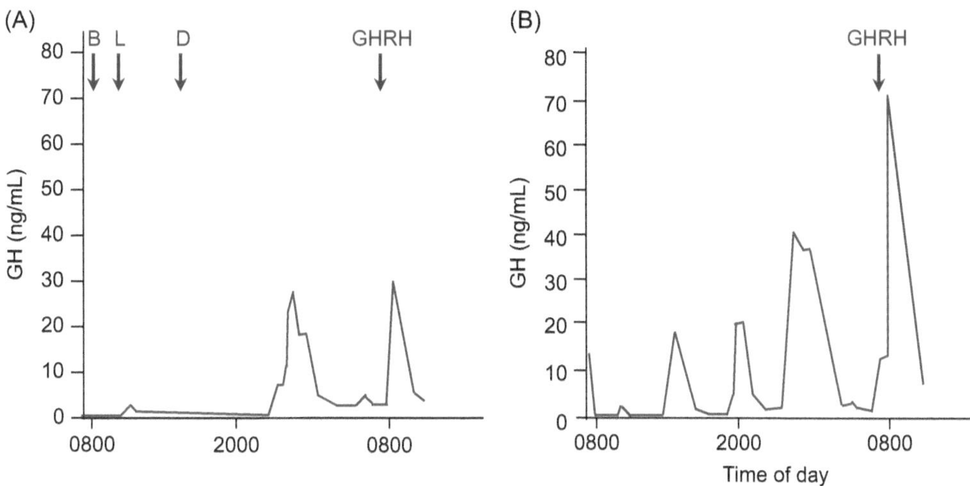

FIGURE 8.25 Effects of 1 day of fasting on GH secretion. (A) Normal fed young man. B, L, D indicate meal times. GHRH (1 μg/kg) was given intravenously at the time indicated by the arrow. (B) GH concentrations in plasma in the same subject after a 24-h fast. Blood was sampled every 20 min. Note that GH secretion is pulsatile and that the amplitudes of the spontaneous secretory bursts and the response to GHRH were increased by fasting. *GH*, Growth hormone; *GHRH*, growth hormone–releasing hormone. Source: *From Ho, K. Y., Veldhuis, J. D., Johnson, M. L., Furlanetto, R., Evans, W. S., Alberti, K. G., et al. (1988). Fasting enhances growth hormone secretion and amplifies the complex rhythms of growth hormone secretion in man.* Journal of Clinical Investigation, *81, 968.*

production of T3 results in an overall decrease in metabolic rate and can be viewed as an adaptive mechanism for conservation of metabolic fuels.

Secretion of GH follows a pulsatile pattern that is exaggerated during starvation (see Chapter 11: Hormonal Control of Growth). Fasting increases both the frequency of secretory pulses and their amplitude (Fig. 8.25).

The values for GH shown in Fig. 8.25 are averages and represent concentrations present in a mixed sample of blood that was continuously drawn at a very slow rate over a 24-hour period. The metabolic changes produced by an increase in GH secretion are like those that result from a decrease in insulin secretion. GH increases lipolysis, decreases glucose utilization in muscle and fat, and increases glucose production by the liver. These effects of GH are relatively small compared to the effects of diminished insulin secretion. However, persons suffering from a deficiency of GH may become hypoglycemic during fasting, and treatment with GH helps to maintain their blood glucose (Fig. 8.26).

In the nonfasting individual, GH stimulates the liver and other tissues to secrete insulin-like growth factor-1 (IGF-1), which stimulates protein synthesis (see Chapter 11: Hormonal Control of Growth). However, the liver becomes insensitive to this effect of GH during fasting, and plasma concentrations of IGF-1 fall dramatically. This, too, may be an adaptive mechanism that maximizes availability of amino acids for gluconeogenesis and replenishment of critical proteins.

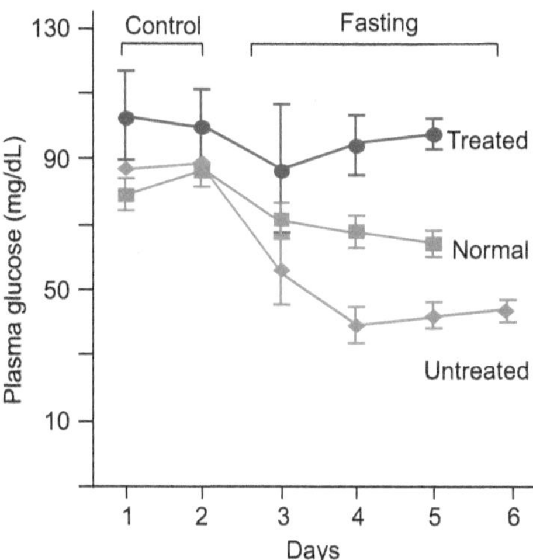

FIGURE 8.26 Plasma concentrations of glucose in normal subjects and patients suffering from isolated deficiency of GH during control days of normal food intake and while fasting. Some GH-deficient patients were untreated and others were given 5 mg of hGH per day (treated). The fast began after the collection of blood on day 2. *GH*, Growth hormone; *hGH*, human growth hormone. *From Merimee, T. J., Felig, P., Marliss, E., Fineberg, S. E., & Cahill, G. F., Jr. (1971). Glucose and lipid homeostasis in the absence of human growth hormone.* Journal of Clinical Investigation, *50, 574–582.*

Hormonal interactions during exercise

During exercise, overall oxygen consumption may increase 10- to 15-fold in a well-trained young athlete. The requirements for fuel are met by mobilization of reserves within muscle cells by increased activity of AMPK, and from extramuscular fuel depots. Rapid uptake of glucose from blood can potentially deplete, or at least dangerously lower, glucose concentrations and hence jeopardize the brain unless some physiological controls are operative. We can consider two forms of exercise: short-term maximal effort, characterized by sprinting for a few seconds, and sustained aerobic work, characterized by marathon running.

Short-term maximal effort

For the few seconds of the 100-yard dash, endogenous ATP reserves in muscle, creatine phosphate, and glycogen are the chief sources of energy. Some ATP also is generated by transfer of high-energy phosphate from one ADP to another, leading to accumulation of AMP and activation of AMPK. For short-term maximal effort, energy must be released from fuel anaerobically before circulatory adjustments can provide the required oxygen. Activation of AMPK leads to increased glucose transport from extracellular fluid. Breakdown of glucose and glycogen to lactate provides the needed ATP. Calcium released from the sarcoplasmic reticulum in response to neural stimulation not only triggers muscle contraction but also activates glycogen phosphorylase. These intrinsic mechanisms are reinforced by epinephrine and norepinephrine released from the adrenal medullae and sympathetic nerve endings in response to central activation of the sympathetic nervous system.

The endocrine system is important primarily for maintaining or replenishing fuel reserves in muscle. Through actions of hormones and the glucose–fatty acid cycle already discussed, glycogen reserves in resting muscle are sustained at or near capacity, so that muscle always is prepared to respond to demands for maximal effort. During the recovery phase, lactate released from working muscles is converted to glucose in liver and can be exported back to muscle in the classic Cori cycle. Accelerated oxidation of fatty acids and increased transport of glucose stimulated by AMPK contribute to restoration of glycogen reserves, and these effects are reinforced by insulin secreted in response to increased dietary intake of glucose or amino acids.

Sustained aerobic exercise

Glucose taken up from the blood or derived from muscle glycogen is also the most important fuel in the early stages of moderately intense exercise, but with continued effort, dependence on fatty acids increases. Although fat is a more efficient fuel than glucose from a storage point of view, glucose is more efficient than fatty acids from the perspective of oxygen consumption and yields about 5% more energy per liter of oxygen. Fig. 8.27 shows the changes in fuel consumption with time in subjects exercising at 30% of their maximal oxygen consumption.

For reasons that are not fully understood, working muscles, even in the trained athlete, cannot derive more than about 70% of their energy from oxidation of fat. Hypoglycemia and exhaustion occur when muscle glycogen is depleted. With sustained exercise the decline in insulin coupled with an increase in all the counterregulatory hormones contributes to supplying fat to the working muscles and maximizing gluconeogenesis (Fig. 8.28).

Anticipation of exercise may be sufficient to activate the sympathetic nervous system, which is of critical importance, not only for supplying the fuel for the working muscles but also for making the cardiovascular adjustments that maintain blood flow to carry fuel and oxygen to muscle, gluconeogenic precursors to liver, and heat to sites of dissipation. Insulin secretion is shut down by sympathetic activity. This removes the major inhibitory influence on the production of glucose by the liver, glycogen breakdown in muscle, and FFA release from adipocytes. At first glance, decreasing insulin secretion might seem deleterious for glucose consumption in muscle. However, the decrease in insulin concentration only decreases glucose uptake by nonworking muscles. Mobilization of GLUT4 and transport of glucose across the sarcolemma are stimulated by AMPK, the activity of which is increased by the increased demand of muscular contractions. Glucose metabolism in working muscles therefore is not limited by membrane transport.

Increased hepatic glucose production results primarily from the combined effects of the fall in insulin secretion and the rise in glucagon secretion augmented with some contribution from catecholamines. The contributions of the increased secretion of GH and cortisol to this effect are unlikely to be important initially, but with sustained exercise the contributions of both are likely to increase. Actions of both hormones increase the output of FFA and glycerol and decrease glucose utilization by adipocytes and nonworking muscles. In addition, the increased cortisol would be expected to increase the expression of gluconeogenic enzymes in the liver.

Glycogen reserves of nonworking muscles may provide an important source of carbohydrate for working muscles during sustained exercise and for restoring muscle glycogen after exercise. Epinephrine and norepinephrine stimulate glycogenolysis in nonworking as well as working muscles. Glucose-6-phosphate produced from glycogen can be broken down completely to carbon dioxide and water in working muscles, but nonworking muscles convert it to pyruvate and lactate, which escape into the blood. Liver then reconverts these 3-carbon acids to glucose, which is returned to the circulation and selectively taken up by the working muscles (Fig. 8.29).

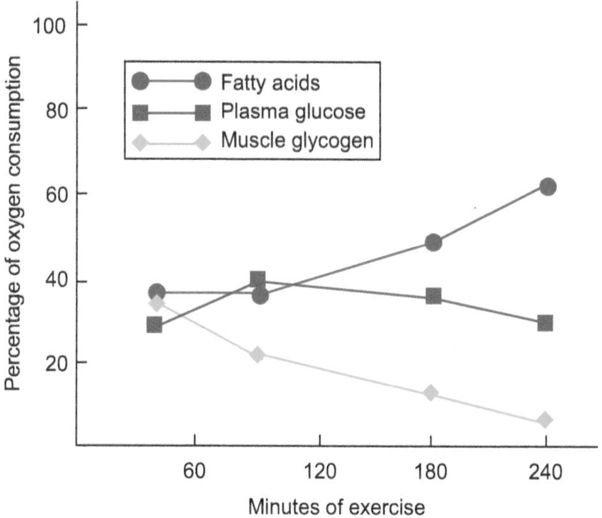

FIGURE 8.27 Changes in sources of fuels utilized during prolonged exercise at 30% of maximal oxygen consumption. Source: *Drawn from the data of Ahlborg, G., Felig, P., Hagenfeldt, L., Hendler, R., & Wahren, J. (1974). Substrate turnover during prolonged exercise in man. Splanchnic and leg metabolism of glucose, free fatty acids, and amino acids.* Journal of Clinical Investigation, 53, *1080–1090.*

Long-term regulation of fuel storage

Long-term regulation of fuel storage is intimately connected with the biology of adipose tissue. Adipose tissue, which is diffusely scattered throughout the body in subcutaneous and intraabdominal (visceral) deposits, has an almost limitless capacity for fuel storage. Increasing or decreasing the total amount of fat stored is achieved primarily by changes in the volume of the fat droplets within each adipocyte by mechanisms of fat deposition and mobilization already discussed. In addition, the number of adipocytes is not fixed and may increase throughout life by multiplication and differentiation of precursor cells. Conversely, when their TAG stores are depleted adipocytes may undergo dedifferentiation and apoptosis.

Although once thought of merely as inert storage depots, it is now recognized that adipocytes not only receive signals to store or mobilize TAGs but also secrete hormones that notify the brain and other parts of the body of their state of fullness. In this way, adipocytes are active participants in the regulation of fuel storage, food

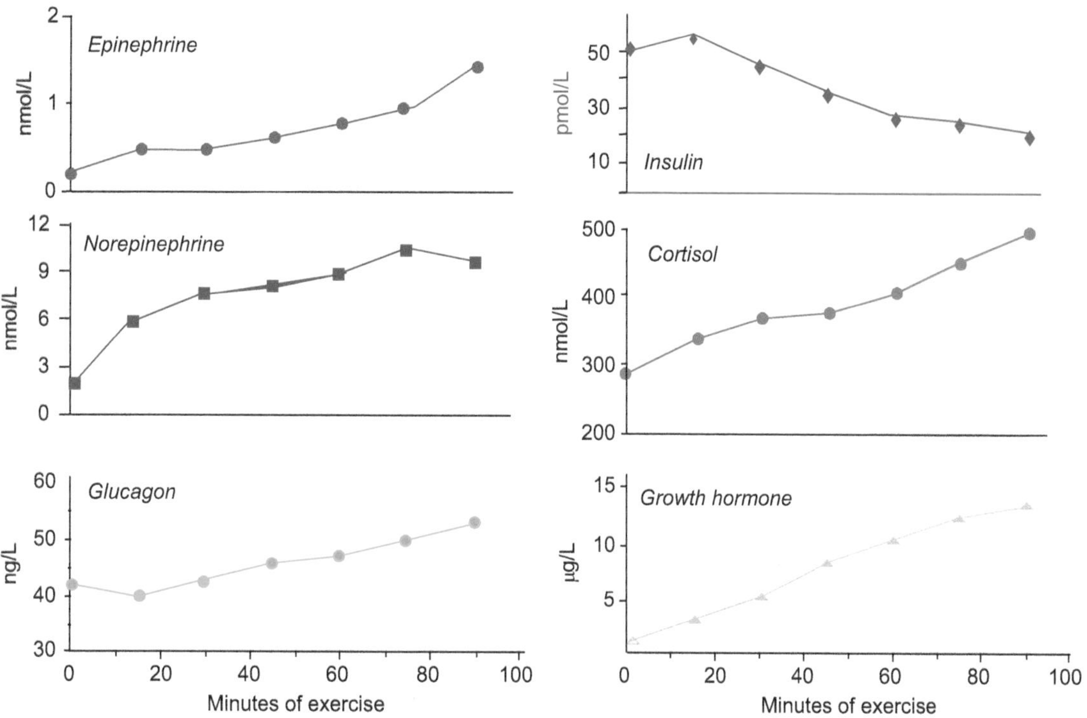

FIGURE 8.28 Changes in concentration of insulin and counterregulatory hormones during prolonged moderate exercise. Values shown are the means obtained for eight young men exercising on a bicycle ergometer at ~50% of maximum oxygen consumption. Source: *Drawn from data of Davis, S. N., Galassetti, P., Wasserman, D. H., & Tate, D. (2000). Effects of gender on neuroendocrine and metabolic counterregulatory responses to exercise in normal man.* The Journal of Clinical Endocrinology and Metabolism, 85, *224–230.*

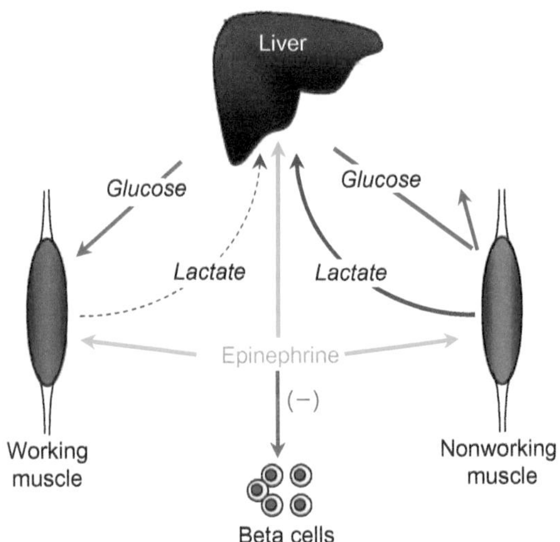

FIGURE 8.29 Postulated interaction between exercising muscle and resting muscle via the Cori cycle. Source: *Redrawn from Ahlborg, G., Wahren, J., & Felig, P. (1986). Splanchnic and peripheral glucose and lactate metabolism during and after prolonged arm exercise.* Journal of Clinical Investigation, *77, 690–699.*

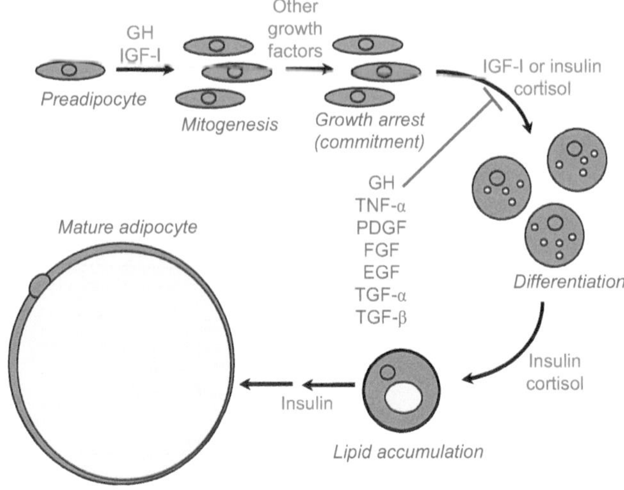

FIGURE 8.30 Adipocyte differentiation. *EGF*, Epidermal growth factor; *FGF*, fibroblast growth factor; *GH*, Growth hormone; *IGF-1*, insulin-like growth factor-1; *PDGF*, platelet-derived growth factor; *TGF-α*, transforming growth factor-α; *TGF-β*, transforming growth factor-β; *TNF-α*, tumor necrosis factor-α.

intake, growth and development, and reproduction. When increased in number and filled to excess with TAGs as occurs in obesity, secretions of adipose tissue play a crucial role in the development of pathological changes, including decreased insulin sensitivity, type II diabetes, hypertension, atherosclerosis, and other characteristics of the so-called metabolic syndrome.

Adipogenesis

Adipocytes are derived from multipotential mesenchymal stem cells present in adipose tissue stroma. Little is known of the factors that commit these pluripotential cells to the adipocyte lineage and the formation of preadipocytes, but it is likely that paracrine signals released from fat cells that have reached their storage capacity trigger the initiation of preadipocyte differentiation into mature fat cells. Terminal differentiation of preadipocytes depends on the expression of key transcription factors that induce the expression of genes that are characteristic of the fat cell, including the enzymatic machinery for fatty acids synthesis, storage, and mobilization.

The crucial nuclear transcription factor required for adipogenesis and maintenance of the adipocyte phenotype is the peroxisome proliferator–activated receptor γ (PPARγ). PPARγ is a member of the nuclear receptor superfamily that also includes receptors for adrenal and thyroid hormones (see Chapter 1: Introduction). Although some arachidonic acid derivatives and pharmacological agents of the thiazolidinedione class can activate PPARγ, its endogenous ligand is not known.

Adipocyte differentiation is influenced heavily by the balance of pro- and antidifferentiation signals delivered by locally produced growth factors, cytokines and circulating hormones (Fig. 8.30).

Insulin and cortisol play prominent roles in promoting differentiation of human preadipocytes. Insulin and the related IGF-1 (see Chapter 11: Hormonal Control of Growth) stimulate proliferation of preadipocytes and directly or indirectly increase the expression of PPARγ. Insulin is essential for the uptake and synthesis of the TAGs that form the lipid droplet that is the central feature of adipocyte morphology and function. Glucocorticoids also increase the expression of PPARγ and other transcription factors that play a role in differentiation. Growth hormone either directly or through the production of its surrogate IGF-1 (see Chapter 11: Hormonal Control of Growth) stimulates preadipocyte proliferation but inhibits differentiation of preadipocytes to mature adipocytes and limits fat storage.

Human preadipocytes also express estrogen receptors and proliferate in response to estrogen, which may account for the differences in adipose mass and distribution in women and men. Estrogens and androgens may also be responsible for regional differences in sensitivity of mature adipocytes to signals for lipolysis.

Chronic actions of insulin and GH on adipogenesis are consistent with their short-term actions as already discussed, but the effects of cortisol are unexpected in light of its short-term effects that promote lipolysis and decrease fatty acid reesterification. However, the importance of cortisol for the formation and maintenance of adipose tissue is underscored by the finding that removal of the adrenal glands in experimental animals prevents or reverses all forms of genetic or experimentally induced obesity. In addition, chronic excess production of glucocorticoids in humans is associated with increased body fat especially in the torso (truncal obesity), the face (moon face), and between the scapulae (buffalo hump).

It is noteworthy that adipocytes and their precursors express the enzyme 11β hydroxysteroid dehydrogenase-I (HSD-I), which catalyzes the reduction of the inactive steroid cortisone to the active hormone cortisol (see Chapter 4: The Adrenal Glands). These cells thus have the capacity to form cortisol locally and are exposed to higher concentrations than prevail in the circulation. Expression of HSD-I is upregulated in differentiating adipocytes and is greater in omental fat than in subcutaneous fat, which may contribute to the preferential deposition of fat at intraabdominal rather than subcutaneous sites in states of cortisol excess.

Hypothalamic control of appetite and food intake

The overall mass of TAG stored in adipose tissue is determined by the balance between metabolic fuel ingested and metabolic fuel consumed, and increases or decreases to compensate for imbalances. Prior to the fast food era, body fat reserves in most people were maintained at a nearly constant level throughout adult life despite enormous variations in daily food consumption and energy expenditure.

Fig. 8.31 summarizes the findings of five independent studies of changes in body weight and fat mass with aging in about 12,000 individuals living in the middle of the 20th century. Although total body fat increased steadily with age, the increase was less than a gram per day when averaged over a period of 50 years and corresponds to a daily positive energy balance of about 6 cal. Assuming that daily energy consumption averaged about 2000 cal, the intake of fuel in a mixed diet matched the rate of energy utilization with an error of only 0.3%, consistent with the operation of rather precise regulatory mechanisms. However, if these studies were repeated in the present era remarkably different results would be found. In the nearly half century that elapsed since these data were collected, there has been a dramatic change, and affluent nations now face an epidemic of obesity. Ready access to high-calorie foods and technology that fosters a sedentary lifestyle have so distorted the balance between caloric intake and energy expenditure that 30% of the adult American population is classified as obese, and an even higher percentage is overweight. Thus mechanisms for maintaining a nearly constant fuel reserve are overwhelmed when caloric supply exceeds demand. It has been argued that evolutionary pressures experienced over millennia of uncertain food supply have equipped us with stronger mechanisms that favor storage than mechanisms that defend against the less likely event of excessive fuel availability.

Understanding of the mechanisms that govern long-term fuel storage requires understanding how energy expenditure and food intake are regulated. For most people, physical activity accounts for only about 30% of daily energy expenditure, and 60% is expended at rest for maintenance of ion gradients, renewal of cellular constituents, neuronal activity, and to support cardiopulmonary work. The remaining 10% is dissipated as the thermogenic effect of feeding and the consequent processes of assimilation. Neither resting nor thermogenic energy expenditure is fixed but is adjustable in a manner that tends to keep body fat reserves constant.

In the experiment illustrated in Fig. 8.32, normal human subjects were overfed or underfed in order to increase or decrease body weight by 10%. They were then given just enough food each day to maintain their new weight at a constant level. Energy utilization increased disproportionately in the overfed subjects

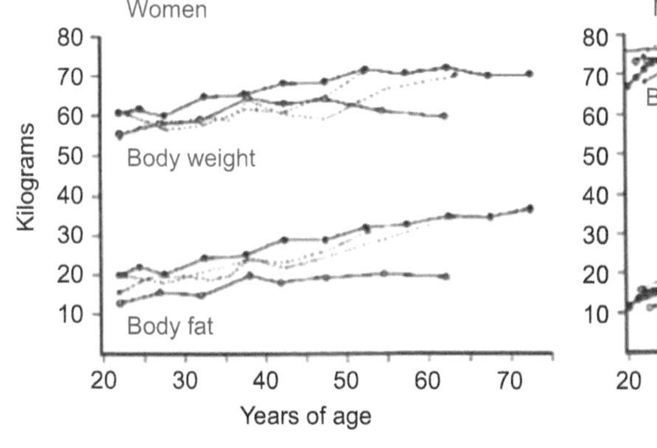

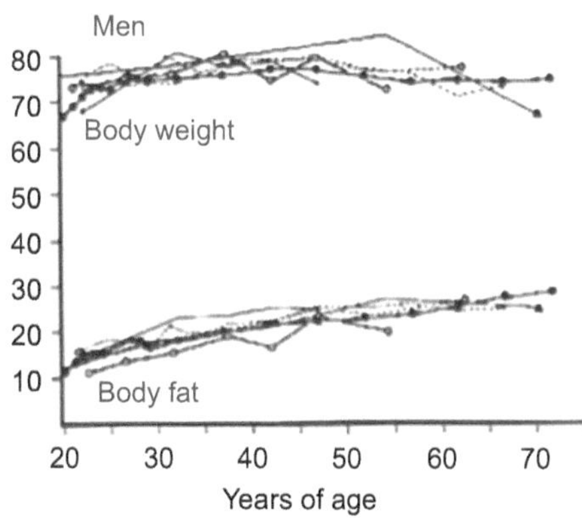

FIGURE 8.31 Data showing changes in body weight and fat content with aging obtained in five independent studies of individuals living in the early-to-middle decades of the 20th century. Source: *From Forbes, G. B., & Reina, J. C. (1970). Adult lean body mass declines with age: Some longitudinal observations.* Metabolism, *19, 653–663.*

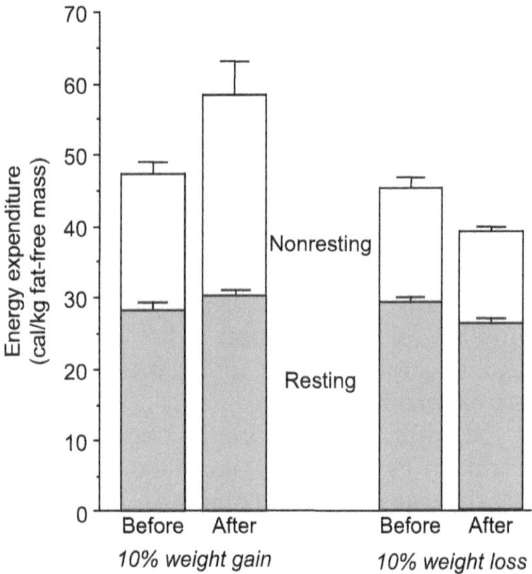

FIGURE 8.32 Changes in energy expenditure after increase or decrease of body weight. Thirteen normal subjects were overfed a defined diet until their body weight increased by 10%. Eleven normal subjects were underfed until their body weight decreased by 10%. Both groups were then fed just enough to maintain their new weights for 2 weeks, at which time energy expenditure and lean body mass were measured. Source: *Drawn from data of Leibel, R. L., Rosenbaum, M., Hirsch, J. (1995). Changes in energy expenditure resulting from altered body weight.* The New England Journal of Medicine, 332, *673–674.*

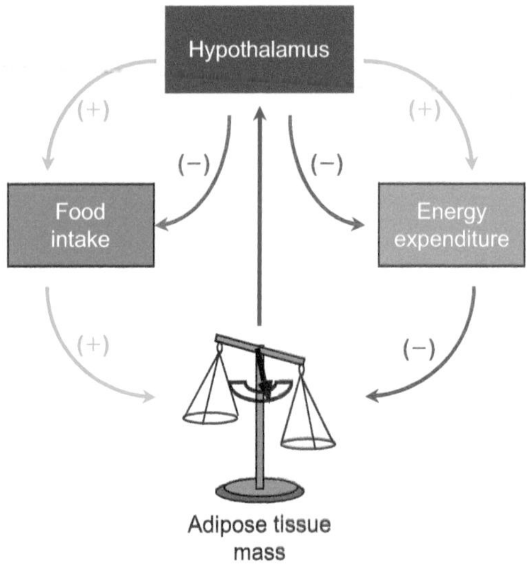

FIGURE 8.33 Hypothetical regulatory system for maintaining constancy of adipose mass by monitoring the mass of stored fat. Adjustments in energy intake and expenditure are made to maintain constancy. Green arrows (+) denote increase; red arrows (−) denote decrease.

and decreased disproportionately in the underfed subjects. These compensatory changes in energy expenditure opposed maintenance of the change from initial body fat content and favored return to the previous set point.

How such changes in energy expenditure are brought about are currently subjects of intensive investigation. One possibility is that metabolic efficiency may be regulated by adjusting the expression of genes that encode proteins that uncouple ATP generation from oxygen consumption (see Chapter 3: Thyroid Gland). Decreased efficiency in maintaining ion gradients, as seen in nonshivering thermogenesis, may also play a role.

Studies like those illustrated in Figs. 8.29 and 8.30 and many older observations gave rise to the idea that the mass of the fat storage depot is monitored and maintained nearly constant by feedback mechanisms that regulate food consumption and energy expenditure (Fig. 8.33).

Clinical observations and studies in experimental animals established that the hypothalamus coordinates the drive for food intake with such energy-consuming processes as temperature regulation, growth, and reproduction. Injuries to a "satiety center" in the ventromedial hypothalamus produce insatiable eating behavior accompanied by severe obesity; and injuries to a "hunger center" in the lateral hypothalamus cause food avoidance and lethal starvation. A complex neural network interconnects these centers to each other, to autonomic integrating centers in the hypothalamus and brain stem, and to neurons in the arcuate and paraventricular nuclei that secrete hypophysiotropic hormones (see Chapter 2: Pituitary Gland). Neurons in the arcuate nuclei are the primary components of the system that regulates food consumption and energy utilization. Neuropeptide transmitters of some of these neurons have been identified along with their receptors and the sites of their expression have been located. Some of the relevant neuropeptides are as follows:

- Neuropeptide Y (NPY) (described in Chapter 6: Hormones of the Gastrointestinal Tract) is a 36-amino acid peptide that is abundantly expressed in arcuate neurons, the axons of which project to the paraventricular nuclei and the lateral hypothalamic area. When delivered to the hypothalamus of rodents, NPY increases food intake, lowers energy expenditure, and with chronic administration may produce obesity. NPY expression is upregulated during fasting. We refer to neurons that express NPY as the NPY neurons.
- Proopiomelanocortin (POMC), the precursor of ACTH in pituitary corticotropes, is also expressed in neurons in the arcuate nucleus where posttranslational processing (see Fig. 2.3 in Chapter 2: Pituitary Gland) gives rise to α-melanocyte-stimulating hormone (MSH), and the neurons that secrete this peptide are called POMC neurons. As a neuropeptide, α-MSH is a potent negative regulator

of food intake and activates melanocortin receptors in neurons in the lateral hypothalamic area, in dorsomedial and paraventricular hypothalamic nuclei, and in the hindbrain (see Fig. 2.7 in Chapter 2: Pituitary Gland).

Pharmacological blockade or genetic depletion of brain melanocortin receptors results in obesity.

- In the skin, α-MSH increases the expression of a black pigment, melanin, in hair follicles. A protein, called agouti, competes with α-MSH for the melanocortin receptor, and under its influence, a yellow pigment is expressed. The observation that a mutation, which results in ubiquitous inappropriate expression of the agouti gene in mice, also produces obesity, led to the discovery that neurons in the arcuate nucleus express a similar protein, the agouti-related protein (AGRP) that competes with α-MSH for binding to melanocortin receptors in hypothalamic neurons. AGRP and NPY are coexpressed in arcuate neurons, and their combined actions provide a strong drive for food intake.
- Another appetite-suppressing peptide is the cocaine- and amphetamine-regulated transcript (CART), the discovery of which arose out of studies of drugs of abuse. It is widely expressed in the brain, including some neurons in the arcuate nuclei that also express α-MSH. Administration of CART inhibits the feeding response to NPY, and mice that are deficient in CART become obese.
- Melanin-concentrating hormone (MCH) originally was described as the factor that opposes the melanophore-dispersing activity of MSH in fish, but MCH also is expressed in neurons in the lateral hypothalamus. When administered to rodents, MCH stimulates feeding behavior and antagonizes the inhibitory effects of α-MSH. Unlike AGRP, MCH does not bind to the same receptor as α-MSH. Fasting increases MCH expression, and absence of the MCH gene in mice results in reduction in body fat content.

Fig. 8.34 illustrates the likely relationship of cells that produce and respond to these neuropeptides. In

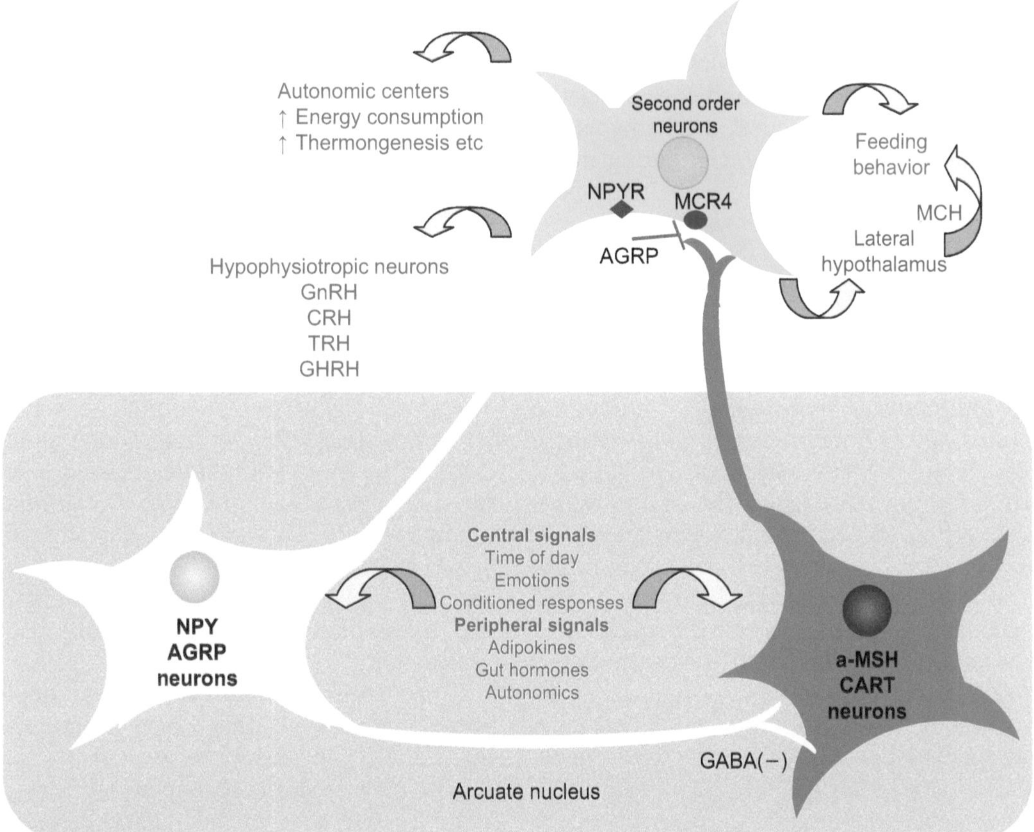

FIGURE 8.34 Schematic drawing of the relationship between the principal neurons in the arcuate nuclei that control fuel consumption and energy utilization to each other and to their up- and downstream effectors. *AGRP*, Agouti-related peptide; *CART*, cocaine- and amphetamine-related transcript; *CRH*, corticotropin-releasing hormone; *GABA*, gamma-amino butyric acid; *GHRH*, growth hormone−releasing hormone; *GnRH*, gonadotropin-releasing hormone; *MCH*, melanin-concentrating hormone; *MCR4*, melanocortin receptor 4 (MSH receptor); *NPY*, neuropeptide Y; *NPYR*, NPY receptor; *TRH*, thyrotropin-releasing hormone; *α-MSH*, α-melanocyte-stimulating hormone.

addition to releasing antagonistic neuropeptides at synapses with second-order neurons, the NPY neurons form synapses with POMC neurons and release the inhibitory neurotransmitter gamma-amino butyric acid (GABA). Other neuropeptides, including corticotropin- (CRH) and thyrotropin-releasing hormone and amine transmitters that originate in the paraventricular nuclei and other brain loci also, coordinate the complex regulation of feeding behavior with such energy-consuming processes as thermogenesis, growth, and reproduction. The actions of CRH are not limited to activating the pituitary–adrenal axis, but CRH also plays an important role in communicating with autonomic centers and the dorsal vagal complex.

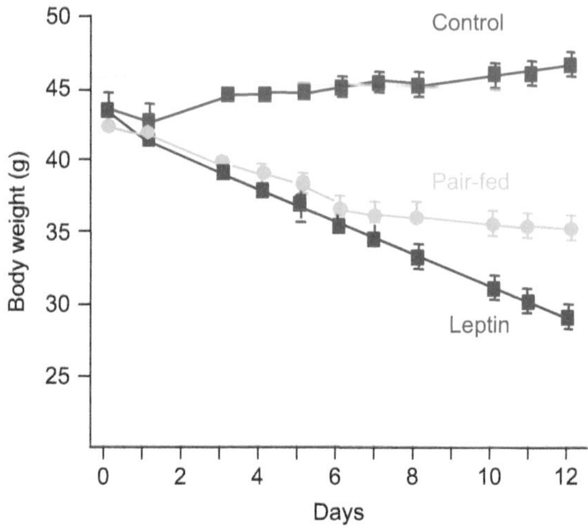

FIGURE 8.35 Effects of leptin in leptin-deficient mice. Body weights of female obese mice treated with saline (control) or 270 μg of leptin/day were compared to body weights of obese mice treated with saline but were fed an amount of food equal to that consumed by the leptin-treated mice (pair-fed). Note that the loss of body weight produced by leptin was not accounted for simply by decreased food intake. Source: *From Levin, N., Nelson, C., Gurney, A., Vandlen, R., & de Sauvage, F. (1996). Pair-feeding studies provide compelling evidence that the* ob *protein exerts adipose-reducing effects in excess of those induced by reductions in food intake.* Proceedings of the National Academy of Sciences of the United States of America, 93, *1726–1730.*

Peripheral input to hypothalamic feeding and satiety neurons

Hypothalamic centers that regulate energy homeostasis receive input from multiple sources, including signals from adipose tissue, the pancreas, the gastrointestinal tract, and circulating nutrients. Hormones, the production and actions of which are associated with monitoring the mass of adipose tissue stores, are called adiposity signals. Fuel intake and disposition also are regulated on a meal-by-meal basis, and the associated gastrointestinal hormones and neural mechanisms are referred to as satiety signals. Finally, circulating nutrients themselves are monitored by hypothalamic neurons and provide input to energy homeostasis.

Adiposity signals

Leptin

Adipocytes communicate their degree of fullness to the hypothalamus and peripheral tissues by secreting a hormone called leptin. Leptin, which means "thin," is expressed primarily, but not exclusively, in adipocytes and was discovered as the missing factor in the ob/ob mouse, an animal model of obesity. Inactivating mutations of the ob gene, which encodes leptin, or the *db* gene, which encodes its receptor, result in hyperphagia (excess food consumption), obesity, diabetes, impaired temperature regulation, and infertility in rodents. In the very rare cases that have been reported in humans, mutation of the genes that code either for leptin or its receptor results in hyperphagia, morbid obesity, and impaired sexual development. When administered to obese, leptin-deficient mice or their human counterparts, leptin decreases body weight by reducing food intake and increasing energy utilization (Fig. 8.35).

Leptin is encoded as a 167-amino acid prohormone in the ob gene located on chromosome 7. Its tertiary structure resembles that of the class of cytokines and hormones that includes GH and prolactin. Leptin synthesis, storage, and mRNA content are highest in large adipocytes and correlate with adipocyte size. The cellular mechanisms that are activated by fat cell enlargement are not understood. Some leptin is stored, perhaps in small submembranous vesicles, but processes of storage and secretion are not typical of endocrine cells and are incompletely understood. Leptin concentrations in blood correlate positively with body fat content (Fig. 8.36) consistent with its role as an indicator of the mass of fat stores. Secretion largely reflects rates of synthesis, augmented by the release of stored leptin in response to insulin. Insulin and cortisol act synergistically to increase leptin mRNA and synthesis, whereas GH, norepinephrine, or increased activity of the sympathetic nervous system decrease leptin production.

Blood levels of leptin also reflect acute changes in nutritional state. Within hours after initiation of fasting, leptin concentrations decrease sharply and are restored by feeding. It is possible that leptin has an acute as well as a chronic function, and that a fall in blood leptin concentration acts as a starvation signal to increase food intake and initiate energy conservation. Plasma concentrations of leptin oscillate in a circadian pattern with highest levels found at night. Frequent spikes in leptin concentration in blood are indicative of

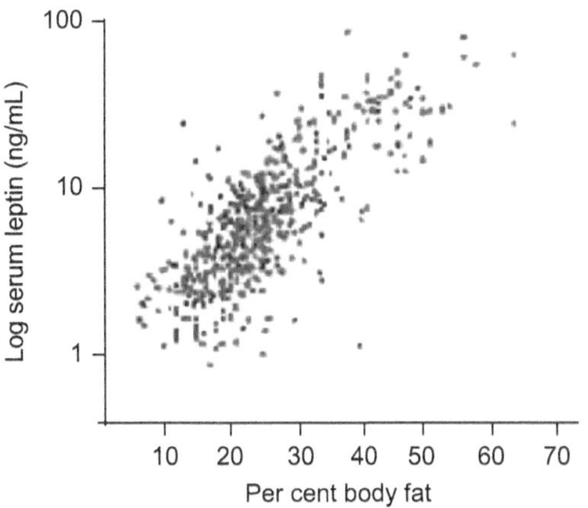

FIGURE 8.36 Leptin concentrations in blood plasma correlate with body fat content in 500 human subjects. Source: *From Caro, J. F., Sinha, M. K., Kolaczynski, J. W., Zhang, P. L., Considine, R. V. (1996). Leptin: The tale of an obesity gene.* Diabetes, *45, 1455–1462.*

synchronized pulsatile secretion, but how secretion by diffusely distributed adipocytes is coordinated is not understood. More than 40% of the leptin in blood is bound to a soluble fragment of the leptin receptor. Leptin is cleared from the blood primarily by the kidney with a half-life of about 4 hours.

The leptin receptor, like receptors for GH and prolactin, belongs to the class of transmembrane cytokine receptors that signal by activating the cytosolic tyrosine kinase JAK2 and regulating gene expression via STAT3, and signal acute events downstream from phosphatidyl inositol-3 kinase (see Chapter 1: Introduction). Multiple splice variants of the leptin receptor mRNA give rise to different isoforms, including one that circulates as a soluble protein bound to leptin. Other isoforms have truncated cytoplasmic domains, but only the form with the full-length cytoplasmic tail appears to be capable of signaling. Truncated forms, which are expressed in vascular endothelium and the choroid plexus, may serve a transport function to facilitate passage of leptin across the blood–brain barrier and thus deliver leptin to target cells in the central nervous system. Neurons in the arcuate nuclei of the hypothalamus are major targets for leptin, but leptin receptors also are found in neurons of the paraventricular, ventromedial, and dorsomedial nuclei of the hypothalamus, in the brainstem, and in the hippocampus. Leptin activates nonspecific ion channels in the membranes of POMC neurons causing them to depolarize and release α-MSH and CART from synaptic terminals. It also stimulates the synthesis of these neuropeptides. Simultaneously leptin suppresses the synthesis of NPY and AGRP in nearby NPY neurons and activates potassium channels. The resulting hyperpolarization of their plasma membranes blocks the synaptic release of NPY and AGRP as well as the inhibitory neurotransmitter GABA. Blockade of GABA release augments the stimulation of POMC neurons by removing a restraining influence in a typical push–pull type of mechanism as described in Chapter 5, Principles of Hormone Integration. Because projections of these arcuate neurons directly or indirectly signal to neurons in the lateral hypothalamus, leptin also indirectly inhibits MCH secretion and further blunts the drive for food intake. Projections to the paraventricular nuclei activate CRH neurons that communicate with autonomic centers to stimulate energy utilizing processes. The overall result of these positive and negative actions is a decrease in food intake and an increase in energy expenditure. Further communication between leptin target neurons and hypophysiotropic neurons in the arcuate and paraventricular nuclei integrates nutritional status with pituitary-dependent process of growth and development, reproduction, lactation, and adrenocortical functions.

Other effects of leptin

Leptin receptors also are found in many cells outside of the central nervous system. Adipocytes express leptin receptors and increase their rates of lipolysis in response to autocrine stimulation. Leptin acts directly on pancreatic beta cells and inhibits insulin synthesis and secretion. Leptin and insulin are participants of a negative feedback arrangement between beta cells and adipocytes in which stimulation of leptin secretion by insulin leads to inhibition of insulin secretion by leptin. This relationship may contribute, albeit weakly, to maintenance of regulation of adipose tissue mass, which increases in response of insulin. In muscle, leptin activates AMPK and thereby increases the oxidation of fatty acids and the uptake of glucose. The presence of leptin receptors in the gonads suggests that peripheral actions of leptin may complement the fertility-promoting effects exerted at the hypothalamic level. Other peripheral effects of leptin include actions in bone marrow to promote hematopoiesis and actions in capillary endothelium to increase angiogenesis (blood vessel formation).

Insulin as an adiposity signal

Until now we have considered insulin as the promoter of fat storage and defender of body fuel reserves. It may therefore seem paradoxical that insulin also acts as an adiposity signal that may limit accumulation of fat reserves. On average, plasma concentrations of insulin, like those of leptin, are proportional to adipose mass, and secretion of both hormones is reduced during fasting and inhibited by sympathetic nervous stimulation. Consistent with other homeostatic negative feedback mechanisms, the increase in insulin secretion evoked by eating might be expected to limit further food intake. It may be recalled that hyperphagia (excessive food intake) is one of the hallmarks of untreated insulin deficiency. Actions of insulin on arcuate neurons virtually duplicate the actions of leptin. Both the NPY and the POMC neurons express insulin receptors and respond to insulin with a decrease in NPY and AGRP release and an increase in α-MSH and CART release. However, insulin cannot substitute for leptin as witnessed by the severe consequences of leptin deficiency even in hyperinsulinemic subjects.

To serve as an adiposity signal, insulin secretion must be influenced by adipose tissue in a way that is proportionate to its mass. Even in the fed state, adipose tissue releases some FFAs and the total amount that enters the bloodstream reflects the overall mass of adipose tissue. FFAs, perhaps acting through G-protein-coupled receptors in the beta cell membrane, or perhaps through effects on beta cell metabolism, amplify insulin secretion in response to circulating concentrations of glucose. At the same time, FFA decreases the sensitivity of muscle and liver to the effects of insulin. Increased availability of FFA limits metabolism of glucose in muscles and stimulates hepatic gluconeogenesis, thereby countering insulin's inhibitory effect on glucose production. In addition, adipose tissue secretes a variety of peptides that further decrease insulin sensitivity. In compensation, and to maintain plasma glucose concentrations within the physiological range (Fig. 8.37), pancreatic beta cells increase their secretion of insulin. Normal homeostatic regulation of metabolism is maintained as long as the beta cells remain competent and can secrete enough insulin to compensate for decreased sensitivity. Failure to keep pace with the decrease in sensitivity results in type II diabetes mellitus.

With the prevalence of obesity in contemporary society, it appears that insulin and leptin are not very effective in maintaining constancy of lipid stores. Two possible explanations have been offered to account for this. The "thrifty gene" hypothesis holds that because mammals evolved in environments of nutrient scarcity, mechanisms for storing excess calories in the rare times of plenty took precedence over maintaining leanness. Traits that promoted nutrient storage are essential for successful reproduction and survival, whereas those that favored leanness had little survival value. Consequently, leptin and insulin may be effective in regulating energy expenditure at the relatively low plasma concentrations produced in circumstances ranging from fasting to what we would consider normal nutrition. Beyond this point, regulatory capacity may be saturated and the higher concentrations produced by the overexpanded adipose mass may have little effect. Alternatively, the high circulating concentrations of leptin and insulin may lead to hormone resistance at the level of the hypothalamus, much like the insulin resistance of peripheral insulin targets. Leptin was discussed earlier in this chapter.

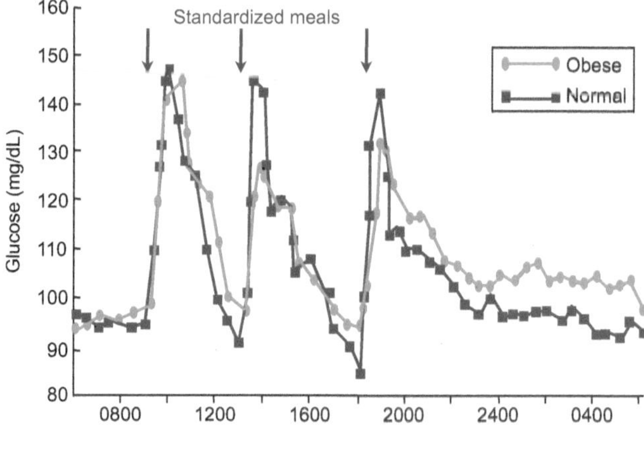

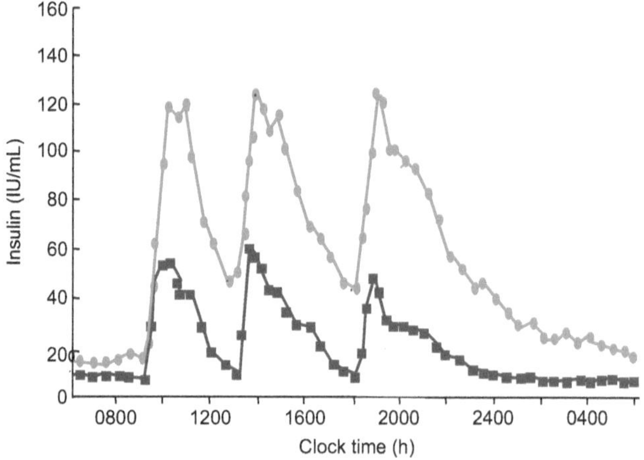

FIGURE 8.37 Twenty-four-hour profiles of plasma concentrations of glucose and insulin in 15 obese and 14 age- and sex-matched normal subjects. The greater excursions of insulin values in the obese despite virtually identical levels of blood glucose are indicative of decreased sensitivity of liver, muscle, and adipose tissue to the actions of insulin. Source: *From Polonsky, K., Given, B. D., & Van Cauter, E. (1988). Twenty-four-hour profiles and pulsatile patterns of insulin secretion in normal and obese subjects.* Journal of Clinical Investigation, *81, 442–448.*

Adipokines

In addition to its role as the body's fuel tank, adipose tissue secretes more than 50 biologically active peptides called adipokines. Some adipokines are produced by the adipocytes themselves; others are secreted by the various stromal and vascular elements, macrophages, and other immune cells that populate the adipose depots. Many of these adipokines are associated with immune responses, inflammation, hemostasis, and blood pressure regulation and have been studied in the context of obesity and its pathological sequelae, which include type II diabetes (see Chapter 7: The Pancreatic Islets) and the metabolic syndrome. Their increased production in obesity may be a reflection of the dysfunctional state of hypertrophied adipocytes and the mild inflammation that is associated with this condition. Adipokines, the elevated plasma levels of which are associated with cardiovascular complications and type II diabetes, seem to be produced in greater abundance by visceral (intraabdominal) adipose tissue depots than by subcutaneous depots. Their roles, if any, in normal physiology and energy homeostasis are not understood. We consider only a few of these peptides, the physiological roles of which are apparent in the context of energy homeostasis.

Adiponectin

Adiponectin is produced exclusively in adipocytes and is more abundant in plasma than any other peptide hormone. It was discovered simultaneously in several different labs and given different names by each, but adiponectin is now its generally accepted name. It is synthesized as a 248-amino acid protein, including a 16-amino acid signal sequence. Prominent structural features include a collagen-like domain and a C-terminal globular domain, the three-dimensional shape of which resembles that of the unrelated cytokine, tumor necrosis factor-α (TNF-α). Adiponectin monomeric units self-assemble into homotrimers, which are the primary secreted form. The trimers in turn assemble into high-molecular-weight complexes of 6, 12, or 18 monomeric units.

Posttranslational processing includes glycosylation and hydroxylation that, along with formation of high-molecular-weight complexes, appear to be required for maximal biological activity. In sharp contrast to the adipokines discussed earlier, adiponectin production and its plasma concentrations are highest when the adipose mass is small and decrease as the adipose mass increases. TNF-α and IL-6 inhibit adiponectin secretion, and their secretion in turn may be inhibited by adiponectin. Adiponectin secretion is increased by the class of drugs called thiazolidinediones, which activate PPARγ, and are used therapeutically for treating type II diabetes.

Adiponectin has both peripheral and central effects on energy metabolism. Peripherally, it is an insulin sensitizer. It activates AMPK in muscle and liver and decreases plasma glucose, and FFA increases their uptake and oxidation in muscle. Because AMPK blocks production and accelerates destruction of malonyl CoA, accumulated lipid metabolites are oxidized and their inhibitory effects on glucose metabolism are reduced. In the liver, adiponectin suppresses the expression of gluconeogenic enzymes and reduces hepatic glucose production. Its autocrine effects on adipocytes include enhanced activity of lipoprotein lipase leading to increased uptake and storage of lipids and decreased plasma TAGs. In combination, these actions increase insulin sensitivity and lower circulating concentrations of insulin.

Adiponectin receptors are present in neurons in the paraventricular nucleus. These neurons receive input from arcuate POMC and NPY neurons as well as direct input from leptin. Paraventricular neurons, including CRH neurons, communicate with autonomic centers implicated in energy utilization. When injected directly into the brains of experimental obese animals, adiponectin excited pathways leading to increased energy expenditure in much the same manner as leptin but did not inhibit or stimulate food intake. Adiponectin and leptin appear to work in concert to increase energy expenditure.

Tumor necrosis factor-α

TNF-α is a cytokine that usually is associated with macrophages and immune and inflammatory responses (see Chapter 4: The Adrenal Glands). It is also expressed in adipocytes and the macrophages that populate adipose tissue. TNF-α is synthesized as a 26 kDa transmembrane protein and is cleaved to release a 17 kDa protein that then trimerizes to its 51 kDa active form. Increased TNF-α is associated with decreased food intake in a variety of pathological states. Although it circulates in blood and can cross the blood–brain barrier, it does not appear to affect hypothalamic feeding centers directly. TNF-α is overexpressed in obesity, and its plasma concentrations correlate with both the mass of adipose tissue and degree of insulin resistance. In normal physiology, adipocyte-derived TNF-α acts mainly in an autocrine or paracrine capacity that can be viewed as protecting against expansion of the adipose tissue depots. It increases basal lipolysis and the release of FFA and decreases uptake and esterification of circulating lipids by downregulating lipoprotein lipase and GLUT4. TNF-α disrupts insulin signaling by promoting phosphorylation and inactivation of insulin receptor substrates. TNF-α indirectly reduces food intake by increasing leptin production and decreasing insulin sensitivity.

Interleukin-6

Interleukin-6 (IL-6) is another cytokine that is produced by immune cells and usually is associated with inflammation. It is a member of the superfamily of cytokines that includes leptin, GH, and prolactin and is produced and secreted in proportion to adipose mass. In obesity as much as one-third of the IL-6 that circulates in plasma arises in adipose tissue. IL-6 is synthesized mainly in the stromal and vascular cells rather than adipocytes and is produced more abundantly in intraabdominal fat depots than in subcutaneous depots. Its production increases acutely in response to eating. IL-6 acts both as a circulating hormone and a local paracrine factor. In adipose tissue, IL-6 increases lipolysis and leptin secretion, decreases the expression of lipoprotein lipase, and interferes with insulin signaling. In the central nervous system, IL-6 increases energy expenditure, but paradoxically, although secretion and plasma concentrations are increased in obesity, concentrations of IL-6 within the brain are decreased in animal models of obesity.

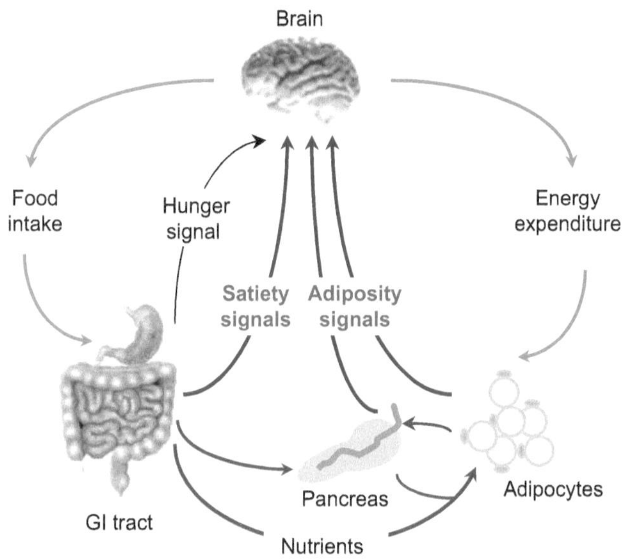

FIGURE 8.38 Overall regulation of energy balance. Ghrelin is the only known hunger signal arising from gut. All other input from the GI tract signal satiety. Leptin and insulin are the principal adiposity signals.

Satiety signals

Adiposity signals by and large operate on a long time scale and monitor accumulation or depletion of fat stores. Storage of excess calories also depends upon the frequency and duration of food intake. Food intake is monitored on a meal-to-meal basis and is reported to the brain by signals that arise from the gastrointestinal tract. Chemo- and mechanosensors in endocrine cells or neurons embedded in the walls of the stomach and intestines monitor volume and composition of luminal contents and generate hormonal or neural signals (Fig. 8.38).

Gastrointestinal hormones that act as satiety signals are discussed in Chapter 6, Hormones of the Gastrointestinal, and are listed in Table 8.1. Ghrelin is the only peripheral orexigenic (promoter of food intake) signal thus far known. Its secretion increases just prior to eating and, although duodenal glucose and fatty acids inhibit its secretion, factors that increase ghrelin secretion are unknown.

Except for ghrelin, peripheral satiety factors, both hormonal and neuronal, operate to limit meal size (Table 8.1).

The sites of integration of satiety signals are in the hindbrain in regions that include the nucleus of the tractus solitarius (NTS), the area postrema, and the dorsal motor nucleus of the vagus nerve. This region also receives input relating to gastric or intestinal distension from vagal and spinal afferents, and information regarding the taste, texture, and smell of food from cranial nerves. There is strong evidence for bidirectional communication between the arcuate and paraventricular nuclei and the NTS, and that adiposity signals modulate responsiveness to satiety signals. Leptin and insulin increase sensitivity to the inhibitory effects of CCK and other hormonal satiety signals on food intake. Neurons in the NTS express receptors for leptin and insulin; these hormones

TABLE 8.1 Peripheral satiety factors.

Hormone	Source	Food intake	Target cells
Ghrelin	Gastric X/A cells	↑	Arcuate NPY cells, dorsal vagal complex, gastric vagal afferent neurons
CCK	Duodenal I cells	↓	Vagal afferent neurons and the area postrema
Glucagon-like peptide 1	Ileal L cells	↓	Paraventricular nucleus, area postrema, nucleus of the tractus solitarius vagal afferent neurons
Oxyntomodulin	Ileal L cells	↓	Arcuate nucleus
Peptide YY	Ileal L cells	↓	Arcuate NPY cells, area postrema
Pancreatic polypeptide	Pancreatic F cells	↓	Area postrema
Amylin	Pancreatic Beta cells	↓	Area postrema

NPY, Neuropeptide Y.

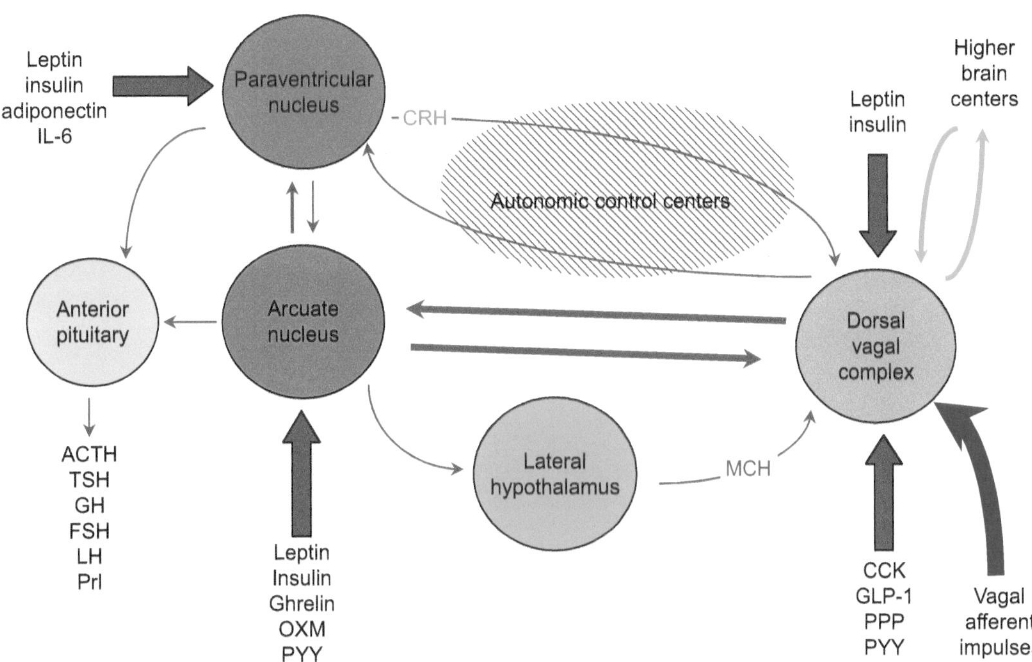

FIGURE 8.39 Major routes of communication in the regulation of energy balance. Cross talk between the hypothalamus and the dorsal vagal complex integrates input from adiposity and satiety signals. The dorsal vagal complex includes the area postrema, the nucleus of the tractus solitarius, and the dorsal motor nucleus of the vagus. *CCK*, Cholecystokinin; *CRH*, corticotropin-releasing hormone; *GLP-1*, glucagon-like peptide-1; *IL-6*, interleukin 6; *MCH*, melanin-concentrating hormone; *OXM*, oxyntomodulin; *PPP*, pancreatic polypeptide; *PYY*, peptide YY.

may modulate satiety responses either through direct actions or by way of projections from hypothalamic neurons. The NTS also receives neural input from α-MSH and GLP-1-secreting neurons, which may be intermediaries between the arcuate and hindbrain feeding centers. Eating is a voluntary act and input from higher brain centers driven by hedonic or emotional impulses converge on the hindbrain feeding center (Fig. 8.39).

Perspective

The obvious importance of controlling obesity from an economic as well as a public health point of view has engendered a frenzy of research in this area. In addition, technological advances that allow targeted knockout, knock in, and knockdown of specific genes provide unprecedented capacity to study both central and peripheral regulatory mechanisms. Nevertheless, much remains to be learned, and new and exciting findings are reported with increasingly frequency.

Summary

This chapter explores the role of hormones in the regulation of glucose and lipids. These body fuels are responsible for normal growth and homeostasis. Of particular interest is the regulation of satiety and its lack thereof in obesity.

Suggested readings

Basic foundations

Cone, R. D., & Elmquist, J. K. (2016). Neuroendocrine control of energy stores. In S. Melmed, K. S. Polonsky, P. R. Larson, & H. M. Kronenberg (Eds.), *Williams textbook of endocrinology* (13th ed., pp. 1608–1632). Philadelphia, PA: Elsevier.

Hall, J. E. (2016). *Lipid metabolism. Guyton and Hall textbook of medical physiology* (13th ed., pp. 863–874). Philadelphia, PA: Elsevier.

Semenkovich, C. F., Goldberg, A. C., & Goldberg, I. (2016). Disorders of lipid metabolism. In S. Melmed, K. S. Polonsky, P. R. Larson, & H. M. Kronenberg (Eds.), *Williams textbook of endocrinology* (13th ed., pp. 1660–1700). Philadelphia, PA: Elsevier.

Shulman, G. I., & Pittersen, K. F. (2017). Metabolism. In W. F. Boron, & E. L. Boulpaep (Eds.), *Medical physiology* (3rd ed., pp. 1170–1192). Philadelphia, PA: Elsevier.

Advanced information

Chait, A., & Goldberg, I. (2017). Treatment of dyslipidemia in diabetes: Recent advances and remaining questions. *Current Diabetes Reports*, *17*(11), 112. Available from https://doi.org/10.1007/s11892-017-0942-8.

Gupta, N., Asi, N., Farah, W., Almasri, J., Barrionuevo, P., Alsawas, M., ... Murad, M. H. (2017). Clinical features and management of non-HIV-related lipodystrophy in children: A systematic review. *The Journal of Clinical Endocrinology & Metabolism*, *102*(2), 363–374. Available from https://doi.org/10.1210/jc.2016-2271.

Hussain, I., & Garg, A. (2016). Lipodystrophy syndromes. *Endocrinology and Metabolism Clinics of North America*, *45*(4), 783–797. Available from https://doi.org/10.1016/j.ecl.2016.06.012.

Quinn, K., & Purcell, S. M. (2017). *Lipodystrophies*. StatPearls [Internet].

CHAPTER

9

Regulation of salt and water balance

Case study—Primary aldosteronism (Conn syndrome)

He was the head of a corporation in his late 40s. He came to his family physician because he was having headaches. A routine blood pressure was attempted, but the systolic could not be read—the diastolic appeared to be 175 mmHg. He was referred to endocrinology and was admitted to the hospital on the basis of his diastolic bp. A call to the local zoo found a blood pressure cuff that went over 300 mmHg, the upper limit of all standard sphygmomanometers. The zoo's cuff was obtained and with it a systolic of 310 mmHg was found. It was amazing that the hypertension this patient had did not rupture a cerebral artery and cause a stroke. There were no other signs of end-organ damage, presumably because the blood pressure build-up was over time rather than suddenly.

The patient was started on intravenous nitroprusside with a small amount of dopamine (dopamine is no longer concurrently with nitroprusside). His blood pressure was reduced to 160 systolic and maintained there while the diagnostic work up was completed.

His blood work showed that he had hypokalemia and hypernatremia. His diet was unremarkable, and he had not ingested any black licorice nor taken glycyrrhizin. Glycyrrhizin is a drug found in black licorice. In China and Europe, it is also used to treat biliary inflammation. Glycyrrhizin acts like aldosterone, and there have been several cases of hypertension with end-organ damage due to this compound.

A CT of the abdominal cavity was taken as such cases are usually indicative of a tumor, either a pheochromocytoma (a neoplasm of the chromaffin cells of the adrenal medulla) or an adenoma of the zona glomerulosa. The CT was similar to the one in Fig. 9.1 except that the tumor was on the left side instead of the right.

To confirm the results of the CT scan the right and left adrenal veins were sampled for aldosterone. Sampling on the left side is comparatively easy as the adrenal vein comes into the left renal vein at an angle and inserting a cannula via a right femoral cutdown is relatively easy (Fig. 9.2).

Visualizing by fluoroscopy, the cannula goes up the right femoral vein which becomes the right external iliac vein, then across the common right iliac vein and into the inferior vena cava. From there it goes into the left renal vein and from thence into the left adrenal vein. However, the right adrenal vein presents a challenge because it enters the inferior vena cava at a right angle, making the insertion of the cannula difficult. The sampling showed very high aldosterone output on the left side, characteristic of a benign adenoma of the glomerulosa tissue.

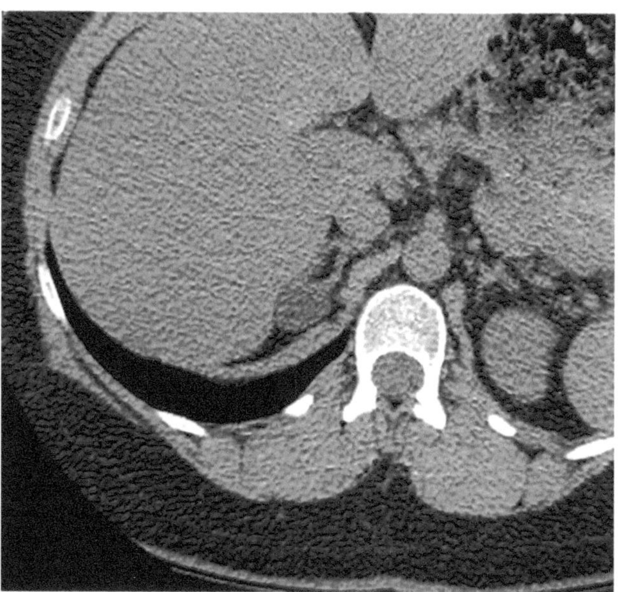

FIGURE 9.1 An aldosterone-secreting adenoma (*blue arrow*). In this patient, a woman in her 40s, the aldosterone sampled from the right adrenal vein was 32,278 ng/dL and from the left adrenal vein 107 ng/dL. The left adrenal is normal (*white arrow*) with its "Y"-shaped image. Source: *From Figure 53.5 in Ho L. M. (2017). Chapter 53:* Adrenal glands. *In John R. Haaga, & Daniel T. Boll (Eds.),* CT and MRI of the whole body *(6th ed.) (p. 1763). Elsevier.*

Goodman's Basic Medical Endocrinology.
DOI: https://doi.org/10.1016/B978-0-12-815844-9.00009-9

(cont'd)

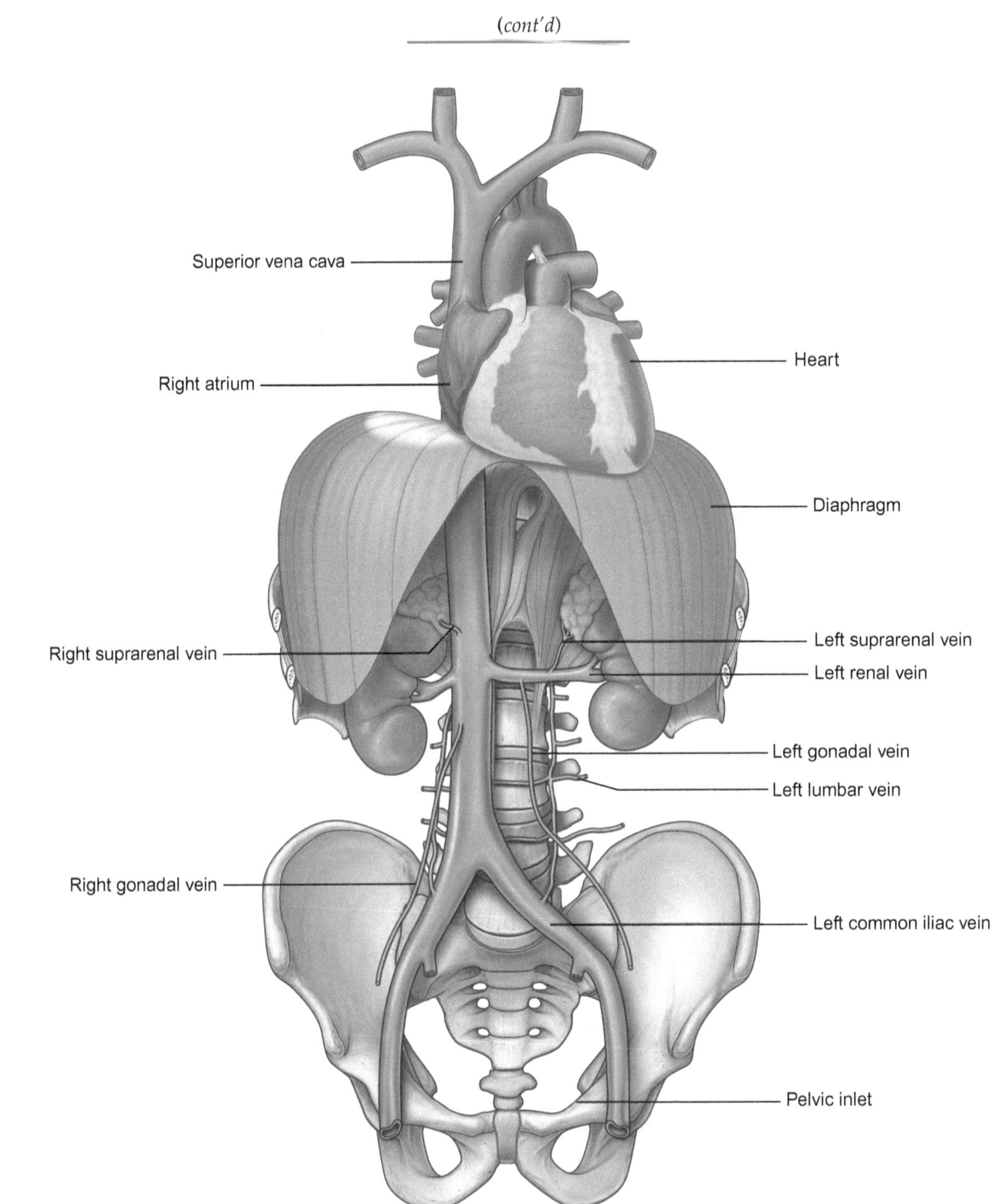

FIGURE 9.2 The right and left adrenal (suprarenal) veins. Note that the right comes off at right angles to the inferior vena cava, whereas the left is angled and ends in the left renal vein which then empties into the inferior vena cava. Source: *From Figure 4.18 in R. L. Drake, A. W. Vogl, & A. W. M. Mitchell. (2015).* Gray's anatomy for students *(3rd ed.) (p. 273). Elsevier.*

Accordingly, a unilateral anterior surgical approach was done to remove the left adrenal gland. As this technique is now outdated, the newer laparoscopic approach will be demonstrated (Figs. 9.3 and 9.4).

The adrenal gland is highly vascular (Fig. 9.5), and despite careful surgery, postoperative bleeding was encountered necessitating reopening the incision and stopping the bleeders.

(cont'd)

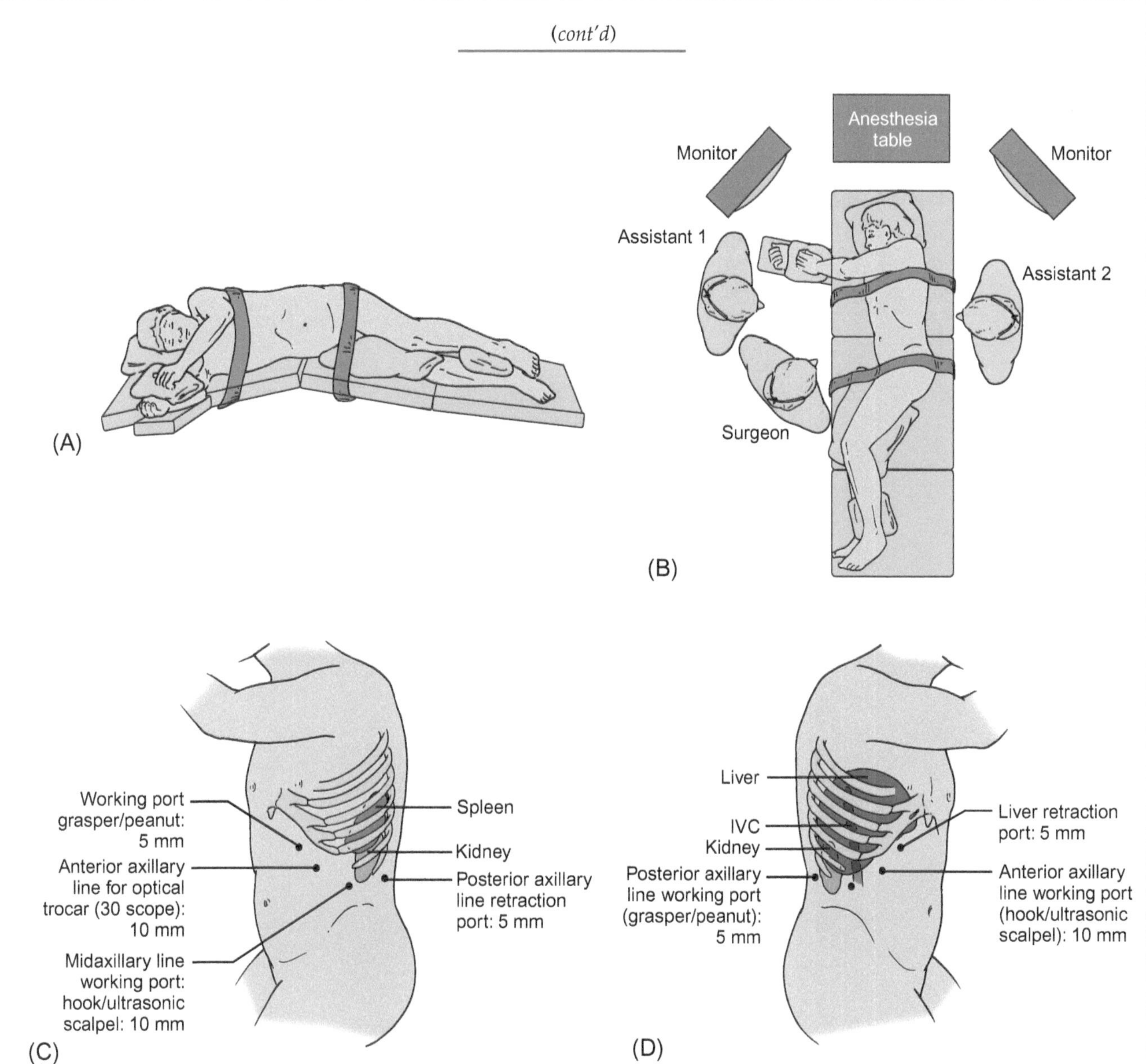

FIGURE 9.3 Positioning for left laparoscopic adrenalectomy. (A) The flexed position of the operating table so that the space is increased between the lower rib cage and the iliac crest. The patient is taped to the table and bean bags placed under the patient as shown. (B) The position of the surgeons and assistants around the table and the placement of the monitors. (C) and (D) The position of the ports for left and right adrenalectomies. Source: *From Figure 129-2, Peng, P., Bischof, D., Ball, D., & Ahuja, N. (2014). Chapter 129: The management of adrenal cortical tumors. In J. L. Cameron, & A. M. Cameron (Eds.),* Current surgical therapy *(11th ed.) (p. 633). Elsevier.*

A biopsy of the excised left adrenal gland revealed four aldosteronomas, one which had grown large enough to be visualized by CT scan.

The patient recovered and his blood pressure returned to normal. He did complain of being more tired than usual, which was due to the general anesthetic agent. The drug goes into the adipose tissue after leaving the brain and takes up to 6 months to be fully released during which time, as it is released, it causes patients to feel sleepy and tired in the afternoon.

He was discharged but came back periodically to have his blood pressure checked. There were no sequelae.

(*cont'd*)

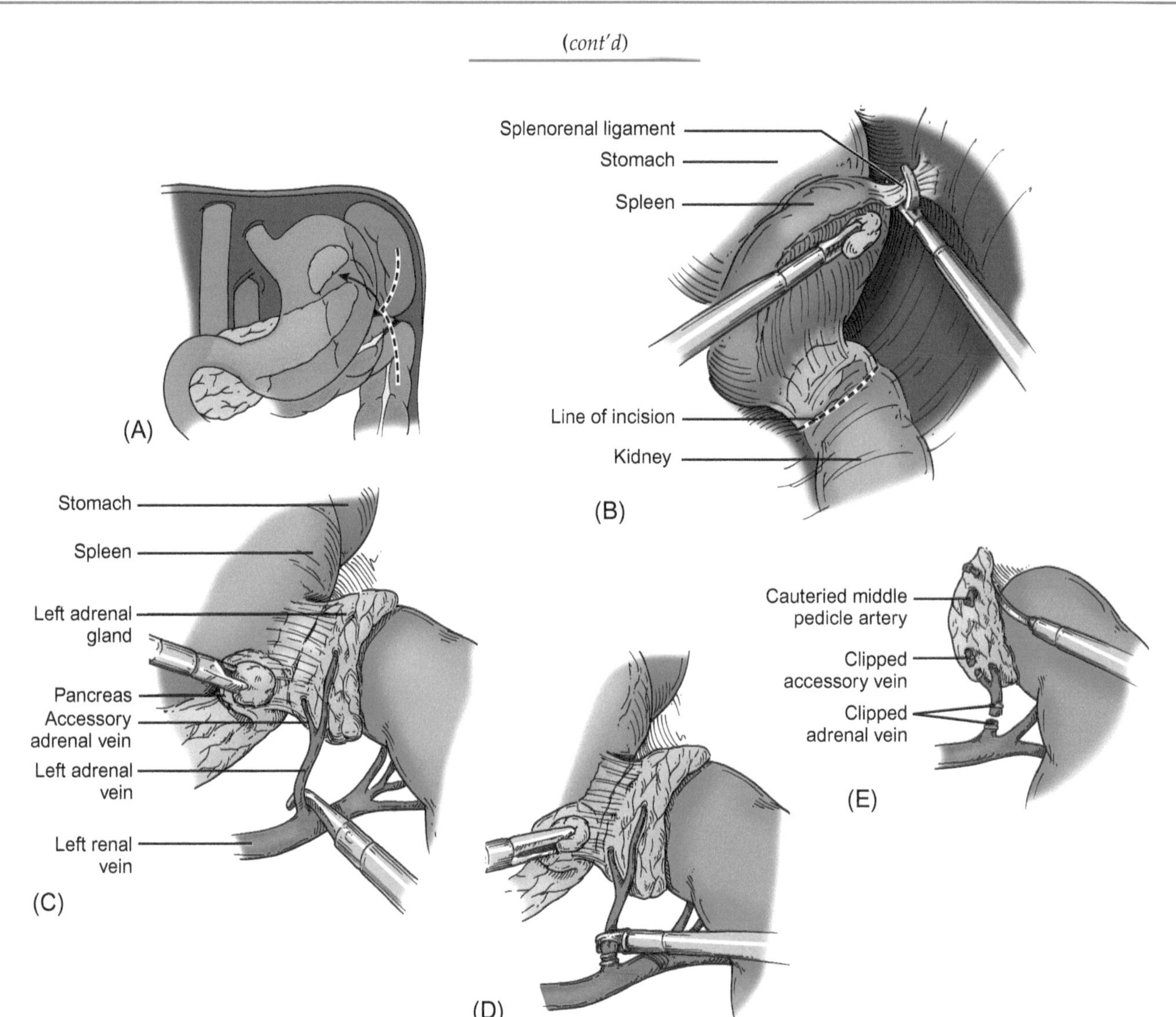

FIGURE 9.4 Procedure for laparoscopic left adrenalectomy. In (A), after induction of general anesthesia and the placement of an orogastric tube to deflate the stomach and duodenum, trochars are placed on either side of the camera port. The splenic flexure of the colon is mobilized inferiorly and the spleen mobilized medially over the body and fundus of the stomach by a fan retractor. In (B), the peritoneum is incised at the tail of the pancreas (not labeled) to expose the adrenal gland. In (C), using a sonic scalpel. the left adrenal vein is exposed (D) and in (E) it is clipped and divided. The adrenal gland is then dissected away from the abdominal wall, the arteries cauterized and other veins clipped. Source: *From Figure 129-3, Peng, P., Bischof, D., Ball, D., & Ahuja, N. (2014). Chapter 129: The management of adrenal cortical tumors. In J. L. Cameron, & A. M. Cameron (Eds.),* Current surgical therapy *(11th ed.) (p. 634). Elsevier.*

(cont'd)

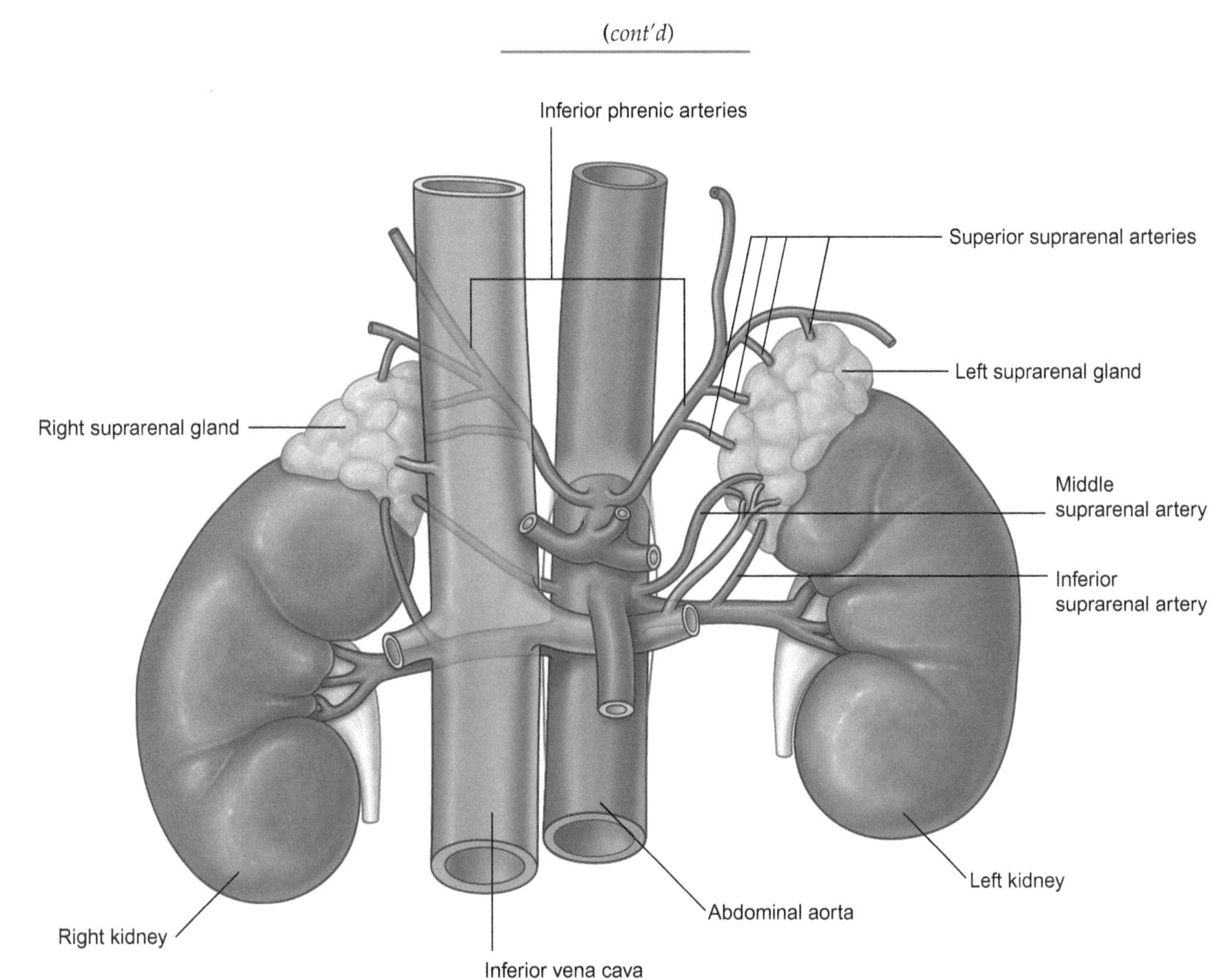

FIGURE 9.5 The arterial system of the adrenal gland. The adrenal glands obtain their arterial blood from three different sources: (1) superior adrenal arteries are branches of the inferior phrenic arteries, (2) the middle adrenal artery comes directly from the abdominal aorta, and (3) the inferior adrenal artery is a branch of the renal artery. Source: *From Figure 4.150 in R. L. Drake, A. W. Vogl, & A. W. M. Mitchell. (2015).* Gray's anatomy for students *(3rd ed.) (p. 386). Elsevier.*

In the clinic

Conn syndrome

Hypertension is one of the most common cardiovascular disorders. It is the third most common cause of death (after heart disease and cancer) in developed countries. Most cases are idiopathic and so are called essential or primary hypertension. Of the causes of secondary hypertension, primary aldosteronism (Conn syndrome) is responsible for 1%–10% of cases. Conn described the first case in 1955 and so the disorder bears his name. Sixty-five percent of those cases are due to unilateral adrenal involvement and 25% are bilateral, with both adrenals being involved.

Signs and symptoms

The patient has hypertension that cannot be well controlled with medication. He or she also has hypokalemia which may cause cardiac arrhythmias. The patient may complain of headaches and cardiac palpitations and be weak from lack of potassium.

(cont'd)

Diagnosis

The diagnosis is made when a CT scan reveals either a tumor, as in the case study, or enlarged adrenals called idiopathic adrenal hyperplasia. As the name implies, the cause of the hyperplasia has never been determined. A careful history will usually establish whether the condition is genetic or not. The diagnosis must be confirmed by sampling each adrenal vein. If only one vein is sampled, for example, only the left vein, a unilateral adrenalectomy will do little good if there is tumor material on the opposite side.

An aldosterone-to-renin ration is one of the most sensitive tests for primary aldosteronism. Several other tests (furosemide, saline infusion, and captopril tests) can also be done to confirm the diagnosis.

Management

Initially, the blood pressure must be quickly brought under control. This can be done pharmacologically. After that, surgical intervention to remove the tumor or hyperplastic adrenal should be done. If both adrenals are removed, adrenal replacement therapy must be instituted. Even if one is removed, aldosterone and cortisol levels should be monitored as the remaining normal adrenal output may have been suppressed. Electrolytes and cardiac function should also be monitored to prevent arrhythmias. If primary aldosteronism is due to bilateral adrenal hyperplasia and surgery cannot be performed, then spironolactone can be used to treat this disorder.

Prognosis

Patients with primary aldosteronism have a higher mortality rate than the normotensive population because the hypertension may have shortened end-organ longevity.

Introduction

Sodium and water balance are precisely regulated by the endocrine system. Osmolality of the extracellular fluid is monitored and adjusted by regulating water excretion by the kidney in response to antidiuretic hormone (ADH), which is secreted by the posterior lobe of the pituitary gland. Constancy of blood osmolality ensures constancy of cellular volume, but if it were attained only by adjusting water retention, the vascular volume would fluctuate widely. Therefore blood volume must also be precisely regulated so that it is sufficient to ensure perfusion of body tissues but not so expanded that blood pressure is increased. Because sodium is the major electrolyte in extracellular fluid, maintenance of vascular volume depends on the maintenance of sodium balance. Renal mechanisms that govern retention or loss of sodium are regulated by the renin–angiotensin–aldosterone system and the atrial natriuretic factor (ANF). ADH also contributes directly to volume regulation, and when demands for constancy of osmolality are in conflict with demands for constancy of volume, the latter prevail. These hormonal mechanisms operate largely by regulating renal function, but they also regulate salt and water intake and vascular tone.

General considerations

All cells of the body have an uninterrupted requirement for nutrients and oxygen, and produce waste materials. In addition, many cells must receive signals from other parts of the body to perform their specialized tasks, which in some cases include the production of some product that must be transported to other specialized cells. The cardiovascular system accommodates these nutritive, excretory, and communicative needs. Blood readily equilibrates with the fluid that bathes each cell and thereby preserves the integrity of the extracellular environment, delivers chemical messages, and transports excretory and secretory products. The integrity of the blood is restored as it flows through organs such as kidneys, lungs, and liver, whose specialized functions renew the blood's composition and maintain its constancy.

Perfusion of tissues is ensured by maintaining both a sufficient volume of arterial blood and adequate pressure to drive it through the capillaries. Blood flow to a region is matched to the changing requirements of cells by locally initiated adjustments in arteriolar tone. Circularly oriented smooth muscle cells in arterioles relax in response to products of cellular metabolism and thus decrease resistance to flow. Increased flow washes away accumulated products, and with removal of the signal for vasodilation, arterioles regain their former tone. The circulatory system can thus be viewed as a central reservoir of pressurized fluid that can be tapped on demand at any locale to provide needed renewal of the cellular environment.

Several factors go into maintenance of the central reservoir of pressure: (1) the contraction of the heart that provides pressure, (2) a high degree of arteriolar tone that slows the dissipation of the energy imparted by each contraction of the heart, (3) low compliance of the arterial tree that allows pressure to build up, and (4) sufficient volume of blood that fills the system. Central control exerted through the autonomic nervous system provides the minute-to-minute adjustments to cardiac function and arteriolar constriction that maintain blood pressure relatively constant. Volume is regulated largely by the endocrine system, but volume and pressure are closely interrelated. Changes in volume can offset changes in arteriolar tone and vice versa to maintain constancy or at least adequacy of the central pressure reservoir. It is not surprising, therefore, that hormones that play decisive roles in regulating blood volume also constrict or dilate arterioles.

Permeability of capillaries to small molecules allows blood in the vascular compartment to equilibrate quickly with interstitial fluid. Blood and interstitial fluid together comprise the extracellular compartment, which contains about one-third of total body water (Fig. 9.6).

Water distributes freely between the vascular compartment and the interstitial compartment, usually in a ratio of 1:3. In some pathological states, however, the interstitial compartment becomes disproportionately enlarged, and edema may be considerable. Major determinants of this distribution are the protein content of plasma (colloid osmotic pressure), principally albumin, and blood pressure within the capillaries. It appears that the volume of the interstitial compartment is not directly monitored or regulated. Rather, control of interstitial volume is achieved indirectly by controlling pressure, composition, and volume of the vascular compartment.

The volumes of fluid in the intracellular and extracellular compartments also are determined by their solute contents. With a few important exceptions in the kidney, biological membranes are freely permeable to water. Net movement of water into or out of cells is determined by the osmotic gradient. Osmotic flow of water is independent of the identity of solutes and responds simply to the discrepancy in number of solute particles (osmolytes) on either side of the cell membrane. Addition or depletion of water in one compartment, therefore, is followed by compensatory changes in the other. Concentrations of particular solutes on the extracellular or intracellular sides of the plasma membrane are different, however, and are determined by the properties of the membrane.

The major intracellular cation is potassium, whose concentration in cellular water is about 30 times higher than that in extracellular water. The major extracellular cation is sodium, which is present at more than 10 times its intracellular concentration. Blood plasma is in osmotic equilibrium with interstitial and intracellular fluids; therefore regulation of plasma osmolality regulates total body osmolality. Because sodium is the major contributor to the osmolality of blood, and because it is largely excluded from the intracellular compartment, changes in sodium balance can change both the distribution of body water and its total volume. Thus homeostatic regulation of blood volume depends on regulation of intake and excretion of sodium as well as water.

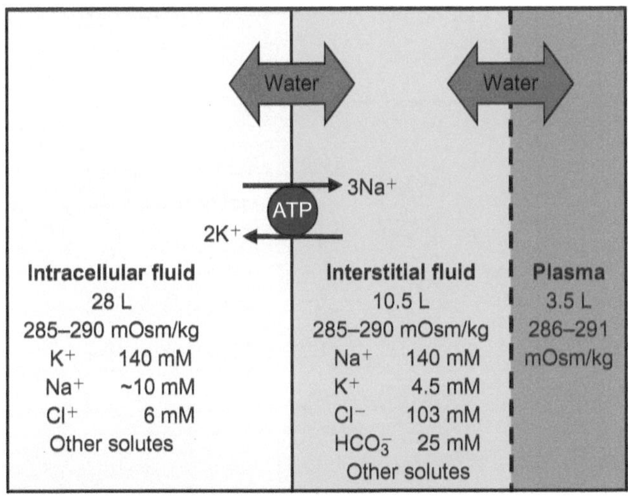

FIGURE 9.6 Distribution of body water and principal electrolytes. Note that water and electrolytes equilibrate freely between plasma and interstitial fluid, but only water equilibrates between the intracellular and extracellular compartments. The electrochemical gradient for sodium is maintained by the activity of the sodium/potassium ATPase.

Salt and water balance

Salt and water balance are maintained remarkably constant despite wide variations in intake and loss of both sodium and water. Intake of sodium may vary from almost none in salt-poor environments to several grams during a binge of potato chips and pretzels. Output is primarily in urine, but smaller losses are also incurred in sweat and feces. Large losses can result from excessive sweating, vomiting, diarrhea, burns, or hemorrhage. The kidney is a powerful regulator of sodium output and can preserve sodium balance even when daily intake varies over the 4000-fold range between 50 mg and 200 g.

Under basal conditions the typical adult turns over about 1.75 L of water each day. Most of it originates in the diet in the form of solid and liquid foods, and the remainder is formed metabolically from the oxidation of carbohydrate and fat. Unavoidable losses occur by evaporation from the lungs and skin, as well as by elimination of wastes in the urine and feces.

Environment, climate, daily activities, and personal habits impose additional needs for either intake or excretion that must be perfectly offset to maintain physiological balance. So long as intake exceeds obligatory losses, balance can be achieved by controlling excretion. Intake, however, is a voluntary act and varies widely. Thirst and salt appetite are increased when intake falls below the amount needed to maintain balance.

Blood volume is monitored indirectly, primarily as a function of pressure. The concentration of sodium, which is the principal osmolyte and electrolyte of plasma and the primary determinant of blood volume, is monitored only indirectly as a function of osmolality. The kidney is the primary effector of regulation, and at least four hormones—ADH, aldosterone, angiotensin II, and ANF (also called atrial natriuretic peptide, ANP)—are used to signal regulatory adjustments. To understand how these hormones regulate water and electrolyte balance, we first consider briefly some aspects of renal function.

The human kidney lies in the abdominal cavity behind the peritoneum (Figs. 9.7–9.9).

Each human kidney contains about 1 million nephrons (Fig. 9.10), which are the functional units that adjust the composition of the urine, and hence the blood, by selective reabsorption or secretion of solutes from the ultrafiltrate of plasma formed at each glomerulus. Each glomerulus (Fig. 9.11) contains a specialized tuft of capillaries situated within the swollen proximal end of the nephron. Glomerular capillaries lie between

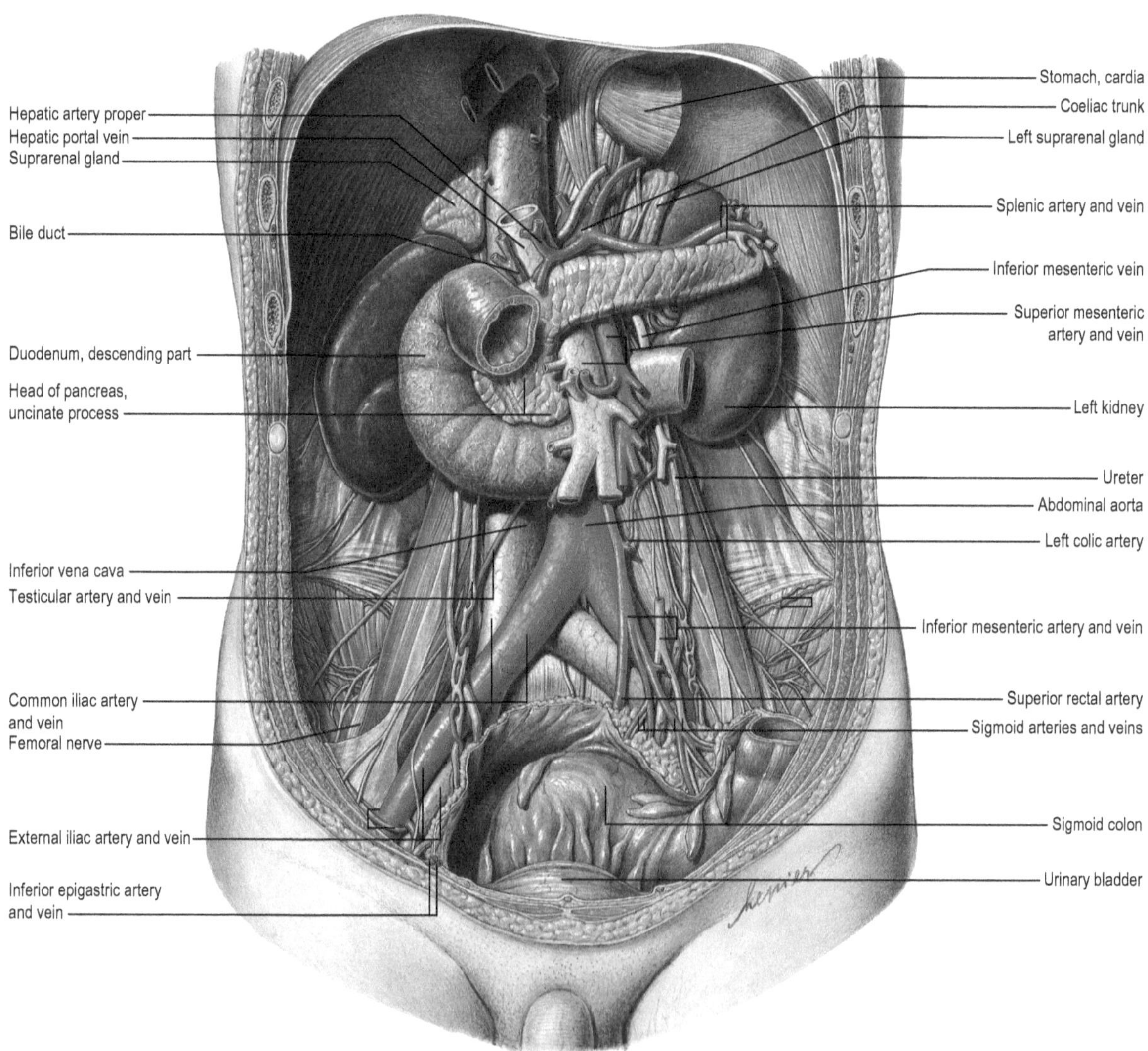

FIGURE 9.7 The kidneys in position at the back of the abdominal cavity. The peritoneum and perirenal fat has been removed so the kidneys can be seen. Note that the right kidney is lower than the left due to the liver. The kidneys formed in the pelvis and moved up. On the right side the liver stopped the upward ascent. Source: *From Figure 74.1 in Susan Standring, editor, (2016).* Gray's anatomy *(41st ed.) (p. 1237). Elsevier.*

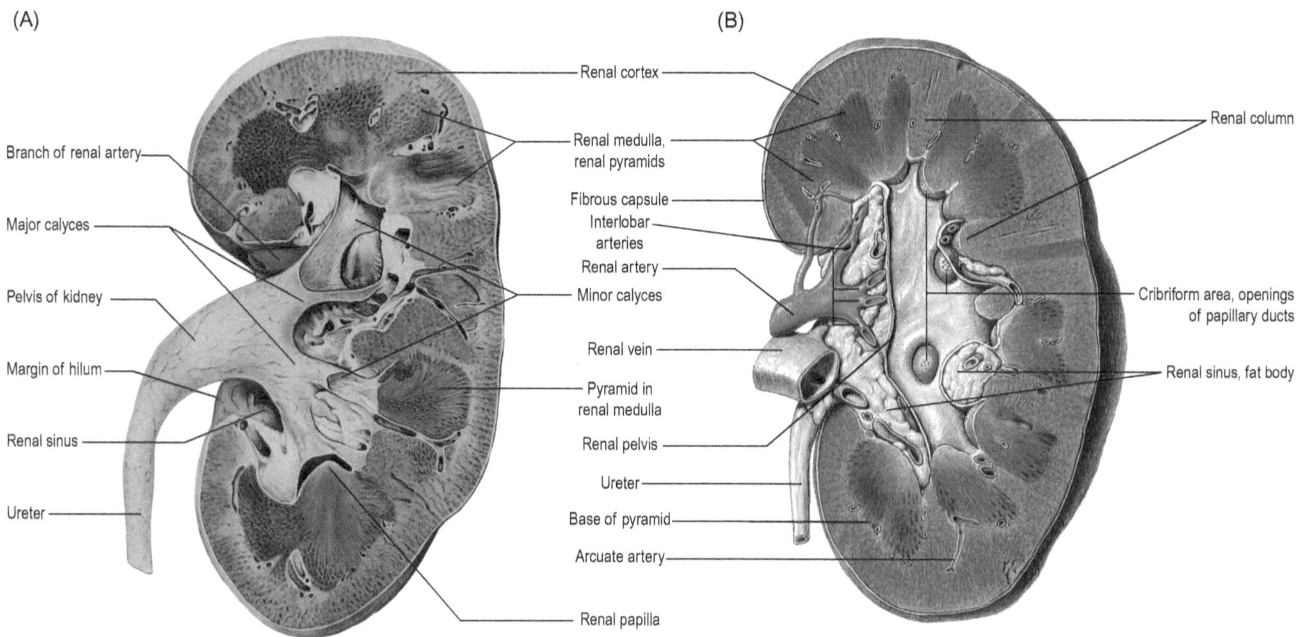

FIGURE 9.8 The left kidney in hemisections so that in (A) the more posterior ureter and pelvis are visible and (B) displays the overlying renal artery and vein as well as the renal sinus fat body. Source: *From Figure 74.9 in Susan Standring, editor. (2016).* Gray's anatomy *(41st ed.) (p. 1242). Elsevier.*

two resistance vessels, an afferent arteriole, which brings blood to them, and an efferent arteriole, which carries blood away. Efferent arterioles give rise to a second capillary network, the peritubular capillaries in the cortex or the vasa recta in the medulla.

Because blood pressure in the glomerular capillaries is relatively high and their endothelium is specialized for filtration, a large volume of nearly protein-free fluid ($\sim$180 L/day) filters through the endothelium to become the precursor of the urine. The increased concentration of proteins in postglomerular blood provides a strong colloid osmotic force for the absorption of interstitial fluid into peritubular capillaries and the vasa recta. About 99% of the glomerular filtrate is reabsorbed, driven through the tubular epithelium by the osmotic forces created by active transport of sodium. Because so large a volume of fluid is processed each day, changes in tubular transport mechanisms that affect reabsorption of only a few percent of the filtered sodium or water are sufficient to maintain homeostasis. Likewise, small changes in intrarenal blood pressure or flow can influence both filtration and reabsorption and provide an additional means of regulating renal function.

Initial processing of the glomerular filtrate takes place in the proximal convoluted tubule where about two-thirds of the sodium and water are reabsorbed isosmotically, driven by sodium-coupled transport of glucose, amino acids, phosphate, bicarbonate, and other solutes. The electrochemical gradient for sodium across the luminal membrane of the tubular cells provides the driving force for sodium-coupled uptake of these compounds. Energy that maintains the sodium gradient is provided by the sodium-potassium ATPase located in the basolateral membranes of these cells. This enzyme "pumps" out three ions of sodium in exchange for two ions of potassium. Passive movements of potassium and other ions maintain electrical neutrality, and the passive movement of water created by accumulation of solutes in the interstitial space drives the reabsorption of water. Although multiple different cotransporters, exchangers, and ion channels are present in different portions of the nephron, the general pattern of passive uptake of sodium at the luminal surface coupled by active sodium/potassium exchange at the basolateral surfaces accounts for virtually all renal tubular renal reabsorptive activity.

The volume of the glomerular filtrate is further reduced by about 20%–25% in the loop of Henle, which is shaped like a hairpin and doubles back on itself in the renal medulla. The loop of Henle consists of three functionally distinct segments: the thin descending limb, which is freely permeable to water; the thin ascending limb, which is permeable to sodium but impermeable to water; and the thick ascending limb, which is also impermeable to water and which actively transports sodium chloride from the tubular

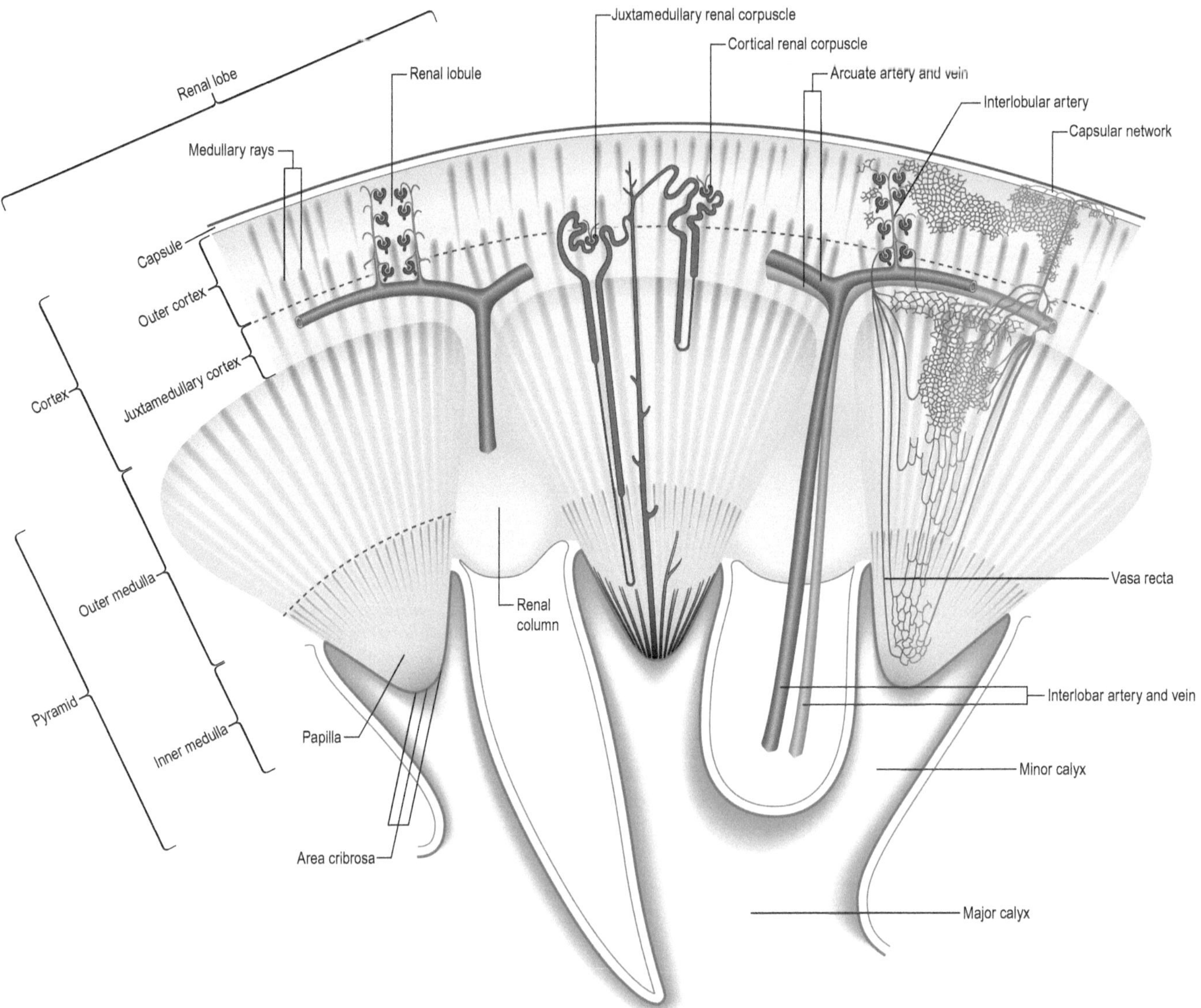

FIGURE 9.9 Detail through a section of the kidney showing the renal lobe and lobule. Human kidneys are multilobular. Source: *From Figure 74.14 in Susan Standring, editor. (2016).* Gray's anatomy *(41st ed.) (p. 1245). Elsevier.*

lumen to the interstitial space. Because sodium chloride is transported while water is held back, the solute concentration of the interstitial space is increased, while the fluid in the thick ascending limb is diluted. Water leaves the thin descending limb and equilibrates rapidly with the sodium chloride-enriched interstitial fluid and hence luminal fluid becomes increasingly concentrated as it flows by the thick ascending limb. Diffusion of sodium, but not water, out of the thin ascending limb increases the sodium concentration in the inner medullary interstitial space. The combination of the geometry of Henle's loop, selective permeability to water, active transport of sodium chloride in the thick ascending limb, and countercurrent flow of fluid through the tubule sets up a countercurrent multiplier effect that produces a gradient of increasing osmolality so that the interstitial sodium concentration in the inner medulla is more than twice that of plasma (Fig. 9.12).

Further reabsorption of solutes in the distal convoluted tubule, the connecting tubule, and the cortical portion of the collecting duct is partially under hormonal control and provides fine-tuning of the ionic composition of the urine, and hence the extracellular fluid. Final steps in the processing of urine take place in the collecting ducts, which extend from the cortex through the deepest reaches of the medulla and empty into the renal pelvis. Fluid in the collecting ducts passes through the interstitial osmotic gradient,

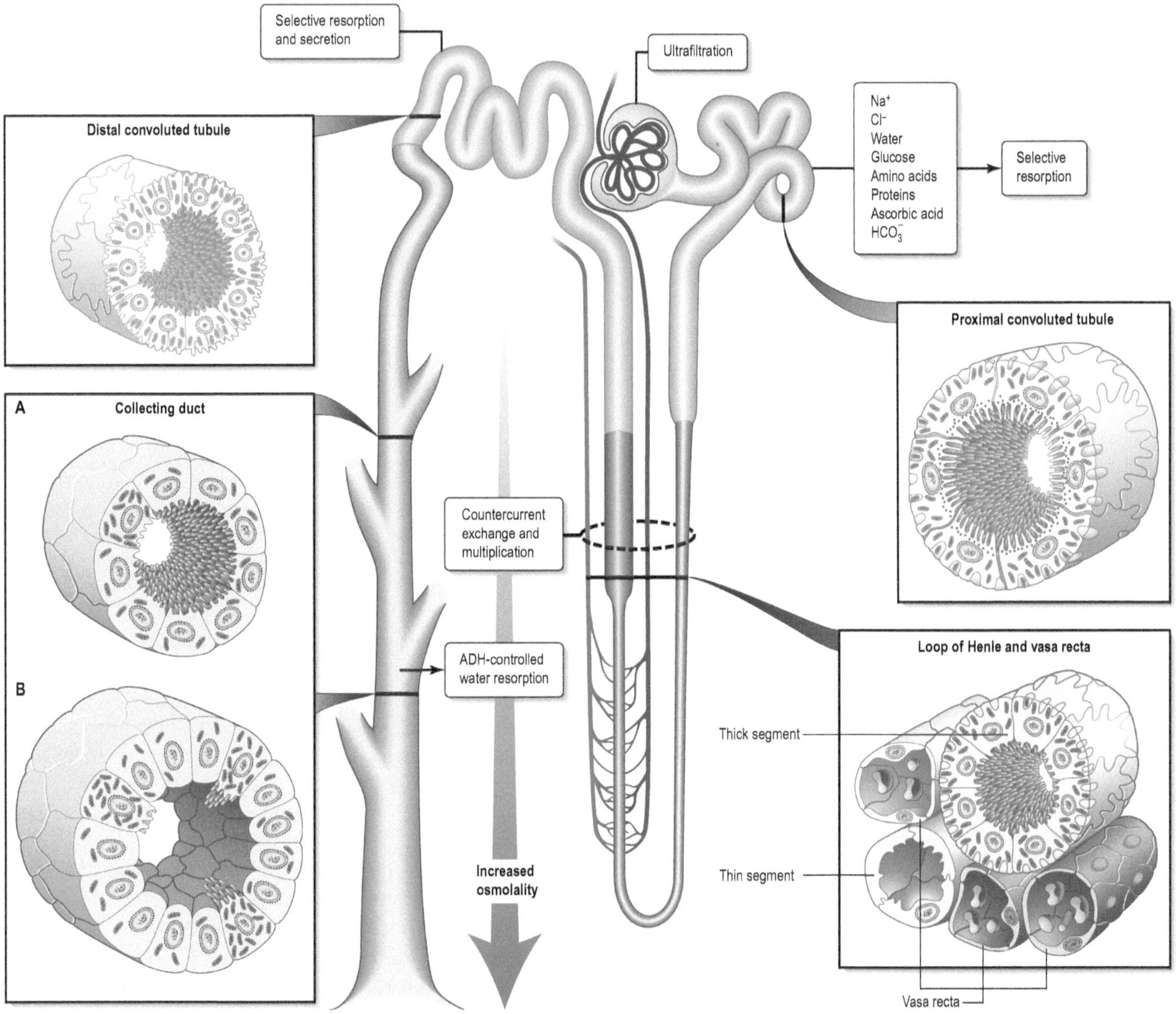

Selective resorption and secretion
Ultrafiltration
Distal convoluted tubule
Na+
Cl−
Water
Glucose
Amino acids
Proteins
Ascorbic acid
HCO_3^-
Selective resorption
Proximal convoluted tubule
A
Collecting duct
Countercurrent exchange and multiplication
ADH-controlled water resorption
B
Loop of Henle and vasa recta
Thick segment
Thin segment
Increased osmolality
Vasa recta

FIGURE 9.10 The nephron in a kidney. Source: *From Figure 74.16 in Susan Standring, editor. (2016).* Gray's anatomy *(41st ed.) (p. 1247). Elsevier.*

Renal corpuscle
Afferent arteriole
Juxtaglomerular apparatus
Efferent arteriole
Glomerular capsule (parietal layer)
Urinary (Bowman's) space
Podocyte of visceral layer of glomerular capsule
Glomerular capillaries
Granular juxtaglomerular cells
Macula densa
Distal convoluted tubule
Efferent arteriole
Parietal wall of glomerular capsule
Afferent arteriole
Smooth muscle cell
Extraglomerular mesangial cells (lacis cells)
"Polar cushion"
Granular juxtaglomerular cells (renin-secreting)
Urinary space
Basal lamina
Podocyte nucleus
Filtration slits
Fenestrated endothelial cell
Mesangial cell

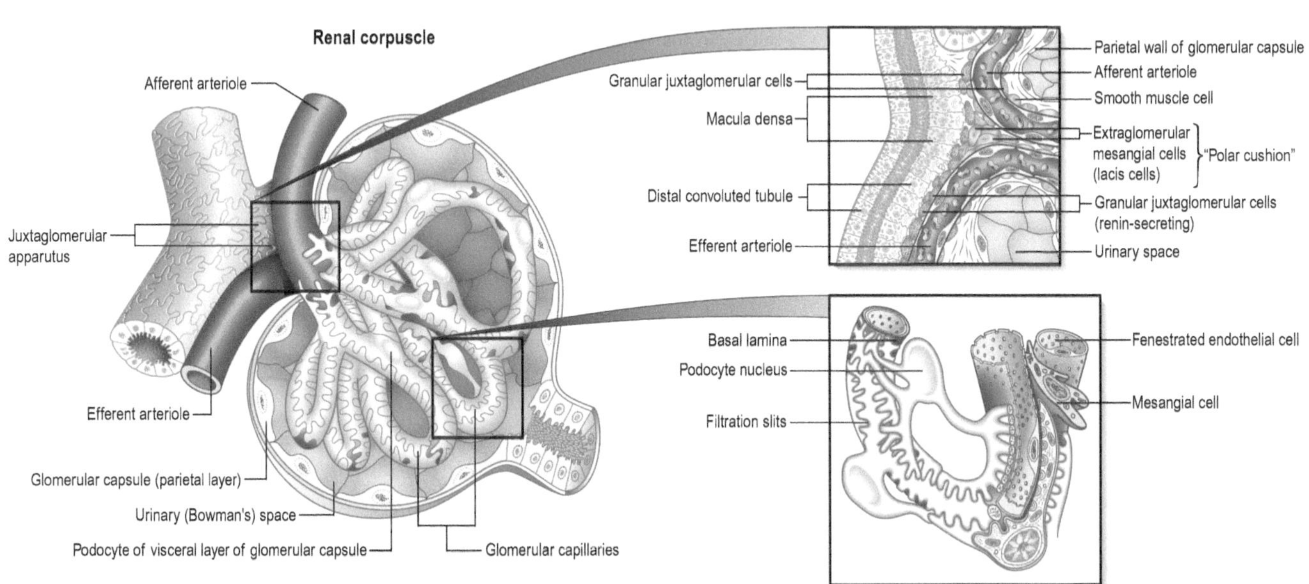

FIGURE 9.11 The glomerulus. The juxtaglomerular apparatus and podocyte are enlarged to the right. Source: *From Figure 74.16 in Susan Standring, editor. (2016).* Gray's anatomy *(41st ed.) (p. 1247). Elsevier.*

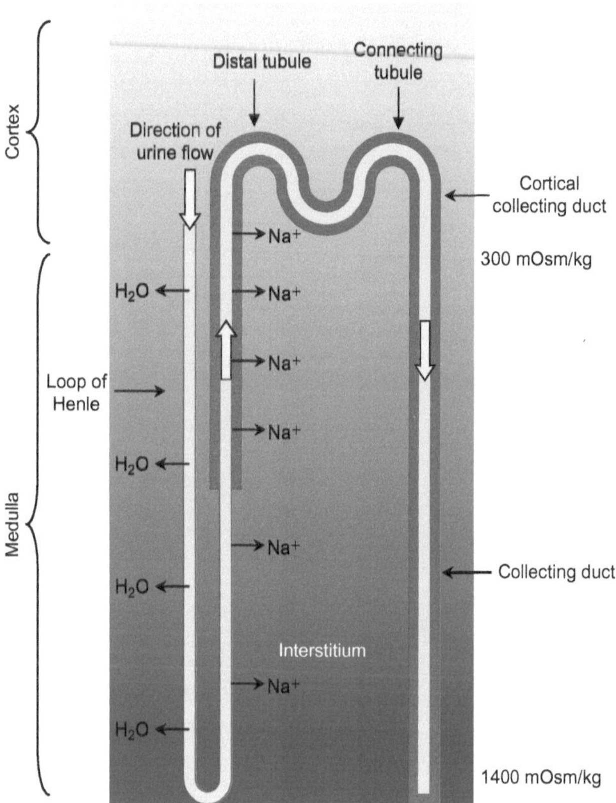

FIGURE 9.12 The countercurrent multiplier in the loop of Henle. Selective permeability of the tubular epithelium and active transport of sodium by the thick ascending limb create osmotic gradients. Tubular to interstitial flow of water concentrates sodium in the descending limb. Sodium movement across the water-impermeable ascending limb creates the osmotic gradient in the interstitium. Yellow arrows indicate the direction of flow. Note that active sodium transport in the thick ascending limb creates the gradient in the interstitium and makes the tubular fluid hypoosmotic by the time it emerges from Henle's loop.

which provides the driving force for water reabsorption and the production of a concentrated urine. Hormonally regulated permeability of the collecting ducts to water and urea determines the final composition of the urine.

Antidiuretic hormone

ADH is another name for vasopressin (arginine vasopressin or AVP), discussed in Chapter 2, Pituitary Gland, and Chapter 4, The Adrenal Glands. ADH is synthesized in magnicellular hypothalamic neurons in the supraoptic and paraventricular nuclei. Axons of these cells pass down the pituitary stalk and terminate in the posterior lobe of the pituitary gland from whence the hormone is secreted. As we have seen, the same peptide also is produced by other hypothalamic neurons and may act as a hypophyseal hormone (see Chapter 4: The Adrenal Glands) or as a neurotransmitter. ADH is the hormone

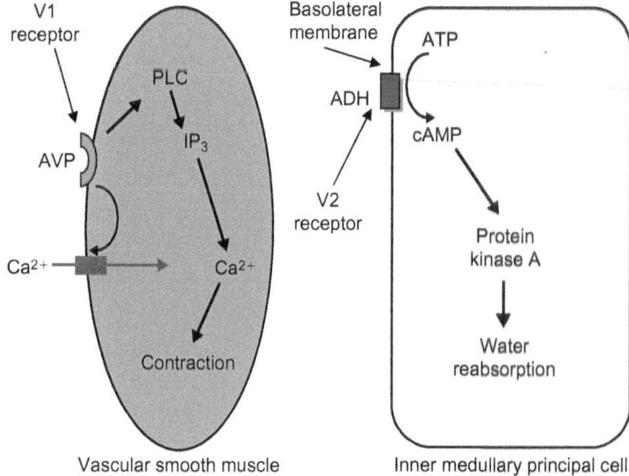

FIGURE 9.13 The V1 receptor mediates the pressor actions of AVP/ADH, and the V2 receptor mediates the water conservation effects. The two receptors signal by way of different G-proteins. *ADH*, Antidiuretic hormone; *AVP*, arginine vasopressin.

that signals the kidney to conserve water when plasma osmolality is increased or when plasma volume is decreased. The name ADH describes the prompt decrease in urine volume that follows hormone administration. The name AVP refers to the acute increase in blood pressure seen as a result of arteriolar constriction produced when the hormone is administered in sufficient dosage.

Antidiuretic effects are seen at lower hormone concentrations than vasoconstrictor effects. The two actions of the hormone are produced by two different G-protein coupled receptors. The V1 receptor is coupled through $G\alpha q\beta\gamma$ to phospholipase B and, therefore, signals through the diacylglycerol/inositol trisphosphate second messenger system (see Chapter 1: Introduction) and produces its vasopressor effect by constricting vascular smooth muscle. The antidiuretic effect is produced by the V2 receptor, which signals through $G\alpha s\beta\gamma$ to activate adenylyl cyclase and cyclic AMP production in renal tubular cells (Fig. 9.13).

Antidiuretic effect

Osmolality of blood plasma can be increased or decreased by adjusting the proportion of water relative to solute that is excreted in the urine and thus produce reciprocal changes in the osmolality of the urine. Water that is reabsorbed or excreted in excess of solute is referred to as free water. Conservation of free water lowers, whereas excretion of free water raises plasma osmolality. As already mentioned, the geometry of the nephron and the permeability characteristics of some segments provide a mechanism for varying water reabsorption without an accompanying change in sodium reabsorption. ADH conserves free water by increasing collecting duct permeability to water. Because of sodium chloride reabsorption by the water-impermeable thick ascending limb and distal tubule, fluid that enters the collecting ducts from Henle's loop is hypoosmolar. As it flows through the cortical and medullary collecting ducts toward the renal pelvis, it passes through the regions of increasing osmolality, but in the absence of ADH, the tubules are impermeable to water and urea so that the low solute concentration is preserved, and a relatively large volume of dilute urine is excreted. In the presence of ADH the collecting ducts in the cortex and outer medulla become permeable to water but remain impermeable to urea. As a consequence of water reabsorption, the concentration of urea in the terminal regions of the collecting ducts may become as high as 700 mM compared to about 15 mM in plasma. In this region, ADH increases the permeability of the principal cells to urea as well as water. Urea can then diffuse out the collecting ducts and into the extracellular space where it provides about half of the total osmolytes at the tip of the medullary papilla.

Plasma membranes of most cells are permeable to water because of the presence of specialized proteins, called aquaporins (AQPs) that form water channels. At least four of these proteins (AQP-1, 2, 3, and 4) are expressed in mammalian kidneys. In the proximal convoluted tubule, water and solute are reabsorbed proportionally because AQP-1 is abundantly expressed in both the apical and basolateral membranes of tubular cells and because the intercellular junctions are leaky. Segments of the nephron that are impermeable to water, such as the ascending limb of the loop of Henle, do not express AQPs on their luminal surfaces. AQP-3 and AQP-4 are expressed by the principal cells of the collecting ducts but only in the basolateral membranes. These cells also express AQP-2, which may be found in their luminal membranes or in submembranous vesicles (Fig. 9.14).

ADH stimulates an exocytosis-like process in which the AQP-2 bearing vesicles fuse with the luminal membrane and thus insert AQP-2 in much the same manner that insulin increases the abundance of GLUT-4 in adipocyte membranes (see Chapter 7: The Pancreatic Islets). In the absence of ADH, AQP-2 is removed from the luminal membrane by endocytosis and stored in vesicular membranes. The presence of AQP-3 and AQP-4 in the basolateral surfaces of the principal cells allows intracellular fluid to equilibrate rapidly with interstitial fluid. Water channels formed by AQP-2 do not allow passage of urea.

Permeability to urea depends upon the presence of specialized urea transport proteins. ADH promotes the insertion of urea transporters into the luminal membranes of the principal cells in the terminal portions of the inner medullary collecting ducts in much the same way that it regulates AQP-2. These effects of ADH depend upon the formation of cyclic AMP. V2 receptors

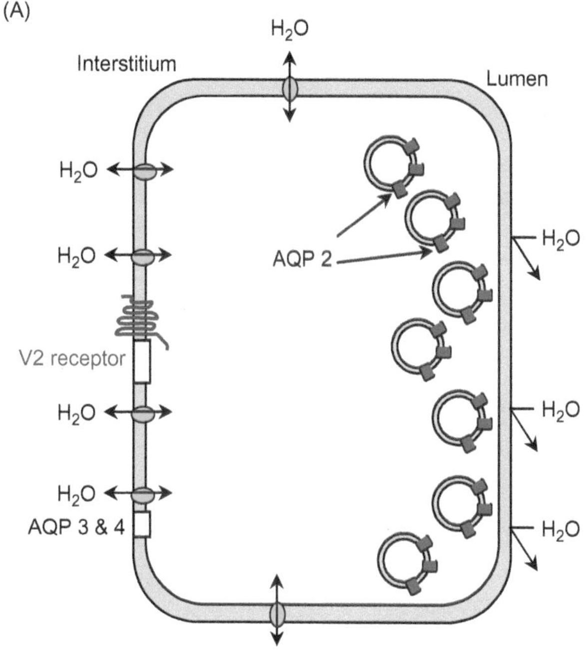

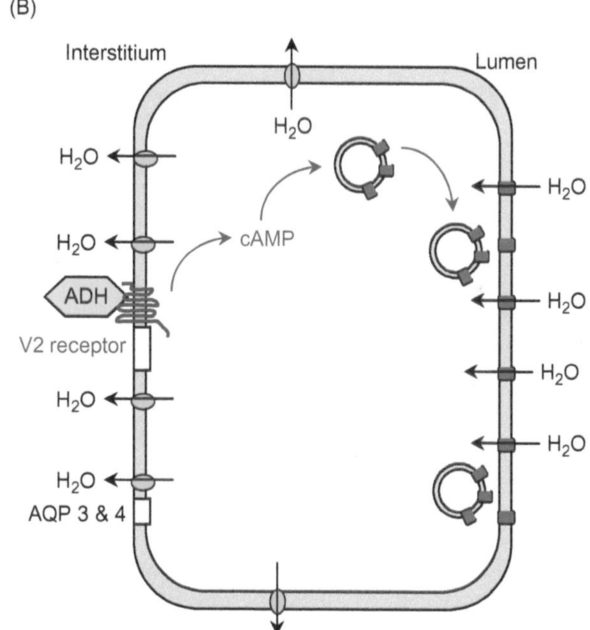

FIGURE 9.14 Principal cells of the collecting duct before (A) and (B) after ADH. ADH binds to V2 receptors to induce formation of cAMP, which promotes insertion of AQP-2 into the luminal membrane making it permeable to water. In the presence of ADH, water can pass through the principal cell from lumen to interstitium driven by the osmotic gradient. Deep in the medulla, urea transporters also are inserted in the luminal membrane in addition to AQP-2. Expression of AQPs-3 and -4 in the basolateral membranes allows osmotic equilibration between intercellular and interstitial water. *ADH*, Antidiuretic hormone; *AQP*, aquaporin; *cAMP*, cyclic AMP.

are found in the basolateral membranes of the principal cells of the collecting ducts and the cells of the thick portion of Henle's loop. Substrates for cyclic AMP-dependent protein kinase in the collecting ducts have not been identified but are thought to include proteins that regulate vesicle trafficking, and perhaps the urea transporters. Stimulation of water and urea permeability is seen in less than 10 minutes after addition of ADH. On a longer time scale, ADH increases transcription of the genes that encode AQP-2, AQP-3, and the urea transporter. In addition, ADH stimulates sodium reabsorption in the thick ascending limb of the loop of Henle and thereby increases the formation of the osmotic gradient that provides the driving force for water reabsorption in the collecting ducts. In these cells protein kinase A catalyzes the phosphorylation and activation of the sodium, potassium, 2-chloride transporter in the luminal membranes. Sodium that enters the cells by this route is extruded into the extracellular fluid by the sodium/potassium ATPase, and chloride passes into the extracellular fluid through chloride channels in the basolateral membranes. Potassium, which is available in luminal fluid at much lower concentrations than sodium or chloride, is recycled back to the lumen by way of ROMK channels (see Chapter 4: The Adrenal Glands) in the luminal membranes. ADH may also stimulate sodium reabsorption at more distal sites in the nephron.

Effects on blood pressure

Vasopressin may be the most potent naturally occurring constrictor of vascular smooth muscle. On a molar basis, it is at least 10 times more active than norepinephrine or angiotensin II in stimulating contraction of isolated strips of artery. Increases in total peripheral resistance are observed at concentrations of ADH that fall within the upper part of the range that promotes water reabsorption. Small increases in peripheral resistance produced by ADH are not accompanied by increased systemic blood pressure, however, because the baroreceptor reflexes mediate compensatory decreases in heart rate and cardiac output and because ADH may decrease cardiac contractility secondary to coronary arteriolar constriction.

Because not all arterioles are equally sensitive to it, ADH does not increase resistance uniformly in all vascular beds. Consequently, there is a redistribution of blood flow, which decreases most profoundly in skin and skeletal muscle. Redistribution can compensate for decreased blood volume by making a disproportionate share of the cardiac output available to essential tissues such as the brain. Arteriolar constriction also changes the distribution of fluid between the vascular and interstitial compartments. It may be recalled that filtration and reabsorption of fluid in the capillaries are balanced largely between the outward hydrostatic force and the inward colloid osmotic force. By constricting arterioles, ADH lowers downstream capillary and venular blood pressure and thereby promotes net reabsorption of interstitial fluid in skin and skeletal muscle. Intravascular volume increases, therefore, at the expense of the interstitial compartment.

Regulation of antidiuretic hormone secretion

Plasma osmolality

The most important stimulus for ADH secretion is an increase in blood osmolality. Little ADH is secreted so long as the osmolality of plasma remains at or below a threshold value of about 280 mOsm/L. Osmoreceptors are exquisitely sensitive and elicit increased secretion of ADH when the osmolality increases by as little as 1%–2%. Above the osmolar threshold the concentration of ADH in plasma changes in direct proportion to the increase in plasma osmolality (Fig. 9.15) and decreases urine volume significantly.

The finding that the injection of a small volume of hyperosmotic fluid into the internal carotid artery elicits ADH secretion even though peripheral osmolality remains unchanged indicated that osmolality is detected in the region of the hypothalamus. In rats, intracarotid injection of concentrated saline increased

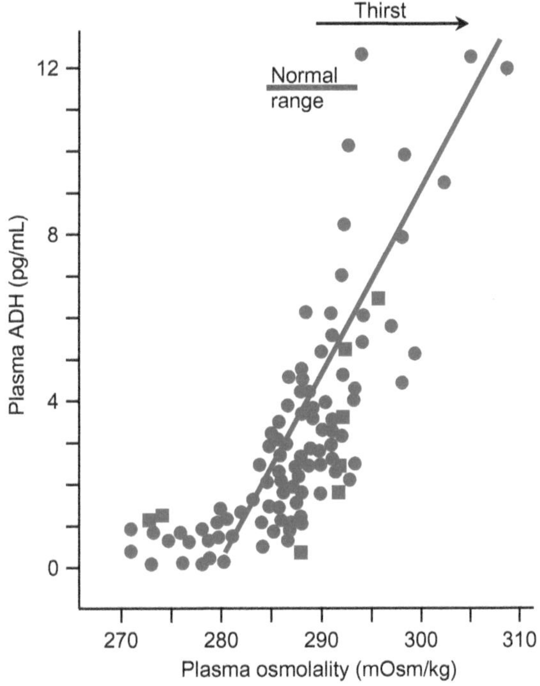

FIGURE 9.15 Relation between ADH and osmolality in plasma of unanesthetized rats. Note the appearance of thirst (increased drinking behavior) when plasma osmolality exceeds 290 mOsm/kg. *ADH*, Antidiuretic hormone. Source: *From Robertson, G. L., & Berl, T. (1996). In B. M. Brenner, & F. Rector, (Eds.),* The kidney *(5th ed.), (p. 881). Saunders, Philadelphia, with permission.*

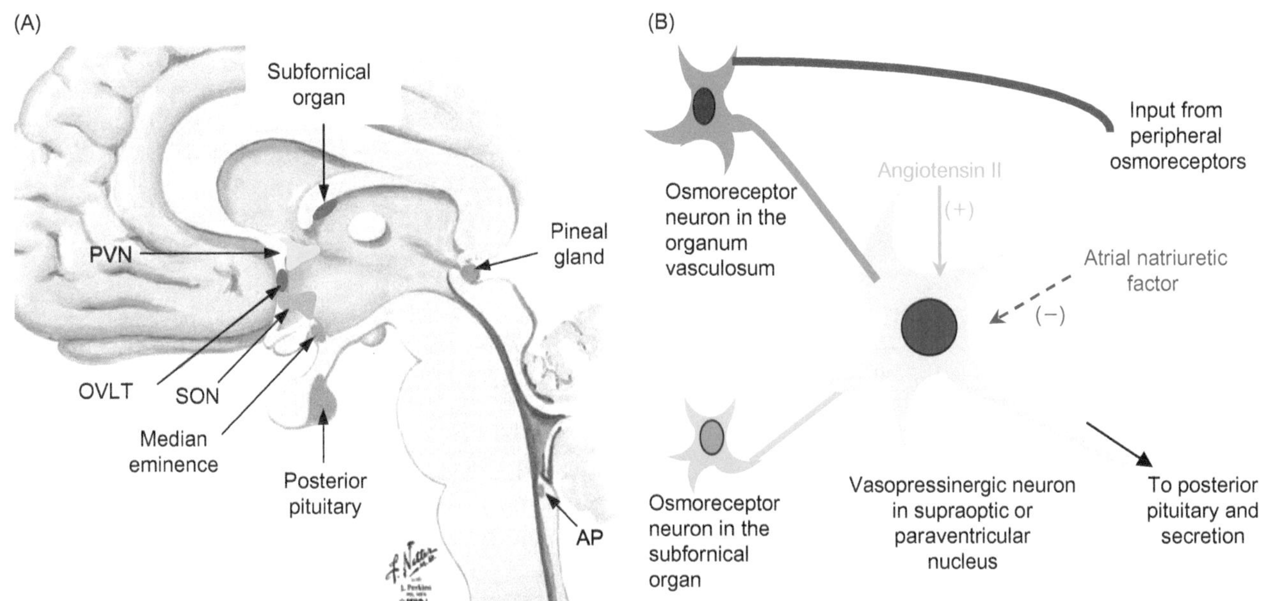

FIGURE 9.16 (A) Sagital view of the brain showing the circumventricular organs and their relation to ADH-producing cells. (B) Neural and hormonal input to ADH-secreting cells. *ADH*, Antidiuretic hormone; *AP*, area postrema; *OVLT*, organum vasculosum of the lamina terminalis; *PVN*, paraventricular nucleus; *SON*, supraoptic nucleus. Source: *Adapted from Netter, F. H. (2003) In D. L. Felten, & R. Jozefowicz (Eds.),* Netter's atlas of human neuroscience. *Teterboro, NJ: Icon Learning Systems.*

the electrical activity of nerve cells in the supraoptic and paraventricular nuclei. Osmoreceptor cells are thought to reside in the circumventricular organs, particularly the organum vasculosum and subfornical organ located near the third ventricle. This region lies outside the blood–brain barrier and derives its blood supply from the internal carotid artery. Axons project from this region to make synaptic connections with ADH-producing cells in the supraoptic and paraventricular nuclei and stimulate them to release hormone from nerve terminals in the posterior pituitary gland. Some evidence also indicates that the ADH-producing neurons themselves may be directly activated by increased osmolality. In addition, peripheral input from cells in the area drained by the mesenteric and portal veins detect changes in osmolality associated with intestinal absorption and stimulate or inhibit ADH secretion through a neural pathway (Figs. 9.16 and 9.18).

Osmolality is detected as a change in volume of the whole cell or specialized vesicular components. Cells bounded by membranes that allow water to pass freely, but restrict movement of most solutes swell in a hypoosmotic environment and shrink when the extracellular fluid is hyperosmotic. Hyperosmolality activates nonselective cation channels and causes the membrane to depolarize and generate an action potential. Conversely closure of these channels when the cell swells results in hyperpolarization. Sodium chloride, which is largely excluded from cells, is perhaps the most potent osmolyte, as judged by its ability to increase ADH secretion; a more permeant molecule such as urea has only a small effect.

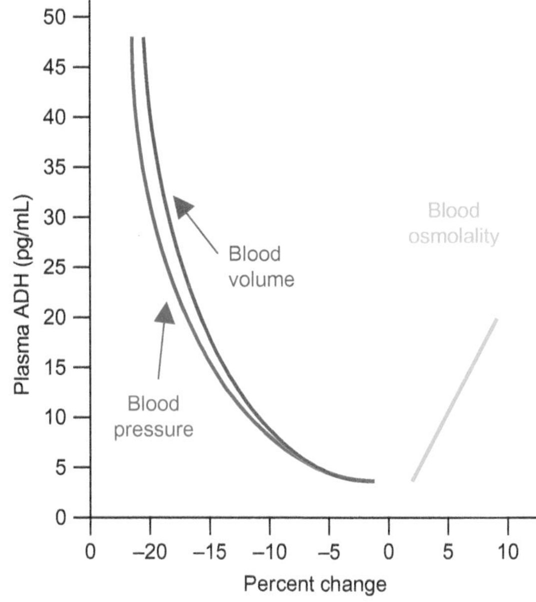

FIGURE 9.17 Relation between changes in blood osmolality, pressure, or volume and ADH concentration in plasma of unanesthetized rats. *ADH*, Antidiuretic hormone. Source: *From Dunn, F. L., Brennan, T. J., Nelson, A. E., & Robertson, G. L. (1973). The role of blood osmolality and volume in regulating vasopressin secretion in the rat.* Journal of Clinical Investigation, *52, 3212, with permission.*

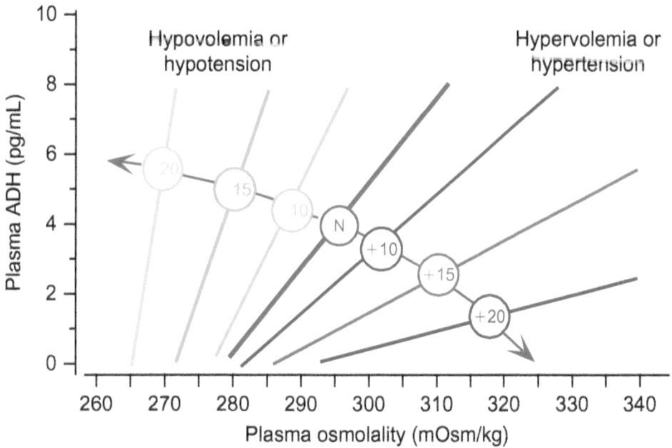

FIGURE 9.18 The effects of increases or decreases in blood volume or blood pressure on the relation between ADH concentrations and osmolality in the plasma of unanesthetized rats. Circled numbers indicate percent change from normal (N). *ADH*, Antidiuretic hormone. Source: *Modified from Robertson, G. L., & Berl, T. (1996). In B. M. Brenner and F. Rector,* The kidney *(5th ed.) (p. 881). Philadelphia, PA: Saunders, with permission.*

Blood volume

Changes in blood volume are sensed by receptors in both arterial (high pressure) and venous (low pressure) sides of the circulation. Volume is monitored indirectly as the tension exerted on stretch receptors located (1) on the arterial side, in the carotid sinuses and aortic arch and (2) on the venous side in the atria and perhaps the thoracic veins. Low pressure receptors monitor central venous pressure, which can vary widely with redistribution of blood, as might occur with changes in posture, physical activity, and ambient temperature. Central venous pressure can fall by as much as 10%–15% when an individual simply rises from a recumbent to an upright posture. Thus there is a wide range over which deviations in venous pressure are not reliable indicators of true variations in volume. Because of the extensive buffering capacity of the baroreceptor reflexes, changes in arterial pressure are seen only after large decreases in blood volume. Changes in volume of a few percent are difficult to detect and do not elicit acute compensatory adjustments in fluid balance.

At normal osmolality, ADH secretion is minimal so long as blood volume remains at or above its physiological threshold or set point. Because volume receptors are not equipped to detect small changes, stimulation of ADH secretion is not initiated until a relatively large depletion has occurred. The minimal change needed for low pressure receptors to signal ADH secretion is a 10%–15% reduction in volume. Similarly, a loss of 10%–15% of the blood volume can occur before the threshold for high volume receptors is reached. Secretion of ADH in response to a decrease in volume is thus an emergency response and not a fine-tuner of blood volume. Retention of free water alone is not an effective means of defending the plasma volume. Because it distributes in all compartments, only about 1 mL of every 12 mL of free water retained remains in the vascular compartment. However, if volume falls below a critical threshold value, a potentially life-threatening event is perceived and vigorous secretion of ADH increases blood levels exponentially (Fig. 9.17).

The ADH-secreting cells of the supraoptic and paraventricular nuclei are stimulated by two inputs: increased osmolality and decreased volume. They must be able to integrate these signals and respond appropriately. Decreases in volume or pressure heighten the sensitivity of the osmoreceptors and lower the threshold for ADH pressure secretion in response to increased osmolality (Fig. 9.18).

Both volume depletion and increased osmolality, as might result from dehydration, for example, stimulate ADH secretion and reinforce each other. Situations can arise, however, when inputs from osmotic and volume receptors are conflicting. As a rule, osmolality is preferentially guarded when volume depletion is small. When volume loss is large, however, osmolality is sacrificed to maintain the integrity of the circulation.

Diseases

The disease state associated with a deficiency of ADH is called diabetes insipidus and is characterized by copious production of dilute urine. With this condition, more than 20 L of water may be excreted per day. If not balanced by water intake, osmolality of body fluids and the concentration of plasma sodium increase dramatically and catastrophically. The term insipidus, meaning tasteless, was adopted to distinguish the consequences of ADH deficiency from those of insulin deficiency (diabetes mellitus, *mellitus* is from the Greek word for honey) in which there is copious production of glucose-laden urine (see Chapter 7: The Pancreatic Islets). Nephrogenic diabetes insipidus is the disease that results from failure of the kidney to respond to ADH and may result from defects in the V2 receptor, AQP-2, or any of the regulatory proteins that govern cellular responses to ADH. In the syndrome of inappropriate secretion of ADH, ADH secretion is increased above baseline despite low plasma osmolality. Neurogenic diabetes insipidus is less common and can be due to head trauma or tumor that affects the posterior pituitary. In this form, ADH is not produced or not produced in sufficient quantities. Death may result from a profound dilution of plasma electrolytes because of excessive reabsorption of free water.

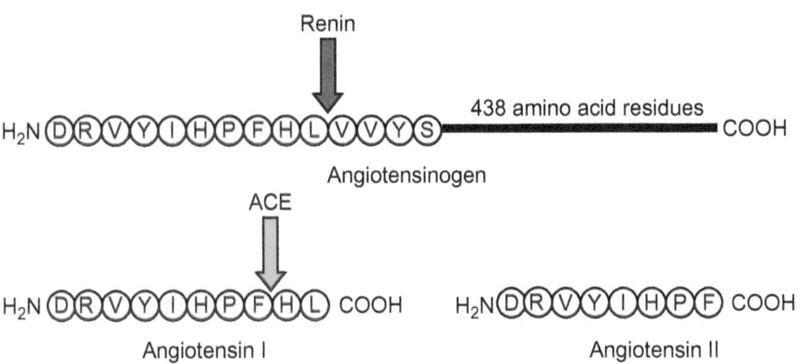

FIGURE 9.19 Two-step formation of angiotensin II. Amino acids are represented by the single letter amino acid code, D is the aspartic acid, F is the phenylalanine, H is the histidine, I is the isoleucine, L is the leucine, P is the proline, R is the arginine, S-serine, V is the valine, Y is the tyrosine.

The renin–angiotensin–aldosterone system

As already described in Chapter 4, The Adrenal Glands, aldosterone is an adrenal steroid that plays a pivotal role in maintaining salt and water balance. Aldosterone is secreted by the cells of the zona glomerulosa and acts primarily on the principal cells in the cortical collecting ducts to promote reabsorption of sodium and excretion of potassium. It may be recalled that aldosterone does not stimulate a simple one-for-one exchange of sodium for potassium in the nephron. Sodium reabsorption exceeds potassium excretion by the principal cells. However, because sodium and potassium reabsorption are governed by additional factors, the net effects of administered aldosterone on sodium and potassium excretion in the urine differ in different physiological states. Retention of sodium obligates simultaneous reabsorption of water by the nephron and expands the interstitial and vascular volume, accordingly. The effects of aldosterone to promote sodium retention by the kidney are augmented by similar effects on sweat and salivary glands and by a poorly understood effect on the brain that increases the appetite for sodium chloride. Aldosterone secretion is controlled by angiotensin II, whose complementary actions on a variety of target tissues play a critical role in maintaining the central pressure: volume reservoir. Angiotensin II is an octapeptide formed in blood by proteolytic cleavage of a circulating precursor, angiotensinogen (Fig. 9.19).

Angiotensinogen is a glycoprotein with a mass of about 60,000–65,000 Da depending upon its degree of glycosylation and belongs to the serine protease inhibitor superfamily of plasma proteins. It is present in blood at a concentration of about 1 μM and is constitutively secreted by the liver, which is the major, though not exclusive, source of angiotensinogen in blood. The hepatic production of angiotensinogen varies in different physiological conditions, but although its rate of cleavage to angiotensin is sensitive to changes in its concentration, it is normally present in adequate amount to satisfy demands for angiotensin production.

The initial cleavage of angiotensinogen, catalyzed by the enzyme renin, releases the amino terminal decapeptide called angiotensin I. Angiotensin I is biologically inactive and is rapidly converted to angiotensin II by the angiotensin converting enzyme, often called ACE, which removes two amino acids from the carboxyl terminus to produce the biologically active octapeptide, angiotensin II. Angiotensin converting enzyme is an ectopeptidase that is anchored to the plasma membranes of endothelial cells by a short tail at its carboxyl terminus. It is widely distributed in vascular epithelium and may also be secreted into the blood as a soluble enzyme. Angiotensin I is converted to angiotensin II mainly during passage through the pulmonary circulation, but some angiotensin II also is produced throughout the circulation including the glomerular capillaries. The reaction appears to be limited only by the concentration of angiotensin I. The rate of angiotensin II formation, therefore, is governed by the rate of release of angiotensin I from angiotensinogen, which in turn is primarily regulated by secretion of renin by the kidneys. Angiotensin II has a very short half-life and may be metabolized further to form angiotensin III and angiotensin IV by successive removal of the N terminal and C terminal amino acids. Some data indicate that these compounds may have biological activity, but their physiological importance has not been established.

Renin is an aspartyl protease that is synthesized and secreted by the juxtaglomerular cells, which are modified smooth muscle cells in the walls of the afferent glomerular arterioles. These cells and cells of the macula densa, which are in the wall of the distal convoluted tubule of the nephron where it loops back to come in contact with its own glomerulus, make up the juxtaglomerular apparatus (Fig. 9.20).

Prorenin is encoded by a single gene located on chromosome 1 and is converted to its enzymatically active form by removal of a 43-amino acid peptide at the N terminus during maturation of its storage granules. Renin is secreted along with some prorenin by an exocytotic process that is activated in response to a

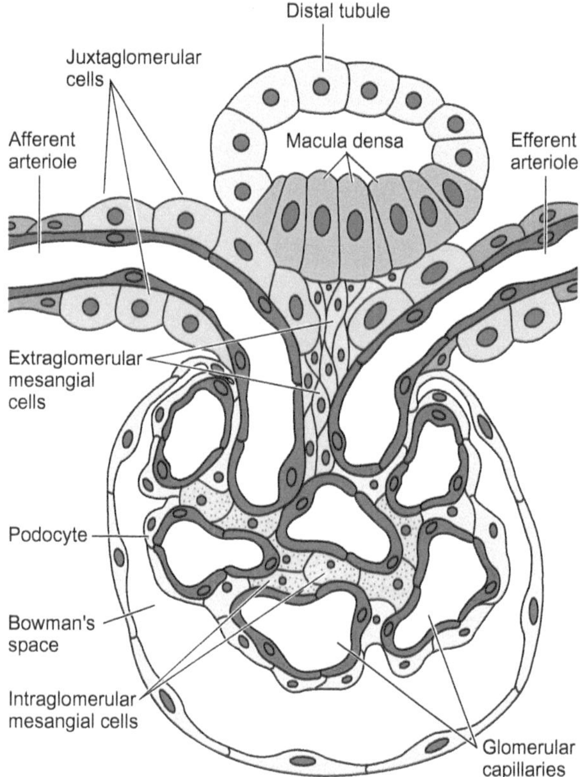

FIGURE 9.20 The juxtaglomerular apparatus is composed of four cell types: The macula densa, the juxtaglomerular cells, the extraglomerular mesangial cells, and the intraglomerular mesangial cells. When the cells of the macula densa detect a decrease in blood pressure, they send a signal to the juxtaglomerular cells to release renin into the circulation. Renin is an enzyme which separates angiotensin I from the precursor molecule angiotensinogen. Angiotensin I then goes to the lung, kidney, and other organs where it becomes converted by ACE to angiotensin II. *ACE*, Angiotensin I converting enzyme. Source: *From Figure 19-14 in Gartner L. P. (2017).* Textbook of histology *(4th ed.) (p. 513). Elsevier.*

decrease in blood volume. At the cellular level, this secretory process is stimulated by cyclic AMP and, contrary to most secretory processes, is inhibited by increased intracellular calcium.

Three different, but related, inputs signal the increased secretion of renin:

- Juxtaglomerular cells are richly innervated by sympathetic nerve fibers. These fibers are activated reflexly by a decrease in arterial pressure that is sensed by baroreceptors in the carotid sinuses, aortic arches, and perhaps the great veins in the chest. Release of norepinephrine from sympathetic nerve terminals stimulates cyclic AMP production in juxtaglomerular cells by activating beta adrenergic receptors and adenylyl cyclase.
- Blood pressure (volume) also is sensed as tension exerted on the smooth muscle cells of the afferent glomerular arterioles. Stretch-activated ion channels in the membranes of juxtaglomerular smooth muscle cells produce partial membrane depolarization, activation of voltage sensitive calcium channels, and increased intracellular calcium concentrations. Conversely, a decrease in pressure lowers intracellular calcium and relieves inhibition of renin secretion.
- Decreased pressure in the afferent glomerular arterioles also results in decreased glomerular filtration, which in turn decreases the rate of sodium chloride delivery to the distal convoluted tubules. Decreased delivery of sodium chloride to the macula densa cells results in increased renin secretion from the juxtaglomerular cells by mechanisms that are not fully understood. Cells in the macula densa take up sodium and chloride in proportion to their availability by way of the sodium/potassium/2 chloride symporter in the luminal membrane. High rates of sodium chloride uptake cause the macula densa cells to release adenosine, which acts as a paracrine mediator that increases intracellular calcium in juxtaglomerular cells and inhibits renin release. A fall in sodium chloride uptake may result in the release of prostaglandins, which increase cyclic AMP in juxtaglomerular cells and increase renin release.

Actions of angiotensin II

Actions on the adrenal cortex

Angiotensin II is the primary signal for increased aldosterone secretion by adrenal glomerulosa cells (see Chapter 4: The Adrenal Glands). Administration of angiotensin II to normal or sodium-deficient humans increases aldosterone concentrations in blood plasma. Conversely, drugs that block angiotensin II receptors or that lower angiotensin II concentration by blocking the angiotensin converting enzyme (ACE inhibitors) decrease the plasma concentrations of aldosterone. On a longer time scale, angiotensin II causes the volume of the zona glomerulosa to increase by stimulating an increase in both cell size (hypertrophy) and cell number (hyperplasia). Such an effect is seen in individuals who maintain high plasma levels of angiotensin II as a result of a sodium-poor diet. These individuals show an increased sensitivity of aldosterone secretion in response to angiotensin II in part because of the upregulation of angiotensin II receptors, and in part because of the increase in both the number of responsive cells and the capacity of their biosynthetic machinery.

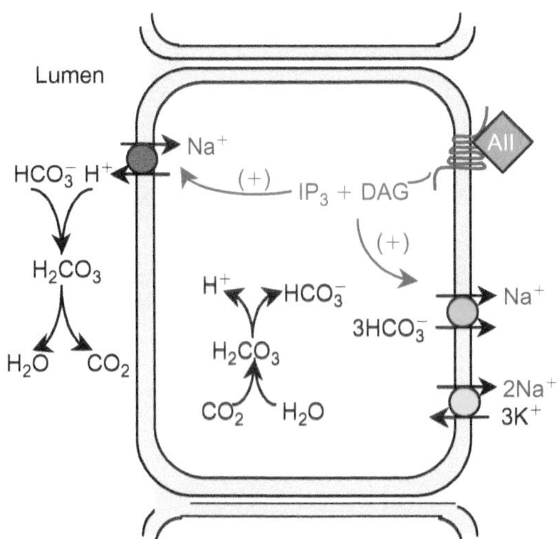

FIGURE 9.21 Angiotensin II increases sodium reabsorption by stimulating sodium proton exchange in the luminal brush border and sodium bicarbonate cotransport in the basolateral membrane. Hydrogen ions and bicarbonate are regenerated in the cell cytosol from CO_2 and water.

Actions on the kidney

In addition to its indirect effects to promote salt and water reabsorption through the stimulation of aldosterone secretion, angiotensin II also defends the vascular volume directly through actions exerted on both vascular and tubular elements of the kidney. By constricting renovascular smooth muscle, it increases vascular resistance in the kidney and hence decreases renal blood flow and glomerular filtration. Glomerular filtration may be decreased further by the constriction of the glomerular mesangial cells, which decreases the effective area for filtration. By selective constriction of efferent arterioles, angiotensin II increases the colloid osmotic pressure and lowers the hydrostatic pressure in the peritubular capillaries, thereby increasing their capability to reabsorb renal interstitial fluid. Because reabsorptive mechanisms are not 100% efficient, a small fraction of the glomerular filtrate is inevitably lost in the urine. Therefore by decreasing glomerular filtration, angiotensin II decreases sodium and water excretion. Angiotensin II also directly increases sodium bicarbonate reabsorption by stimulating sodium–proton exchange in the luminal membranes of proximal tubular cells and activating the sodium bicarbonate cotransporter in the basolateral membrane of these cells (Fig. 9.21).

Cardiovascular effects

Angiotensin II produces profound long- and short-term effects on the cardiovascular system. Stimulation of angiotensin II receptors in vascular smooth muscle activates the diacylglycerol/inositol trisphosphate second messenger system (see Chapter 1: Introduction) and results in increased intracellular calcium concentrations and sustained vasoconstriction. These direct effects on smooth muscle tone are reinforced by the activation of vasomotor centers in the brain to increase sympathetic outflow to vascular smooth muscle and decrease vagal inhibitory input to the heart. Angiotensin II also acts directly on cardiac myocytes to increase calcium influx and, therefore, cardiac contractility. The combination of these effects and the expansion of vascular volume markedly increase blood pressure and make angiotensin II the most potent pressor agent known. Vasoconstrictor effects are not uniformly expressed in all vascular beds, however, probably because of differences in receptor abundance. In addition to increasing volume and pressure, angiotensin II also redistributes blood flow to the brain, heart, and skeletal muscle at the expense of skin and visceral organs. However, at high concentrations it may also constrict the coronary arteries and compromise cardiac output. Chronically high concentrations of angiotensin can lead to remodeling of cardiac and vascular muscle as angiotensin II may act as a growth factor.

Central nervous system effects

Angiotensin II, acting both as a hormone and as a neurotransmitter, stimulates thirst, appetite for sodium, and secretion of ADH through actions exerted on the hypothalamus and perhaps other regions of the brain. Blood-borne angiotensin II can interact with receptors present on hypothalamic cells in the subfornical organ and the organum vasculosum of the lamina terminalis, which project to the supraoptic and paraventricular nuclei and other hypothalamic sites, including vasomotor regulatory centers (Fig. 9.16A). In addition, ADH-producing cells in the paraventricular nuclei express receptors for angiotensin II and release ADH when angiotensin II is presented to them experimentally by intraventricular injection or when released from impinging axons. These diverse actions of angiotensin II are summarized in Fig. 9.22.

Regulation of the renin–angiotensin–aldosterone system

The renin–angiotensin–aldosterone system is regulated by negative feedback, but neither the concentration of aldosterone, nor angiotensin II, nor the concentration of sodium per se is the controlled variable. Although preservation of body sodium is the central theme of aldosterone action, the concentration of sodium in blood does not appear to be monitored

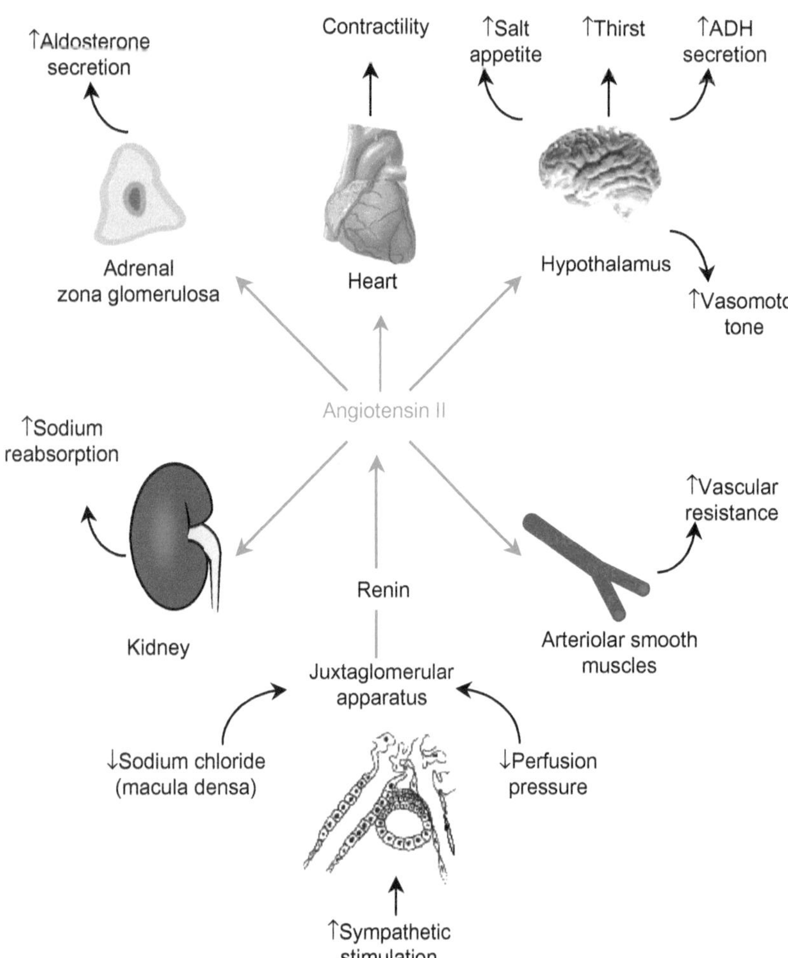

FIGURE 9.22 Actions of angiotensin.

directly, and fluctuations in plasma concentrations have little direct effect on the secretion of renin. Reabsorption of sodium by the kidney results in reabsorption of a proportionate volume of water. Increased blood volume, which is the ultimate result of sodium retention, provides the negative feedback signal for regulation of renin and aldosterone secretion (Fig. 9.23).

It is noteworthy that even though angiotensin II directly increases sodium reabsorption and exerts a variety of complementary actions that contribute to the maintenance of the central pressure-volume reservoir, it cannot sustain an adequate vascular volume to ensure survival in the absence of aldosterone. Despite apparent redundancies in their actions, both aldosterone and angiotensin II are critical for maintaining salt and water balance.

The kidney is the primary regulator of the angiotensin II concentration in blood, but angiotensin II also is produced locally in a variety of other tissues including walls of blood vessels, adipose tissue, and brain, where it functions as a neurotransmitter. These extrarenal tissues synthesize angiotensinogen as well as renin and ACE and may form angiotensin II intracellularly. Locally produced angiotensin II may serve a paracrine function to stimulate prostaglandin production and, in some instances, may act as a local growth factor. The extent to which such localized production of angiotensin II contributes to the regulation of sodium and water balance is unclear.

Atrial natriuretic factor

ANF as its name implies promotes the excretion of sodium (natrium in Latin) in the urine. It is synthesized, stored in membrane-bound granules, and secreted by exocytosis from cardiac atrial myocytes (Fig. 9.24).

A second natriuretic peptide originally isolated from pig brain, and, therefore, called brain natriuretic peptide (BNP), is also produced in the atria and to a greater extent in ventricles of the human heart. ANF and BNP are the products of separate genes but have similar structures and actions. A third gene in this family encodes CNP, which is expressed in the central nervous system and in endothelial cells. ANF is a 28-amino-acid peptide that corresponds to the carboxyl terminus of a 126-amino-acid prohormone that is the principal storage form. BNF

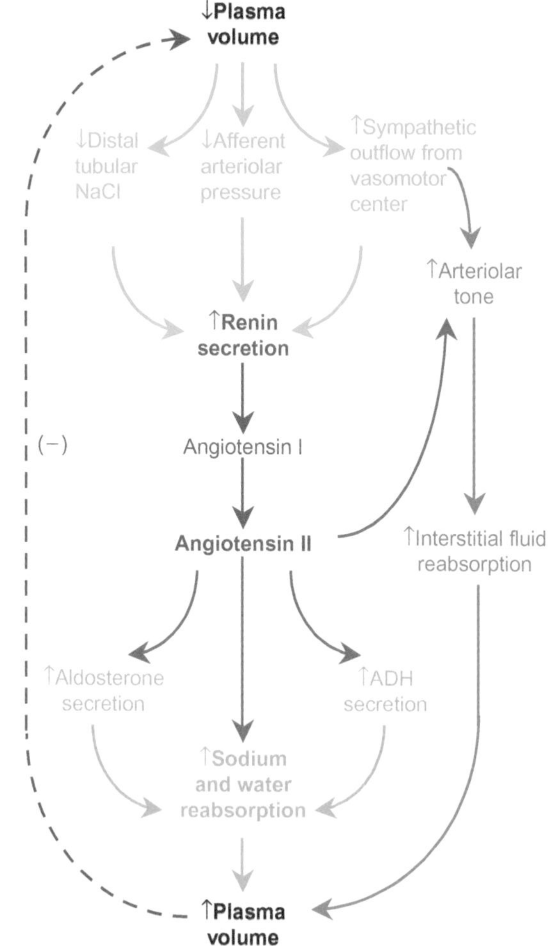

FIGURE 9.23 Negative feedback control of renin and angiotensin secretion. The monitored variable is blood volume detected as decreases in sodium chloride at the macula densa; decreased pressure in the afferent arterioles; and decreased pressure in the carotid sinuses, aortic arch, and thoracic low pressure receptors. Coordinated actions of angiotensin restore plasma volume and abolish the stimuli for renin secretion. Note that angiotensin II contributes directly and indirectly to the maintenance of blood volume, but its influence in this regard is inadequate in the absence of aldosterone (see Chapter 4: The Adrenal Glands).

contains 32 amino acids. A 17-amino acid loop structure formed by disulfide linkage of two cysteines is essential for biological activity of all three peptides (Fig. 9.25).

The biological actions of both ANF and BNP are mediated by natriuretic peptide receptor-A (NPR-A), which forms dimers or tetramers in the membranes of target cells. Each NPR-A peptide strand has a single membrane-spanning region and an extracellular hormone-binding domain. The cytosolic portion contains a noncatalytic ATP binding region, which may have a regulatory function, and a C terminal enzymatic domain, which catalyzes the formation of cyclic guanosine monophosphate (cGMP) from GTP. The closely related NPR-B receptor mediates the actions of CNP and also contains a C terminal guanylyl cyclase. A third receptor, NPR-C, binds all three peptides but has only a short cytosolic tail that lacks both ATP binding and guanylyl cyclase activity. Its internal domain binds and activates the inhibitory G-protein inhibitory alpha subunit, although it does not belong to the superfamily of G-protein coupled receptors.

NPR-C receptors are abundant and widely distributed. In addition to their signaling role in some tissues, they may function as "clearance" receptors that remove ANF, BNP, and CNP from blood and extracellular fluid and deliver them to the lysosomes for degradation. However, recent observations suggest that NPR-C may also interact with the inhibitory alpha G-protein subunit G-proteins and have a signaling function. ANF disappears from plasma with a half-life of about 3 minutes due in part to the action of the clearance receptors and in part to proteolytic cleavage at the brush border of renal proximal tubular cells. BNP, which is bound less avidly by NPR-C, has a half-life of about 20 minutes.

ANF and BNF produce their biological effects by stimulating the formation of cGMP, which may modify cellular functions through at least three mechanisms. cGMP binds to and activates cGMP-dependent protein kinase (PKG), which catalyzes the phosphorylation of key regulatory proteins. cGMP also binds to and regulates the activity of cyclic nucleotide phosphodiesterases and may, therefore, lower cellular concentrations of cyclic AMP. Finally, cGMP may bind directly to ion channel proteins and regulate their activity.

Physiological actions

The physiological role of ANF is to protect against volume overload. Through its combined effects on the cardiovascular system, the kidneys, and the adrenal glands, it lowers mean arterial blood pressure and decreases the effective blood volume. Its physiological effects are essentially opposite to those of angiotensin II (Fig. 9.26).

Cardiovascular actions

Increased concentrations of ANF in blood produce a prompt decrease in mean arterial blood pressure through modulation of autonomic input and through direct actions on vascular smooth muscle. ANP causes resistance vessels to relax by increasing cGMP production, which activates PKG, and the subsequent decrease in availability of intracellular calcium and sensitivity of the contractile apparatus to calcium. Protein kinase G-dependent phosphorylation activates potassium channels, hyperpolarizing the cell membrane and thereby preventing entry of extracellular calcium through voltage sensitive calcium channels. Phosphorylation of a regulatory protein associated

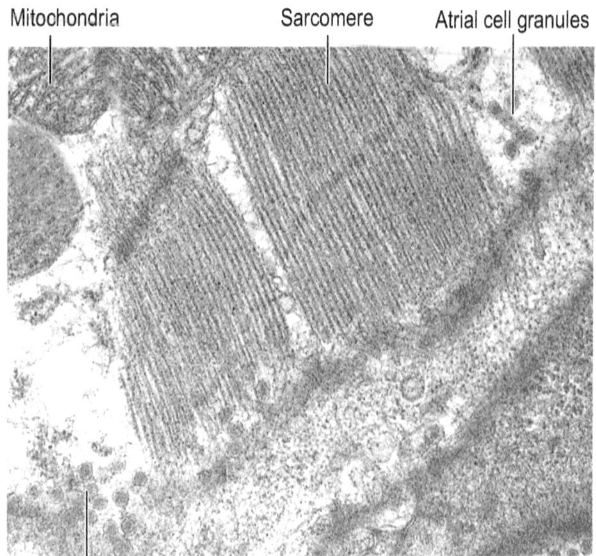

Atrial cardiocytes store membrane-bound granules whose density can be altered by varying the intake of salt and water.

Atrial cell granules contain the precursor of **atrial natriuretic peptide (ANP)**, a potent polypeptide hormone that stimulates **diuresis** (Greek *diourein*, to urinate) and **natriuresis** (Latin *natrium*, sodium + Greek *diourein*). Once outside the atrial cell, the ANP precursor undergoes a rapid enzymatic cleavage to produce circulating ANP.

ANP binding to **natriuretic peptide receptors NPR1, NPR2,** and **NPR3** (with guanylyl cyclase activity) causes the conversion of guanosine triphosphate (GTP) to cyclic guanosine monophosphate (cGMP). Then, cGMP activates a cGMP-dependent kinase that phosphorylates specific serine and threonine residues in target proteins.

ANP antagonizes the actions of **vasopressin**, a polypeptide released from the neurohypophysis, and **angiotensin II (ANG II)**. ANG II is a peptide derived from the **renin**-induced breakdown of **angiotensinogen (AGT)**, produced in liver and released into the systemic blood.

ANP prevents sodium and water reabsorption from causing **hypervolemia** (abnormal increase in the volume of circulating fluid in the body) and **hypertension** that can result in cardiac failure.

FIGURE 9.24 Granules from cardiac atria that contain atrial natriuretic peptide. Source: *From Figure 12-3 in Kierszenbaum, A. L., & Tres, L. L.(2020).* Histology and cell biology: An introduction to pathology *(5th ed.) (p. 424). Elsevier.*

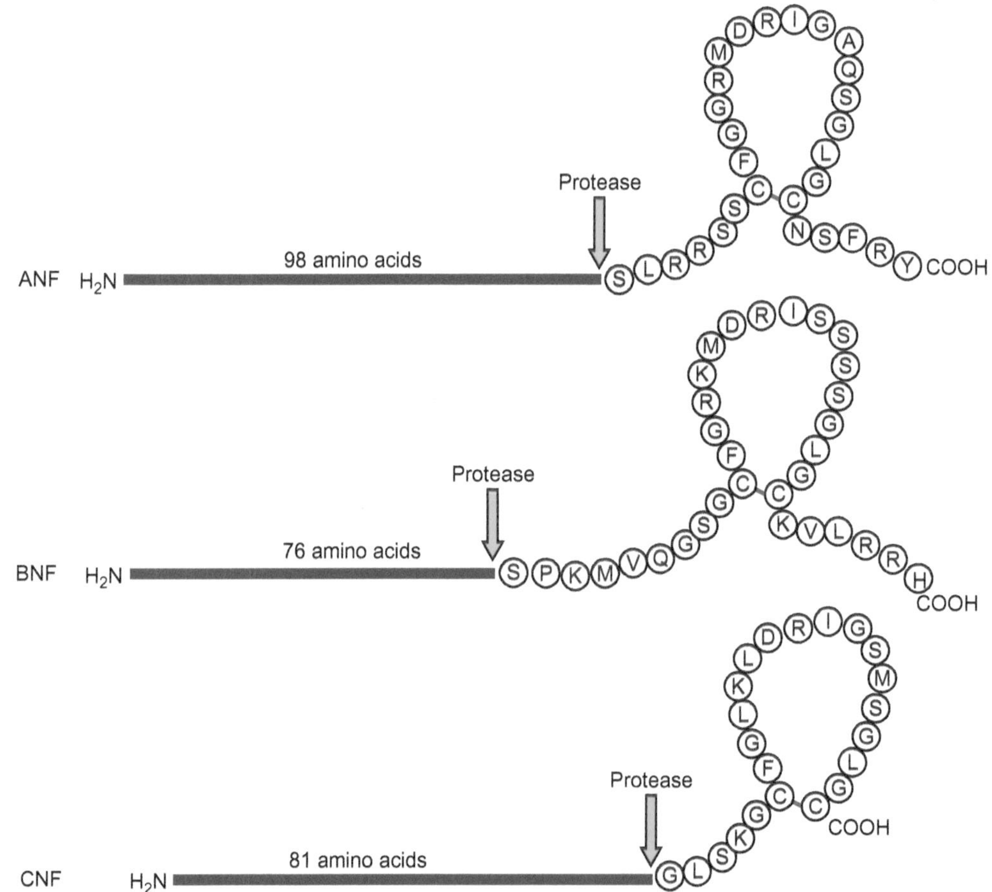

FIGURE 9.25 The natriuretic peptides. Amino acids are represented by the single letter amino acid code. Amino acids are represented by the single amino acid code: A is the alanine, C is the cysteine, D is the aspartic acid, F is the phenylalanine, G is the glycine, H is the histidine, I is the isoleucine, K is the lysine, L is the leucine, M is the methionine, N is the asparagine, Q is the glutamine, R is the arginine, S is the serine, and V is the valine.

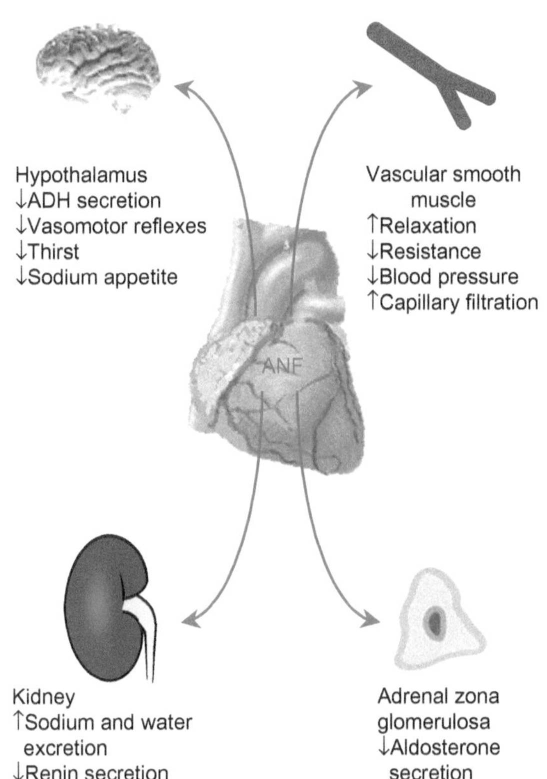

FIGURE 9.26 The actions of ANP. *ANP*, Atrial natriuretic peptide.

with the IP3 receptor inhibits release of calcium from the endoplasmic reticulum. Dephosphorylation of a key contractile protein by PKG-dependent activation of an associated phosphatase further contributes to the decrease in vascular tone.

Some evidence indicates that ANF may decrease calcium-dependent release of norepinephrine from sympathetic nerve endings and the adrenal medullae. An overall decrease in sympathetic input to vascular smooth muscle attenuates the pressor responses that might otherwise counteract vasodilatory effects of ANF. The decrease in arteriolar tone results in increased capillary pressure and favors net filtration of fluid from the vascular to the interstitial compartment and thus decreases vascular volume.

Decreased sympathetic stimulation of the juxtaglomerular cells combined with direct inhibitory effects of ANF on renin secretion lowers circulating levels of angiotensin II. Renin secretion is increased by cyclic AMP-dependent reactions. The direct inhibition of renin secretion by ANF probably results from cGMP activation of phosphodiesterase and the consequent reduction in cyclic AMP in juxtaglomerular cells. This effect may be augmented, by CNF inhibition of adenylyl cyclase. The reduction in sympathetic activity and in renin secretion enable the decrease in blood pressure to be sustained. Cardiac rate and contractility are also reduced as a consequence of decreased

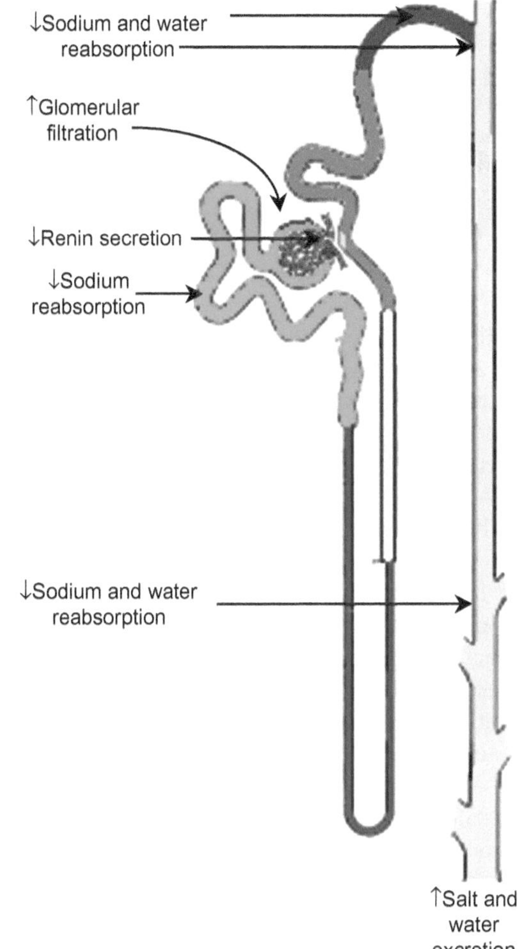

FIGURE 9.27 Direct and indirect actions of ANF on the kidney. *ANF*, Atrial natriuretic factor.

sympathetic stimulation of the heart and by direct actions of the natriuretic peptides on cardiac muscle.

Renal actions

Vascular volume is decreased further by actions on the kidney that promote excretion of water and sodium (Fig. 9.27).

ANF relaxes afferent glomerular arterioles and glomerular mesangial cells while constricting efferent arterioles. The resulting increase in capillary hydrostatic pressure and surface area amplifies glomerular filtration and accounts in large measure for increased urinary loss of salt and water. ANF also decreases sodium reabsorption in the proximal tubule by inhibiting the effects of angiotensin II on sodium bicarbonate reabsorption and perhaps by directly inhibiting the sodium–proton antiporter. As a consequence of these actions, increased amounts of salt and water reach the loop of Henle and partially "wash out" the osmotic gradient that provides the driving force for water reabsorption in the collecting ducts (see the section on ADH). In addition, ANF acts directly on the collecting ducts to decrease salt and water reabsorption, probably through its ability to decrease cyclic AMP levels. The net result increased sodium excretion in a large volume of diluted urine and a reduction in blood volume and total body sodium.

Effects on aldosterone secretion

As already discussed in Chapter 4, The Adrenal Glands, ANF receptors are present in adrenal glomerulosa cells where ANF directly inhibits aldosterone synthesis and secretion. ANF blocks the stimulatory effects of angiotensin II and high potassium on aldosterone secretion, possibly through PKG-dependent antagonism of the required increase in intracellular calcium. ANF also decreases aldosterone secretion indirectly by inhibiting renin secretion and hence the production of angiotensin II. Finally, ANF decreases ACTH secretion and antagonizes its action by activating a phosphodiesterase that degrades cyclic AMP. These actions deprive glomerulosa cells of the supportive effects of ACTH on the steroid synthetic apparatus. Although the consequences of the cardiovascular and renal actions of ANF are apparent immediately, the decrease in blood volume that follows from inhibition of aldosterone secretion is slower in onset and depends on the rapidity of cellular degradation of aldosterone-induced proteins.

Other effects

Acting on the hypothalamus through mechanisms that are not yet understood, ANF inhibits the secretion of ADH. This effect on hypothalamic neurons is reinforced by the decrease in circulating angiotensin II. Other hypothalamic effects include the suppression of thirst and salt seeking behavior. All these effects are opposite to those of angiotensin II.

Regulation of atrial natriuretic factor secretion

Like most other hormones, secretion of ANF is under negative feedback control, and like the renin–angiotensin–aldosterone system, it is the physiological consequences of its actions, rather than a humoral signal, that provides the negative input. Under normal physiological circumstances expansion of vascular volume increases the rate of right atrial filling and hence atrial pressure. The principal stimulus for secretion of ANF is an increased stretch of atrial muscle fibers produced by increased atrial pressure. Stretch-activated ion channels allow entry of cations and trigger ANF secretion. Increased secretion of ANF reduces the effective blood volume as described earlier, and when blood volume is restored to the normal range, secretion returns to basal levels (Fig. 9.28).

Integrated compensatory responses to changes in salt and water balance

The three hormones—ADH, angiotensin II, and aldosterone—collaborate to maintain or increase the effective volume of the blood plasma. Their properties and characteristics are summarized in Table 9.1.

In addition to reinforcing each other's effects, each of these hormones acts at multiple sites to reinforce its own effects. Physiological responses to these hormones are countered by the natriuretic peptides, which act at many of the same target sites. To some extent all these hormones are present in the circulation simultaneously, though in different relative amounts. Such target cells as vascular smooth muscle and the principal cells of the cortical collecting ducts must integrate these and other conflicting and reinforcing signals. The following discussion focuses on the endocrine adjustments that play decisive roles in maintaining salt and water balance. Students should be aware, however, that the sympathetic nervous system and a variety of locally produced paracrine factors, some of which are listed in Table 9.2, make important contributions, particularly by adjusting arteriolar tone.

To gain some understanding of how the various endocrine pathways interact, we consider several examples of perturbations in salt and water balance and the hormonal mechanisms that restore homeostasis. Volume changes can take several forms and may or may not be accompanied by changes in osmolality (sodium balance), as shown in Table 9.3.

Hemorrhage

With hemorrhage the vascular volume is decreased without a change in osmolality. To cope with blood loss, especially if it is large, a three-part strategy usually is followed: prevention of further fluid loss, redistribution of remaining fluid to maximize its usefulness, and replacement of the water and sodium losses. The sympathetic nervous system is indispensable for survival during the initial moments after hemorrhage. Hormonal contributions may augment the initial sympathetic reactions and are largely responsible for mediating the later aspects of recovery.

The immediate response to hemorrhage is massive vasoconstriction driven by the sympathetic nervous system. This response sustains arterial pressure and redistributes the cardiac output to ensure adequate blood flow to essential tissues. Renal blood flow and glomerular filtration are markedly reduced. Although slower in onset, hormonal responses nevertheless may contribute to maintenance of arterial blood pressure through vasoconstrictor actions of angiotensin II, ADH, and adrenomedullary hormones. The sum of these responses transfers extracellular water to the vascular

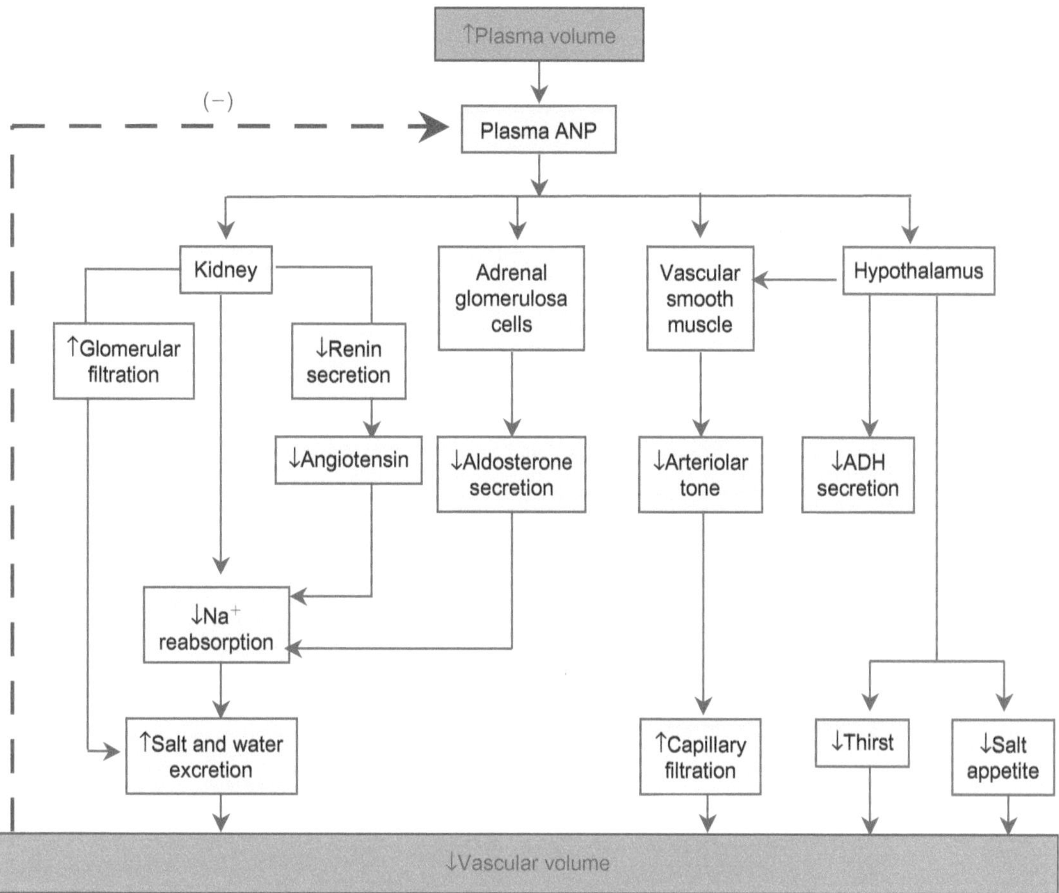

FIGURE 9.28 Negative feedback regulation of ANF secretion. *ANF*, Atrial natriuretic factor.

compartment by promoting net fluid absorption by capillaries and venules. Fig. 9.29 shows the pathways that eventually lead to restoration of blood volume.

Initially, hemorrhage, especially if it is severe (30% of blood volume), decreases venous return and thereby reduces right atrial pressure. Cardiac output, thus, is decreased, which at least transiently decreases arterial blood pressure and triggers the sympathetic response.

Response of the renin angiotensin system

Decreased arterial pressure is one of the signals for renin secretion and is sensed directly by the juxtaglomerular cells in the afferent arterioles. This input is nullified if arterial pressure is fully restored by the increase in total peripheral resistance, but direct sympathetic stimulation of the juxtaglomerular cells also increases renin secretion. In addition, decreased renal blood flow and glomerular filtration decrease sodium chloride flux through the distal tubule, which acts as yet another stimulus for renin secretion. Redundant pathways for evoking renin secretion, and therefore angiotensin production, ensure that this crucial system is activated by hemorrhage.

Angiotensin II has a wide variety of temporally and spatially separate actions that summate to restore plasma volume and compensate for hemorrhage. This situation is a good example of how different actions of a hormone expressed in different target cells reinforce each other to produce a cumulative response. They were discussed earlier and, therefore, are summarized here only in terms of the temporal sequence. Constriction of arteries and arterioles occurs within seconds, but the consequent mobilization of extravascular fluid requires several minutes. Also on the order of minutes may be direct stimulation of salt and water reabsorption by the proximal tubule by angiotensin II. The concentration of angiotensin II required to activate this mechanism is considerably below that required for vasoconstriction, but obviously this action is of little consequence when hemorrhage is so severe that renal blood flow is nearly completely shut down.

Other results of angiotensin action are considerably slower to appear. Consequences of stimulating adrenal glomerulosa cells to secrete aldosterone are not seen for almost an hour. Because aldosterone is not stored, it must be synthesized de novo, and as long as 10–15 minutes may be required to achieve peak

TABLE 9.1 Properties of the principle hormones that regulate water and sodium balance.

Hormone	Chemistry	Mode of action	Major target cells	Major cellular actions	Physiological responses
ADH	Peptide	cAMP (V2 receptors)	Principal cells of collecting ducts	↑Water and urea permeability	Water conservation
		DAG and IP3 (V1 receptors)	Vascular smooth muscle	Vasoconstriction	↑Blood pressure
Aldosterone	Steroid	Gene transcription (primarily)	Principal cells of cortical collecting duct	↑Na^+ reabsorption	Expand vascular volume
				↑K^+ excretion	
ANF	Peptide	cGMP	Vascular smooth muscle	Vasodilation	↓Blood pressure
					↓Blood volume
			Glomerular mesangial cells	Relaxation	↑GFR natriuresis, diuresis
			Proximal tubule cells	↓Na^+ reabsorption	
			Adrenal glomerulosa	↓Aldosterone secretion	
			Hypothalamic neurons	↓Vasomotor reflexes	
				↓ADH secretion	
Angiotensin II	Peptide	DAG and IP3 (AT1 receptors)	Adrenal glomerulosa	↑Aldosterone secretion	(See above)
			Vascular smooth muscle	Vasoconstriction	↑Blood pressure
					↓GFR
			Proximal tubule cells	↑Na + /H1 exchange	Na^+ retention
				↑$NaHCO_3$ reabsorption	
			Hypothalamic neurons	↑ADH secretion	(see above) Salt and water ingestion
				↑Thirst and salt appetite	

ADH, Antidiuretic hormone; *cAMP*, cyclic AMP; *cGMP*, cyclic guanosine monophosphate; *GFR*, glomerular filtration rate.

TABLE 9.2 Some locally produced hormone-like agents that affect cardiovascular functions related to salt and water balance.

Agent	Chemistry	Source	Relevant actions
Nitric oxide	Gas	Vascular endothelium	Relax vascular smooth muscle
Adrenomedullin	Peptide	Ubiquitous	Relax vascular smooth muscle
Endothelin	Peptide	Ubiquitous	Constrict vascular smooth muscle
Bradykinin	Peptide	Plasma, many tissues	Relax vascular smooth muscle
			Natriuresis and diuresis
Prostaglandins	Arachidonic acid derivatives	Ubiquitous	Constrict or relax vascular smooth muscle
			Increase capillary
			Permeability

production rates. Furthermore, aldosterone, like other steroid hormones, requires a lag period of at least 30 minutes before its effects are evident.

The final contribution of angiotensin II is stimulation of salt appetite, thirst, and fluid absorption by the colon. Depending on the severity of the blood loss and the availability of water and salt, many hours or even days may pass before the renin–angiotensin system can restore the plasma volume to prehemorrhage levels.

Response of the antidiuretic hormone system

Even though osmolality is unchanged, decreased pressure sensed by receptors in the atria, aorta, and carotid sinuses stimulate ADH secretion. In addition,

TABLE 9.3 Examples of changes in fluid volume.

	Expansion	Contraction
Isosmolar	↑Salt and water ingestion	Hemorrhage
	Hyperaldosteronism	Hypoalbuminemia
	Heart failure	
Hypoosmolar	Excessive water intake	Excessive sweating followed by water intake
	Syndrome of inappropriate ADH secretion	
Hyperosmolar	Excessive salt intake	Dehydration

ADH, Antidiuretic hormone.

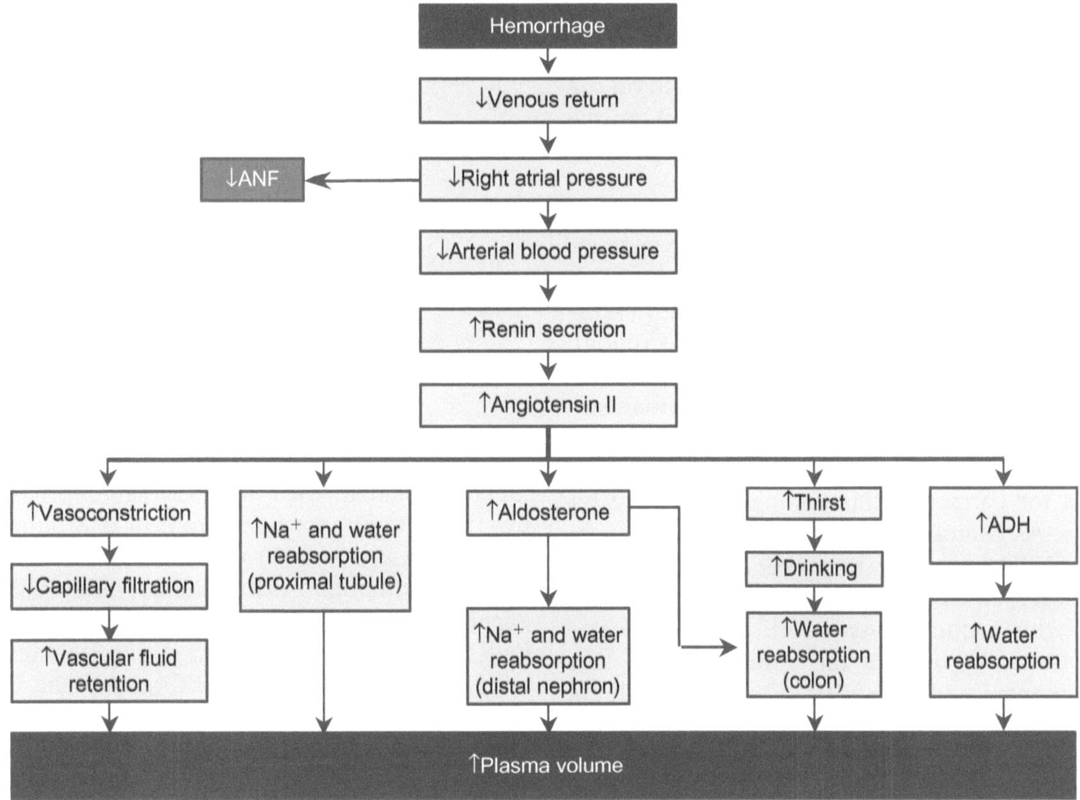

FIGURE 9.29 Hormonal responses to hemorrhage.

ADH secretion also is increased by angiotensin II. Here we have another case of redundancy, as ADH and angiotensin II have overlapping actions on arteriolar smooth muscle. These hormones also reinforce each other's actions at the level of the renal tubule, as they increase water reabsorption at different sites and by different mechanisms. Although ADH is secreted almost instantaneously in response to hemorrhage, its physiological importance for the early responses is questionable because vascular smooth muscle may already be maximally constricted by sympathetic stimulation, which is even faster. In addition, when renal shutdown is severe, little urine reaches the collecting ducts and hence even maximal antidiuresis can conserve little water. ADH, however, is an indispensable component of the recovery phase. Thirst and salt-conserving mechanisms would be of little benefit without ADH to promote renal retention of water.

Response of aldosterone

Like ADH, aldosterone is of little consequence for the immediate reactions to hemorrhage. It acts too slowly. Furthermore, decreased glomerular filtration is far more important quantitatively in conserving sodium. Increased secretion of aldosterone, which is initiated promptly by the renin–angiotensin system and reinforced by increased ACTH secretion, can be regarded as an anticipatory response to ensure sodium conservation when renal blood flow is restored. Aldosterone is indispensable for replenishing blood volume by conserving sodium ingested during recovery and probably by stimulating sodium intake.

Response of atrial natriuretic factor

It almost goes without saying that depleted vascular volume reduces or eliminates signals for the secretion of ANF. This situation is the converse of that depicted in Fig. 9.28. We thus have a push–pull mechanism wherein the secretion of an inhibitory influence on the actions of angiotensin II and ADH is shut off by the same events that increase secretion of these hormones.

Dehydration

Dehydration (water deficit) is a commonly encountered derangement of homeostasis and may result from severe sweating, diarrhea, vomiting, fever, excessive alcohol ingestion (which inhibits ADH secretion), or simply insufficient fluid intake. Because dehydration usually involves a greater deficit of water than solute, both intracellular and extracellular osmolality increase. Consequently, the ADH pathway is the principal means for correcting this derangement in water homeostasis. As osmolality increases above its threshold value, ADH secretion promptly increases, and water is reabsorbed in excess of solute until osmolality is restored. This action prevents further loss of water in urine, but cannot restore the volume deficit that usually accompanies dehydration. Decreased volume stimulates the renin–angiotensin–aldosterone system to facilitate vascular adjustments, stimulates thirst, and prepares for replenishment from increased intake of salt and water. Decreased volume also reinforces osmotic stimulation of ADH secretion. Again, ANF secretion is not activated and the actions of ADH and angiotensin II are unopposed. Fig. 9.30 illustrates the endocrine responses to dehydration and the series of events that restore osmolality and volume to normal.

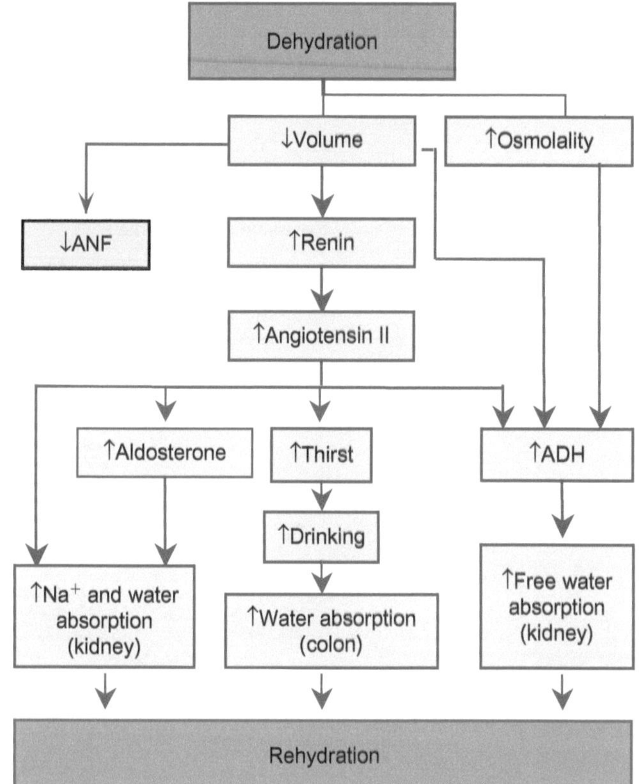

FIGURE 9.30 Hormonal responses to dehydration.

Salt loading and depletion

Although sodium chloride is scarce in many regions of the world, it is in oversupply in most Western diets. The endocrine system plays a pivotal role in maintaining homeostasis and normal blood pressure in the face of salt loading or depletion. Fig. 9.31 shows the responses of normal human subjects who volunteered to consume diets that contained high, low, or standard amounts of sodium.

Salt-loaded subjects excreted more than 10 times as much sodium in their urine as salt-deprived subjects, but the concentration of sodium in plasma and systolic blood pressure was nearly identical in all the three groups. Although extracellular fluid volume was expanded on the high salt diet and contracted on the low salt diet, osmolality and sodium concentration of body fluids remained remarkably constant. Changes in blood concentrations of angiotensin II (as reflected in renin levels), aldosterone, ADH, and ANF elicited by different amounts of sodium intake are shown in Fig. 9.26. Plasma renin activity and aldosterone secretion decreased as sodium intake increased. The high rate of sodium loss by subjects on the high sodium diet may be explained by decreased reabsorption of sodium in the proximal tubule as a result of decreased angiotensin II and increased ANF, and in the cortical collecting ducts as a result of decreased aldosterone. As might be expected, the ANF concentration was increased when sodium intake was increased and decreased when sodium intake was low. The reciprocal relation between ANF and angiotensin II acts as a push–pull mechanism to promote sodium loss in the sodium-loaded individual and sodium conservation in the salt-deprived subject. ADH secretion was also increased in subjects on high salt intake, probably in response to the small increase in plasma osmolality. The plasma sodium

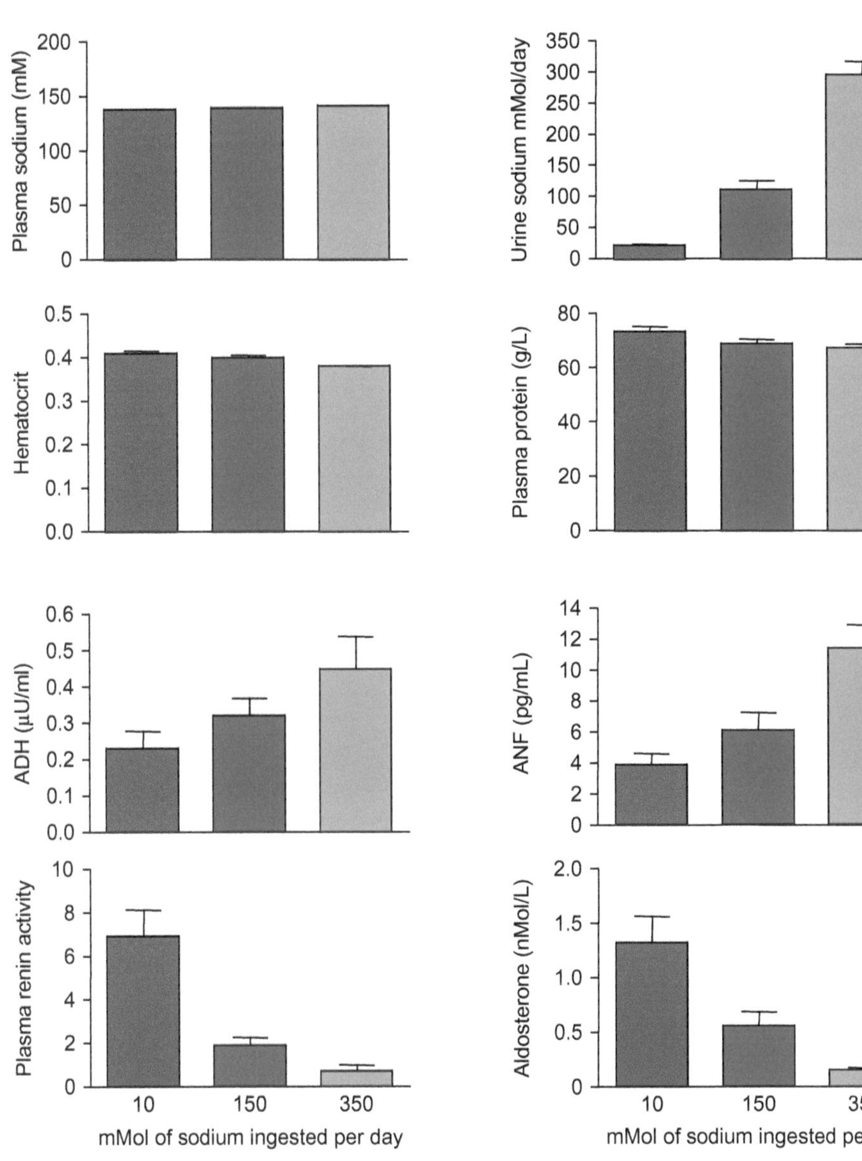

FIGURE 9.31 Responses of normal subjects to low or high intake of sodium chloride for 5 days. Plasma sodium concentrations were maintained within less than 2% by compensating rates of sodium excretion. The small increases or decreases in hematocrit and plasma protein concentrations indicate the contraction of the plasma volume in the low sodium group and expansion in the high sodium group. The changes in hormone concentrations are in response to the small changes in osmolality and volume. Plasma renin activity is a measure of renin concentration expressed as ng of angiotensin I formed per mL of plasma in 1 h. Source: *Drawn from the data of Sagnella, G. A., Markandu, N. D., Shore, A. C., Forsling, M. L., MacGregor, G. A. (1987). Plasma atrial natriuretic peptide: Its relationship to changes in sodium intake, plasma renin activity and aldosterone secretion in man.* Clinical Science 72, *25–30.*

concentration in these subjects was 2% higher than in subjects on the low sodium diet and 1.4% higher than in subjects on the normal diet. ADH secreted in response to the osmotic stimulus prevented the loss of water that might otherwise have accompanied increased amounts of sodium in urine.

Summary

As land animals we must preserve the milieu interior which is believed to be the same as that of the ancient seas. To do so, aldosterone from the adrenal gland regulates sodium while ADH from the hypothalamus regulates water. The various interactions with the target structures and the feedback to maintain salt and water concentrations within very narrow parameters have been discussed in this chapter.

Suggested reading

Basic foundations

Giebisch, G., Windhager, E. E., & Aronson, P. S. (2017). Transport of sodium and chloride. In W. F. Boron, & E. L. Boulpaep (Eds.), *Medical physiology* (3rd ed., pp. 754–769). Philadelphia, PA: Elsevier.

Stewart, P. M., & Newell-Price, J. D. C. (2017). The adrenal cortex. In S. Melmed, K. S. Polonsky, P. R. Larsen, & H. M. Kronenberg (Eds.), *Williams textbook of endocrinology* (13th ed., pp. 490–555). Philadelphia, PA: Elsevier.

Young, W. F. J. (2017). Endocrine hypertension. In S. Melmed, K. S. Polonsky, P. R. Larsen, & H. M. Kronenberg (Eds.), *Williams textbook of endocrinology* (13th ed., pp. 556–588). Philadelphia, PA: Elsevier.

Advanced information

Farrugia, F.-A., Zavras, N., Martikos, G., Tzanetis, P., Charalampopoulos, A., Misiakos Evangelos, P., ... Koliakos, N. (2018). A short review of primary aldosteronism in a question and answer fashion. *Endocrine Regulations, 52*, 27.

Kline, G. A., Prebtani, A. P. H., Leung, A. A., & Schiffrin, E. L. (2017). Primary aldosteronism: a common cause of resistant hypertension. *Canadian Medical Association Journal, 189*(22), E773.

Li, J., Fan, X., & Wang, Q. (2018). Hypertensive crisis with 2 target organ impairment induced by glycyrrhizin: A case report. *Medicine, 97*(11), e0073. Available from https://doi.org/10.1097/md.0000000000010073.

Monticone, S., Buffolo, F., Tetti, M., Veglio, F., Pasini, B., & Mulatero, P. (2018). Genetics in Endocrinology: The expanding genetic horizon of primary aldosteronism. *European Journal of Endocrinology, 178*(3), R101–R111. Available from https://doi.org/10.1530/eje-17-0946.

Parikh, P. P., Rubio, G. A., Farra, J. C., & Lew, J. I. (2017). Nationwide review of hormonally active adrenal tumors highlights high morbidity in pheochromocytoma. *Journal of Surgical Research, 215*, 204–210. Available from https://doi.org/10.1016/j.jss.2017.04.011.

Prada, E. T. A., Burrello, J., Reincke, M., & Williams, T. A. (2017). Old and new concepts in the molecular pathogenesis of primary aldosteronism. *Hypertension, 70*(5), 875.

Vilela, L. A. P., & Almeida, M. Q. (2017). Diagnosis and management of primary aldosteronism. *Archives of Endocrinology and Metabolism, 61*, 305–312.

Historical information

Conn, J. W., & Louis, L. H. (1955). Primary aldosteronism: A new clinical entity. *Transactions of the Association of American Physicians, 68*, 215–231.

Streeten, D. H. P. (1999). Orthostatic intolerance. A historical introduction to the pathophysiological mechanisms. *The American Journal of the Medical Sciences, 317*(2), 78–87. Available from https://doi.org/10.1016/S0002-9629(15)40481-1.

CHAPTER

10

Hormonal regulation of calcium balance

Case study: primary hyperparathyroidism

Patient is a 58-year-old female with a history of hypertension and osteopenia who presented to the outpatient endocrine clinic for hypercalcemia that was incidentally noted on routine laboratory evaluation performed by her primary care doctor. She reports a history of recurrent nephrolithiasis. In the past, she had three kidney stones but never had a kidney stone analysis performed so their composition is unknown. She has never had a clinical fracture as an adult. She admits to constipation but denies any nausea, vomiting, or abdominal pain. On physical examination, her vital signs were normal. She appeared well and did not have any costovertebral angle tenderness.

Laboratory evaluation revealed hypercalcemia (serum calcium 11.5 mg/dL; normal 8.6–10.4), hyperparathyroidism [intact parathyroid hormone (iPTH) 186 pg/mL; normal 10–69], 25-hydroxyvitamin D 29 ng/mL, hypophosphatemia (serum phosphorus 1.7 mg/dL; normal range 2.5–4.5), normal renal function, and an elevated 1,25-dihydroxyvitamin D level (112 pg/mL; normal 18–72). Further evaluation revealed hypercalciuria with a 24-h urine calcium level of 399 mg (upper limit of normal 250 mg) and a normal urinary creatinine of 1.62 g.

Her DXA (dual-energy X-ray absorptiometry) scan (bone density scan) showed osteopenia of the lumbar spine, femoral neck, total hip, and the forearm (Table 10.1).

TABLE 10.1 Dual-energy X-ray absorptiometry scan of the lumbar spine, left hip, and forearm.

Site	*T*-score	WHO classification
L1–L3 vertebrae	− 1.1	Osteopenia
Left femoral neck	− 1.7	Osteopenia
Left total hip	− 1.2	Osteopenia
Forearm	− 1.7	Osteopenia

Osteopenia is noted at these three sites.

Based on her biochemical evaluation, which showed hypercalcemia with an inappropriately elevated iPTH as well as hypercalciuria, a diagnosis of primary hyperparathyroidism (PHPT) was made. The fractional excretion of calcium was calculated to be 0.02, which is consistent with a diagnosis of PHPT. A history of nephrolithiasis is a clinical indication for surgical intervention with a parathyroidectomy. Thus the patient was referred to an endocrine surgeon and had a single parathyroid adenoma resected. Her repeat DXA scan 2 years after this procedure showed significant improvements of 13%, 8%, and 5% at her spine, total hip, and forearm, respectively. After parathyroidectomy a patient's bone density typically improves, as it did in this case.

In the clinic:

Primary hyperparathyroidism

Introduction

Primary hyperparathyroidism (PHPT) is a condition in which there is an inappropriately high parathyroid hormone level in the setting of hypercalcemia. The most common cause of PHPT is a single parathyroid adenoma. Less common causes are double adenomas and multigland parathyroid hyperplasia. Multigland parathyroid hyperplasia may be seen in familial syndromes

Goodman's Basic Medical Endocrinology.
DOI: https://doi.org/10.1016/B978-0-12-815844-9.00010-5

(cont'd)

such as multiple endocrine neoplasia 1 (MEN1) and multiple endocrine neoplasia 2A (MEN2A). Rarely, parathyroid carcinomas can be found.

Signs and symptoms

The most common clinical presentation of PHPT is asymptomatic hypercalcemia. Patients with more severe disease can exhibit clinical symptoms of hypercalcemia such as fatigue, nausea, vomiting, abdominal pain, constipation, and polyuria. Severe hypercalcemia may also lead to dehydration, worsening hypercalcemia, and mental status changes. Additional symptoms that may be seen in PHPT include bone pain, fragility fractures, nephrolithiasis, anxiety, and changes in mood. As biochemical screening has become more common, severe presentations of PHPT are uncommon. It is important to note that patients with asymptomatic PHPT can still have the skeletal sequelae of osteopenia or osteoporosis as well as the presence of asymptomatic kidney stones and nephrocalcinosis.

Diagnosis

The diagnosis of PHPT is made biochemically if a patient has hypercalcemia and an elevated or inappropriately normal iPTH level. It is not physiologically appropriate for a patient to have an iPTH in the normal range in the setting of hypercalcemia. Normally, hypercalcemia should suppress the iPTH level.

Of note, normocalcemic PHPT is a variant of this condition in which the serum calcium level is normal but the iPTH level is elevated.

It is also important to rule out familial hypocalciuric hypercalcemia (FHH), a condition that can also show hypercalcemia but is due to a mutation in the calcium-sensing receptor (CASR). Patients with FHH usually have a fractional excretion of calcium of less than 0.01.

The laboratory evaluation of patients with PHPT should include serum calcium, albumin, serum phosphate, creatinine, and 25-hydroxyvitamin D level. In addition, one should check a 24-hour urinary calcium level since these patients typically have hypercalciuria and thus are at increased risk of nephrolithiasis. If the patient's urinary calcium level is greater than 400 mg, another 24-h urine test is performed to check the full kidney stone risk profile looking for other risk factors for kidney stone development. Renal imaging should be performed to check for kidney stones or nephrocalcinosis. These studies may include a kidney ultrasound, abdominal X-ray, or CT scan.

DXA (dual-energy X-ray absorptiometry) scan should be performed to measure the patient's bone density at the lumbar spine, hip, and the forearm. X-rays of the spine may be performed to evaluate for vertebral compression fractures.

Management

Management of PHPT may include either surgical management with a parathyroidectomy or medical management. Parathyroidectomy is recommended for patients with symptomatic disease. Parathyroidectomy is also indicated in patients with asymptomatic PHPT if they meet any of the following criteria: (1) age <50 years old, (2) serum calcium $\geq$ 1 g/dL above the upper limit of normal, (3) *T*-score -2.5 or lower (osteoporosis) or vertebral fracture seen on imaging, (4) creatinine clearance of <60 mL/min, increased risk of kidney stones based on a 24-h stone risk analysis, and kidney stones or nephrocalcinosis on imaging. Preoperative localization of the enlarged parathyroid gland is typically performed with neck ultrasound, sestamibi parathyroid scan, or a 4DCT scan.

Medical management of PHPT includes assuring adequate fluid intake to avoid dehydration and to decrease the risk of kidney stones. In addition, if osteoporosis is present, it may be treated with antiresorptive therapy to decrease the risk of fragility fractures. Monitoring of PHPT includes checking serum calcium and creatinine/estimated glomerular filtration rate once yearly, and performing DXA scans every 1–2 years. Cinacalcet, a CASR agonist, may be used in patients with severe hypercalcemia but who cannot undergo parathyroidectomy.

Prognosis

After a successful parathyroidectomy, patients have normalization of serum calcium and iPTH levels and typically their bone density improves. For patients who opt for medical management or who are unable to undergo a parathyroidectomy, they will be monitored for sequelae of PHPT, including worsening hypercalcemia, a decline in bone density, and nephrolithiasis. In one natural history, study of patients with asymptomatic PHPT who were followed for 15 years, 37% of patients developed a sequela that would meet criteria for parathyroidectomy.

Hormonal regulation of calcium balance

Adequate amounts of calcium in its ionized form, Ca^{2+}, are needed for normal function of all cells. Calcium ion regulates a wide range of biological processes and is one of the principal constituents of bone. In terrestrial vertebrates, including humans, maintenance of adequate concentrations of calcium ion in the extracellular fluid requires the activity of two hormones, parathyroid hormone (PTH) and a derivative of vitamin D called 1,25-dihydroxycholecalciferol [1,25 $(OH)_2D3$] or calcitriol. In more primitive vertebrates living in a marine environment, guarding against excessively high concentrations of calcium requires another hormone, calcitonin. These three hormones collectively are called calciotropic hormones. In addition, calcium behaves like a hormone and acts through cell surface receptors that directly or indirectly regulate the calcium concentration in plasma.

Body calcium is ultimately derived from the diet, and daily intake is usually offset by urinary loss. The skeleton acts as a major reservoir of calcium and can buffer the concentration of calcium in extracellular fluid by taking up or releasing calcium phosphate. PTH promotes the transfer of calcium from bone, the glomerular filtrate, and intestinal contents into the extracellular fluid. It acts on bone cells to promote calcium mobilization and on renal tubules to reabsorb calcium and excrete phosphate. It promotes intestinal transport of calcium and phosphate indirectly by increasing the formation of $1{,}25(OH)_2D3$, which increases calcium uptake by intestinal cells. This vitamin D metabolite also promotes calcium mobilization from bone and reinforces the actions of PTH on this process. In addition, $1{,}25(OH)_2D3$ promotes reabsorption of calcium by renal tubules. The secretion of PTH is inversely related to the concentration of blood calcium. If the blood calcium level is low, then PTH is released to increase the calcium level. If the blood calcium level is high, then this directly inhibits PTH secretion by the chief cells of the parathyroid glands.

Calcitonin helps regulate blood calcium in fish but its role in humans is not clear. If pharmacologic calcitonin is given to a patient, it inhibits the activity of bone-resorbing cells and thereby blocks inflow of calcium to the extracellular fluid compartment. Thus this can be used as a temporary treatment of hypercalcemia (high blood calcium level) in some patients.

General features of calcium balance

Calcium plays a role in a wide range of cellular and molecular processes. Changes of its concentration within cells regulate enzymatic activities and fundamental cellular events such as cell division, secretion, and muscular contraction. As already discussed (see Chapter 1: Introduction), calcium and calmodulin also act as intracellular mediators of hormone action. In the extracellular compartment, calcium is vital for blood clotting and maintenance of normal membrane function. In addition, calcium may act in a hormone-like way as an extracellular regulator of a variety of cellular responses through the stimulation of membrane calcium receptors. Calcium is the basic mineral of bones and teeth and thus plays a structural as well as a regulatory role. Not surprisingly, its concentration in extracellular fluid must be maintained within narrow limits. Deviations in either direction are not readily tolerated and, if severe, may be life-threatening. Electrical excitability of cell membranes increases when the extracellular concentration of calcium is low, and the threshold for triggering action potentials may be lowered almost to the resting potential, which results in spontaneous, asynchronous, and involuntary contractions of skeletal muscle called tetany. A typical attack of tetany involves muscular spasms in the face, known as Chvostek's sign, and characteristic contortions of the arms and hands. Laryngeal spasm and contraction of respiratory muscles may compromise breathing. Severe hypocalcemia (low blood calcium) may produce more generalized muscular contractions and convulsions.

Increased concentrations of calcium in blood (hypercalcemia) may cause calcium salts to precipitate out of solution because of their low solubility at physiological pH. Kidney stones may form and can cause severe pain (renal colic) and renal damage, which may lead to renal failure and hypertension.

Distribution of calcium in the body

The adult human body contains approximately 1000 g of calcium, about 99% of which is sequestered in bone, primarily in the form of hydroxyapatite crystals $[Ca_{10}(PO_4)_6(OH)_2]$. In addition to providing structural support, bone serves as an enormous reservoir for calcium. Each day, about 500 mg of calcium is exchanged between bone mineral and the extracellular fluid. Much of this exchange reflects resorption and reformation of bone as the skeleton undergoes constant remodeling.

Most of the calcium that is not in bone crystals is found in cells of soft tissues bound to proteins within the sarcoplasmic reticulum, mitochondria, and other organelles. Energy-dependent transport of calcium by these organelles and the cell membrane maintains the resting concentration of free calcium in cytosol at low levels of about 0.1 μM. Cytosolic calcium can increase 10-fold or more, however, with just a brief change in membrane permeability or affinity of intracellular-binding proteins. The rapidity and magnitude of changes in cytosolic calcium are consistent with its role as a biological signal.

The concentration of calcium in interstitial fluid is about 1.5 mM. Interstitial calcium consists mainly of free, ionized calcium, but about 10% is complexed with anions such as citrate, lactate, or phosphate. Ionized and complexed calcium pass freely through capillary membranes and equilibrate with calcium in blood plasma. The total calcium concentration in blood is nearly twice that of interstitial fluid because calcium is avidly bound by albumin and other proteins. Total calcium in blood plasma is normally about 9–10 mg/dL (4.5–5 mEq/L or 2.2–2.5 mM), but only the ionized component appears to be monitored and regulated. Since most of the blood calcium is protein-bound, diseases that produce substantial changes in albumin concentrations may produce striking abnormalities in total plasma calcium concentrations, even though the concentration of ionized calcium may be normal.

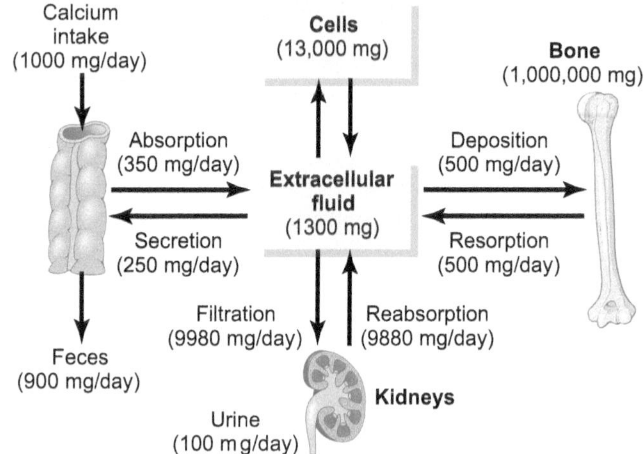

FIGURE 10.1 An overview of calcium exchange between various tissues. Source: *From Figure 80-3 in J. Hall. (2016).* Guyton and Hall's textbook of medical physiology *(13th ed.) (p. 1003). Elsevier.*

Calcium balance

Normally, adults are in calcium balance; that is, on average, daily intake equals daily loss in urine and feces. Except for lactation and pregnancy, deviations from balance reflect changes in the metabolism of bone. Immobilization of a limb, bed rest, weightlessness, and malignant disease are examples of circumstances that produce negative calcium balance, whereas growth of the skeleton produces positive calcium balance. Dietary intake of calcium in the United States typically varies between 500 and 1500 mg/day, primarily in the form of dairy products. For example, an 8-oz glass of milk contains about 300 mg of calcium. Calcium absorbed from the intestine exchanges with the various body pools and ultimately is lost in the urine so that there is no net gain or loss of calcium in the extracellular pool in young adults. These relations are illustrated in Fig. 10.1 (Blaine et al., 2015).

It is noteworthy that the entire extracellular calcium pool turns over many times in the course of a day. Hence, even small changes in any of these calcium fluxes can have profound effects.

Intestinal absorption

Calcium is taken up along the entire length of the small intestine, but uptake is greatest in the duodenum and jejunum. Secretions of the gastrointestinal tract are rich in calcium and add to the minimum load that must be absorbed to maintain balance. Net uptake is usually in the range of 100–200 mg/day. Absorption of calcium requires metabolic energy and the activity of specific carrier molecules in the luminal membrane (brush border) of intestinal cells. Although detailed understanding is not yet at hand, it appears that carrier-mediated transport across the brush border determines the overall rate. Calcium is carried down by its concentration gradient into the cytosol of intestinal epithelial cells and is extruded from the basolateral surfaces in exchange for sodium, which must then be pumped out at metabolic expense. Overall transfer of calcium from the intestinal lumen to interstitial fluid proceeds against a concentration gradient and is largely dependent on $1{,}25(OH)_2D3$ (see later). Although some calcium is taken up passively, simple diffusion is not adequate to meet the body's needs even when the concentration of calcium in the intestinal lumen is high.

Bone

Understanding the regulation of calcium balance requires at least a rudimentary understanding of the physiology of bone. Metabolic activity in bone must satisfy two needs. The skeleton must attend to its own structural integrity through continuous remodeling and renewal, and it must respond to systemic needs for adequate amounts of calcium in the extracellular fluid. By and large, maintenance of adequate concentrations of calcium in blood takes precedence over maintenance of structural integrity of bone. However, it must be recognized that these two homeostatic functions, though driven by different forces, are not completely independent. Diseases of bone that disrupt skeletal homeostasis may have consequences for overall calcium balance; and, conversely, inadequacies of calcium balance lead to inadequate mineralization of bone.

Bone consists of an outer cortical and an inner trabecular component (Fig. 10.2).

Cortical (compact) bone is the most prevalent form and is found in the shafts of long bones and on the surfaces of the pelvis, skull, and other flat bones. The basic unit of cortical bone is called an osteon (haversian system) and consists of concentric layers, or lamellae, of bone arranged around a central channel (haversian canal), which contains the capillary blood supply. Osteons are usually 200–300 mm in diameter and several hundred millimeters long. They are arranged with their long axes oriented in parallel with the shaft of bone. Other canals, called Volkmann's canals, which run roughly perpendicularly, connect the longitudinal haversian canals and osteons (Fig. 10.3).

Within each osteon are numerous holes called lacunae (lacuna, singular, Latin for small lake or pool or a pit—our word "lagoon" comes from this), which is where bone cells called osteocytes reside. Radiating out from each lacuna are numerous small channels called canaliculi, which contain processes of the osteocytes that connect to the processes of other osteocytes in other lacunae (Fig. 10.4). Between the processes of two different osteocytes, there is a gap junction.

The canal network extends to the haversian canal in the center. Nutrients, calcium, and metabolic products diffuse into and out of the capillaries in the haversian canal (Fig. 10.5).

Surrounding the haversian canal are rings called lamellae (from *lamina*, Latin for thin plate). Collagen

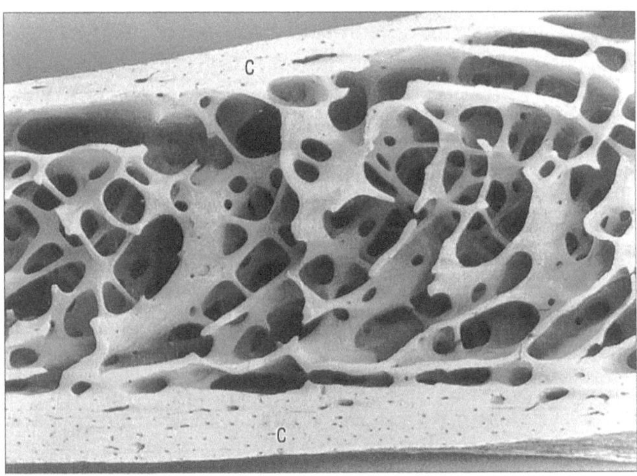

FIGURE 10.2 Cortical (C) bone and trabecular bone inside. This is a section through the iliac crest of a 42-year-old female. The small dots in the cortical bone are haversian canals (named after Clopton Havers, the English physician who first described them in 1691). Trabecular bone is so named because of the trabeculae, which means "little beams" (from Latin: the diminutive form of *trabs*, a beam or timber). This provides structural support for the bone. Its other name is spongy bone because of its resemblance to natural sponges. The space between the trabeculae is normally filled with red marrow and is the site of blood formation. In older adults, red marrow leaves the long bones and is replaced by fat so is called yellow marrow. Source: *From Figure 5.8 in S. Standring. (2016).* Gray's anatomy *(41st ed.) (p. 85). Elsevier.*

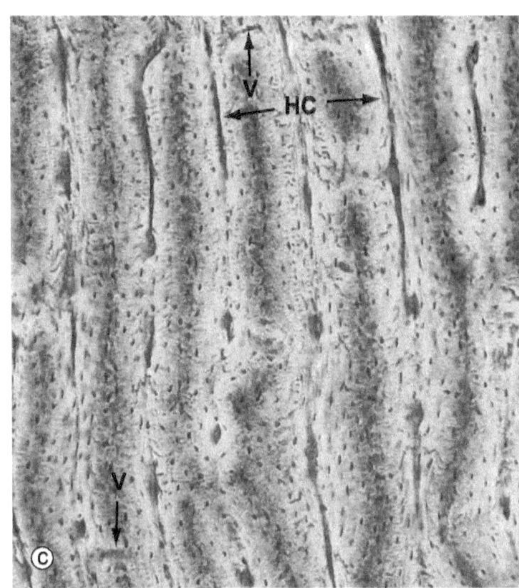

FIGURE 10.3 A longitudinal section through cortical bone. It illustrates the longitudinal haversian canals (HC) and the Volkmann's canals (V) running at right angles to the HC. *HC*, Haversian canals. Source: *From Fig. 10.11C in Young, B., O'Dowd, G., & Woodford, P. (2014).* Wheater's functional histology *(6th ed.) (p. 186). Elsevier.*

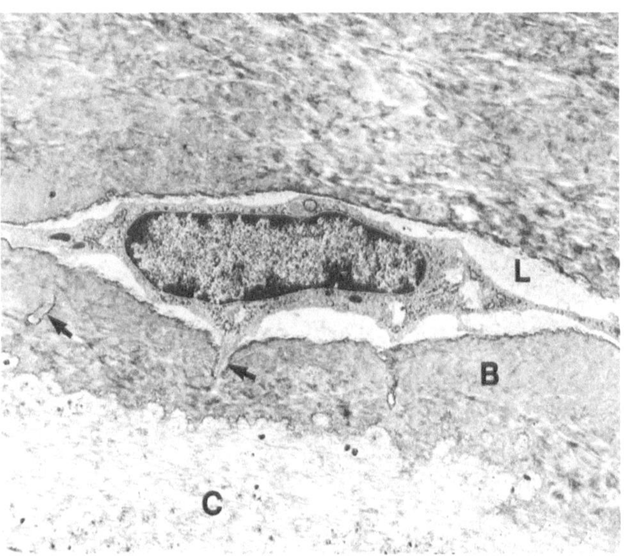

FIGURE 10.4 An osteocyte in its lacuna. It has a large nucleus, the black edge of which is composed of heterochromatin composed of tightly coiled DNA that the cell is not using, while in the center the DNA is lighter because it is largely uncoiled and is being used, and is called euchromatin. Note the osteocytic processes (*arrows*) extending into the canaliculus. *B*, Bone; *C*, cartilage; *L*, lacuna. This image was taken from a growing bone in which the cartilage becomes bone. Source: *From Figure 7-7B in Gartner, L. P. (2017).* Textbook of histology *(4th ed.) (p. 157). Elsevier.*

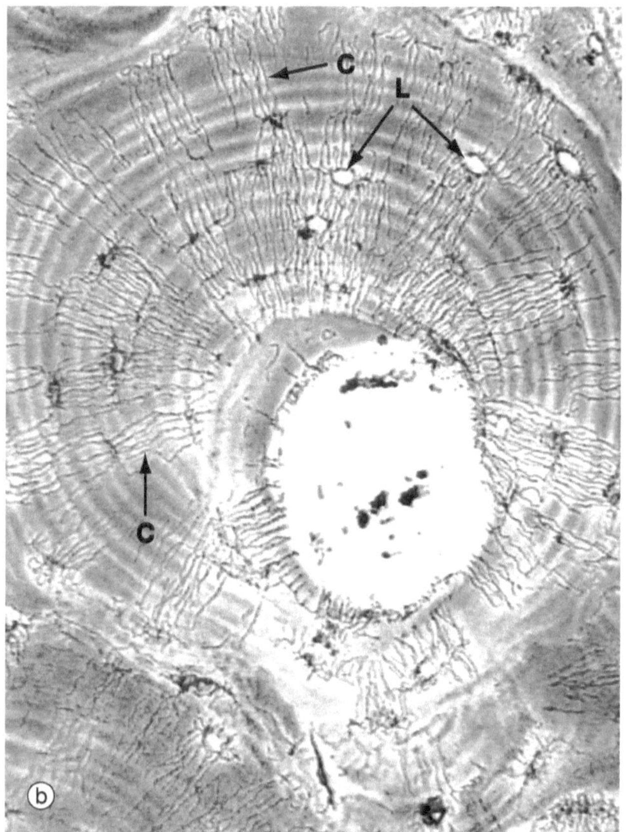

FIGURE 10.5 An osteon. L is the lacunae where osteocytes reside (osteocytes not shown here); C is the canaliculi that connect lacunae to each other and to the haversian canal, the large space in the center. The lamellae are the rings that surround the haversian canal. Source: *From Fig. 10.11b in Young, B., O'Dowd, G., & Woodford, P. (2014).* Wheater's functional histology *(6th ed.) (p. 186). Elsevier.*

fibers make up the rings and within each ring the collagen fibers are oriented in a different direction (Fig. 10.6).

If the lamellae were parallel in each ring, the bone would not be very strong. Since the lamellae are oriented in different directions, this gives the bone strength. This is analogous to wood in plywood: the more layers in which the wood grains in each layer are at a different angle, the stronger the plywood. If they are all arranged going the same way as in a regular piece of wood, it will not be very strong and bends more easily than a piece of plywood having the same dimensions. Likewise, the number of lamellae also determines the strength of bone. The more lamellae there are, the stronger the bone.

Cancellous (trabecular) bone is found at the ends of the long bones, in the vertebrae, sternum, and in the pelvis, skull, and other flat bones. It is also called spongy bone, a term that well describes its appearance in section (Fig. 10.2).

The extracellular matrix is the predominant component of bone. One-third of the bony matrix is organic matrix called osteoid, while the remaining two-thirds comprise highly ordered hydroxyapatite, a geological term referring to its calcium phosphate crystalline structure.

Bone formation begins with osteoblasts, which are thought to differentiate from mesenchymal precursors in the perichondrium or periosteum. The osteoblasts secrete collagen, which is then mineralized by vesicles. These vesicles can be either exosomes or ectosomes (Fig. 10.7).

About 10%–20% of osteoblasts wall themselves in and become osteocytes. The rest remain as a layer of quiescent cells on the matrix surface.

Although only about 20% of the skeleton comprises trabecular bone, its sponge-like organization provides at least five times as much surface area for metabolic exchange as compact bone. The trabeculae of spongy bone are not penetrated by blood vessels, but the spaces between them are filled with blood sinusoids, which are highly vascular marrow. Each trabecula is completely surrounded by endosteum.

The periosteocytic space, which is in the lacunae and canaliculi, lies between the osteocytes and the bone matrix. This space is filled with extracellular fluid. The surface area of bone matrix that is in contact with this pool of extracellular fluid has been estimated to be between 1000 and 5000 m^2 square meters and therefore represents a major site for mineral exchange between soluble and crystallized calcium phosphate.

Crystallization or solubilization of bone mineral is determined by physicochemical equilibria related to the concentrations of calcium, phosphate, hydrogen, and other constituents in bone water. The fluxes of calcium and phosphate into or out of the bone extracellular fluid involve active participation osteoblasts and osteocytes. Hormones regulate the calcium concentration in the extracellular fluid compartment and the mineralization of bone by regulating the activities of these cells.

Osteoblasts are the cells responsible for the formation of bone and form a continuous sheet on the surface of newly forming bone. When actively laying down bone, osteoblasts are cuboidal or low columnar in shape. They have a dense rough endoplasmic reticulum consistent with synthesis and secretion of collagen and other proteins of bone matrix. Osteoblasts also promote mineralization. Under physiological conditions, calcium and phosphate are in metastable solution. That is, their concentrations in extracellular fluid would be sufficiently high for them to precipitate out of solution were it not for other constituents, particularly pyrophosphate, which stabilize the solution. During mineralization, osteoblasts secrete alkaline phosphatase, which cleaves pyrophosphate and thus removes a stabilizing influence, and at the same time increases local

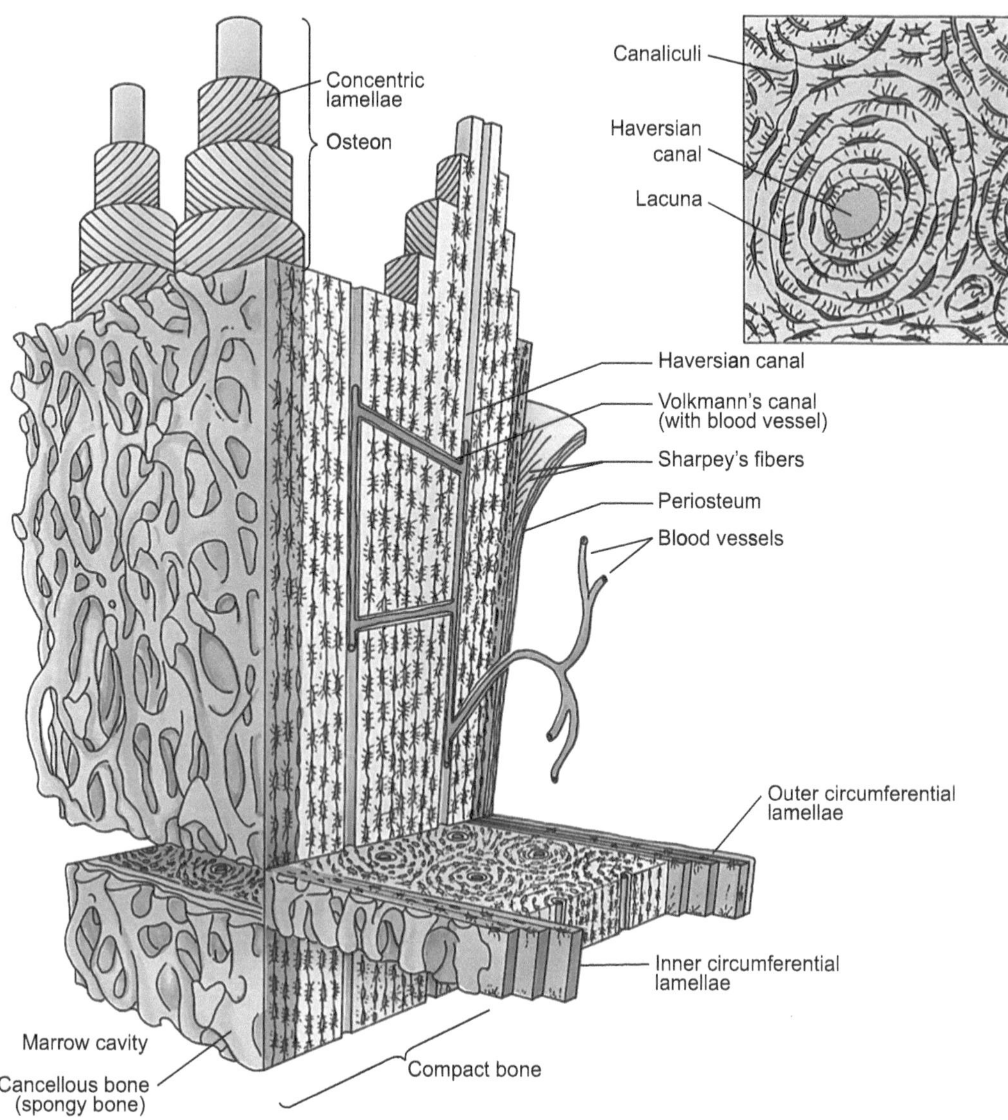

FIGURE 10.6 A schematic drawing showing that the collagen in each lamella is oriented in a different direction to provide strength to the bone. Surrounding the entire cortex are several outer circumferential lamellae. These lie just underneath the periosteum (blue). Source: *From Figure 7–10 in Gartner, L. P. (2017).* Textbook of histology *(4th ed.) (p. 162). Elsevier.*

concentrations of phosphate, which promotes crystallization. In addition, during bone growth and remodeling of mature bone, osteoblasts secrete apatite-rich vesicles into the calcifying osteoid.

During growth or remodeling of bone, 10%–20% of osteoblasts become entrapped in matrix and differentiate into osteocytes. Osteocytes are the most abundant cells in bone and make up 90%–95% of bone cells. In comparison, osteoblasts make up 4%–6% and osteoclasts make up 1%–2% of bone cells. Upon completion of growth or remodeling, surface osteoblasts dedifferentiate to become the flattened, spindle-shaped cells of the endosteum that lines most of the surface of bone. These cells may be reactivated in response to stimuli for bone formation. Thus osteoblasts, osteocytes, and quiescent lining cells represent three stages of the same cellular lineage (Fig. 10.8).

In subsequent discussion, these cells along with their stromal and periosteal precursors are referred to as osteoblastic cells (Rosen et al., 2013).

Osteoclasts, which arise from hematopoietic progenitor cells, resorb bone (Fig. 10.8). They are large cells that arise by fusion of mononucleated hematopoietic cells and thus may have 20–40 nuclei. Precursors of osteoclasts originate in bone marrow and migrate through the circulation from thymus and other reticuloendothelial tissues to sites of bone destined for resorption. Differentiation and activation of osteoclasts require proximity to osteoblastic cells that govern these processes by producing at least two indispensable

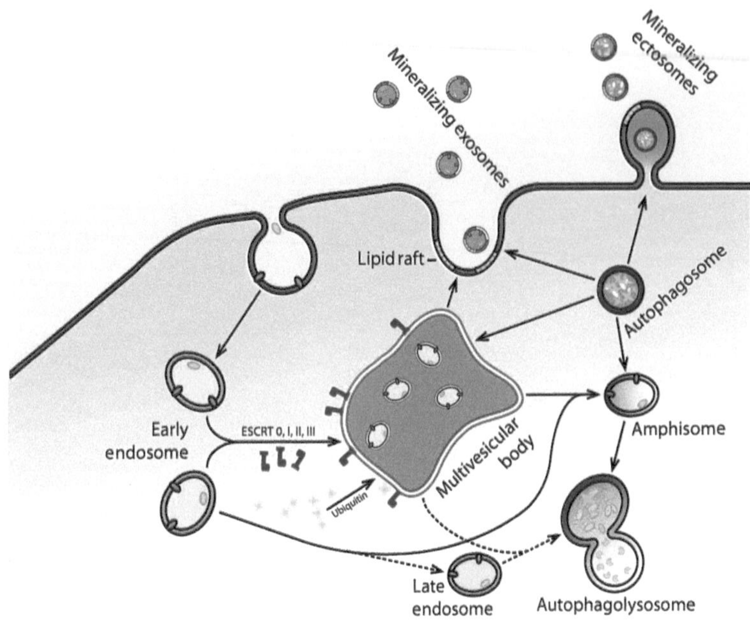

FIGURE 10.7 The formation of mineralizing exosomes or ectosomes from the surface of the osteoblast. These vesicles already contain hydroxyapatite crystals that are then expelled in order to seed the formation of hydroxyapatite on the collagen fibers. This process is still in the early stages of being fully elucidated. Source: *From Figure 4 from I. M. Shapiro, W. J. Landis, & M. V. Risbud. (2015). Matrix vesicles: Are they anchored exosomes?* Bone *79, 29–36.*

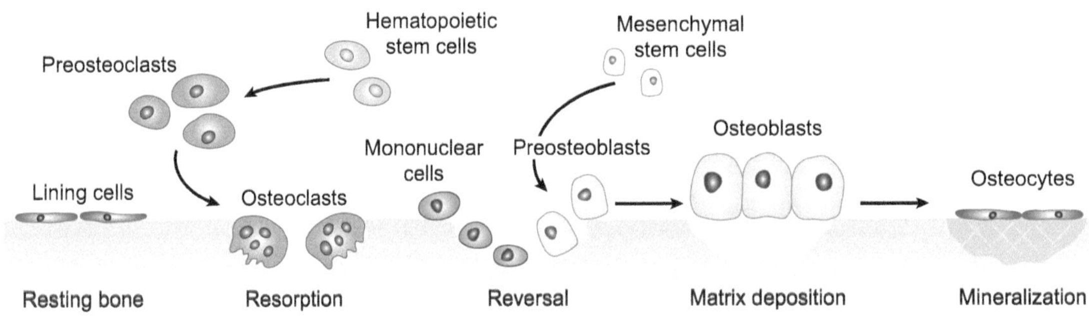

FIGURE 10.8 The BMU of bone. A number of 10–20 osteoclasts resorb old, weak, or damaged bone tissue. The osteoclasts recruit 1000–2000 osteoblasts, which produce new bone matrix. The osteoblasts become osteocytes that complete mineralization of the bone. The osteocytes also help regulate serum calcium by depositing and reabsorbing calcium from labile (soft) bone surrounding them. The rate of movement is 20–40 μm/day and exists for 6 months. *BMU*, Basic multicellular unit. Source: *From Figure 243-4 from Weber, T. J. (2016). Chapter 243: Osteoporosis. In Goldman* et al. *(Eds.),* Goldman-cecil medicine *(25th ed.) (p 1639). Elsevier.*

cytokines: macrophage colony-stimulating factor (M-CSF) and receptor activator of nuclear factor-kB ligand (RANKL). These cytokines may be membrane-bound and soluble. Nuclear factor-kB (NF-kB) is a transcription factor that translocates from the cytosol to the nucleus upon activation (Fig. 10.9).

RANKL belongs to the tumor necrosis factor (TNF) superfamily of cytokines. On osteoclasts, RANK is the receptor for RANKL (Fig. 10.10). Thus RANKL binds to and activates RANK on the surface of osteoclasts or their precursors that come in contact with osteoblastic cells. Steps in the differentiation of osteoclasts are illustrated in Fig. 10.9.

Another receptor of the TNF receptor family exerts negative control over osteoclast formation and activity. This compound, called osteoprotegerin (OPG), binds RANKL with high affinity. Unlike typical members of the TNF receptor family, OPG lacks a transmembrane domain and is secreted as a soluble protein. OPG, which is produced by many different cells, is a "decoy receptor" that competes with RANK for RANKL on the surface of osteoblastic cells and thereby limits osteoclast formation and activity (Fig. 10.11).

An unusual and confusing aspect of osteoclast regulation is the seemingly inverted participation of a membrane-bound ligand (RANKL) and a soluble receptor (OPG). Although the factors that regulate expression of RANK and M-CSF are known (see later), the factors that regulate expression of OPG are still being studied.

In histological sections, osteoclasts are usually found on the surface of bone in pits, called Howship's lacunae, created by their erosive action. Integrins on

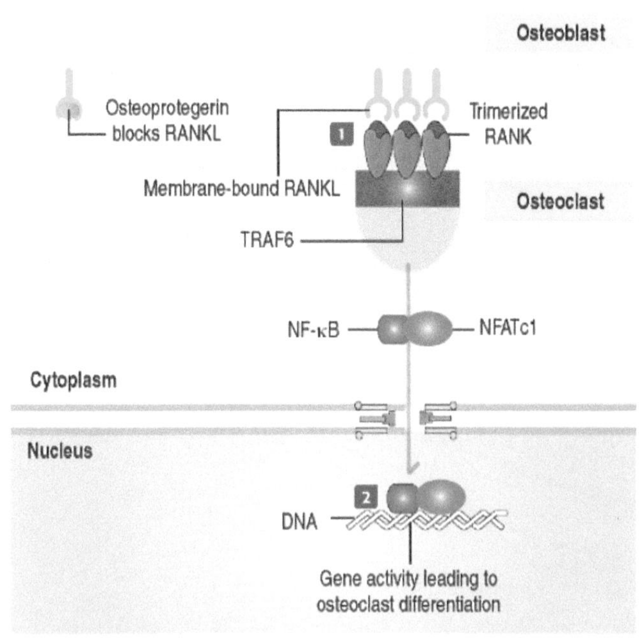

FIGURE 10.9 RANK–RANKL signaling in an osteoclast precursor causes differentiation into an osteoclast. Source: *From Figure 10.4–24 in Kierszenbaum, A. L. and Tres, L. L. (2020). Histology and cell biology: An introduction to pathology (5th ed.) (p. 170). Elsevier.*

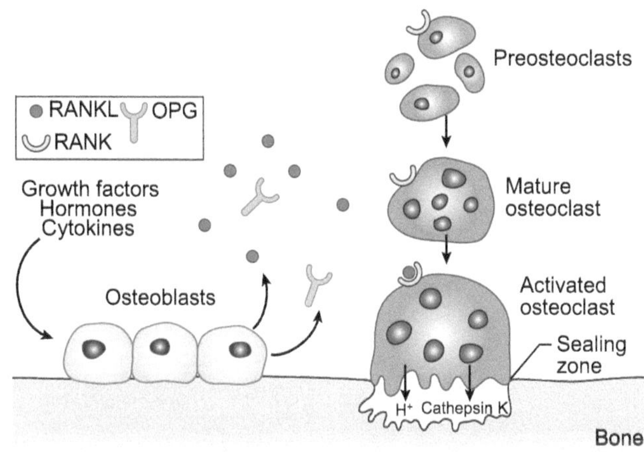

FIGURE 10.10 RANK is a receptor on preosteoclasts and mature osteoclasts. The ligand for that receptor is RANKL, which is produced by osteoblasts. Osteoblasts also produce OPG, which is a "decoy receptor" that binds to RANKL and thus prevents RANKL from combining with RANK on the osteoclast. *OPG*, Osteoprotegerin. Source: *From Figure 243-3 from Weber, T. J. (2016). Chapter 243: Osteoporosis. In Goldman* et al. *(Eds.),* Goldman-Cecil textbook of medicine *(25th ed.) (p 1638). Elsevier. (Adapted from Lewiecki EM. New Targets for intervention in the treatment of postmenopausal osteoporosis. Nat Rev Rheumatol. 2011;7;631–638).*

the surface of osteoclasts form tight bonds with osteocalcin, osteopontin, and other proteins of the bone matrix and create a sealed off region of extracellular space between the osteoclasts and the surface of the bony matrix (Fig. 10.12).

The specialized part of the osteoclast that faces the bony surface bone is thrown into many folds called the ruffled border. The ruffled border sweeps over the surface of bone, continuously changing its configuration as it releases acids and hydrolytic enzymes that dissolve the mineral crystals and the protein matrix. Small bone crystals often are seen in phagocytic vesicles deep in its folds. Upon completion of resorption, osteoclasts are inactivated and lose some of their nuclei. Complete inactivation involves fission of the giant, polynucleated cell back to mononuclear cells, which may undergo apoptosis, but some multinuclear cells remain quiescent on the bone surface interspersed among the lining cells.

Resorption of bone is precisely coupled with bone formation. The pattern of events in bone remodeling typically begins with differentiation and activation of osteoclasts followed sequentially by bone resorption, osteoblast activation and migration to the site of bone resorption, and finally bone formation. Details of the signaling mechanisms that couple bone formation with bone resorption are not yet known, but it appears that bone resorption releases growth factors stored in the bone matrix, which then attract osteoblast precursors. In addition, these growth factors promote differentiation of new osteoblasts from progenitor cells that are attracted to the site by peptide fragments of partially degraded osteoid. Osteoclastogenesis is summarized in Fig. 10.13.

Kidney

Ionized and complexed calcium pass freely through glomerular membranes. Normally, 98%–99% of the 10,000 mg of calcium filtered by the glomeruli each day is reabsorbed by the renal tubules. About two-thirds of the reabsorption occur in the proximal tubule, tightly coupled to sodium reabsorption and, for the most part, dragged passively along with water. Much of the remaining calcium is resorbed in the loop of Henle and is also tightly coupled to sodium reabsorption. Reabsorption of calcium in this part of the nephron is subject to regulation by the plasma calcium concentration and to a limited extent by hormones.

Normally, only about 10% of the filtered calcium reaches the distal nephron. Reabsorption of calcium in the vicinity of the junction of the distal convoluted

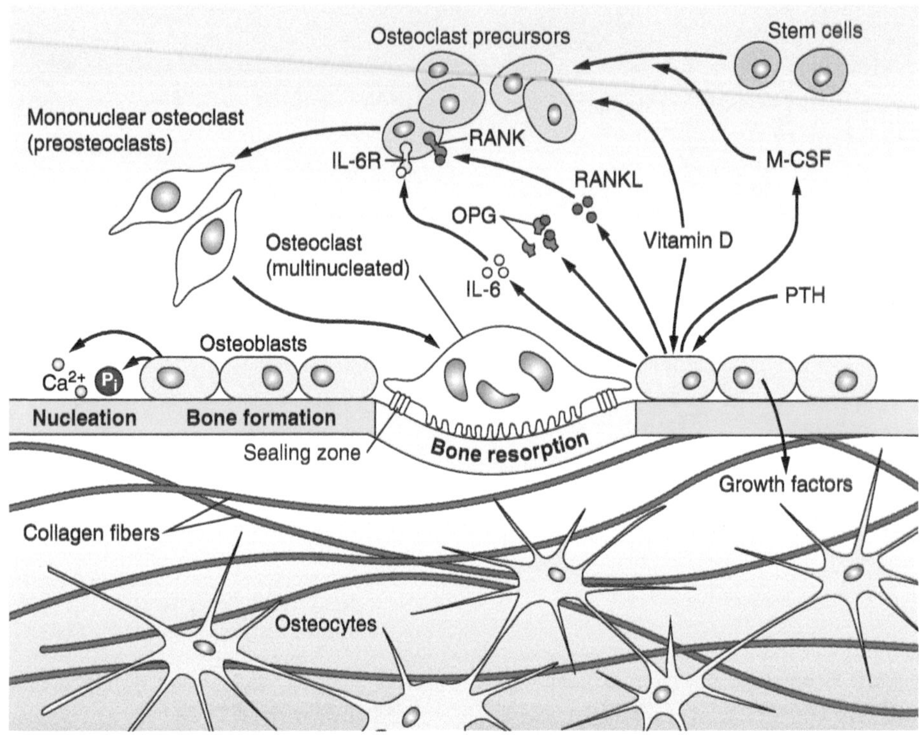

FIGURE 10.11 An overview of bone resorption. Source: *Redrawn from Figure 52.4 in Barrett, E. J., & Barrett, P. Q. (2017). Chapter 52: The parathyroid glands and Vitamin D. In W. F. Boron, & E. L. Boulpaep (Eds.),* Medical physiology *(3rd ed.) (p. 1058). Elsevier.*

tubules and the collecting ducts is governed by an active, saturable process that is independent of sodium reabsorption. Active transport of calcium in this region is the principal target of hormonal regulation by PTH to allow for calcium excretion (Fig. 10.14).

Phosphorus balance

Because of their intimate relationship, the fate of calcium cannot be discussed without also considering phosphorus. Calcium usually is absorbed in the intestines accompanied by phosphorus, and deposition and mobilization of calcium in bones always occurs in conjunction with phosphorus. Phosphorus is as ubiquitous in its distribution and physiological role as calcium. The high-energy phosphate bond of ATP and other metabolites is the source of energy for the cell. Phosphorus is indispensable for biological information transfer. It is a component of nucleic acids and second messengers such as cyclic AMP (cAMP) and IP3 and can be the addition that increases or decreases enzymatic activities or guides protein–protein interactions.

About 90% of the 500–800 g of phosphorus in the adult human is deposited in the skeleton. Much of the remainder is incorporated into organic phosphates distributed throughout soft tissues in the form of phospholipids, nucleic acids, and soluble metabolites. Daily intake of phosphorus is in the range of 700–2000 mg, mainly in dairy products. Organic phosphorus is digested to inorganic phosphate before it is absorbed in the small intestine by both active and passive processes. Net absorption is linearly related to intake and appears not to saturate. The concentration of inorganic phosphate in blood is about 2.5–4.5 mg/dL. About 55% is present as free ions, about 35% is complexed with calcium or other cations, and 10% is protein-bound.

Ionized and complexed phosphate pass freely across glomerular and other capillary membranes. Phosphate in the glomerular filtrate is actively reabsorbed by a sodium-coupled cotransport process in the proximal tubule. These relations in daily phosphorus balance are shown in Figs. 10.15 and 10.16.

Parathyroid glands and parathyroid hormone

Parathyroid glands are located on the posterior side of the thyroid gland (Fig. 10.17).

Human beings typically have four parathyroid glands, but this number may vary. Each gland is a flattened ellipsoid measuring about 6 mm in its longest diameter. The normal mass of an adult parathyroid glands is about 30–40 mg. These glands adhere to the posterior surface of the thyroid gland or occasionally

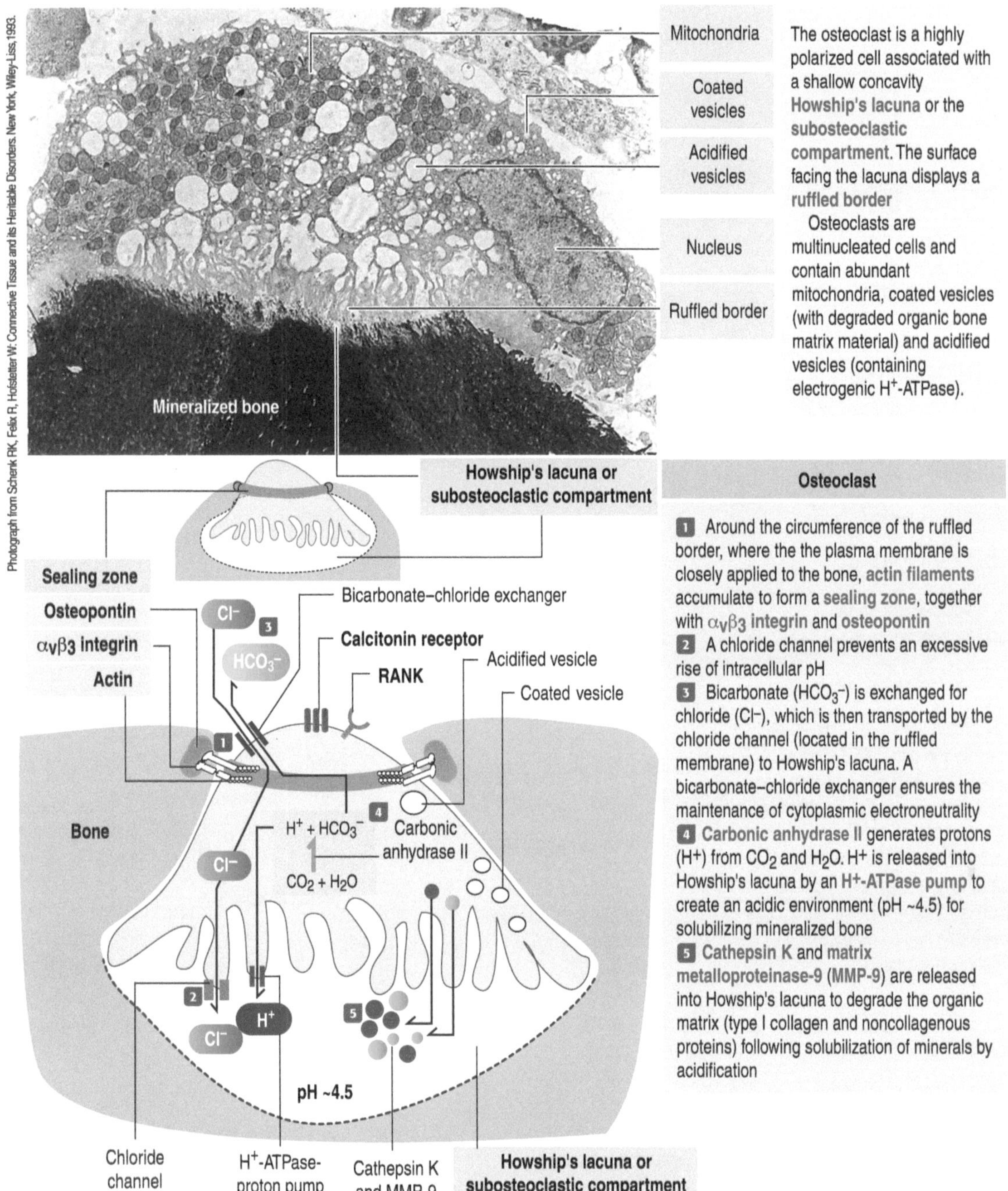

FIGURE 10.12 Details of the action of an osteoclast in bone remodeling. Source: *From Figure 10.4–22 in Kierszenbaum, A., & Tres, L. (2016).* Histology and cell biology: An introduction to pathology *(5th ed.) (p. 153). Elsevier.*

are embedded within thyroid tissue. They are well vascularized and derive their blood supply mainly from the inferior thyroid arteries. Parathyroid glands comprise two cell types (Fig. 10.18).

Chief cells predominate and are arranged in clusters or cords. They are the source of PTH and have all the cytological characteristics of cells that produce protein hormones: rough endoplasmic reticulum, prominent Golgi apparatus, and some membrane-bound storage granules. The calcium receptor on the chief cell is shown in Fig. 10.19. Oxyphil cells, which appear singly or in small groups, are larger than chief cells and contain a remarkable number of mitochondria. Oxyphil cells have no known function. Their cytological properties are not characteristic of secretory cells.

PTH is the principal regulator of the extracellular calcium pool. It increases the calcium concentration and decreases the phosphate concentration in blood by various

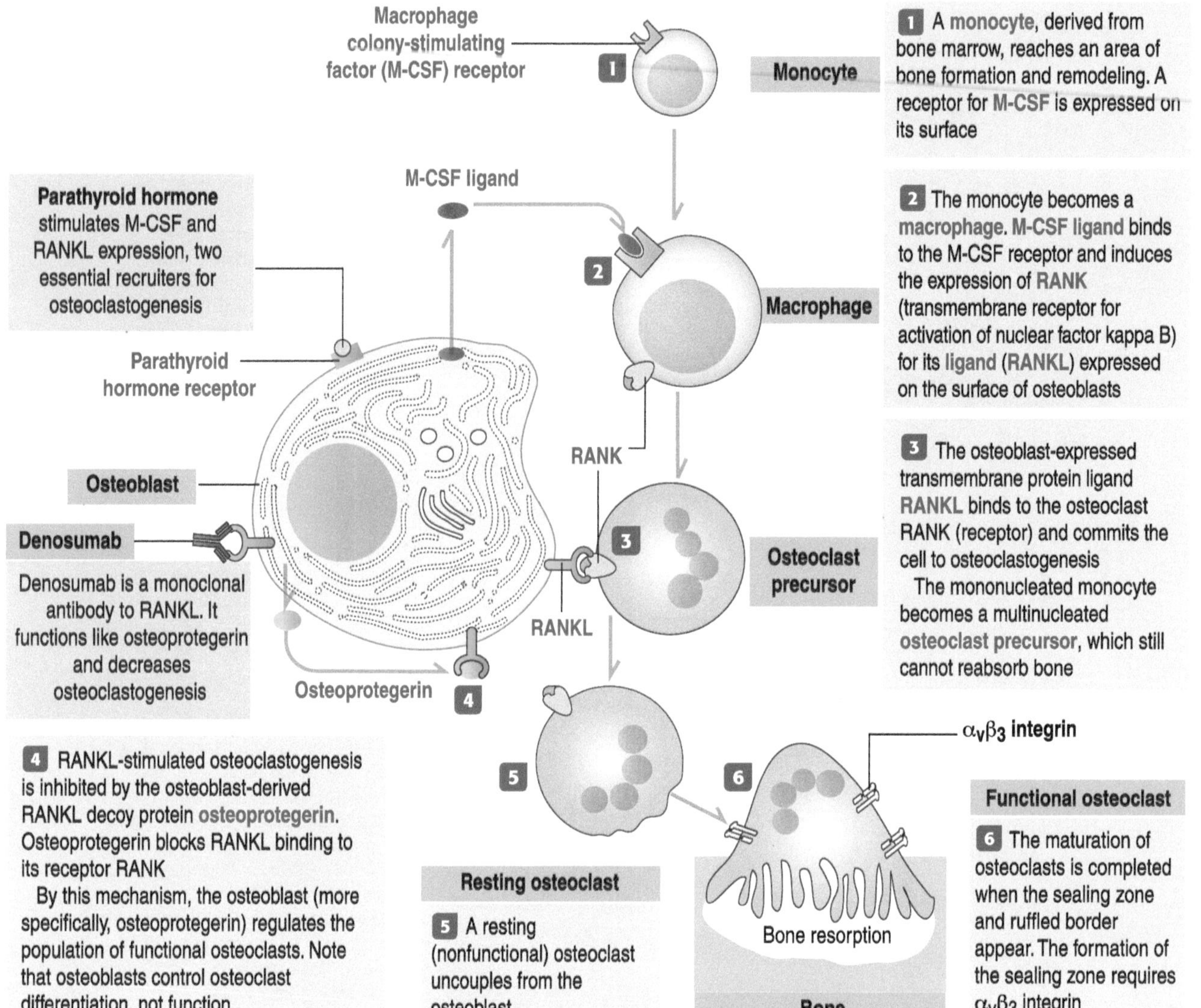

FIGURE 10.13 Osteoblasts regulate osteoclastogenesis. Source: *Figure 4–27 in Kierszenbaum, A., & Tres, L. (2016).* Histology and cell biology: An introduction to pathology *(4th ed.) (p. 154). Elsevier.*

direct and indirect actions on bone, kidney, and intestine. If PTH is lacking, which is termed hypoparathyroidism, the concentration of calcium in blood decreases dramatically, while the concentration of phosphate increases. Hypoparathyroidism may result from insufficient production of active hormone or defects in the responses of target tissues. In acute hypoparathyroidism, all of the symptoms of hypocalcemia may be seen, including tetany and even seizures or laryngospasm if severe (Fig. 10.20).

In chronic hypoparathyroidism, additional findings of neurological (basal ganglia calcifications), ocular (cataracts), and dental abnormalities (dental hypoplasia, defective enamel and root formation) may also be seen. If excess PTH is present, which is the case in primary hyperparathyroidism, sequelae of kidney stones and osteoporosis may develop.

Although peptides closely related to PTH are found in bony fish, it appears that discrete clusters of cells forming parathyroid glands arose relatively recently in vertebrate evolution, coincident with the emergence of ancestral forms onto dry land. Parathyroid glands are seen in amphibians such as the salamander only after metamorphosis to the land-dwelling form. The importance of the parathyroids in normal calcium economy was established during the latter part of the nineteenth century when it was found that parathyroidectomy resulted in lethal tetany. Diseases may arise in the parathyroid glands and result in overproduction or underproduction of PTH (primary hypoparathyroidism or hyperparathyroidism). In addition, low or high PTH levels may be seen as an appropriate response to an underlying condition. For example, secondary

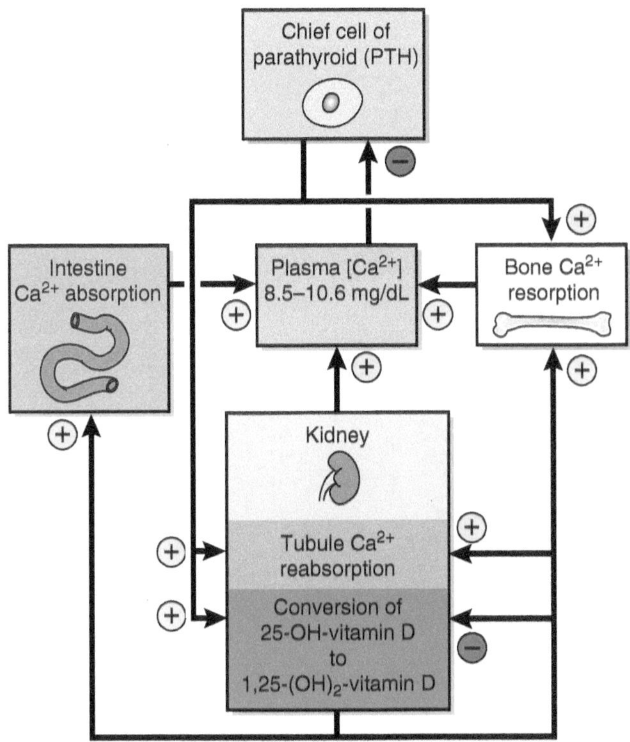

FIGURE 10.14 Feedback loops in the control of calcium level. Source: *Redrawn from Figure 52-8A in Barrett, E. J., & Barrett, P. Q. (2017). Chapter 52: The parathyroid glands and Vitamin D. In W. F. Boron, & E. L, Boulpaep (Eds.),* Medical physiology *(3rd ed.) (p. 1061). Elsevier.*

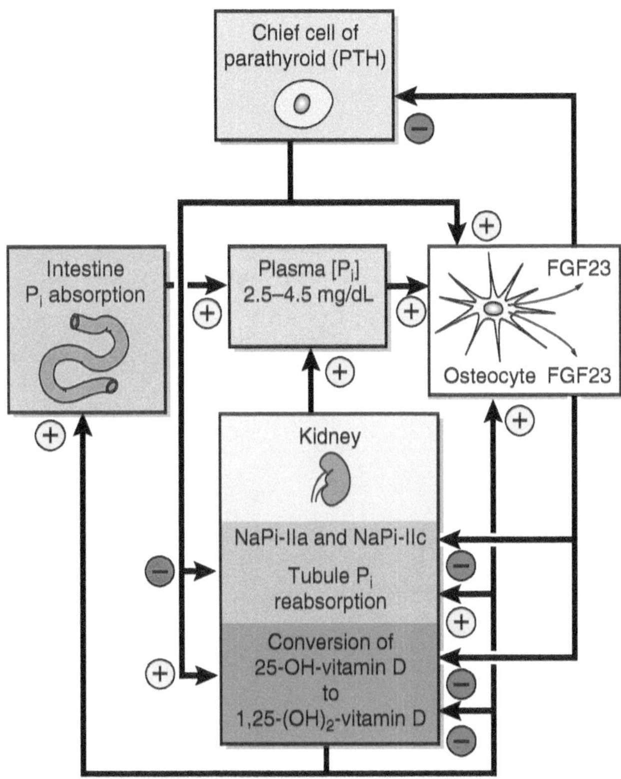

FIGURE 10.16 Feedback loops in the control of phosphate. Source: *Redrawn from Figure 52-8B in Barrett, E. J., & Barrett, P. Q. (2017). Chapter 52: The parathyroid glands and Vitamin D. In W. F. Boron, & E. L. Boulpaep (Eds.),* Medical physiology *(3rd ed.) (p. 1061). Elsevier.*

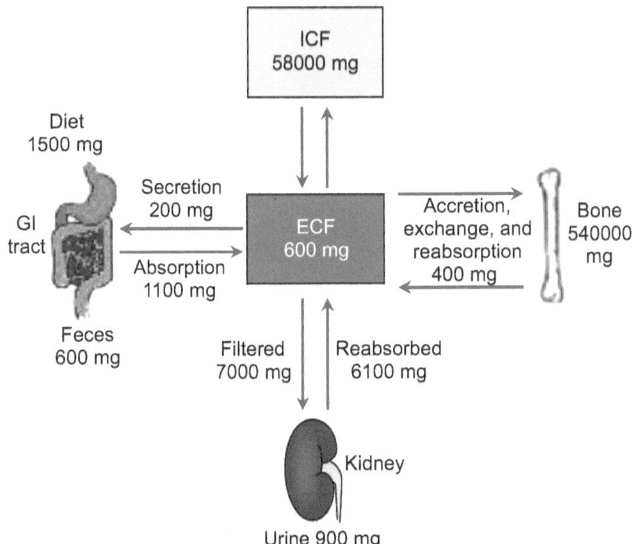

FIGURE 10.15 Daily phosphorus balance in an adult.

hyperparathyroidism may be seen in chronic kidney disease patients due to the lack of 1,25-dihydroxyvitamin D. Secondary hyperparathyroidism may also be seen in the setting of calcium malabsorption, which may occur after a gastric bypass procedure.

Biosynthesis, storage, and secretion of parathyroid hormone

PTH is a simple straight-chain peptide of 84 amino acids. It is the product of a single copy gene located on chromosome 11 and is expressed as a larger 115 amino acid preprohormone (Fig. 10.21).

Initial processing includes the cotranslational removal of the 25-amino acid leader sequence in the endoplasmic reticulum followed by cleavage of the adjacent hexapeptide after transfer to the Golgi apparatus. PTH then is packaged into secretory granules along with proteolytic enzymes, called cathepsins that are normally found in lysosomes. Synthesis of PTH is regulated at both transcriptional and at posttranscriptional sites. cAMP, acting through the cAMP response element–binding protein (CREB), upregulates PTH gene transcription, whereas vitamin D (and high levels of intracellular calcium) downregulates transcription.

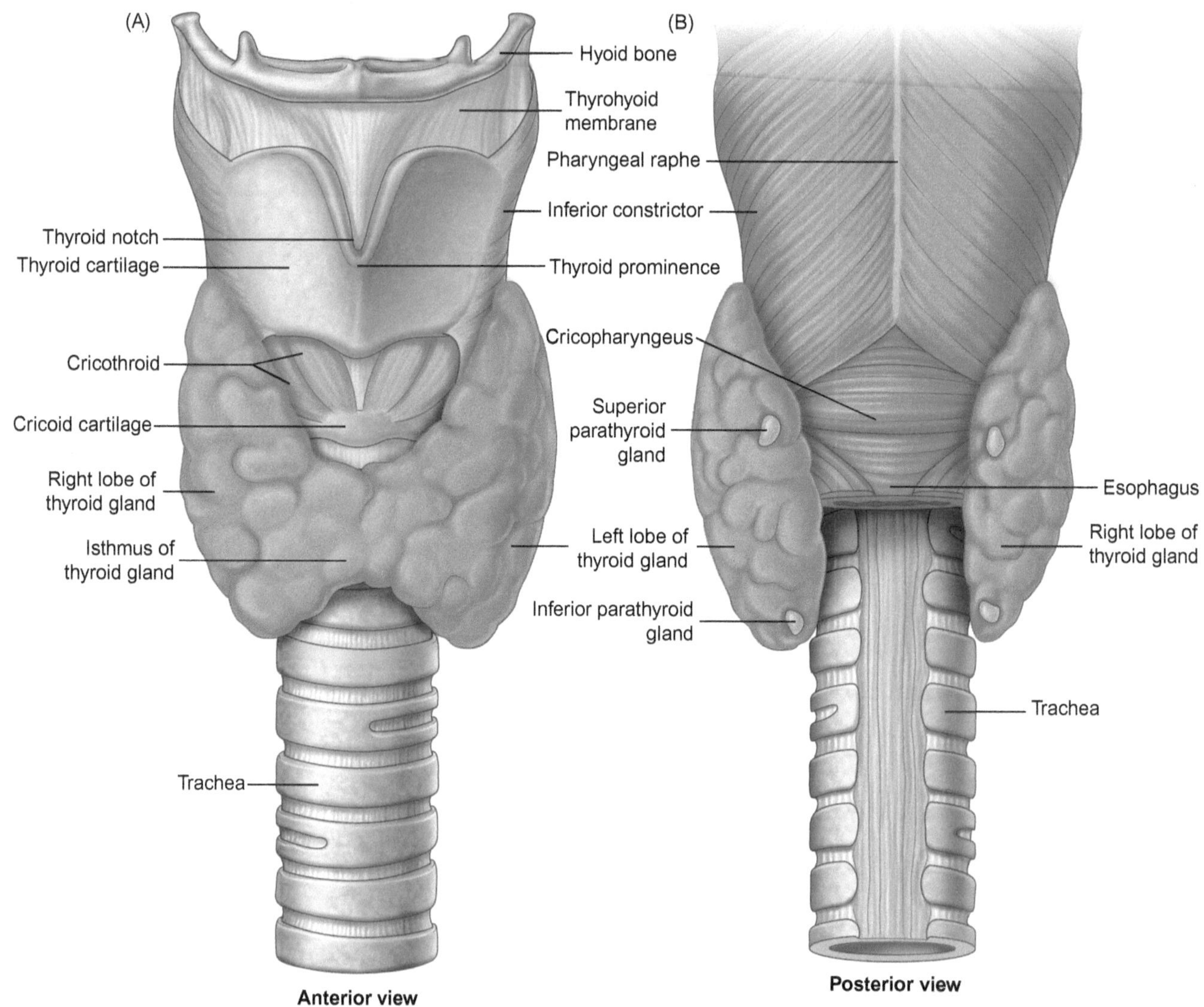

FIGURE 10.17 The parathyroid glands are located on the posterior side of the thyroid. There are typically four parathyroid glands but this number may vary. Source: *From R. L. Drake, A. W. Vogl, A. W. M. Mitchell, R. M. Tibbitt, & P. E. Richardson. (2015). Thyroid gland. In* Gray's atlas of anatomy *(2nd ed.) (p. 563). Elsevier.*

Low plasma calcium concentrations prolong the survival time of the mRNA transcript, whereas low concentrations of plasma phosphate accelerate message degradation. PTH is synthesized continuously, but the glands store little hormone, only enough to sustain maximal secretion rates for about 90 minutes.

Parathyroid cells are unusual in the respect that hormone degradation as well as synthesis is adjusted according to physiological demand. As much as 90% of the hormone synthesized may be metabolized within the chief cells, which cleave PTH into fragments at an accelerated rate when plasma calcium concentrations are high. Cleavage by cathepsins at different residues results in a complex mixture of fragments containing the carboxyl terminus that are present along with intact PTH in the secretory granules. The amino terminal fragments produced in this way appear to be completely degraded in lysosomes. In addition, a short stretch of amino acids is clipped from the amino terminus of PTH 1–84 to produce a PTH derivative that lacks the first six amino acids (PTH 7–84). The ratio of fragments to intact hormone released into the circulation increases when plasma calcium is high and decreases when it is low. Similar fragments also are produced by the metabolism of PTH in the liver and released into the blood. PTH fragments are cleared from blood by filtration at the glomeruli but remain in the circulation hours longer than intact hormone, which has a half-life of only about 2–4 minutes. As a result, less than 20% of the PTH peptides circulating in blood are the intact hormone. Intact PTH and PTH 7–84 are also

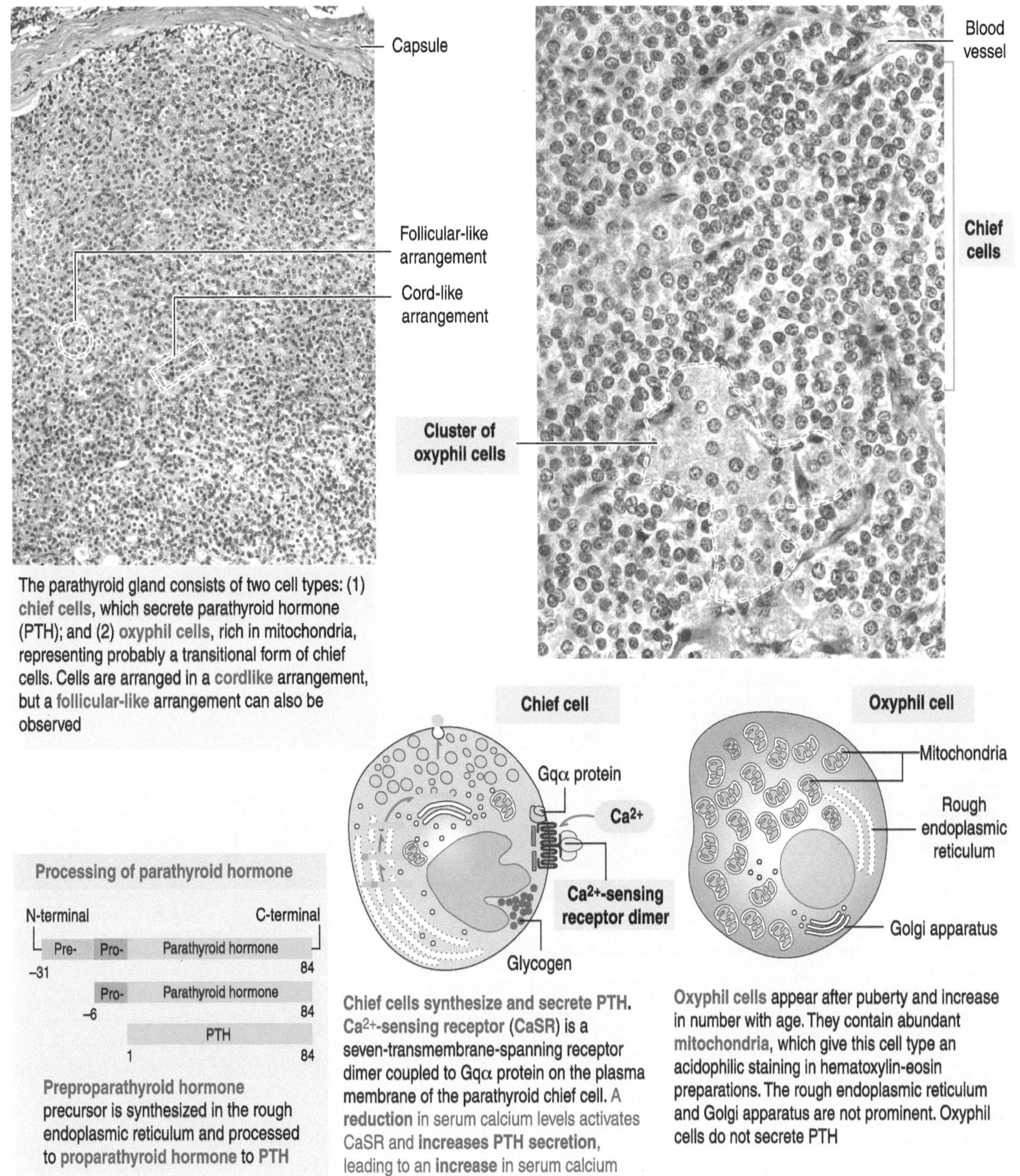

FIGURE 10.18 Structure and function of the parathyroid gland. The chief and the oxyphil cells are the two cell types in the parathyroid gland. Source: *From Figure 19-5 in Kierszenbaum, A., & Tres, L. (2016).* Histology and cell biology: An introduction to pathology *(5th ed.) (p. 588). Elsevier.*

degraded in target cells following receptor-mediated endocytosis.

Homeostatic regulation of calcium balance by the actions of PTH described next appears to be attributable to the intact 84-amino acid peptide, which is the only form secreted with its amino terminus intact. The amino terminus is critical for the function of PTH. Removal of just the serine at the amino

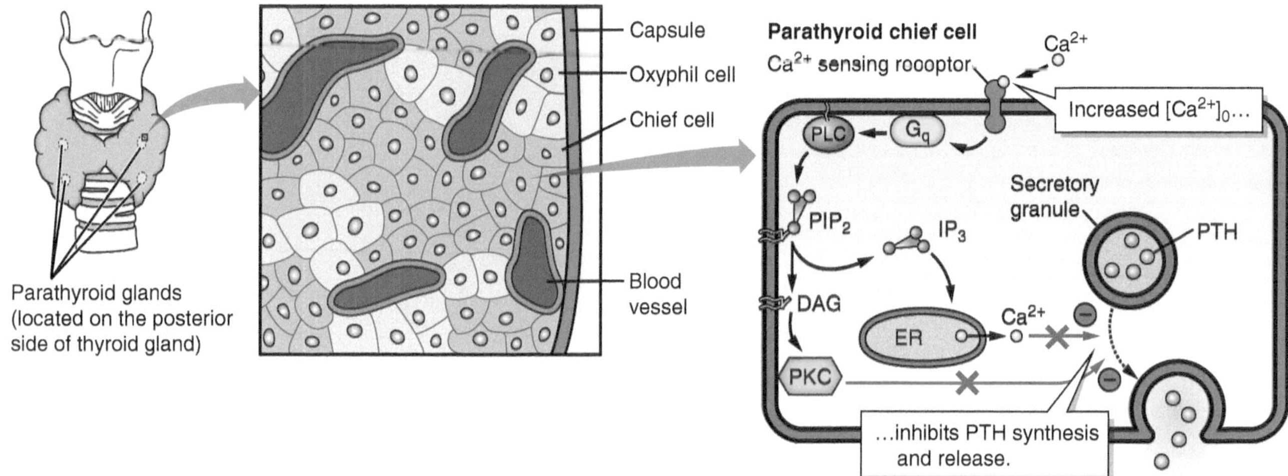

FIGURE 10.19 The calcium receptor on the chief cells of the parathyroid gland. High ionized calcium concentrations inhibit PTH synthesis and release. *PTH*, Parathyroid hormone. Source: *Redrawn from Figure 52-7A in Barrett, E. J., & Barrett, P. Q. (2017). Chapter 52: The parathyroid glands and Vitamin D. In W. F. Boron, & E. L. Boulpaep (Eds.),* Medical physiology *(3rd ed.) (p. 1060). Elsevier.*

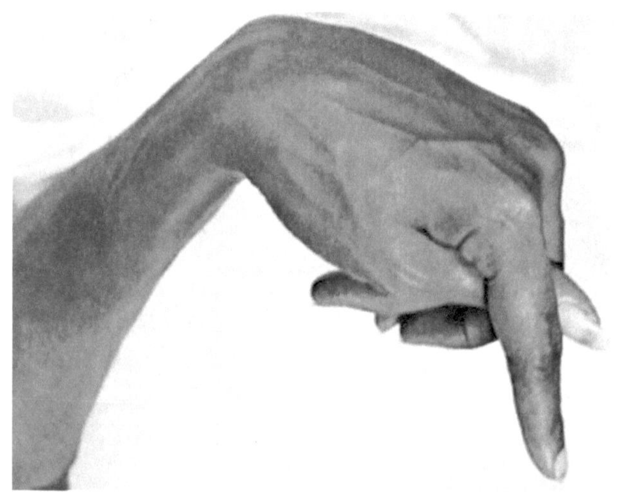

FIGURE 10.20 Carpopedal spasm (tetany) observed when a blood pressure cuff is inflated on the upper arm, stopping arterial flow and, with it, calcium, to the muscles of the forearm that control the movements of the wrist and hand. If the calcium is borderline low, there is not enough calcium to cause muscle relaxation and the muscles contract. Source: *From Figure 80-2 in Hall, J. E. (2016).* Guyton and Hall's textbook of medical physiology *(13th ed.) (p. 1002). Elsevier.*

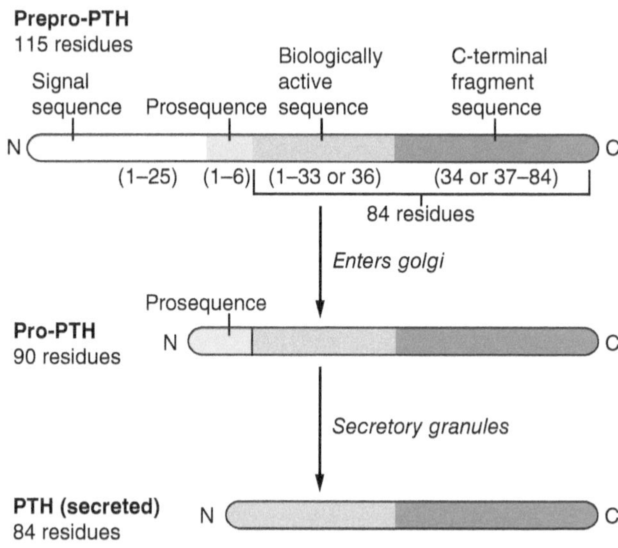

FIGURE 10.21 The biosynthesis of PTH. *PTH*, Parathyroid hormone. Source: *Redrawn from Figure 52-6 in Barrett, E. J., & Barrett, P. Q. (2017). Chapter 52: The parathyroid glands and Vitamin D. In W. F. Boron, & E. L. Boulpaep (Eds.),* Medical physiology *(3rd ed.) (p. 1060). Elsevier.*

terminus severely inactivates the hormone and removal of the first two amino acids completely inactivates it. Consequently, synthetic PTH consisting of amino acids 1–34 has been used both experimentally and therapeutically as a surrogate of PTH on the assumption that the 60% of the molecule at the carboxyl end is irrelevant. Recent observations, however, indicate that the middle and carboxyl portions of the PTH molecule may not be biologically inert and may modulate or even antagonize the actions of the intact form of PTH.

The complex mixture of intact PTH and its fragments in the circulation has confounded immunoassays. Any particular antibody detects only a short sequence of amino acids called an epitope. The mixture of antibodies in any serum detects a mixture of epitopes scattered throughout the PTH molecule. Consequently, early radioimmunoassays of PTH with antibodies that recognized epitopes in the central or carboxyl parts of the molecule failed to distinguish fragments from intact hormone and overestimated the concentration of active PTH in blood. Subsequent immunoassays revealed the abundant presence of C-terminal fragments, but true intact PTH assays were developed later with the introduction of a two-site immunometric or "sandwich" assay (see Chapter 1: Introduction) that recognizes only the epitope that contains the serine, valine, and serine tripeptide at the amino terminus (Fig. 10.22).

It has become evident that long, N-terminally truncated PTH molecules also circulate in blood. Although understanding of the importance of PTH fragments for calcium homeostasis is still evolving, it is now evident that these fragments are not irrelevant as was long believed.

Mechanisms of parathyroid hormone actions

Binding of PTH to G-protein-coupled receptors on the surfaces of target cells increases the formation of the second messengers, cAMP, IP3, and diacylglycerol (see Chapter 1: Introduction). The PTH receptor is coupled to adenylyl cyclase through a stimulatory G-protein (Gαs) and to phospholipase C through Gαq. Consequently, protein kinases A and C also are activated. Rapid responses result from protein phosphorylation, and delayed responses result from altered expression of genes regulated by CREB (cAMP response element–binding protein). It is likely that the two second messenger pathways activated by PTH are redundant and reinforce each other. The critical role of cAMP for the action of PTH is underscored by the occurrence of a rare disease called pseudohypoparathyroidism, in which patients are unresponsive to PTH. About one-half of the reported cases of unresponsiveness to PTH are attributable to a genetic defect in the GTP-binding protein (Gαs) that couples the hormone receptor with adenylyl cyclase. These patients also have decreased responses to some other cAMP–dependent signals, but because there are four distinct genes for Gαs, each expressed with particular receptors, not all cAMP–dependent responses are affected.

Physiological actions of parathyroid hormone

Actions on bone

Increases in PTH concentration in blood result in mobilization of calcium phosphate from the bone matrix due primarily, and perhaps exclusively, to increased osteoclastic activity.

The initial phase is seen within 1–2 hours and results from activation of preformed osteoclasts already present on the bone surface. A later and more pronounced phase becomes evident after about 12 hours and is characterized by widespread resorption of both mineral and organic components of bone matrix particularly in trabecular bone. Evidence of osteoclastic activity is reflected by not only calcium phosphate mobilization but also increased urinary excretion of hydroxyproline and other products of collagen breakdown. Although activity of all bone cell types is affected by PTH, it appears that only cells of osteoblastic lineage express receptors for PTH. Osteoclasts and their precursors are thus not direct targets for PTH.

Activation, differentiation, and recruitment of osteoclasts in response to PTH result from increased expression of at least two cytokines by cells of osteoblastic lineage. PTH induces osteoblastic cells to synthesize and secrete M-CSF and to express RANKL on their surfaces (Fig. 10.23).

These cytokines stimulate the differentiation and activity of osteoclasts and protect them from apoptosis. In addition, PTH appears to decrease osteoblastic expression of OPG, the soluble protein that binds to RANKL to competitively inhibit the activation of RANK.

Synthesis and secretion of collagen and other matrix proteins by osteoblasts are inhibited in the early phases

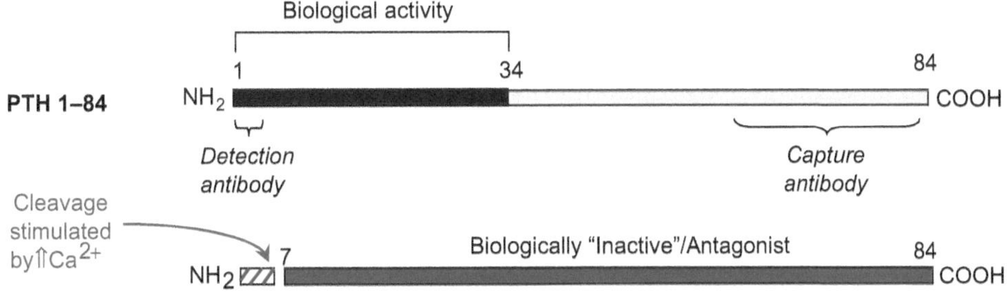

FIGURE 10.22 The known biologically active portion of PTH, the epitopes required for detection and assay of the intact hormone. Detection antibodies that recognize sequences downstream from the amino terminal tripeptide cannot distinguish between the intact active hormone and its truncated antagonist. *PTH*, Parathyroid hormone.

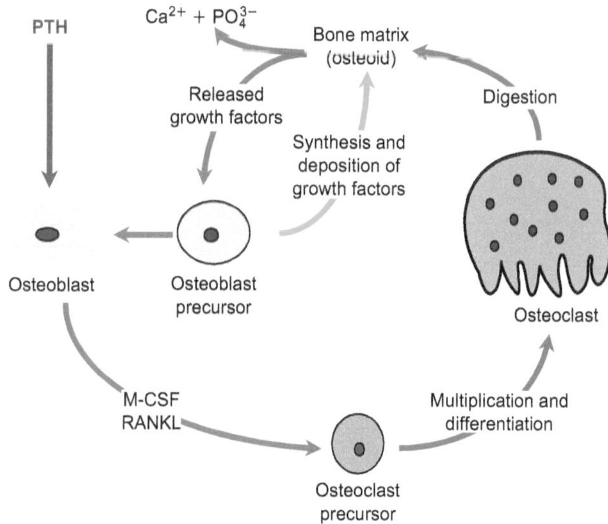

FIGURE 10.23 Effects of PTH on bone. PTH acts on cells of osteoblastic lineage to stimulate production of *M-CSF* (macrophage colony-stimulating factor) and *RANKL* (receptor activator of N-kappa B ligand), which results in osteoclast formation and activation. Digestion of the bone matrix releases calcium and phosphorus and growth factors that were deposited by osteoblasts when the matrix was laid down. Growth factors stimulate osteoblast precursors to multiply, differentiate, and lay down new bone matrix. *PTH*, Parathyroid hormone.

of PTH action but are reactivated subsequently as a result of biological coupling discussed earlier, and new bone is laid down. At this stage, PTH stimulates osteoblasts to synthesize and secrete growth factors, including insulin-like growth factors I and II (IGF-I and IGF-II) and transforming growth factor-β (TGF-β) that are sequestered in the bone matrix and also act in an autocrine or paracrine manner to stimulate osteoblast progenitor cells to divide and differentiate. At least part of the stimulus for osteoblastic activity that follows osteoclastic activity may come from liberation of growth factors that were sequestered in the bone matrix when the bone was laid down. With prolonged continuous exposure to high concentrations of PTH, as seen with hyperparathyroidism, osteoclastic activity is greater than osteoblastic activity, and bone resorption predominates. However, a therapeutic regimen of intermittent stimulation with PTH leads to net formation of bone by mechanisms that are incompletely understood. In addition to its critical role in maintaining the blood calcium concentration, PTH is also important for skeletal homeostasis. As already mentioned, bone remodeling continues throughout life. Remodeling of bone not only ensures renewal and maintenance of strength but also adjusts bone structure and strength to accommodate the various stresses and strains of changing demands of daily living. Increased stress leads to bone formation strengthening the affected area, and weightlessness or limb immobilization leads to mineral loss. Osteocytes entrapped in the bony matrix are thought to function as mechanosensors that signal remodeling through the release of prostaglandins, nitric oxide, and growth factors. In animal studies, these actions are facilitated and enhanced by PTH.

Actions on kidney

In the kidney, PTH produces three distinct effects, each of which contributes to the maintenance of calcium homeostasis. In the distal nephron, it promotes the reabsorption of calcium, and in the proximal tubule, it inhibits reabsorption of phosphate and promotes activation of 25-hydroxyvitamin D to 1,25-dihyroxyvitamin D. In producing these effects, PTH binds to G-protein-coupled receptors in both the proximal and distal tubules and stimulates the production of cAMP, diacylglycerol, and IP3. Some cAMP escapes from renal tubular cells and appears in the urine. About one-half of the cAMP found in urine arises in the kidney and is attributable to the actions of PTH.

Calcium reabsorption

The kidney reacts quickly to changes in PTH concentrations in blood and is responsible for minute-to-minute adjustments in blood calcium. PTH acts directly on the distal portion of the nephron to decrease urinary excretion of calcium well before significant amounts of calcium can be mobilized from bone. Because about 90% of the filtered calcium is reabsorbed before the filtrate reaches distal reabsorptive mechanisms, PTH can only provide fine-tuning of calcium excretion. Even small changes in the fraction of calcium reabsorbed from the glomerular filtrate, however, can be of great significance. Hypoparathyroid patients whose blood calcium is maintained in the normal range excrete about three times as much urinary calcium as normal subjects.

PTH stimulates calcium reabsorption by the principal cells located primarily in the distal convoluted tubules and the connecting tubules (see Chapter 9: Regulation of Salt and Water Balance in Fig. 9.10). These cells express an abundance of PTH receptors in their basolateral membranes. Transfer of calcium across the tubular epithelium is energy-dependent and occurs by secondary active transport that can best be described in three steps. Calcium passes through the luminal membranes of the principal cells through two closely related isoforms of calcium channels called TRPV5 and TRPV6, or more simply, epithelial calcium channels (ECaC). Entry into the principal cells is driven by the steep electrochemical gradient that exists between the filtrate and the cytoplasm. Principal cells are protected from the harmful effects of increased intracellular free calcium by a cytosolic protein called calbindin-28, which associates with ECaC and binds calcium as it enters (Fig. 10.24).

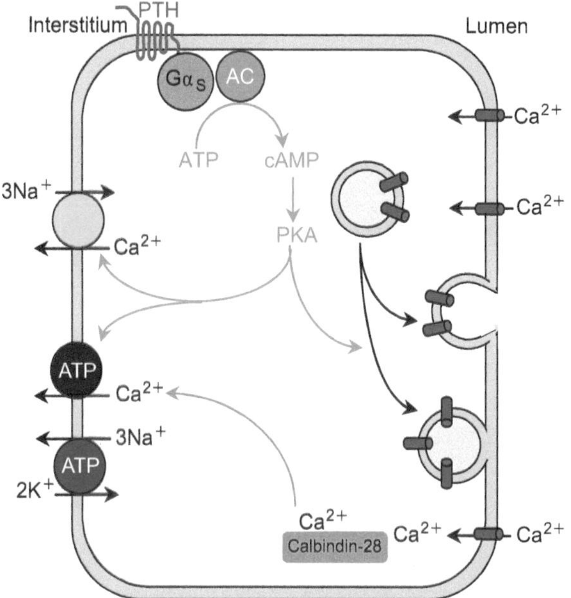

FIGURE 10.24 Effects of PTH on the principal cells in the distal nephron. PTH stimulates insertion of epithelial calcium channels in the luminal membrane and calcium extrusion mechanisms in the basolateral membrane. *AC*, Adenylyl cyclase; *cAMP*, cyclic adenosine monophosphate; *GαS*, the stimulatory G-protein; *PKA*, protein kinase A; *PTH*, parathyroid hormone.

The loaded calbindin diffuses across the cell and delivers its calcium to the basolateral surface for export to the extracellular space. Extrusion of calcium against its concentration gradient is accomplished by the actions of calcium ATPases and sodium/calcium exchangers in the basolateral membrane.

The sodium/calcium exchanger is powered by the sodium gradient, which is maintained by the activity of the sodium/potassium ATPase.

PTH stimulates calcium reabsorption by accelerating both the uptake at the luminal surface and extrusion at the basolateral surface (Fig. 10.23). PTH rapidly increases the insertion of ECaC containing vesicles into the luminal membrane and simultaneously stimulates the activity of the sodium/calcium exchanger and the calcium ATPase. It may also stimulate the activity of the sodium/potassium ATPase. These actions are mediated by protein kinases A and C activated by cAMP and the DAG/IP3 second messengers. On a longer time scale, PTH increases the synthesis of both isoforms of ECaC, calbindin-28, the sodium/calcium exchanger, and the calcium ATPase. These actions are reinforced by 1,25-dihydroxy vitamin D, the synthesis of which is also stimulated by PTH.

To a modest extent, PTH may also contribute to the passive reabsorption of calcium in the thick ascending limb of Henle's loop. In this part of the nephron, calcium passes from tubular fluid to the extracellular space through intercellular junctions driven by the lumen-positive electrochemical potential created by the sodium reabsorptive mechanism (see Chapter 9: Regulation of Salt and Water Balance). Cells in this portion of the nephron express PTH receptors and respond to PTH with increased production of cAMP. Phosphorylation of the sodium/potassium/2 chloride transporter in the luminal membrane increases transport of these three ions. Back leakage of positively charged potassium to the lumen through renal outer medullary potassium (ROMK) channels produces the positive potential of the lumen (see Chapter 9: Regulation of Salt and Water Balance).

Paradoxically, an increase in urinary calcium is seen in late phases of PTH action. PTH increases plasma calcium concentrations in blood and therefore increases the concentration of calcium in the glomerular filtrate. Consequently, the rate at which calcium reaches the distal tubule may increase dramatically and exceed the limited capacity for reabsorption, even when maximally stimulated by PTH. Calcium that cannot be reabsorbed passes into the urine. Regardless of the absolute amount excreted, however, PTH decreases the fraction of filtered calcium that escapes in the urine.

Phosphate excretion

PTH powerfully inhibits tubular reabsorption of phosphate and thus increases the amount excreted in urine. This effect is seen within minutes after injection of PTH and is exerted on the proximal tubules, where the bulk of phosphate reabsorption occurs. Proximal tubule cells contain an abundance of PTH receptors on both their apical and basolateral surfaces. PTH reaches its receptors via diffusion from the peritubular capillaries and is also present in the glomerular filtrate. Phosphate ions (HPO_4^{2-}) cross the luminal membranes of proximal tubule cells on carrier molecules that cotransport three ions of sodium with each ion of phosphate. Phosphate ions then are extruded across the basolateral membrane by unknown mechanisms, and the sodium gradient is restored by the activity of the sodium–potassium ATPase. Decreased reabsorption of phosphate results from decreased abundance of sodium phosphate cotransporters in luminal membranes of tubular cells. PTH decreases the number of sodium phosphate cotransporters in the brush border of proximal tubule cells by stimulating their internalization and transfer to lysosomes (Fig. 10.25).

Replenishment of the cotransporters depends upon de novo synthesis and insertion in the membrane.

Sodium phosphate–coupled cotransporters are stabilized in the luminal membrane by their attachment to a submembranous protein called the sodium–hydrogen exchange regulatory factor (NERF or NHERF).

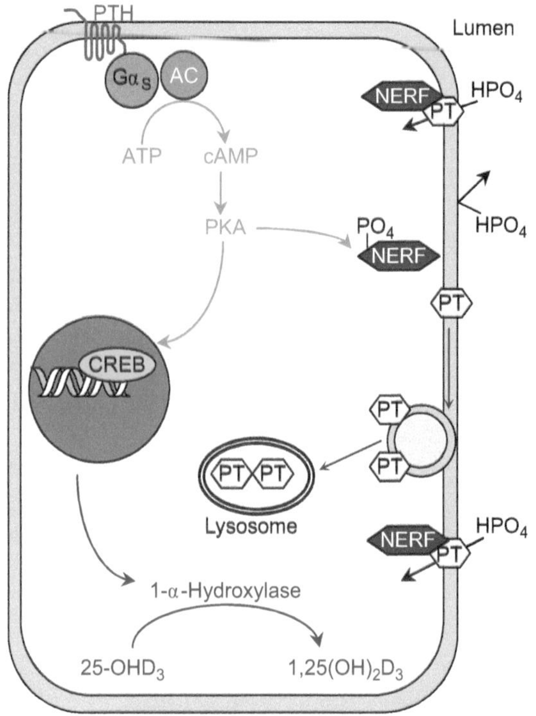

FIGURE 10.25 Effects of PTH on proximal tubule cells. Phosphorylation of *NERF* (sodium–hydrogen exchange regulatory factor) releases *PT* (sodium phosphate cotransporter) from anchoring sites in the membrane. PTs migrate in the plane of the membrane to clathrin-coated pits where they are internalized and transferred to lysosomes and degraded. PTH also stimulates the expression and activation of the enzyme (P450 1α-hydroxylase) that converts *25-0HD*$_3$ to *1,25(OH)*$_2$*D*$_3$, the active form of vitamin D (see Fig. 10.16). *AC*, Adenylyl cyclase; *cAMP*, cyclic adenosine monophosphate; *CREB*, cyclic AMP response element–binding protein; *G*α_S, α subunit of the stimulatory G-protein; *PKA*, protein kinase A; *PTH*, parathyroid hormone.

Phosphorylation of NERF by protein kinases A and C releases the cotransporters, allowing them to migrate in the plane of the membrane to clathrin-coated pits where they are internalized by endocytosis. PTH that acts through receptors on the basolateral surfaces primarily stimulates the formation of cAMP and the activation of protein kinase A. PTH that reaches receptors in the luminal membrane acts predominately through phospholipase C and the activation of protein kinase C by DAG and calcium.

Effects on intestinal absorption

Calcium balance ultimately depends on intestinal absorption of dietary calcium. Calcium absorption is severely reduced in hypoparathyroid patients and dramatically increased in those with hyperparathyroidism. Within a day or two after treatment of hypoparathyroid subjects with PTH, calcium absorption increases. Intestinal uptake of calcium is stimulated by an active metabolite of vitamin D. PTH stimulates the renal enzyme that converts vitamin D to its active form, 1,25-dihydroxyvitamin D, but has no direct effects on intestinal transport of either calcium or phosphate (Figs. 10.26 and 10.27).

Parathyroid hormone fragments

As already mentioned, an intact amino terminus is required for PTH binding to its receptor and the activation of adenylyl cyclase. PTH molecules devoid of the first three amino acid residues are not just inactive but actually inhibit the effects of the intact molecule on plasma calcium and phosphate. For example, PTH 7–84 does not bind efficiently to the PTH receptor to which intact PTH binds. Instead, PTH 7–84 is felt to bind to a C-terminal specific PTH receptor. Effects of this may include inhibiting calcium release and bone resorption. The former effect was demonstrated in neonatal mouse calvariae, where human PTH 7–84 reduced the release of preincorporated ^{45}Ca (Divieti et al., 2002).

Parathyroid hormone–related peptide

A substance closely related to PTH, called PTH–related peptide (PTHrP), is found in the plasma of patients suffering from certain malignancies and accounts for the accompanying hypercalcemia. The gene for PTHrP was isolated from some tumors and found to encode a peptide, the first 13 amino acid residues of which are remarkably similar to the first 13 amino acids of PTH; thereafter, the structures of the two molecules diverge. The similarities of the N-terminal primary sequence and presumably the secondary structure of subsequent segments allow PTHrP to bind with high affinity to the PTH receptor and therefore produce the same biological effects as PTH. PTH and PTHrP are immunologically distinct and do not cross-react in immunoassays, but both appear to be the natural ligands for the PTH receptor. PTHrP is synthesized in a wide range of tissues and acts locally as a paracrine factor to regulate processes that are largely unrelated to regulation of calcium concentrations in extracellular fluid. PTHrP causes vascular smooth muscle to relax, causes chondrocytes in developing bone to grow and differentiate, and regulates placental calcium transport. Except during lactation (see Chapter 14: Hormonal Control of Pregnancy and Lactation), little or no PTHrP is found in blood plasma of normal individuals. PTHrP thus appears to function in calcium homeostasis during lactation when secretion of milk may drain as much as 300 mg of calcium from the mother's body each day.

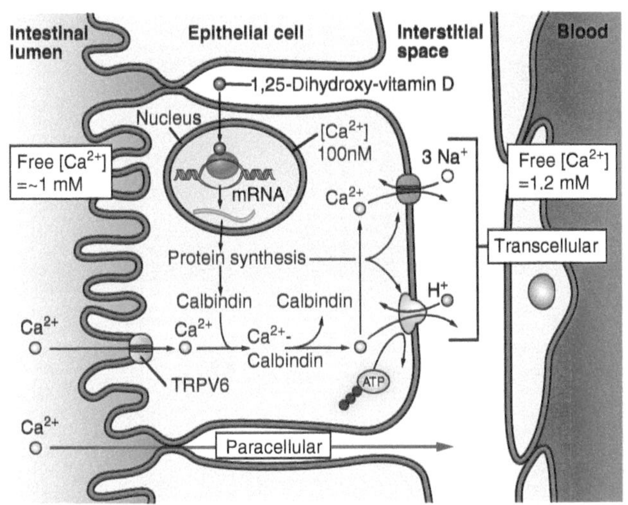

FIGURE 10.26 Intestinal absorption of calcium is dependent on 1,25-dihydroxyvitamin D. Source: *Redrawn from Figure 52.10A in Barrett, E. J., & Barrett, P. Q. (2017). Chapter 52: The parathyroid glands and Vitamin D. In W. F. Boron, & E. L. Boulpaep (Eds.),* Medical physiology *(3rd ed.) (p. 1066). Elsevier.*

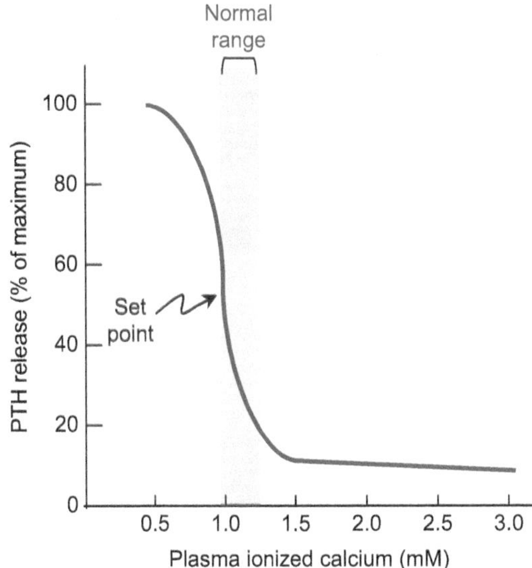

FIGURE 10.28 Relation between plasma ionized calcium concentration and PTH secretion. *PTH,* Parathyroid hormone. Source: *Redrawn and modified from Brown, E. B. (1983). Four parameter model of the sigmoidal relationship between parathyroid hormone release and extracellular calcium concentration in normal and abnormal parathyroid tissue.* The Journal of Clinical Endocrinology and Metabolism 56, *572–581.*

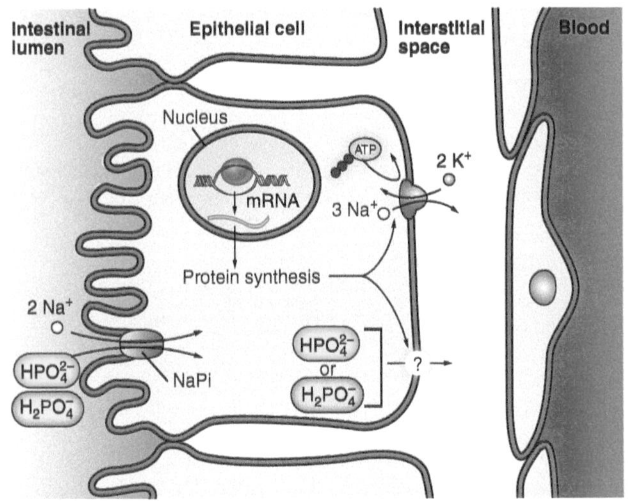

FIGURE 10.27 Intestinal absorption of phosphate. Source: *Redrawn from Figure 52.10 B in Barrett, E. J., & Barrett, P. Q. (2017). Chapter 52: The parathyroid glands and Vitamin D. In W. F. Boron, & E. L. Boulpaep (Eds.),* Medical physiology *(3rd ed.) (p. 1066). Elsevier.*

Regulation of parathyroid hormone secretion

Chief cells of the parathyroid glands are exquisitely sensitive to changes in extracellular calcium and rapidly adjust their rates of PTH secretion in a manner that is inversely related to the concentration of ionized calcium (Fig. 10.28).

The resulting increases or decreases in blood levels of PTH produce either positive or negative changes, respectively, in the plasma calcium concentration. When PTH increases, there is a rise in serum calcium and activated vitamin D concentrations, which then provide negative feedback signals to regulate PTH secretion (Fig. 10.29).

In addition, FGF-23, which is a phosphaturic hormone, inhibits PTH synthesis and secretion. Magnesium deficiency can inhibit PTH release and thus this may be seen in patients with celiac disease who have malabsorption. *PTH,* Parathyroid hormone.

Hyperphosphatemia is felt to increase PTH mRNA stability and also lead to parathyroid cell growth. This may be due to the fact that the increased serum phosphate level decreases the serum calcium concentration.

Chief cells are programed to synthesize and secrete PTH unless inhibited by extracellular calcium, but secretion may not be completely suppressed even when plasma concentrations of calcium are very high. Through mechanisms that are not understood, normal individuals secrete PTH throughout the day in bursts of 1–3 pulses/hour. Blood levels of PTH also follow a diurnal pattern with peak values seen shortly after midnight and minimal values seen in late morning. Diurnal fluctuations appear to arise from endogenous events in the chief cells and may promote anabolic responses of bone to PTH. The cellular mechanisms by which extracellular calcium regulates PTH secretion are poorly understood. These cells are equipped with

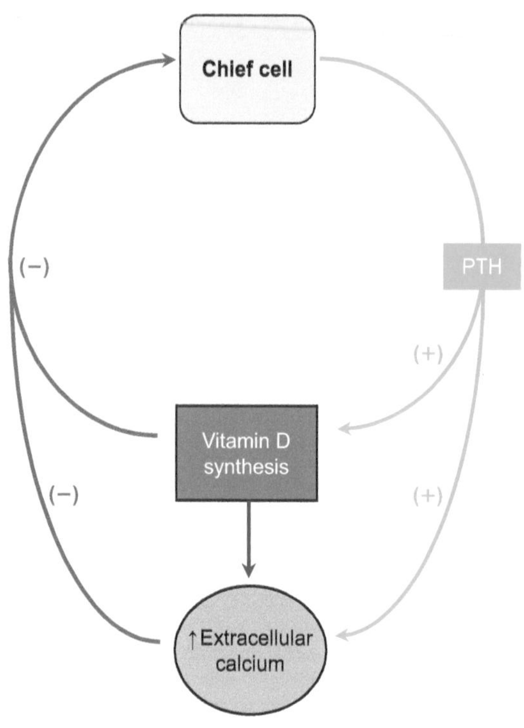

FIGURE 10.29 Regulation of PTH secretion. (−), Decrease; (+), increase.

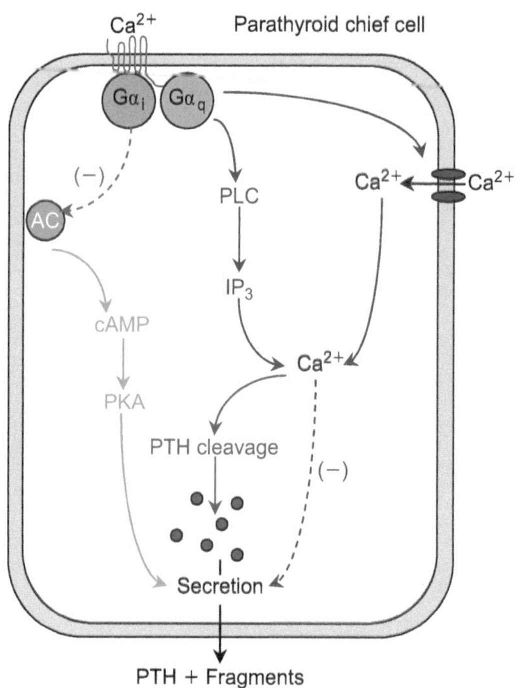

FIGURE 10.30 Regulation of parathyroid hormone secretion by calcium (Ca^{2+}). Heptahelical calcium receptors on the surface of chief cells communicate with Ca^{2+} channels, *AC*, and *PLC* by way of guanosine nucleotide–binding proteins ($G\alpha_i$ and $G\alpha_q$). The resulting increase in Ca^{2+} and decrease in cAMP concentration decreases **PKA**–mediated events that lead to secretion. The increase in calcium also accelerates cleavage of PTH to C-terminal fragments. *AC*, Adenylyl cyclase; *cAMP*, cyclic AMP; *IP3*, inositol trisphosphate; *PLC*, phospholipase C; *PTH*, parathyroid hormone; *PKA*, protein kinase A.

calcium-sensing receptors (CASRs) in their plasma membranes and can adjust secretion in response to as little as a 2% or 3% change in extracellular calcium concentration. CASRs are members of the G-protein-coupled receptor superfamily (see Chapter 1: Introduction) and bind calcium in proportion to its concentration in extracellular fluid. Because they are coupled to adenylyl cyclase through Gαi, activation of these receptors decreases constitutive production of cAMP. These receptors also signal through phospholipase C, and stimulate production of DAG and IP3 through activation of Gαq, and perhaps also directly activate membrane calcium channels. Cytosolic calcium rises as a result of IP3-mediated release from intracellular stores and influx through membrane channels.

Paradoxically, in chief cells, unlike most other secretory cells, increased intracellular calcium inhibits rather than stimulates hormone secretion. Inhibition of PTH secretion coincides with the decline in cAMP and the activity of protein kinase A. Increased extracellular calcium also increases cleavage of PTH to the C-terminal fragments described earlier. Thus, as the secretion of PTH peptides decreases, the proportion of C-terminal peptides increases. These events are summarized in Fig. 10.30.

Calcitonin

Cells of origin

Calcitonin is sometimes also called thyrocalcitonin to describe its origin in the parafollicular cells of the thyroid gland. These cells, which are also called C cells, occur singly or in clusters in or between thyroid follicles. They are larger and stain less densely than follicular cells in routine preparations (Fig. 10.31), and like other peptide hormone-secreting cells, contain membrane-bound storage granules. Parafollicular cells arise embryologically from neuroectodermal cells that migrate to the last branchial pouch and, in submammalian vertebrates, give rise to the ultimobranchial glands. In addition to producing calcitonin, parafollicular cells can take up and decarboxylate amine precursors and thus have some similarity to pancreatic alpha cells and cells of the adrenal medulla. Parafollicular cells may give rise to a unique neoplasm, medullary carcinoma of the thyroid, which may secrete large amounts of calcitonin.

Biosynthesis, secretion, and metabolism

Calcitonin consists of 32 amino acids and has a molecular weight of about 3400 Da. Except for a seven-member disulfide ring at the amino terminus, calcitonin has no remarkable structural features. Immunoreactive circulating forms are heterogeneous in size, reflecting the presence of precursors, partially degraded hormone, and disulfide-linked dimers and polymers. The active hormone has a half-life in plasma of about 5–10 minutes and is cleared from the blood primarily by the kidney. The gene that encodes calcitonin also encodes a neuropeptide called calcitonin gene–related peptide (CGRP). This gene contains six exons, but only the first four are represented in the mRNA transcript that codes for the precursor of calcitonin. As a result of alternate splicing, the portion of the RNA transcript corresponding to exon 4 is deleted and replaced by exons 5 and 6 in the mRNA that codes for CGRP. Since the first exon codes for a nontranslated region, and the peptide corresponding to exons 2 and 3 is removed in posttranslational processing, the mature products have no common amino acid sequences (Fig. 10.32).

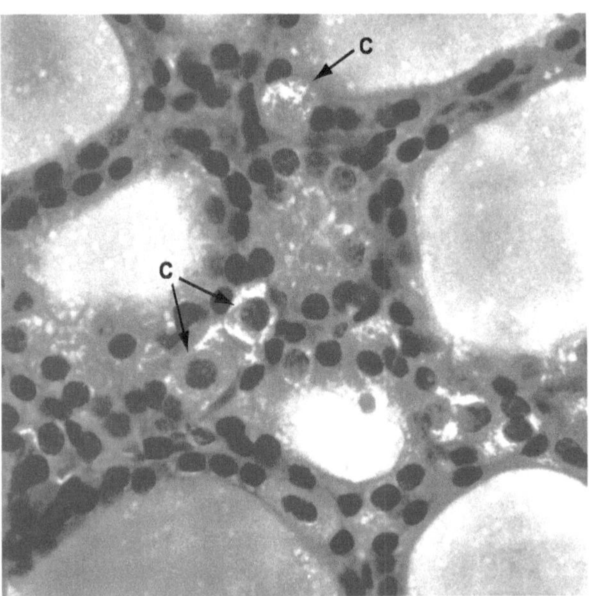

FIGURE 10.31 The location of the C cells in the thyroid gland. Source: *Figure 19-6 in Kierszenbaum, A., & Tres, L. (2016).* Histology and cell biology: An introduction to pathology *(4th ed.) (p. 590). Elsevier.*

Physiological actions of calcitonin

Calcitonin escaped discovery for many years because no obvious derangement in calcium balance or other homeostatic function results from deficient or excessive production. Thyroidectomy does not produce a tendency toward hypercalcemia, and thyroid tumors that secrete massive amounts of calcitonin do not cause hypocalcemia. Attention was drawn to the possibility of a calcium-lowering hormone by the experimental finding that directs injection of a concentrated solution of calcium into the thyroid artery in dogs causing a more rapid fall in blood calcium than parathyroidectomy. Indeed, calcitonin promptly and dramatically lowers the blood calcium concentration in many experimental animals. Calcitonin is not a major factor in calcium homeostasis in humans, however, and does not participate in minute-to-minute regulation of blood calcium concentrations. Rather, the importance of calcitonin may be limited to protection against excessive bone resorption.

Actions on bone

Calcitonin lowers blood calcium and phosphate primarily, and perhaps exclusively, by inhibiting osteoclastic activity. The decrease in blood calcium produced by calcitonin is greatest when osteoclastic bone resorption is most intense and is least evident when osteoclastic activity is minimal. Interaction of calcitonin with receptors on the osteoclast surface promptly increases cAMP formation, and within

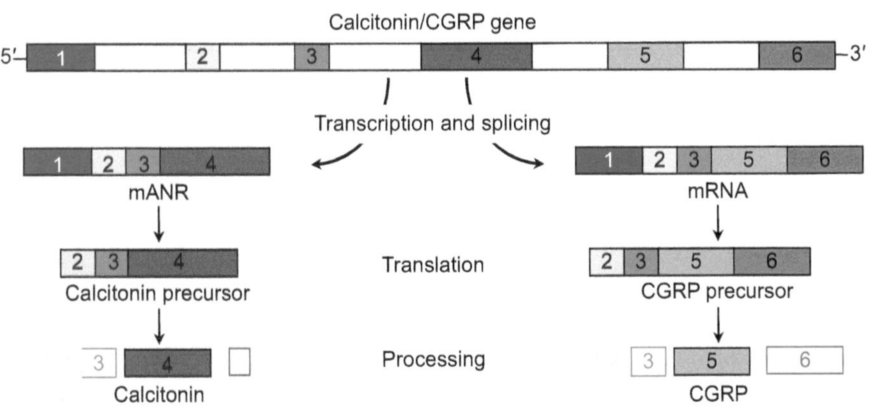

FIGURE 10.32 Alternate splicing of calcitonin/CGRP mRNA gives rise to either calcitonin or CGRP, with no shared sequences of amino acids. *CGRP*, Calcitonin gene–related peptide.

minutes the expanse and activity of the ruffled border diminishes. Osteoclasts pull away from the bone surface and begin to dedifferentiate. Synthesis and secretion of lysosomal enzymes is inhibited. In less than an hour, fewer osteoclasts are present, and those that remain have decreased bone-resorbing activity.

Osteoclasts are the principal, and probably only, target cells for calcitonin in bone. Osteoblasts do not have receptors for calcitonin and are not directly affected by it. Curiously, although they mediate opposite effects on osteoclast activity, receptors for PTH and calcitonin are closely related and have about a third of their amino acid sequences in common, suggesting they evolved from a common ancestral receptor molecule. Because of the coupling phenomenon in the cycle of bone resorption and bone formation discussed earlier, inhibition of osteoclastic activity by calcitonin eventually decreases osteoblastic activity as well. All cell types appear quiescent in histological sections of bone that was chronically exposed to high concentrations of calcitonin. Although they express an abundance of receptors for calcitonin, osteoclasts quickly become insensitive to the hormone because continued stimulation results in massive downregulation of receptors.

Actions on kidney

At high concentrations, calcitonin may increase urinary excretion of calcium and phosphorus, probably by acting on the proximal tubules. In humans, these effects are small, last only a short while, and are not physiologically important for lowering blood calcium. Renal handling of calcium is not disrupted in patients with thyroid tumors that secrete large amounts of calcitonin. Kidney cells "escape" from prolonged stimulation with calcitonin and become refractory to it, probably as a result of downregulation of receptors.

Regulation of secretion

Circulating concentrations of calcitonin are quite low when blood calcium is in the normal range or below. High concentrations of calcium stimulate calcitonin secretion. Parafollicular cells respond directly to ionized calcium in blood and express the same G-protein-coupled CASR in their surface membranes as the parathyroid chief cells. Both cell types respond to extracellular calcium over the same concentration range, but their secretory responses are opposite, presumably because of differences in the secretory apparatus. Although little information is available concerning intracellular mechanisms in parafollicular cells, the relation between stimulation and secretion is typical of endocrine cells.

In addition to the direct stimulation by high concentrations of calcium, calcitonin secretion may also increase after eating. Gastrin, produced by the gastric mucosa (see Chapter 6: Hormones of the Gastrointestinal Tract), stimulates parafollicular cells to secrete calcitonin. Other gastrointestinal hormones, including cholecystokinin, glucagon, and secretin, have similar effects, but gastrin is the most potent of these agents. Secretion of calcitonin in anticipation of an influx of calcium from the intestine is a feedforward mechanism that may guard against excessive concentrations of plasma calcium after calcium ingestion by decreasing osteoclastic activity. Although the importance of this response in humans is not established, sensitivity of parafollicular cells to gastrin has been exploited clinically as a provocative test for diagnosing medullary carcinoma of the thyroid.

Vitamin D hormone

A derivative of vitamin D3, 1,25-dihydroxycholecalciferol (1,25$(OH)_2$D3), is indispensable for maintaining adequate concentrations of calcium in the extracellular fluid and adequate mineralization of bone matrix. Vitamin D deficiency leads to inadequate calcification of bone matrix manifested as severe softening of the skeleton, called osteomalacia, and may result in bone deformities and fractures. Osteomalacia in children is called rickets and may produce permanent deformities of the weight-bearing bones (bowed legs).

One important distinction between hormones and vitamins is that hormones are synthesized within the body from simple precursors, but vitamins must be provided in the diet. Vitamin D3 is unique because it can be synthesized endogenously in humans, but the rate is limited by a nonenzymatic reaction that requires UV light from the Sun. The immediate precursor for vitamin D3, 7-dehydrocholesterol, is synthesized from acetyl coenzyme A and is stored in skin. Conversion of 7-dehydrocholesterol to vitamin D3 proceeds spontaneously in the presence of sunlight that penetrates the epidermis to the outer layers of the dermis. Vitamin D deficiency became a significant public health problem as a by-product of industrialization. Urban living, smog, and increased indoor activity limit exposure of the population to sunshine and hence endogenous production of vitamin D3. This problem is readily addressed by adding vitamin D supplementation to food or drink, particularly to milk.

1,25-Dihydroxy-vitamin D3 also fits the description of a hormone in the respect that it travels through the blood in small amounts from its site of production to affect cells at distant sites. 1,25$(OH)_2$D3 produces many of its biological effects in a manner characteristic of steroid hormones (see Chapter 1: Introduction). It binds to a specific receptor that is a member of the nuclear receptor superfamily.

Synthesis and metabolism

The form of vitamin D produced in mammals is called cholecalciferol or vitamin D3. Vitamin D2 is produced in plants and differs from vitamin D3 due to different side chains. Exposure of the skin to ultraviolet light results in photolysis of the bond that links carbons 9 and 10 in 7-dehydrocholesterol and thus opens the B ring of the steroid nucleus (Fig. 10.33).

The resultant cholecalciferol is biologically inert but, unlike its precursor, has a high affinity for a vitamin D–binding protein in plasma.

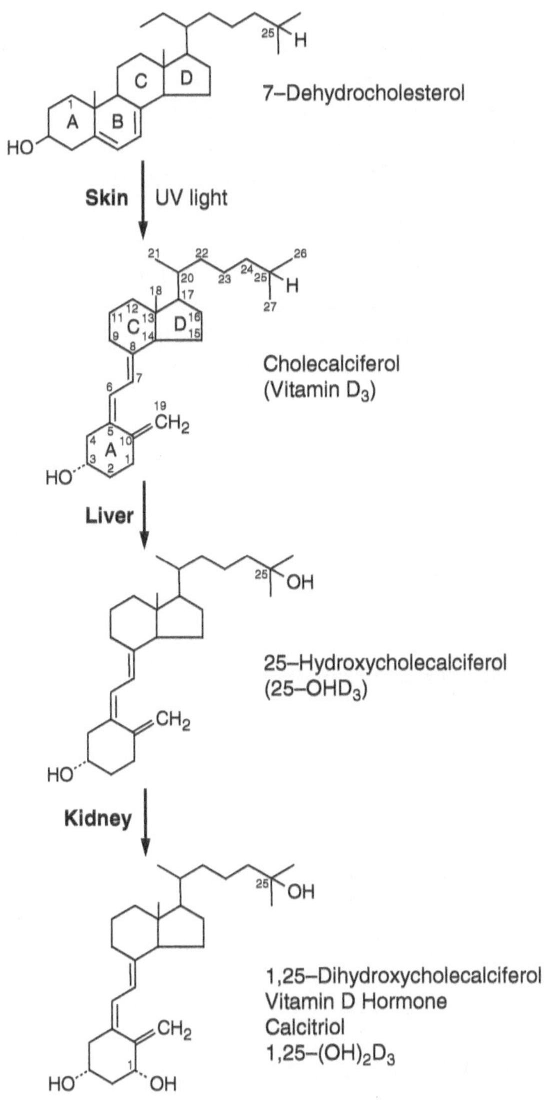

FIGURE 10.33 Synthesis of vitamin D hormone from 7-dehydrocholesterol in the skin. The active vitamin D hormone is produced in the kidney. This active form of vitamin D is called 1,25-dihydroxycholecalciferol or calcitriol. Source: *Redrawn from Figure 52.9 in Barrett, E. J., & Barrett, P. Q. (2017). Chapter 52: The parathyroid glands and Vitamin D. In W. F. Boron, & E. L. Boulpaep (Eds.),* Medical physiology *(3rd ed.) (p. 1064). Elsevier.*

Vitamin D3 is transported by the blood to the liver, where it is oxidized to form 25-hydroxy-cholecalciferol (25-OH-D3) by 25-hydroxylase, a P450 mitochondrial enzyme. This reaction appears to be controlled only by the availability of substrate. 25-OH-D3 has high affinity for the vitamin D–binding protein and is the major circulating form of vitamin D. In the proximal tubules of the kidney, a second hydroxyl group is added by 1-α-hydoxylase, to yield the compound 1,25-$(OH)_2$D3, which is about 1000 times as active as 25-OH-D3, and probably accounts for all the biological activity of vitamin D. 1,25-$(OH)_2$D3 is considerably less abundant in blood than its precursor 25-OH-D3 and binds less tightly to vitamin D–binding globulin than 25-OH-D3. Consequently, 1,25-$(OH)_2$D3 has a half-life in blood of 15 hours compared to 15 days for 25-OH-D3.

Physiological actions of 1,25-$(OH)_2$D3

Overall, the principal physiological actions of 1,25-$(OH)_2$D3 increase calcium and phosphate concentrations in extracellular fluid. These effects are exerted primarily on intestine and bone. Vitamin D receptors are widely distributed, however, and a variety of other actions that are not obviously related to calcium balance have been described or postulated. Since these latter effects are not germane to regulation of calcium balance they are not discussed further here.

Actions on intestine

Uptake of dietary calcium and phosphate depends on active transport by epithelial cells lining the small intestine. Vitamin D deficiency severely impairs intestinal transport of both calcium and phosphorus. Although calcium uptake usually is accompanied by phosphate uptake, the two ions are transported by independent mechanisms, both of which are stimulated by 1,25-$(OH)_2$D3. Increased calcium uptake is seen about 2 hours after 1,25-$(OH)_2$D3 is given to deficient subjects and is maximal within 4 hours. A much longer time is required when vitamin D is given, presumably because of the time needed for sequential hydroxylations in liver and kidney. Calcium uptake by intestinal epithelial cells is illustrated in Fig. 10.34.

Calcium enters passively down its electrochemical gradient through the same two forms of ECaC that are expressed in the principal cells of the kidney. Upon entry into the cytosol, calcium is bound virtually instantaneously by calcium-binding proteins, mainly calbindin-9 and carried through the cytosol to the basolateral membrane where it is extruded into the extracellular space by calcium ATPase and sodium/calcium exchangers.

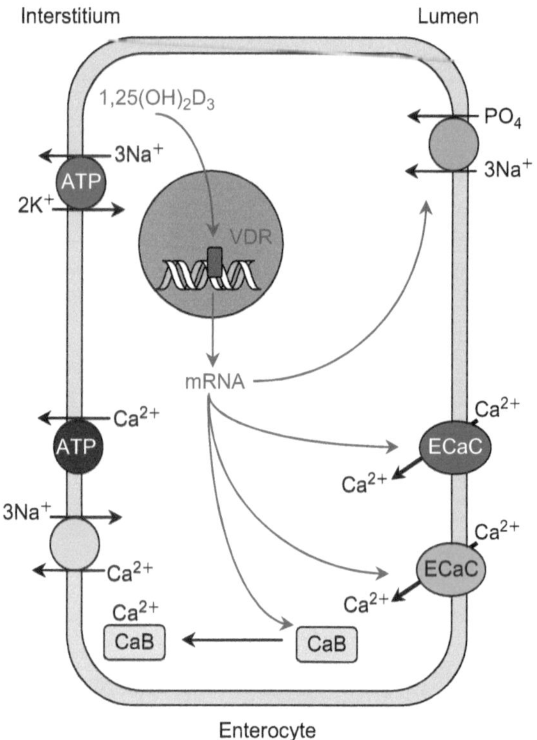

FIGURE 10.34 Effects of 1,25(OH)$_2$D$_3$ on intestinal transport of calcium. *CaB*, Calbindin-9; *ECaC*, epithelial calcium channels (also called TRPV5 and TRPV6); *VDR*, vitamin D receptor.

In addition to shuttling calcium across cells, calbindin keeps the cytosolic calcium concentration low and thus maintains a gradient favorable for calcium influx while affording protection from deleterious effects of high concentrations of free calcium. 1,25-(OH)$_2$D3 increases the expression of ECaCs and calbindin by activating gene transcription and increases the amount or activity of calcium ATPase and sodium/calcium exchangers in the basolateral membranes.

Some evidence obtained in experimental animals and in cultured cells indicates that 1,25-(OH)$_2$D3 may also produce rapid actions that are not mediated by altered genomic expression. Among these are rapid transport of calcium across the intestinal epithelium and activation of membrane calcium channels. The physiological importance of these rapid actions of 1,25-(OH)$_2$D3 is not known.

Actions on bone

The most obvious consequence of vitamin D deficiency is decreased mineralization of bone, which is known as osteomalacia. The major effect of 1,25-(OH)$_2$D3 is to allow calcium and phosphate absorption in the intestine, thereby providing these necessary components for deposition in osteoid. Without these essential components, osteomalacia may develop due to calcium and/or phosphate deficiency.

Paradoxically, 1,25-(OH)$_2$D3 acts on bone to promote resorption in much the same manner as PTH and appears to be redundant. As seen for PTH, osteoblasts rather than mature osteoclasts have receptors for 1,25-(OH)$_2$D3. 1,25-(OH)$_2$D3 stimulates osteoblastic cells to express RANK ligand and decreases OPG. Thus 1,25-(OH)$_2$D3 increases the osteoclastogenesis mediated by RANKL–RANK.

Actions on kidney

When given to vitamin D–deficient subjects, 1,25 (OH)$_2$D3 increases reabsorption of both calcium and phosphate from the glomerular filtrate. The effects on phosphate reabsorption are probably indirect. PTH secretion is increased in vitamin D deficiency (see later); hence, tubular reabsorption of phosphate is restricted. Replenishment of 1,25-(OH)$_2$D3 decreases the secretion of PTH and thus allows proximal tubular reabsorption of phosphate to increase. Effects of 1,25-(OH)2D3 on calcium reabsorption are probably direct.

Specific receptors for 1,25(OH)$_2$D3 are found in the distal nephron, probably in the same cells in which PTH stimulates calcium uptake. These cells express the same vitamin D–dependent proteins as found in intestinal cells and are likely to respond to 1,25-(OH)2D3 in the same manner as intestinal epithelial cells. These effects and distal tubular calcium reabsorption also seem to overlap with the actions of PTH. However, it is unlikely that 1,25-(OH)$_2$D3 regulates calcium balance on a minute-to-minute basis. Instead, it may support the actions of PTH, which is the primary regulator.

Actions on the parathyroid glands

The chief cells of the parathyroid glands are physiological targets for 1,25-(OH)$_2$D3 and respond to it in a manner that is characteristic of negative feedback. In this case, negative feedback is exerted at the level of synthesis rather than secretion. The promoter region of the PTH gene contains a vitamin D response element. Binding of the liganded receptor suppresses transcription of the gene and produces a decline in preproPTH mRNA. Because the chief cells store relatively little hormone, decreased synthesis rapidly leads to decreased secretion. In a second negative feedback action, 1,25(OH)$_2$D3 indirectly decreases PTH secretion by its actions to increase plasma calcium concentration. Consistent with the crucial role of calcium in regulating PTH secretion, the negative feedback effects of 1,25-(OH)$_2$D3 on PTH synthesis are modulated by the plasma calcium concentration. In responses mediated through the CASR, nuclear receptors for 1,25-(OH)$_2$D3 are upregulated when the plasma calcium concentration is high and downregulated when it is low.

Regulation of 1,25-(OH)$_2$D3 production

As true of any hormone, the concentration of 1,25-(OH)$_2$D3 in the blood must be appropriate for prevailing physiological circumstances if it is to exercise its proper role in maintaining homeostasis. Production of 1,25-(OH)$_2$D3 is subject to feedback regulation in a fashion quite like that of other hormones (Fig. 10.35).

PTH increases the synthesis of 1,25-(OH)$_2$D3, which exerts a powerful inhibitory effect on PTH gene expression in the parathyroid chief cells. The most important regulatory step in 1,25(OH)$_2$D3 synthesis is the hydroxylation of 25-OH-vitamin D by 1α-hydroxylase in the proximal tubules of the kidney. The rate of this reaction is determined by the availability of the 1α-hydroxylase enzyme, which has a half-life of only about 2–4 hours. In the absence of PTH the concentration of 1α-hydroxylase in renal cells quickly falls. PTH regulates transcription of the gene that encodes the 1α-hydroxylase by increasing production of cAMP. Several cAMP response elements (CREs) are present in its promoter region.

Through a "short" feedback loop, 1,25-(OH)$_2$D3 also acts as a negative feedback inhibitor of its own production by rapidly downregulating 1α-hydroxylase expression. At the same time, 1,25-(OH)D3 upregulates expression of the enzyme that hydroxylates vitamin D metabolites on carbon 24 to produce 24,25-(OH)$_2$D3 or 1,24,25-(OH)$_3$D3. Hydroxylation at carbon 24 is the initial reaction in the degradative pathway that culminates in the production of calcitroic acid, the principal biliary excretory product of vitamin D. Upregulation of the 24-hydroxylase by 1,25 (OH)$_2$D3 is not only confined to the kidney but also seen in all 1,25-(OH)$_2$D3 target cells. Finally, the actions of 1,25-(OH)$_2$D3 result in increased calcium and phosphate concentrations in blood, which directly or indirectly silence the two activators of 1,25(OH)$_2$D3 production, PTH and low phosphate.

Calcium regulation of plasma calcium concentrations

PTH, calcitonin, and vitamin D generally have been referred to as calciotropic hormones. The growth of information about the CASR and its role in normal calcium homeostasis highlight the hormone-like actions of calcium itself as a fourth calciotropic hormone. At high concentrations, calcium plays more of a hormone-like role than calcitonin in lowering its plasma concentrations. Reabsorption of calcium in the kidney is at least partially controlled by the plasma calcium concentration (Fig. 10.36).

About 25% of the filtered calcium is reabsorbed by the thick ascending limb of Henle, driven by the positive luminal voltage created because of active reabsorption of sodium chloride. Sodium chloride enters these tubular cells along with potassium on the neutral sodium/potassium/2 chloride cotransporters in the luminal membranes. Sodium chloride exits through the basolateral membranes, but potassium ions carrying their positive charge recycle back into the lumen through ROMK (renal outer medullary potassium) channels. The positive voltage thus created drives luminal calcium ions across intercellular junctions, and into the extracellular space.

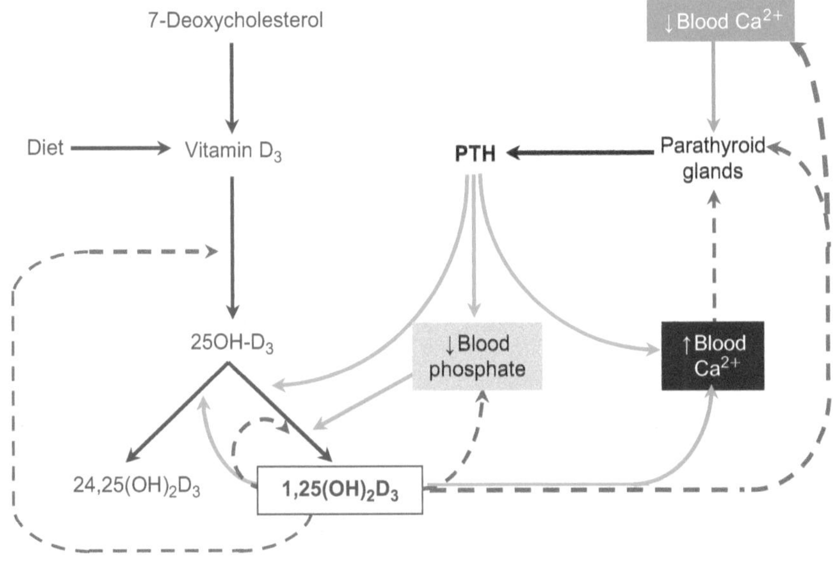

FIGURE 10.35 Multiple negative feedback loops in the regulation of 1α,25-dihydroxycholecalciferol synthesis. Solid arrows indicate stimulation; dashed red arrows represent inhibition.

The basolateral surfaces of cells of the thick ascending limb of Henle express the same CASRs as the parathyroid chief cells. The CASR coupled with both Gαi and Gαq, and when activated, decreases cAMP formation and increases production of DAG and IP3. The resulting diminution of protein kinase A activity lowers its stimulatory actions on the sodium/potassium/2 chloride cotransporter. The increase in DAG activates protein kinase C, which phosphorylates and decreases the activity of ROMK channels. The combination of effects decreases reabsorption of both sodium chloride and calcium. Because of the limited capacity of downstream calcium reabsorbing mechanisms, more calcium is lost in urine, and plasma calcium levels fall.

We already have discussed how high concentrations of calcium act as receptor-mediated signals to decrease PTH secretion and to increase secretion of calcitonin. The CASR is also expressed in luminal membranes of renal proximal tubules and moderates the effects of PTH on phosphate reabsorption. Although physiological roles have not been defined, the calcium receptor is also found in intestinal cells and in bone cells, the other principal targets of the calciotropic hormones. The importance of receptor-mediated effects of calcium to the overall calcium balance is underscored by the human diseases that result from activating or inactivating mutations in the CASR that lead to hypocalcemia and hypercalcemia, respectively.

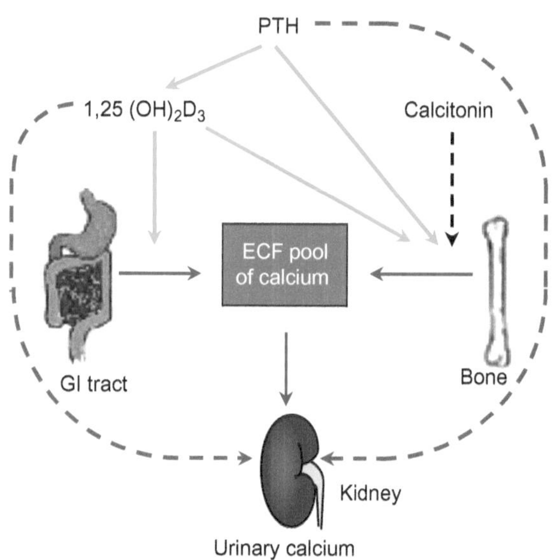

FIGURE 10.36 Overall regulation of calcium balance by PTH, calcitonin, and 1,25(OH)$_2$D$_3$. Solid green arrows indicate stimulation; dashed arrows represent inhibition. *PTH*, Parathyroid hormone.

Integrated actions of calciotropic hormones

Response to a hypocalcemic challenge

Since some calcium is always lost in urine, even a short period of total fasting can produce a mild hypocalcemic challenge. More severe challenges are produced by a chronic diet deficient in calcium or anything that might interfere with calcium absorption by renal tubules or the intestine. The parathyroid glands are exquisitely sensitive to even a small decrease in ionized calcium and promptly increase PTH secretion (Fig. 10.37).

Effects of PTH on calcium reabsorption from the glomerular filtrate coupled with some calcium mobilization from bone are evident after about an hour, providing the first line of defense against a hypocalcemic challenge. These actions are adequate only to compensate for a mild or brief challenge. When the hypocalcemic challenge is large and sustained, additional

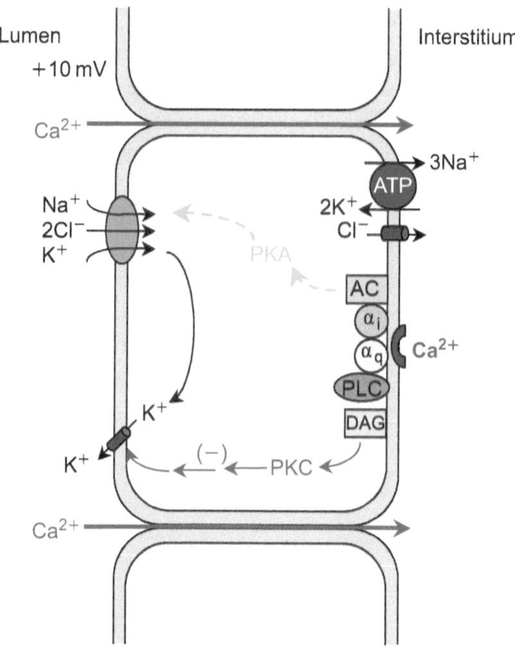

FIGURE 10.37 Increased plasma calcium concentrations regulate calcium reabsorption in the thick ascending limb of Henle's loop. In this portion of the nephron, calcium passes through the cellular junctions driven by a positive luminal voltage. The calcium receptor signals through the guanosine nucleotide–binding protein $G\alpha_q$ to activate *PLC* and form *DAG*, which activates *PKC*. Back diffusion of potassium through renal outer medullary potassium (ROMK) channels is inhibited, which decreases the positive potential of luminal fluid and limits reabsorption of sodium and chloride. The receptor also signals through $G\alpha_i$, thus inhibiting AC reducing any cyclic AMP–dependent stimulation of the sodium/potassium/2 chloride cotransporter. *AC*, Adenylyl cyclase; *DAG*, diacylglycerol; *PKA*, protein kinase A; *PKC*, protein kinase C; *PLC*, phospholipase C.

delayed responses to PTH are needed. After about 12–24 hours, increased formation of 1,25-$(OH)_2D3$ increases the efficiency of calcium absorption from the gut. Osteoclastic bone resorption in response to both PTH and 1,25-$(OH)_2D3$ taps the significant reserves of calcium in the skeleton. If calcium intake remains inadequate, skeletal integrity may be sacrificed in favor of maintaining blood calcium concentrations.

Response to a hypercalcemic challenge

Hypercalcemia may be a complication of a variety of pathological conditions and may be accompanied by increased blood concentrations of PTH or PTHrP. An example of hypercalcemia that might arise under physiological circumstances is the case of a person who has been living for some time on a low calcium diet and then ingests a large amount of calcium-rich food. Under the influence of high concentrations of PTH and 1,25-$(OH)_2D3$ that would result from calcium insufficiency, osteoclastic transfer of bone mineral to the extracellular fluid and calcium absorptive mechanisms in the intestine and renal tubules are stimulated to their maximal efficiency. Consequently, ingested calcium is absorbed efficiently and blood calcium is increased by a few tenths of a milligram per deciliter. PTH secretion promptly decreases and its effects on calcium and phosphate transport in renal tubules quickly diminish. The proportion of PTH fragments released from the glands increases promptly, but several hours pass before hydroxylation of 25-OH-D3 and osteoclastic bone resorption diminish. Even after its production is shut down, many hours are required for some responses to 1,25-$(OH)_2D3$ to decrease.

Although some calcium phosphate may crystallize in demineralized osteoid, renal loss of calcium is the principal means of lowering blood calcium. The rate of renal loss by PTH-sensitive mechanisms, however, is limited to only about 10% of the calcium present in the glomerular filtrate, or about 40 mg/h, even after maximum shutdown of PTH secretion. Decreased reabsorption of calcium in the thick ascending limb triggered by the CASR, however, would quickly facilitate further calcium excretion.

The effects of the calciotropic hormones and calcium are summarized in Table 10.2.

TABLE 10.2 Comparison of the major effects of calcitropic hormones and calcium.

Effects	PTH	PTHrP	D_3	Calcium
Intestine				
Calcium absorption			↑	↑
Phosphate absorption			↑	
Kidney				
Proximal tubule				
Phosphate reabsorption	↓	↓	↑	
1α-Hydroxylase activity	↑		↓	↓
Thick ascending limb				
Calcium reabsorption	↑	↑		↓
Distal tubule				
Calcium reabsorption	↑	↑	↑	
Bone				
Osteoblasts' production of osteoclast differentiation factors	↑	↑	↑	
Precursor multiplication and development	↑	↑	↑	
Matrix formation and mineralization	↑	↑		↑
Chondrocytes				
Multiplication and differentiation		↑		
Parathyroid chief cells				
PTH synthesis			↓	↓
PTH secretion			↓	↓
PTH metabolism to fragments				↑

PTH, Parathyroid hormone; *PTHrP*, parathyroid hormone–related peptide.

Other hormones that influence calcium balance

In addition to the primary endocrine regulators of calcium balance just discussed, many other endocrine and paracrine factors influence calcium balance. Most of the calcium reabsorbed from the glomerular filtrate is by passive processes driven by active reabsorption of sodium. Therefore renal conservation of calcium is intimately related to sodium balance, and adjustments of sodium reabsorption discussed in Chapter 9, Regulation of Salt and Water Balance, are accompanied by changes in renal calcium reabsorption. For example, volume expansion results in increased glomerular filtration and decreased sodium reabsorption in the proximal tubule. The proximal tubule accounts for the bulk of the calcium reabsorbed, and hence even small changes at this level can result in significant calcium loss.

Bone remodeling profoundly affects the flux of calcium into or out of the mineralized matrix and is controlled by a still incompletely understood interplay of local and circulating factors in addition to the calciotropic hormones discussed earlier. Insulin-like growth factor-I, growth hormone (see Chapter 11: Hormonal Control of Growth), the cytokines interleukin-1 (see Chapter 4: The Adrenal Glands), interleukin-6, and interleukin-11, TNF α, TGF-β, prostaglandins, and doubtless many others play a role.

Many of the systemic hormones directly or indirectly affect calcium balance. Obviously, special demands are imposed on overall calcium balance during growth, pregnancy, and lactation. All the hormones that govern growth—namely, growth hormone, the insulin-like growth factors, thyroid and gonadal hormones (see Chapter 11: Hormonal Control of Growth)—directly or indirectly influence the activity of bone cells and calcium balance. The gonadal hormones, particularly estrogens, play a critical role in maintaining bone mass, which decreases in their absence, leading to osteoporosis. This condition is common in postmenopausal women. Osteoblastic cells express receptors for estrogens that stimulate proliferation of osteoblast progenitors and inhibit production of cytokines such as interleukin-6, which activates osteoclasts. Consequently, in the absence of estrogens, osteoclastic activity is increased and osteoblastic activity is decreased, and there is net loss of bone (Fig. 10.38).

Defects in calcium metabolism also are seen in hyperthyroidism and in conditions of excess or deficiency of adrenocortical hormones. Excessive thyroid hormone accelerates activity of both the osteoclasts and osteoblasts and often results in net bone resorption and a decrease in bone density. This action may produce a mild hypercalcemia and secondarily suppress PTH secretion and hence also decrease 1,25-$(OH)_2D3$ production. These hormonal changes result in increased urinary loss of calcium and decreased intestinal absorption. Excessive glucocorticoid concentrations also cause osteoporosis. The use of supraphysiologic doses of glucocorticoids is known to decrease bone formation and increase the risk of fractures. In addition, glucocorticoids inhibit calcium uptake in the intestine and

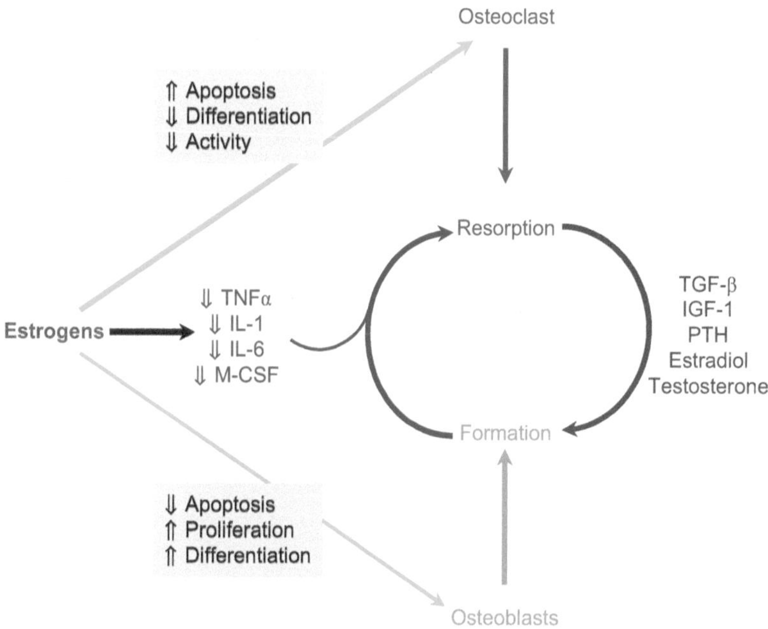

FIGURE 10.38 Relation of estrogens to cytokines and growth factors in the overall economy of bones.

increase renal calcium excretion. Conversely, adrenal insufficiency may lead to hypercalcemia due largely to decreased renal excretion of calcium.

Summary

Even in the ancient seas, animals had to concentrate calcium in order to grow bones, clot blood, and maintain normal neuronal function. On land, animals developed an elaborate sequence of hormonal interactions and feedback to absorb calcium and phosphate and yet maintain serum calcium levels while building and rebuilding bone. These processes and pathways are explored in this chapter.

References

Blaine, J., Chonchol, M., & Levi, M. (2015). Renal control of calcium, phosphate, and magnesium homeostasis. *Clinical Journal of the American Society of Nephrology: CJASN, 10*(7), 1257–1272, *PMC*. Web. 1 Oct. 2018.

Divieti, P., John, M. R., Jüppner, H., & Bringhurst, F. R. (2002). Human PTH-(7–84) inhibits bone resorption *in vitro* via actions independent of the type 1 PTH/PTHrP receptor. *Endocrinology, 143*(1), 171–176. Available from https://doi.org/10.1210/endo.143.1.8575, 1 January.

Rosen, C. J., Bouillon, R., Compston, J. E., & Rosen, V. (Eds.), (2013). *Primer of the metabolic bone disease and disorders of mineral metabolism* (8th Ed). John Wiley & Sons, Inc. ASBMR, Chapter 4. Osteocytes.

Suggested readings

Basic foundations

Barrett, E. J., & Barrett, P. Q. (2017). The parathyroid glands and vitamin D. In W. F. Boron, & E. L. Boulpaep (Eds.), *Medical physiology* (3rd ed., pp. 1054–1069). Philadelphia, PA: Elsevier.

Bringhurst, F. R., Demay, M. B., & Kronenberg, H. M. (2016). Hormones and disorders of mineral metabolism. In S. Melmed, K. S. Polonsky, P. R. Larsen, & H. M. Kronenberg (Eds.), *Williams textbook of endocrinology* (pp. 1254–1322). Philadelphia, PA: Elsevier.

De Paula, F. J. A., Black, D. M., & Rosen, C. J. (2016). Osteoporosis and bone biology. In S. Melmed, K. S. Polonsky, P. R. Larsen, & H. M. Kronenberg (Eds.), *Williams textbook of endocrinology* (pp. 1323–1364). Philadelphia, PA: Elsevier.

Schmitz, M. R., DeHart, M. M., Qazi, Z., & Shuyler, F. D. (2016). Basic sciences. In M. D. Miller, & S. R. Thompson (Eds.), *Miller's review of orthopaedics* (7 ed., pp. 1–83). Philadelphia, PA: Elsevier.

Advanced information

Bozec, A., & Zaiss, M. M. (2017). T regulatory cells in bone remodelling. *Current Osteoporosis Reports, 15*(3), 121–125. Available from https://doi.org/10.1007/s11914-017-0356-1.

Cervantes-Diaz, F., Contreras, P., & Marcellini, S. (2017). Evolutionary origin of endochondral ossification: the transdifferentiation hypothesis. *Development Genes and Evolution, 227*(2), 121–127. Available from https://doi.org/10.1007/s00427-016-0567-y.

Golden, N. H., & Abrams, S. A. (2014). Optimizing bone health in children and adolescents. *Pediatrics, 134*(4), e1229–e1243. Available from https://doi.org/10.1542/peds.2014-2173.

Hofbauer, L. (1999). Osteoprotegerin ligand and osteoprotegerin: novel implications for osteoclast biology and bone metabolism. *European Journal of Endocrinology, 141*(3), 195–210. Available from https://doi.org/10.1530/eje.0.1410195.

Khosla, S., & Hofbauer, L. C. (2017). Osteoporosis treatment: Recent developments and ongoing challenges. *The lancet. Diabetes & endocrinology, 5*(11), 898–907. Available from https://doi.org/10.1016/S2213-8587(17)30188-2.

Salmon, P. (2014). Non-linear pattern formation in bone growth and architecture. *Frontiers in Endocrinology, 5*, 239. Available from https://doi.org/10.3389/fendo.2014.00239.

Sandberg, O. H., & Aspenberg, P. (2016). Inter-trabecular bone formation: a specific mechanism for healing of cancellous bone: A narrative review. *Acta Orthopaedica, 87*(5), 459–465. Available from https://doi.org/10.1080/17453674.2016.1205172.

Shapiro, I. M., Landis, W. J., & Risbud, M. V. (2015). Matrix vesicles: Are they anchored exosomes? *Bone, 79*, 29–36. Available from https://doi.org/10.1016/j.bone.2015.05.013.

Wang, C., Meng, H., Wang, X., Zhao, C., Peng, J., & Wang, Y. (2016). Differentiation of bone marrow mesenchymal stem cells in osteoblasts and adipocytes and its role in treatment of osteoporosis. *Medical Science Monitor: International Medical Journal of Experimental and Clinical Research, 22*, 226–233. Available from https://doi.org/10.12659/MSM.897044.

Xiong, Q., Zhang, L., Ge, W., & Tang, P. (2016). The roles of interferons in osteoclasts and osteoclastogenesis. *Joint Bone Spine, 83*(3), 276–281. Available from https://doi.org/10.1016/j.jbspin.2015.07.010.

Yang, L., Tsang, K. Y., Tang, H. C., Chan, D., & Cheah, K. S. E. (2014). Hypertrophic chondrocytes can become osteoblasts and osteocytes in endochondral bone formation. *Proceedings of the National Academy of Sciences United States of America, 111*(33), 12097–12102. Available from https://doi.org/10.1073/pnas.1302703111.

Zhao, N., Wang, X., Qin, L., Zhai, M., Yuan, J., Chen, J., & Li, D. (2016). Effect of hyaluronic acid in bone formation and its applications in dentistry. *Journal of Biomedical Materials Research Part A, 104*(6), 1560–1569. Available from https://doi.org/10.1002/jbm.a.35681.

Zigdon-Giladi, H., Rudich, U., Michaeli Geller, G., & Evron, A. (2015). Recent advances in bone regeneration using adult stem cells. *World Journal of Stem Cells, 7*(3), 630–640. Available from https://doi.org/10.4252/wjsc.v7.i3.630.

CHAPTER

11

Hormonal control of growth

Case study: suprasellar teratoma

He was 17-years-old and in high school, but his bone age was that of a 10-year-old and he had not yet entered puberty. Serum values for growth hormone, gonadotropin, T3, and T4 were very low as was his cortisol level. He had panhypopituitarism. A suprasellar mass was detected by CT and confirmed by MRI which extended into the pituitary stalk. It was similar to the one seen in Fig. 11.1.

Because of the extensive tumor, neurosurgeons decided to do a frontotemporal approach. This was done and the mass excised and biopsies taken. The mass was a mature teratoma.

Teratomas are 0.5% of all intracranial tumors. Most teratomas are usually found along the midline. Most often they arise in the coccygeal area (Fig. 11.2) with a female predominance.

Other common sites are the anterior mediastinum, gonads of either sex, and within the cranium (pineal, parapineal, and suprasellar locations) intracranial teratomas occur almost exclusively in males. In some cases the teratoma completely replaces normal structures in the fetus, as in Fig. 11.3.

Teratomas arise from germ cells that are haploid and usually migrate to the gonads of the individual from the yolk sac (Fig. 11.4).

If they do not become haploid germ cells in the gonads, the cells divide and become diploid and if a mature teratoma, form structures with all three germ layers (ectoderm, mesoderm, and endoderm) from which are formed many tissue and organ structures (Figs. 11.5–11.8).

Teratomas are not a malformed twin, and they have no sentience as a fetal twin would have. These haploid cells become diploid and are always XX regardless of the sex of the host. They are immunologically privileged, meaning that they do not initiate an immune response on the part of the host. Germ cells, because they are undifferentiated and multipotent, are a form of stem cells. Mature teratomas are benign but can cause clinical problems because of compression of other structures. Immature teratomas—in which there are less than the three basic layers of tissues—can become malignant and should be treated as such until examined histologically.

Stem or germ cells injected into another animal can form teratomas, which is the major reason why stem cell therapy is not currently being used.

After the excision of the teratoma the patient in this case was placed on replacement hormone therapy. He was also referred to a psychologist, as individuals who go through puberty very rapidly need psychological support.

Goodman's Basic Medical Endocrinology.
DOI: https://doi.org/10.1016/B978-0-12-815844-9.00011-7

(*cont'd*)

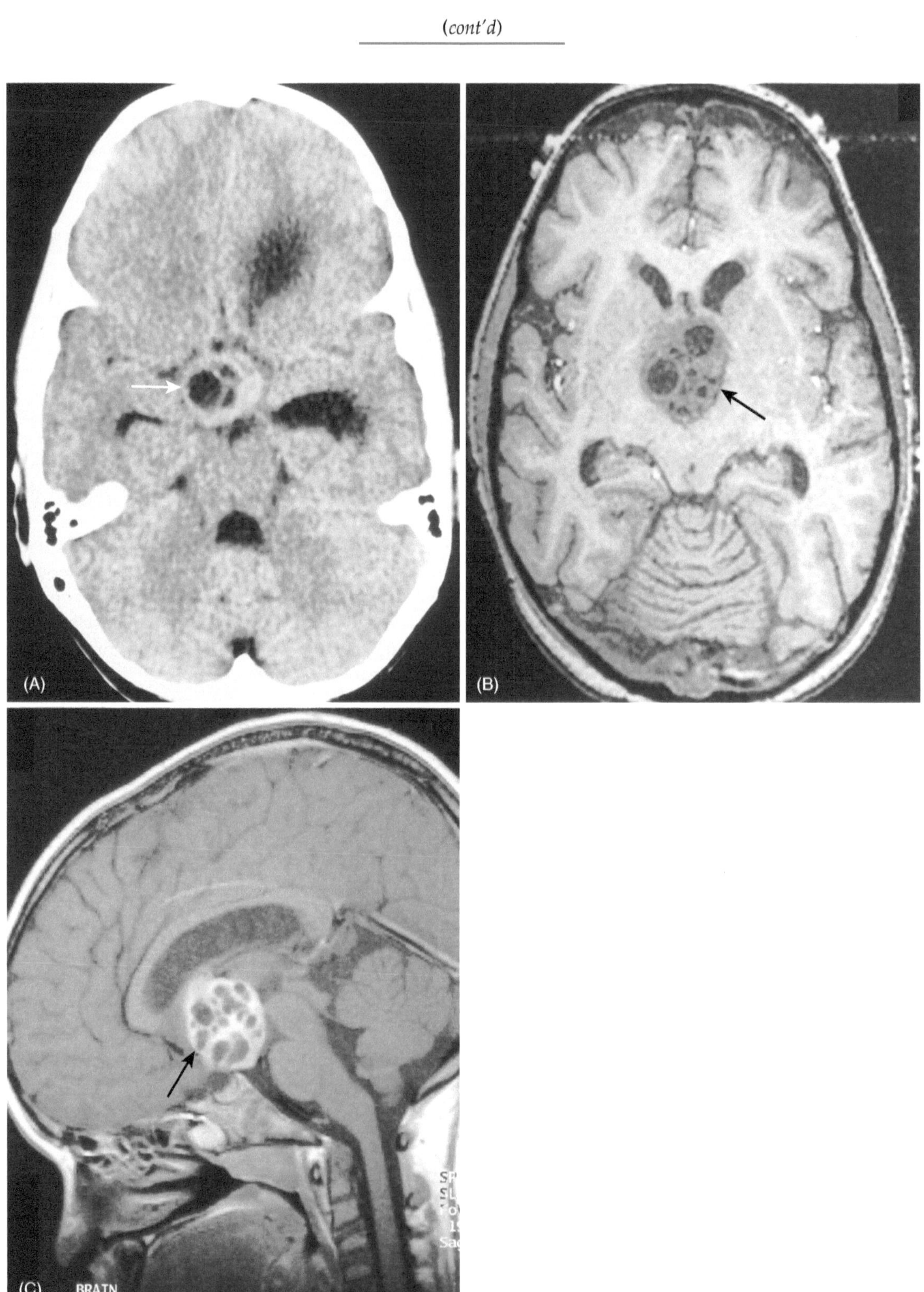

FIGURE 11.1 Suprasellar teratoma on (A) axial CT noncontrast scan, (B) axial T1 weighted MRI, and (C) sagittal T1 weighted MRI following 3cc of IV gadolinium to enhance contrast. The cystic nature of mature teratomas is evident here. Source: *From Figure 9-51 in Blackham, K. A., Montagnese, J., Kieffer, S. A., & Brace, J. R. (2017). Chapter 9: Intracranial neoplasms. In J. R. Haaga, & D. T. Boll (Eds.),* CT and MRI of the whole body *(6th ed.) (p. 230). Elsevier.*

(cont'd)

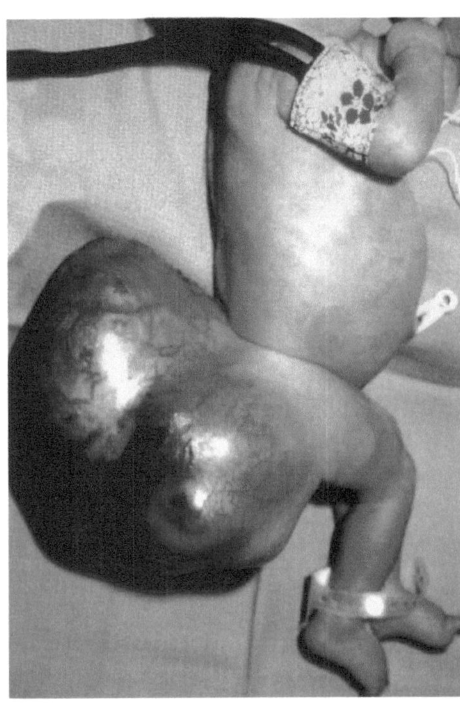

FIGURE 11.2 An infant with a sacrococcygeal teratoma. This location is the most common site for teratomas and is a site more often occurring in females. Source: *From Figure 1-1E, Schoenwolf, Bleyl, Brauer, & Francis-West. (2015).* Larson's human embryology *(5th ed.) (p. 17). Elsevier.*

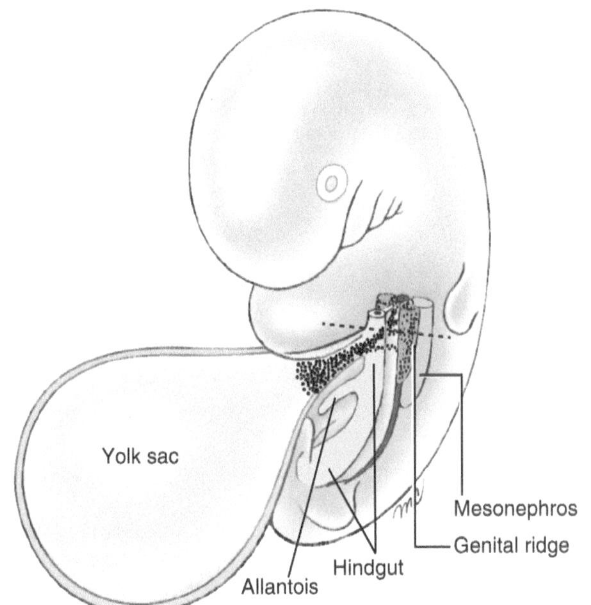

FIGURE 11.4 Migration of germ cells to the genital ridge where the gonads form. Migration is by pseudopodia on the germ cells. Unfortunately, some migrate to other areas of the body, usually along the midline. Source: *From Figure 1-1E, Schoenwolf, Bleyl, Brauer, & Francis-West. (2015).* Larson's human embryology *(5th ed.) (p. 17). Elsevier.*

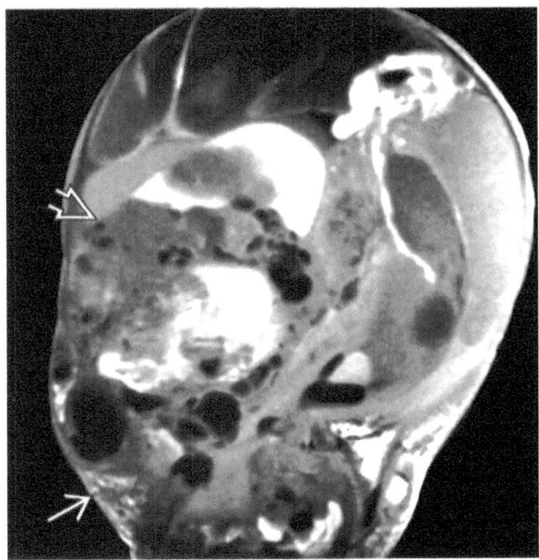

FIGURE 11.3 MRI of stillborn infant showing an immature teratoma which has completely replaced normal brain tissue and facial structures. Large arrow points to some of the soft tissue of the teratoma and the thinner arrow where the face should have been. Source: *From (No figure number) Osborn, A., & Thurnher, M. (2016). Teratoma. In Osborn, Salzman, & Jhaveri.* Diagnostic imaging: Brain *(3rd ed.) (p. 585). Elsevier.*

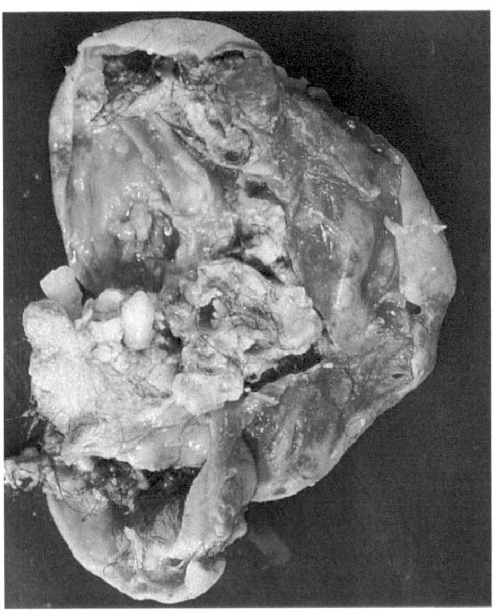

FIGURE 11.5 Mature ovarian teratoma. Teeth, blood vessels, and hair can be seen. Source: *From Figure 4-11 Damjanov, I. (2017).* Pathology for the health professions *(5th ed.) (p. 79). Elsevier.*

(cont'd)

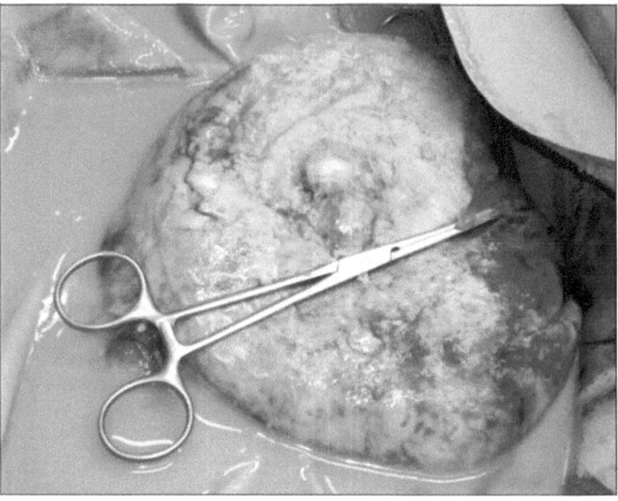

FIGURE 11.6 A ruptured mature cystic ovarian teratoma showing the liquid keratin that is the cystic fluid. Source: *From Figure 1, Hackethal, A., et al. (2008).* Lancet Oncology *9(12). (An Elsevier publication).*

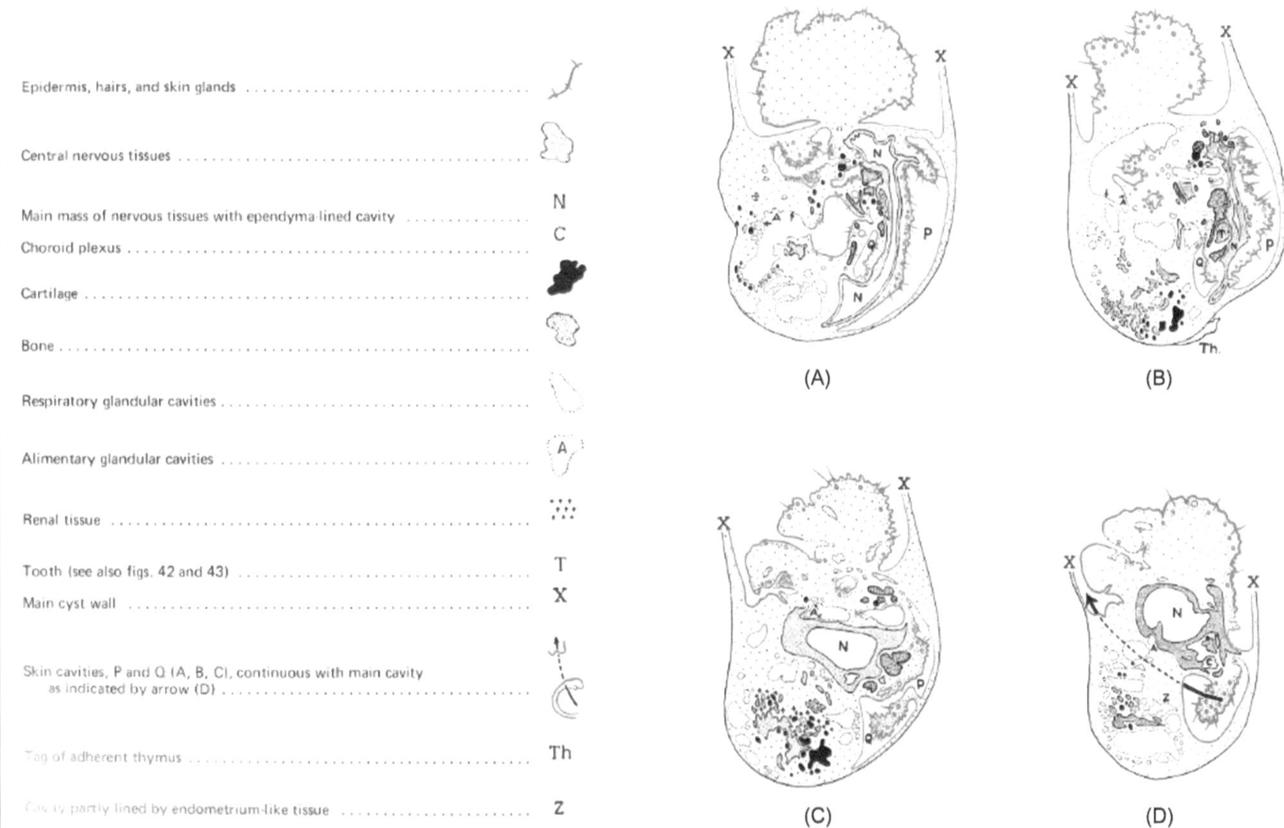

FIGURE 11.7 A drawing of an anterior mediastinal teratoma showing the different tissues. The teratoma was 10 cm. (A) through (D) Extragonadal teratomas. Source: *By Gonzales-Crussi, F. (1982). Armed Forces Institute of Pathology, Washington (pp. 84–85).*

(*cont'd*)

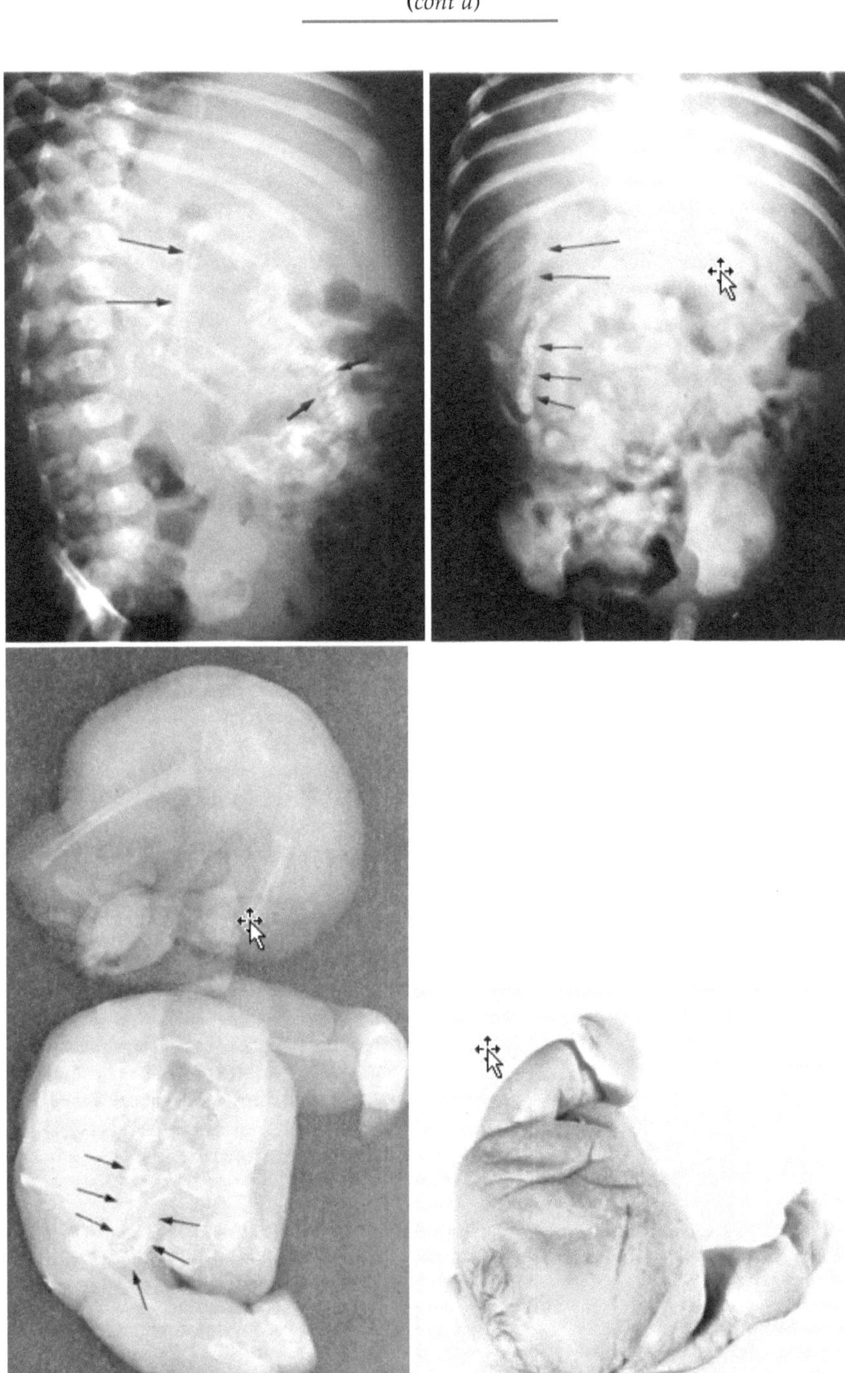

FIGURE 11.8 A large mature teratoma excised from a 6-week-old male child. Such large teratomas are sometimes called *fetus in fetu* teratomas. The long arrows in the top pictures point out long bones, while the short arrows denote the spine formations of the teratoma. The arrows in the lower picture show the outline of a primitive digestive tract using barium as the contrast medium. The excised teratoma is shown in the lower right. Source: *From Grosfeld, J.L., et al. (1974).* Annals of Surgery, 180, *80–84.*

In the clinic: sellar tumors

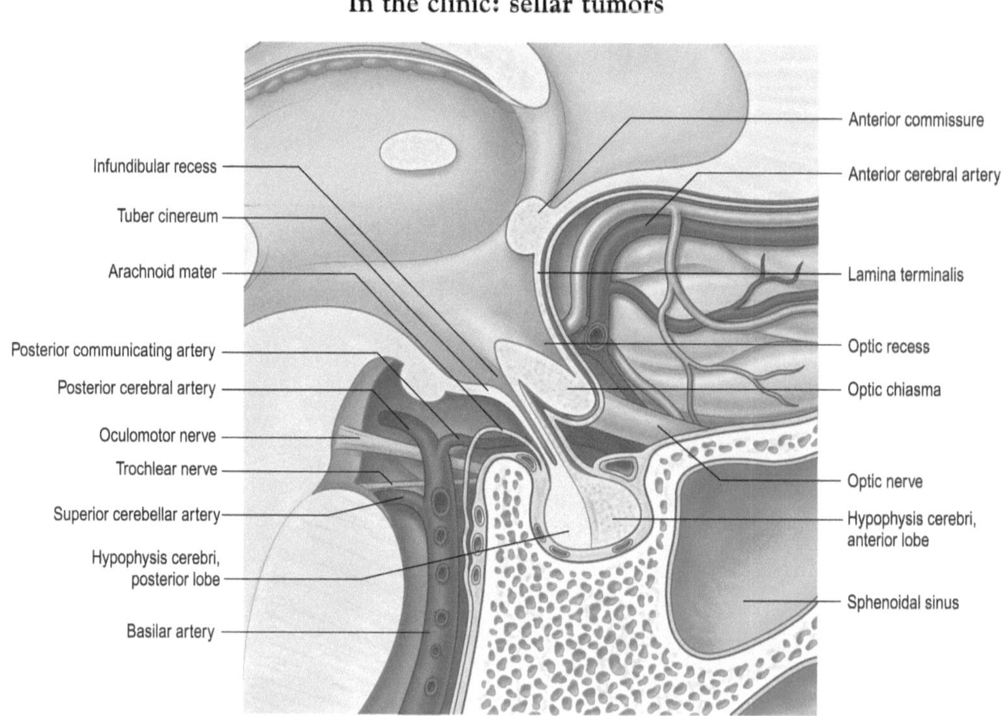

FIGURE 11.9 Sagittal section showing the two parts of the pituitary. Source: *From Figure 23-10, Standring. (2016).* Gray's anatomy *(41st ed.) (p. 360). Elsevier.*

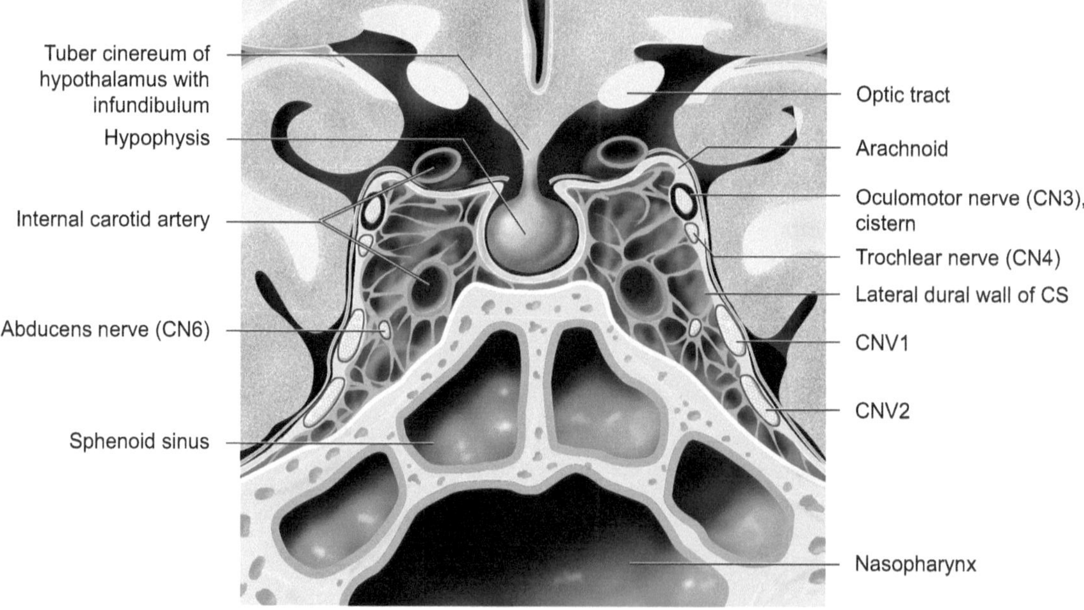

FIGURE 11.10 A coronal section shows the pituitary surrounded by the cavernous sinus and the tissues within. Source: *From (No figure number) Osborn, Salzman, & Jhaveri. (2016). Sella and pituitary.* Diagnostic imaging: Brain *(3rd ed.) (p. 1022). Elsevier.*

Introduction

The pituitary lies below the hypothalamus (hence its alternative name, hypophysis cerebri—Greek and Latin for "undergrowth of the brain"). It is surrounded by the venous cavernous sinus through which traverse the carotid artery and several cranial nerves (Figs. 11.9–11.11).

(cont'd)

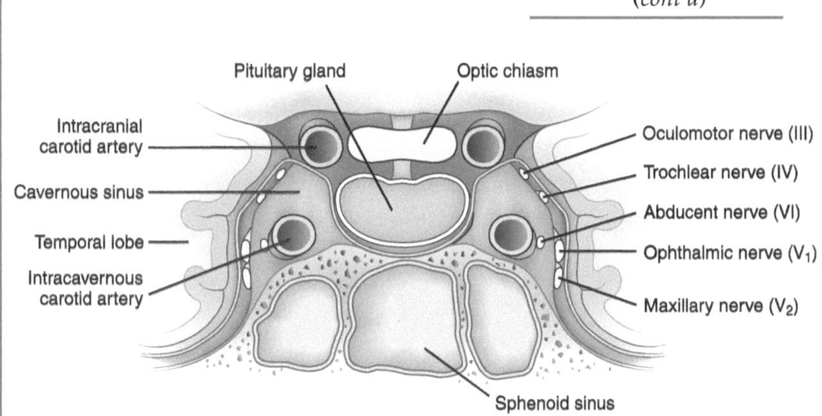

FIGURE 11.11 Another coronal view through the pituitary showing the surrounding structures in the cavernous sinus. Source: *From Figure 9-4 in Melmed, S., & Kleinberg, D. (2016). Chapter 9: Pituitary masses and tumors. In Melmed, Polonsky, Larsen, & Kronenberg (Eds.),* Williams' textbook of endocrinology *(13th ed.) (p. 237). Elsevier.*

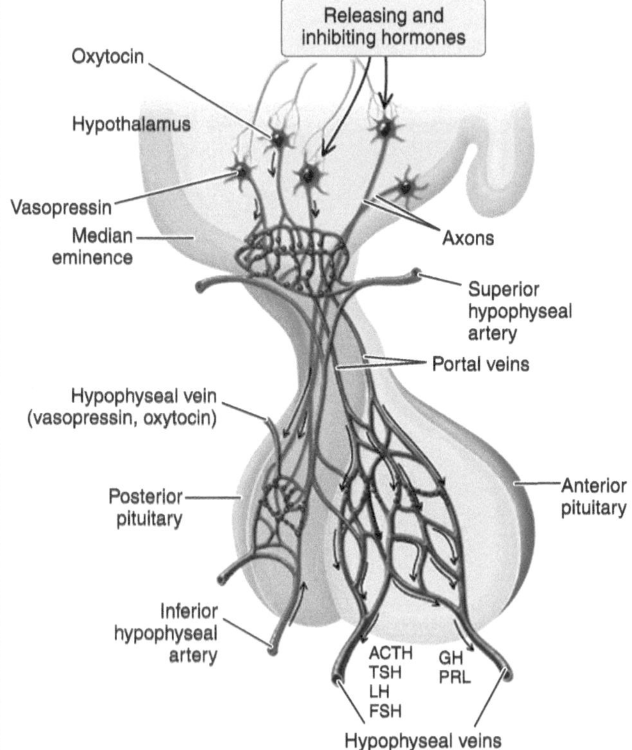

FIGURE 11.12 The connections of the pituitary to the hypothalamus. Source: *Figure 224-1 from Molitch, M. E. (2016). Chapter 224: Anterior pituitary. In Goldman, & Schafer (Eds.),* Goldman-Cecil medicine *(25th ed.) (p. 1480). Elsevier.*

The pituitary lies below the hypothalamus and is connected by the infundibulum (pituitary stalk). The posterior pituitary is an extension of the hypothalamus and is connected to it by the hypothalamic–hypophyseal tract. The anterior pituitary receives hormonal releasing or inhibitory hormones from the hypothalamus via the hypothalamic hypophyseal portal system (Fig. 11.12).

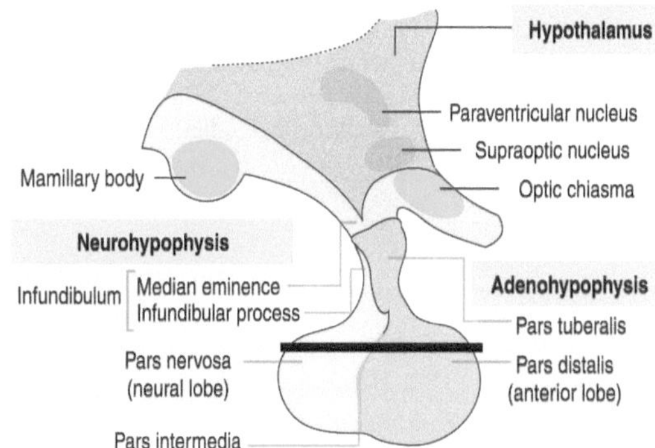

FIGURE 11.13 Parts of the pituitary. The heavy black line is the section through which the image below (Fig. 11.14) was taken but from the horizontal plane and not the sagittal plane. Source: *From Figure 18.1 in Kierszenbaum, & Tres. (2016).* Histology and cell biology: An introduction to pathology *(4th ed.) (p. 559). Elsevier.*

The anterior pituitary comprises 70%–80% of the total pituitary mass (Fig. 11.13 and 11.14).

For physiological and clinical purposes the horizontal section of the anterior pituitary is divided into two wings and a central wedge portion. The wings contain acidophilic cells and produce prolactin and growth hormone (GH) while the central area contains basophilic cells and produces corticotropin (ACTH) and thyrotropin (TSH) (Fig. 11.15). FSH and LH are produced throughout the anterior pituitary.

The sellar, suprasellar, and parasellar regions are among the most common sites for intracranial neoplasms. These can be of two physiological types: null or active and two histological types: microadenomas or macroadenomas. Microadenomas are usually active and secrete hormones. These tumors will be found where its cell type is normally located. Macroadenomas are usually null but grow and displace normal tissue. Null tumors are composed of cells that either are

(*cont'd*)

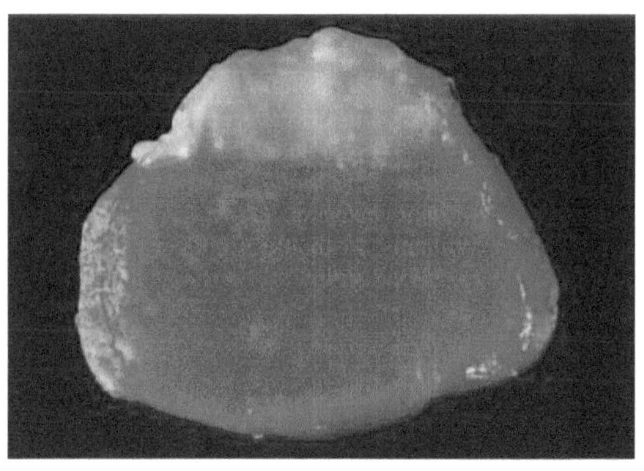

FIGURE 11.14 A horizontal section (*black band* in Fig. 11.13) of an unfixed adult pituitary showing a lighter posterior pituitary (top) and a more vascular red anterior pituitary (bottom) with a few cells from the pars intermedia which is nonfunctional in humans. Source: *From Figure 12.1 in Lopes, Pernicone, Scheithauer, Horvath, & Kovacs. (2012). Chapter 12: Pituitary and sellar region. In S. Mills (Ed.),* Histology for pathologists *(4th ed.) (p. 344). Wolters Kluwer.*

undifferentiated or lack specific receptors to cause the release of hormones. Null neoplasms can occur in any region of the anterior pituitary. Most neoplasms in the sellar area are null and only cause clinical problems because of a mass effect in which adjacent structures are compressed. The progression of tumor formation is shown in Fig. 11.16 and at the molecular level in Fig. 11.17.

Table 11.1 lists some of the factors that predispose a patient to a pituitary tumor and Table 11.2 indicates some of the genes that are involved.

Signs and symptoms

Neurological, endocrinological, and visual disturbances are the hallmarks of tumors in this area. Neurological manifestations include headaches, irritability, seizures (rare), and, if cranial nerves are involved, deficits of their functions. Endocrinological manifestations

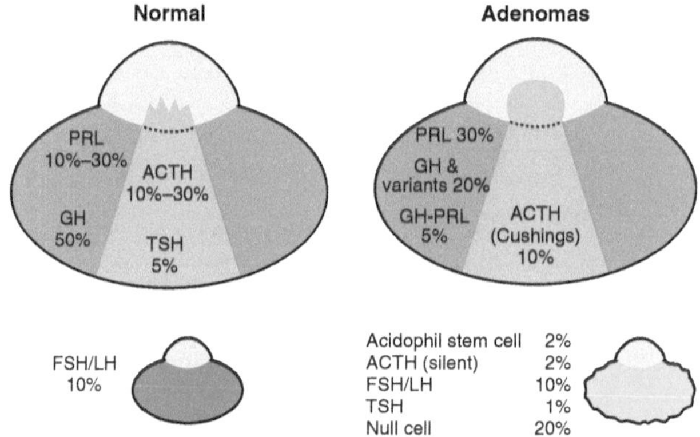

FIGURE 11.15 The schematic location of normal cells in the anterior pituitary and the location of adenomas. The posterior pituitary is the yellow structure atop the anterior pituitary. The microadenomas are usually in the same location as the normal cells.

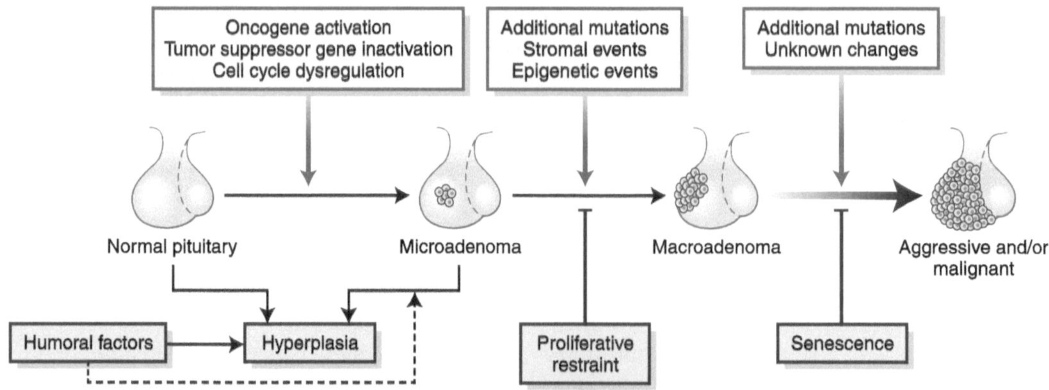

FIGURE 11.16 The progression of tumor formation. Source: *From Figure 9-16 in Melmed, S., & Kleinberg, D. (2016). Chapter 9: Pituitary masses and tumors. In Melmed, Polonsky, Larsen, & Kronenberg (Eds.),* Williams' textbook of endocrinology *(13th ed.) (p. 254). Elsevier.*

(cont'd)

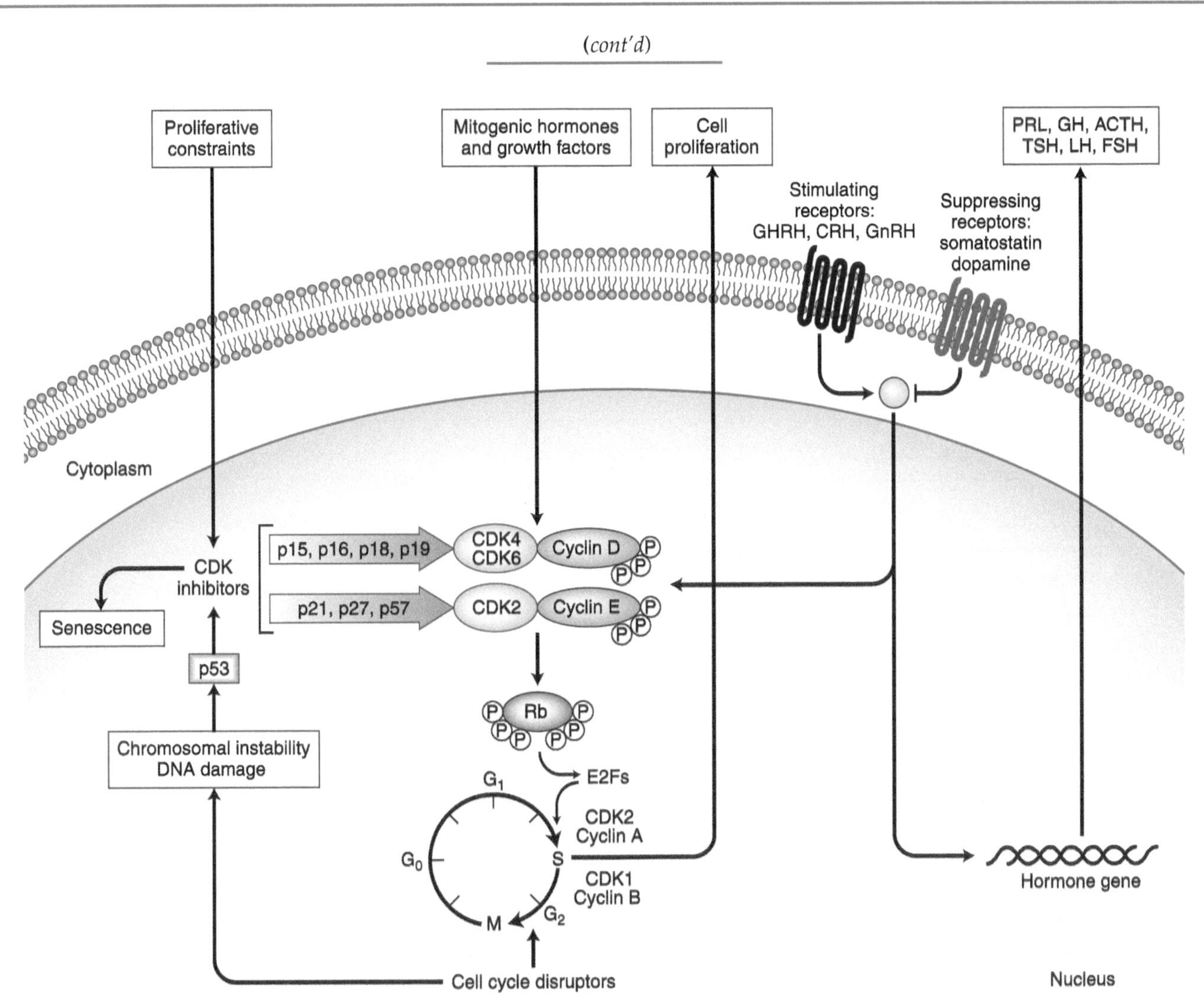

FIGURE 11.17 The transformation of a cell from normal to abnormal at the molecular level. Source: *From Figure 9-17 in Melmed, S., & Kleinberg, D. (2016). Chapter 9: Pituitary masses and tumors. In Melmed, Polonsky, Larsen, & Kronenberg (Eds.),* Williams' textbook of endocrinology *(13th ed.) (p. 254). Elsevier.*

depend on whether the cell is active or null. If active, the effects of hypersecretion of the hormone, such as GH, will become clinically manifest as, for example, in Robert Wadlow, the clinical case in Chapter 1, Introduction. If it is a null macroadenoma, this tumor can compress normal pituitary cells so that they are nonfunctional or even destroyed resulting, for example, in a pituitary dwarf if GH is suppressed from birth or if there is a discordinance between bone age and chronologic age, as with the case at the beginning of this chapter (however, the patient in that case did not have a macroadenoma, but a teratoma). Visual disturbances are the result of the proximity of the optic chiasma (Fig. 11.18).

Compression of the optic chiasma itself results in bitemporal hemianopia as well as in visual field fusion failure (Figs. 11.19 and 11.20).

Diagnosis

MRI is best because CT often misses small tumors. MRI should be T1 weighted and preferably with a contrast IV infusion with gadolinium which will enhance the contrast

(cont'd)

TABLE 11.1 Factors involved in pituitary tumor pathogenesis.

Hereditary
MEN1 Transcription factor defect (e.g., PROP1 excess) Carney complex AIP mutations
Hypothalamic
Excess GHRH or CRH production Receptor activation Dopamine deprivation
Pituitary
Signal transduction mutations or constitutive activation (e.g., GSP, CREB, and McCune-Albright syndrome) Disrupted paracrine growth factor or cytokine action (e.g., FGF2, FGF4, LIF, BMP, and EGF) Activated oncogene or cell cycle disruption (e.g., PTTG, RAS, P27, and HMG) Intrapituitary paracrine hypothalamic hormone action (e.g., GHRH and TRH) Loss of tumor suppressor gene function with LOH (11q13, 13, and GADD45γ)
Environmental
Estrogens Irradiation
Peripheral
Target failure (ovary, thyroid, adrenal) Ectopic hypothalamic hormone secretion
Evidence for an intrinsic pituitary defect in the pathogenesis of pituitary tumors
Pituitary adenomas are monoclonal There is no hyperplasia surrounding the adenomas Surgical resection of well-circumscribed small adenomas leads to control in ~75% of patients Unrestrained pituitary hormonal hypersecretion persists independently of feedback regulation by elevated target hormones Hormonal pulsatility pattern is often restored after adenoma resection

CRH, corticotropin releasing hormone; *GHRH*, growth-hormone-releasing hormone.
Source: *Modified from Melmed S. (2009). Acromegaly pathogenesis and treatment.* Journal of Clinical Investigation *119, 3189–3202; and Melmed, S. (2011). Pathogenesis of pituitary tumors.* Nature Reviews Endocrinology *7, 257–266. Table 9-11, in Melmed, S., & Kleinberg, D. (2016). Chapter 9: Pituitary masses and tumors. In Melmed, Polonsky, Larsen, & Kronenberg (Eds.),* Williams' textbook of endocrinology *(13th ed.) (p. 253). Elsevier.*

between soft tissue and spaces. In addition, serum levels of pituitary hormones should be obtained as well as documenting bone age with standard radiographs of the patient's hands. Any macroadenoma or other sellar, parasellar, or suprasellar tumor will also affect the optic chiasm as was noted previously.

Management

Transsphenoidal is the most common unless it is suprasellar or parasellar in which case a lateral incision is made through the fontal bone. Transsphenoidal hypophyseal resection is not new, being first performed in 1907 and refined by Harvey Cushing from 1910 to 1925. He did a sublabial approach entering the nose by going above the upper lip (Fig. 11.21).

Newer techniques with less morbidity involve an endonasal endoscopic microsurgical approach which goes completely through the nasal cavity, thus avoiding oral microorganisms and the need for packing the nasal cavity (Fig. 11.22).

Prognosis

With a skilled neurosurgical team, there should be an excellent recovery unless the tumor was malignant and the prognosis would then depend on the type and extent of the malignancy. There may be some short-term side effects due to the surgery, such as transient diabetes insipidus or inappropriate ADH secretion which are the most commonly encountered.

(*cont'd*)

TABLE 11.2 Selected genes associated with molecular pathogenesis of pituitary adenomas.

Gene	Function	Mode of activation or inactivation	Clinical context
GNAS	Oncogene	Activating, imprinting	Nonfamilial, syndromic or sporadic
CREB	Transcription factor	Constitutive phosphorylation	Sporadic
AIP	Tumor suppressor	Inactivating	Familial, syndromic
MEN1	Tumor suppressor	Inactivating	Familial, syndromic
PRKAR1A	Tumor suppressor	Inactivating	Familial, syndromic
H-Ras	Oncogene	Activating	Invasive or malignant
CCNB2	Cyclin	Induced by *HMGA*	Sporadic
CCND1	Oncogene	Overexpression	Sporadic
CDKNIB	Cyclin-dependent kinase inhibitor	Inactivating	Sporadic, syndromic
HMGA2	Oncogene	Overexpression	Sporadic
FGFR4	Oncogene	Alternative transcription	Sporadic
PTTG	Securin	Overexpression	Sporadic
Rb	Tumor suppressor	Epigenetic silencing	Sporadic
CDKN2A	Cyclin-dependent kinase inhibitor	Epigenetic silencing	Sporadic
BRG1	Tumor suppressor	Glucocorticoid receptor function	Sporadic
GADD45G	Proliferation inhibitor	Epigenetic silencing	Sporadic
MEG3	Proliferation inhibitor	Epigenetic silencing	Sporadic

Table 9.12 modified from Melmed, S. (2009). Acromegaly pathogenesis and treatment. Journal of Clinical Investigation *119(11), 3189–3202; used with permission of the American Society for Clinical Investigation. in Melmed, S., & Kleinberg, D. (2016). Chapter 9: Pituitary masses and tumors. In Melmed, Polonsky, Larsen, & Kronenberg (Eds.),* Williams' textbook of endocrinology *(13th ed.) (p. 255). Elsevier.*

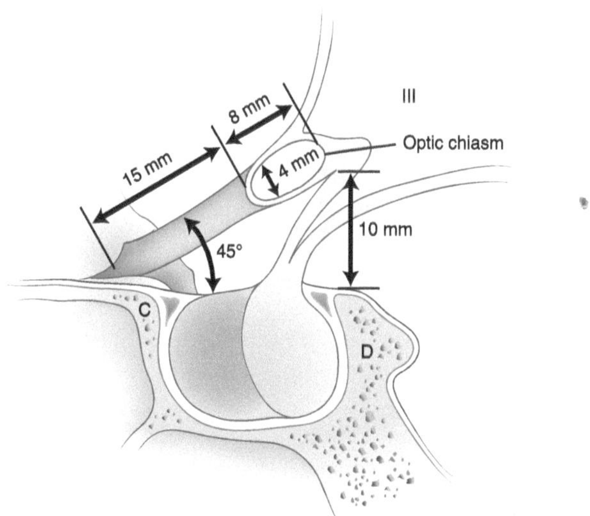

FIGURE 11.18 A sagittal view showing the angles and associations with structures above the pituitary. Source: *From Figure 9-5 in Melmed, S., & Kleinberg, D. (2016). Chapter 9: Pituitary masses and tumors. In Melmed, Polonsky, Larsen, & Kronenberg (Eds.),* Williams' textbook of endocrinology *(13th ed.) (p. 237). Elsevier.*

(cont'd)

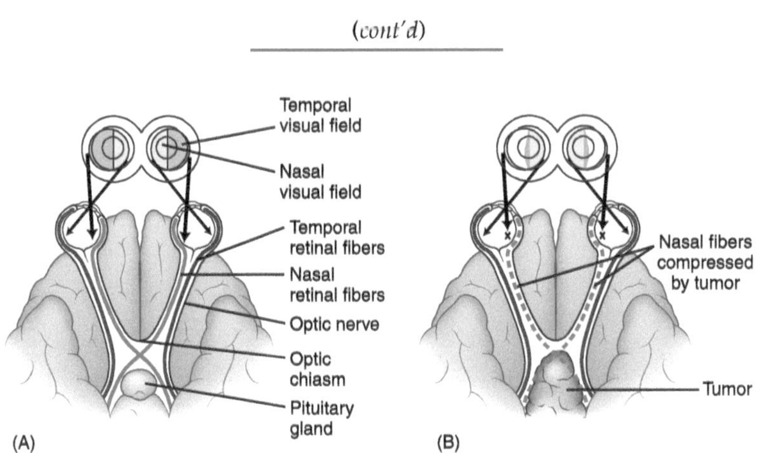

FIGURE 11.19 The visual pathway that is (A) normal and (B) compromised because a tumor at the optic chiasm has affected the visual pathway from both nasal retinas resulting in bitemporal hemianopia (literally, in Greek, "half no vision") in which the patient has limited or no vision from either temporal visual field resulting in limited or no peripheral vision (i.e., tunnel vision). Source: *From Figure 9-6A and C in Melmed, S., & Kleinberg, D. (2016). Chapter 9: Pituitary masses and tumors. In Melmed, Polonsky, Larsen, & Kronenberg (Eds.),* Williams' textbook of endocrinology *(13th ed.) (p. 238). Elsevier.*

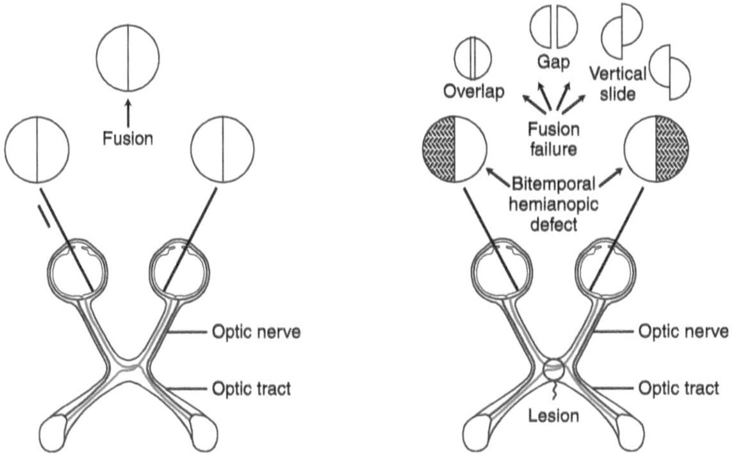

FIGURE 11.20 Fusion failure due to a lesion compressing the optic chiasm. Source: *From Figure 9-6 B and C in Melmed, S., & Kleinberg, D. (2016). Chapter 9: Pituitary masses and tumors. In Melmed, Polonsky, Larsen, & Kronenberg (Eds.),* Williams' textbook of endocrinology *(13th ed.) (p. 238). Elsevier.*

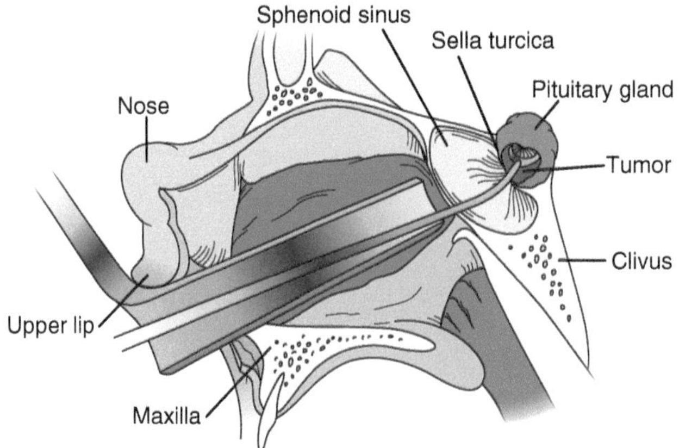

FIGURE 11.21 Sublabial approach for endonasal approach to resecting a pituitary tumor. The perpendicular plate of the ethmoid bone is partly removed and nasal cartilage pushed aside. The surgeon goes through the palatine process of the maxillary bone. A curette is shown inserted in the speculum to remove the tumor.

(*cont'd*)

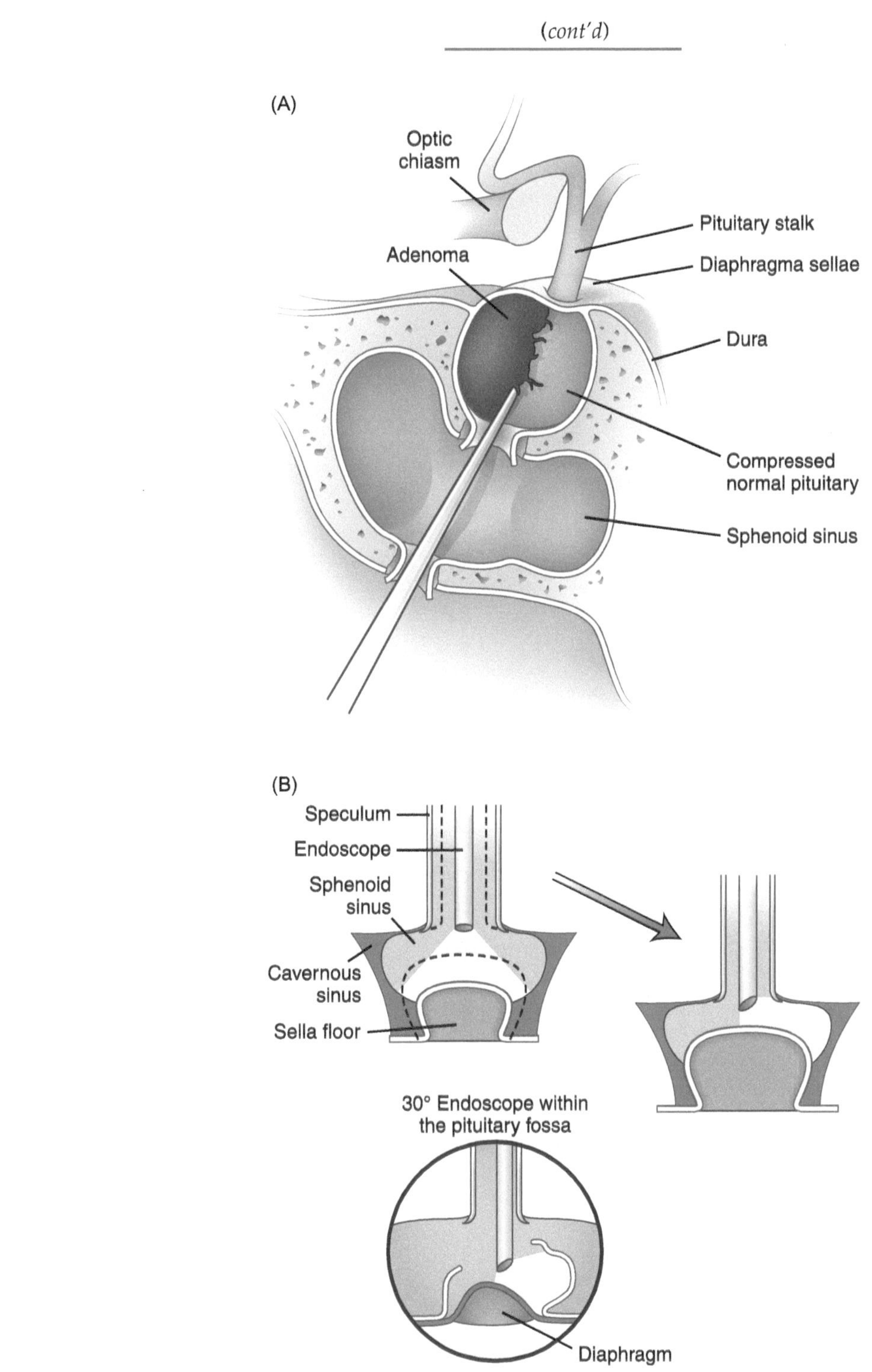

FIGURE 11.22 Endonasal endoscopic microsurgical transsphenoidal approach to removing a tumor. Source: *From Figures 9-9 and 9-10 in Melmed, S., & Kleinberg, D. (2016). Chapter 9: Pituitary masses and tumors. In Melmed, Polonsky, Larsen, & Kronenberg (Eds.),* Williams' textbook of endocrinology *(13th ed.) (p. 238). Elsevier.*

Hormonal control of growth

The simple word "growth" describes a variety of processes, both living and nonliving, that share the common feature of increase in mass. For purposes of this chapter, we limit the definition of growth to mean the organized addition of new tissue that occurs normally in development from infancy to adulthood. This process is complex and depends on the interplay of genetic, nutritional, and environmental influences as well as actions of the endocrine system. Growth of an individual or an organ involves increases both in cell number and cell size, differentiation of cells to perform highly specialized functions, and tissue remodeling that may require apoptosis as well as new cell formation. Most of these processes depend on locally produced growth factors that operate through paracrine or autocrine mechanisms. Many continue to operate throughout life providing not only for cell renewal but also for adaptations to meet changing physiological demands. Dozens of families of growth factors have been described, and an unknown number of others await discovery. Regulation of growth by the endocrine system can be viewed as the coordination of local growth processes with the overall development of the individual and with external environmental influences. This chapter describes the major hormones that play important roles in growth and their interactions at critical times in development.

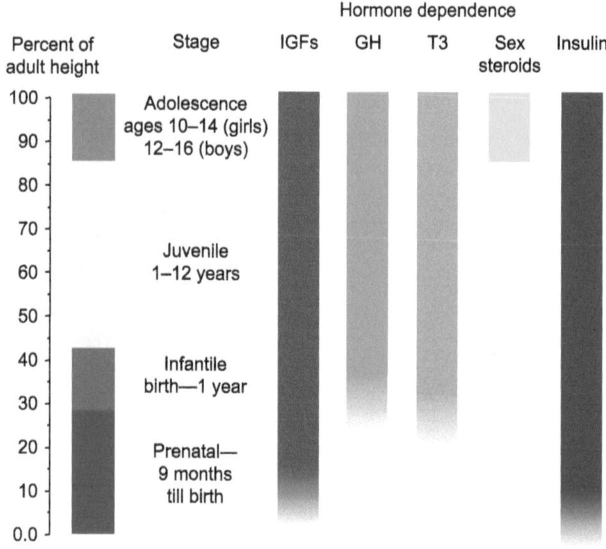

FIGURE 11.23 Hormonal regulation of growth at different stages of life. *GH*, Growth hormone; *IGFs*, insulin-like growth factors; *T3*, triiodothyronine.

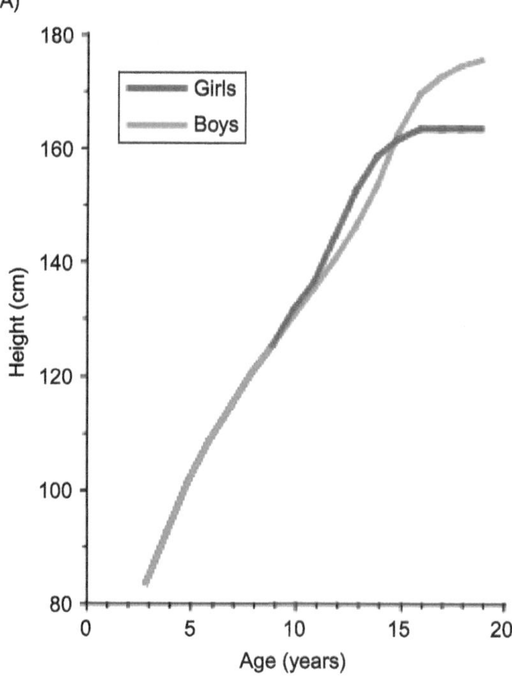

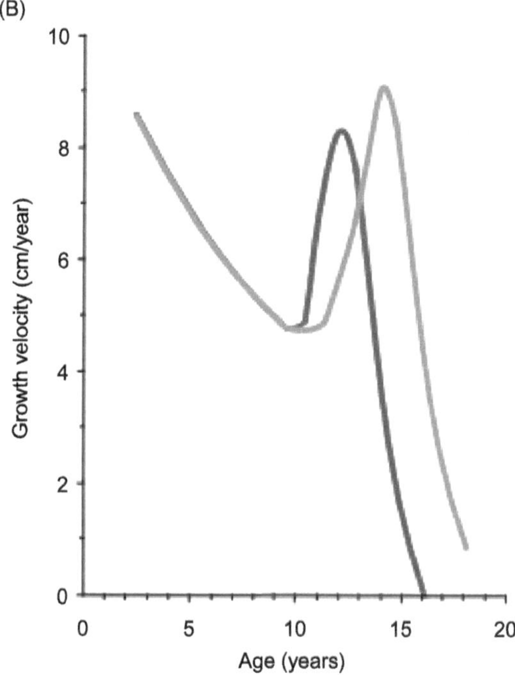

FIGURE 11.24 (A) Typical growth curves for young males and females. Note that growth is not linear and that it proceeds at the same rate in juvenile boys and girls. At puberty, which begins earlier in girls than in boys, there is a spurt in growth that immediately precedes growth arrest. (B) Nonlinearity of growth is more clearly evident when plotted as changes in growth velocity over time. Note that growth, which is very rapid in the newborn, slows during the juvenile period and accelerates at puberty.

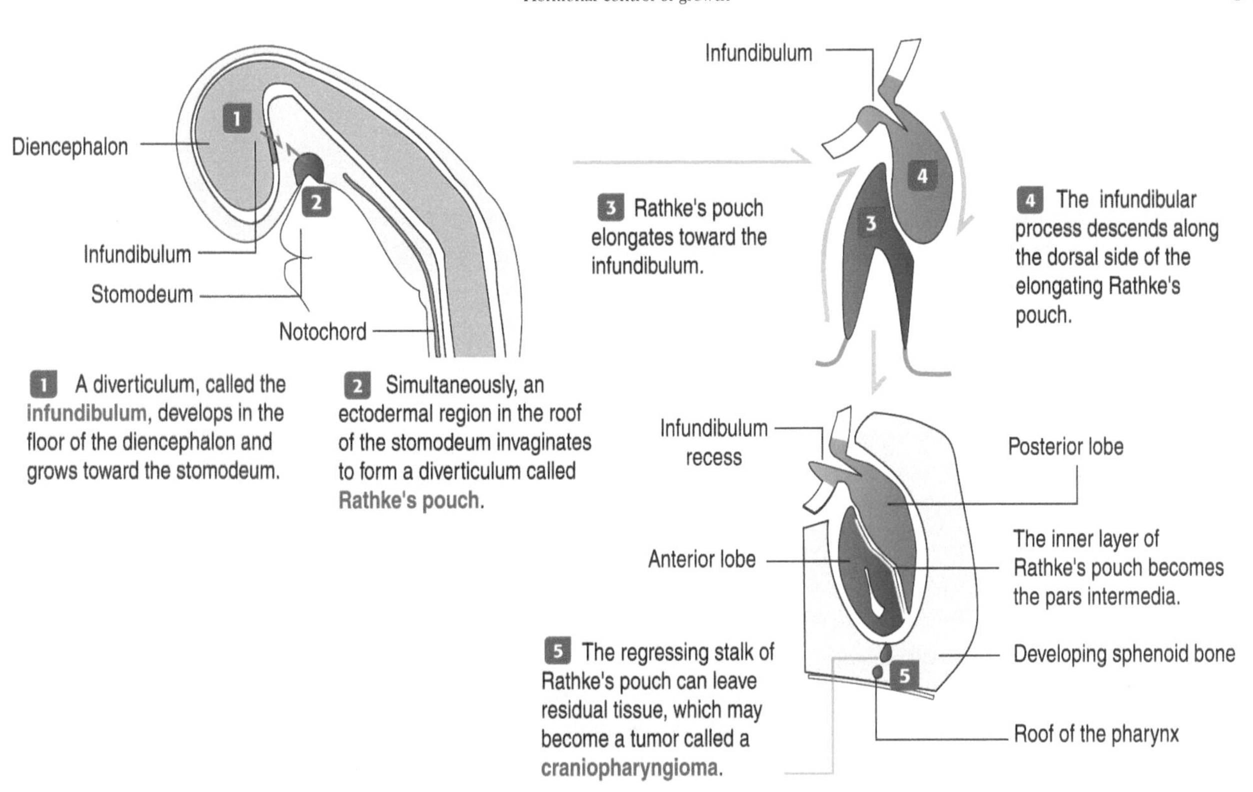

FIGURE 11.25 The development of the pituitary gland from the nasopharynx and an extension of the hypothalamus. Source: *From Figure 18-2 in Kierszenbaum, & Tres. (2016).* Histology and cell biology: An introduction to pathology *(4th ed.) (p. 560). Elsevier.*

Growth is most rapid during prenatal life. In only 9 months, body length increases from just a few micrometers to almost 30% of final adult height. The growth rate decelerates after birth but during the first year of life is rapid enough that the infant increases half again in height to about 45% of final adult stature. Thereafter growth decelerates and continues at a slower rate, about 2 in./year until puberty. Steady growth during this juvenile period contributes the largest fraction, about 40%, to final adult height. With the onset of sexual development, growth accelerates to about twice the juvenile rate and contributes about 15%–18% of final adult height before stopping altogether (Figs. 11.23 and 11.24).

Our understanding of hormonal influences on growth is limited largely to the juvenile and adolescent periods, but emerging information is providing insight into the regulation of prenatal growth, which is largely independent of the classic hormones. During the juvenile period the influence of growth hormone (GH) is preeminent, but appropriate secretion of thyroid and adrenal hormones and insulin is essential for optimal growth. The adolescent growth spurt reflects the added input of androgens and estrogens, which speed up growth, and the maturation of bone that brings it to a halt.

The pituitary and growth

The pituitary gland exerts the greatest influence on growth. Embryologically, it is formed from both nasal and nervous tissue. A fingerlike projection of nasal tissue, Rathke's pouch, juts upward to envelop an infundibulum (funnel) of nervous tissue which descends downward (Fig. 11.25).

The hypothalamus has complete control over the secretions of the pituitary gland, as was described in Chapter 2, Pituitary Gland, and can be seen in Fig. 11.26.

GH, also called somatotropin (STH), is the most important hormone required for normal growth. Attainment of adult size is dependent on GH; in its absence, growth is severely limited (Fig. 11.49). GH does not act directly on tissues but instead stimulates the liver to produce insulin growth factor-1 (IGF-1, formerly called somatomedin C) which then stimulates tissues (Fig. 11.27).

GH does act on tissues to actively on cells to take up certain amino acids. GH secretion is inhibited by somatostatin (Fig. 11.28).

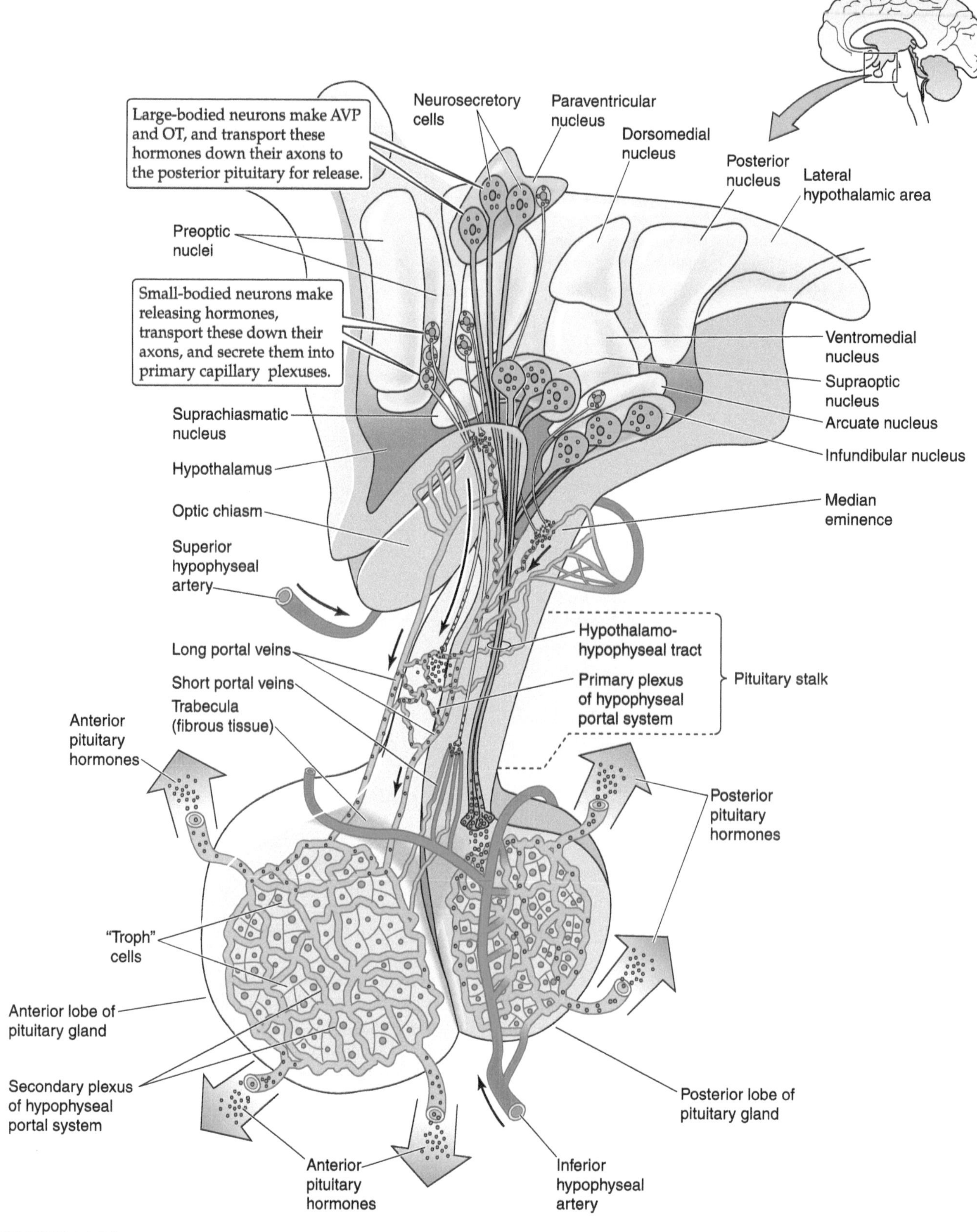

FIGURE 11.26 Pituitary–hypothalamus relationship. The anterior pituitary is regulated by releasing or inhibitory hormones released into the blood by hypothalamic nuclei; the posterior pituitary releases hormones synthesized in the hypothalamus. Source: *From Figure 47-3 in Barrett, E. J. (2017). Chapter 47: Organization of endocrine control. In W. F. Boron, & E. L. Boulpaep (Eds.),* Medical physiology *(3rd ed.) (p. 980). Elsevier.*

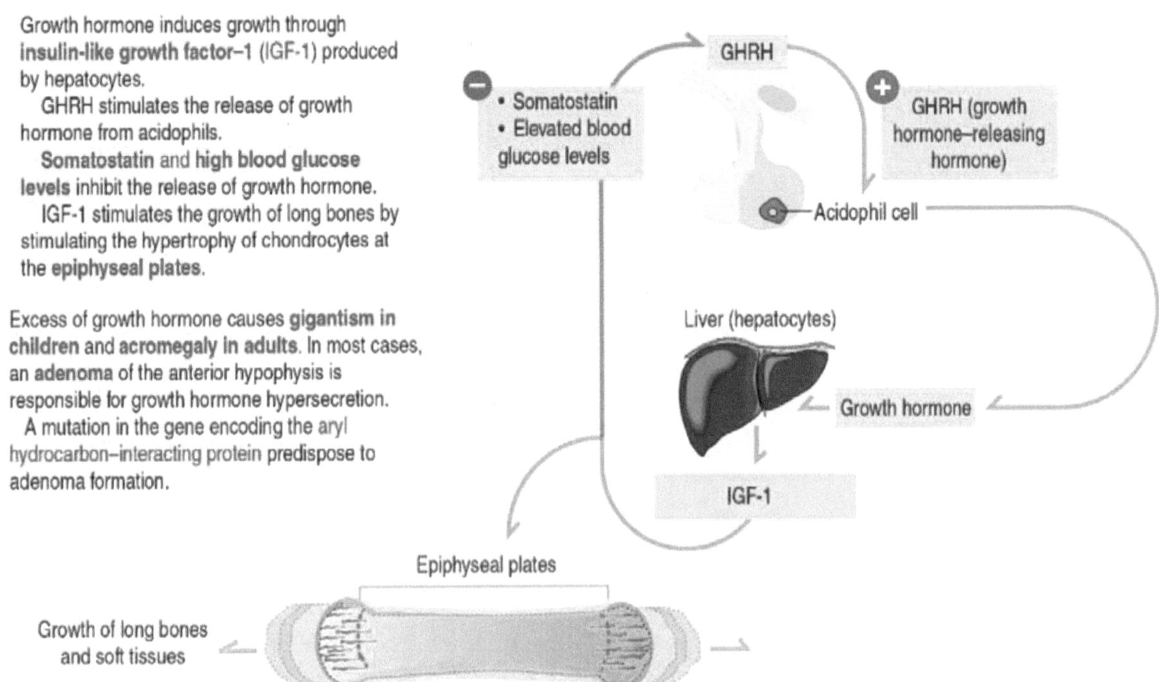

FIGURE 11.27 Production of GH is initiated by growth-hormone-releasing hormone. GH stimulates the liver to produce IGF-1 (also called somatomedin C) which stimulates the elongation of the epiphyseal plates of bones. IGF-1 feeds back to stimulate somatostatin, which inhibits the release of growth-hormone-releasing hormone. *GH*, Growth hormone. Source: *From Figure 18-6 in Kierszenbaum, & Tres. (2016).* Histology and cell biology: An introduction to pathology *(4th ed.) (p. 564). Elsevier.*

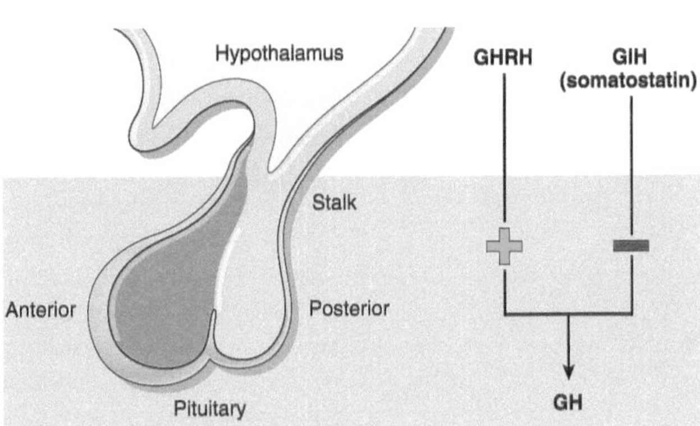

FIGURE 11.28 The hypothalamic hormones that stimulate and inhibit the secretion of GH by the anterior pituitary. *GH*, Growth hormone. Source: *From Figure 24-1, Maitra, A. (2015). Chapter 24: The endocrine system. In Kumar, Abbas, & Aster (Eds.),* Robbins and cotran pathologic basis of disease *(9th ed.) (p. 107). Elsevier.*

At the molecular level—boxed material for additional information

Growth hormone (GH), like other peptide hormones, is synthesized as a preprohormone in the rough ER. This is reduced to the prohormone and to the final hormone in the Golgi Complex where two products emerge one with 191 amino acids and another with 176 amino acids (Fig. 11.29).

Both forms (the 191 and 176 amino acid forms) of GH act on the same receptors but the 176-amino acid version may not exert all the effects on tissues that the larger version does. GH is secreted by somatotrophs (the pituitary cells that secrete GH) in bursts throughout a 24-h period (Fig. 11.30).

(*cont'd*)

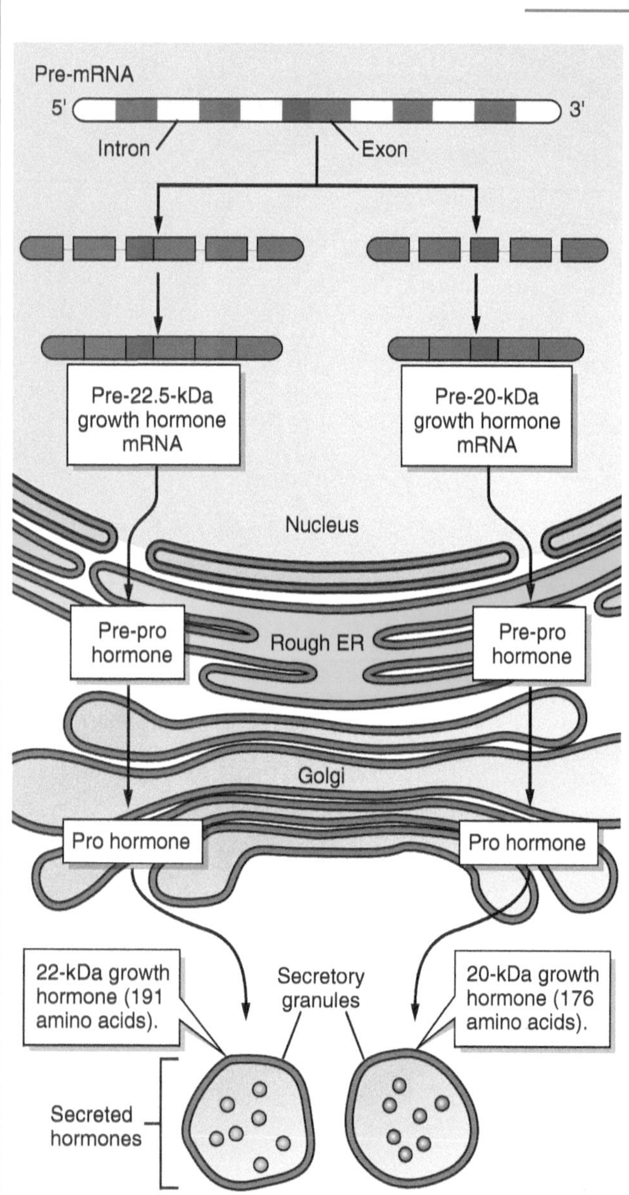

FIGURE 11.29 Synthesis of growth hormone.

GH secretion is controlled primarily by the hypothalamus (Fig. 11.31).

And there is feedback from insulin-like growth factor (IGF-1), also called somatomedin C, which is produced by the liver in response to GH (Fig. 11.32).

Because IGF-1 secretion is dependent on GH stimulation, IGF-1 levels in plasma are used to indirectly determine GH secretion.

IGF-1 (somatomedin C)

IGF-1[1] is a blood-borne substance that activates chondrogenesis and perhaps other GH-dependent growth processes in other tissues. This substance was originally named somatomedin C (somatotropin mediator—chondrogenesis) and, upon purification, was found to consist of two closely related substances that also produce an insulin-like activity that persists in plasma after insulin is removed by immunoprecipitation. These substances now are called insulin-like growth factors, or IGF-1 and IGF-2. Of the two, IGF-1 is the more important mediator of the actions of GH and has been studied more thoroughly. The crucial role of IGF-1 as an intermediary in the growth-promoting action of GH is now firmly established.

In general, plasma concentrations of IGF-1 reflect the availability of GH on the rate of growth. They are higher than normal in blood of persons suffering from acromegaly and are very low in GH-deficient individuals. Children whose growth is more rapid than average have higher than average concentrations of IGF-1, whereas children at the lower extreme of normal have lower values. When GH is injected into GH-deficient patients or experimental animals, IGF-1 concentrations increase after a delay of about 4–6 h and remain elevated for more than a day. Children or adults who are resistant to GH because of a receptor defect have low concentrations of IGF-1 in their blood despite high concentrations of GH. Growth of these children is restored to nearly normal rates following daily the administration of IGF-1 (Fig. 11.33).

Disruption of the IGF-1 gene in mice causes severe growth retardation despite high concentrations of GH in their blood. Daily treatment with even large doses of GH does not accelerate their growth. Similarly, a child with a homozygous deletion of the IGF-1 gene suffered severe pre- and postnatal growth retardation that was partially corrected by daily treatment with IGF-1.

Although overwhelming evidence indicates that IGF-1 stimulates cartilage growth in the epiphyseal plates and many other tissues, production of IGF-1 is not limited to the liver and may be increased by GH in many tissues including cells in the epiphyseal growth plate. Direct infusion of small amounts of GH into epiphyseal cartilage of the proximal tibia in one leg of hypophysectomized

(*cont'd*)

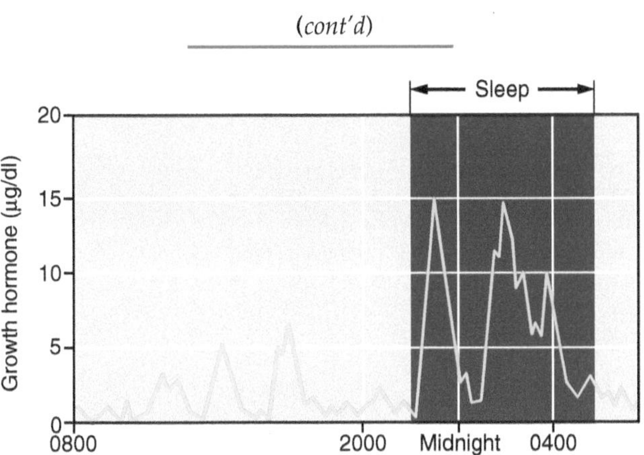

FIGURE 11.30 The pulsatile secretion of GH over a 24-h period. *GH*, Growth hormone.

rats was found to stimulate tibial growth of that limb but not of the contralateral limb. Only a direct action of GH on osteogenesis can explain such localized stimulation of growth, because IGF-1 that arises in the liver is equally available in the blood supply to both hind limbs.

GH stimulates prechondrocytes and other cells in the epiphyseal plates to synthesize and secrete IGFs, which act locally in an autocrine or paracrine manner to stimulate cell division, chondrocyte maturation, secretion of extracellular matrix proteins, and bone growth. Further evidence to support this conclusion includes findings of receptors for both GH and IGF-1 in chondrocytes in the epiphyseal plates along with the GH-dependent increase in mRNA for IGFs and IGF-1 receptors.

Growth of the long bones might be stimulated by IGF-1 that reaches them either through the circulation or by diffusion from local sites of production or a combination of the two. A genetic engineering approach was adopted to evaluate the relative importance of locally produced and blood-borne IGF-1. A line of mice was developed in which the IGF-1 gene was selectively disrupted only in hepatocytes. Concentrations of IGF-1 in the blood of these animals were severely reduced, but their growth and body proportions were no different from those of control animals that produced normal amounts of IGF-1 in their livers and had normal blood levels of IGF-1. These findings indicate that locally produced IGF-1 may be sufficient to account for normal growth and that IGF-1 in the circulation plays only a minor role in stimulating growth. However, the average concentration of GH in the blood of these genetically altered mice was considerably increased, consistent with the negative feedback effect of IGF-1 on GH secretion.

The current view of the relationship between GH and IGF-1 is summarized in Fig. 11.34.

GH acts directly on both the liver and its peripheral target tissues to promote IGF-1 production. Liver is the principal source of IGF in blood, but target tissues also make some contributions to circulating IGF. Stimulation of longitudinal growth is provided primarily by locally produced IGF-1 acting in an autocrine/paracrine manner, but circulating IGF-1 produced primarily in liver also contributes to overall bone growth, particularly in increasing bone diameter and thickening of the cortical region. A major function of blood-borne IGF is to regulate GH secretion.

Properties of the insulin-like growth factors

IGF-1 and IGF-2 are small, unbranched peptides that have molecular masses of about 7500 Da. They are encoded in separate genes located on chromosomes 12 and 11, respectively, and are expressed in a wide variety of cells. Although the regulatory elements and exon/intron architecture of their genes differ significantly, protein structures of the IGFs are very similar to each other and to proinsulin (see Chapter 7: The pancreatic islets), both in terms of amino acid sequence and in the arrangement of disulfide bonds (S–S) (Fig. 11.35). The IGFs share about 50% amino acid identity with the corresponding A and B chains of insulin (Fig. 11.36).

Where they differ is the receptor for IGF-1 and IGF-2. The IGF-1 receptor has tyrosine kinase which broadens the effect, whereas tyrosine kinase is absent in the IGF-2 receptor, indicating a more limited effect (Fig. 11.37). Both IGF-1 and IGF-2 can bind to the insulin receptor and the IGF-2 can bind to the IGF-1 receptor, but the affinity is not as great as when it binds to its own receptor.

(cont'd)

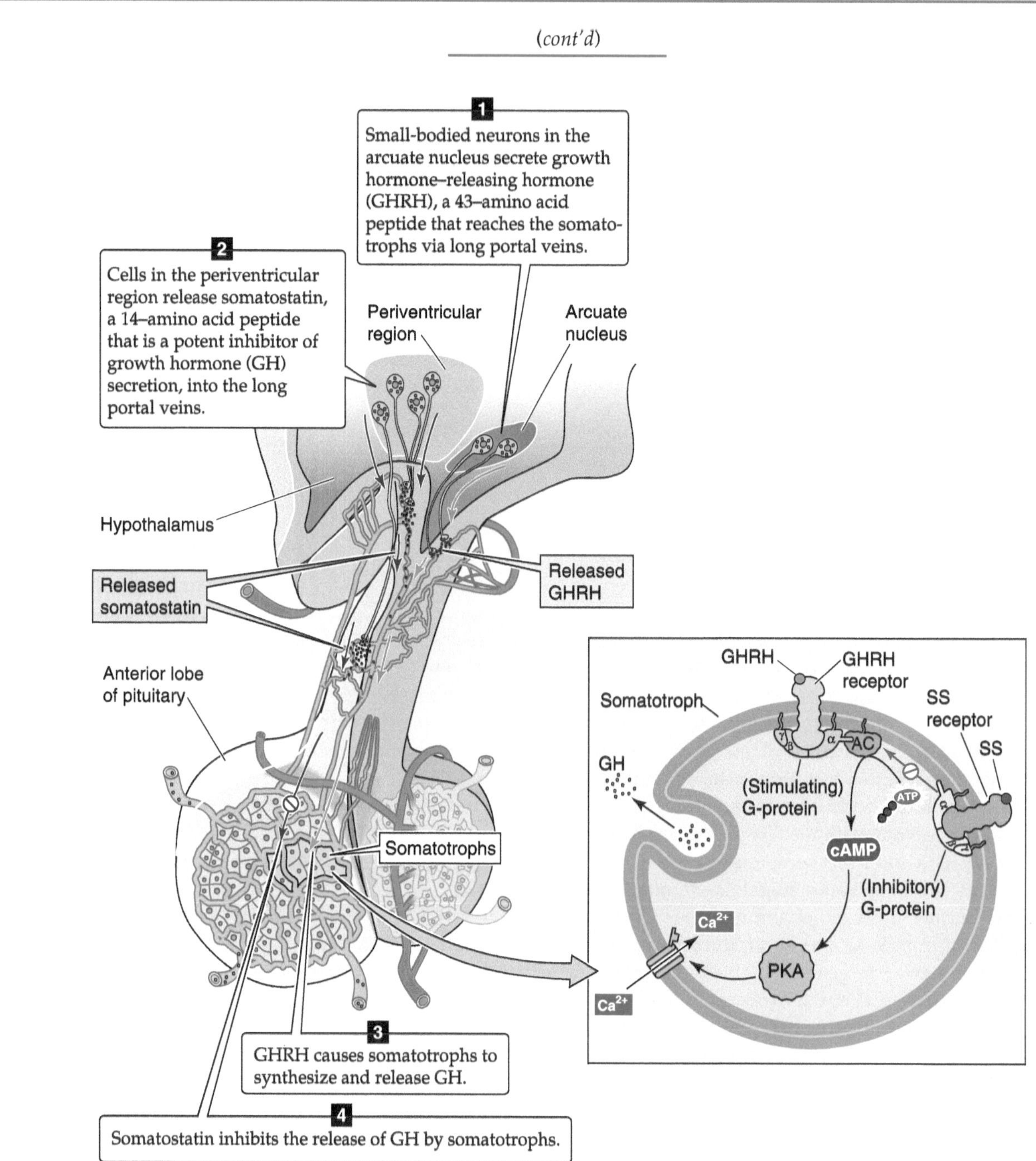

FIGURE 11.31 The hypothalamic hormones that stimulate and inhibit the release of growth hormone. Source: *From Figure 48-3 in Barrett, E. J. (2017). Chapter 48: Endocrine regulation of growth and body mass. In W. F. Boron, & E. L. Boulpaep (Eds.),* Medical physiology *(3rd ed.) (p. 993). Elsevier.*

(cont'd)

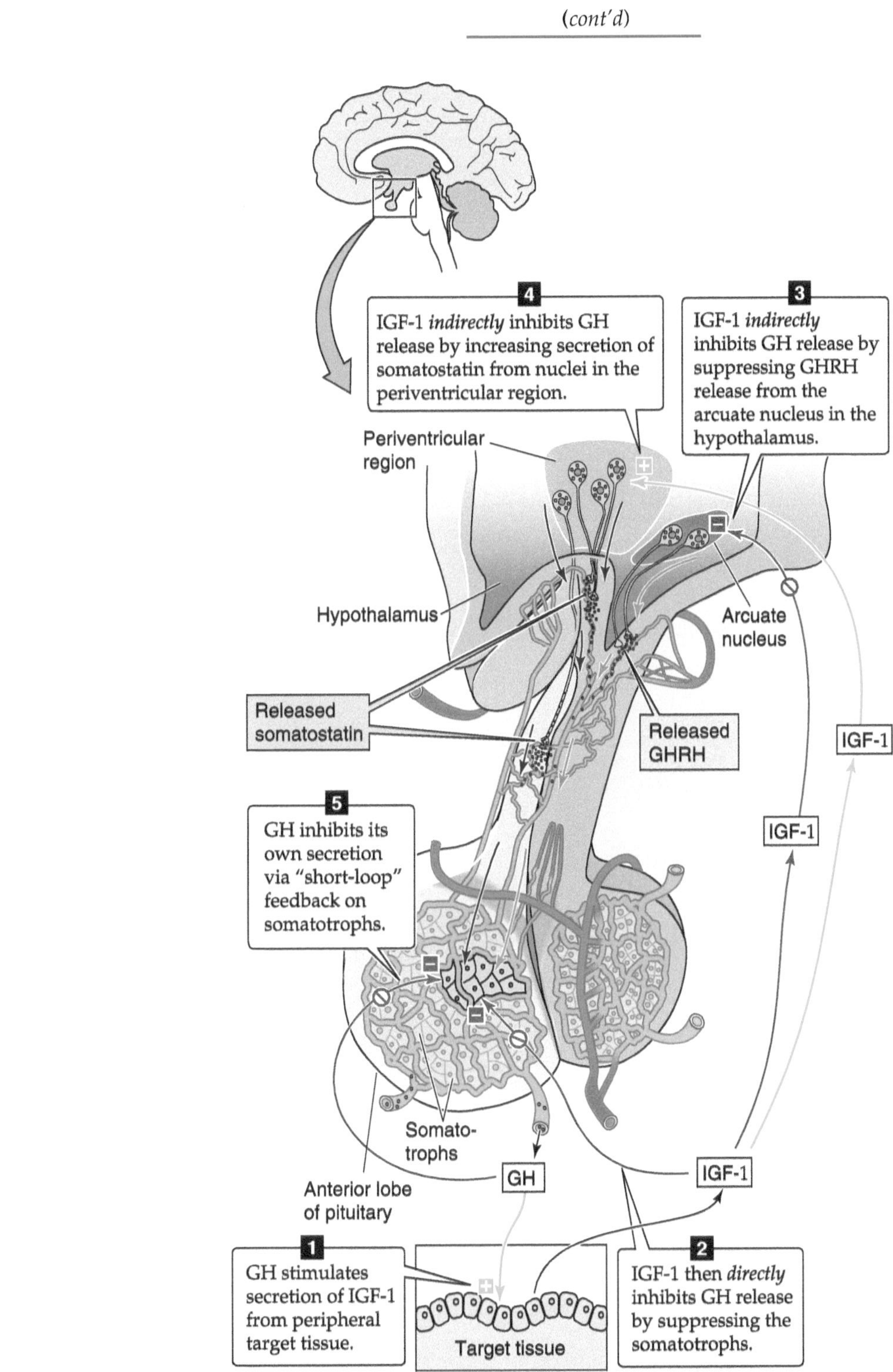

FIGURE 11.32 Feedback inhibition by both IGF-1 and GH help regulates the secretion of growth hormone. *GH*, Growth hormone. Source: *From Figure 48-4 in Barrett, E. J. (2017). Chapter 48: Endocrine regulation of growth and body mass. In W. F. Boron, & E. L. Boulpaep (Eds.),* Medical physiology *(3rd ed.) (p. 995). Elsevier.*

(cont'd)

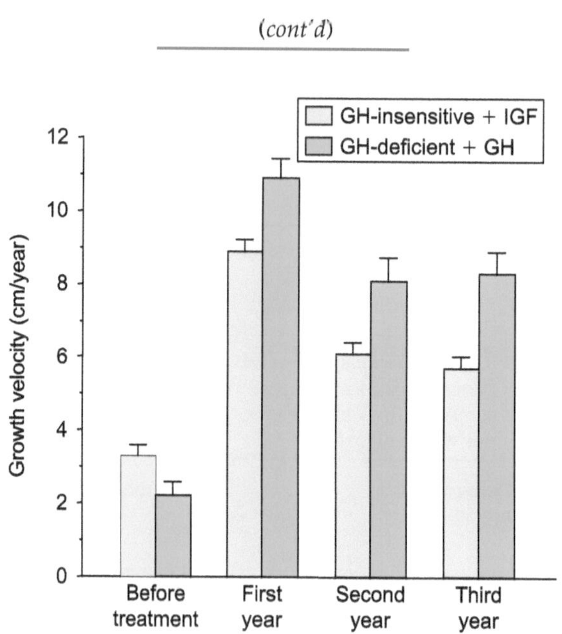

FIGURE 11.33 IGF-1 treatment of children with GH insensitivity due to a receptor deficiency compared to GH treatment of children with GH deficiency. *GH*, Growth hormone; *IGF-1*, insulin-like growth factor-I. Source: *Plotted from data of Guevara-Aguirre, J., Rosenbloom, A. L., Vasconez, O., Martinez, V, Gargosky, S., Allen, L., & Rosenfeld, R. (1997). Two-year treatment of growth hormone (GH) receptor deficiency with recombinant insulin-like growth factor-I in 22 children: Comparison of two dosage levels to GH-treated deficiency.* The Journal of Clinical Endocrinology and Metabolism 82, *629–633.*

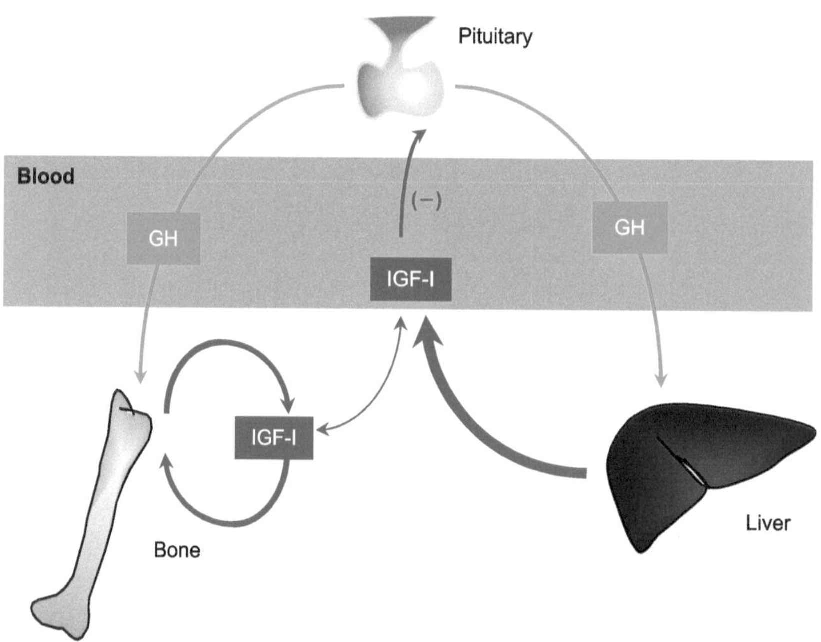

FIGURE 11.34 The roles of *GH* and insulin-like growth factor-I (*IGF-1*) in promoting growth. GH stimulates IGF-1 production in liver and epiphyseal growth plates. Epiphyseal growth is stimulated primarily by autocrine/paracrine actions of IGF-1. IGF-1 produced by the liver accounts for growth in diameter of bones and acts as a negative feedback regulator of GH secretion. Liver is the principal source of IGF-1 in blood, but other GH target organs may also contribute to the circulating pool. *GH*, Growth hormone.

(*cont'd*)

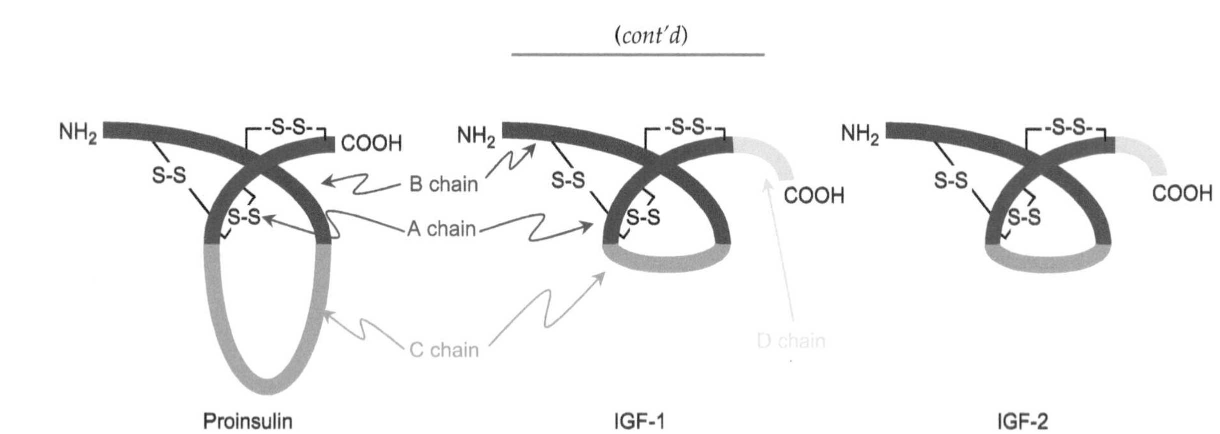

FIGURE 11.35 Proinsulin, insulin-like growth factor-1 (IGF-1) and insulin-like growth factor-2 (IGF-2). Structures are drawn to emphasize similarities. Amino acid sequences show about 50% identity in the regions corresponding to the A and B chains of all three compounds, and more than 74% identity in the IGFs. The C chain regions have the most variability.

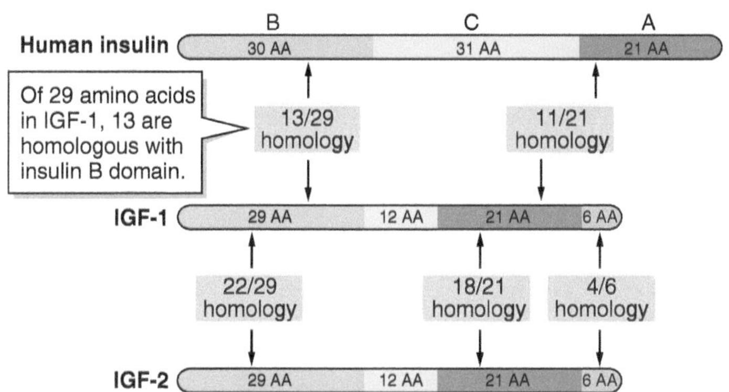

FIGURE 11.36 Homology between human insulin, IGF-1 and IGF-2. Source: *Redrawn from Figure 48-5 in Barrett, E. J. (2005). Chapter 48: Endocrine regulation of growth and body mass. In W. F. Boron, & E. L. Boulpaep (Eds.),* Medical physiology *(3rd ed.) (p. 996). Elsevier.*

Although the anterior pituitary gland produces at least six hormones, more than one-third of its cells synthesize and secrete GH. In humans the 5–10 mg of stored GH make it the most abundant hormone in the pituitary, accounting for almost 10% of the dry weight of the gland. More than 10 times as much GH is produced and stored there than any other pituitary hormone. Ninety percent of the GH produced by somatotropes comprise 191 amino acids and has a molecular weight of about 22,000. The remaining 10%, called 20K GH, has a molecular weight of 20,000 and lacks the 15-amino acid sequence corresponding to residues 32–46. Both forms are the products of the same gene and result from alternate splicing of the RNA transcript. Both forms of hormone are secreted and have similar growth-promoting activity, although metabolic effects of the 20K form are reduced.

About half the GH in blood circulates bound to a protein that has the same amino acid sequence as the extracellular domain of the GH receptor (see later). In fact, the plasma GH binding protein is a product of the same gene that encodes the GH receptor and originates by proteolytic cleavage of the receptor at the outer surface of target cells. It is thought that the binding protein provides a reservoir of GH that prolongs its half-life and buffers changes in free hormone concentration. Free GH can readily cross capillary membranes, but bound hormone is restricted to the vascular compartment. The half-life of GH in blood is about 20 minutes. GH that crosses the glomerular membrane is reabsorbed and destroyed in the kidney, which is the major site of GH degradation. Less than 0.01% of the hormone secreted each day reaches the urine in recognizable form. GH also is degraded in its various target cells following uptake by receptor mediated endocytosis.

In contrast to insulin, however, the region corresponding to the connecting peptide (the C chain) is retained in the mature form of the IGFs, which also have a C-terminal extension referred to as the D chain. Both IGF-1 and IGF-2 are present in blood at relatively high

(cont'd)

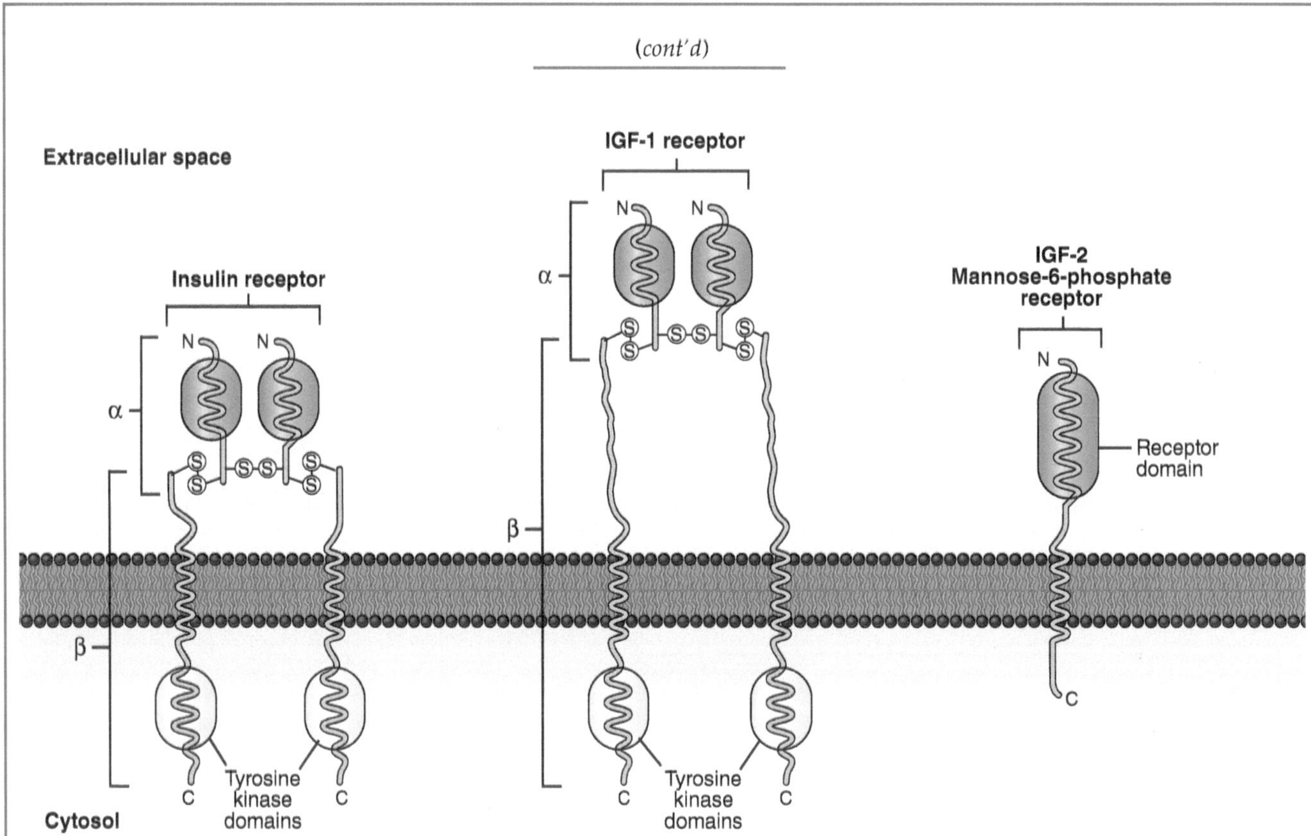

FIGURE 11.37 Comparison of insulin, IGF-1 and IGF-2 receptors. The first two have tyrosine kinase domains but the receptor for IGF-2 does not, suggesting a limited effect.

concentrations throughout life although the absolute amounts differ at different stages of life. The concentration of IGF-2 is usually about three times higher than that of IGF-1.

Two receptors for the IGFs have been identified. The IGF-1 receptor, which binds IGF-1 with greater affinity than IGF-2, is remarkably similar to the insulin receptor. Like the insulin receptor (see Fig. 5.18 and Fig. 11.35) it is a tetramer that consists of two membrane-spanning β subunits connected by disulfide bonds to two extracellular α subunits, which contain the IGF binding domain.

As in the insulin receptor, the β subunits have intrinsic protein tyrosine kinase activity that is activated by ligand binding and catalyzes the phosphorylation of some of its own tyrosine residues and tyrosines on many of the same proteins that mediate the intracellular responses to insulin: the insulin receptor substrates, phosphatidylinositol-3-kinase, and so on (see Fig. 7.19).

Cells that coexpress both insulin and IGF-1 receptors may also produce "hybrid receptors" that have one α and one β subunit of the insulin receptor coupled to one α one β subunit of the IGF-1 receptor. These receptors behave more like IGF-1 receptors than like insulin receptors. Their physiological importance has not been established. Both IGF-1 and IGF-2 can combine with the IGF-1 receptor.

The IGF-2 receptor is structurally unrelated to the IGF-1 receptor and binds IGF-2 with a very much higher affinity than IGF-1. It consists of a single membrane-spanning protein with a short cytosolic domain that has a novel signaling mechanism. Curiously, the IGF-2 receptor is identical to the mannose-6-phosphate

(cont'd)

receptor that binds mannose-6-phosphate groups on newly synthesized lysosomal enzymes and transfers them from the *trans*-Golgi vesicles to the endosomes and thence to lysosomes. It may also transfer mannose-6-phosphate containing glycoproteins from the extracellular fluid to the lysosomes by an endocytic process. The IGF-2 receptor plays an important role in clearing IGF-2 from extracellular fluids.

The insulin-like growth factor binding proteins

The IGFs circulate in blood tightly bound to IGF binding proteins (IGFBPs). Six different closely related IGFBPs, each the product of a separate gene, are found in mammalian plasma and extracellular fluids. Their affinities for both IGF-1 and IGF-2 are considerably higher than the affinity of IGF-1 receptors for either IGF-1 or IGF-2. The circulating IGFBPs act both as reservoirs for these growth factors and as regulators of their delivery across capillary endothelia. The combined binding capacity of all the plasma IGFBPs is about twice than that needed to bind all the IGFs in blood and, therefore, there is essentially no "free" IGF in plasma. Because of its small molecular size, free IGF could readily cross capillary endothelia and potentially produce indiscriminate, unregulated multiplication of the wide variety of cells that express its receptors. In addition, by stimulating either IGF or insulin receptors, IGFs produce hypoglycemia. The IGFBPs provide mechanisms for controlled delivery of IGF to discreet cellular populations. The same binding proteins also are produced and secreted along with the IGFs by extrahepatic cells and are, therefore, found in extracellular fluid in various tissues where they act as regulators of IGF bioavailability. IGFBP-3 is the most abundant of the IGFBPs in blood and has the highest affinity for the IGFs. Its concentration in plasma is somewhat lower than the sum of the concentrations of IGF-1 and IGF-2, and hence its binding capacity is normally saturated. IGFBP-3 and its cargo of IGF form a large 150 kDa ternary complex that includes an 88 kDa glycoprotein called the acid-labile subunit (als).[2] GH stimulates the synthesis of all the three components of this complex in the liver, and consequently, their concentrations are quite low in the blood of GH-deficient subjects and increase upon treatment with GH. The complex, which is too large to cross capillary endothelia, readily has a half-life of about 15 hours.

About 25% of the IGFs in plasma are distributed among the other IGFBPs, which, except for IGFBP-5, do not bind to acid-labile subunits and hence form complexes that are small enough to escape across the capillary endothelium. Of these, IGFBP-2 is the most important quantitatively. Its concentration in blood is increased in plasma of GH-deficient patients and is decreased by GH but rises dramatically after administration of IGF-1. Plasma levels of IGFBP-1, the next in importance quantitatively, are regulated by insulin, which suppresses its formation. Although the binding capacity of IGFBP-3 is saturated, the other IGFBPs have free binding sites and readily associate with IGFs that are released from IGFBP-3 after proteolytic "clipping" by proteases present in plasma lowers its binding affinity. IGFs complexed with other IGFBPs escape to the extracellular fluid and remain sequestered until destroyed or targeted to specific locales.

The IGFBPs are synthesized locally in conjunction with IGF in a wide variety of cells and are distributed extensively in extracellular fluid. Their biology is complex and not completely understood. It may be recalled that the IGFs mediate localized growth in response to a variety of signals in addition to GH. Many different cells both produce and respond to IGF-1, which is a small and readily diffusible molecule. The IGFBPs in interstitial fluid may provide a means of restricting the extent of cell growth to the precise location dictated by physiological demand. Because their affinity for both IGFs is so much greater than the affinity of the IGF-1 receptor, the IGFBPs can compete successfully for binding free IGF and thus restrict its bioavailability. Conversely, IGFBPs may also enhance the actions of IGF-1. Some of the IGFBPs bind to extracellular matrices where they may provide a localized reservoir of IGFs that might be released by proteolytic modification of the IGFBPs.

Binding to the cell surface lowers the affinity of some of the IGFBPs and thus provides a means of targeted delivery of free IGF-1 to receptive cells. The affinities of the IGFBPs also are modified by phosphorylation and partial proteolysis, both of which may provide mechanisms for local control IGF bioavailability. Some evidence also suggests that IGFBPs may produce biological effects that are independent of the IGFs. The complex physiology of the IGFBPs continues to be a subject of active research.

(cont'd)

Insulin-like growth factors and prenatal growth

In addition to serving as mediators of GH-induced growth postnatally, IGF-1 and IGF-2 appear to be the major regulators of GH-independent growth during fetal life, whereas human infants or mouse pups born with inactivating mutations of GH or the GH receptor are of normal birth weight, absence of IGF-1, IGF-2, or the IGF-1 receptor results in severe prenatal growth retardation that persists through postnatal life. Both IGFs acting through the IGF-1 receptor stimulate cell division and differentiation in fetal tissues and their actions in these regards appear to be modulated by the IGFBPS. Studies in rodents suggest that IGF-2 is critical for growth of the placenta, which in turn affects growth of the fetus through its influence on nutrient availability. Although the IGFs and their binding proteins play a central role in stimulating fetal growth, little is known of how their production and actions are regulated.

Effects of growth hormone/IGF-1 on body composition

The bodies of GH-deficient animals and human subjects have a relatively high proportion of fat, compared to water and protein, in their bodies. Treatment with GH changes the proportion of these bodily constituents to resemble the normal juvenile distribution. Body protein stores increase, particularly in muscle, and there is a relative decrease in fat. Despite their relatively higher fat content, subjects who are congenitally deficient in GH or unresponsive to it have fewer total adipocytes than normal individuals. Their adiposity is due to an increase in the amount of fat stored in each cell. Treatment with GH restores normal cellularity by increasing proliferation of fat cell precursors through autocrine stimulation by IGF-1. Curiously, however, GH also restrains the differentiation of fat cell precursors into mature adipocytes. The overall decrease in body fat produced by GH results from decreased deposition of fat, accelerated mobilization, and increased reliance of fat for energy production (see Chapter 8: Hormonal Regulation of Fuel Metabolism).

Most internal organs grow in proportion to body size, except liver and spleen, which may be disproportionally enlarged by prolonged treatment with GH. The heart may also be enlarged in acromegalic subjects, in part from stimulation of cardiac myocyte growth by GH or IGF, and in part from hypertension, which is frequently seen in these individuals. Conversely, GH deficiency beginning in childhood is associated with decreased myocardial mass due to the decreased thickness of the ventricular walls. Treatment of these individuals with GH leads to increased myocardial mass and improved cardiac performance. Skin and the underlying connective tissue also increase in mass, but GH does not influence growth of the thyroid, gonads, or reproductive organs.

Changes in body composition and organ growth have been monitored by studying changes in the biochemical balance of body constituents (Fig. 11.38).

When human subjects or experimental animals are given GH repeatedly for several days, there is net retention of nitrogen, reflecting increased protein synthesis. Urinary nitrogen is decreased, as is the concentration of urea in blood. Net synthesis of protein is increased without an accompanying change in the net rates of protein degradation. Increased retention of potassium reflects the increase in intracellular water that results from increased cell size and number. An increase in sodium retention and the consequent expansion of extracellular volume is characteristic of GH replacement, but understanding of the mechanisms involved remains elusive. Increased phosphate retention reflects the expansion of the cellular and skeletal mass and is brought about in part by the activation of sodium phosphate cotransporters in the proximal tubules and activation of the 1α-hydroxylase that catalyzes production of calcitriol (see Chapter 10: Hormonal Regulation of Calcium Balance).

Comparison of the growth promoting actions of growth hormone and IGF-1

Although IGF-1 figures prominently as an intermediary in the actions of GH, not all the effects of GH are mediated by the IGFs. Clinical experience indicates that IGF-1 is less effective than GH in promoting skeletal growth (Fig. 11.36), but more effective than GH in stimulating growth of some soft tissues. In muscle, GH appears to promote growth primarily by stimulating protein synthesis with little effect on protein degradation, whereas IGF-1 strongly inhibits protein degradation. Whether these observations reflect intrinsic differences in the actions of GH and IGF or simply inadequate emulation of local production of IGF by systemic administration of IGF remains to be resolved. Some aspects of growth stimulated by GH are independent of IGF-1, although their physiological importance is unknown. It is important to recognize that treatment with IGF-1 reproduces most of the effects of GH on body size and composition in patients who are insensitive to GH because of a receptor defect.

(cont'd)

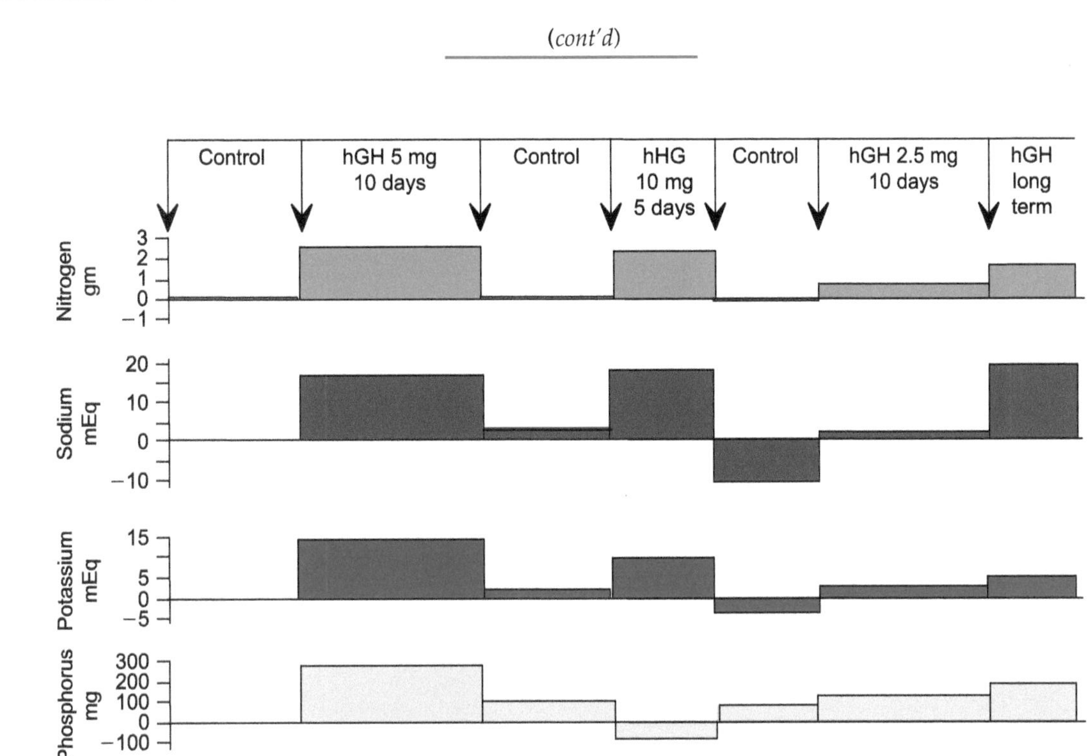

FIGURE 11.38 Effects of human growth hormone (hGH) on nitrogen, sodium, potassium, and phosphorus balances in an 11.5-year-old girl with pituitary dwarfism. Changes above the control baseline represent retention of the substance and changes below the line represent loss. *hGH*, Human growth hormone. Source: *From Hutchings, J. J., Escamilla, R. F., Deamer, W. C., et al. (1959). Metabolic changes produced human growth hormone in a pituitary dwarf.* The Journal of Clinical Endocrinology and Metabolism 19, *759–764.*

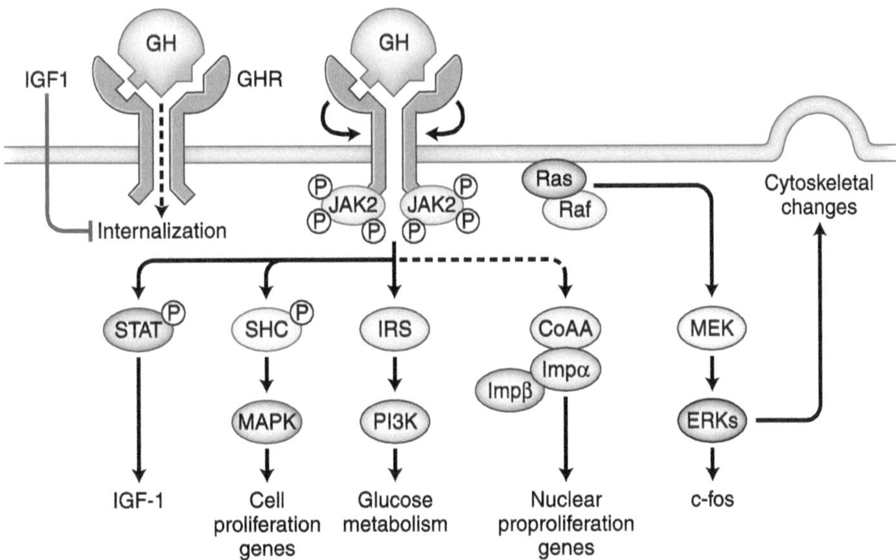

FIGURE 11.39 Action of GH on receptors. The growth hormone receptor is a dimer which undergoes internal rotation to form JAK-2 phosphorylation (P). This results in several different effects. *CoAA*, Coactivator signaling; *ERK*, extracellular signal-related kinase; *GH*, growth hormone; *impα and impβ*, importin alpha and beta; *IRS*, insulin receptor substrate; *JAK-2*, Janus kinase-2; *MAPK*, mitogen-activated protein kinase; *MEK*, dual specifying mitogen-activated kinase 2. Source: *From Figure 8-15 in Kaiser, U., & Ho, K. K. Y. (2016). Chapter 8: Pituitary physiology and diagnostic evaluation. In Melmed, Polonsky, Larsen, & Kronenberg (Eds.),* Williams' textbook of endocrinology *(13th ed.) (p. 192). Elsevier.*

(*cont'd*)

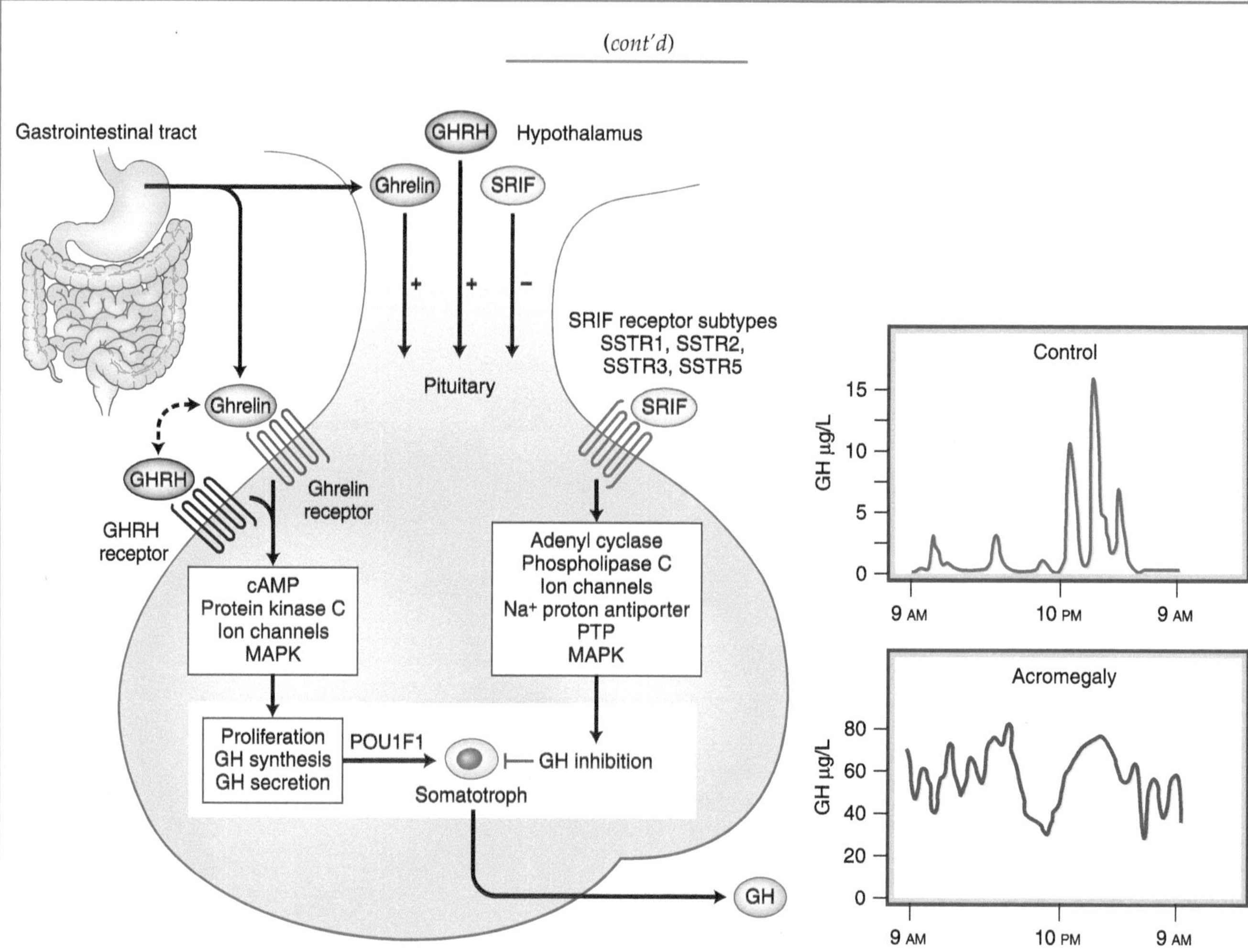

FIGURE 11.40 Some of the factors that affect normal and abnormal GH output—which can also be the targets of therapy. *GH*, Growth hormone; *GHRH*, growth-hormone-releasing hormone; *MAPK*, mitogen activated protein kinase; *PTP*, protein tyrosine phosphatase; *SRIF*, somatotropin (GH) releasing inhibitory factor, better known as somatostatin; *SSTR*, somatostatin receptor subtypes. Source: *From Figure 9-27 in Melmed, S., & Kleinberg, D. (2016). Chapter 9: Pituitary masses and tumors. In Melmed, Polonsky, Larsen, & Kronenberg (Eds.),* Williams' textbook of endocrinology *(13th ed.) (p. 270). Elsevier.*

In other respects, clear differences in the actions of GH and IGF-1 are apparent. For example, hepatocytes and mature adipocytes lack IGF-1 receptors, but GH nevertheless modifies expression of a variety of their genes. GH increases lipolysis in adipocytes (see Chapter 8: Hormonal Regulation of Fuel Metabolism), but IGF-1, when present at concentrations high enough to activate insulin receptors, inhibits lipolysis. Although treatment with either GH or IGF-1 decrease body fat, they do so by different mechanisms. GH acts directly on adipocytes to mobilize free fatty acids. IGF-1 decreases adipocyte fat content probably due to its inhibitory effects on insulin secretion. In contrast, GH increases insulin secretion and decreases insulin sensitivity, whereas IGF-1 behaves as an insulin sensitizer.

Mechanism of action

Like other peptide and protein hormones GH binds to its receptor on the surface of target cells. The GH receptor is a glycoprotein that has a single membrane-spanning region and a relatively long intracellular tail that neither has catalytic activity nor interacts with G-proteins. The GH receptor binds to a cytosolic enzyme called Janus kinase-2 (JAK-2), which catalyzes the phosphorylation of the receptor and other proteins on tyrosine residues (see Chapter 1: Introduction). GH activates a signaling cascade by binding sequentially to two GH receptor molecules to form a receptor dimer that sandwiches the hormone between the two receptor molecules. Such dimerization of receptors also is seen for

(cont'd)

other hormone and cytokine receptors of the super family to which the GH receptor belongs. Dimerization of receptors brings the bound JAK-2 enzymes into favorable alignment to promote tyrosine phosphorylation and activation of their catalytic sites. In addition, dimerization may also recruit JAK-2 molecules to unoccupied binding sites on the receptors. Tyrosine phosphorylation provides docking sites for other proteins and facilitates their phosphorylation. One group of target proteins, called STATs (signal transduction and activation of transcription), migrate to the nucleus and activate gene transcription (see Chapter 1: Introduction). Another target group, the mitogen-activated protein kinases (MAPK), also promotes gene transcription (Figs. 11.39 and 11.40).

Other proteins include the insulin receptor substrates and their downstream kinases, including PI3 kinase and protein kinase B (see Chapter 7: The Pancreatic Islets).

Activation of the GH receptor also results in an influx of extracellular calcium through voltage regulated channels and may further promote transcription of target genes. GH produces its effects in various cells by stimulating the transcription of specific genes.

Growth hormone secretion

Growth is a slow, continuous process that takes place over more than a decade. It might be expected, therefore, that concentrations of GH in blood would be fairly static. In contrast to such expectations, however, frequent measurements of GH concentrations in blood plasma throughout the day reveal wide fluctuations indicative of multiple episodes of secretion. Because the rate of degradation of GH is thought to be invariant, changes in plasma concentration imply changes in secretion. In male rats, GH is secreted in regular pulses every 3.0–3.5 hours in what has been called an ultradian rhythm. In humans, GH secretion is also pulsatile, but the pattern of changes in blood concentrations is usually less obvious than in rats. Frequent bursts of secretion occur throughout the day, with the largest being associated with the early hours of sleep (Fig. 11.41).

Effects of stress

Stressful changes in the internal and external environment can produce brief episodes of hormone secretion. Little information or diagnostic insight can, therefore, be obtained from a single random measurement of the GH concentration in blood. Because secretory episodes last only a short while, multiple, frequent measurements are needed to evaluate functional status or to relate GH secretion to physiological events. Alternatively, it is possible to withdraw small amounts of blood continuously over the course of a day, and by measuring GH in the pooled sample, to obtain a 24-hour integrated concentration of GH in blood.

The possible physiological significance of intermittent as compared to constant secretion of GH much attention experimentally. Pulsatile administration of GH to hypophysectomized rats is more effective in stimulating growth than continuous infusion of the same daily dose. However, similar findings have not been made in human subjects, whose rate of growth, like that of experimental animals, can be restored to normal or near normal with single daily or every other day injections of GH. Although expression of some hepatic genes appears to be sensitive to the pattern of changes in plasma GH concentrations in rodents, there is neither evidence for comparable effects in humans nor an obvious relationship of the affected genes to growth of rodents. In normal human adults the same total amount of GH given either as a constant infusion or in eight equally spaced brief infusions over 24 hours increased expression IGF-1 and IGFBP-3 to the same extent.

Effects of age

Using the continuous sampling method, it was found that GH secretion, though most active during the adolescent growth spurt, persists throughout life, long after the epiphyses have fused and growth has stopped (Fig. 11.42).

In mid-adolescence the pituitary secretes between 1 and 2 mg GH/day. Between ages 20 and 40 years the daily rate of secretion gradually decreases in both men and women, but remarkably, even in middle age the pituitary continues to secrete about 0.1 mg GH/day. Low rates of GH secretion in the elderly may be related to the loss of lean body mass in later life. Changes in GH secretion with age primarily reflect changes in magnitude of secretory pulses (Fig. 11.43).

Regulation of growth hormone secretion

In addition to spontaneous pulses, secretory episodes are induced by such metabolic signals as a rapid

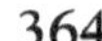

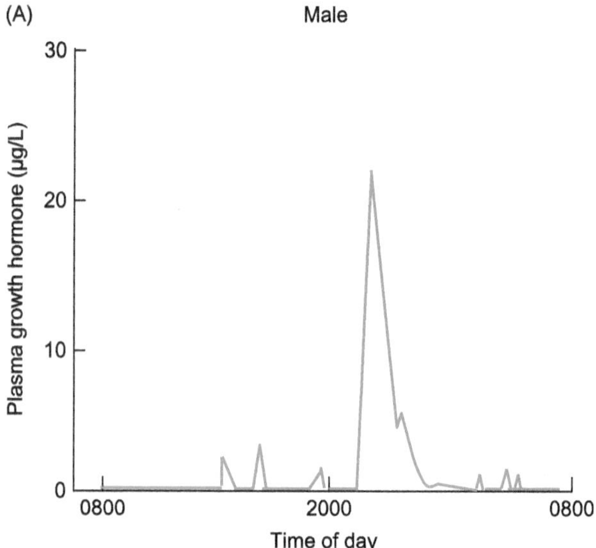

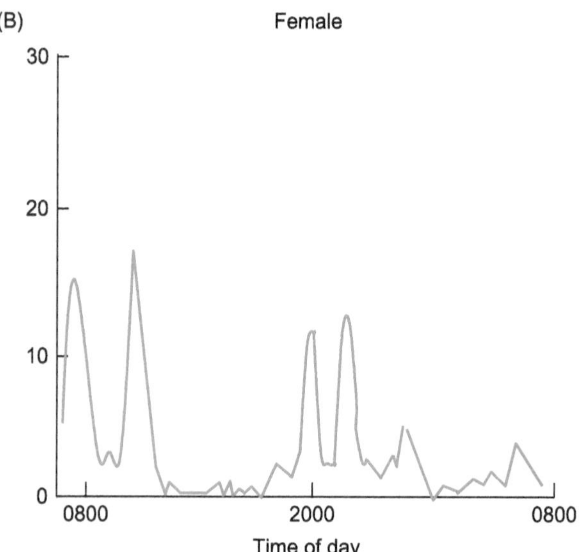

FIGURE 11.41 Growth hormone concentrations in blood sampled at 10-min intervals over a 24-h period in a normal man (A) and a normal woman (B). The large pulse in A coincides with the early hours of sleep. Note that the pulses of secretion are more frequent and of greater amplitude in the woman. Source: *From Asplin, C. M., Faria, H. C. S., Carlsen, E. C., et al. (1989). Alterations in the pulsatile mode of growth hormone release in men and women with insulin-dependent diabetes mellitus.* The Journal of Clinical Endocrinology and Metabolism 69, *239–245.*

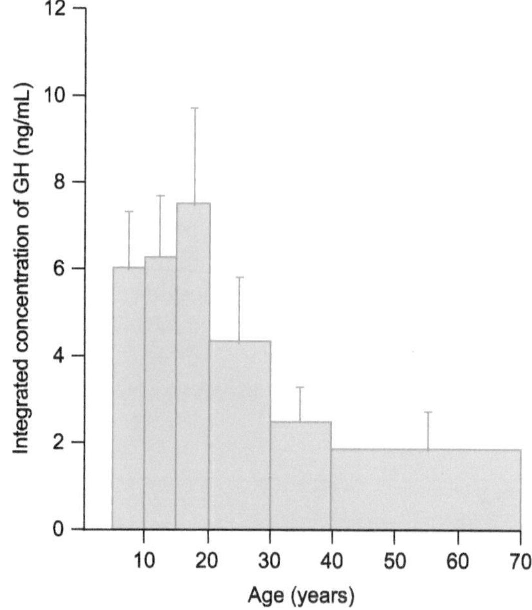

FIGURE 11.42 Relation between the integrated plasma concentration of GH and age in 173 normal males and females. *GH*, Growth hormone. Source: *From Zadik, Z., Chalew, S. A., McCarter, R. J. Jr, Meistas, M., & Kowarski, A. A. (1985). The influence of age on the 24-hour integrated concentration of growth hormone in normal individuals.* The Journal of Clinical Endocrinology and Metabolism 60, *513–516.*

fall in blood glucose concentration or an increase in certain amino acids, particularly arginine and leucine. The physiological significance of these changes in GH secretion is not understood, but provocative tests using these signals are helpful for judging the competence of the GH secretory apparatus (Fig. 11.44).

Traumatic and psychogenic stresses are also powerful inducers of GH secretion in humans and monkeys, but whether increased secretion of GH is beneficial for coping with stress is not established and is not universally seen in mammals. In rats, for example, GH secretion is inhibited by the same signals that increase it in humans. However, regardless of their significance, these observations indicate that GH secretion is under minute-to-minute control by the nervous system. That control is expressed through the hypothalamic-hypophyseal portal circulation, which delivers GH-releasing hormone (GHRH) and somatostatin to the somatotropes (see Chapter 2: Pituitary Gland). A third hormone, ghrelin (see Chapter 2: Pituitary Gland, and Chapter 6: Hormones of the Gastrointestinal Tract), which is produced in arcuate neurons and the gastric mucosa, is also involved in regulating GH secretion. Somatotropes express receptors for many neurohormones (Fig. 11.45)

Growth-hormone-releasing hormone provides the primary drive for GH synthesis and secretion. It is a 44-amino acid polypeptide member of the secretin/glucagon family (see Chapter 6: Hormones of the Gastrointestinal Tract). In the absence of GHRH, or when a lesion interrupts hypophyseal portal blood flow, secretion of GH ceases. Defective hypothalamic production or secretion of GHRH may be a more common cause of GH deficiency than defects in the pituitary gland. GH concentrations in plasma are restored to normal in many GH-deficient individuals after treatment with GHRH, suggesting that their somatotropes

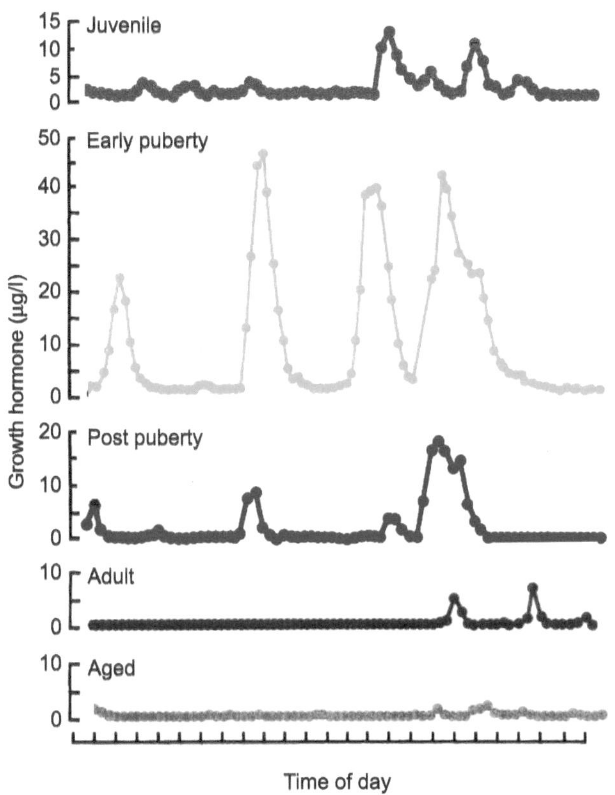

FIGURE 11.43 Changing patterns of GH secretion with age. *GH*, Growth hormone. Source: *Modified from Robinson, I. C. A. F., & Hindmarsh, P. C. (1999). The growth hormone secretory pattern and statural growth. In Kostyo, J. L. (Ed.),* Handbook of physiology, *Section 7, The Endocrine System, Vol. V Hormonal Control of Growth (pp. 329–396). Oxford University Press, New York.*

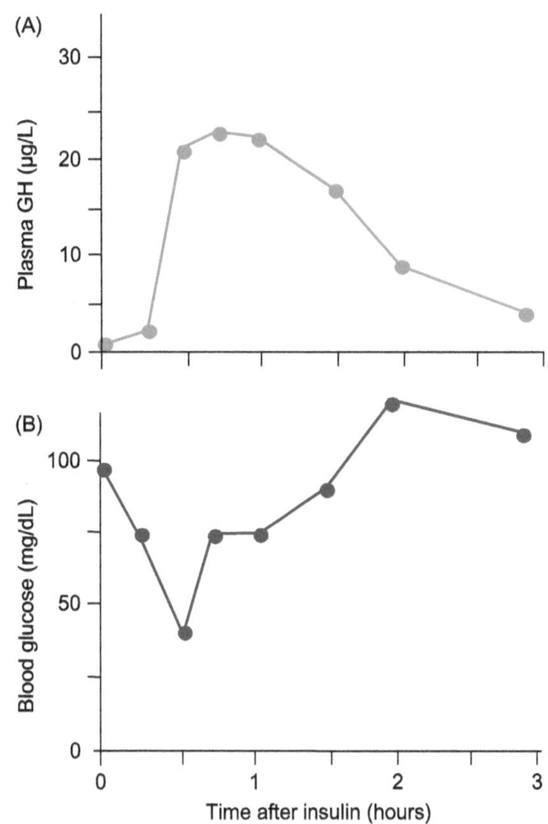

FIGURE 11.44 Acute changes in plasma growth hormone concentration (A) in response to insulin-induced hypoglycemia (B). Source: *From Roth, J., Glick, S. M., Yalow, R. S., & Berson, S. (1963). Hypoglycemia: A potent stimulus to secretion of growth hormone.* Science, *140, 987–989.*

are competent but not adequately stimulated. Release of somatostatin from neurons in the periventricular and paraventricular nuclei into the hypophyseal portal circulation reduces or blocks secretion of GH in response to GHRH, but has little or no influence on GH synthesis. Nearly constant secretion of somatostatin restrains secretion of GH throughout most of the day. Periodic interruptions in secretion or sudden withdrawal of somatostatin produces a rebound release of GH and may contribute to the pulsatile nature of GH secretion. Defects in somatostatin synthesis or secretion are not known to be responsible for disease states, but acromegaly is sometimes associated with an inactivating mutation of the somatostatin receptor. Long-acting analogs of somatostatin are used to decrease GH secretion in patients with acromegaly.

Ghrelin secreted by neurons in the arcuate nuclei reaches the pituitary by way of the hypophyseal portal circulation and augments responses of somatotropes to GHRH. Ghrelin, or synthetic peptides that stimulate the same receptor, increase GH secretion by somatotropes in tissue culture, but in vivo stimulation of GH secretion by ghrelin requires costimulation by GHRH. In addition to their expression by somatotropes, ghrelin receptors are also expressed by GHRH secreting neurons suggesting that ghrelin may increase GHRH as well as GH secretion. Fluctuations in ghrelin concentrations in the general circulation reflect its secretion mainly by the gastric mucosa and do not coincide with changes in plasma GH concentrations. It is unlikely that ghrelin of gastric mucosal origin participates in regulating GH secretion.

In addition to neuroendocrine mechanisms that adjust secretion in response to changes in the internal or external environment, secretion of GH is under negative feedback control. As with other negative feedback systems, products of GH action, principally IGF-1, act as inhibitory signals (Fig. 11.46).

IGF-1 acts on the pituitary to decrease GH synthesis and secretion in response to GHRH. Increased plasma concentrations of FFA or glucose, which are related to GH's metabolic action, exert inhibitory effects on GH secretion, probably by increasing somatostatin secretion, but fasting, which also is associated with increased FFA, inhibits somatostatin secretion. GH also inhibits its own secretion by a short loop negative

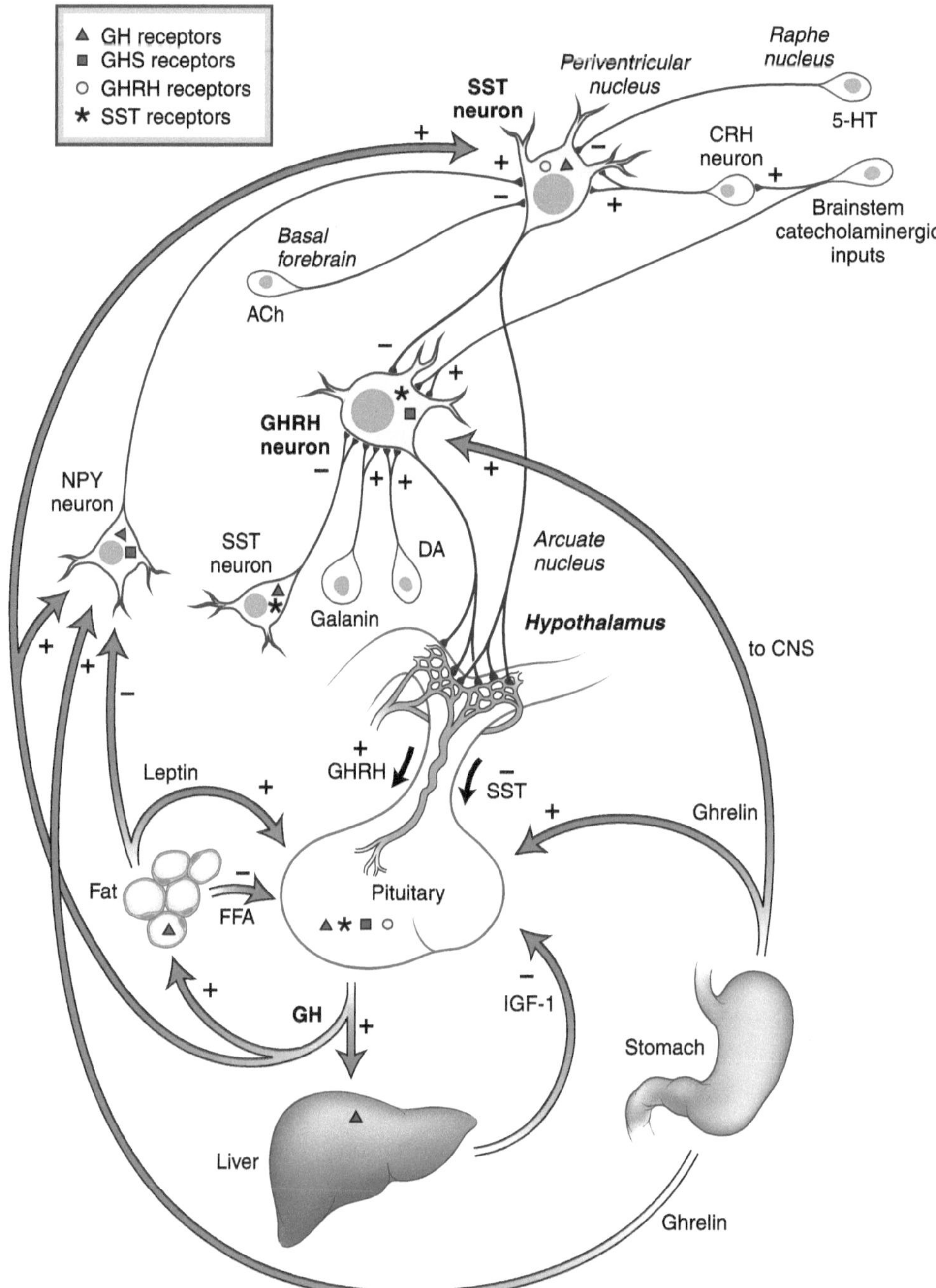

FIGURE 11.45 Many different hormones affect the somatotrophs in the anterior pituitary that secrete growth hormone. Not shown are the effects of thyroid, adrenal, and gonadal hormones on GH secretion. *5-HT*, 5-Hydroxytryptamine (serotonin); *ACh*, acetylcholine; *CRH*, corticotropin releasing hormone; *DA*, dopamine; *FFA*, free fatty acids; *GH*, growth hormone; *GHRH*, growth-hormone-releasing hormone; *IGF-1*, insulin-like growth factor-1; *NPY*, neuropeptide Y; *SST*, somatostatin. Source: *From Figure 7-22 in M. J. Low. (2016). Chapter 7: Neuroendocrinology. In Melmed, Polonsky, Larsen, & Kronenberg (Eds.),* Williams' textbook of endocrinology *(13th ed.) (p. 141). Elsevier.*

feedback effect that involves inhibition of GHRH secretion and stimulation of somatostatin secretion. These effects are illustrated in Fig. 11.47.

Negative feedback control sets the overall level of GH secretion by regulating the amounts of GH secreted in each pulse. The phenomenon of pulsatility and the circadian variation that increases the magnitude of the secretory pulses at night are entrained by neural mechanisms. Pulsatility appears to be the result of reciprocal intermittent secretion of both GHRH and somatostatin. It appears that bursts of GHRH secretion are timed to coincide with interruptions in

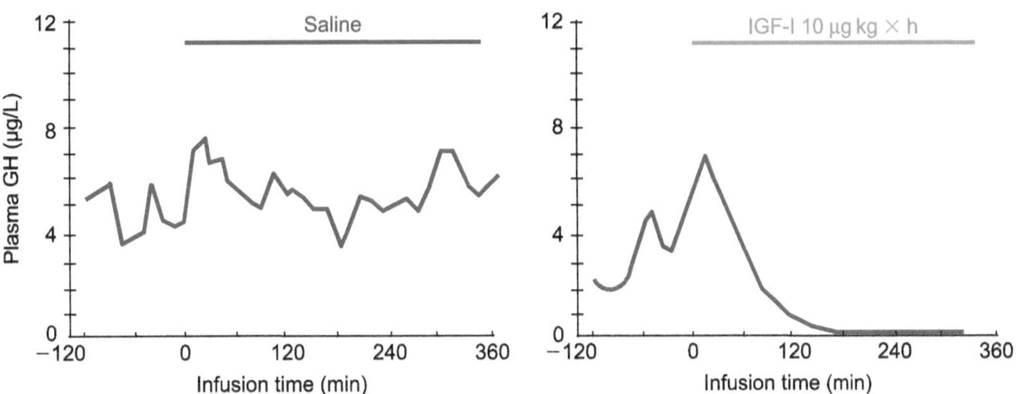

FIGURE 11.46 Effects of insulin-like growth factor-I (IGF-1) on GH secretion in normal fasted men. Values shown are averages for the same 10 men given infusions of either physiological saline (control) or IGF-1 for the periods indicated. Note: IGF-1 completely blocked GH secretion after a lag period of 1 hour. *GH*, Growth hormone. Source: *Redrawn from Hartman, M. L., Clayton, P. E., Johnson, M. L., Celniker, A., Perlman, A. J., Alberti, K. G., & Thorner, M. O. (1993). A low dose euglycemic infusion of recombinant human insulin-like growth factor-I rapidly suppresses fasting-enhanced pulsatile growth hormone secretion in humans.* Journal of Clinical Investigation *91, 2453–2462.*

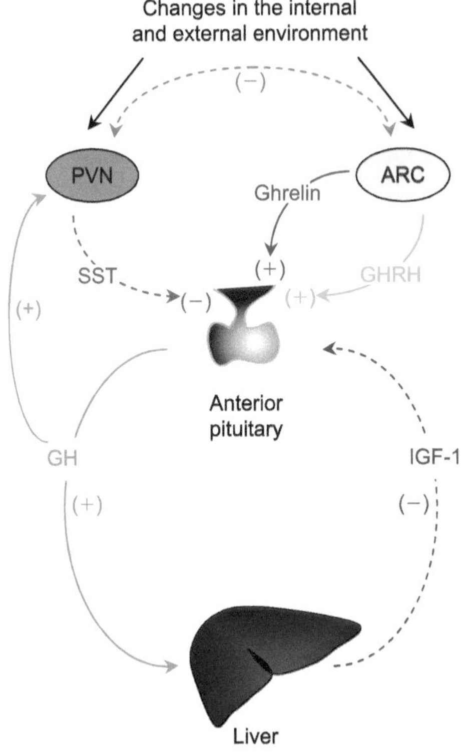

FIGURE 11.47 Regulation of growth hormone (GH) secretion. (−), Inhibition; (+), stimulation; *ARC*, arcuate nuclei; *GH*, growth hormone; *GHRH*, growth-hormone-releasing hormone; *IGF-1*, insulin-like growth factor-I; *PVN*, periventricular nuclei; *SST*, somatostatin.

somatostatin secretion. Experimental evidence obtained in rodents indicates that GHRH secreting neurons in the arcuate nuclei communicate with somatostatin secreting neurons in the periventricular nuclei either directly or through interneurons, and conversely, somatostatinergic neurons communicate with GHRH neurons. However, understanding of how reciprocal changes in secretion of these two neurohormones are brought about is still incomplete.

Actions of growth-hormone-releasing hormone, somatostatin, IGF-1, and ghrelin on the somatotrope

The complex interplay of GHRH, somatostatin, ghrelin, and IGF-1 on somatotropes is illustrated in Fig. 11.48.

Receptors for GHRH and somatostatin are coupled to several G-proteins and express their antagonistic effects on GH secretion in part through their opposing influences on cyclic AMP production, cyclic AMP action, and cytosolic calcium concentrations. GHRH activates adenylyl cyclase through a typical Gαs-linked mechanism (see Chapter 1: Introduction). Cyclic AMP activates protein kinase A, and phosphorylation of the cyclic AMP response element binding protein (CREB). Activation of CREB promotes the expression of the transcription factor, Pit 1, which, in turn, increases transcription of genes for both GH and the GHRH receptor. In addition, cyclic AMP-dependent phosphorylation of voltage-sensitive calcium channels is thought to lower their threshold and increase their probability of opening. Voltage-sensitive calcium channels are activated by a G-protein-dependent mechanism that depolarizes the somatotrope membrane by activating sodium channels and inhibiting potassium channels. The resulting increase in cytosolic calcium concentration triggers exocytosis of GH. These effects of GHRH are augmented by ghrelin, whose receptors also are coupled to G-proteins and increase intracellular calcium through activation of phospholipase C and the DAG/IP3 second messenger system.

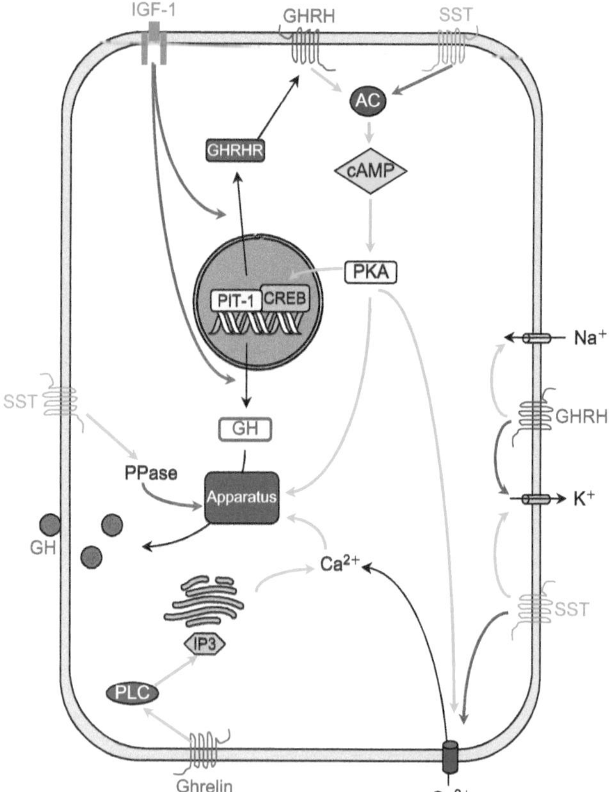

FIGURE 11.48 14 Effects of GHRH, IGF-1, SST, and ghrelin on the somatotrope. Green arrows indicate activation; red arrows indicate inhibition. Opposing effects of GHRH and SST on Na + and K + lead to depolarization and activation of voltage-sensitive Ca^{2+} channels (GHRH) or hyperpolarization (SST) and prevention of Ca2 + channel activation. See text for discussion. *cAMP*, Cyclic adenosine monophosphate; *CREB*, cAMP response element binding protein; *GHRH*, growth-hormone-releasing hormone; *GHRHR*, GHRH receptor; *IGF-1*, insulin-like growth factor-I; *IP3*, inositol trisphosphate; *PIT-1*, pituitary-specific transcription factor-1; *PKA*, protein kinase A; *PLC*, phospholipase C; *PPase*, protein phosphatase.; *SST*, somatostatin.

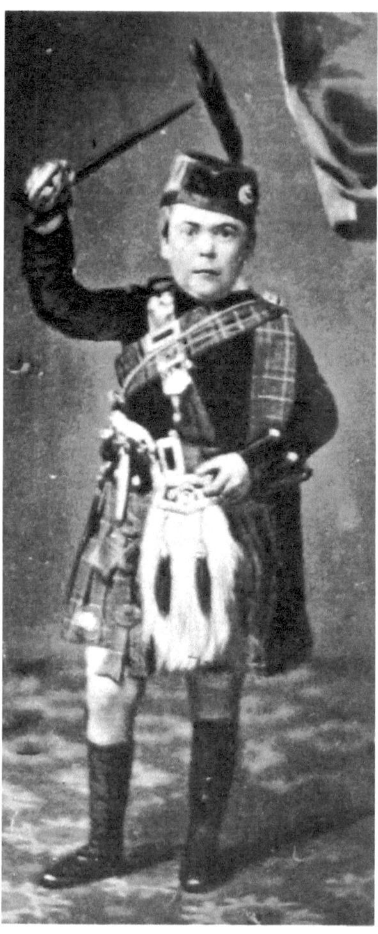

FIGURE 11.49 Charles Stratton (General Tom Thumb) in 1861, at age 23 but less than a meter in height. He performed as part of the PT Barnum tour company. He died in 1883, age 45, of a stroke. Unlike many people with unusual deformities, he became very wealthy. *From* Wikipedia. *Image is in the public domain.*

Somatostatin acts through the inhibitory guanine nucleotide binding protein (Gi) to antagonize activation of adenylyl cyclase and activates a protein phosphatase through a G-protein-dependent mechanism. The inhibitory effects of somatostatin on GH secretion are not limited to reduction of the cyclic AMP pathway of activating of the secretory apparatus. Somatostatin also inhibits calcium channels and activates potassium channels through G-protein mediated mechanisms. Activation of potassium channels hyperpolarizes the plasma membrane and prevents the activation of voltage-sensitive calcium channels. In a similar manner the increased intracellular calcium concentration each secretory event by activating calcium-sensitive potassium channels, which restores the resting membrane potential and closes voltage-sensitive calcium channels.

The negative feedback effects of IGF-1 are slower in onset than the G-protein–mediated effects of GHRH and somatostatin and require tyrosine phosphorylation-initiated changes in gene expression that downregulate GHRH receptors and GH synthesis.

Pituitary dwarfism is the failure of growth that results from the lack of GH during childhood. Pituitary dwarfs, such as Charles Stratton (better known as General Tom Thumb), who was less than a meter in height (Fig. 11.49).

Typically pituitary dwarfs are of normal weight and length at birth and grow rapidly and nearly normally during early infancy. Before the end of the first year, however, growth is noticeably below normal and continues slowly for many years. Left untreated, they may reach heights of 4 ft or less. The pituitary dwarf usually retains a juvenile appearance because of the retention of "baby fat" and the disproportionately small size of maxillary and mandibular bones.

Pituitary dwarfism is not a single entity and may encompass a range of defects. The deficiency in GH may be accompanied by deficiencies of several or all other anterior pituitary hormones (panhypopituitarism) as might result from defects in pituitary development (see Chapter 2: Pituitary Gland). Alternatively, traumatic injury to the pituitary gland or a tumor that either destroys pituitary cells or their connections to the hypothalamus also might interfere with normal pituitary function. These individuals do not mature sexually and suffer from inadequacies of thyroid and adrenal glands as well. The lack of GH also might be an isolated inherited defect, with no abnormalities in other pituitary hormones. Aside from their diminutive height, such individuals are normal in all respects and can reproduce normally. Causes of isolated GH deficiency are multiple and include derangements in synthesis, secretion, and end-organ responsiveness.

Overproduction of GH may occur either as a result of some derangement in mechanisms that control secretion by normal pituitary cells or from tumor cells that secrete GH autonomously (Fig. 11.50).

Overproduction of GH before the epiphyseal plates fuse results in gigantism, in which adult heights more than 8 ft have been reported (See case study for Chapter 1: Introduction) (Fig. 11.51).

Overproduction of GH after the epiphyseal plates of long bones have fused (see later) produces growth in thickness, but not in length. There is thickening of the cranium, the mandible, and widening of some facial bones and bones in the hands and feet called acromegaly (Greek, *akron*, end or extremity; *megas*, large) bones. There is also growth in soft tissues and organs (Fig. 11.52).

Persistence of responsive cartilage progenitor cells in the costochondral junctions leads to elongation of the ribs to give a typical barrel-chested appearance. In acromegalic patients, there is also thickening of the skin and disproportionate growth of some soft tissues, including spleen and liver.

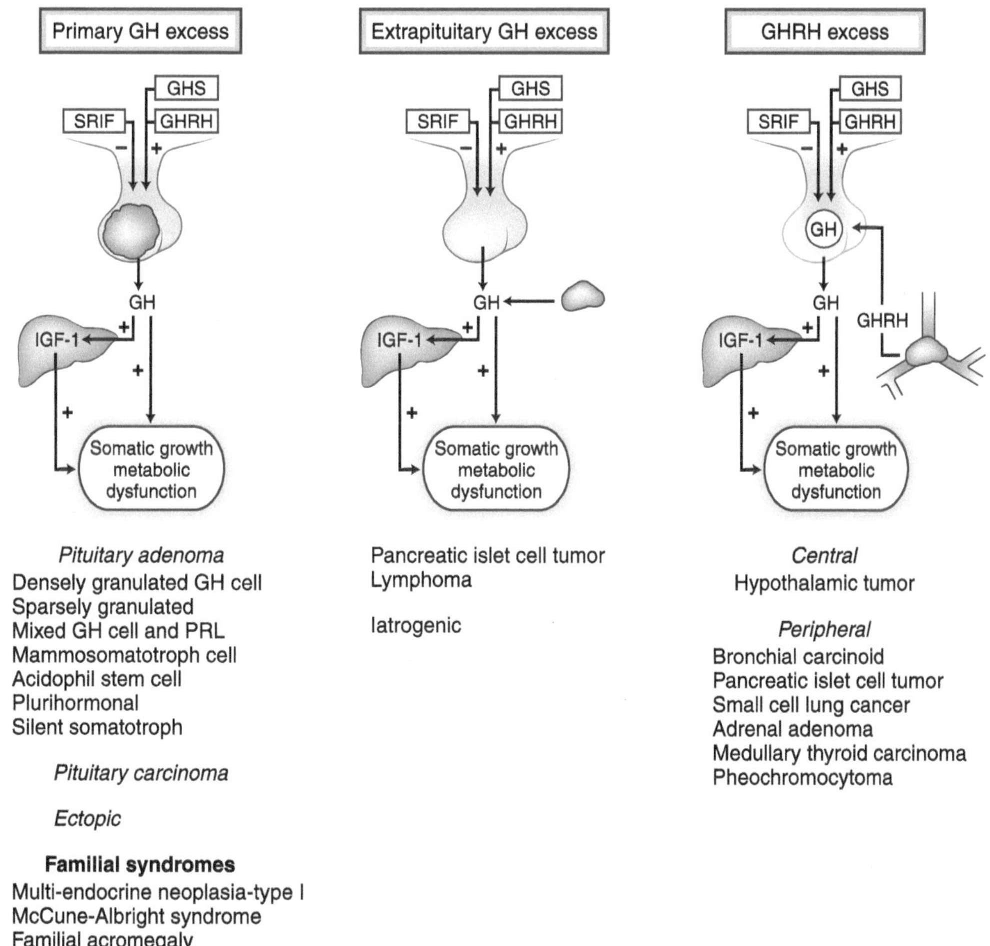

FIGURE 11.50 Causes and effects of GH excess. *GH*, Growth hormone. Source: *From Figure 9-26 in Melmed, S., & Kleinberg, D. (2016). Chapter 9: Pituitary masses and tumors. In Melmed, Polonsky, Larsen, & Kronenberg (Eds.),* Williams' textbook of endocrinology *(13th ed.) (p. 238). Elsevier.*

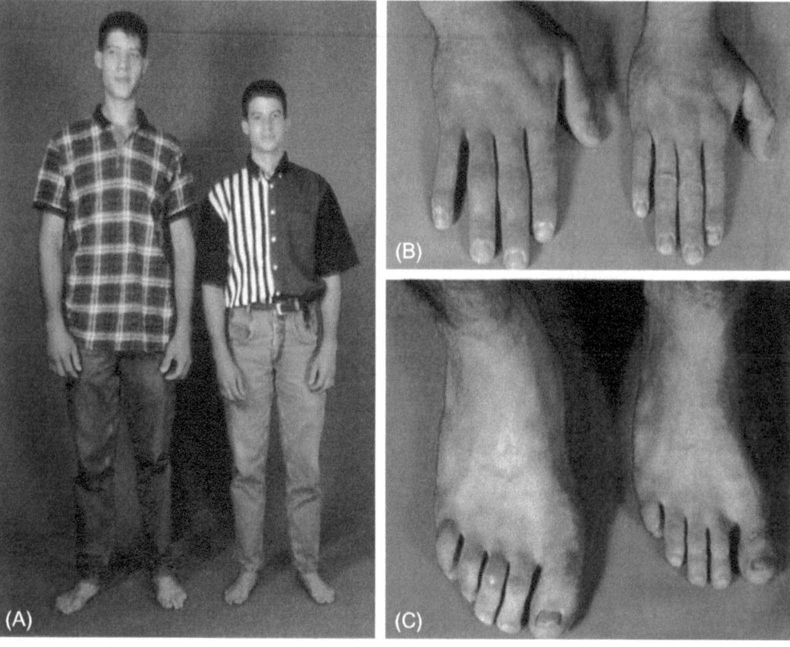

FIGURE 11.51 Giantism in an identical twin. The relative heights are compared in (A), the fingers in (B), and the feet in (C). Note also the elongated face in (A). Source: *From Figure 9-29 in Melmed, S., & Kleinberg, D. (2016). Chapter 9: Pituitary masses and tumors. In Melmed, Polonsky, Larsen, & Kronenberg (Eds.),* Williams' textbook of endocrinology *(13th ed.) (p. 273). Elsevier.*

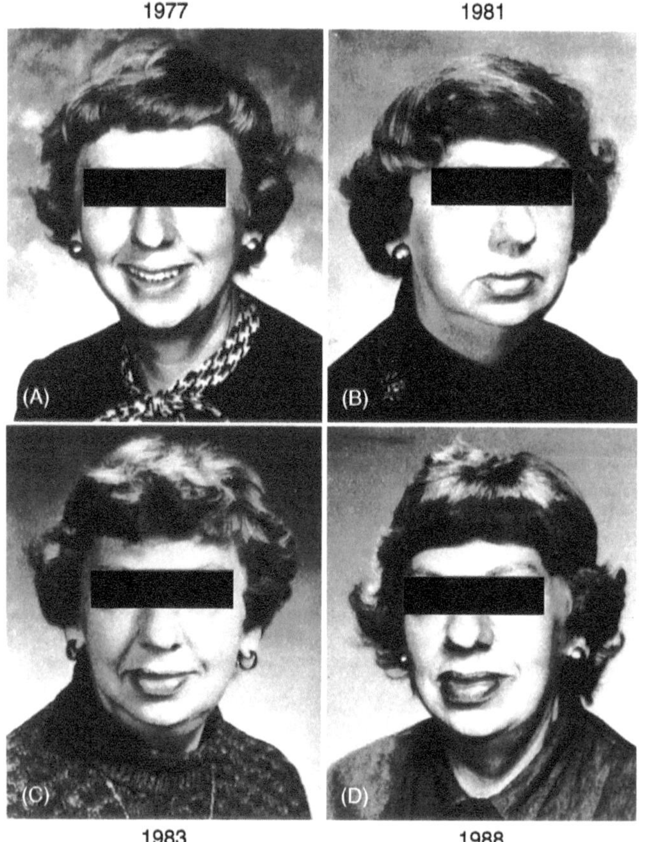

FIGURE 11.52 Development of acromegaly over an 11-year period. (A) through (D) Note the coarsening and enlargement of facial features over this period. Source: *From Figure 224-5 in M. E. Molitch. (2016). Chapter 224: Anterior pituitary. In L. Goldman, & A. I. Schafer (Eds.),* Goldman-Cecil textbook of medicine *(25th ed.) (p. 1486). Elsevier.*

There are limitations of GH action. The pediatric literature makes frequent use of the term genetic potential in discussions of diagnosis and treatment of disorders of growth. GH is a facilitator of expression of genetic potential for growth rather than as the primary determinant. The entire range over which GH can influence adult stature is only about 30% of the genetic potential. A person destined by genetic makeup to attain a final height of 6 ft will attain a height of about 4 ft even in the absence of GH and is unlikely to exceed 8 ft in height even with massive overproduction of GH from birth. It is not understood what determines genetic potential for growth, but it is clear that, although both arise from a single cell, a hypopituitary elephant is enormously larger than a giant mouse. Within the same species, something other than aberrations in GH secretion accounts for the large differences in the size of miniature and standard poodles or Chihuahuas and Great Danes.

Actions of growth hormone on skeletal structure

The ultimate height attained by an individual is determined by the length of the skeleton especially the vertebral column and long bones of the legs. Growth of these bones occurs by a process called endochondral ossification, in which proliferating cartilage is replaced by bone (Fig. 11.53).

The growing ends of long bones are called epiphyses and arise from ossification centers that are separate from those responsible for ossification of the diaphysis,

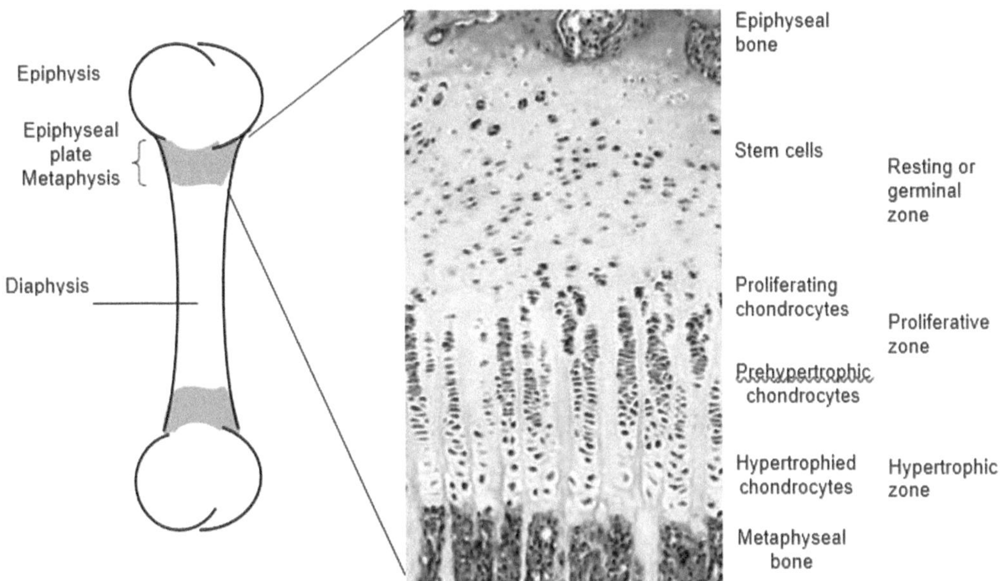

FIGURE 11.53 Schematic representation of the tibial epiphyseal growth plate. Source: *Modified from Nilsson, O., Marino, R., De Luca, F., Phillip, M., & Baron, J. (2005). Endocrine regulation of the growth plate.* Hormone Research, *64, 157.*

or shaft. In the growing individual the epiphyses are separated from the diaphysis by cartilaginous regions called epiphyseal plates, in which continuous production of chondrocytes provides the impetus for diaphyseal elongation. Chondrocytes in epiphyseal growth plates are arranged in orderly columns in parallel with the long axis of the bone reflecting the vectoral nature of their mitotic divisions. Frequent division of small, flattened chondrocyte precursors in the germinal zone at the distal end of the growth plate provides for continual elongation of columns of chondrocytes. As they grow and mature, chondrocytes produce the mucopolysaccharides and collagen that constitute the cartilage matrix. Cartilage cells hypertrophy become heavily vacuolated and degenerate as the surrounding matrix becomes calcified. Ingrowth of blood vessels and migration of osteoblast progenitors from the marrow results in the replacement of calcified cartilage with true bone.

Proliferation of chondrocytes at the epiphyseal border of the growth plate is balanced by cellular degeneration at the diaphyseal end, so in the normally growing individual, the thickness of the growth plate remains constant as the epiphyses are pushed further and further outward by the elongating shaft of bone. Eventually, progenitors of chondrocytes are either exhausted or lose their capacity to divide. As remaining chondrocytes go through their cycle of growth and degeneration, the epiphyseal plates become progressively narrower and ultimately are obliterated when diaphyseal bone fuses with the bony epiphyses. At this time the epiphyseal plates are said to be closed, and the capacity for further growth is lost.

In the absence of GH there is severe atrophy of the epiphyseal plates, which become narrow as proliferation of cartilage progenitor cells slows markedly. Conversely, after GH is given to a hypopituitary subject, resumption of cellular proliferation causes columns of chondrocytes to elongate and epiphyseal plates to widen. This characteristic response has been used as the basis of a biological assay for GH in experimental animals.

Growth of bone requires that diameter as well as length increase. Thickening of long bones is accomplished by proliferation of osteoblastic progenitors from the connective tissue sheath (periosteum) that surrounds the diaphysis. As it grows, bone is also subject to continual reabsorption and reorganization, with the incorporation of new cells that originate in both the periosteal and endosteal regions. Remodeling, which is an intrinsic property of skeletal growth, is accompanied by destruction and replacement of calcified matrix, as is described in Chapter 10, Hormonal Regulation of Calcium Balance. Treatment with GH often produces a transient increase in urinary excretion of calcium, phosphorus, and hydroxyproline, reflecting bone remodeling. Hydroxyproline derives from breakdown and replacement of collagen in bone matrix.

Effect of thyroid hormone on growth

As already mentioned in Chapter 3, Thyroid Gland, growth is stunted in children suffering from unremediated deficiency of thyroid hormones. Treatment of hypothyroid children with thyroid hormone results in rapid "catch up" growth and accelerated maturation of bone. Conversely, hyperthyroidism in children increases their rate of growth, but because of early epiphyseal closure, the maximum height attained is not increased. Thyroidectomy of juvenile experimental animals produces nearly as drastic an inhibition of growth as hypophysectomy, and restoration of normal amounts of triiodothyronine (T3) or thyroxine (T4) promptly reinitiates growth. Young mice grow somewhat faster than normal after treatment with thyroxine, but although attained earlier, adult size is no greater than normal.

The effects of thyroid hormones on growth are intimately entwined with GH. T3 and T4 have little, if any, growth-promoting effect in the absence of GH. Plasma concentrations of both GH (Fig. 11.54) and IGF-1 (Fig. 11.55) are reduced in hypothyroid children and adults and restored by treatment with thyroid hormone. This decrease is due to decreased amplitude of secretory pulses of GH and possibly also to a decrease in frequency consistent with impairments at both the hypothalamic and pituitary levels. Insulin-induced hypoglycemia and other stimuli for GH secretion produce abnormally small increases in the concentration of GH in the plasma of hypothyroid subjects. Such blunted responses to provocative signals probably reflect decreased sensitivity to GHRH as well as depletion of GH stores. Curiously, GH secretion in response to a test dose of GHRH is decreased when there is either a deficiency or an excess of thyroid hormone (Fig. 11.56).

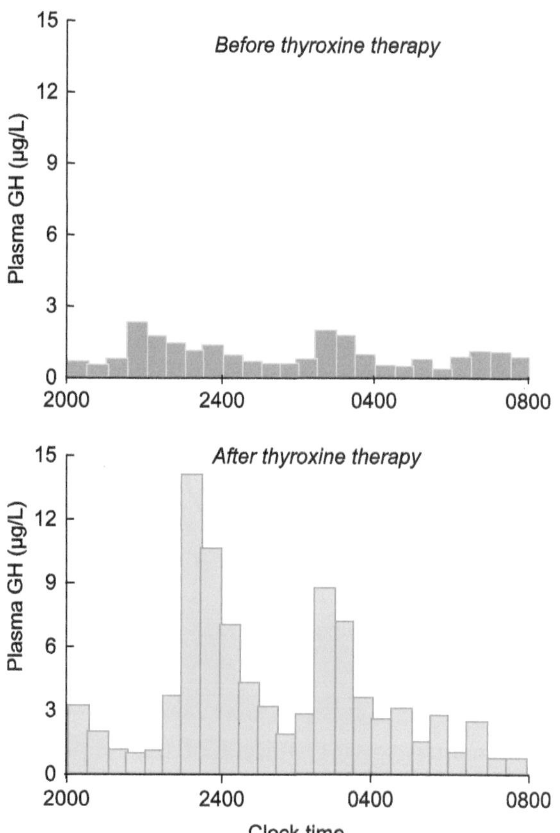

FIGURE 11.54 Nocturnal plasma concentrations of growth hormone in a hypothyroid boy in the early stages of puberty before and 2 months after treatment with thyroxine. Each bar represents the average plasma GH concentration during a 30-min period of continuous slow withdrawal of blood. Plasma IGF-1 was increased more than fourfold during treatment. Source: *From Chernausek, S. D., & Turner, R. (1989). Attenuation of spontaneous nocturnal growth hormone secretion in children with hypothyroidism and its correlation with plasma insulin-like growth factor I concentrations.* The Journal of Pediatrics 114, *965–972.*

Dependence of growth hormone synthesis and secretion on T3

The promoter region of the rodent GH gene contains a thyroid hormone response element and its transcriptional activity is enhanced by T3. Furthermore, T3 increases the stability of the GH messenger RNA transcripts. GH synthesis comes to an almost complete halt and the somatotropes become severely depleted of GH only a few days after thyroidectomy. The human GH gene lacks the thyroid hormone response element, and its transcription is not directly activated by T3. However, thyroid hormones affect synthesis of human GH indirectly. Blunted responses to GHRH in hypothyroid children and adults probably result from decreased expression GHRH receptors by somatotropes. Thyroidectomy also decreases the abundance of GHRH receptors in rodent somatotropes, and hormone replacement increases GHRH mRNA and restores both receptors. Similarly, thyroid hormones increase the expression of ghrelin receptors by rat somatotropes.

Importance of T3 for expression of growth hormone actions

Failure of growth in thyroid-deficient individuals is due largely to a deficiency of GH, which may be compounded by a decrease in sensitivity to GH. Treatment of thyroidectomized animals with GH alone can reinitiate growth, but even large amounts cannot sustain a normal rate of growth unless some thyroid hormone also is given. In rats that were both hypophysectomized and thyroidectomized, T4 decreased the amount of GH needed to stimulate growth (increased sensitivity) and exaggerated the magnitude of the response (increased efficacy). Thyroid hormone receptors are expressed by chondrocytes in the reserve and proliferating zones of the growth plate and mediate increased synthesis of matrix proteins. These cells also express the type 2 deiodinase and can convert T4 to T3 (see

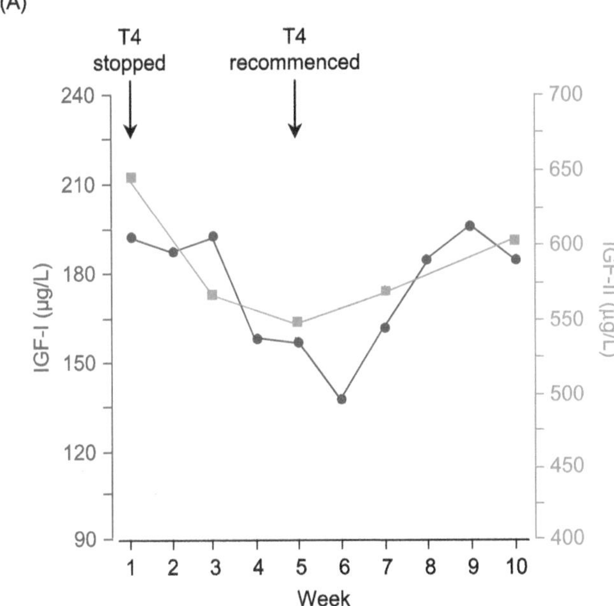

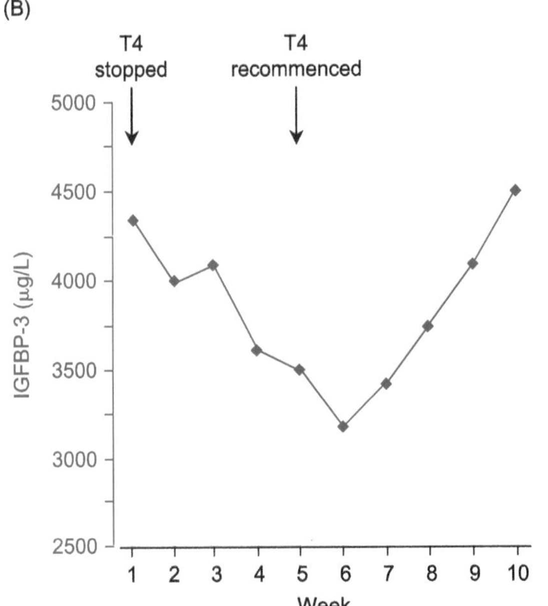

FIGURE 11.55 Effects of thyroxine on the plasma concentrations of IGF-1 and IGF-2 (panel A) and IGF binding protein-3 (panel B) in 10 thyroidectomized subjects following cessation and resumption of thyroxine (T4) treatment. Note the long delay in responses to both hormone deprivation and recommenced treatment. Source: *From Miell. J. P., Zini, M., Quin, J. D., Jones, J., Portioli, I., & Valcavi, R. (1994). Reversible effects of cessation and recommencement of thyroxine treatment on insulin- like growth factors (IGFs) and IGF-binding proteins in patients with total thyroidectomy.* The Journal of Clinical Endocrinology and Metabolism 79, *1507–1512.*

Chapter 3: Thyroid Gland). Treatment of thyroid deficient animals with T3 or T4 increases the expression of GH and IGF-1 receptors in growth plate cartilage and other tissues. The decrease in concentration of IGF-1 seen in the blood of hypothyroid individuals is due in

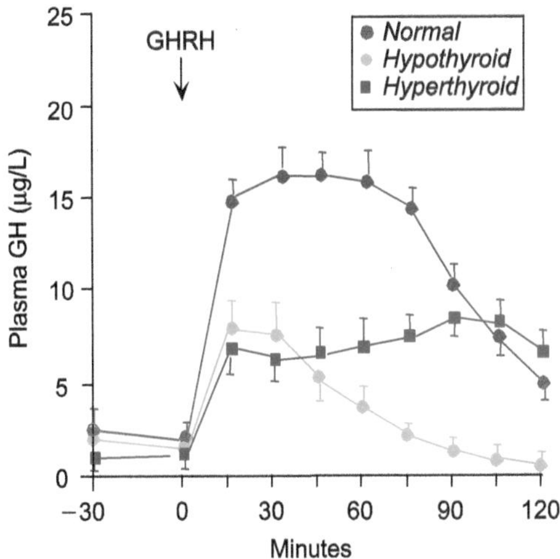

FIGURE 11.56 Decreased GH secretion in response to a test dose of GHRH in hypothyroid, normal, and hyperthyroid individuals. Data shown represent average responses from 30 normal, 25 hypothyroid, and 38 hyperthyroid adult patients. *GH*, Growth hormone; *GHRH*, growth-hormone-releasing hormone. Source: *From Valcavi, R., Zini, M., & Portioli, M. (1992). Thyroid hormones and growth hormone secretion.* Journal of Endocrinological Investigation 15, *313–330.*

part to decreased circulating GH and in part to decreased hepatic responsiveness to GH. In hypothyroid humans the extremities fail to develop to their full length and the individual remains small. Epiphyses in the hands fail to close and remain open (Fig. 11.57).

Effect of insulin on growth

Although neither GH nor thyroxine appears to be important determinants of fetal growth, many investigators have suggested that insulin may serve as a growth-promoting hormone during the fetal period. Infants born of diabetic mothers often are larger than normal, especially when the diabetes is poorly controlled. Because glucose readily crosses the placenta, high concentrations of glucose in maternal blood increases fetal blood glucose and stimulate the fetal pancreas to secrete insulin. In the rare cases of congenital deficiency of insulin that have been reported, fetal size is below normal. Structurally, insulin is closely related to IGF-1 and IGF-2 (Figs. 11.35 and 11.36) and when present in adequate concentrations can activate IGF-1 receptors. It is likely that at least some of the effects of insulin on fetal growth are mediated by IGF-1 receptors or by hybrid insulin/IGF-1 receptors.

Optimal concentrations of insulin in blood are required to maintain normal growth during postnatal life, but it has been difficult to obtain a precise definition of the role of insulin. Because life cannot be maintained for long without insulin, dramatic effects of

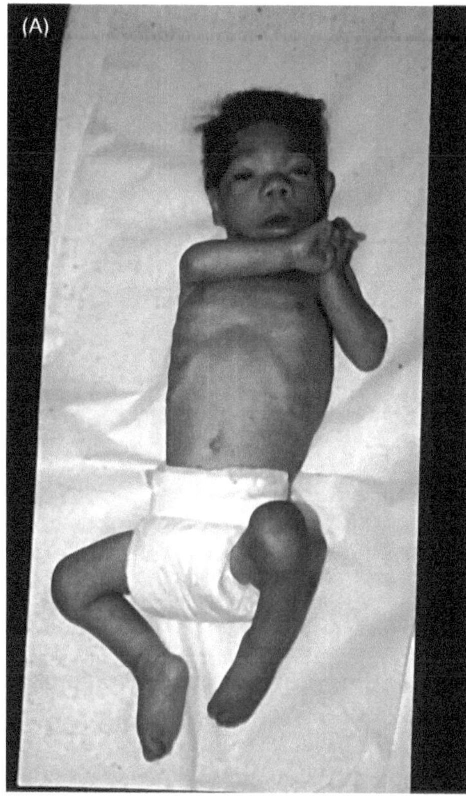

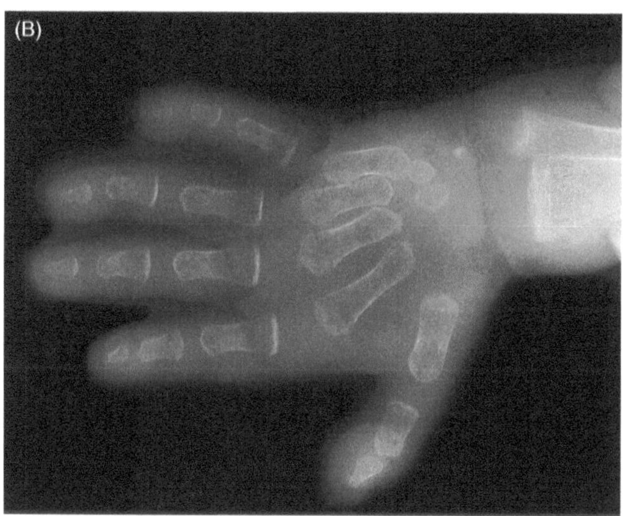

FIGURE 11.57 (A) A 17-year-old female who was found to be hypothyroid at birth but was not treated. Note the short limbs with respect to the trunk. (B) A radiograph of her hands shows that the epiphyses have no closed. Source: *From Figures 13-3 and 13-4 in Brent, G. A., & Weetman, A. P. (2016). Chapter 13: Hypothyroidism and thyroiditis. In Melmed, Polonsky, Larsen, & Kronenberg (Eds.),* Williams' textbook of endocrinology *(13th ed.) (p. 421). Elsevier.*

sustained deficiency on final adult size are not seen. However, growth often is retarded in insulin-dependent diabetic children, particularly in the months leading up to the diagnosis of full-blown disease.

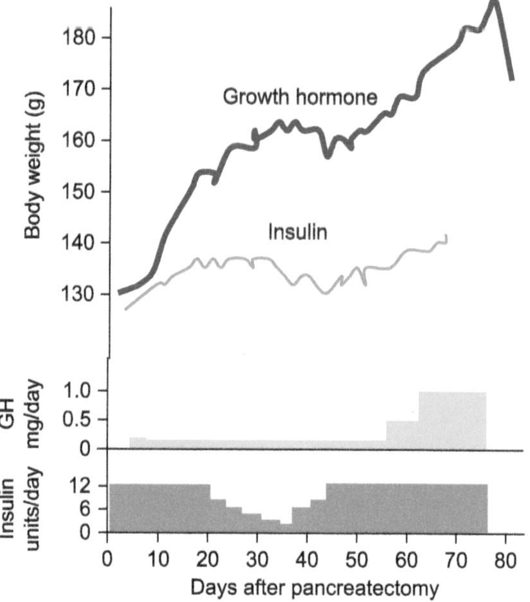

FIGURE 11.58 Requirement of insulin for normal growth in response to GH. Rats were pancreatectomized 3–7 weeks before the experiment was begun. Each rat was fed 7 g food/day. The treated group was injected with the indicated amounts of GH daily. Note the failure to respond to GH in the period between 20 and 44 days, coincident with the decrease in daily insulin dose, and the resumption of growth when the daily dose of insulin was restored. *GH,* Growth hormone. Source: *From Scow, R. O., Wagner, E. M., & Ronov, E. (1958). Effect of growth hormone and insulin on body weight and nitrogen retention in pancreatectomized rats.* Endocrinology, *62, 593–604.*

Studies in pancreatectomized rats indicate a direct relation between the effectiveness of GH and the dose of insulin administered. Treatment with GH sustained a rapid rate of growth so long as the daily dose of insulin was adequate, but growth progressively decreased as the dose of insulin was reduced (Fig. 11.58). Conversely, insulin cannot sustain a normal rate of growth in the absence of GH.

The effects of insulin on postnatal growth cannot be attributed to changes in GH secretion, which, if anything, is increased in human diabetics. Although insulin sometimes was used diagnostically to provoke GH secretion, it is the resulting hypoglycemia, rather than insulin per se, that stimulates GH release. Expression of IGF-1 mRNA in liver and other tissues is decreased in diabetes and in low insulin states such as fasting or caloric restriction, consistent with the possibility that insulin is permissive for growth. Insulin stimulates protein synthesis and inhibits protein degradation and, in its absence, protein breakdown is severe. Consequently, without insulin, normal responses to GH are not seen. The anabolic effects of GH on body protein either cannot be expressed or are masked by simultaneous, unchecked catabolic processes.

Effect of gonadal hormones on growth

Awakening of the gonads at the onset of sexual maturation is accompanied by a dramatic acceleration of growth. The adolescent growth spurt, like other changes at puberty, is attributable to steroid hormones of the gonads and perhaps the adrenals. Because the development of pubic and axillary hair at the onset of puberty is a response to increased secretion of adrenal androgens, this initial stage of sexual maturation is called adrenarche. The physiological mechanisms that trigger the increased secretion of adrenal androgens and the awakening of the gonadotropic secretory apparatus are poorly understood. They are considered further in Chapter 12, Hormonal Control of Reproduction in the Male. At the same time that gonadal steroids promote linear growth, they accelerate closure of the epiphyses and therefore limit the final height that can be attained. Children who undergo early puberty and hence experience their growth spurt while their contemporaries continue to grow at the slower prepubertal rate are likely to be the tallest and most physically developed in grade school or junior high but among the shortest in their high school graduating class. Deficiency of gonadal hormones, if left untreated, delays epiphyseal closure, and despite the absence of a pubertal growth spurt, such hypogonadal individuals tend to be tall and have unusually long arms and legs.

In considering the relationship of the gonadal hormones to the pubertal growth spurt, it is important to understand that

- androgens and estrogens are produced and secreted by both the ovaries and the testes,
- androgens are precursors of estrogens and are converted to estrogens in a reaction catalyzed by the enzyme P450 aromatase in the gonads and extragonadal tissues (see Chapter 4: The Adrenal Glands), and
- estrogens produce their biological effects at hormone concentrations that are more than 1000 times lower than the concentrations at which androgens produce their effects.

Until recently it was generally accepted that androgens produce the adolescent growth spurt in both sexes. This idea was rooted in the observations that even at the relatively low doses used therapeutically in women, administration of estrogens inhibits growth, whereas administration of androgens stimulates growth. Some "experiments of nature" that have come to light in recent years have challenged this idea and lead to the opposite conclusion. Girls with ovarian agenesis (congenital absence of ovaries) have short stature and do not experience an adolescent growth surge. Their growth is increased by treatment with very low doses of estrogen, below the threshold needed to cause breast development. In normal girls the adolescent growth spurt usually occurs before estrogen secretion is sufficient to initiate growth of breasts.

Patients of either sex who have a homozygous disruption of the P450 aromatase gene do not experience a pubertal growth spurt despite supranormal levels of androgens and continue to grow at the juvenile rate well beyond the time of normal epiphyseal fusion unless estrogens are given. Although sexual development cannot occur in girls with this extremely rare defect, affected males develop normally. A man with a homozygous disruption of the α estrogen receptor similarly had normal sexual development but failed to experience an adolescent growth spurt (Fig. 11.59).

At age 28, when he was diagnosed, he was 6 ft 8 in. tall and his epiphyses had still not closed. In contrast, patients with nonfunctional androgen receptors experience a normal pubertal growth spurt and their epiphyses close at the normal time. These observations established that estrogen rather than androgen is responsible for both acceleration of growth at puberty and maturation of the epiphyseal plates.

It is noteworthy that estrogen concentrations increase in the plasma of both boys and girls early in puberty and reach similar concentrations at the onset of the growth spurt. The well-established growth promoting the effect of androgens administered to children whose epiphyses are not yet fused is likely attributable to their conversion to estrogen. Synthetic androgens that are chemically modified in ways that prevent aromatization produce only a small and brief stimulation of linear growth even though other aspects of androgen activity (see Chapter 12: Hormonal Control of Reproduction in the Male) are fully evident.

Effects of estrogens on epiphyseal growth plates

Cartilage progenitor cells in the epiphyseal plates express receptors for estrogens, which respond initially with increased rates of differentiation and hypertrophy. In what has been called accelerated senescence, estrogen stimulation of stem cell maturation depletes the pool of cartilage stem cells, perhaps by interfering with their replacement in response to GH, or perhaps by directly causing them to lose their capacity to divide. In any case, with continued stimulation, the growth plate becomes progressively narrower and is ultimately obliterated when the bony epiphysis fuses with the metaphysis.

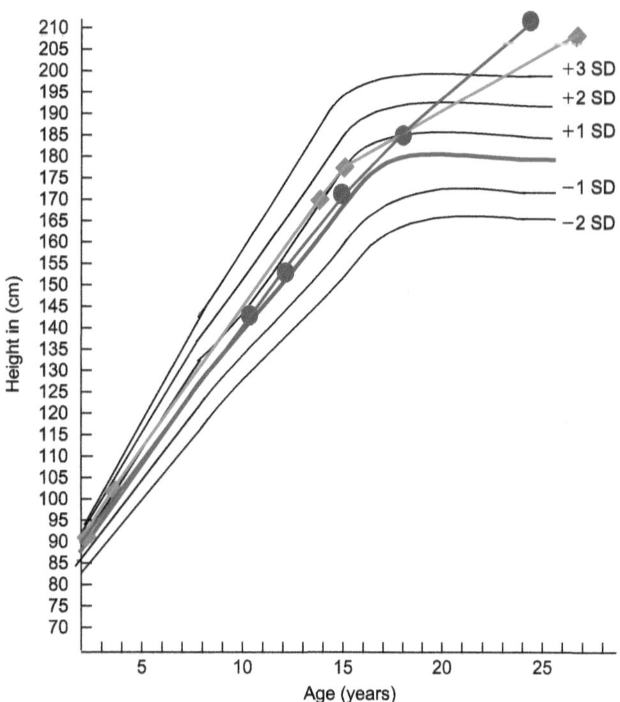

FIGURE 11.59 Growth curves of men with inactivating mutations of the alpha estrogen receptor (*red line*) or P450 aromatase (*green line*). Compared to normal (*blue line*). Standard deviations above and below normal are shown. Source: *From Smith, E. P., Boyd, J., Frank, G. R., Takahashi, H., Cohen, R. M., Specker, B., Williams, T. C., Lubahn, D. B., & Korach, K. S. (1994). Estrogen resistance caused by a mutation in the estrogen-receptor gene in a man.* The New England Journal of Medicine 331, *1056–1061; and Morishima, A., Grumbach, M. M., Simpson, E. R., Fisher, C., & Qin, K. (1995) Aromatase deficiency in male and female siblings caused by a novel mutation and the physiological role of estrogens.* The Journal of Clinical Endocrinology and Metabolism 80, *3689–3698.*

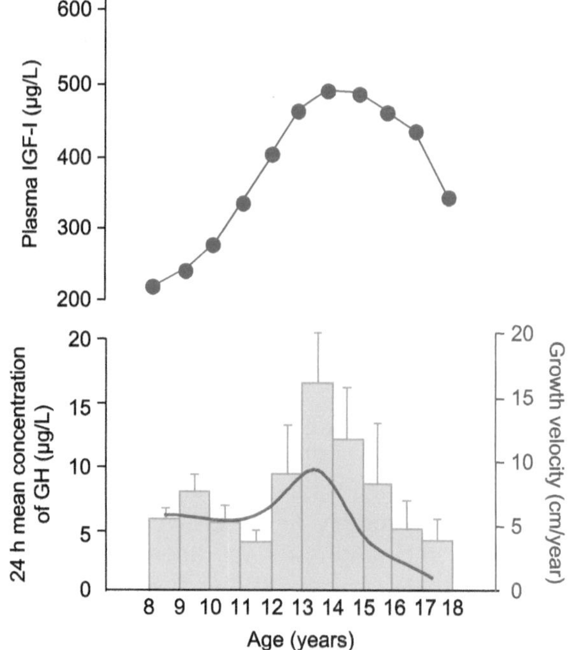

FIGURE 11.60 Changes in plasma IGF-1 and GH concentrations in the peripubertal period in normal boys. Bars in the lower panel indicate 24 h integrated concentrations of GH. The blue curve is the idealized growth velocity curve for North American boys. *GH*, Growth hormone. Source: *Upper panel from Juul, A., Dalgaard, P., Blum, W. F., Bang, P., Hall, K., Michaelsen, K. F., Muller, J., & Skakkebaek, N. E. (1995) Serum levels of insulin-like growth factor (IGF)–binding protein-3 (IGFBP-3) in healthy infants, children, and adolescents: The relation to IGF-1, IGF-2, IGFBP-1, IGFBP-2, age, sex, body mass index, and pubertal maturation.* The Journal of Clinical Endocrinology and Metabolism 80, *2534–2542. Lower panel from Martha, P. M. Jr., Rogol, A. D., Veldhuis, J. D., Kerrigan. J. R., Goodman, D. W., Blizzard, R. M. (1989) Alterations in pulsatile properties of circulating growth hormone concentrations during puberty in boys.* The Journal of Clinical Endocrinology and Metabolism 69, *563–570.*

Effects on growth hormone secretion and action

Most, and possibly all, of the increase in height stimulated by estrogens or androgens at puberty is due to increased secretion of GH, which coincides with maximal growth velocity in mid to late puberty (Fig. 11.60).

This increase in growth velocity is accompanied by increased plasma concentrations of IGF-1 presumably in response to increased GH. During the pubertal growth spurt or when androgens are given to prepubertal children, there is an increase in amplitude, duration, and sometimes frequency of secretory pulses of GH reflecting increased the release of GHRH by arcuate neurons (Fig. 11.61).

Increased secretion of GH at puberty, like the maturation of the growth plate, is triggered by estrogens but not androgens. Aromatase activity is detectable in the hypothalamus and may explain the findings that only estrogens and aromatizable androgens can produce the pubertal increase in GH secretion.

The complexities of the interactions of estrogens and GH are not fully understood. At the same concentrations that estrogens increase GH secretion, they inhibit responses to GH (Fig. 11.7), and plasma concentrations of GH are higher in women than in men. In addition, the GH secretory apparatus tends to be more sensitive to environmental influences in women than in men. Circulating concentrations of GH tend to rise more readily in women in response to provocative stimuli. Estrogens appear to interfere with the actions of GH at the level of its target cells. Estrogens, which are not catabolic, antagonize the effects of GH on nitrogen retention and minimize the increase in IGF-1 in blood of hypophysectomized or hypopituitary individuals treated with GH.

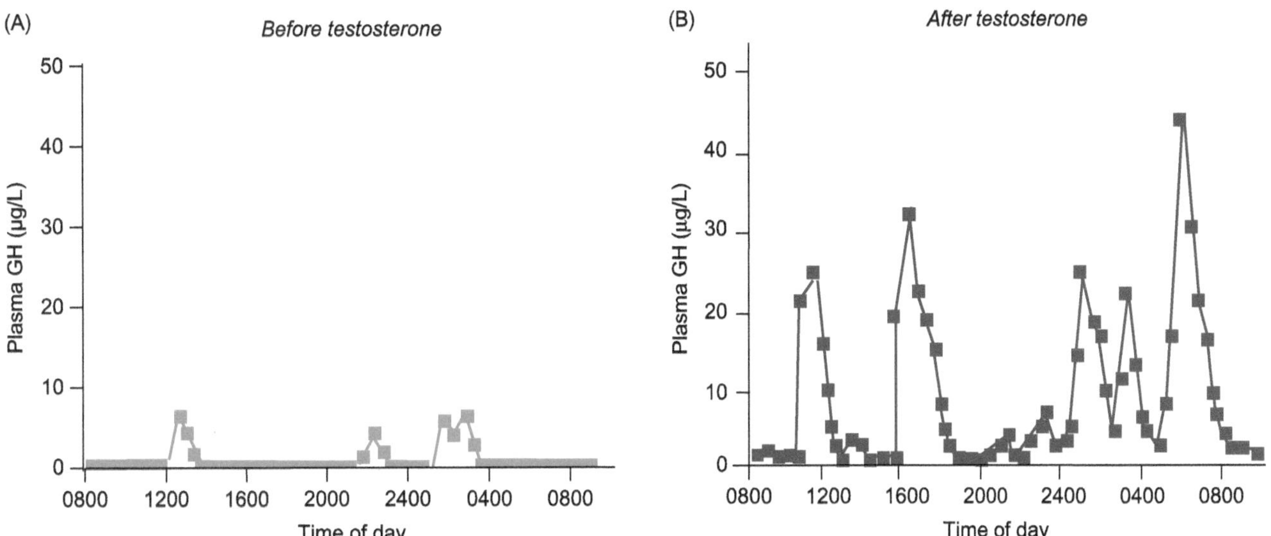

FIGURE 11.61 Effects of testosterone in a boy with short stature and delayed puberty. (A) Before testosterone. (B) During therapy with long-acting testosterone. Note the increase in frequency and amplitude of growth hormone secretory episodes in the treated subjects. Source: *From Link, K., Blizzard, R. M., Evans, W. S., Kaiser, D. L., Parker, M. W., & Rogol, A. D. (1986). The effect of androgens on the pulsatile release and the twenty-four-hour mean concentration of growth hormone in peripubertal males.* The Journal of Clinical Endocrinology and Metabolism 62, *159–164.*

Effects of androgens

Although most of the growth-promoting effects of androgens result from the activation of estrogen receptors following aromatization to estrogen, some stimulation of growth is attributable to activation of androgen receptors.

On average, men are taller and have larger skeletons than women. The greater height of males is due in part to the later onset of puberty in boys, and to the greater maximal rate and duration of growth achieved in adolescence. Cartilage cells in all zones of human tibial growth plates express androgen receptors whose activity may modulate estrogenic effects on epiphyseal closure. Androgens also increase bone diameter and thickening of cortical bone by stimulating periosteal intramembranous bone formation. This may account for the larger diameter of bones in men.

Androgens stimulate growth of muscle, particularly in the upper body. Androgen secretion during puberty in boys produces a doubling of muscle mass by increasing the size and number of muscle cells. Such growth of muscle can occur in the absence of GH or thyroid hormones and is mediated by the same androgen receptors that are expressed in other androgen-sensitive tissues (see Chapter 12: Hormonal Control of Reproduction in the Male). Stimulation of muscle growth by androgens is most pronounced in androgen-deficient or hypopituitary subjects, and only small effects, if any, are seen in men with normal testicular function except when very large doses of anabolic steroids are used. It is this action of androgens that lead to their abuse by athletes seeking to enhance performance.

Effect of glucocorticoids on growth

Normal growth requires the secretion of glucocorticoids, whose widespread effects promote optimal function of a variety of organ systems (see Chapter 4: The Adrenal Glands), a sense of health and well-being, and normal appetite. Glucocorticoids are required for the synthesis of GH and have complex effects on GH secretion. When given acutely, they may enhance GH gene transcription and increase responsiveness of somatotropes to GHRH. However, GH secretion is reduced by excessive glucocorticoids, probably as a result of increased somatostatin production. Children suffering from overproduction of glucocorticoids (Cushing's disease) experience some stunting of their growth. In a recently reported case involving identical twins the unaffected twin was 21 cm taller at age 15 than her sister whose disease was untreated until around the time of puberty. Similar impairment of growth is seen in children treated chronically with high doses of glucocorticoids to control asthma or inflammatory disorders. Consistent with their catabolic effects in muscle and lymphoid tissues, glucocorticoids also antagonize the actions of GH. Hypophysectomized rats grew less in response to GH when cortisone was given simultaneously (Fig. 11.62). Glucocorticoids similarly blunt the response to GH administered to hypopituitary children. The cellular mechanisms for this antagonism are not yet understood.

Hepatic production of IGF-1 may be reduced by treatment with glucocorticoids.

Glucocorticoid receptors are present in the growth plates and are most abundant in the hypertrophic zone. Glucocorticoids inhibit the division of stem cells and increase apoptosis of hypertrophied chondrocytes. In animal studies, glucocorticoids also decrease expression of GH and IGF-1 receptors. Curiously, the suppression of growth during exposure of the growth plates to excessive amounts of glucocorticoids is followed by a period of supranormal growth when glucocorticoid concentrations are restored to normal. This so-called catch-up growth has been explained with the proposal that the potential for growth at the epiphyseal plates may be determined by the cumulative number of stem cell divisions. By suppressing stem cell proliferation, excessive glucocorticoids may delay the age-related decrease in the capacity to proliferate so that rapid cell division follows the release of suppression. Catch-up growth is rarely complete. It is

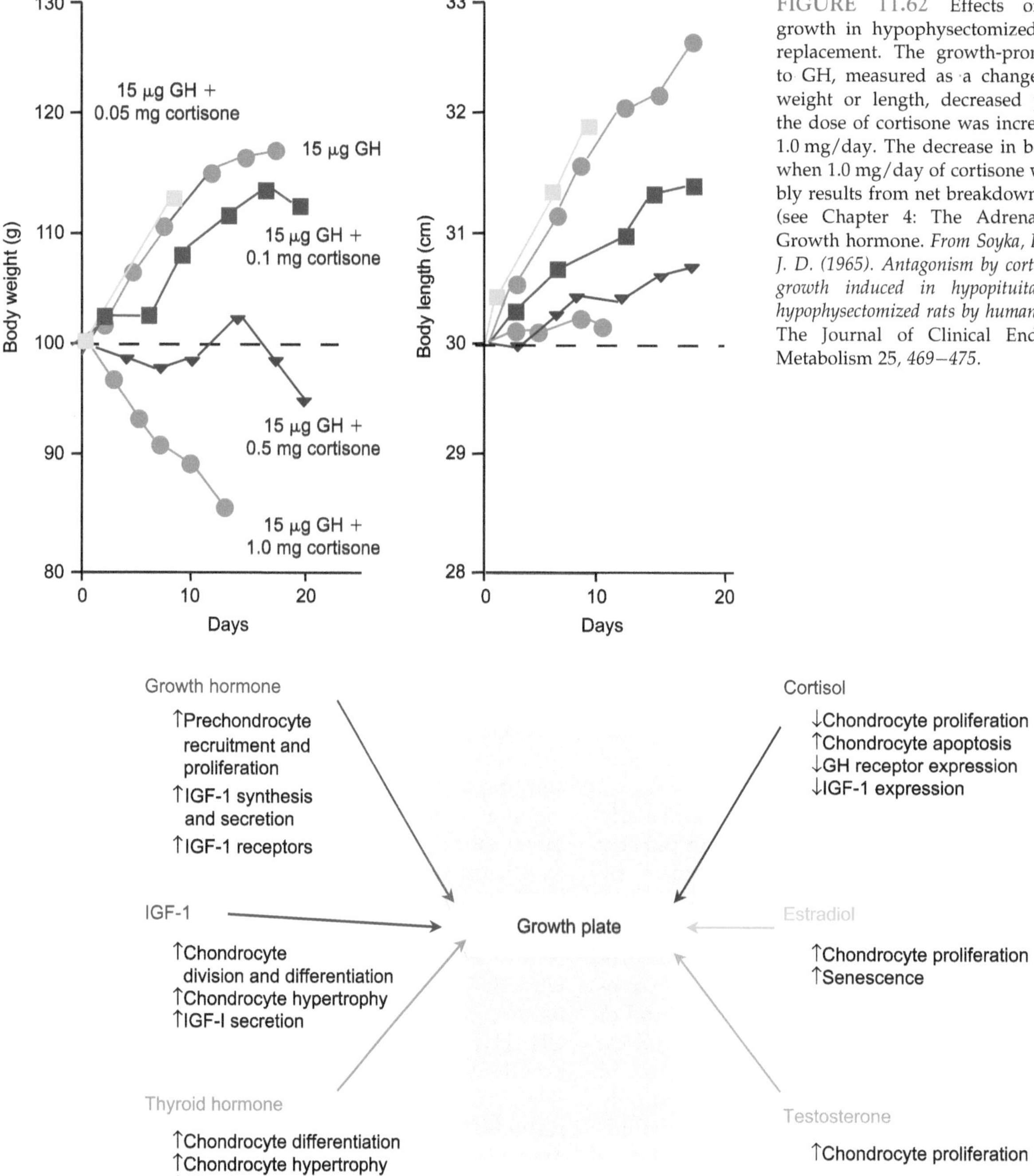

FIGURE 11.62 Effects of cortisone on growth in hypophysectomized rats given GH replacement. The growth-promoting response to GH, measured as a change in either body weight or length, decreased progressively as the dose of cortisone was increased from 0.1 to 1.0 mg/day. The decrease in body weight seen when 1.0 mg/day of cortisone was given probably results from net breakdown of muscle mass (see Chapter 4: The Adrenal Glands). *GH*, Growth hormone. *From Soyka, L. F., & Crawford, J. D. (1965). Antagonism by cortisone of the linear growth induced in hypopituitary patients and hypophysectomized rats by human growth hormone.* The Journal of Clinical Endocrinology and Metabolism 25, *469–475.*

FIGURE 11.63 Effects of hormones on the epiphyseal growth plate.

not limited to relief from glucocorticoid excess, but also is seen after the correction of GH or thyroid hormone deficiency or malnutrition. Effects of the various hormones on the epiphyseal growth plates are summarized in Fig. 11.63.

Summary

Building on previous chapters which discussed the regulation of fuel and the absorption of calcium, this chapter discusses the hormonal interactions that are involved in growth. The diversity of hormones and their target structures reflects the importance of this process. It involves the interactions of the nervous system, liver, digestive system, as well as the endocrine system as initiators of growth.

Suggested reading

Basic foundations

Barrett, E. J. (2017). Endocrine regulation of growth and body mass. In W. F. Boron, & E. L. Boulpaep (Eds.), *Medical physiology* (3rd ed., pp. 990–1005). Philadelphia, PA: Elsevier.

Cooke, D. W., DiVall, S. A., & Radovick, S. (2016). Normal and aberrant growth in children. In S. Melmed, K. S. Polonsky, P. R. Larsen, & H. M. Kronenberg (Eds.), *Williams textbook of endocrinology* (13th ed., pp. 964–1073). Philadelphia, PA: Elsevier.

Keane, V. (2016). Assessment of growth. In R. M. Kliegman, B. F. Stanton, J. W. St. Geme, III, & N. F. Schor (Eds.), *Nelson textbook of pediatrics* (20th ed., Vol. 1, pp. 84-91). Philadelphia, PA: Elsevier.

Additional information

Chiloiro, S., Giampietro, A., Bianchi, A., & De Marinis, L. (2016). Clinical management of teratoma, a rare hypothalamic-pituitary neoplasia. *Endocrine, 53*(3), 636–642. Available from https://doi.org/10.1007/s12020-015-0814-4.

Ibrahim Abdalla, M. M. (2015). Ghrelin – Physiological functions and regulation. *European Endocrinology, 11*(2), 90–95. Available from https://doi.org/10.17925/EE.2015.11.02.90.

Li, Z., Ke, N., Liu, X., & Gong, S. (2018). Mature cystic teratoma of the pancreas with 30 years of clinical course: A case report. *Medicine, 97*(15), e0405. Available from https://doi.org/10.1097/md.0000000000010405.

Magliocca, J. F., Held, I. K. A., & Odorico, J. S. (2006). Undifferentiated murine embryonic stem cells cannot induce portal tolerance but may possess immune privilege secondary to reduced major histocompatibility complex antigen expression. *Stem Cells and Development, 15*(5), 707–717. Available from https://doi.org/10.1089/scd.2006.15.707.

Mohib, K., Allan, D., & Wang, L. (2010). Human embryonic stem cell-extracts inhibit the differentiation and function of monocyte-derived dendritic cells. *Stem Cell Reviews and Reports, 6*(4), 611–621. Available from https://doi.org/10.1007/s12015-010-9185-7.

Quon, J. L., Hwang, P. H., & Edwards, M. S. B. (2016). 201 Transnasal endoscopic approach for pediatric skull base tumors: a case series. *Neurosurgery, 63*(CN_suppl_1), 179-179. Available from https://doi.org/10.1227/01.neu.0000489770.74513.3e.

Saeger, W., Ebrahimi, A., Beschorner, R., Spital, H., Honegger, J., & Wilczak, W. (2017). Teratoma of the sellar region: A case report. *Endocrine Pathology, 28*(4), 315–319. Available from https://doi.org/10.1007/s12022-016-9465-0.

Shim, K.-W., Kim, D.-S., Choi, J.-U., & Kim, S.-H. (2007). Congenital cavernous sinus cystic teratoma. *Yonsei Medical Journal, 48*(4), 704–710. Available from https://doi.org/10.3349/ymj.2007.48.4.704.

Yakar, S. Insulin-like growth factors: Actions on the skeleton. Journal of Molecular Endocrinology, JME-17-0298. https://doi.org/10.1530/JME-17-0298.

CHAPTER

12

Hormonal control of reproduction in the male

Case study: A case of infertility

She came into the clinic seeking medical advice. She had been happily married for 5 years and could not get pregnant. She felt that her biological clock was ticking—after all, she was into her early 30s.

Many of us in the clinic knew her—as she was also a professional in health care. Friendly, hardworking, and down to earth, she commanded—and got—respect and admiration.

Her menstrual cycles were 3–4 months apart, unusual but not uncommon. A pelvic exam did not disclose anything abnormal. In habitus, she was a well-developed female with sparse pubic and axillary hair, similar to Fig. 12.1.

However, subclinical salpingitis could cause adhesions that would prevent pregnancy. A laparoscopic examination would usually be able to confirm such a condition.

According to the World Health Organization, infertility affects approximately 50 million couples worldwide and is on the increase as a percent of the population. This includes couples that have had one child but cannot have a second one. The age range for fertility concerns in females is from 20 to 44 and she must have been in a relationship for 5 years. There is no age limit for males. The top three causes of infertility are ovulatory problems, male reproductive issues, and tubal disorders.

A careful workup was done on her husband. His sperm count, number of normal sperm, and amount of ejaculate were normal.

An exploratory laparoscopy was done. The uterus and uterine (fallopian) tubes were small. The ovaries were in the right location but they looked strange. A biopsy was done and sent down to the lab. The results came back that they were not ovaries but testes. These were removed as there is a high risk of malignancy in undescended testes.

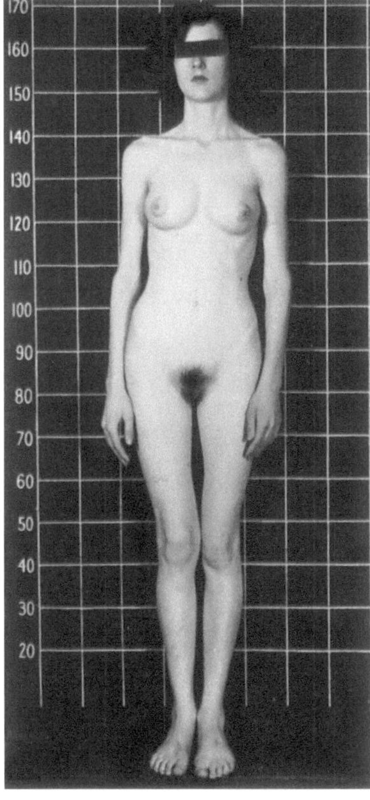

FIGURE 12.1 A 17-year-old patient with a female habitus and a case similar to the one described in the case study. Source: *From Figure 12-41 Moore, K. L., Persaud, T. V. N., & Torchia, M. G. (2016).* The developing human *(10th ed.) (p. 272). Elsevier.*

Subsequent blood studies were done. The serum levels of luteinizing hormone and follicle-stimulating hormone were high, so was the androgen level. Examination of neutrophils in the metaphase of mitosis presented a 46, XY karyotype. It was also found that she was not secreting anti-Müllerian hormone (also called

Goodman's Basic Medical Endocrinology.
DOI: https://doi.org/10.1016/B978-0-12-815844-9.00012-9

(*cont'd*)

Müllerian inhibitory substance), which would have caused the uterus and uterine tubes as well as the vagina to regress during embryonic development.

The patient was genetically, gonadally, and hormonally a male (46, XY), but the receptors for androgen were defective or lacking throughout her body, so she developed as a female and thought of herself as a female. She had androgen insensitivity syndrome (AIS) formerly called testicular feminization. It is a rare condition, affecting approximately 1 in 15,000 male births.

The question then became what to tell the patient. The literature of the time indicated that many AIS patients that were told of their diagnosis committed suicide. Not wanting that result, the gynecologist decided to simply say that she could not have children and suggested that she and her husband adopt a child. They did so.

However, being in the health-care profession, the answer did not satisfy the patient and she began to look at her results and to question the gynecologist. Eventually, she discerned the true nature of her disorder and correctly identified her condition. The gynecologist concurred with her findings. He also asked her what she planned to tell her husband. She elected never to tell him.

Today, many years later, with a team approach, which includes psychologists, surgeons, endocrinologists, and gynecologists as part of that team, the patient is told of their condition and what can be done to either enhance the phenotype, such as enlarging the vagina for intercourse, or to change the phenotype to match the genotype.

In the clinic:

Disorders of sexual development in the male

There are three main causes of male sexual development resulting in a female phenotype. These are disorders due to testis development, androgen synthesis, and androgen action, most commonly due to mutations in the androgen receptor, as the patient in the case study had.

Disorders due to testis development: crossover

Only one disorder will be discussed here and that concerns mutations due to crossover. The crossover mutation begins with meiosis. Normally, in interphase I of meiosis I the chromosomes are replicated. During the pachytene phase of prophase I of meiosis I, there is crossover with the exchange of genes between the homologous pairs of chromosomes and the X and Y chromosomes (one originally of maternal origin and the other of paternal origin). This crossover continues through the diplotene phase and then through metaphase I stage. During the anaphase I stage, the chromosomes pull apart with the exchanged genes remaining on the recipient chromosomes. At the end of meiosis I the pairs separate into two different cells but each member of a pair within those cells still has a duplicate of itself Fig. 12.2.

Although the number of chromosomes has been halved (the cells are haploid), the amount of deoxyribonucleic acid (DNA) is still the same as before meiosis began because the replicated chromosomes are still present. In meiosis II, these replicated pairs are separated into two more cells. At the end of meiosis II, there are four haploid cells with half the chromosome number and half the DNA when compared to the one that underwent meiosis I (Fig. 12.3).

The Y chromosome has a long and short arm (Fig. 12.4).

Sometimes, in meiosis I of an XY male sperm, there can be genes exchanged, which have to do with sexual development (Fig. 12.5).

If in meiosis II the Y chromatid of meiosis II is lacking the *SRY/TDF* gene and if this haploid sperm (Y) then combines with a haploid ovum, the individual will develop as a female because the *SRY/TDF* is absent even though the genotype is XY. Conversely, if the SRY/TDF is on an X chromosome which then combines with a haploid ovum, the phenotype will be male even though the genotype is female (Fig. 12.6).

Signs and symptoms of complete androgen insufficiency syndrome

The signs and symptoms of the above disorders of sex development (and the many more that were not mentioned) are highly varied. Only those pertaining to complete androgen insufficiency syndrome will be discussed.

In the infant, an inguinal enlargement indicates the location of undescended testes. However, in many cases,

(*cont'd*)

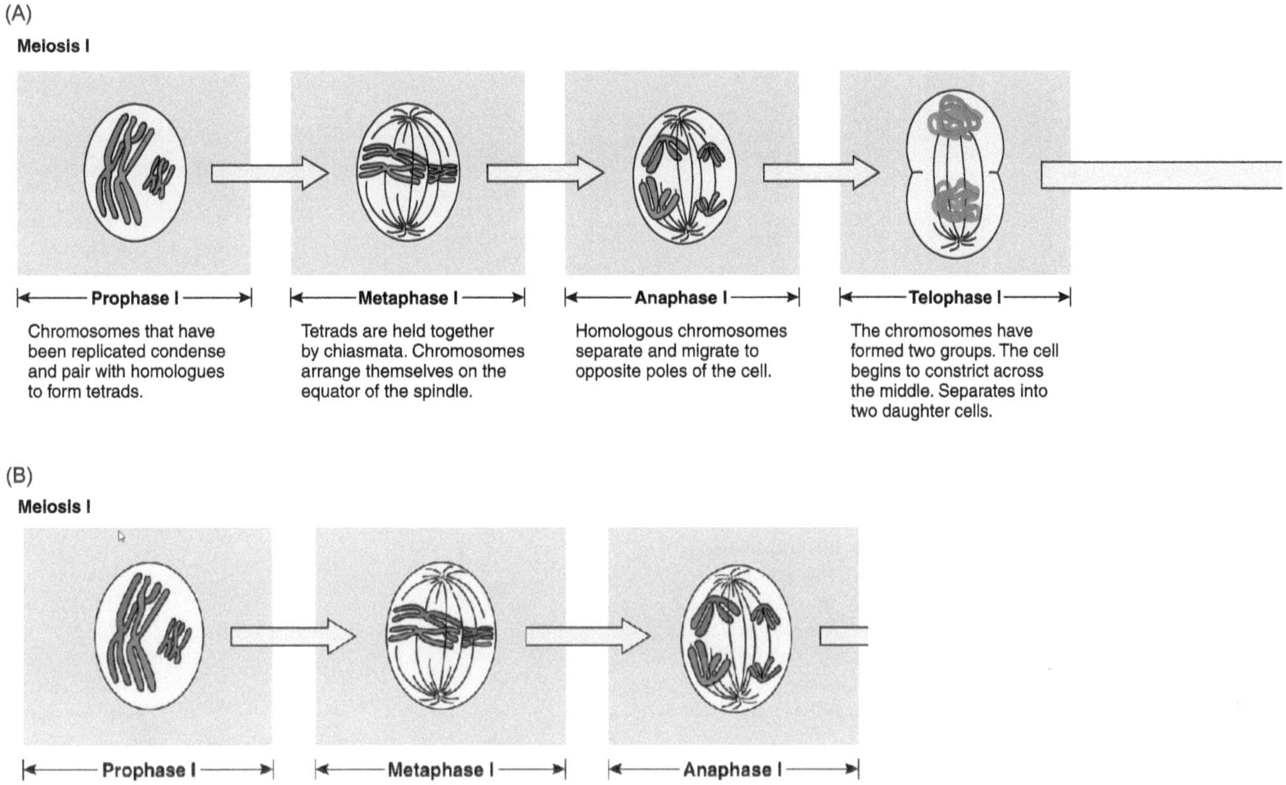

(A)
Meiosis I
Prophase I
Chromosomes that have been replicated condense and pair with homologues to form tetrads.
Metaphase I
Tetrads are held together by chiasmata. Chromosomes arrange themselves on the equator of the spindle.
Anaphase I
Homologous chromosomes separate and migrate to opposite poles of the cell.
Telophase I
The chromosomes have formed two groups. The cell begins to constrict across the middle. Separates into two daughter cells.
(B)
Meiosis I
Prophase I
Metaphase I
Anaphase I

FIGURE 12.2 (A) Meiosis I sequence. (B) Enlargement to show the crossover, which occurs during the leptotene phase of prophase I and continues until anaphase I. In older men and women, there may be abnormalities in the crossover and subsequent separation resulting in genetic disorders in their children. Source: *From Figure 3.18 in Gartner, L. P. (2017).* Textbook of histology *(4th ed.) (p. 76). Elsevier.*

Meiosis II
Prophase II
The chromosomes of the two daughter cells condense again in preparation for a second meiotic division.
Metaphase II
The chromosomes then migrate to the equator.
Anaphase II
The newly separated chromosomes of the two daughter cells move to opposite poles of their spindle.
Telophase II
The cells constrict across the nuclear membrane. Four haploid nuclei are formed, each with one member of each pair of chromosomes from the original nucleus.

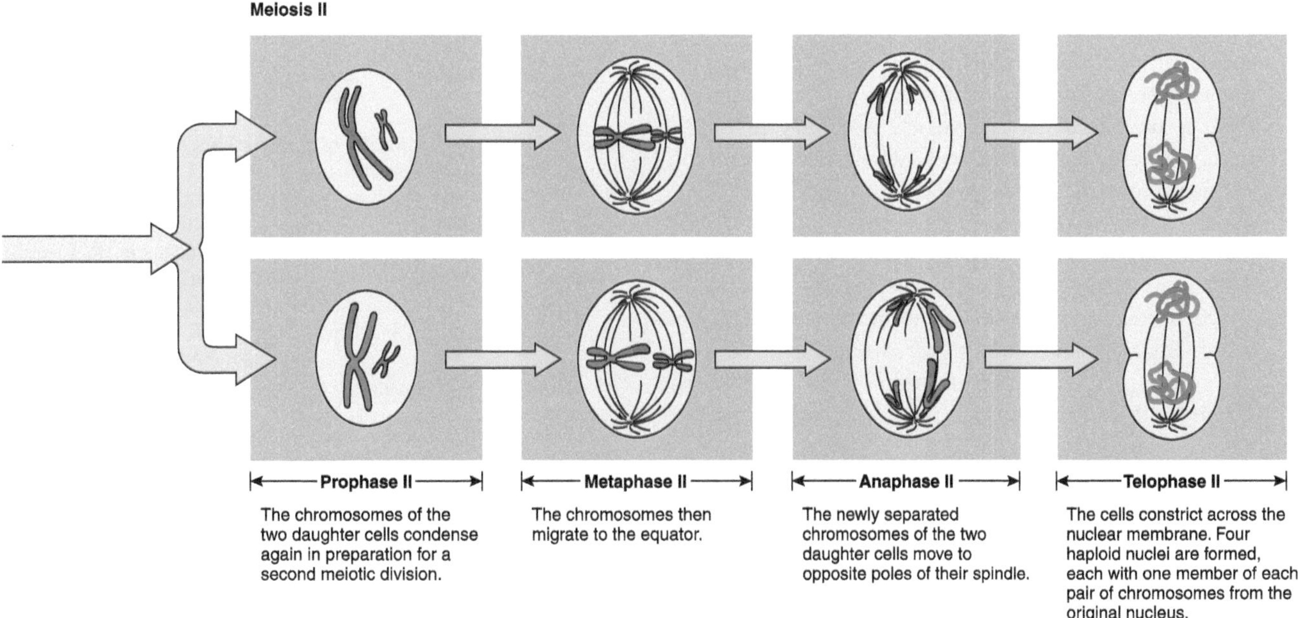

FIGURE 12.3 Meiosis II showing how at the end of telophase II, there are four haploid cells. Source:*From Figure 3.18 in Gartner, L. P. (2017).* Textbook of histology *(4th ed.) (p. 77). Elsevier.*

(cont'd)

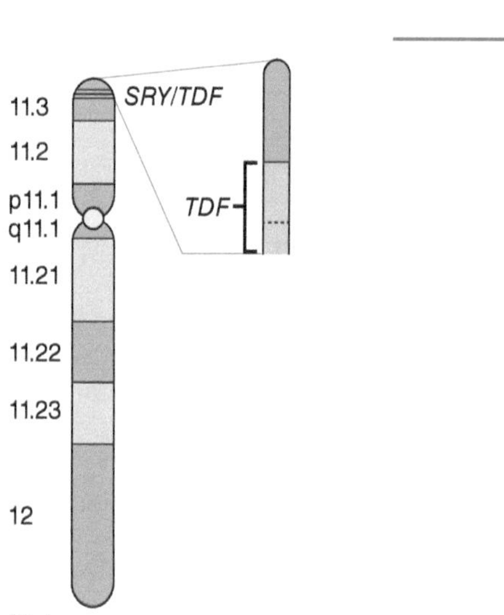

FIGURE 12.4 The Y chromosome showing the end of the p arm where the SRY gene is located. To the right, this end is magnified. The top part is often exchanged, but the TDF region where the SRY gene is located is rarely exchanged. If it is exchanged, the result is seen in Fig. 12.5. Source: *Redrawn from Figure 53.3 in Mesiano, S., & Jones, E. E. (2017). Chapter 53: Sexual differentiation. In W. F. Boron, & E. L. Boulpaep (Eds.),* Medical physiology *(3rd ed.) (p. 1076). Elsevier.*

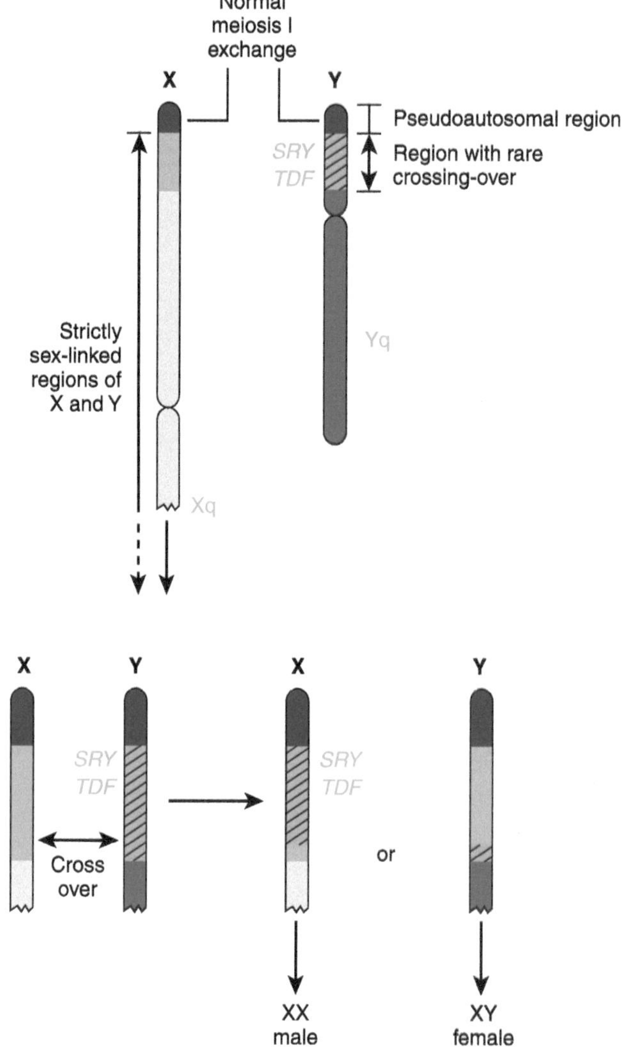

FIGURE 12.5 The results of gene exchange between X and Y chromosomes during meiosis I. If the *SRY* (Sex-determining Region of the Y chromosome) gene that also has the *t*estis-*d*etermining *f*actor (*TDF*) gene is translocated to the X chromosome, then that Y chromosome will not be able to form a normal testis. If the Y chromatid without most of the SRY/TDF region becomes the Y chromosome in an individual, the result will be an XY female. Source: *From Figure 6–11 in R. L. Nussbaum, R.R. McInnes, & H.F. Willard. (2016).* Thompson and Thompson genetics in medicine *(8th ed.) (p. 90). Elsevier.*

the testes remain intraabdominal. In unusual cases – as in the case at the beginning of this chapter, they may be located where the ovaries normally are found. At puberty, the patient will have normal breast development and body habitus as a result of the androgens being converted to estrogens. Axillary and pubic hair is sparse or nonexistent. Because of anti-Müllerian hormone, there is usually no uterus or uterine tubes so there is no menarche. The vagina may vary in length from normal to none at all with merely a dimple in the perineum to mark the place where it should be. At birth, infants are the same size as normal infants. Adult patients tend to be taller than most females, but shorter than most males. Testosterone levels are normal or above normal and luteinizing hormone levels are elevated. Estrogen levels are higher than in men or boys due to the peripheral aromatization of the testosterone, which is added to the normal production of estrogen by the testes. The combined estrogen level is still lower than in a normal female.

Diagnosis

The sex of a fetal child is now usually known before birth by a variety of methods, the least risky of which is analyzing maternal blood for circulating free fetal DNA. At birth, androgen insensitivity syndrome (AIS) can be diagnosed when there is a mismatch between the prenatal sex determination and the birth phenotype. However, as noted previously, complete AIS is not the only syndrome where female genitalia appear in a 46, XY newborn.

(cont'd)

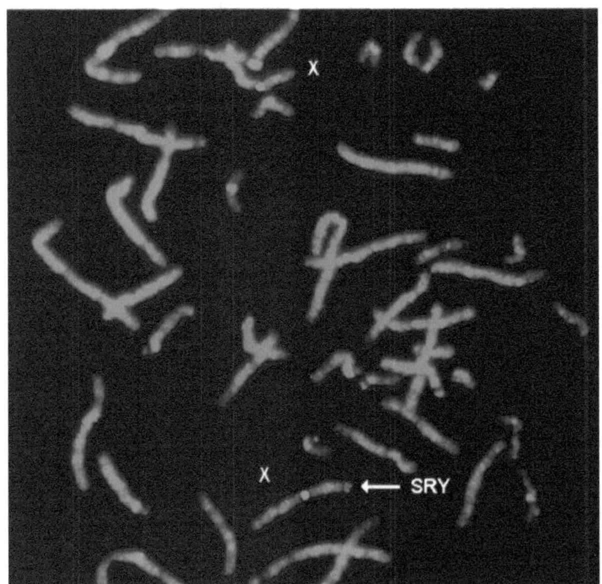

FIGURE 12.6 A patient with a 46, XX genotype but, the phenotype of which is male because of the SRY/TDF region on the X chromosome that was exchanged with a Y chromosome in meiosis I. The arrows point to green dots that are the centromeres of both X chromosomes. The red is the SRY/TDF locus on one X chromosome. Source: *From C-41 in R L Nussbaum, R R McInnes, & H F Willard. (2016).* Thompson and Thompson genetics in medicine *(8th ed.) (p. 472). Elsevier.*

Management

In cases where phenotype does not follow genotype, an MRI can disclose where the testes are located. If intraabdominal, they should be removed because there is a risk of malignancy in patients with cryptorchidism. If the individual prefers to remain a female, then there may be a need to enlarge the vagina or make one if it is not present.

The big challenge in such cases is the psychosocial aspect of sex determination. In the past the gender of the newborn was surgically changed to the phenotype. However, at present, this approach is not considered to be the correct one. Over time, with the guidance of psychologists, many parents are advised to use a wait-and-see approach. That is, the patient will be the one who should make the ultimate decision.

Prognosis

There is no data as to whether the lifespan of patients with 46, XY is different from that of the normal population.

AT THE MOLECULAR LEVEL—FOR A MORE IN-DEPTH UNDERSTANDING—DISORDERS OF SEXUAL DEVELOPMENT IN THE MALE

In addition to crossover, there are also mutations involving the SRY protein itself. Furthermore, a closely associated protein, SOX9, is also a testis-determining protein. Both proteins have mutations rendering them ineffective in their actions on the deoxyribonucleic acid (DNA) (Fig. 12.7).

Mutations that affect androgen synthesis

Androgens are synthesized from cholesterol in the Leydig cells of the testes and in the adrenal cortex (Fig. 12.8).

The adrenal cortex and the gonads do not synthesize the same steroid hormones. These differences and similarities are reflected in Figs. 12.9 and 12.10.

Mutations of the luteinizing hormone receptor

Mutations can occur in the luteinizing hormone receptor on the Leydig cell (Fig. 12.11).

StAR and $P450_{scc}$ deficiency

An essential regulator of the production of androgens is the steroidogenic acute regulatory protein (StAR) that is present in the mitochondrial intermembrane space where it facilitates the movement of 86% of cholesterol from the outer membrane to the inner membrane where it can be modified into androgens. More than 40 different mutations of this protein have been reported. On the mitochondrial inner membrane is cytochrome $P450_{scc}$ that cleaves the side chain of cholesterol, the first step in the production of pregnenolone. The effect of either

(cont'd)

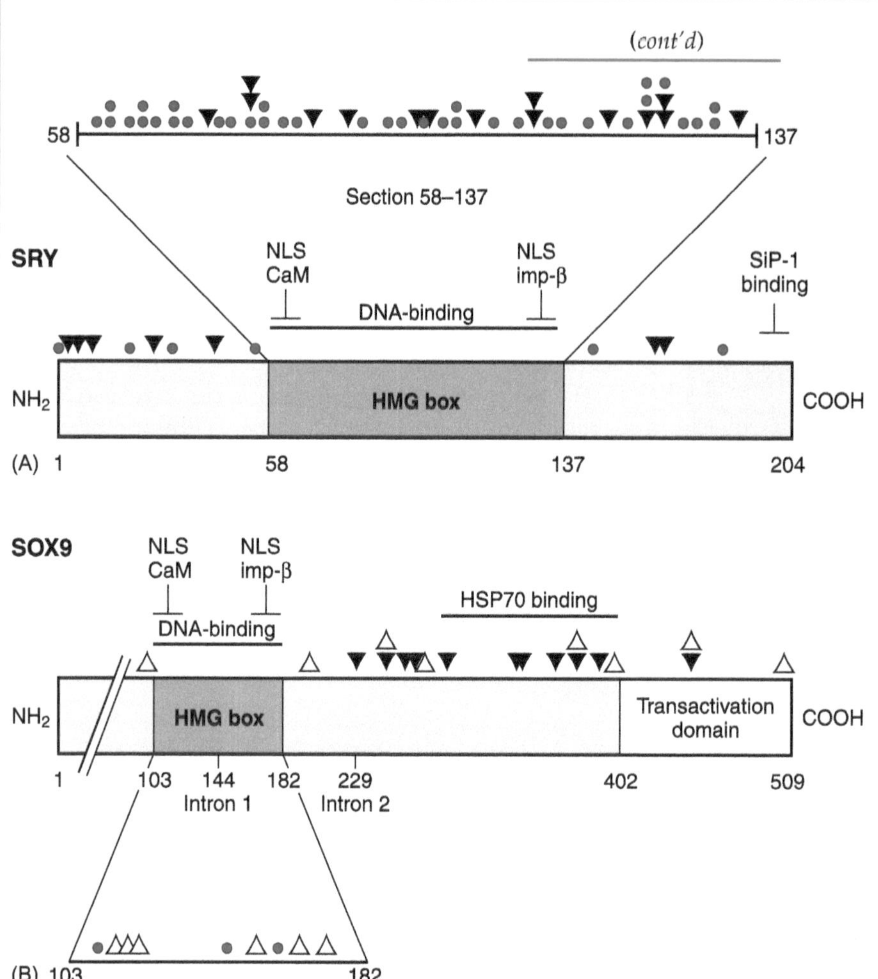

FIGURE 12.7 Some of the mutations (*solid triangles* and *solid circles*) affecting the SRY (A) and SOX9 (B) proteins. The solid triangles are nonsense and frameshift mutations while the solid circles are missense mutations. The open triangles are mutations that cause mutations in bone in both sexes. HMG box is a high-mobility group (movement by electrophoresis) that binds to the DNA. The numbers refer to the amino acid number sequence in the protein. SRY has 204 amino acids while SOX9 has 509 amino acids. *CaM*, Calmodulin; *DNA*, deoxyribonucleic acid; *HSP70*, heat-shock protein seventy; *imp-beta*, importin beta that enables the protein to be imported into the nucleus; *NLS*, nuclear localization signals that locate the DNA before binding. Source: *From Figure 23-20 in Achermann, J., & Hughes, I. A. (2016). Chapter 23: Pediatric disorders of sex development. In S. Melmed, K. S. Polonsky, P. L., Reed, & H. M. Kronenberg (Eds.),* William's textbook of endocrinology *(13th ed.) (p. 920). Elsevier.*

defect is to cause a buildup of cholesterol in the cell, which affects the function of the cell (Figs. 12.12 and 12.13).

Patients with a mutation in StAR eventually develop adrenal insufficiency and hypogonadism. In males, this can result in female genitalia. Originally, most of the mutations were reported in Japan, Korea, Switzerland, Saudi Arabia, and Palestine. More recently, mutations are being recorded for other countries. Fig. 12.14 shows the location of some of these mutations.

3β-Hydroxysteroid dehydrogenase deficiency

3β-Hydroxysteroid dehydrogenase deficiency prevents the conversion of pregnenolone to progesterone and androgens. This deficiency can cause female genitalia in a 46, XY male. This is illustrated stepwise in the pathway shown in Fig. 12.15 and some of the defects are illustrated in Fig. 12.16.

$P450_{c17}$ deficiency

Mutations in the CYP17 gene cause $P450_{c17}$ (17a-hydroxylase/17,20-lyase/17,20 desmolase) deficiency. Despite the many names, they are the same enzyme. Their products are in the pathway of testosterone production (Fig. 12.17) and some of the mutations are illustrated in Fig. 12.18.

Androgen receptor mutations

The gene for the androgen receptor (AR) is on the X chromosome. The receptor has 920 amino acids divided into three domains (parts) (Fig. 12.19).

The first domain binds to the ligand (androgen), a middle domain binds to DNA, and an N-terminal domain, which is composed of polyglycine and polyglutamine repeats, that modulates the activity of the receptor. There is a hinge region between the first and middle domain. When dihydrotestosterone or other androgen

(cont'd)

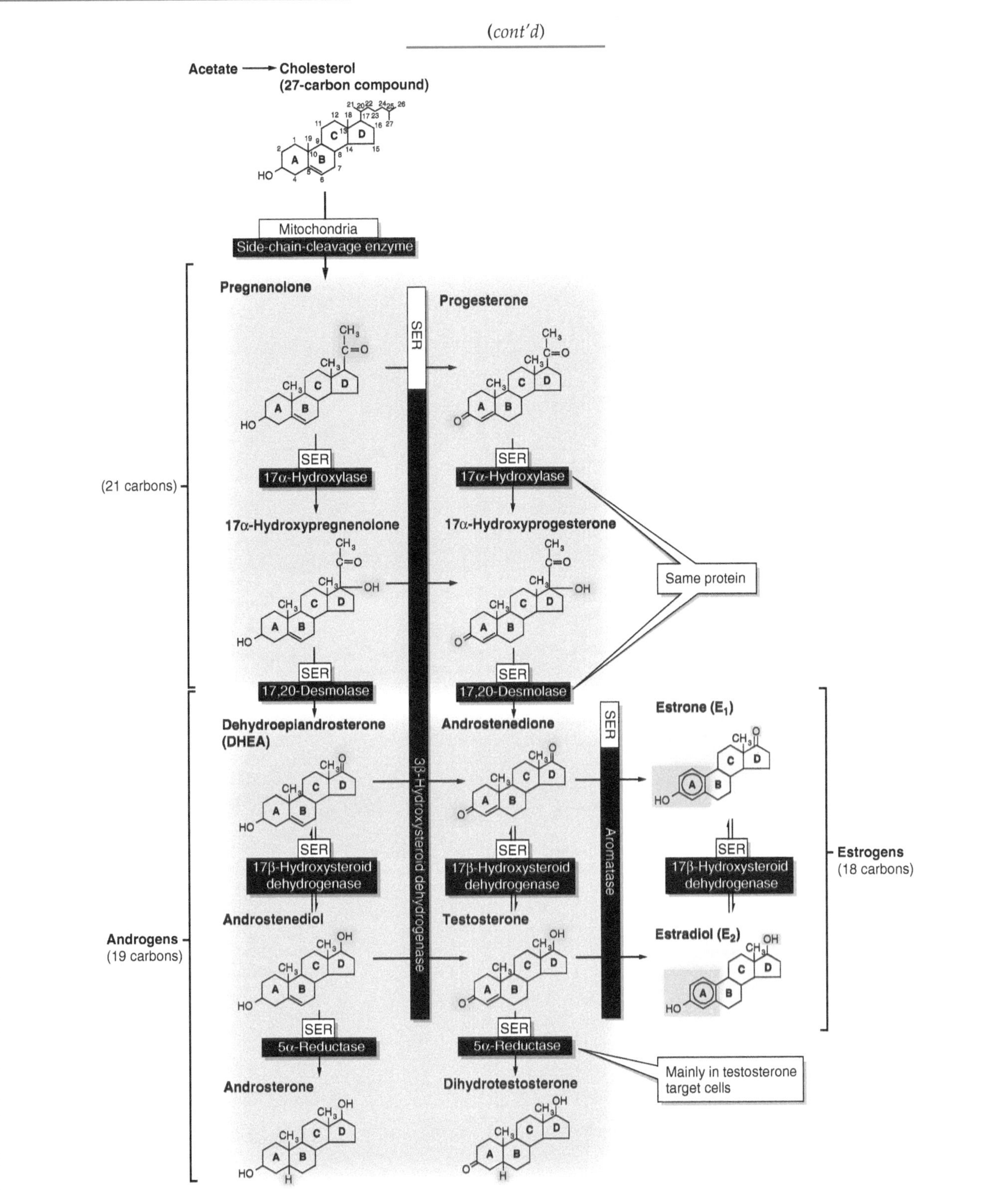

FIGURE 12.8 Pathway of androgen synthesis in the Leydig cell of the testis. This is the same pathway in the adrenal cortex, but some enzymes are not present in the testis, which are present in the adrenal cortex so that in the latter structure, glucocorticoids and mineralocorticoids can be produced. Source: *Redrawn from Figure 54-6 in Mesiano, S., & Jones, E. E. (2017). Chapter 54: The male reproductive system. In W. F. Boron, & E. L. Boulpaep (Eds.),* Medical physiology *(3rd ed.) (p. 1098). Elsevier.*

(cont'd)

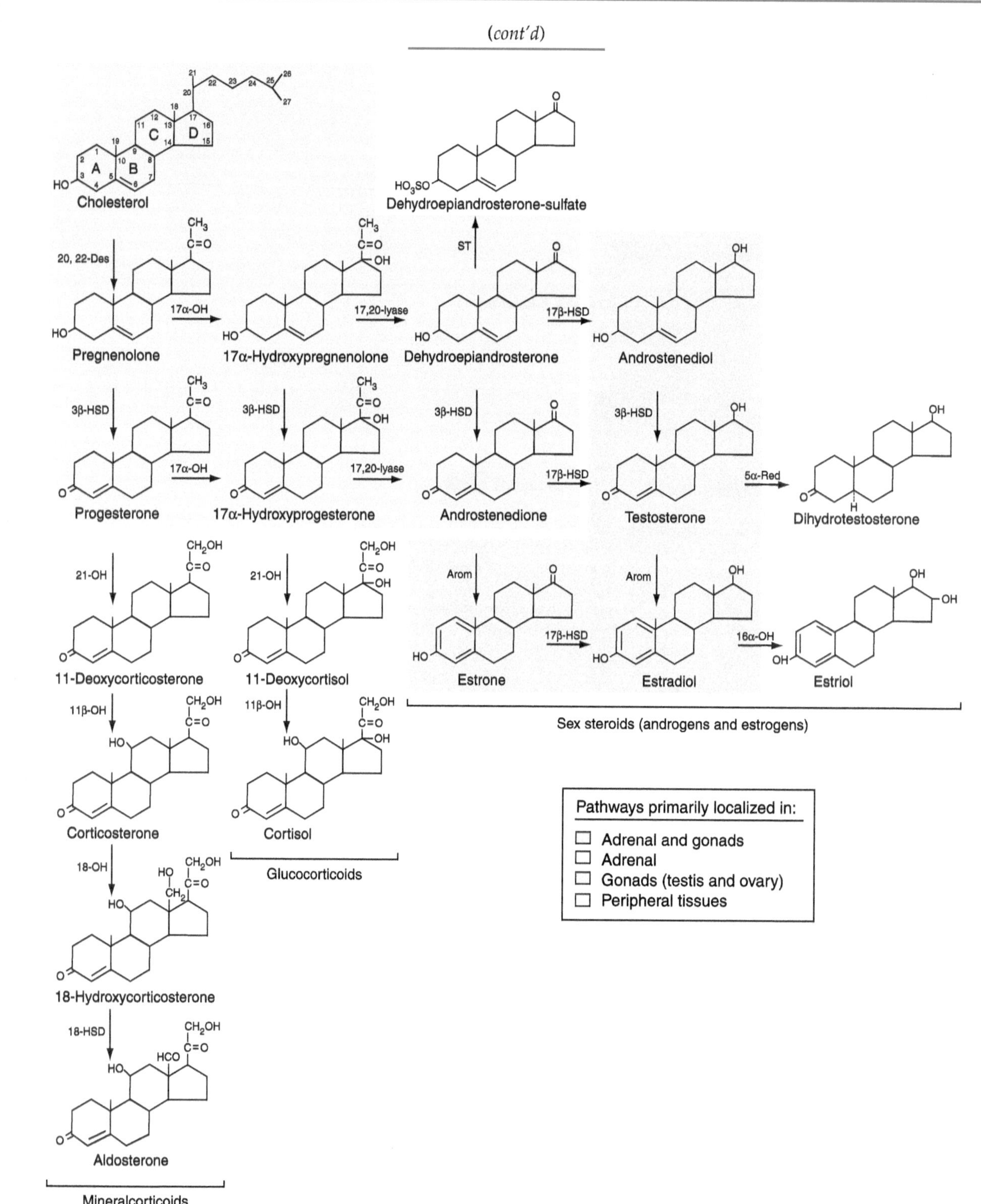

FIGURE 12.9 The steroids outlined in blue are synthesized only in the adrenal cortex; those in purple are synthesized in the adrenal cortex and gonads, while those in pink are synthesized only in the gonads. Those with a light green are formed in the peripheral tissues from either testosterone or estradiol, depending on the target tissue. Source: *From Figure 25-1 in Jeelani, R., & Bluth, M. H. (2017). Chapter 25: Reproductive function and pregnancy. In R. A. McPherson, & M. R. Pincus (Eds.) (p. 401),* Henry's clinical diagnosis and management by laboratory methods *(23rd ed.). Elsevier.*

(cont'd)

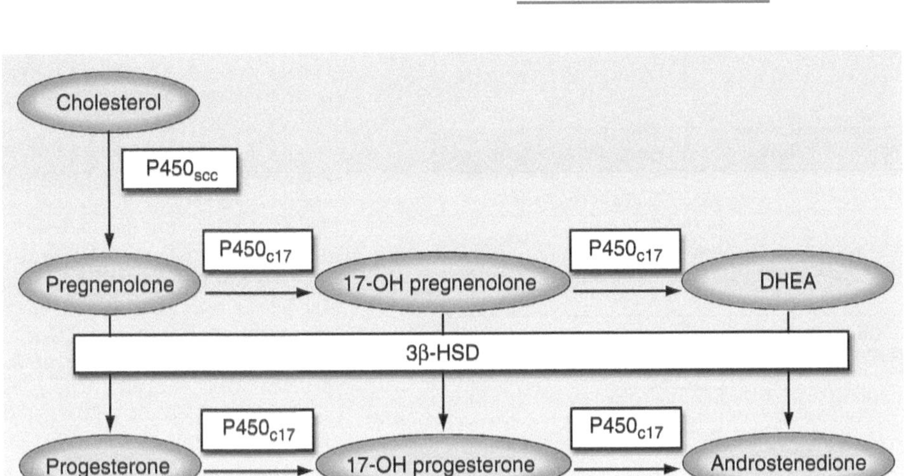

FIGURE 12.10 The initial part of the normal pathway of steroid production in gonads. Source: *Modified from Figure 24-13 in Guber, H. A., & Farag, A. F. (2017). Chapter 24: Evaluation of endocrine function. In R. A. McPherson, & M. R. Pincus (Eds.),* Henry's clinical diagnosis and management by laboratory methods *(23rd ed.) (p. 387). Elsevier.*

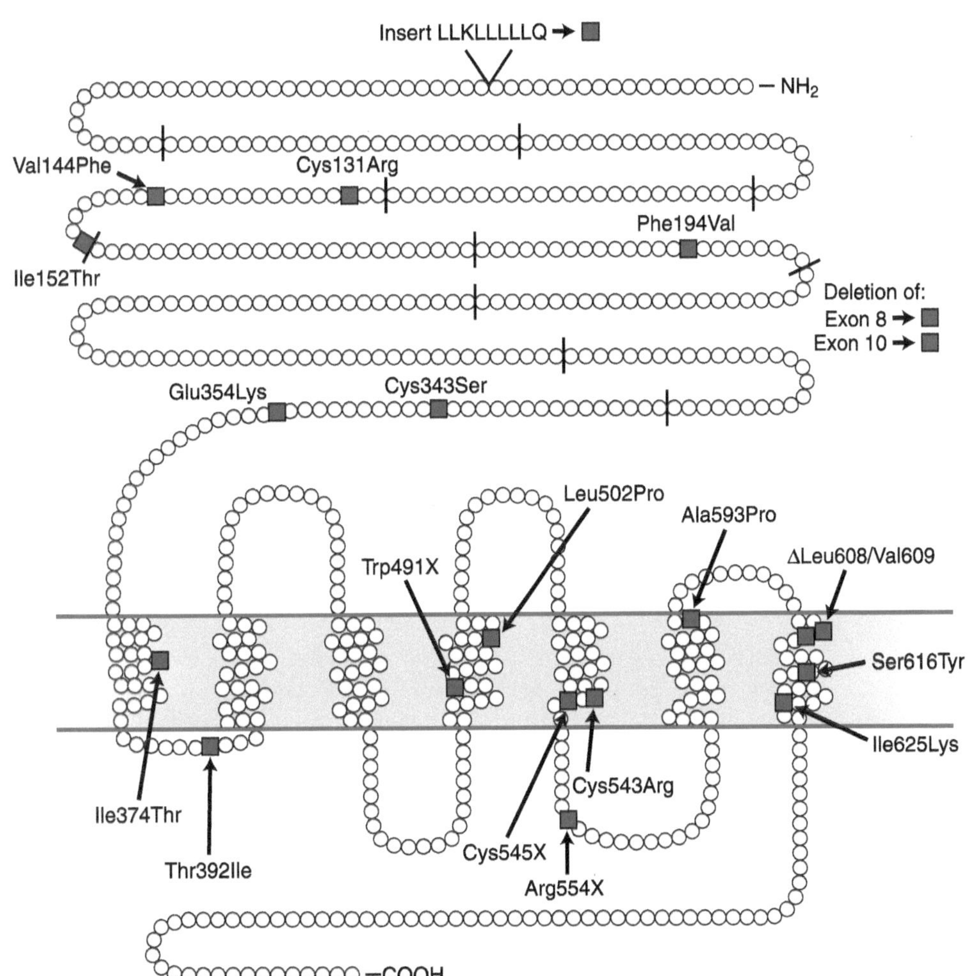

FIGURE 12.11 Diagram of the LH receptor showing the seven transmembrane portions as well as the extracellular and intracellular domains. The dark squares are some of the reported mutations in the LH receptor. *LH*, Luteinizing hormone. Source: *From Figure 23-21 in Achermann, J., & Hughes, I. A. (2016). Chapter 23: Pediatric disorders of sex development. In S. Melmed, K. S. Polonsky, P. L., Reed, & H. M. Kronenberg (Eds.),* William's textbook of endocrinology *(13th ed.) (p. 922). Elsevier.*

(cont'd)

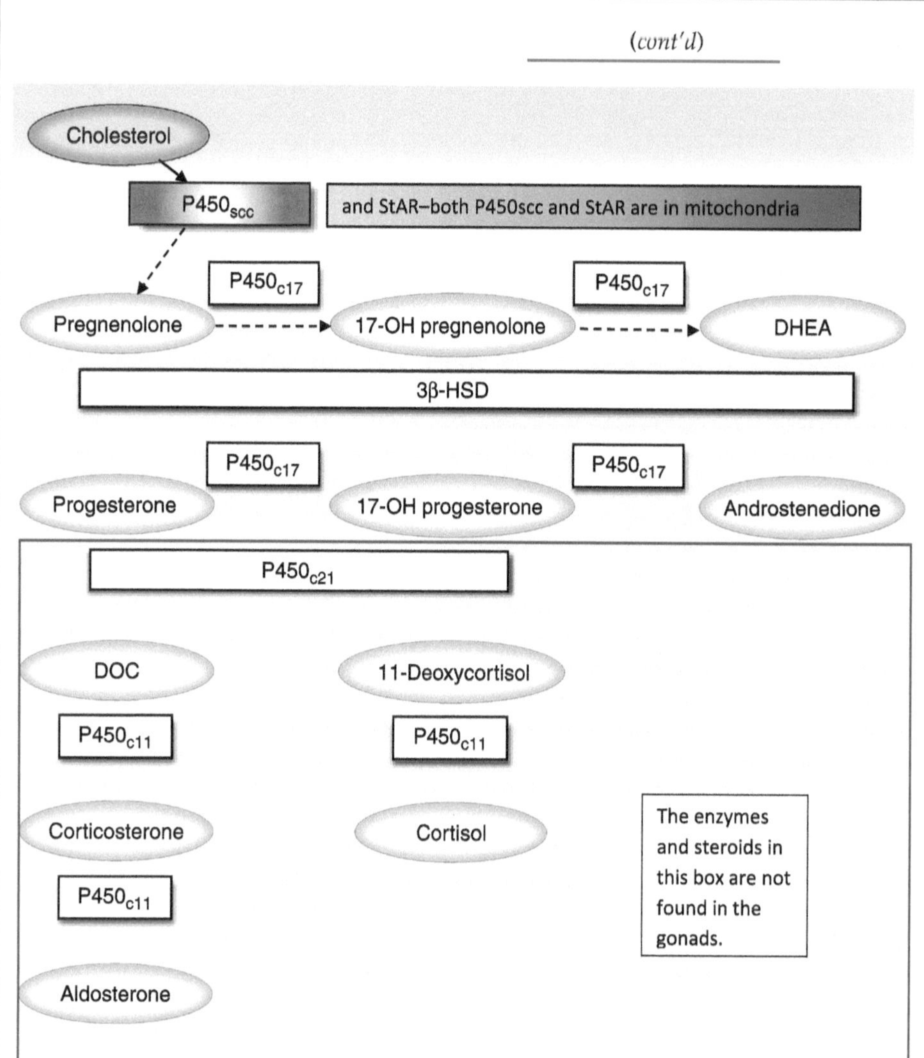

FIGURE 12.12 Defective $P450_{scc}$ (for side-chain cleavage of cholesterol) or defective steroidogenesis acute regulatory (StAR) protein prevents cholesterol from being processed further. It builds up in the cell and produces lipoid hyperplasia illustrated in Fig. 12.11. The more intense color of the substrate (cholesterol in this case) indicates that it builds up in the cell. The intense color of the enzyme indicates that it is defective. Dashed arrows indicate the direction of the pathway that normally would be taken but is not because of the defect. The lack of arrows indicates that the pathway does not progress. DOC is not produced in gonads but is produced in the normal adrenal cortex. *DHEA,* Dehydroepiandrosterone; *DOC,* deoxycorticosterone. Source: *From Figure 24-16 in Guber, H. A., & Farag, A. F. (2017). Chapter 24: Evaluation of endocrine function. In R. A. McPherson, & M. R. Pincus (Eds.),* Henry's clinical diagnosis and management by laboratory methods *(23rd ed.) (p. 390). Elsevier.*

binds to the first domain, the ligand-binding domain, it causes the molecule to fold so that the androgen does not escape thus enhancing and prolonging the effect (Fig. 12.20).

The DNA-binding domain contains two zinc fingers, one proximal (P box) and one distal (D box) where some of the more common mutations occur (Fig. 12.21). These mutations are usually missense ones where one amino acid is substituted for another, but they make a large difference in the syndrome. If phenylalanine is substituted for valine, there is complete loss of function and the patient has complete androgen insensitivity syndrome (AIS). If leucine is substituted for valine, there is not quite as much loss of function and the patient has partial AIS.

There are more than 400 mutations in the AR (Fig. 12.22).

(cont'd)

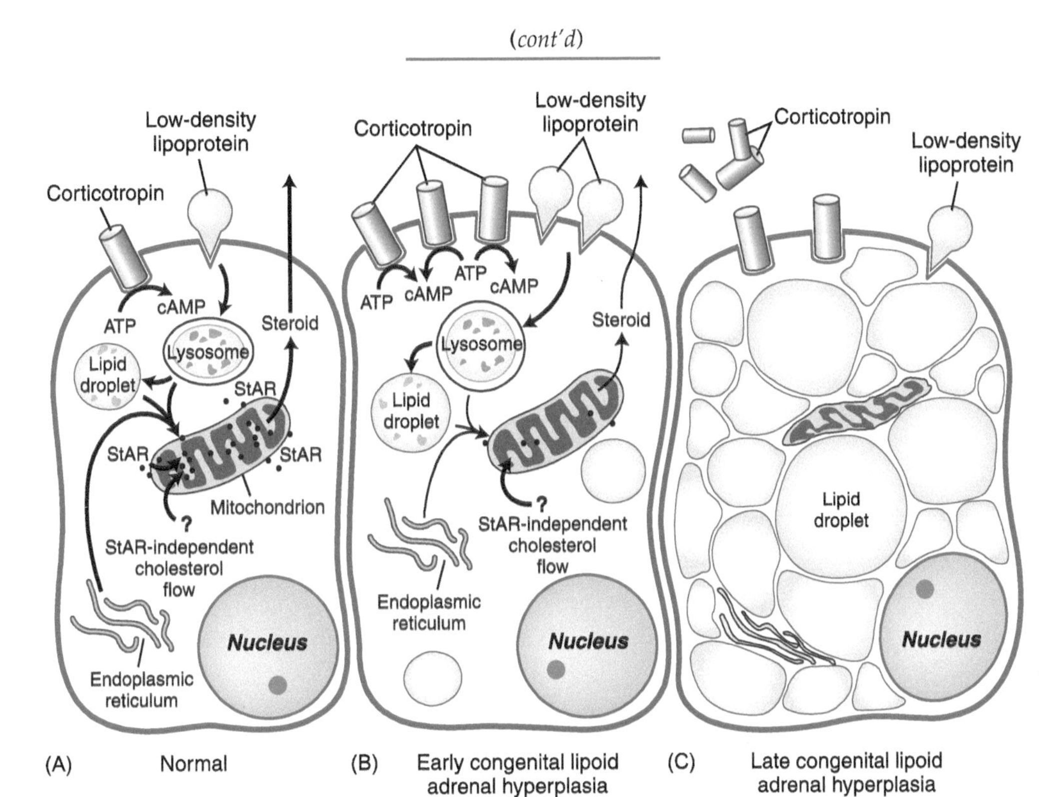

FIGURE 12.13 Buildup of lipids in an adrenal cell due to a mutation in the $P450_{scc}$ (side-chain cleavage of cholesterol) or StAR (steroidogenesis acute regulatory) proteins—only StAR is labeled in this figure. (A) Cholesterol is carried on LDL, which upon corticotropin (ACTH) stimulation enters the cell and is transported by steroidogenic acute regulatory protein (StAR) from the outer mitochondrial membrane to the inner membrane where its side chain is cleaved by $P450_{scc}$ on the mitochondrial inner membrane. If cholesterol cannot enter or be broken down in the mitochondria, it is stored as a lipid droplet in the cell. With defective $P450_{scc}$ or StAR, this does not happen (B), but the lack of adrenal hormone stimulates the pituitary to release more corticotropin, so that more cholesterol is taken up and stored. Eventually (C) the adrenal cell becomes so filled with cholesterol that it no longer functions properly. *cAMP*, Cyclic adenosine monophosphate; *LDL*, low-density lipoprotein. Source: *From Figure 23-22 in Achermann, J., & Hughes, I. A. (2016). Chapter 23: Pediatric disorders of sex development. In S. Melmed, K. S. Polonsky, P. L., Reed, & H. M. Kronenberg (Eds.),* William's textbook of endocrinology *(13th ed.) (p. 924). Elsevier.*

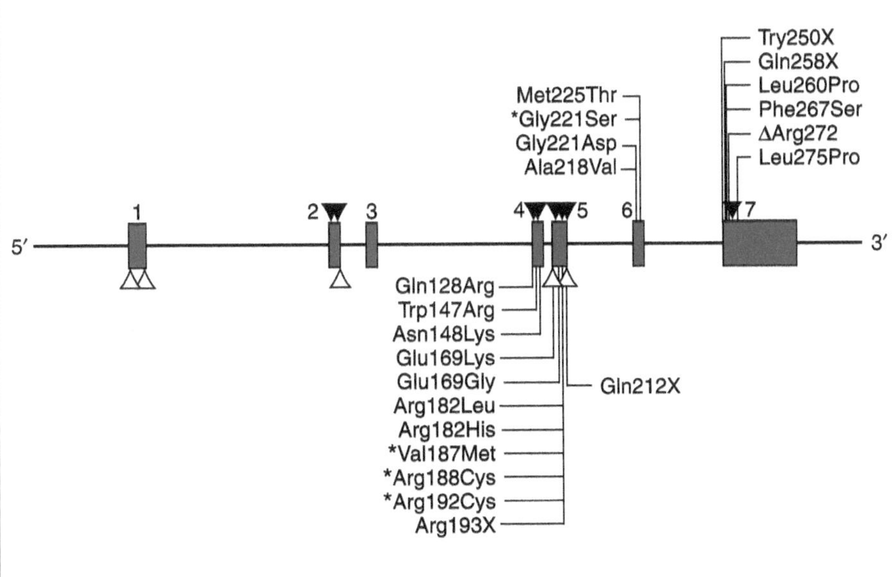

FIGURE 12.14 Mutations in the StAR gene. The numbers refer to the exons. Mutations with an asterisk are missense mutations that are found in late-onset forms of adrenal insufficiency. Source: *From Figure 23-23 in Achermann, J., & Hughes, I. A. (2016). Chapter 23: Pediatric disorders of sex development. In S. Melmed, K. S. Polonsky, P. L., Reed, & H. M. Kronenberg (Eds.),* William's textbook of endocrinology *(13th ed.) (p. 924). Elsevier.*

(*cont'd*)

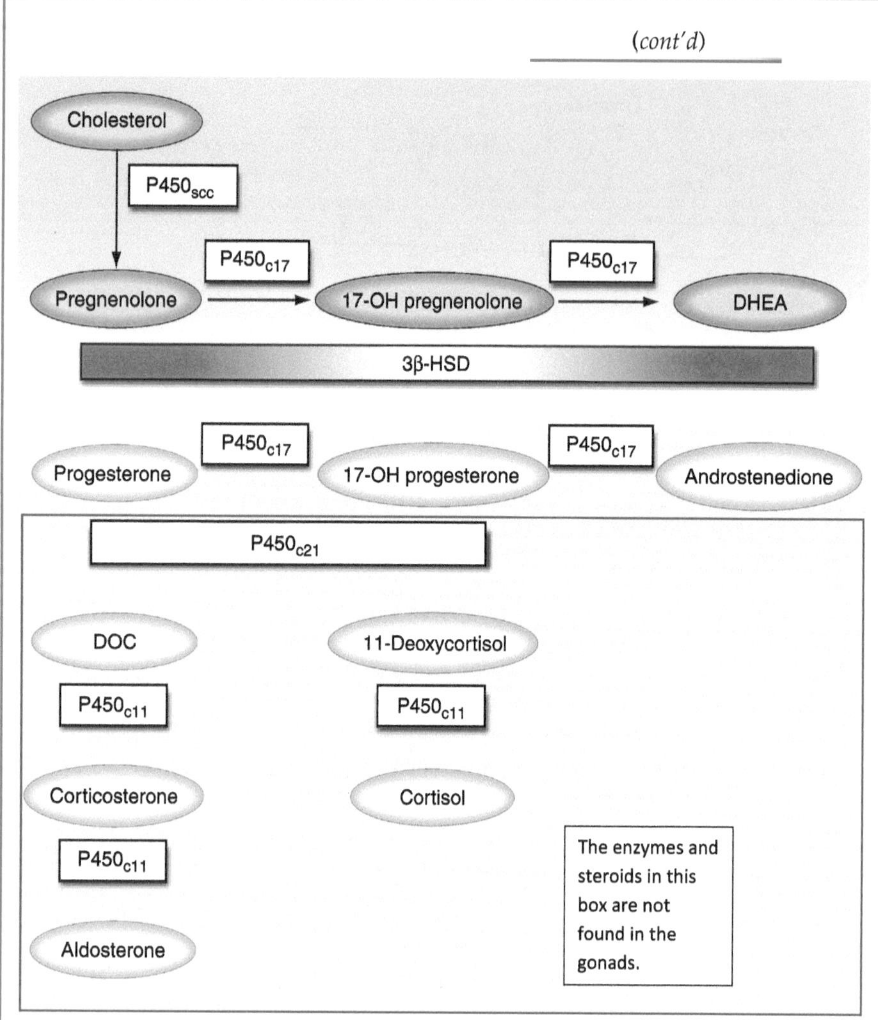

FIGURE 12.15 Defective 3β-hydroxysteroid dehydrogenase synthesis blocks the production of testosterone by the testis. This is a rare disorder. *DHEA*, Dehydroepiandrosterone; *DOC*, deoxycorticosterone. Source: *From Figure 24-14 in Guber, H. A., & Farag, A. F. (2017). Chapter 24: Evaluation of endocrine function. In R. A. McPherson, & M. R. Pincus (Eds.),* Henry's clinical diagnosis and management by laboratory methods *(23rd ed.) (p. 388). Elsevier.*

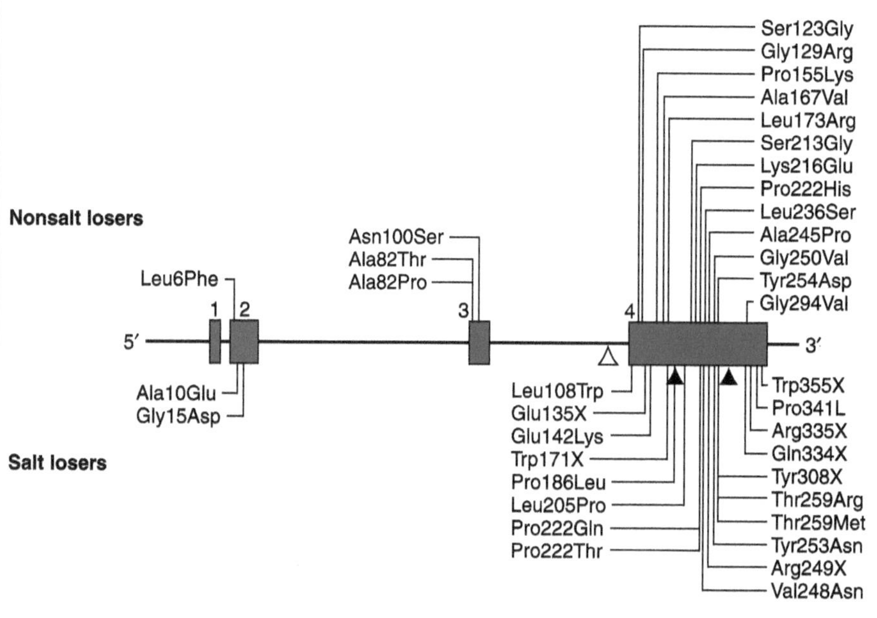

FIGURE 12.16 Some of the mutations in the 3β-hydroxysteroid dehydrogenase type 2 gene. The protein from which goes into the mitochondria and removes a hydrogen from any one of four steroids, one of the products being testosterone. The X on a mutation refers to a stop (nonsense) mutation. The solid triangles refer to insertions or deletions resulting in frameshift mutations. The open triangles indicate splice site mutations. The chart is divided into those patients that have salt losing adrenal insufficiency as a result and those that do not lose salt. Source: *From Figure 23–24 in Achermann, J., & Hughes, I. A. (2016). Chapter 23: Pediatric disorders of sex development. In S. Melmed, K. S. Polonsky, P. L., Reed, & H. M. Kronenberg (Eds.),* William's textbook of endocrinology *(13th ed.) (p. 926). Elsevier.*

(*cont'd*)

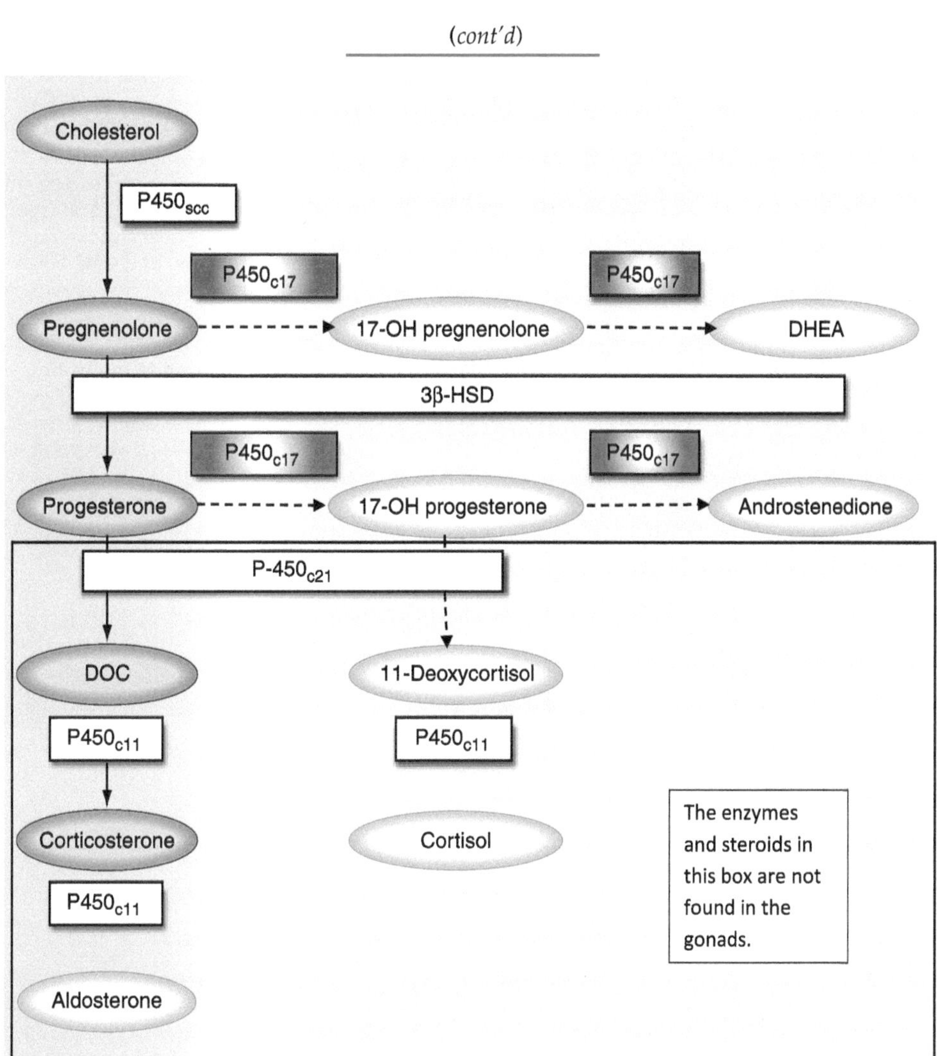

FIGURE 12.17 The effect of mutations in $P450_{c17}$. Solid arrow is the direction of the progression of the steroid formation. Dashed arrows indicate a blockage. The dark ovals indicate that products are present, while the light ovals indicate that the steroids are not present. The highlighted enzyme is the one that is defective. Source: *From Figure 24-15 in Guber, H. A., & Farag, A. F. (2017). Chapter 24: Evaluation of endocrine function. In R. A. McPherson, & M. R. Pincus (Eds.),* Henry's clinical diagnosis and management by laboratory methods *(23rd ed.) (p. 389). Elsevier.*

(cont'd)

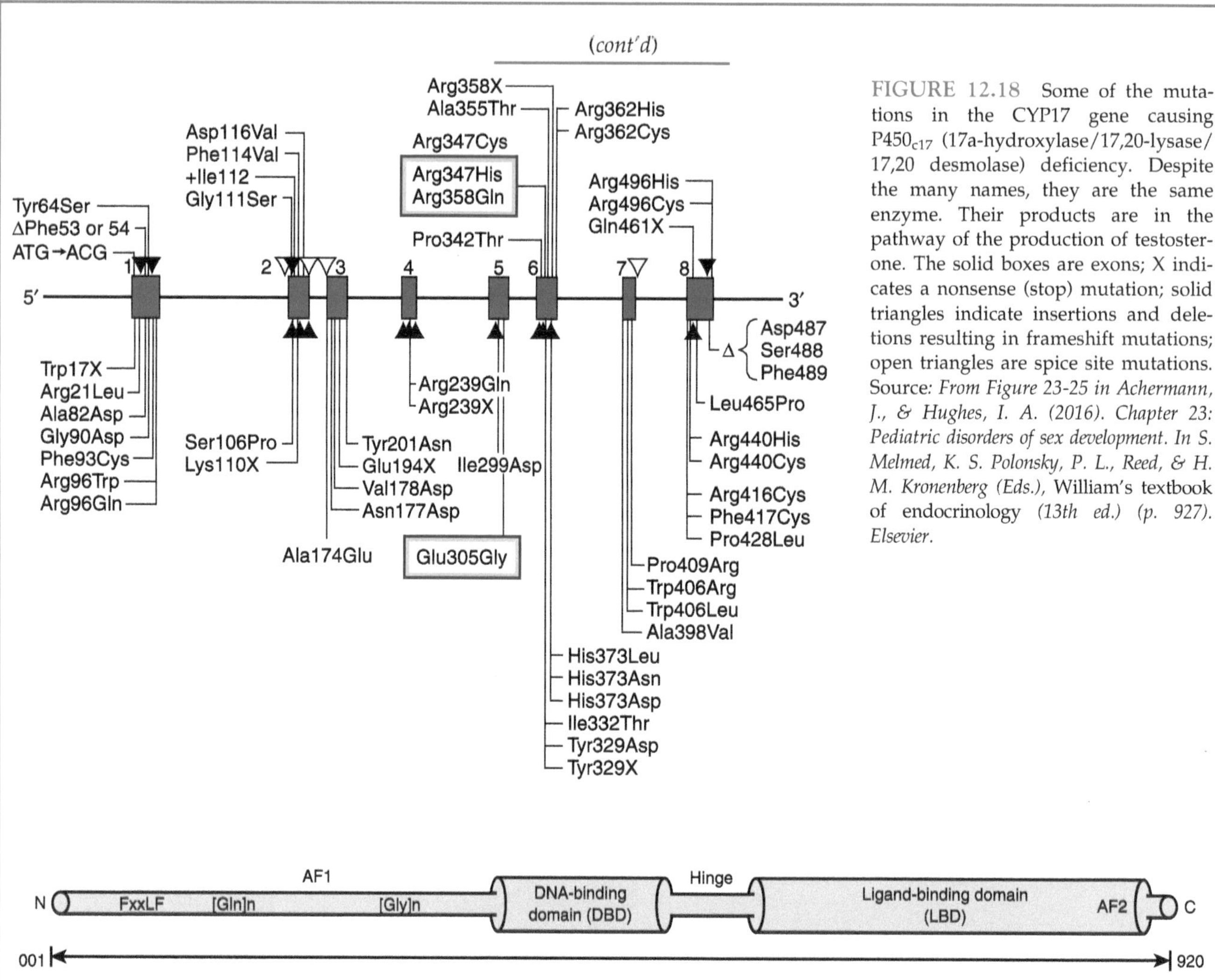

FIGURE 12.18 Some of the mutations in the CYP17 gene causing $P450_{c17}$ (17a-hydroxylase/17,20-lysase/17,20 desmolase) deficiency. Despite the many names, they are the same enzyme. Their products are in the pathway of the production of testosterone. The solid boxes are exons; X indicates a nonsense (stop) mutation; solid triangles indicate insertions and deletions resulting in frameshift mutations; open triangles are spice site mutations. Source: *From Figure 23-25 in Achermann, J., & Hughes, I. A. (2016). Chapter 23: Pediatric disorders of sex development. In S. Melmed, K. S. Polonsky, P. L., Reed, & H. M. Kronenberg (Eds.),* William's textbook of endocrinology *(13th ed.) (p. 927). Elsevier.*

FIGURE 12.19 The androgen receptor with the three domains. It is 920 amino acids long. Source: *From Figure 23.29 in Achermann, J., & Hughes, I. A. (2016). Chapter 23: Pediatric disorders of sex development. In S. Melmed, K. S. Polonsky, P. L., Reed, & H. M. Kronenberg (Eds.),* William's textbook of endocrinology *(13th ed.) (p. 932). Elsevier.*

(cont'd)

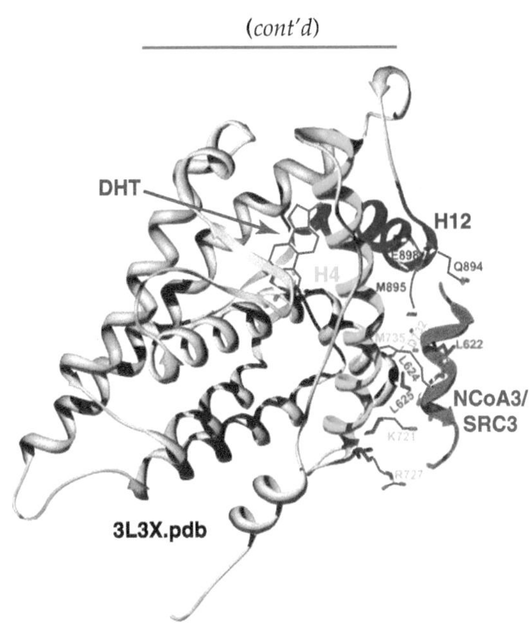

FIGURE 12.20 The androgen receptor combined with DHT, its ligand. This causes folding of the molecule at its hinge, trapping DHT, and prolonging the effect. *DHT*, Dihydrotestosterone. Source: *From Figure 23.29 in Achermann, J., & Hughes, I. A. (2016). Chapter 23: Pediatric disorders of sex development. In S. Melmed, K. S. Polonsky, P. L., Reed, & H. M. Kronenberg (Eds.),* William's textbook of endocrinology *(13th ed.) (p. 932). Elsevier.*

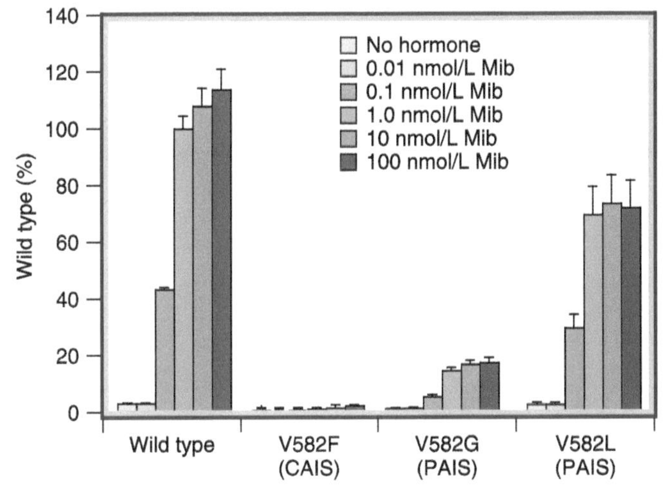

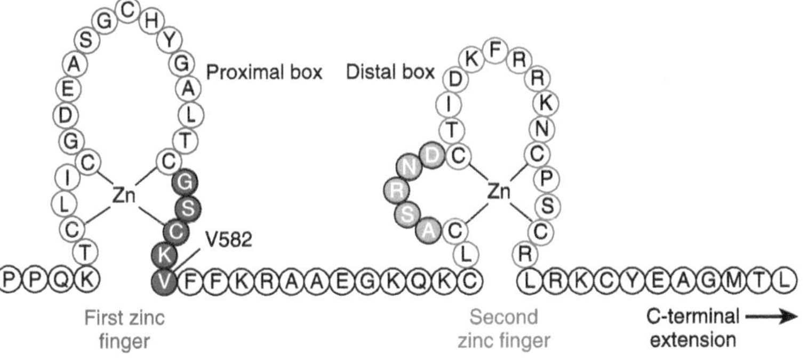

FIGURE 12.21 The two zinc fingers and some of the amino acids that are substituted in mutations. For example, if phenylalanine is substituted for valine in the proximal box at position 582 (written V582F), this results in CAIS, whereas if glycine is substituted for valine (V582G), this causes partial loss of function, called PAIS. Another cause of PAIS is the substitution of leucine for valine; however, this substitution permits greater function so the patient is not as compromised. *CAIS*, Complete androgen insensitivity syndrome; *PAIS*, partial androgen insensitivity syndrome; *wild type*, normal development. Source: *From Figure 23-31 in Achermann, J., & Hughes, I. A. (2016). Chapter 23: Pediatric disorders of sex development. In S. Melmed, K. S. Polonsky, P. L., Reed, & H. M. Kronenberg (Eds.),* William's textbook of endocrinology *(13th ed.) (p. 935). Elsevier.*

(cont'd)

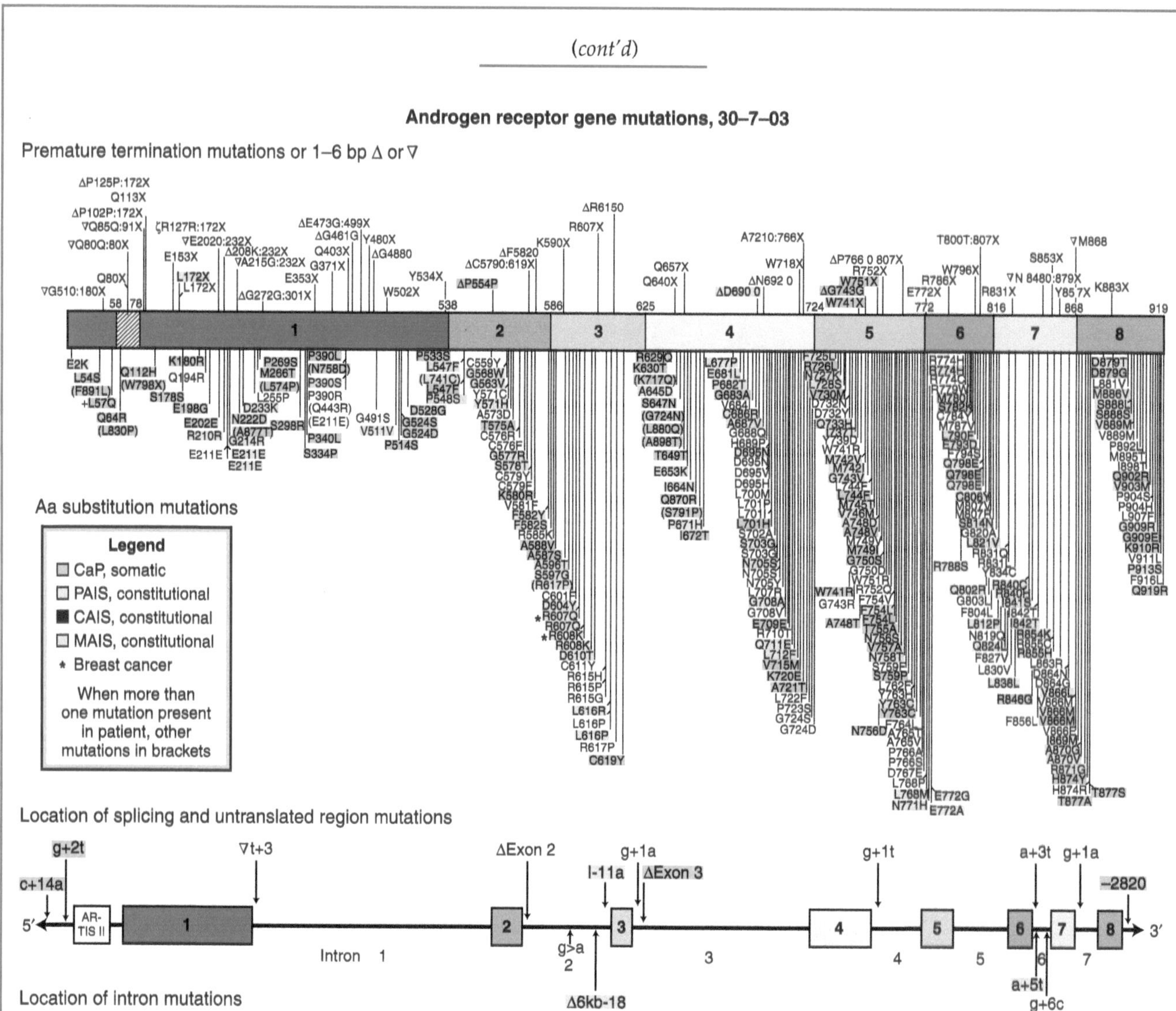

FIGURE 12.22 Some of the over 400 mutations that have been found to date in the androgen receptor protein. Source: *From Figure 23.30 in Achermann, J., & Hughes, I. A. (2016). Chapter 23: Pediatric disorders of sex development. In S. Melmed, K. S. Polonsky, P. L., Reed, & H. M. Kronenberg (Eds.),* William's textbook of endocrinology *(13th ed.) (p. 934). Elsevier.*

Introduction

The gonads are derived from the gonadal ridge, a bilateral thickening of the coelom of the developing embryo. Germ cells migrate (by pseudopodia—so they move like amoeba) from the yolk sac and become embedded in the gonadal ridge (Figs. 12.23–12.25). The formation of the gonads from these structures is shown in Fig. 12.26 and summarized in Fig. 12.27.

The development of the gonads is also dependent on two duct systems: Wolffian and Müllerian, named after the two German physiologists who discovered them: Caspar Friedrich Wolff in 1759 and Johannes Peter Müller in 1830. (Interestingly, there are no known paintings or portraits of Wolff—we have no idea what he looked like).

The Wolffian duct is derived from the mesonephric duct, a duct that formed the equivalent of ureters for the mesonephric kidney and is a continuation of the duct used for the pronephric kidney. The pronephric kidney is the first embryonic kidney and is nonfunctional in humans but is the kidney of scaleless fish, such as the

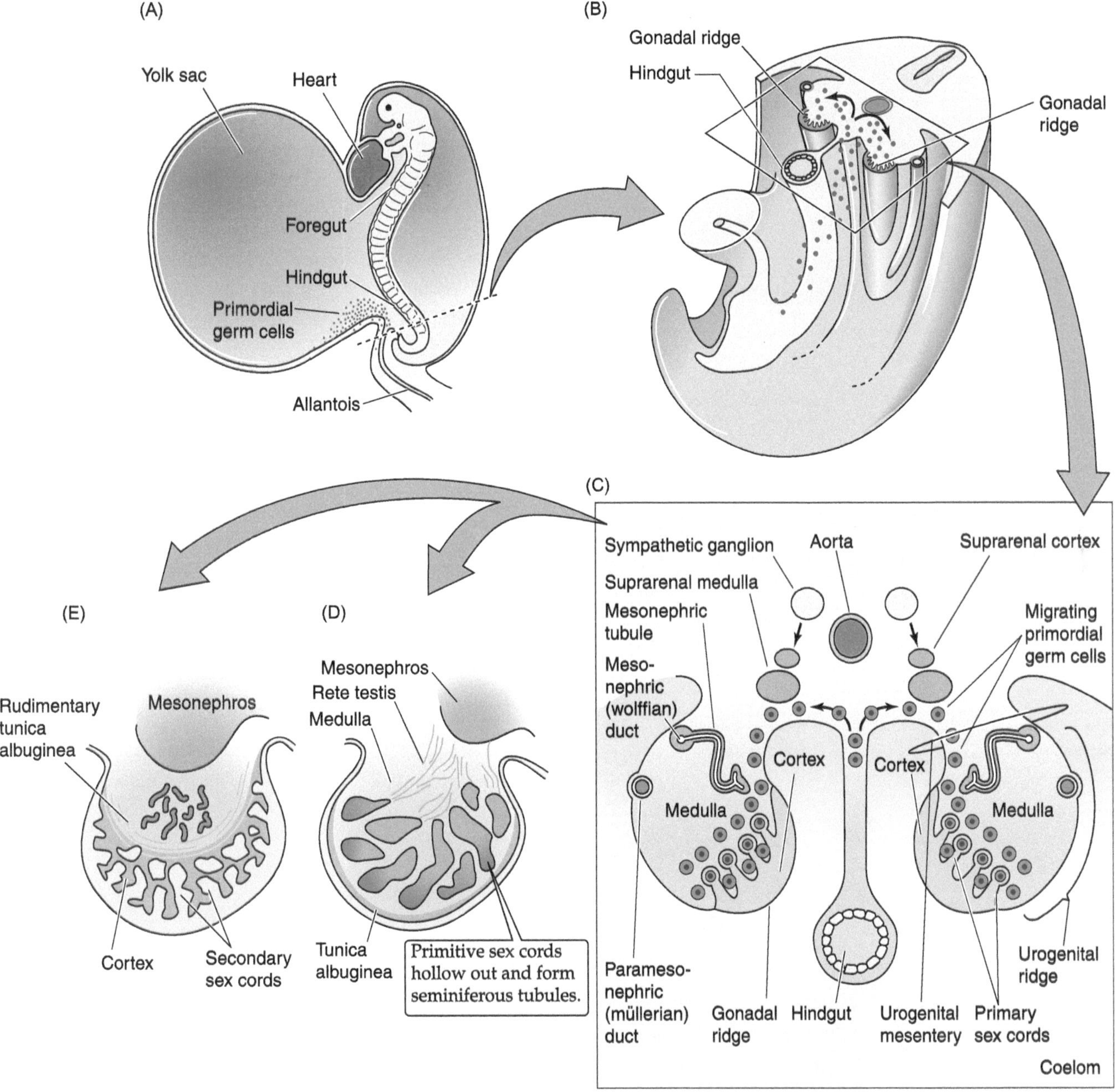

FIGURE 12.23 The development of the gonads. The ovaries develop from the cortex (outside) of the gonadal ridge, while the testes arise from the medulla (inner layer). (A) Early embryo (fifth week), (B) migration of germ cells to gonadal ridges, (C) indifferent or primordial gonad, (D) developing testis, (E) developing ovary. Source: *From Figure 53-4 in Mesiano, S., & Jones, E. E. (2017). Chapter 53: Sexual differentiation. In W. F. Boron, & E. L. Boulpaep (Eds.),* Medical physiology *(3rd ed.) (p. 1077). Elsevier.*

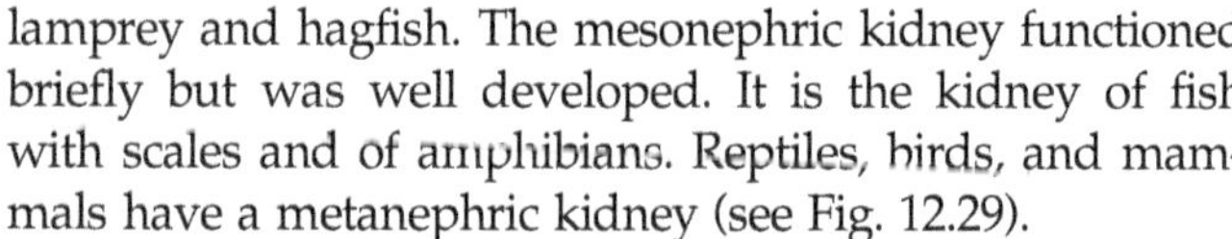
lamprey and hagfish. The mesonephric kidney functioned briefly but was well developed. It is the kidney of fish with scales and of amphibians. Reptiles, birds, and mammals have a metanephric kidney (see Fig. 12.29).

The testes develop in the abdominal cavity adjacent to the mesonephric kidneys but must descend into the scrotum for normal spermatogenesis to take place. The testes—like the ovaries—lie behind the peritoneum. They begin their descent in the eighth week, pulled down by the gubernaculum (Fig. 12.28).

As they descend, a pouch, the vaginal process, forms in the lower peritoneal cavity and the testes are pulled down into this recess. The peritoneum is divided into that portion that covers organs (visceral peritoneum) and forms the wall of the cavity (parietal peritoneum). As the testes are behind the parietal peritoneum, they are considered to be retroperitoneal. As they move into the vaginal recess, the peritoneum is renamed tunica (Latin, coat) vaginalis because it "coats" the testes. The part that covers the testes is called the visceral layer of the tunica vaginalis. The outer layer is then called the parietal layer of the tunica vaginalis.

Testicular descent occurs in two stages, an initial transabdominal movement to the inguinal ring, and a later migration through the inguinal canal into the scrotum. As the primordial gonad develops into a testis, it is held in place by the cranial suspensory ligament, which links its upper pole to the dorsal abdominal wall and a second ligament, the gubernaculum testis, that links the lower pole of the testis to the scrotum. At about the 12th week after fertilization, involution of the cranial

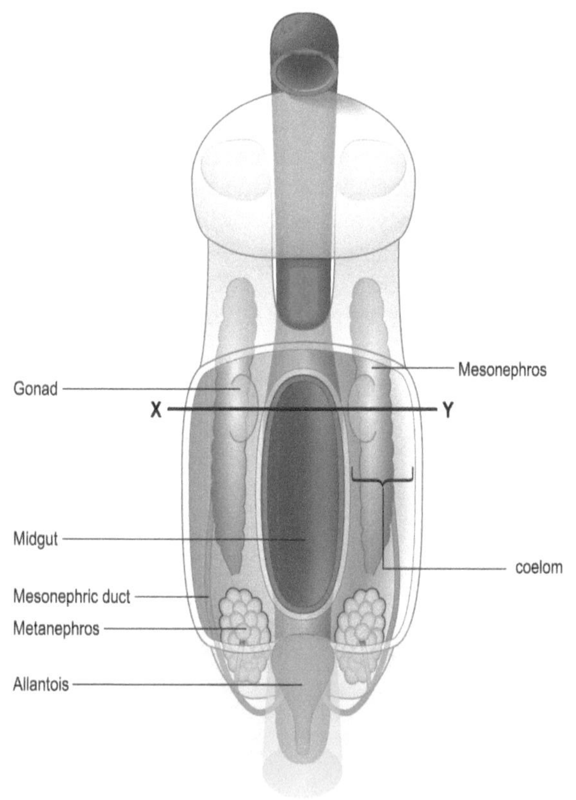

FIGURE 12.24 Another view of the gonadal ridge being developed alongside the mesonephros in the embryo. XY is the line representing the cross section in Fig. 12.25. Source: *From Figure 72.12A in Standring, et al. (2016).* Gray's anatomy *(41st ed.) edited by S. Standring (p. 1209). Elsevier.*

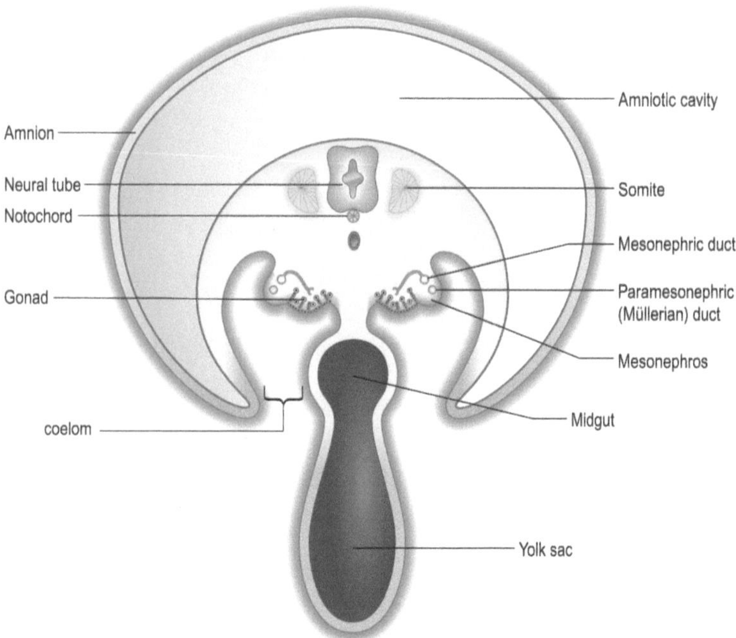

FIGURE 12.25 A cross section of the embryo at the X–Y line in Fig. 12.24. Source: *From Figure 72.12B in Standring, et al. (2016).* Gray's anatomy *(41st ed.) edited by S. Standring (p. 1209). Elsevier.*

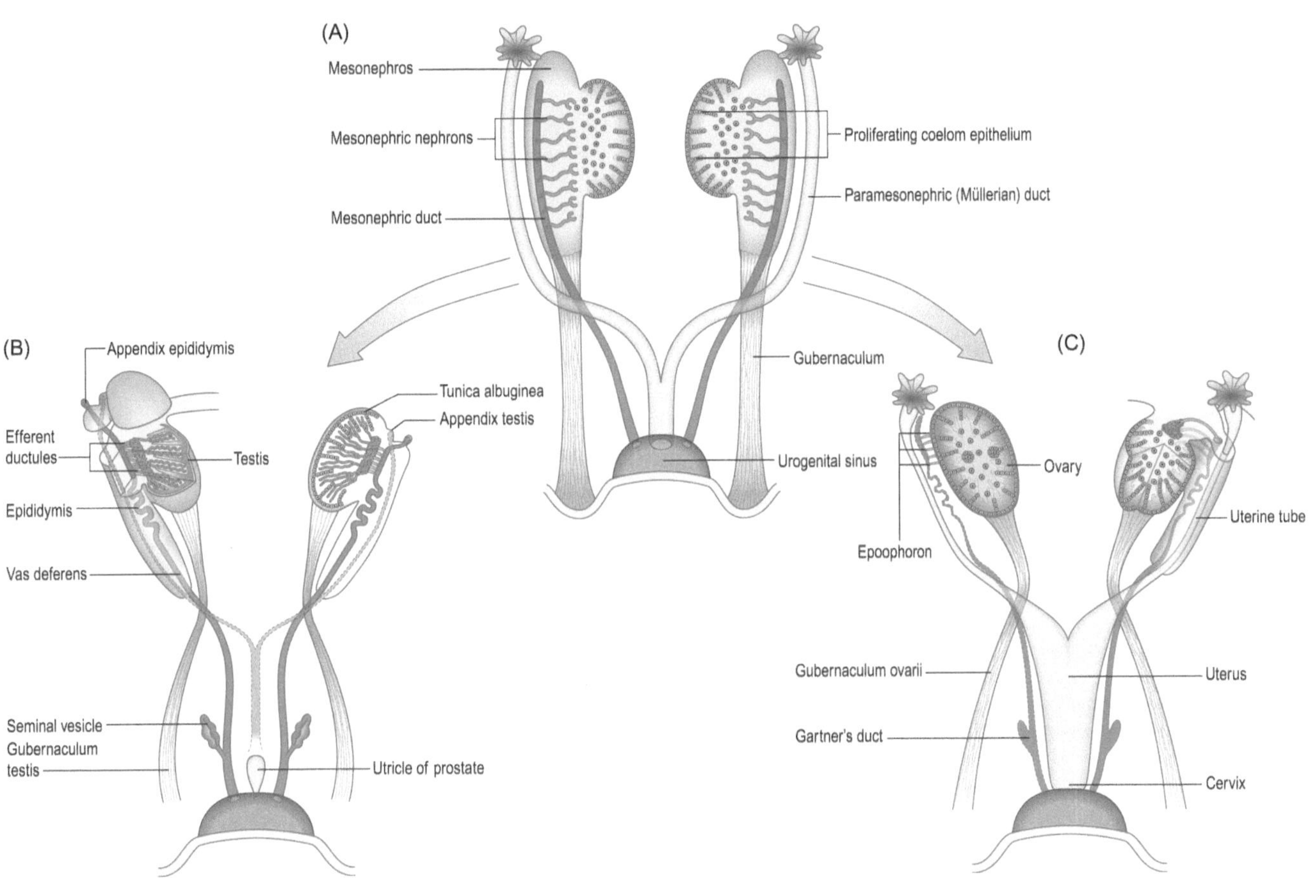

FIGURE 12.26 How the gonads and Wolffian and Müllerian duct structures differentiate in the male and female. In (A) the structures are undifferentiated; in (B) the structures have differentiated into male structures; and, in (C) they have differentiated into female structures. Source: *From Figure 72.13 in Standring, et al. (2016).* Gray's anatomy *(41st ed.) edited by S. Standring (p. 1209). Elsevier.*

suspensory ligament allows the gubernaculum, which is shortening and thickening, to pull the testis down to the inguinal ring where it remains until shortly before birth. The cranial suspensory ligament regresses in response to androgen, but in female fetuses, it develops further to retain the ovary in the abdominal cavity and support the ovarian vasculature. Developmental changes in the gubernaculum are orchestrated by a peptide called insulin-like factor 3 (INSL3). As its name implies INSL3 is structurally related to insulin. It is secreted by the Leydig cells. Final passage of the testis through the inguinal canal and into the scrotum depends upon remodeling of the gubernaculum and is also dependent upon testosterone.

Sexual differentiation

Regardless of its chromosomal makeup, the early embryo has the potential to form either testes or ovaries and develop either the male or female phenotype. By about 5 weeks after fertilization, primordial gonads and the precursors of both male and female reproductive tracts have differentiated from cells of the primitive mesonephros (Fig. 12.29).

Differentiation of the primitive tubular structures into male or female genital tracts depends upon stimulation or repression by humoral factors arising in the primitive testes.

Differentiation of the testes from the ambipotential gonadal primordia depends upon the transient expression of a single gene on the Y chromosome (Fig. 12.9). The sex-determining gene (called SRY, for sex-determining region of the Y chromosome) has no homologous counterpart on the X chromosome. It encodes a transcription factor that elicits expression of some genes and repress expression of others. SRY is expressed only in the primitive indifferent gonads in those cells that are destined to become Sertoli cells. It initiates a differentiation program that channels these cells to the Sertoli development pathway and away from the potential alternate fate of differentiation into ovarian granulosa cells (see Chapter 13: Hormonal Control of Reproduction in the Female: The Menstrual).

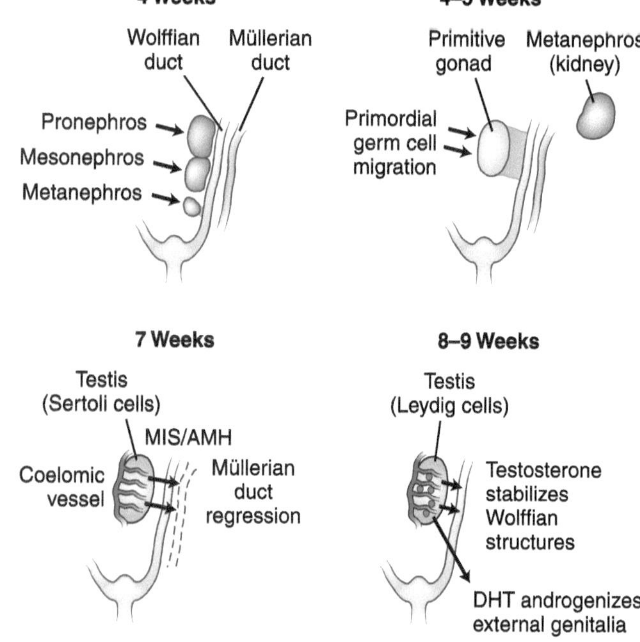

FIGURE 12.27 Summary of the development of the male reproductive system. Source: *From Figure 23-6 in Achermann, J., & Hughes, I. A. (2016). Chapter 23: Pediatric disorders of sex development. In S. Melmed, K. S. Polonsky, P. L., Reed, & H. M. Kronenberg (Eds.),* William's textbook of endocrinology *(13th ed.) (p. 898). Elsevier.*

Understanding of how SRY brings about Sertoli cell differentiation is still incomplete and is based largely upon studies in rodents, which may be different than what happens in humans. One of the primary downstream effects of the SRY gene product is the expression of a related transcription factor called SOX9, which plays a crucial role in regulating expression of other genes in the differentiation pathway. Early in testicular differentiation Sertoli cells release extracellular signals, including prostaglandin D2, which recruits additional cells to the Sertoli cell differentiation pathway, and fibroblast growth factor-9 (FGF9), which acts as a positive feedback activator of SOX9 expression. At around the seventh week after fertilization, developing Sertoli cells aggregate around clusters of primordial germ cells and arrange themselves into cords that will become the seminiferous tubules.

In response to cues from the Sertoli cells, the rapidly proliferating primordial germ cells stop dividing and differentiate into prospermatogonia, which do not resume mitotic activity until after birth. Under the influence of paracrine signals released from the developing Sertoli cells, nearby cells proliferate and give rise to precursors of peritubular myoid (smooth muscle) cells, endothelial cells that form the male-specific vasculature, and Leydig cells. Secretions of Sertoli cells that induce differentiation into Leydig and peritubular cells include FGF9, platelet-derived growth factor, desert hedgehog, and other factors that are not yet identified. Human chorionic gonadotropin

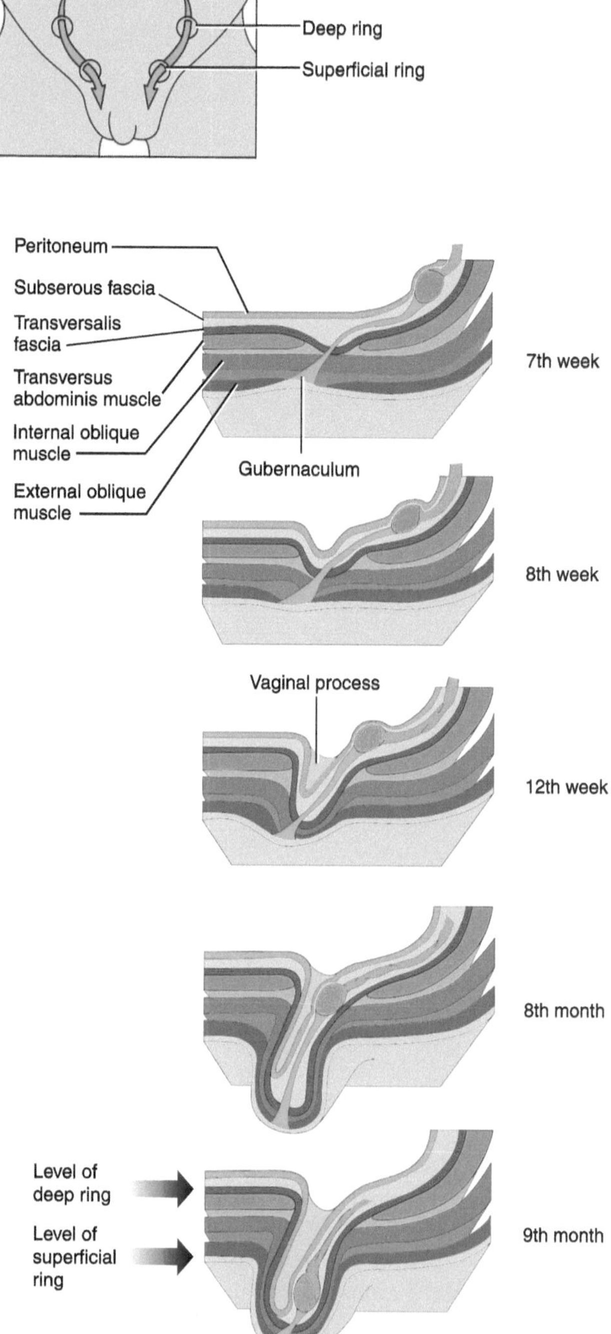

FIGURE 12.28 The descent of the testes. Note how the testes always lie behind the peritoneum. Source: *From Figure 16-25E in Schoenwolf, Bleyl, Brauer, & Francis-West. (2015).* Larsen's human embryology *(5th ed.) (p. 420). Elsevier.*

(hCG) produced in great abundance by the placenta at this time (see Chapter 14: Hormonal Control of Pregnancy and Lactation) probably also participates in Leydig cell differentiation and stimulates the newly differentiated cells to secrete testosterone.

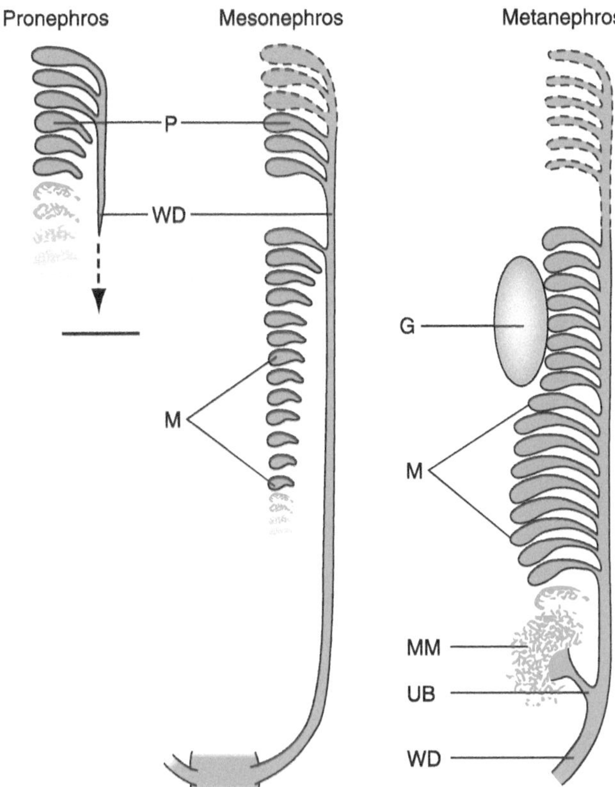

FIGURE 12.29 The Wolffian duct is derived from the mesonephric duct of the embryo. In this sequence that covers days 24–26, the pronephric kidney disintegrates and the mesonephric kidney becomes functional while the metanephric kidney is being formed. *G*, Gonad; *M*, mesonephros; *MM*, metanephric mesenchyme (from which will come the metanephros); *P*, pronephros; *UB*, ureteric bud epithelium; *WD*, Wolffian duct. Source: *From Figure 1.1 in R. P. Scott, et al. (2016). Chapter 1: Embryology of the kidney. In K. Skorecki, et al. (Eds.),* Brenner and Rector's the kidney *(10th ed.) (p. 3). Elsevier.*

The differentiation program that transforms the indifferent gonad to an ovary unfolds in the absence of the SRY gene product and its downstream effectors. Although some signaling pathways are known, the steps that lead to ovarian development are not yet fully understood. Development of ovaries is delayed relative to testicular development. Seminiferous cords are fully formed by 7 weeks and Leydig cells are fully competent by 9 weeks after conception, but primordial follicles that become the functional units of the ovary only start to appear after the 11th week of gestation. Germ cells continue to divide and folliculogenesis continues until the seventh month. Differentiation into primary oocytes begins with mitotic arrest and entry into the first phase of meiosis, at which time the oocytes become surrounded by a single layer of follicular cells to form primordial follicles. Oocytes in primordial follicles remain arrested at the diplotene stage of meiosis until ovulation, which for some follicles may not occur for a half century. In contrast with spermatogonia, which divide thousands of times between puberty and senescence, oogonia complete their proliferation before they are incorporated into primordial follicles and do not multiply after birth.

Development of internal reproductive ducts and their derivatives

The Wolffian ducts, which originate as excretory ducts of the pronephros and mesonephros (Fig. 12.29), appear in the vicinity of the gonadal primordia of both sexes shortly after their formation. The mesonephric ducts become the Wolffian ducts and are the progenitors of the upper male genital tract and give rise to the epididymis, ductus deferens, and seminal vesicles. Soon after the Wolffian ducts appear, a second pair of ducts, called the Müllerian ducts, form in the adjacent space (refer back to Fig. 12.25) as an infolding of the coelom, or internal body cavity. The Müllerian ducts are the progenitors of the upper female genital tract and develop into the uterine (fallopian) tubes at their cranial ends and fuse to form the uterus and upper part of the vagina at their caudal ends (see Chapter 13: Hormonal Control of Reproduction in the Female: The Menstrual). The lower portions of the genital tract, which include the prostate gland, the penis, and scrotum in males, and the lower portion of the vagina, clitoris, and labia in the female, arise from the urogenital sinus and genital tubercle, which are present in both sexes. Thus, regardless of its genetic sex, the embryo has the potential to develop outwardly either as male or female. As for the primordial gonads, the female pattern of development of the internal and external genitalia is expressed unless overridden by secretions of the fetal testis. At around the time the seminiferous cords form in the testes, the Sertoli cells begin to secrete the anti-Müllerian hormone (AMH), which, as its name implies, causes epithelial cells of the Müllerian ducts to undergo apoptosis. Under its influence the Müllerian ducts degenerate and are completely resorbed. A similar fate awaits the Wolffian ducts unless they are rescued by testosterone produced by the developing Leydig cells. Testosterone not only protects the Wolffian duct cells from degeneration but also stimulates them to differentiate into male reproductive structures. Both AMH and testosterone reach their target cells in the Müllerian and Wolffian ducts by the paracrine rather than the endocrine route. It is possible that some testosterone travels through the tubular lumina to reach target cells near the distal ends of the Wolffian ducts. In experiments in which only one testis was removed from embryonic rabbits, the Müllerian duct regressed only on the side with the remaining gonad, indicating that AMH must act locally as a paracrine factor. The Wolffian duct regressed on the opposite side suggesting that testosterone too must act locally to sustain the adjacent Wolffian duct, as the amounts that reached the contralateral duct through the circulation were inadequate to prevent its regression (Fig. 12.30).

Sertoli cell production of AMH is not limited to the embryonic period but continues into adulthood. AMH is present in adult blood and in seminal plasma where it binds to sperm and may increase their motility. Plasma concentrations of AMH are highest in the prepubertal period and fall as testosterone concentrations rise. Its secretion is stimulated by follicle-stimulating hormone (FSH) and strongly inhibited by testosterone. In the testis, AMH inhibits Leydig cell differentiation and expression of steroidogenic enzymes, particularly $P450_{c17}$. AMH also is expressed in the adult ovary and is found in the plasma of women as well as men. No extragonadal role for AMH in adults has yet been established.

AMH is a member of the transforming growth factor-β (TGF-β) family of growth factors. As for other members of the TGF-β family, AMH signals by way of membrane receptors that have intrinsic enzymatic activity that catalyzes phosphorylation of proteins on serine and threonine residues. The AMH receptor consists of two nonidentical subunits, each of which has a single membrane-spanning region and an intracellular kinase domain. After binding with AMH the specific primary receptor forms a complex with and phosphorylates a secondary signal transducing subunit that may also be a component of receptors for other agonists of the TGF-β family. The activated receptor complex associates with and phosphorylates cytosolic proteins called Smads, which enter the nucleus and activate transcription of specific genes (Fig. 12.31).

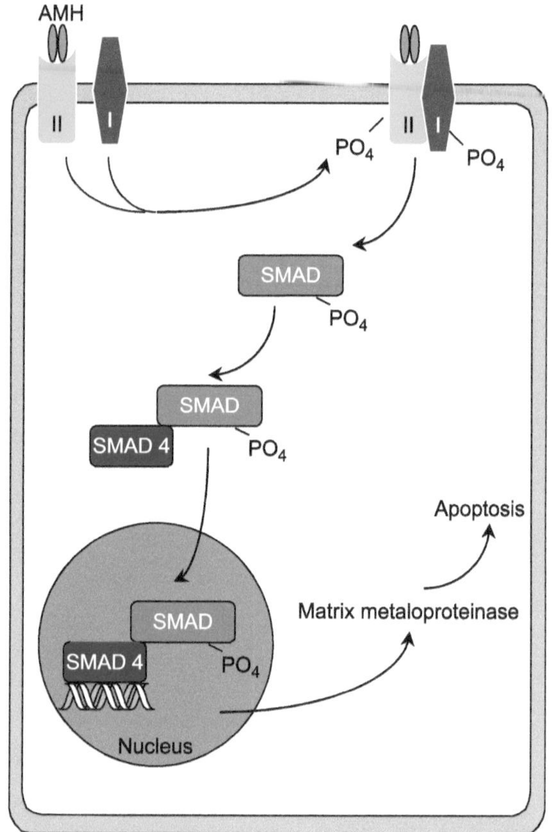

FIGURE 12.31 *AMH*) signaling pathway. AMH binds to its specific primary receptor (*II*), which then forms a heterodimer with and phosphorylates the secondary signal transducing subunit (*I*). The activated receptor complex then catalyzes phosphorylation of *Smad* proteins on serine and threonine residues causing them to bind *Smad 4*, which carries them into the nucleus where transcription of specific genes results in the expression of an apoptotic program and resorption of the Müllerian duct cells. *AMH*, Anti-Müllerian hormone.

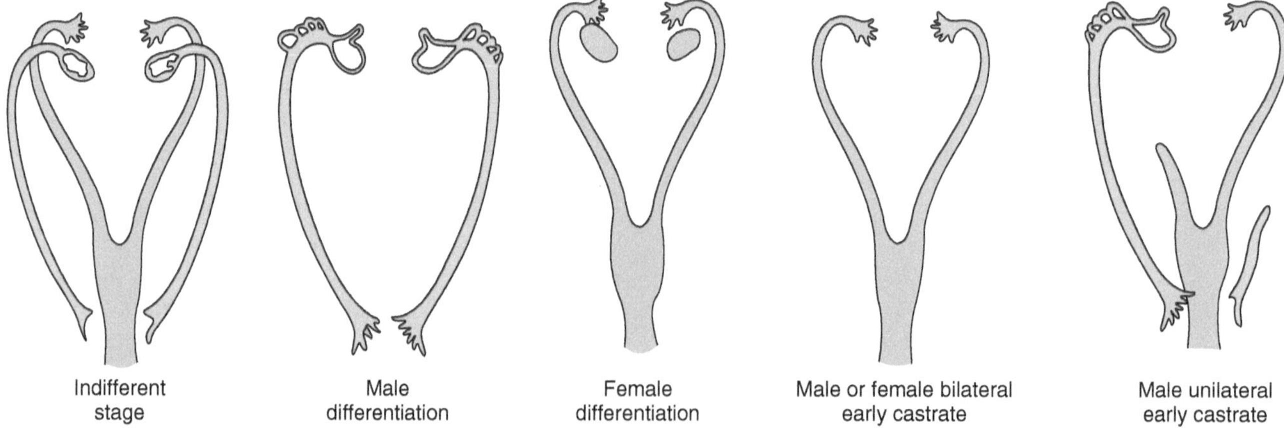

FIGURE 12.30 Normal development of the male and female reproductive tracts. Tissues destined to form the male tract are shown in blue; tissues that develop into the female tract are shown in pink. Bilateral castration of either male or female embryos results in development of the female pattern. Early unilateral castration of male embryos results in development of the normal male duct system on the side with the remaining gonad, but female development on the contralateral side. This pattern develops because both testosterone and anti-Müllerian hormone act as paracrine factors. Source: *Modified from Jost, A. (1971). Embryonic sexual differentiation. In H. W. Jones, & W. W. Scott (Eds.),* Hermaphroditism, genital anomalies and related endocrine disorders *(2nd ed.) (p. 16). Baltimore, MD: Williams & Wilkins, Baltimore.*

Development of the external genitalia

The urogenital sinus and the genital tubercle give rise to the external genitalia in both sexes. Masculinization of these structures to form the penis, scrotum, and prostate gland depends on secretion of testosterone by the fetal testis and its conversion to 5α-dihydrotestosterone (DHT) in these target cells (Fig. 12.32).

Unless stimulated by androgen these structures develop into female external genitalia. When there is insufficient androgen in male embryos, or too much androgen in female embryos, differentiation is incomplete and the external genitalia are ambiguous. Differentiation of the masculine external genitalia depends on the more potent DHT rather than testosterone. The 5α-reductase type II responsible for conversion of testosterone to 5α-DHT is present in tissues destined to become external genitalia even before the testis starts to secrete testosterone. In contrast, this enzyme does not appear in tissues derived from the Wolffian ducts until after they differentiate, indicating that testosterone rather than DHT is the signal for differentiation of the Wolffian derivatives.

The importance of androgen action in sexual development is highlighted by androgen insensitivity syndrome, which can be traced to an inherited defect in the single gene on the X chromosome that encodes the androgen receptor (AR). For more information about this disorder, see the "Case study" at the beginning of this chapter. Afflicted individuals have the normal female phenotype but have sparse pubic and axillary hair and no menstrual cycles (unless, as in the case study, the patient did not produce AMH, in which case she did have menstrual periods, but separated by months). Genetically, they are male and have intraabdominal testes and circulating concentrations of testosterone and estradiol that are within the range found in normal men, but their tissues are totally unresponsive to androgens. Their external genitalia are female because the embryonic tissues develop in the female pattern unless stimulated by androgen. In most cases, because AMH production and responsiveness are normal and their Wolffian ducts are unable to respond to androgen, both of these duct systems regress and neither male nor female internal genitalia develop. Secondary sexual characteristics, including breast development, appear at puberty in response to unopposed action of estrogens formed mainly in the liver by the action of enzymes on testosterone.

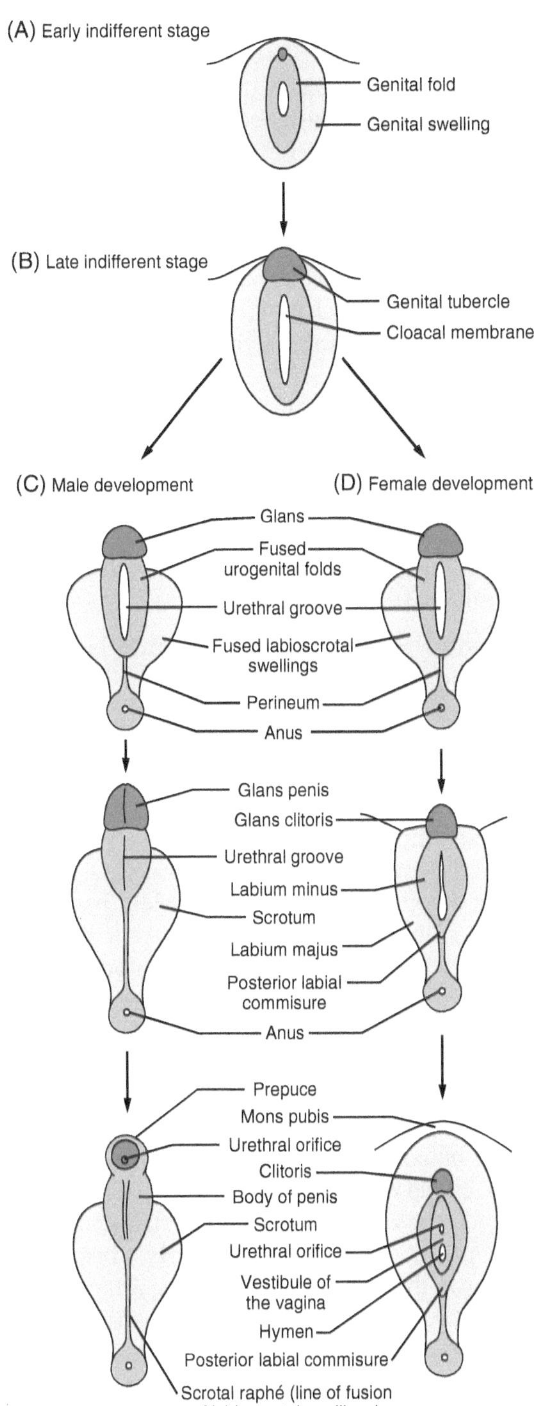

FIGURE 12.32 The differentiation of the external genitalia. The basic pattern of development in the absence of testosterone or the receptor for testosterone is female. To form the male external genitalia, the labia minora fuse to extend the urethral opening from near the entrance of the vagina to the tip of the penis. The labia majora fuse to form the scrotum in the male. Where the labia minora fuse, there is a line of fusion, the median raphe on the underside of the penis, and where the labia majora fuse, there is a line of fusion also called the median raphe, on the scrotum. Source: *Redrawn from Figure 53-8 in Mesiano, S., & Jones, E. E. (2017). Chapter 53: Sexual differentiation. In W. F. Boron, & E. L. Boulpaep (Eds.),* Medical physiology *(3rd ed.) (p. 1083). Elsevier.*

Testes

The testes serve the dual function of producing sperm and hormones. The principal testicular hormone is the steroid testosterone, which has an intratesticular role in sperm production and an extratesticular role in promoting delivery of sperm to the female genital tract. In this respect, testosterone promotes development and maintenance of accessory sexual structures responsible for nurturing gametes and ejecting them from the body and the development of secondary sexual characteristics.

Testicular function is driven by the pituitary through the secretion of two gonadotropic hormones: FSH and luteinizing hormone (LH). Secretion of these pituitary hormones is controlled by the central nervous system through intermittent secretion of the hypothalamic hormone gonadotropin-releasing hormone (GnRH), and by the testes through the secretion of testosterone and inhibin (Fig. 12.33).

Testosterone, its potent metabolite 5α-DHT, and an additional testicular secretion called AMH also function as determinants of sexual differentiation during fetal life (Fig. 12.34).

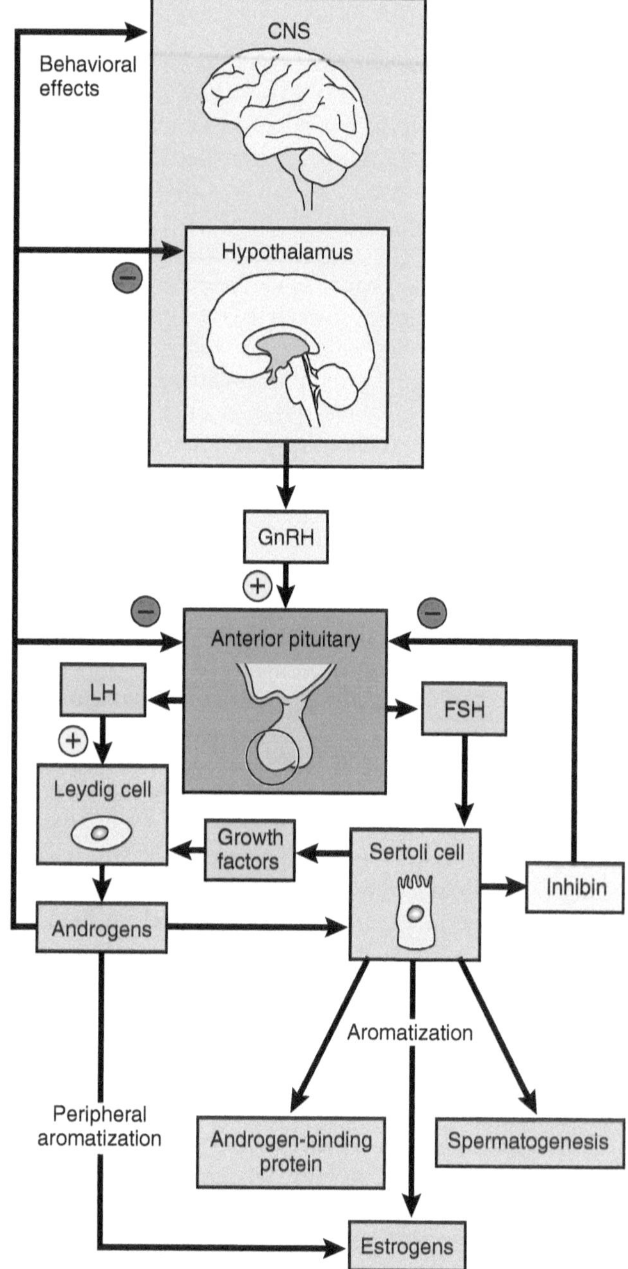

FIGURE 12.33 Schematic diagram of the central role growth hormone releasing hormone has on the male reproductive system. Source: *Redrawn from Figure 54-2 in Mesiano, S., & Jones, E. E. (2017). Chapter 54: The male reproductive system. In W. F. Boron, & E. L. Boulpaep (Eds.),* Medical physiology *(3rd ed.) (p. 1094). Elsevier.*

Morphology of the testes

The testes are paired ovoid organs located in the scrotal sac outside the body cavity (Fig. 12.35).

The extraabdominal location coupled with a vascular countercurrent heat exchanger (the pampiniform plexus) and muscular reflexes (cremaster and dartos muscles) (Figs. 12.36 and 12.37) that lower the testes when too warm and retract the testes toward the abdomen when they are too cold permits testicular temperature to be maintained constant at about 2°C below body temperature. For reasons that are not understood, this small reduction in temperature is crucial for normal spermatogenesis (sperm production). Failure of the testes to descend into the scrotum results in failure of spermatogenesis, although production of testosterone is maintained. Blood reaches the testes primarily through paired testicular arteries and is cooled by heat exchange with returning blood in the pampiniform venous plexus. This complex tangle of blood vessels is formed by highly tortuous and convoluted venules that surround and come in close apposition to the testicular artery before converging to form the testicular vein. This arrangement provides a large surface area for warm arterial blood to transfer heat to cooler venous blood across thin vascular walls. Rewarmed venous blood returns to the systemic circulation primarily through the testicular veins.

Leydig cells, seminiferous tubules, and Sertoli cells

The two principal functions of the testis, sperm production and steroid hormone synthesis, are carried out in morphologically distinct compartments. Sperm are formed and develop within seminiferous tubules, which comprise the bulk of testicular mass. Testosterone is produced by the interstitial cells of Leydig, which lie in clusters between the seminiferous tubules (Fig. 12.38).

Leydig cells

Leydig cells are embedded in loose connective tissue that fills the spaces between seminiferous tubules. They are large polyhedral cells with an extensive smooth endoplasmic reticulum characteristic of steroid-secreting cells. Although extensive at birth, Leydig cells virtually disappear after the first 6 months of postnatal life, only to

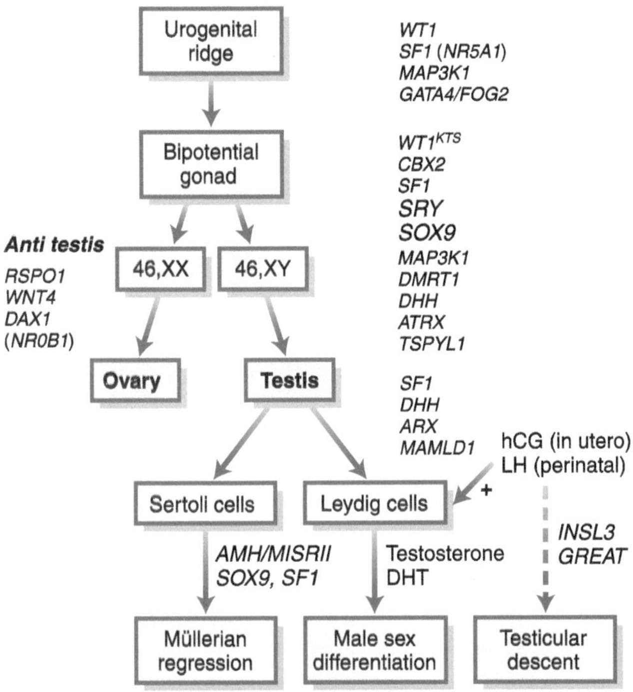

FIGURE 12.34 Flowchart of sexual development showing the AMH and DHT effects. *AMH*, Anti-Müllerian hormone; *DHT*, dihydrotestosterone. Source: *From Figure 23-7 in Achermann, J., & Hughes, I. A. (2016). Chapter 23: Pediatric disorders of sex development. In S. Melmed, K. S. Polonsky, P. L., Reed, & H. M. Kronenberg (Eds.),* William's textbook of endocrinology *(13th ed.) (p. 898). Elsevier.*

reappear more than a decade later with the onset of puberty. In the adult, Leydig cells comprise 10%–20% of testicular mass. Leydig cells cross-talk via hormones with Sertoli cells (Fig. 12.39).

The principal role of Leydig cells is the synthesis and secretion of testosterone in response to stimulation by LH. Testosterone is an important paracrine regulator of intratesticular functions as well as a hormonal regulator of a variety of extratesticular cells. In addition to stimulating steroidogenesis, LH controls the availability of its own receptors (downregulation) and governs growth and differentiation of Leydig cells. After hypophysectomy of experimental animals, Leydig cells atrophy and lose their extensive smooth endoplasmic reticulum where the bulk of testosterone synthesis takes place. LH restores them to normal and can produce frank hypertrophy if given in excess. Leydig cells, which are abundant in newborn baby boys, regress and die shortly after birth. Secretion of LH at the onset of puberty causes dormant Leydig cell precursors to proliferate and differentiate into mature steroidogenic cells. In the fetus, growth and development of Leydig cells and secretion of testosterone depend initially on the placental hormone, chorionic gonadotropin, which is present in high concentrations in early pregnancy. Later, after development of the pituitary, testosterone secretion and maintenance of Leydig cell function are taken over by LH secreted by the fetal pituitary gland. LH and hCG stimulate the same receptors.

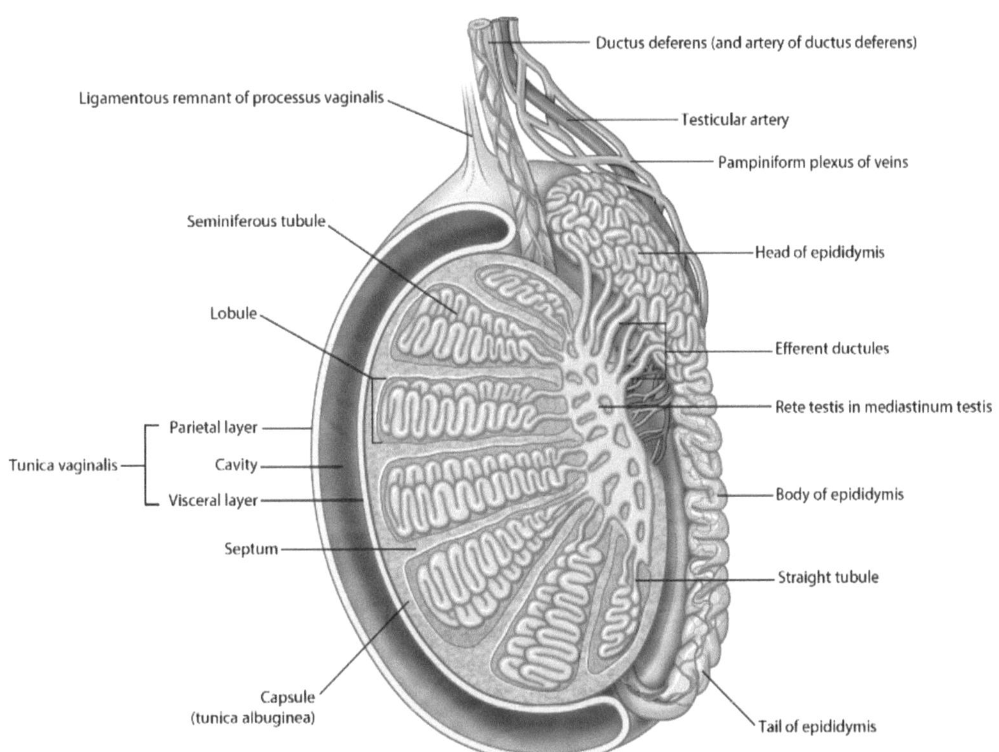

FIGURE 12.35 Cross section of a testis. Source: *From R. L. Drake, A. W. Vogl, A. W. M. Mitchell, R. M. Tibbitts and P. E. Richardson. (2015). Section on pelvis and perineum. In* Gray's atlas of anatomy *(2nd ed.) (p. 239). Elsevier.*

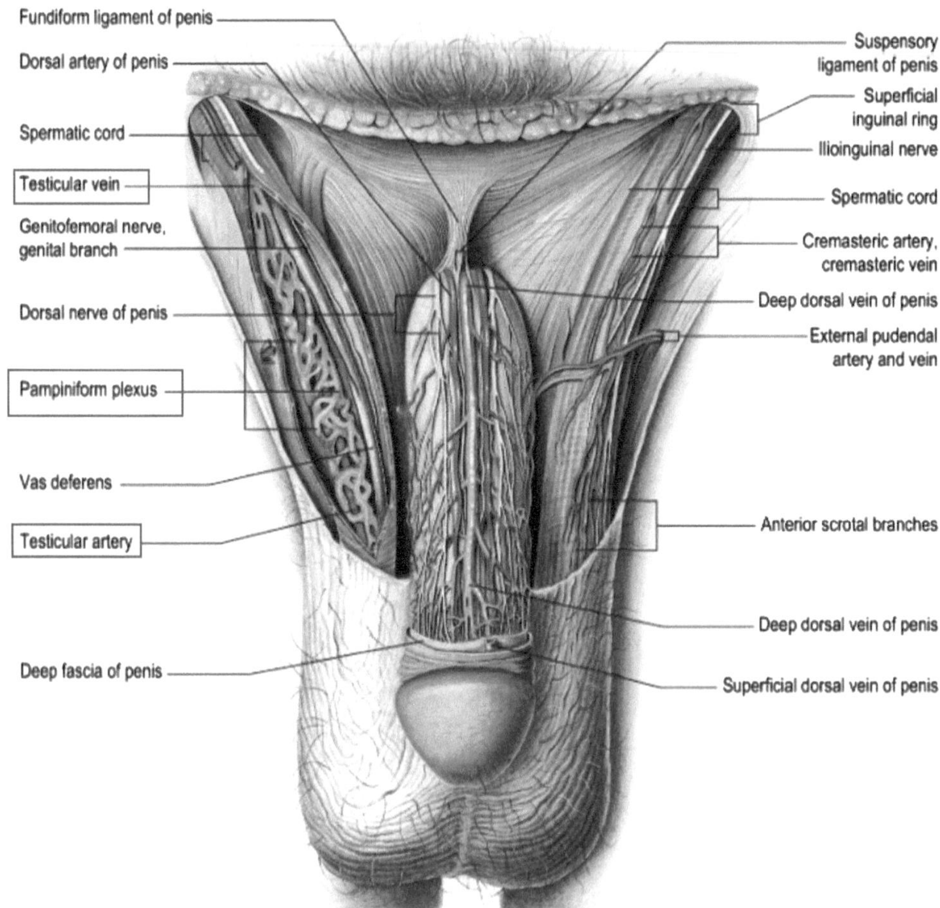

FIGURE 12.36 The pampiniform venous plexus (boxed) surrounding the testicular artery (boxed) cools the blood before it reaches the testes. This is one of three methods of keeping the testes cooler than the abdominal body temperature. The pampiniform plexus becomes the testicular vein (boxed) that returns venous blood from the right testis to the inferior vena cava on the right side and from the left testis to the left renal vein that then empties into the inferior vena cava. Source: *From Figure 75.2 in S. Standring, et al. (2016).* Gray's anatomy *(41st ed.) (p. 1273). Elsevier.*

The LH receptor is a member of the superfamily of receptors that are coupled to heterotrimeric G-proteins. LH stimulates the formation of cyclic AMP (see Chapter 1: Introduction), which in turn activates protein kinase A and the subsequent phosphorylation of proteins that promote steroidogenesis, gene transcription, and other cellular functions (Fig. 12.40).

As with the adrenal cortex (see Chapter 4: The Adrenal Glands), the initial step in the synthesis of testosterone is the conversion of cholesterol to pregnenolone. This reaction requires mobilization of cholesterol from storage droplets and its translocation from cytosol to the intramitochondrial compartment, where cleavage of the side chain occurs. Access of cholesterol to the $P450_{scc}$ enzyme in the mitochondria is governed by the action of the steroid acute regulatory protein (StAR), the expression and phosphorylation of which are accelerated by cyclic AMP. Stored cholesterol may derive either from de novo synthesis within the Leydig cell or from circulating cholesterol, which enters the cell by receptor-mediated endocytosis of low-density lipoproteins.

The biochemical pathway for testosterone biosynthesis was shown in Figs. 12.8 and 12.9. Neither LH nor cyclic AMP appears to accelerate the activity of any of the four enzymes responsible for conversion of the 21-carbon pregnenolone to testosterone. It may be recalled that the rate of steroid hormone synthesis and secretion is determined by the rate of conversion of cholesterol to pregnenolone. In maintaining the functional integrity of the Leydig cells, LH maintains the levels of all steroid-transforming enzymes. Transcription of the gene that encodes $P450_{c17}$, the enzyme responsible for the two-step conversion of 21-carbon steroids to 19-carbon steroids, appears to be especially sensitive to cyclic AMP. Testosterone released from Leydig cells may diffuse into nearby capillaries for transport in the general circulation, or it may diffuse into nearby seminiferous tubules where it performs its essential role in spermatogenesis (Fig. 12.40).

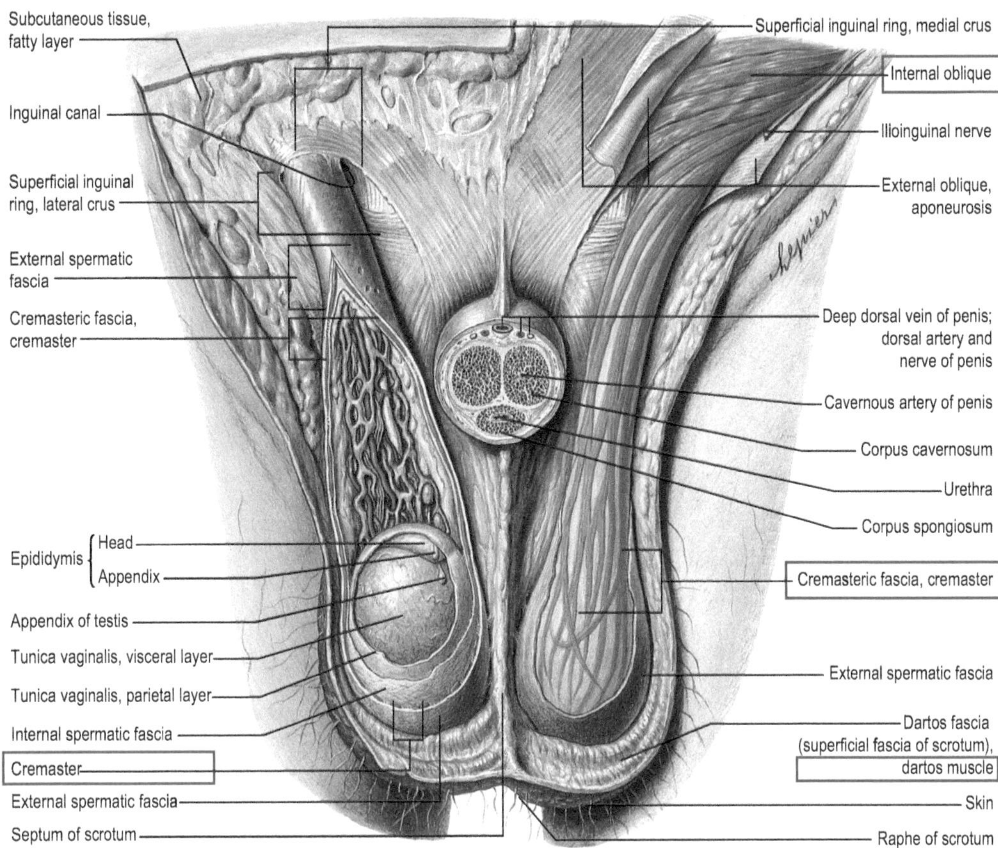

FIGURE 12.37 The cremaster muscle (boxed), an extension of the internal oblique muscle (boxed), relaxes to lower the testes if they get too warm and contracts to bring them closer to the abdominal cavity if they get too cold. The dartos muscle (boxed), part of the skin musculature, will contract and relax for the same reasons. Source: *From Figure 76.3 in S. Standring, et al. (2016).* Gray's anatomy *(41st ed.) (p. 1273). Elsevier.*

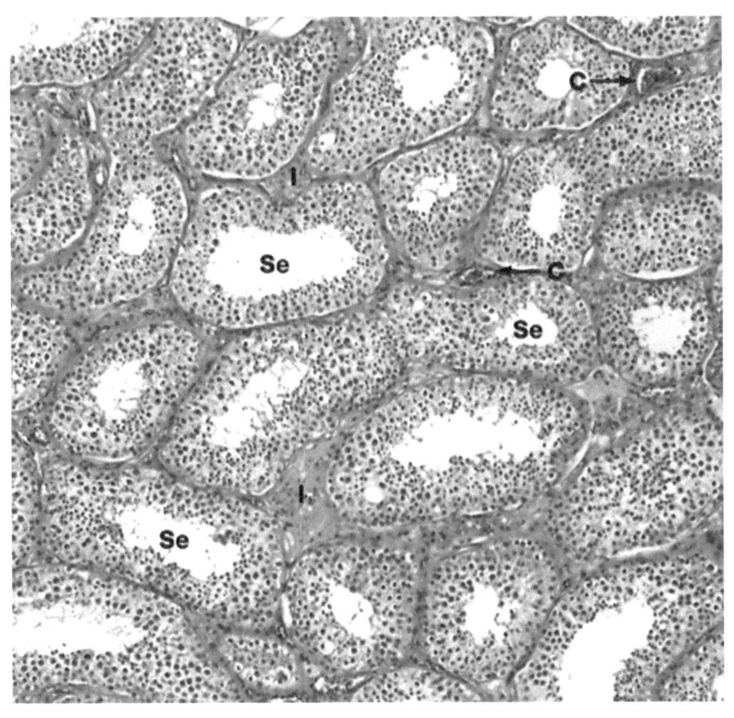

FIGURE 12.38 The location of the interstitial cells (I) of Leydig (Leydig cells) between the seminiferous tubules (Se). Capillaries (C) are also observed. The stain is periodic acid – Schiff (PAS), a stain composed of an iodine-based acid and Schiff's reagent, the latter developed by Hugo Schiff (1834-1915) in 1866. It stains for carbohydrates. Source: *From Wheater's Functional Histology, 6th ed., by Young, O'Dowd and Woodford, Elsevier, 2014, p. 339.*

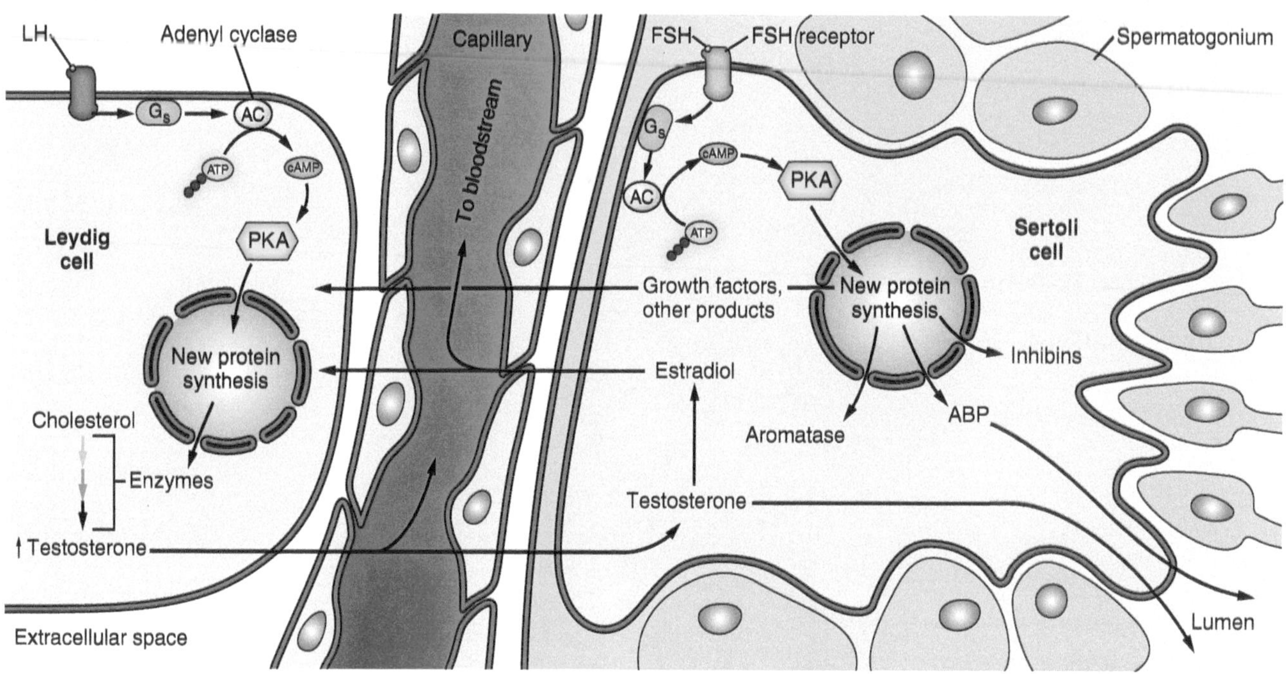

FIGURE 12.39 The relationship between Leydig and Sertoli cells. *ABP*, androgen-binding protein—this is secreted near developing sperm cells to keep local testosterone levels high; *AC*, adenyl cyclase; *Gs*, G-protein receptor—stimulatory; *PKA*, protein kinase A. Source: *Redrawn from Figure 54-4 in Mesiano, S., & Jones, E. E. (2017). Chapter 54: The male reproductive system. In W. F. Boron, & E. L. Boulpaep (Eds.),* Medical physiology *(3rd ed.) (p. 1096). Elsevier.*

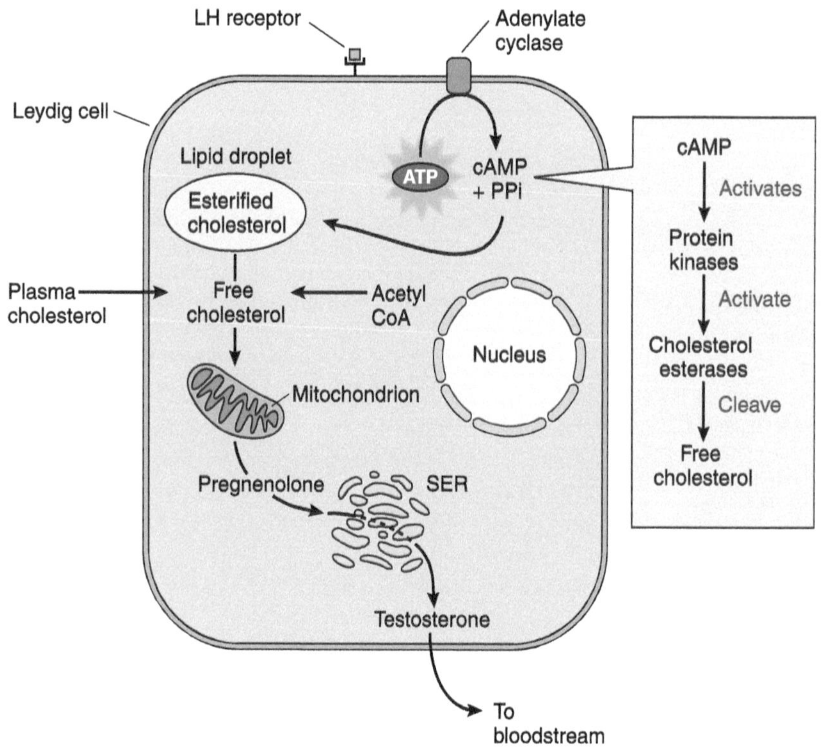

FIGURE 12.40 A schematic diagram of the effect of LH stimulation on the Leydig cell. *LH*, Luteinizing hormone. Source: *Figure 21-13 in Gartner, L. P. (2017).* Textbook of histology *(4th ed.) (p. 571). Elsevier.*

The testes also secrete small amounts of estradiol and some androstenedione, which serves as a precursor for extratesticular synthesis of estrogens. Leydig cells are the chief source of testicular estrogens, but immature Sertoli cells have the capacity to convert testosterone to estradiol. In addition, developing sperm cells express the enzyme $P450_{arom}$ (aromatase) and also convert androgens to estrogens. Estradiol is present in seminal fluid and is essential for fluid reabsorption in the rete testis. The presence of estrogen receptors in the epididymis and several testicular cells, including Leydig cells, suggests that estradiol may have other important actions in normal sperm formation and maturation.

Seminiferous tubules

Seminiferous tubules (Fig. 12.35 and cross section in Fig. 12.41) are highly convoluted loops that range from about 120 to 300 μm in diameter and from 30 to 70 cm in length (schematic in Fig. 12.42).

They are arranged in lobules bounded by fibrous connective tissue. Each testis has hundreds of such tubules that are connected at both ends to the rete testis (Fig. 12.30). It has been estimated that, if laid end to end, the seminiferous tubules of the human testis would extend more than 500 m. The seminiferous epithelium that lines the tubules consists of three cell types: spermatogonia, which are stem cells; spermatocytes, which are in the process of becoming sperm; and Sertoli cells, which nurture developing sperm and secrete a variety of products into the blood and the lumina of seminiferous tubules. Seminiferous tubules are surrounded by a several layers of peritubular myoid epithelial cells, which are contractile and help propel the nonmotile sperm through the tubules toward the rete testis.

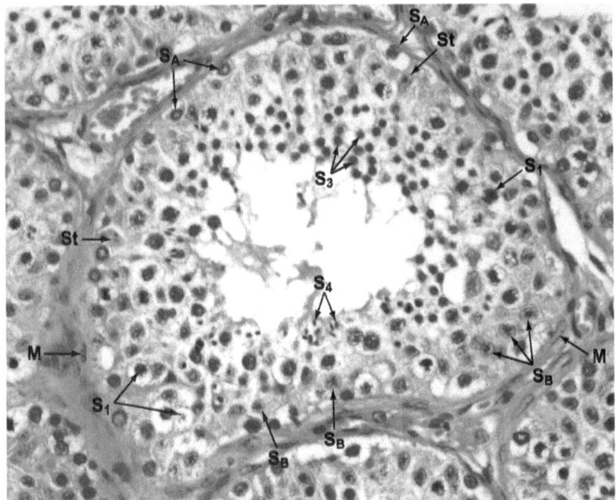

FIGURE 12.41 Micrograph illustrates an adult seminiferous tubule cut in transverse section. The processes of spermatogenesis and spermiogenesis are synchronised, with waves of activity occurring sequentially along the length of each tubule. Thus in a single cross-section of a tubule, not all development phases will be represented. The undifferentiated diploid germ cells, found in the basal compartment of the seminiferous tubule, are called type A spermatogonia. These go through several cycles of mitosis to produce further type A spermatogonia, which maintain the germ cell pool, and type B spermatogonia, which are committed to production of spermatozoa. Spermatogonia type A SA are characterised by a large round or oval nucleus with condensed chromatin; peripheral nucleoli and a nuclear vacuole may be prominent. Spermatogonia type B SB have dispersed chromatin, central nucleoli, and no nuclear vacuole. Both types of spermatogonia have sparse poorly stained cytoplasm. Type B spermatogonia undergo further mitotic divisions to produce primary spermatocytes. These migrate to the adluminal compartment of the seminiferous tubule before commencing the first meiotic division. Primary spermatocytes S1 are readily recognised by their copious cytoplasm and large nuclei containing coarse clumps or thin threads of chromatin; dividing cells may be seen. In humans, the first meiotic division cycle takes approximately 3 weeks to complete, after which time the daughter cells become known as secondary spermatocytes. The smaller secondary spermatocytes rapidly undergo the second meiotic division and are therefore seldom seen. Source: *From Figure 18.5a in Wheater's Functional Histology 6th ed., by Young, Woodford, and O'Dowd. Elsevier, 2014, page 340.*

Spermatogenesis goes on continuously from puberty to senescence along the entire length of the seminiferous tubules. Though a continuous process, spermatogenesis can be divided into three discrete phases:

1. mitotic divisions that maintain a stem cell population of spermatogonia and provide the cells destined to become mature sperm;
2. meiotic divisions that reduce the chromosome number and produce a cluster of haploid spermatids; and
3. transformation of spermatids into mature spermatozoa (spermiogenesis), a process involving the loss of most of the cytoplasm and the development of flagella (Figs. 12.43 and 12.44).

The fully formed spermatozoa (Figs. 12.45–12.47) are then released into the tubular lumina (the relatively straight seminiferous tubules) a process called spermiation.

These events occur along the length of the seminiferous tubules in a definite temporal and spatial pattern. A spermatogenic cycle includes all the transformations from spermatogonium to spermatozoan and requires 64–72 days. As the cycle progresses, germ cells move from the basal portion of the germinal epithelium toward the lumen. Successive cycles begin before the previous one has been completed, so that different stages of the cycle are seen at any given point along a tubule at different depths of the epithelium. Spermatogenic cycles are synchronized in adjacent groups of cells, but the cycles are slightly advanced in similar groups of cells located immediately upstream, so that cells at any given stage of the spermatogenic cycle are spaced at regular intervals along the length of the tubules.

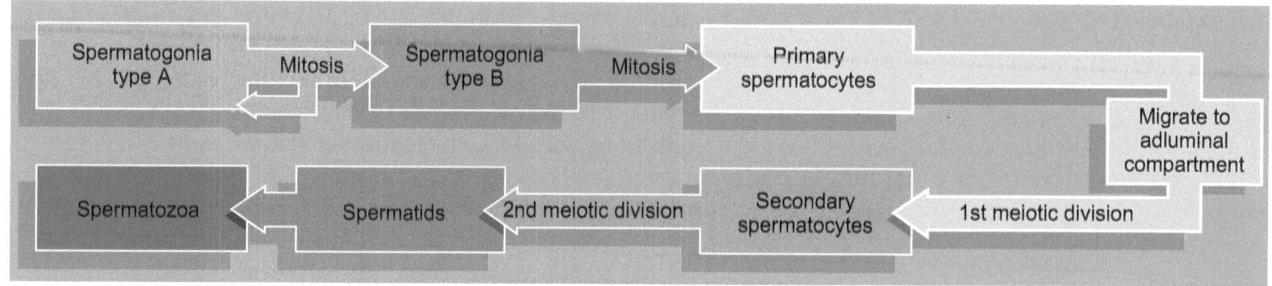

FIGURE 12.42 Schematic diagram of spermatogenesis within a seminiferous tubule Source: *Figure 18.5b in Wheater's Functional Histology 6th ed., by Young, Woodford, and O'Dowd. Elsevier, 2014, page 340.*

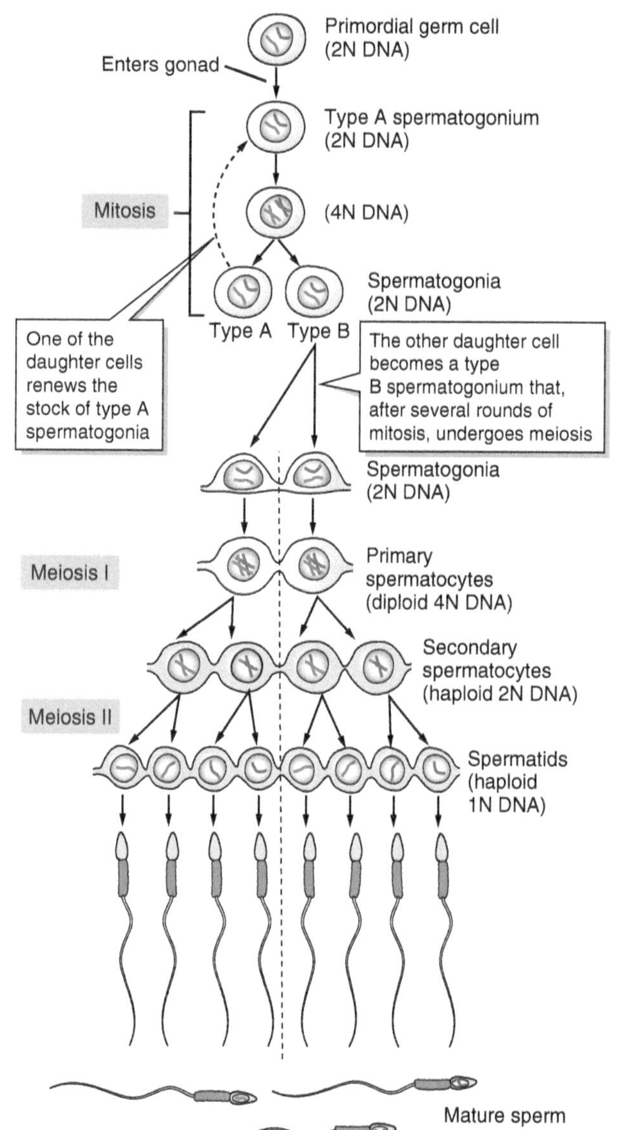

FIGURE 12.43 Spermatogenesis showing the mitotic and meiotic divisions. It takes about 64–72 days to form sperm. Source: *Redrawn from Figure 54-7 in Mesiano, S., & Jones, E. E. (2017). Chapter 54: The male reproductive system. In W. F. Boron, & E. L. Boulpaep (Eds.),* Medical physiology *(3rd ed.) (p. 1101). Elsevier.*

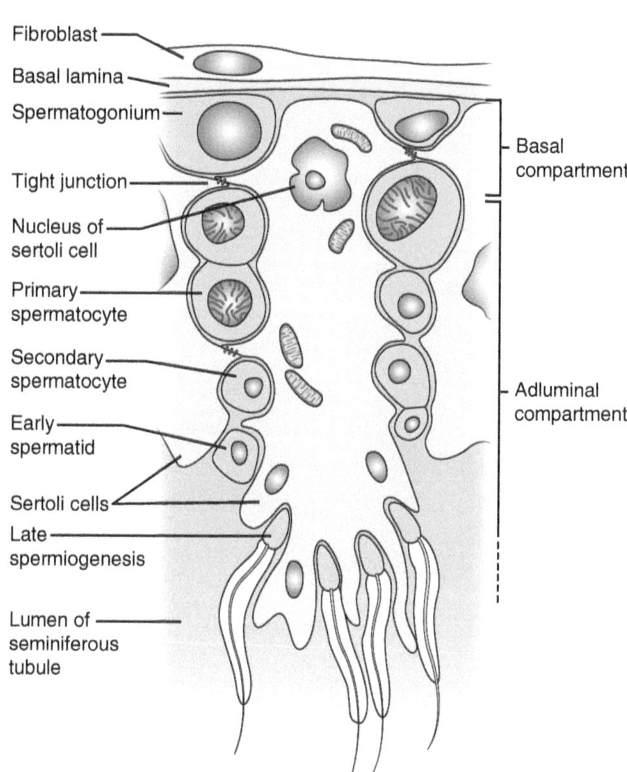

FIGURE 12.44 The Sertoli cell is a nurse cell for the developing sperm. Source: *Redrawn from Figure 54-8 in Mesiano, S., & Jones, E. E. (2017). Chapter 54: The male reproductive system. In W. F. Boron, & E. L. Boulpaep (Eds.),* Medical physiology *(3rd ed.) (p. 1102). Elsevier.*

This complex series of events ensures that mature spermatozoa are produced continuously. About 2 million spermatogonia, each giving rise to 64 sperm cells, begin this process in each testis every day. More than 200 million spermatozoa are produced daily, or about 6×10^{14} in the six or more decades of reproductive life. Table 12.1 gives some normal values for semen.

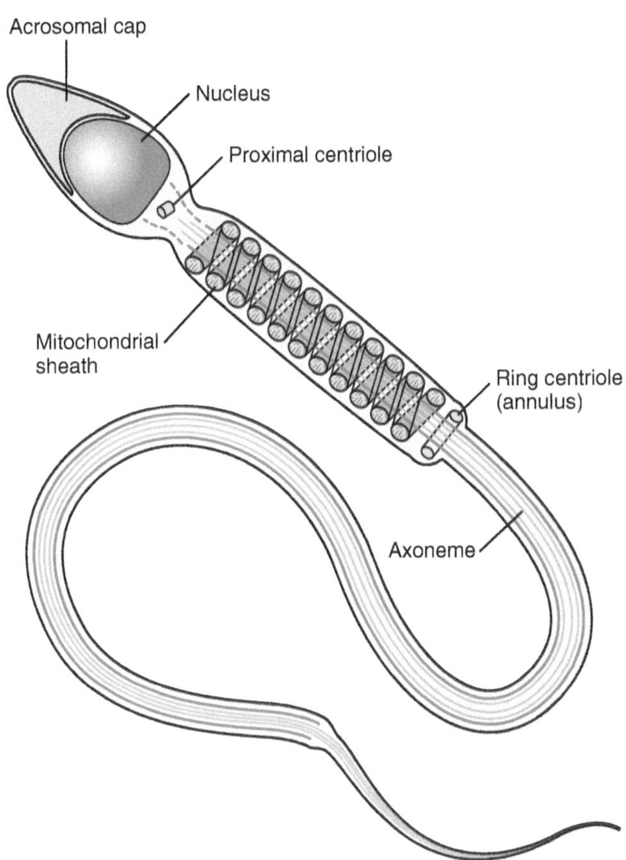

FIGURE 12.45 A spermatozoon. Source: *Redrawn from Figure 54.9 in Mesiano, S., & Jones, E. E. (2017). Chapter 54: The male reproductive system. In W. F. Boron, & E. L. Boulpaep (Eds.),* Medical physiology *(3rd ed.) (p. 1103). Elsevier.*

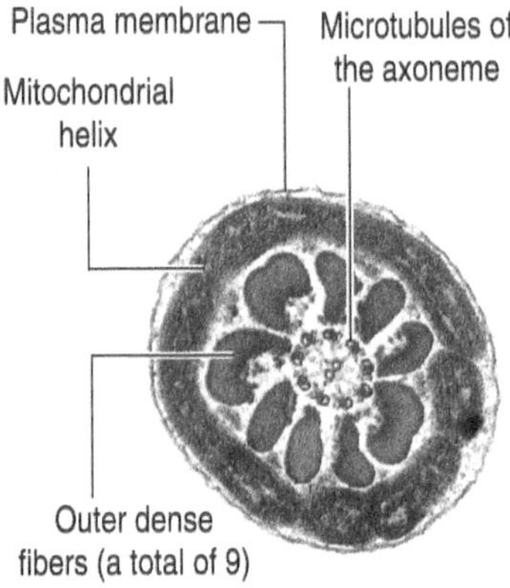

FIGURE 12.46 Cross section through the mitochondrial helix of a sperm as viewed under the electron microscope. The axoneme (Ax) is the collective name for the microtubules that make up the tail of the sperm. The outer dense fibers (F) lie inside the mitochondria (Mi). x48,000. Source: *From Figure 18-7c in Wheater's Functional Histology 6th ed., by Young, O'Dowd and Woodford. Elsevier, 2014, p. 342.*

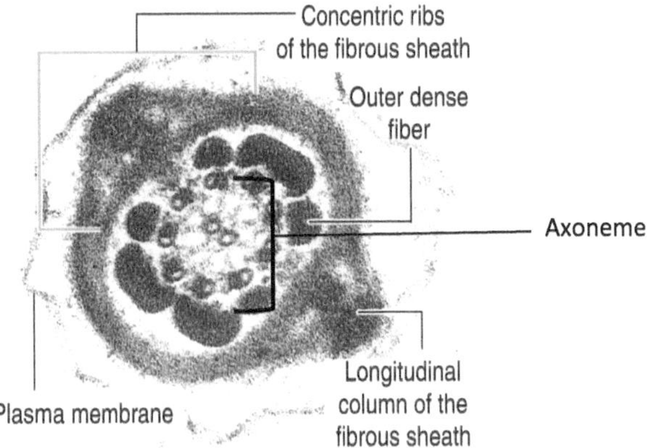

FIGURE 12.47 An electron microglraph cross section of a sperm tail showing the microtubular central core of the axoneme (Ax)—it has the same structure of cilia—and surrounding structures. The axoneme is also called the axial filament. It is composed of a central pair of microtubules surrounded by nine pair of microtubules. Spermatozoa are the only human cell to have flagella. Mi=mitochondria; Rn = fibrous rings; Cy=cytoplasm; F= outer dense fibers; Mi=mitochondria; An= annulus; Rb= fibrous ribs. X17,000. Source: *From Figure 18-7b in Wheater's Functional Histology 6th ed., by Young, O'Dowd and Woodford. Elsevier, 2014, p. 342.*

TABLE 12.1 Normal parameter values for semen.

Parameter	Value
Volume of ejaculate	2–6 mL
Viscosity	Liquefaction in 1 h
pH	7–8
Count	≥ 20 million/mL
Motility	≥ 50%
Morphology	60% normal

From Table 54-3 in Mesiano, S., & Jones, E. E. (2017). Chapter 54: The male reproductive system. In W. F. Boron, & E. L. Boulpaep (Eds.), Medical physiology *(3rd ed.) (p. 1103). Elsevier.*

Sertoli cells

Sertoli cells are remarkable polyfunctional cells, the activities of which are intimately related to many aspects of the formation and maturation of spermatozoa. They extend through the entire thickness of the germinal epithelium from basement membrane to lumen and in the adult take on exceedingly irregular shapes determined by the changing conformations of the 10–12 developing sperm cells embedded in their cytoplasm (Figs. 12.38 and 12.48 and schematically in Fig. 12.44). Differentiating sperm cells are isolated from the bloodstream and interstitial fluid and must rely on Sertoli cells for their sustenance. Adjacent Sertoli cells arch above the clusters of spermatogonia that nestle between them at the level of the basement membrane. A series of tight junctions binds each Sertoli cell to the

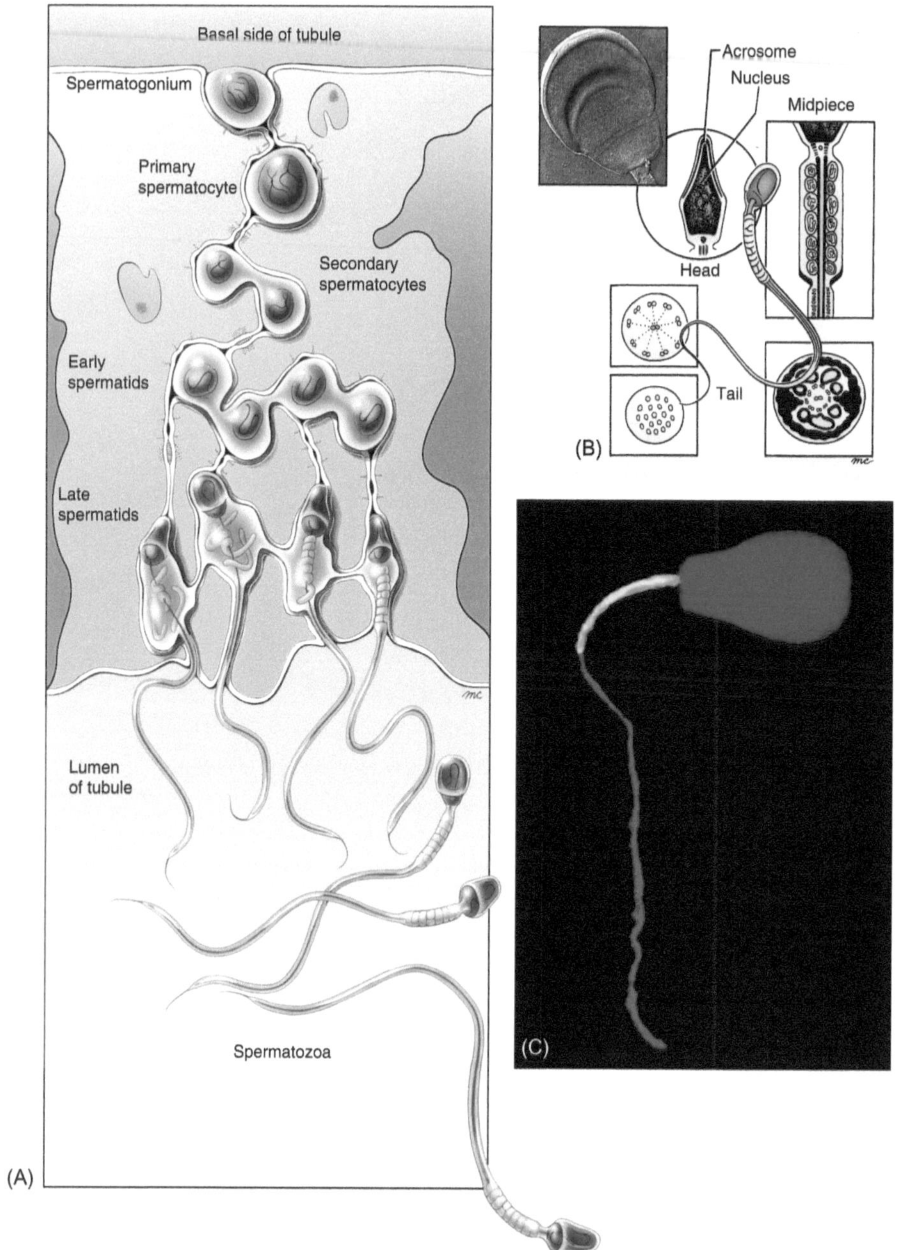

FIGURE 12.48 Spermatogenesis and spermiogenesis. *A*, Schematic section through the wall of the seminiferous tubule. Spermatogonium just under the outer surface of the tubule wall (basal side) undergoes mitosis to produce daughter cells, which may continue to divide by mitosis (thus renewing the spermatogonial stem cell population) or may commence meiosis as primary spermatocytes. As spermatogenesis and spermiogenesis occur, the differentiating cell is translocated between adjacent Sertoli cells to the tubule lumen. Daughter spermatocytes and spermatids remain linked by cytoplasmic bridges. The entire clone of spermatogonia derived from each primordial germ cell is linked by cytoplasmic bridges. *B*, Structure of the mature spermatozoon. The head contains the nucleus capped by the acrosome; the midpiece contains coiled mitochondria; the tail contains propulsive microtubules. The inset micrograph shows the head of a human sperm. *C*, Bull sperm labeled with fluorescent markers to reveal its nucleus (blue) in its head, mitochondria (green) in its midpiece, and microtubules (red) in its tail. The red labeling around the perimeter of the head is background labeling. Source: *From Figure 1-4A-C in Larsen's Human Embryology, 5th ed., by Schoenwolf, Bleyl, Brauer, Francis-West, p. 23.*

six adjacent Sertoli cells and limits passage of physiologically relevant molecules into or out of seminiferous tubules (Figs. 12.48 and 12.49).

The blood–testis barrier has selective permeability that allows rapid entry of testosterone, for example, but virtually excludes cholesterol and completely excludes antibodies. The physiological significance of the blood–testis barrier has not been established, but it is probably of some importance that spermatogonia are located on the blood side of the barrier, whereas developing spermatids are restricted to the luminal side. In addition to harboring and nurturing developing sperm, Sertoli cells secrete the watery fluid that transports spermatozoa through the seminiferous tubules and into the epididymis, where 99% of the fluid is reabsorbed.

Germinal epithelium

The function of the germinal epithelium is to produce large numbers of sperm that are capable of fertilization. The Sertoli cells, which are interposed between the developing sperm and the vasculature, harbor and nurture sperm as they mature. Sertoli cells are the only cells known to express FSH receptors in human males and therefore are the only targets of FSH. FSH increases Sertoli cell proliferation and differentiation in the immature testis and maintains the functional state

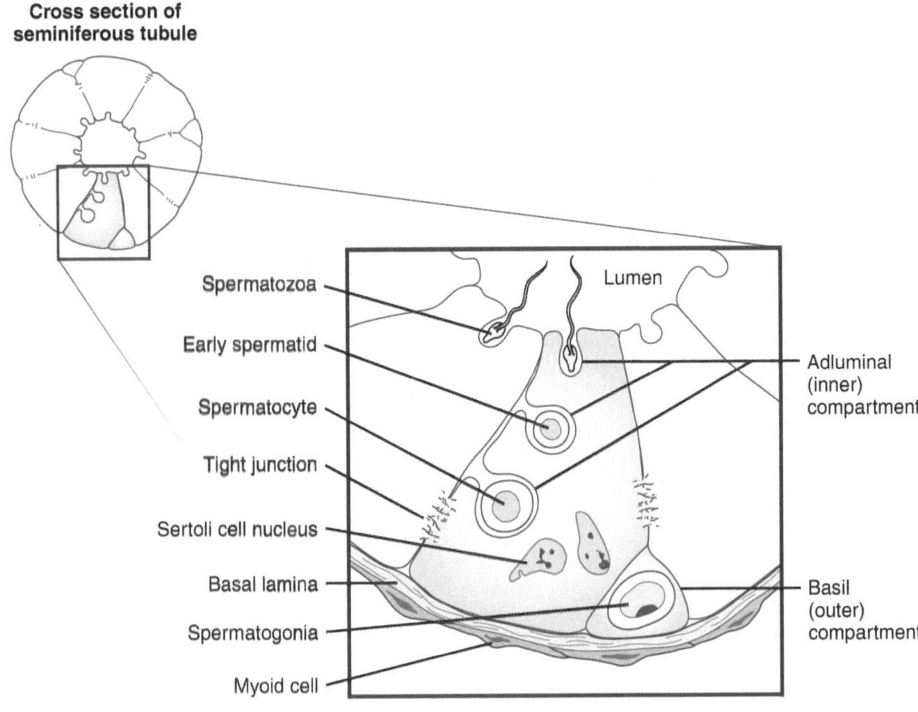

FIGURE 12.49 Schematic diagram of the cells in the seminiferous tubule (top). The seminiferous tubule consists of Sertoli cells that surround developing germ cells (middle). Sertoli cells extend from the basal lamina to the lumen. Tight junctions between adjoining Sertoli cells separate the seminiferous tubule into basal and adluminal compartments and are the anatomic basis for the blood-testis barrier (bottom). The basal compartment, which contains spermatogonia lining the basal lamina and peritubular myoid cells, is exposed to the interstitial compartment, which contains Leydig cells and blood vessels that deliver endocrine regulators of testis function (e.g., gonadotropins). The adluminal compartment contains developing spermatocytes, spermatids, and mature spermatozoa that are released into the lumen of the seminiferous tubule. Source: *(From Matsumoto AM. The testis. In: Felig P, Frohman LA, eds. Endocrinology and Metabolism, 4th ed. New York, NY: McGraw-Hill; 2001:635-705.) From Figure 19.2 in Williams Textbook of Endocrinology, 13th ed., 2016, Elsevier, page 696.*

of the stable population of Sertoli cells in the mature testis. In its absence, testicular size is severely reduced and sperm production, which is limited by Sertoli cell availability, is severely restricted.

It has been known for many years that FSH, LH, and testosterone all play vital roles in spermatogenesis. It is likely that FSH indirectly regulates development and multiplication of spermatogonia by stimulating Sertoli cells to produce both growth and survival factors that prevent germ cell apoptosis. Withdrawal of FSH and LH arrests spermatogonial development, which is the major rate-limiting step in spermatogenesis. Once formed, spermatocytes progress through meiosis normally in the absence of gonadotropic support. Although both FSH and testosterone are required for initiation of normal rates of spermatogenesis, sperm formation can be maintained indefinitely with very high doses of testosterone alone or with sufficient LH to stimulate testosterone production.

Sertoli cells lack receptors for LH but are richly endowed with ARs, indicating that the actions of LH on Sertoli cell function are indirect, and are mediated by testosterone, which reaches them in high concentration by diffusion from nearby Leydig cells (Fig. 12.50).

Testosterone readily passes through the blood–testis barrier and is found in high concentrations in seminiferous fluid. However, the absence of ARs in the developing human sperm cells indicates that support of sperm cell development by testosterone also is exerted indirectly by way of the Sertoli cells. Peritubular myoid epithelial cells express ARs and may secrete peptide factors that may also mediate indirect effects of LH and testosterone on the seminiferous epithelium.

Although testosterone is critically important for spermatogenesis, it is ineffective in this regard when administered to testosterone-deficient individuals in amounts sufficient to restore normal blood concentrations. For reasons that are not understood, the intratesticular concentration of testosterone needed to support spermatogenesis is many times higher than needed to saturate ARs. The concentration of testosterone in testicular venous blood is 40 to 50 times that found in peripheral blood and its concentration in aspirates of human testicular fluid is more than 100 times higher than the concentration found in peripheral blood plasma.

The FSH receptor is closely related to the LH receptor and, when stimulated, activates adenylyl cyclase through the agency of the stimulatory alpha G-protein (Gαs; see Chapter 2: Pituitary Gland). The resulting activation of protein kinase A catalyzes phosphorylation of proteins that regulate the cytoskeletal elements that enable developing spermatids to migrate through the Sertoli cytoplasm toward the lumen. Cyclic AMP–dependent activities also regulate production of the membrane glycoproteins that govern adherence to developing sperm and expression of proteins that directly and indirectly regulate germ cell development (Fig. 12.40). Some of the proteins secreted by Sertoli cells into the seminiferous tubules are thought to facilitate germ cell maturation in the epididymis and perhaps more distal portions of the

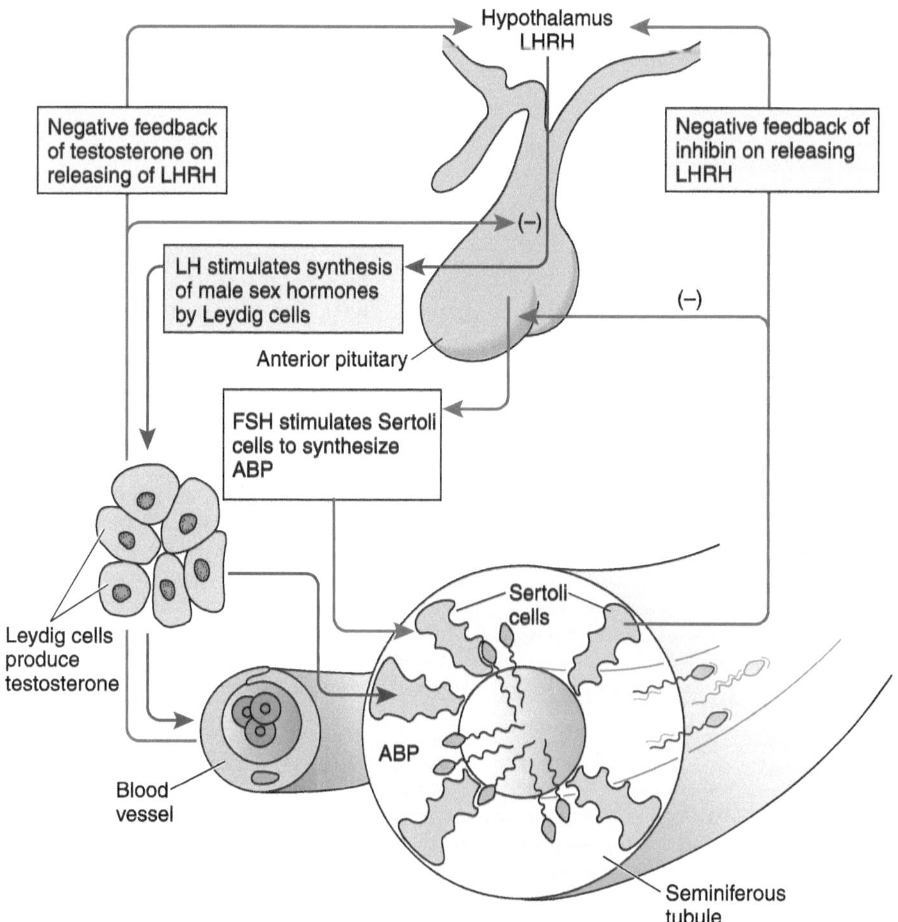

FIGURE 12.50 The relationship between the Leydig and Sertoli cells. The Sertoli cell produces ABP in response to FSH. ABP keeps testosterone levels higher in the seminiferous tubules. This enhances spermatozoa maturation. *ABP*, Androgen-binding protein; *FSH*, Follicle-stimulating hormone. Source: *From Figure 21-14 in Gartner, L. P. (2017).* Textbook of histology *(4th ed.) (p. 572). Elsevier.*

reproductive tract. Upon stimulation by FSH, Sertoli cells may also secrete paracrine factors that enhance Leydig cell responses to LH.

FSH and testosterone have overlapping actions on Sertoli cells and act synergistically, but the precise actions of each remain unknown. Some evidence implicates testosterone in the adherence of developing sperm cells to the Sertoli cell membrane and their release during spermiation. Recently described "experiments of nature" have shed some light on the relative importance of FSH and testosterone in spermatogenesis. Inactivating mutations of the β subunit of LH in humans or rodents result in total failure of spermatogenesis, despite normal prenatal sexual development (see later), suggesting that testosterone is indispensable. In contrast, inactivating mutations of the gene for the FSH receptor did not prevent affected men or mice from fathering offspring. FSH is not absolutely required for spermatogenesis, but the patients and rodents with inactive FSH receptors had small testes, low sperm counts, and a preponderance of defective sperm. Thus stimulation by FSH at some period of life is required for the production of normal quantity and quality of sperm.

Male reproductive tract

The remaining portion of the male reproductive tract consists of modified mesonephric excretory ducts that ultimately deliver sperm to the exterior along with secretions of accessory glands that promote sperm survival and fertility. Sperm never move within the male reproductive system but are always passively carried. Once out of the male reproductive system they become motile. Sperm leave the testis through multiple efferent ductules, the ciliated epithelium of which facilitates passage from the rete testis into the highly convoluted and tortuous duct of the epididymis. Passage through the epididymis requires about 10 days, during which the sperm acquire increased capacity for motility and fertilization. The epididymis is the primary area for storage of sperm, which may remain viable within its confines for months.

Sperm are advanced through the epididymis, particularly during sexual arousal, by rhythmic contractions of circular smooth muscle surrounding the duct. At ejaculation, they are expelled into the ductus deferens and ultimately through the urethra (Figs. 12.51 and 12.52).

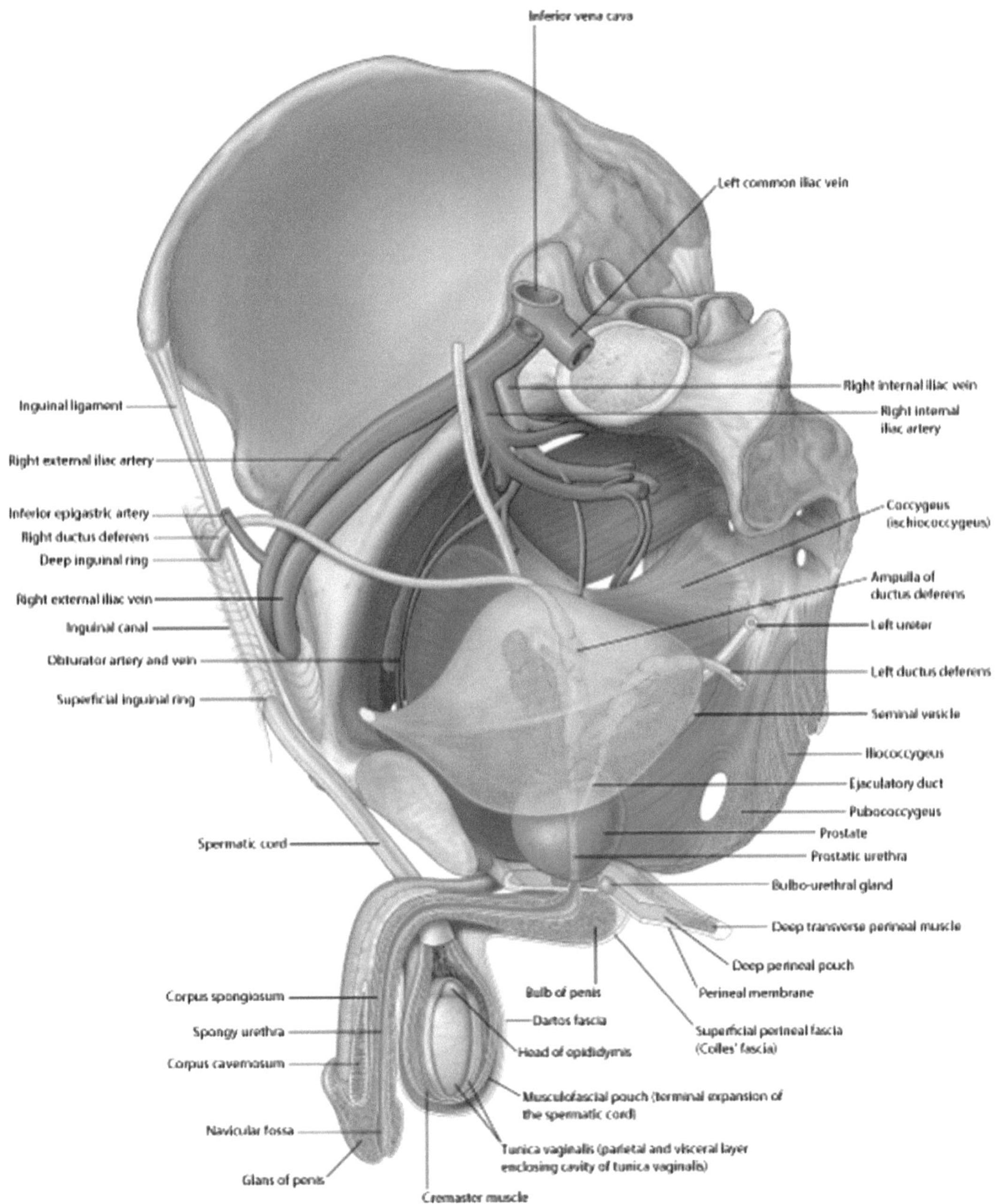

FIGURE 12.51 The male reproductive system. The spermatic cord contains the ductus deferens, testicular artery and vein, and testicular nerve fibers. The spermatic cord enters the superficial inguinal ring and exits in the deep inguinal ring (superficial and deep refer to the depth from the skin surface) into the peritoneal cavity. It then goes posterior to the bladder and enlarges to form the ampulla of the ductus deferens just before receiving the duct from the seminal vesicle. The union of the ampulla of the ductus deferens and the seminal vesicle duct forms the ejaculatory duct which enters the prostate gland and ends by joining the prostatic portion of the urethra. Source: *From R. L. Drake, A. W. Vogl, A. W. M. Mitchell, R. M. Tibbitts and P. E. Richardson. (2015). Section on pelvis and perineum. In* Gray's atlas of anatomy *(2nd ed.) (p. 234). Elsevier.*

An accessory storage area for sperm lies in the ampulla of the ductus deferens, posterior to the seminal vesicles. These elongated, hollow evaginations of the ductus deferens and the seminal vesicles secrete an alkaline fluid rich in fructose that provides nourishment and the energy for sperm motility after ejaculation. The seminal vesicles produce 60%–70% of the seminal fluid. Citrate and a variety of enzymes are added to the ejaculate by the prostate, which is the largest of the accessory secretory glands but produces only 30%–40% of the seminal fluid (Fig. 12.52).

Sperm and the combined secretions of the accessory glands make up the semen, of which less than 10% is sperm. The normal ejaculate contains 20

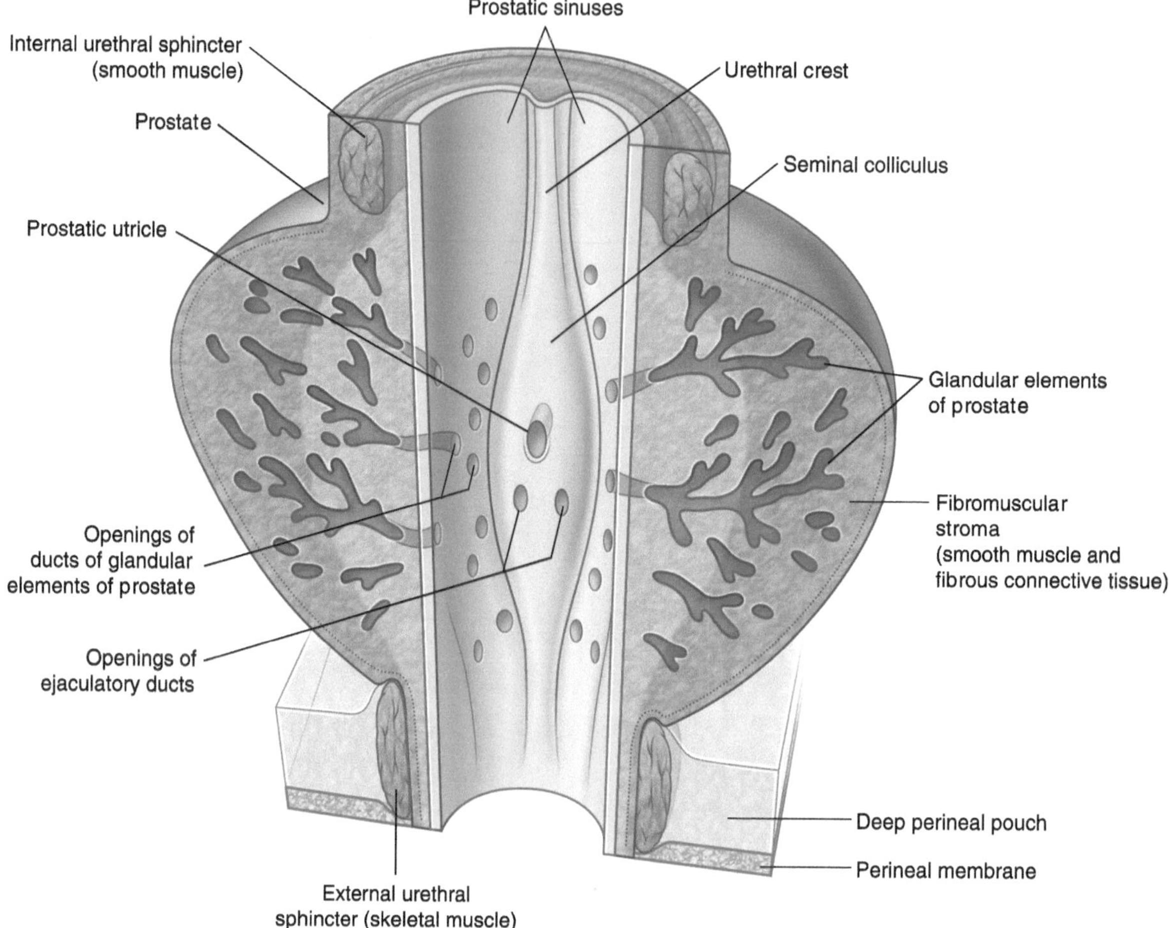

FIGURE 12.52 The human prostate gland. Semen enters the prostatic urethra (blue) through two openings of the ejaculatory ducts (one from each testis). The prostatic utricle is the remains of the Müllerian duct and represents the vagina and part of the cervix of the uterus. Source: *From Figure 5.44 from R. L. Drake, A. W. Vogl, A. W. M. Mitchell, R. M. Tibbitts and P. E. Richardson. (2015).* Gray's anatomy for students *(3rd ed.) (p. 468). Elsevier.*

million sperm/mL and the normal ejaculate is 2–5 mL in volume.

Regulation of testicular function I

Physiological activity of the testis is governed by two pituitary gonadotropic hormones, FSH and LH (see Chapter 2: Pituitary Gland). The same gonadotropic hormones are produced in pituitary glands of men and women, but because their physiology has been studied more extensively in women, the names that have been adopted for them describe their activity in the ovary (see Chapter 13: Hormonal Control of Reproduction in the Female: The Menstrual). FSH and LH are closely related glycoprotein hormones that consist of a common α subunit and unique β subunits that confer FSH or LH specificity. The three subunits are the products of three genes that are regulated independently. Both gonadotropins are synthesized and secreted by a single class of pituitary cells, the gonadotrophs. Their sites of stimulation of testicular function, however, are discrete: LH acts on the Leydig cells and FSH acts on the Sertoli cells in the germinal epithelium. There are many regulatory hormones that also affect the hypothalamic–pituitary–gonadal axis (Fig. 12.53).

Testosterone

Secretion and metabolism

Testosterone is the principal androgen secreted by the mature testis. Normal young men produce about 7 mg each day, of which less than 5% is derived from adrenal secretions. This amount decreases somewhat with age, so that by the seventh decade and beyond, testosterone production may have decreased to 4 mg/day, but in the absence of illness or injury, there is no sharp drop in testosterone production akin to the abrupt cessation of estrogen production in the

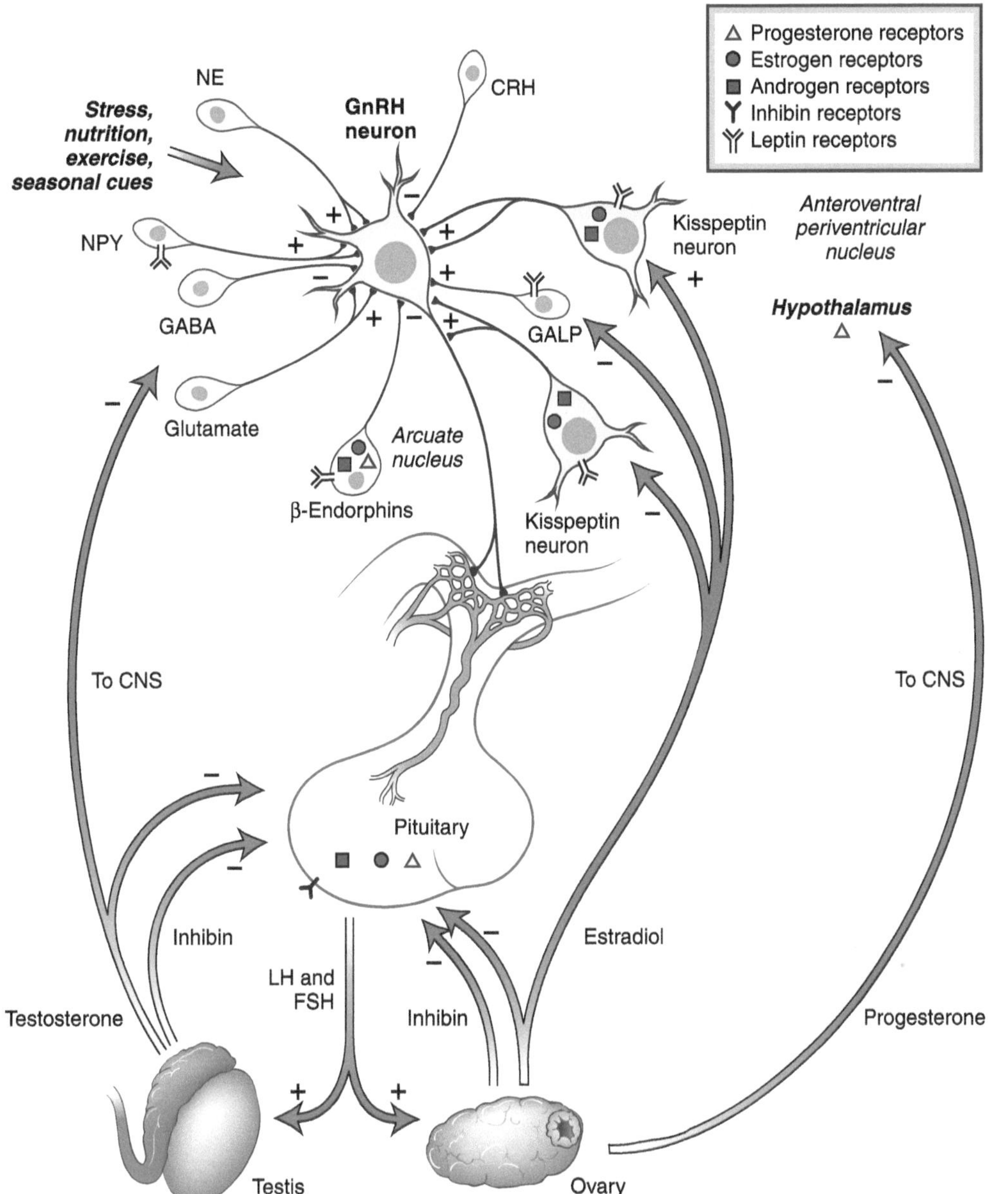

FIGURE 12.53 Some of the hormones that affect the hypothalamic–pituitary–gonadal axis. Source: *From Figure 7-30 in Low, M. J. (2016). Chapter 7: Neuroendocrinology. In S. Melmed, K. S. Polonsky, P. R. Larson, & H. M. Kronenberg (Eds.),* William's textbook of endocrinology *(13th ed.) (p. 156). Elsevier.*

postmenopausal woman. As with the other steroid hormones, testosterone in blood is largely bound to plasma protein, with only about 2%–3% present as free hormone. It is only the free (unbound) hormone that can enter cells. About half is bound to albumin, and slightly less to sex hormone–binding globulin (SHBG), which is also called testosterone–estradiol-binding globulin (Fig. 12.54).

SHBG glycoprotein binds both estrogen and testosterone, but its single binding site has a higher affinity for testosterone. Its concentration in plasma is decreased by androgens. Consequently, SHBG is more than twice as abundant in the circulation of women than men. In addition to its functions as a carrier protein, SHBG may also act as an enhancer of hormone action. Persuasive evidence has been amassed to indicate that SHBG binds to specific receptors on cell membranes and increases the formation of cyclic AMP when its steroid binding site is occupied. The nature of the receptor has not been characterized, nor has the physiological importance of this action been established. Although testosterone decreases expression of SHBG in hepatocytes, both testosterone and FSH increase transcription of the

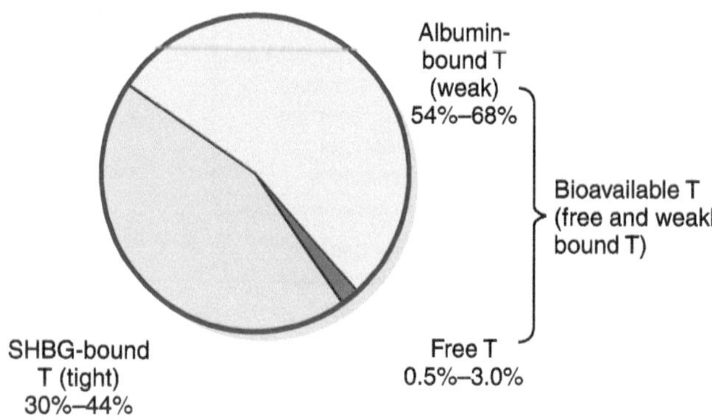

FIGURE 12.54 The transport of testosterone (T) in plasma and the percent carried on each protein. Only a small percentage is free in plasma. Testosterone is tightly bound to SHBG that serves as a reservoir of plasma testosterone. The binding of testosterone to an albumin fraction is weak so it can easily be displaced so that it becomes free. Free testosterone can enter cells and exert its effect. *SHBG*, Sex hormone–binding globulin. Source: *From Figure 19-10 in Matsumoto, A. M., & Bremner, W. J. (2016). Chapter 19: Testicular disorders. In S. Melmed, K. S. Polonsky, P. R. Larson, & H. M. Kronenberg (Eds.),* William's textbook of endocrinology *(13th ed.) (p. 709). Elsevier.*

same gene in Sertoli cells where its protein product was given the name androgen-binding protein (ABP) before its identity with SHBG was known. ABP is secreted into the lumens of seminiferous tubules.

Testosterone that is not bound to plasma proteins diffuses out of capillaries and enters nontarget as well as target cells. In some respects, testosterone can be considered a prohormone, because it is converted in extratesticular tissues to other biologically active steroids. Testosterone may be reduced to the more potent androgen, 5α-DHT, in the liver in a reaction catalyzed by the enzyme 5α-reductase type I and returned to the blood. This enzyme is a component of the steroid hormone degradative pathway and also reduces 21-carbon adrenal steroids. Testosterone also is reduced to 5α-DHT in the cytoplasm of its target cells mainly through the catalytic activity of 5α-reductase type II, the abundance of which is upregulated by is testosterone in these cells. DHT is only about 5% as abundant in blood as testosterone and is derived primarily from

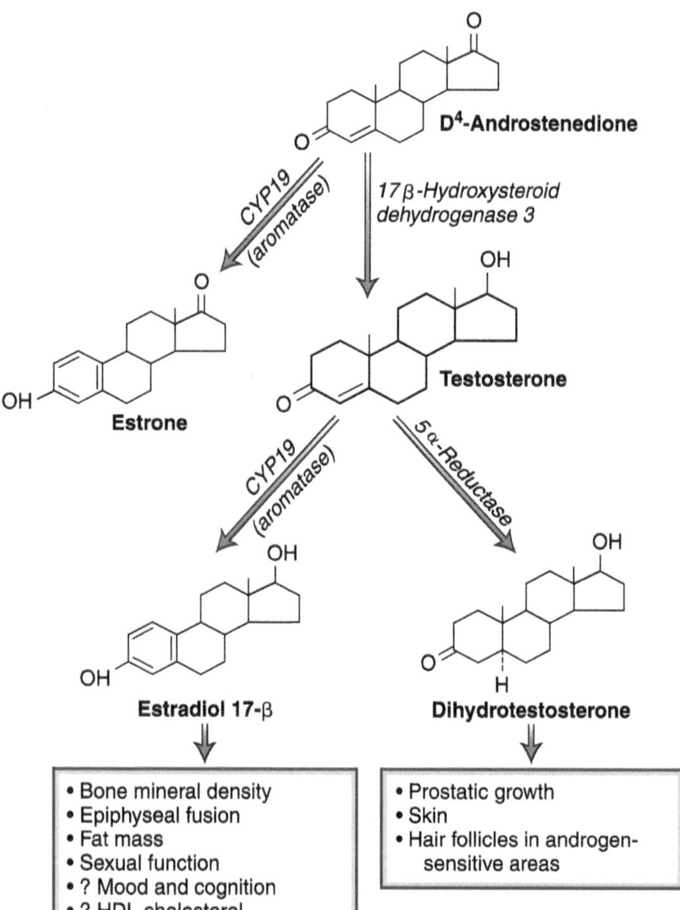

FIGURE 12.55 Metabolism of testosterone and androstenedione. Source: *From Figure 19-11 in Matsumoto, A. M., & Bremner, W. J. (2016). Chapter 19: Testicular disorders. In S. Melmed, K. S. Polonsky, P. R. Larson, & H. M. Kronenberg (Eds.),* William's textbook of endocrinology *(13th ed.) (p. 710). Elsevier.*

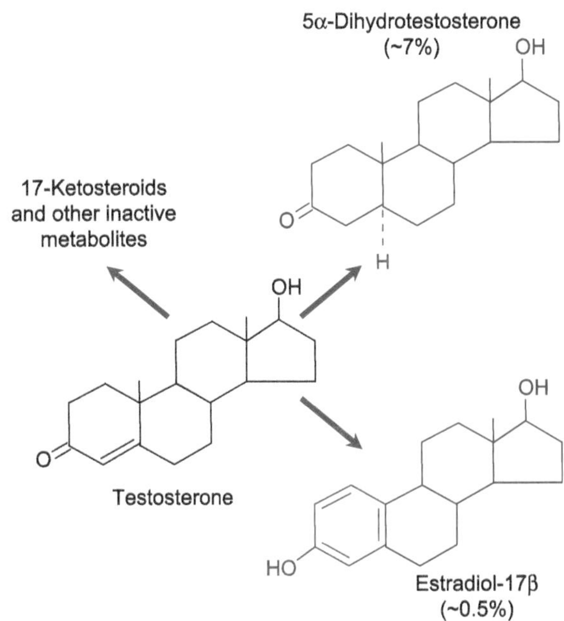

FIGURE 12.56 Metabolism of testosterone. Most of the testosterone secreted each day is degraded in the liver and other tissues by reduction of the A ring, oxidation of the 17 hydroxyl group, and conjugation with polar substituents. Conversion to 5α-dihydrotestosterone takes place in target cells catalyzed mainly by the type II dehydrogenase and in nontarget cells mainly but not exclusively by the type I dehydrogenase. Aromatization of testosterone to estradiol may occur directly or after conversion to androstenedione. Note that 5α-dihydrotestosterone cannot be aromatized or reconverted to testosterone.

extratesticular metabolism. Some testosterone is also metabolized to estradiol (Figs. 12.8 and 12.55) in both androgen target and nontarget tissues.

In the testes, Leydig and Sertoli cells will produce β-estradiol from testosterone. Nontesticular cells can also make this conversion that happens mainly in adipose tissue but also in brain, breast, bone, blood vessels, and liver. These tissues can convert testosterone and androstenedione to estradiol and estrone, respectively (Fig. 12.9), which produce cellular effects that are different from, and sometimes opposite to, those of testosterone. The concentration of estrogens in blood of normal men is similar to that of women in the early follicular phase of the menstrual cycle (see Chapter 13: Hormonal Control of Reproduction in the Female: The Menstrual). About two-thirds of these estrogens are formed from androgen outside of the testis. Although less than 1% of the peripheral pool of testosterone is converted to estrogens, it is important to recognize that estradiol produces its biological effects at concentrations that are far below those needed for androgens to produce their effects.

In other tissues, including liver, reduction catalyzed by 5β-reductase destroys androgenic potency. Liver is the principal site of metabolism of testosterone and releases water-soluble sulfate or glucuronide conjugates into blood for excretion in the urine (Fig. 12.56).

Mechanism of action

Like other steroid hormones, testosterone penetrates the target cells, the growth and function of which it stimulates (Fig. 12.58). Androgen target cells generally convert testosterone to 5α-DHT before it binds to the AR. The AR is a ligand-dependent transcription factor that belongs to the nuclear receptor superfamily (see Chapter 1: Introduction). It binds both testosterone and DHT, but the dihydro form dissociates from the receptor much more slowly than testosterone and therefore is the predominant androgen associated with deoxyribonucleic acid (DNA). It is likely that the higher affinity of DHT for the AR accounts for its greater biological potency compared to testosterone. Upon binding testosterone or DHT, liganded receptors shed their associated proteins and form homodimers that

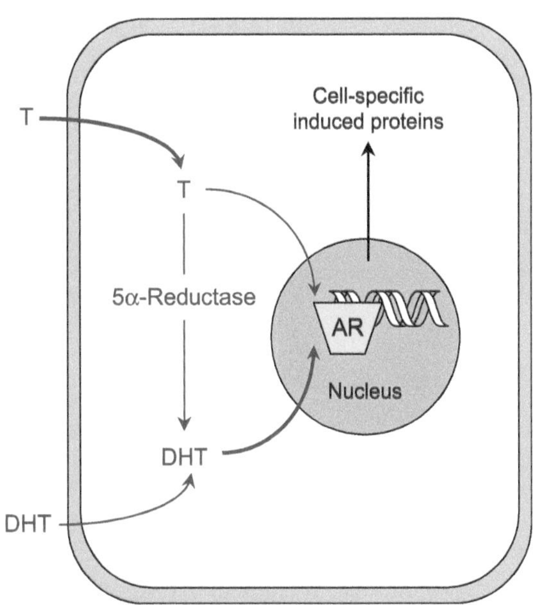

FIGURE 12.57 Action of testosterone. Testosterone (*T*) enters its target cell and binds to its nuclear *AR* either directly or after it is converted to 5α-*DHT*. The thickness of the arrows reflects the quantitative importance of each reaction. The hormone–receptor complex binds to DNA along with a variety of cell-specific nuclear regulatory proteins to induce formation of the RNA that encodes the proteins that express effects of the hormone. Not shown: testosterone may also bind to membrane receptors and initiate rapid ionic changes that may reinforce its genomic effects. Testosterone may also produce rapid changes in cyclic AMP production through the binding of the SHBG to surface receptors. *AMP*, Adenosine monophosphate; *AR*, androgen receptor; *DHT*, dihydrotestosterone; *DNA*, deoxyribonucleic acid; *SHBG*, sex hormone–binding globulin.

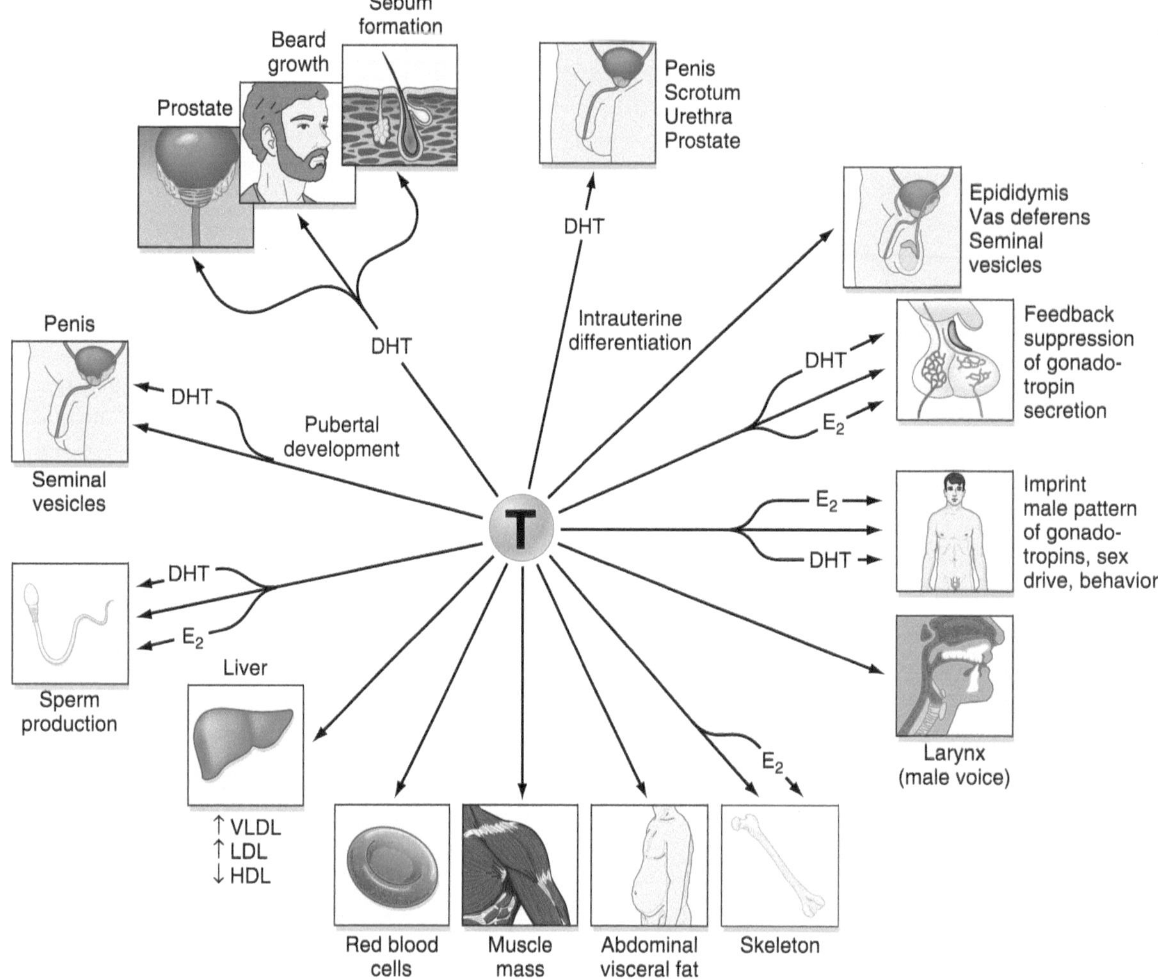

FIGURE 12.58 Some of the many effects of testosterone (T) or its derivatives, DHT or estradiol (E_2). *DHT*, Dihydrotestosterone. Source: *From Figure 44.9 in Koeppen, B. M., & Stanton, B. A. (2018).* Berne and Levy physiology *(7th ed.) (p. 794). Elsevier.*

bind to androgen response elements in specific target genes. In conjunction with a cell-specific array of transcription factors and coactivators, ARs regulate expression of cadres of genes that are characteristic of each particular target cell. These events are summarized in Figs. 12.57 and 12.58.

Some "nongenomic" actions of testosterone also have been described and include rapid increases in intracellular calcium. We do not understand the cellular mechanisms of these effects or their physiological importance. One of the proteins, the expression of which in the prostate is stimulated by DHT, is the prostate-specific antigen (PSA), which is found in blood in high concentrations in patients afflicted with prostate cancer. Its abundance in plasma is now widely used diagnostically as a marker of prostate cancer. PSA is a serine protease that is synthesized in the columnar cells of the glandular epithelium and secreted into the semen. Cleavage of seminogelin by PSA causes liquefaction of the ejaculate and is thought to increase sperm mobility.

Effects on the male genital tract

Testosterone promotes growth, differentiation, and function of accessory organs of reproduction. Its effects on growth of the genital tract begin early in embryonic life (see later) and are not completed until adolescence, after an interruption of more than a decade. Maintenance of normal reproductive function in the adult also depends on continued testosterone secretion. The secretory epithelia of the seminal vesicles and prostate atrophy after castration can be restored with injections of androgen. Prolonged stimulation of the prostate epithelium leads to continued growth of the prostate and in many older men results in a condition known as benign prostatic hyperplasia (BPH). It may be recalled that the prostate is located just below the urinary bladder and completely surrounds the urethra. Benign prostate hyperplasia may partially obstruct the urethra, interfering with the flow of urine and creating difficulty in emptying the bladder. In extreme cases, urine flow may be completely obstructed. Inhibition of 5α-hydroxylase provides successful pharmacologic treatment for BPH in some men.

Effects on secondary sexual characteristics

In addition to its effect on organs directly related to transport and delivery of sperm, testosterone affects a variety of other tissues and thus contributes to the morphological and psychological components of masculinity. During early adolescence, androgens that arise from the adrenals and later from the testes stimulate growth of pubic hair. Growth of chest, axillary, and facial hair is also stimulated, but scalp hair is affected in the opposite manner. Recession of hair at the temples is a typical response to androgen, which also allows expression of genes for baldness. Growth and secretion of sebaceous glands in the skin are also stimulated, a phenomenon undoubtedly related to the acne of adolescence. DHT is the important androgen for recession of scalp hair and stimulation of the sebaceous glands.

Androgen secretion at puberty stimulates growth of the larynx and thickening of the vocal chords and thus lowers the pitch of the voice. At this time, the characteristic adolescent growth spurt results from the interplay of testosterone and growth hormone (see Chapter 11: Hormonal Control of Growth) that promotes growth of the vertebrae and long bones. Development of the shoulder girdle is pronounced. This growth is self-limiting, as androgens, after extragonadal conversion to estrogens, accelerate epiphyseal closure (see Chapter 11: Hormonal Control of Growth). Androgens promote growth of muscle, especially in the upper torso so that men have almost half again as much muscle mass as women. Growth and nitrogen retention, of course, are also related to stimulation of appetite and increased food intake. Accordingly, androgens bring about increased physical vigor and a feeling of well-being. Testosterone also stimulates red blood cell production by direct effects on bone marrow and by stimulating secretion of the hormone erythropoietin from the kidney. This action of androgens accounts for the higher hematocrit in men than women. In both men and women, androgens increase sexual drive (libido).

Male reproductive development

Aside from a brief surge in androgen production during the immediate neonatal period, the Leydig cells regress, and testicular function enters a period of quiescence (Fig. 12.59).

Further development of the male genital tract is arrested until the onset of puberty and the reappearance of Leydig cells. Increased production of testosterone at puberty promotes growth of the penis and

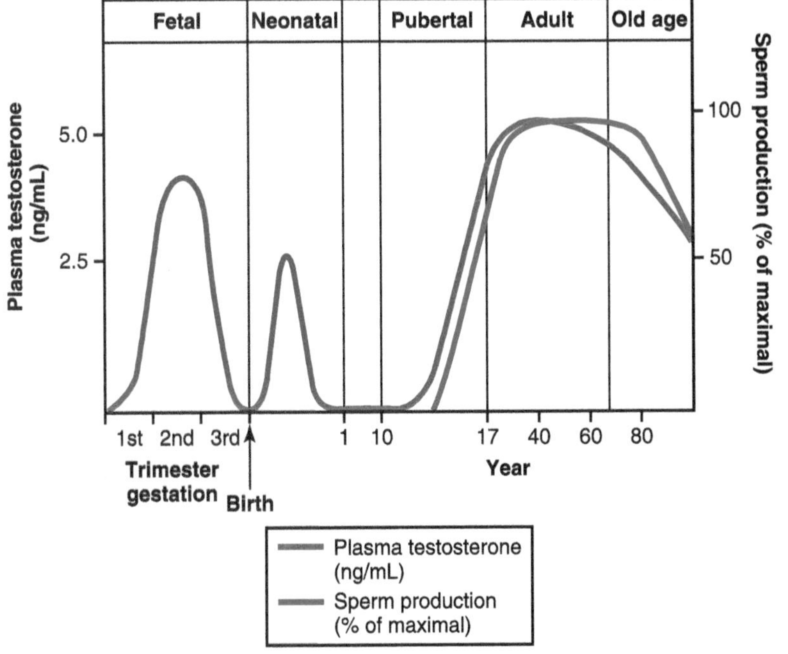

FIGURE 12.59 The serum level of testosterone through the life span. Source: *Figure 81-9 in Hall, J. E. (2016).* Guyton and Hall medical physiology *(13th ed.) (p. 1029). Elsevier.*

scrotum and increases pigmentation of the genitalia as well as the depth of rugal folds in scrotal skin. Further growth of the prostate, seminal vesicles, and epididymis also occurs at this time. Although differentiation of the epididymis and seminal vesicles is independent of DHT during the early fetal period, later acquisition of 5α-reductase type II makes this more active androgen the dominant form that stimulates growth and secretory activity during the pubertal period. At puberty, FSH stimulates a transient burst of proliferation by Sertoli cells, and in the mature testis, it maintains their functional integrity. In response to FSH the Sertoli cells begin to secrete fluid, which opens lumens in the seminiferous cords and converts them to the seminiferous tubules.

The importance of some of the foregoing information is highlighted by another interesting genetic disorder that has been described as penis at 12. Affected individuals have a deletion or inactivating mutation in the gene that codes for 5α-reductase type II; hence, they cannot convert testosterone to 5α-DHT in derivatives of the genital tubercle. Although testes and Wolffian derivatives develop normally, the prostate gland is absent, and at birth external genitalia are ambiguous or overtly feminine. Affected children have been raised initially as females. With the onset of puberty, testosterone production increases dramatically. Testosterone is converted to 5α-DHT by 5α-reductase type I in liver and skin and released into the plasma. Though delayed by a decade or more, stimulation of the underdeveloped penis accounts for its growth.

Prenatal and postnatal

Testicular function is critical for the development of the normal masculine phenotype early in the prenatal period. All the elements of the control system are present in the early embryo. GnRH and gonadotropins are detectable at about the time that testosterone begins stimulating Wolffian duct development. The hypothalamic GnRH pulse generator and its negative feedback control are functional in the newborn. Both the frequency and amplitude of GnRH and LH pulses are similar to those observed in the adult. After about the sixth month of postnatal life and for the remainder of the juvenile period, the GnRH pulse generator is restrained and gonadotropin secretion is low. The amplitude and frequency of GnRH pulses decline but do not disappear, and responsiveness of the gonadotrophs to GnRH diminishes. It is evident that negative feedback regulation remains operative, however, because blood levels of gonadotropins increase after gonadectomy in prepubertal subjects and fall with gonadal hormone administration.

The system is extremely sensitive to feedback inhibition during this time, but suppression of the pulse generator cannot be explained simply as a change in the set point for feedback inhibition. The plasma concentration of gonadotropins is high in juvenile subjects whose testes failed to develop and who consequently lack testosterone but rise even higher when these subjects reach the age when puberty would normally occur. Thus restraint of the GnRH pulse generator imposed by the central nervous system diminishes at the onset of puberty.

Puberty

Early stages of puberty are characterized by the appearance of high-amplitude pulses of LH during sleep (Fig. 12.60).

Testosterone concentrations in plasma follow the gonadotropins, and there is a distinct day–night pattern. As puberty progresses, high-amplitude pulses are distributed throughout the day at the adult frequency of about one every 2 hours. Sensitivity of the pituitary gland to GnRH increases during puberty possibly as a result of a self-priming effect of GnRH on gonadotrophs. GnRH increases both the abundance of its receptors on the gonadotroph surface and the amount of releasable FSH and LH in the gonadotrophs.

The underlying neural mechanisms for suppression of the GnRH pulse generator in the juvenile period are not understood. Increased inhibitory input from neuropeptide Y and γ-amino butyric acid secreting neurons

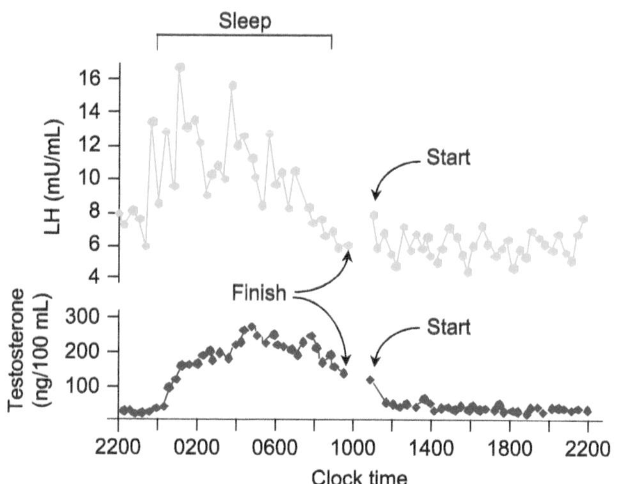

FIGURE 12.60 Plasma LH and testosterone measured every 20 minutes reveal nocturnal pulsatile secretion of GnRH in a pubertal 14-year-old boy. Source: *From Boyer, R. M., Rosenfeld, R. S., Kapen, S., Finkelstein, J. W., Roffwarg, H. P., Weitzman, E. D., et al. (1974). Simultaneous augmented secretion of luteinizing hormone and testosterone during sleep.* Journal of Clinical Investigation, *54, 609.*

has been observed, but neither the factors that produce nor terminate such input are understood. Recently it was found that some individuals with hypogonadotropic hypogonadism who fail to undergo puberty carry a mutation in the gene for a G-protein-coupled receptor called GPR54. The ligand for this receptor was found to be a 54-amino acid peptide called kisspeptin, which had been studied earlier as a possible suppressor of tumor metastasis. Kisspeptin is expressed in abundance in neurons in the arcuate nuclei, and its receptors are expressed in GnRH neurons. It now appears likely that kisspeptin-secreting neurons provide positive input to GnRH neurons and that it is activation of these neurons that awakens and sustains the GnRH pulse generator (Fig. 12.63). It is likely that kisspeptinergic neurons may also be the targets of the negative feedback effects of gonadal steroids. However, the factors that lead to awakening of these neurons are not understood.

Clearly, the onset of reproductive capacity is influenced by, and must be coordinated with, metabolic factors and attainment of physical size. In this regard, as we have seen (see Chapter 11: Hormonal Control of Growth), puberty is intimately related to growth. Onset of puberty, especially in girls has long been associated with adequacy of body fat stores, and it appears that adequate circulating concentrations of leptin (see Chapter 8: Hormonal Regulation of Fuel Metabolism) are permissive for the onset of puberty. Nevertheless, we still do not understand how genetic, developmental, and nutritional factors are integrated to signal readiness for reproductive development and function and how that readiness is transmitted to kisspeptinergic neurons.

Anomalies of sexual differentiation

Anomalies of sexual differentiation result from inactivating mutations in genes that are critical for normal sexual differentiation. As already stated, in the absence of a functional testis the female phenotype develops in embryos carrying either XX or XY chromosomes. Mutations in genes that code for transcription factors that are critical for gonadal differentiation result in the birth of apparently normal girls whose XY genotype and gonadal dysgenesis are not apparent until puberty or in some cases, a clinical workup for infertility. In individuals with a single X chromosome, primordial

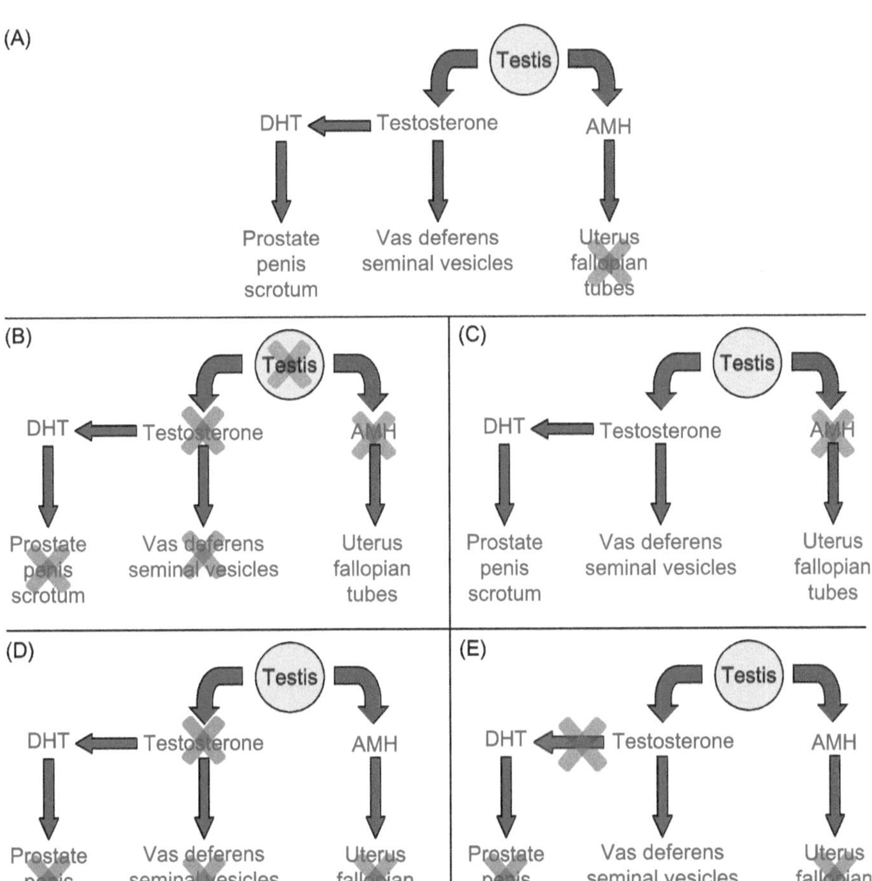

FIGURE 12.61 Anomalies in male sexual development due to single gene mutations. (A) Normal production of AMH, testosterone, and 5α-*DHT* results in regression of the female internal organs and the development of internal and external male organs. (B) Absence or defect in *SRY* (sex-determining region of the Y chromosome) leads to ovarian agenesis and the otherwise normal development of female internal and external genitalia and the absence of any male characteristics. (C) Absence of AMH leads to the development of both male and female internal genitalia and normal male external genitalia except that in some cases the presence of the female organs interferes with normal testicular descent into the scrotum. (D) Absence of 17α-hydroxylase or the androgen receptor results in an individual without an internal male or female reproductive tract, and with female external genitalia. (E) Absence of 5α-dehydrogenase II results in normal development of male internal organs, except the prostate, and normal regression of female internal sex organs. The external organs may be overtly female or ambiguous. *AMH*, Anti-Müllerian hormone; *DHT*, dihydrotestosterone.

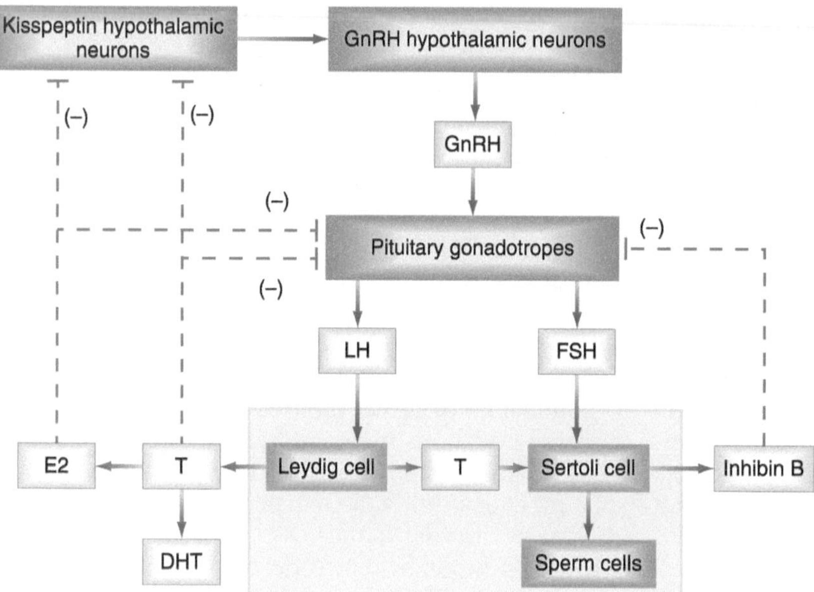

FIGURE 12.62 The effect of GnRH on the male reproductive system. Source: *From Figure 44.10 in Koeppen, B. M., & Stanton, B. A. (2018).* Berne and Levy physiology *(7th ed.) (p. 794). Elsevier.*

follicles usually degenerate before birth. Mutations in either AMH or its receptor result in persistence of Müllerian derivatives in an otherwise normal male. Inactivating mutations of $P450_{c17}$, the LH receptor, or the AR result in total absence of both Wolffian and Müllerian duct derivatives and female external genitalia, because Wolffian duct development requires androgen stimulation, and AMH secretion induces regression of the Müllerian ducts. Finally, as we have seen, the boy who lacks the 5α dehydrogenase II will have normal internal genital development except for the prostate, and ambiguous or feminine external genitalia until puberty when sufficient 5α-DHT can be produced to induce growth and development of male genitalia. These phenomena are summarized in Fig. 12.61.

As indicated in Chapter 4, The Adrenal Glands, anomalies of sexual development may also result from defects in the synthesis of 21-carbon adrenal steroids. The resulting overproduction of adrenal androgens can masculinize the external genitalia of female babies and cause overdevelopment of the genitalia in male infants.

Regulation of testicular function II

Testicular function, as we have seen, depends on stimulation by two pituitary hormones, FSH and LH. Without them the testes lose spermatogenic and steroidogenic capacities, and either atrophy or fail to mature. Secretion of these hormones by the pituitary gland is driven by the central nervous system through its secretion of the GnRH (Fig. 12.62), which reaches the pituitary by way of the hypophyseal portal blood vessels (see Chapter 2: Pituitary Gland).

Separation of the pituitary gland from its vascular linkage to the hypothalamus results in total cessation of gonadotropin secretion and testicular atrophy. The central nervous system and the pituitary gland are kept apprised of testicular activity by signals related to each of the testicular functions: steroidogenesis and gametogenesis. Characteristic of negative feedback, signals from the testis are inhibitory. Castration results in a prompt increase in secretion of both FSH and LH. The central nervous system also receives and integrates other information from the internal and external environments and modifies GnRH secretion accordingly.

Gonadotropin-releasing hormone and the hypothalamic pulse generator

Gonadotropin-releasing hormone is a decapeptide produced by a diffuse network of about 2000 neurons, the perikarya of which are located primarily in the arcuate nuclei in the medial basal hypothalamus, and the axons of which terminate in the median eminence in the vicinity of the hypophyseal portal capillaries. GnRH-secreting neurons also project to other parts of the brain and may mediate some aspects of sexual

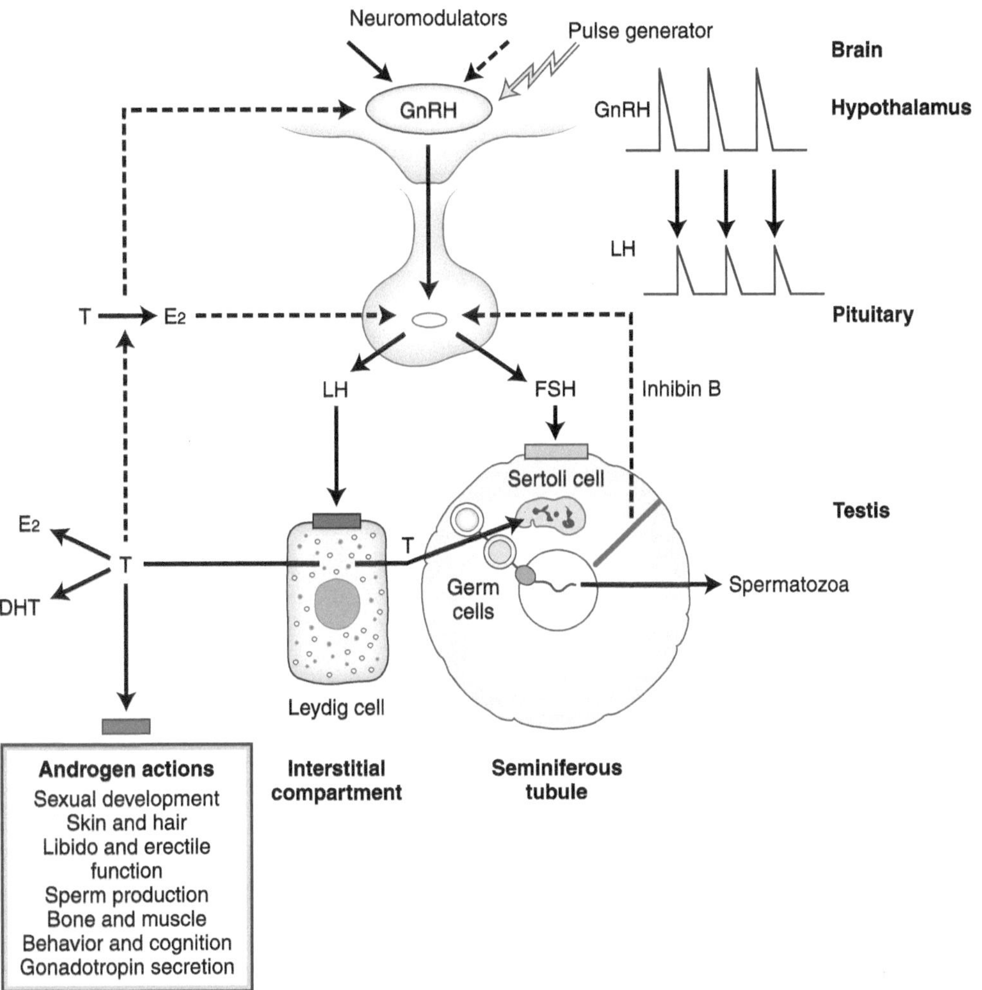

FIGURE 12.63 The pulse generation of GnRH followed by the pulse generation of LH by the anterior pituitary. *GnRH*, Gonadotropin-releasing hormone; *LH*, luteinizing hormone. Source: *From Figure 19-6 in Matsumoto, A. M., & Bremner, W. J. (2016). Chapter 19: Testicular disorders. In S. Melmed, K. S. Polonsky, P. R. Larson, & H. M. Kronenberg (Eds.),* William's textbook of endocrinology *(13th ed.) (p. 702). Elsevier.*

behavior. GnRH is released into the hypophyseal portal circulation in discrete pulses at regular intervals ranging from about one every hour to one every 3 hours or longer (Figs. 12.63 and 12.64).

Each pulse lasts only a few minutes and the secreted GnRH disappears rapidly with a half-life of about 4 minutes. GnRH secretion is difficult to monitor directly because hypophyseal portal blood is inaccessible and because its concentration in peripheral blood is too low to measure even with the most sensitive assays. The pulsatile nature of GnRH secretion has been inferred from results of frequent measurements of LH concentrations in peripheral blood (Fig. 12.40). FSH concentrations tend to fluctuate much less, largely because FSH has a longer half-life than LH, 2–3 hours compared to 20–30 minutes.

Pulsatile secretion requires synchronous firing of many neurons, which therefore must be in communication with each other and with a common pulse generator. Because pulsatile secretion of GnRH continues even after experimental disconnection of the medial basal hypothalamus from the rest of the central nervous system, the pulse generator must be located within this small portion of the hypothalamus. Pulsatile secretion of GnRH by neurons maintained in tissue culture indicates that episodic secretion is an intrinsic property of GnRH neurons. There is good correspondence between electrical activity in the arcuate nuclei and LH concentrations in blood as determined in rhesus monkeys fitted with permanently implanted electrodes. The frequency and amplitude of secretory pulses and corresponding electrical activity can be modified experimentally (Fig. 12.65) and are regulated physiologically by gonadal steroids and probably by other information processed within the central nervous system.

The significance of the pulsatile nature of GnRH secretion became evident in studies of reproductive function in rhesus monkeys whose arcuate nuclei had been destroyed. Secretion of LH and FSH therefore came to a halt. When GnRH was given as a constant infusion in an effort to replace hypothalamic secretion, gonadotropin secretion was restored, but only for a short while. FSH and LH secretion soon decreased and stopped even though the infusion of GnRH continued. Only when GnRH was administered intermittently for a few minutes of each hour was it possible to sustain normal gonadotropin secretion in these monkeys. Similar results have been obtained in human patients. Persons who are deficient in GnRH fail to experience pubertal development and remain sexually juvenile. Treating GnRH deficiency with the aid of a pump that delivers GnRH under the skin in intermittent pulses every 2 hours induces pubertal development and normal reproductive function. Treating them with a long-acting analog of GnRH that provides constant stimulation to the pituitary is ineffective in restoring normal function. Treatment with a long-acting analog of GnRH desensitizes the pituitary gland and blocks gonadotropin secretion. This regimen has been used successfully to arrest premature sexual development in children with precocious puberty.

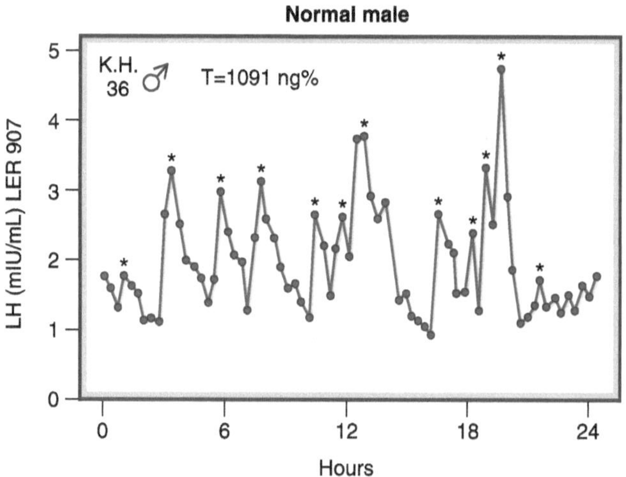

FIGURE 12.64 The 24-h pulsatile secretion of LH from a normal 36-year-old man. There is increased secretion at night. The star above the peaks indicates that it is statistically significant. T, testosterone levels; ng%, nanograms per 100 mL. *LH*, Luteinizing hormone. Source: *From Figure 19-7A in Matsumoto, A. M., & Bremner, W. J. (2016). Chapter 19: Testicular disorders. In S. Melmed, K. S. Polonsky, P. R. Larson, & H. M. Kronenberg (Eds.),* William's textbook of endocrinology *(13th ed.) (p. 702). Elsevier.*

The cellular mechanisms that account for the complex effects of GnRH on gonadotrophs are not fully understood. The GnRH receptor is a G-protein-coupled heptahelical receptor that activates phospholipase C through Gαq (see Chapter 1: Introduction). The resulting formation of inositol trisphosphate and diacylglycerol results in mobilization of intracellular calcium and activation of protein kinase C. Transcription of genes for FSH-β, LH-β, and the common α-subunit depends upon increased cytosolic calcium and several protein kinases, the activation pathways of which are not understood. Secretion of gonadotropins depends upon the increase in cytosolic calcium achieved by mobilizing calcium from intracellular stores and by activating membrane calcium channels. Desensitization of gonadotrophs after prolonged uninterrupted exposure to

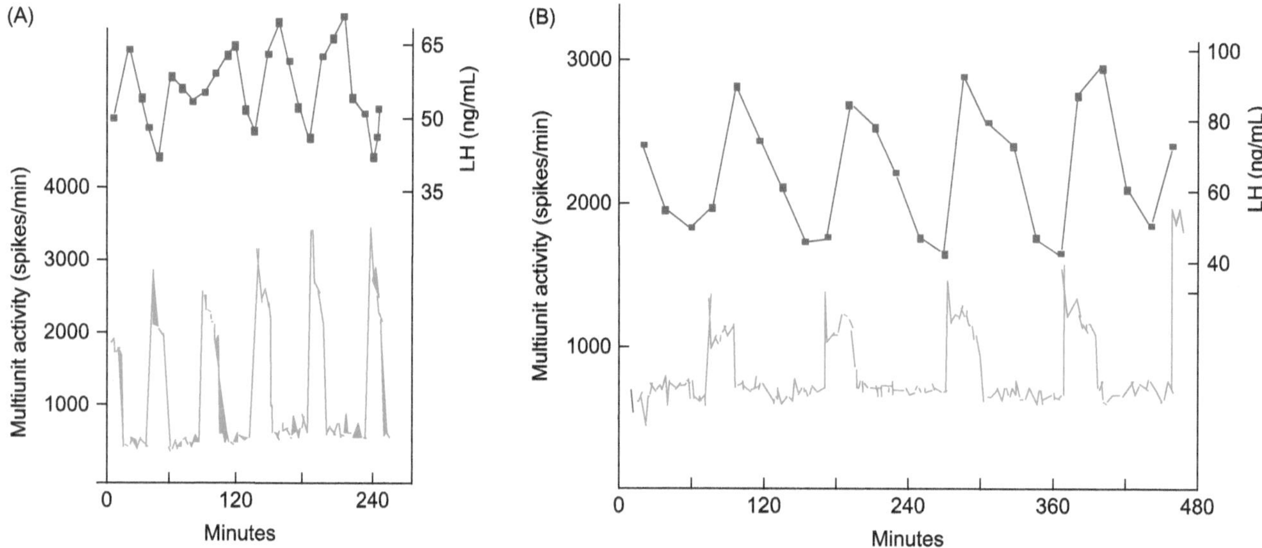

FIGURE 12.65 Recording of MUA in the arcuate nuclei of conscious (A) and anesthetized (B) monkeys fitted with permanently implanted electrodes. Simultaneous measurements of LH in peripheral blood are shown in the upper tracings. *LH*, Luteinizing hormone; *MUA*, multiple unit activity. Source: *From Wilson, R. C., Kesner, J. S., Kaufman, J. N., Uemura, T., Akema, T., Knobil, E. (1984). Central electrophysiologic correlates of pulsatile luteinizing hormone secretion in the rhesus monkey.* Neuroendocrinology, 39, 256.

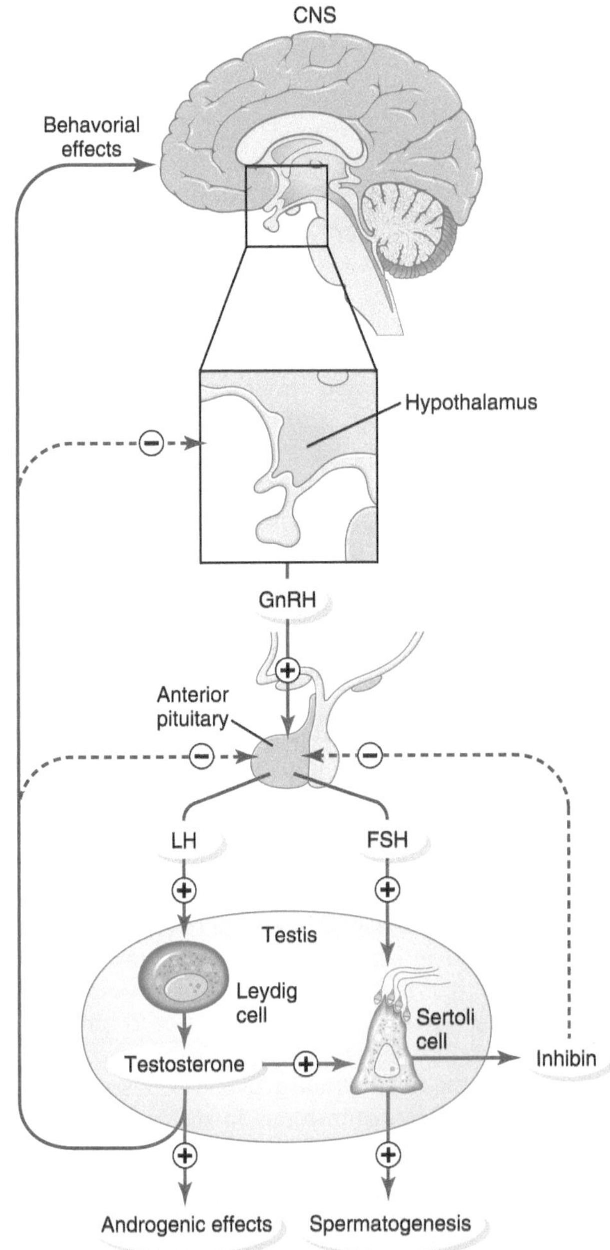

FIGURE 12.66 Feedback regulation of the testicular hormones. Source: *From Figure 81-10 in Hall, J. E. (2016).* Guyton and Hall medical physiology *(13th ed.) (p. 1032). Elsevier.*

GnRH appears to result from the combined effects of downregulation of GnRH receptors and calcium channels associated with secretion and a decrease in the releasable storage pool of gonadotropin.

Negative feedback regulators

The hormones FSH and LH originate in the same pituitary cell, the secretory activity of which is stimulated by the same hypothalamic hormone, GnRH. Secretion of FSH is controlled independently of LH secretion by negative feedback signals that relate to the separate functions of the two gonadotropins (Fig. 12.66).

Although castration is followed by increased secretion of both FSH and LH, only LH is restored to normal when physiological amounts of testosterone are given. Failure of testicular descent into the scrotum (cryptorchidism) may result in destruction of the germinal epithelium without affecting Leydig cells. With this condition, blood levels of testosterone and LH are normal, but FSH is elevated. Thus testosterone, which is secreted in response to LH, acts as a feedback regulator of LH and hence of its own secretion. By this reasoning, we would expect that spermatogenesis, which is stimulated by FSH, might be associated with secretion of a substance that reflects gamete production. Indeed, FSH stimulates the Sertoli cells to synthesize and secrete a glycoprotein called inhibin, which acts as a feedback inhibitor of FSH.

Inhibin and testosterone

Inhibin, which originally was purified from follicular fluid of the pig ovary, is a disulfide-linked heterodimer comprised an α subunit and either of two forms of a β subunit, βA or βB (Fig. 12.67).

The physiologically important form of inhibin secreted by the human testis is the $\alpha\beta$B dimer called inhibin B. Its concentration in blood plasma is reflective of the number of functioning Sertoli cells and spermatogenesis. Both inhibin A and inhibin B are produced by the ovary (see Chapter 13: Hormonal Control of Reproduction in the Female: The Menstrual). Little is known about the significance of alternate β subunits or the factors that determine when each form is produced. The three subunits are encoded in separate genes and presumably are regulated independently. They are members of the same family of growth factors that includes AMH and TGF-β.

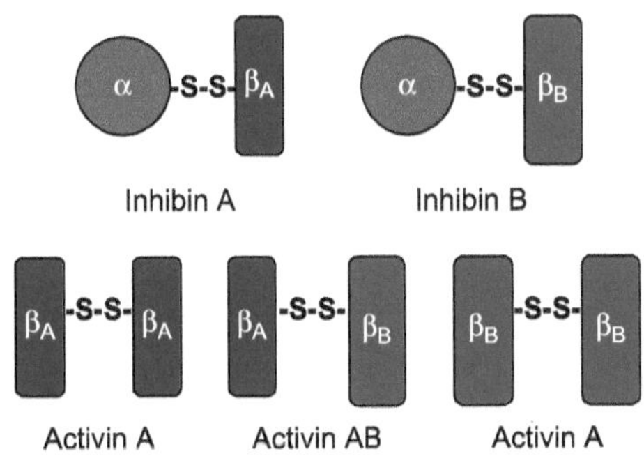

FIGURE 12.67 The activins and inhibins are disulfide-bonded dimers of the products of three separate genes. Inhibin B is the major circulating form in the human male and comprises an alpha subunit and the beta B subunit. Activins comprise two beta subunits.

Of additional interest is the finding that dimers formed from two β subunits produce effects that are opposite those of the αβ dimer and stimulate FSH release from gonadotrophs maintained in tissue culture. These compounds are called activins and function in a paracrine mode in the testis and many other tissues. Although the production of the α subunit is confined largely to male and female gonads, β subunits are produced in many extragonadal tissues where activins mediate a variety of functions that are unrelated to FSH secretion. Activins produced in the pituitary appear to play a supportive role in FSH production. The pituitary, ovaries, and other tissues also produce an unrelated protein called follistatin, which binds activins and blocks their actions.

The feedback relations that fit best with current understanding of the regulation of testicular function in the adult male are shown in Fig. 12.53. Pulses of GnRH originating in the arcuate nuclei evoke secretion of both FSH and LH by the anterior pituitary. FSH and LH are positive effectors of testicular function and stimulate release of inhibin and testosterone, respectively.

Testosterone has an intratesticular action that reinforces the effects of FSH. It also travels through the circulation to the hypothalamus, where it exerts its negative feedback effect primarily by slowing the frequency of GnRH pulses. Because secretion of LH decreases with frequency of stimulation (see Fig. 13.14), decreases in GnRH pulse frequency lower the ratio of LH to FSH in the gonadotropic output. In the castrate monkey the hypothalamic pulse generator discharges once per hour and slows to once every 2 hours after testosterone is replaced. This rate is about the same as that seen in normal men. The higher frequency in the castrate triggers more frequent bursts of gonadotropin secretion, resulting in higher blood levels of both FSH and LH.

Testosterone also exerts its negative feedback effects at the pituitary level by decreasing the amount of LH secreted in each pulse, probably as a result of decreasing sensitivity of the gonadotrophs to GnRH (Fig. 12.68).

In high enough concentrations, testosterone may inhibit GnRH release sufficiently to shut off secretion of both gonadotropic hormones. The negative feedback effects of testosterone on the pituitary depend in large measure on its aromatization to estradiol by the gonadotrophs. DHT, which cannot be aromatized, has little feedback effect, and men who lack aromatase have abnormally high circulating amounts of LH. The negative feedback effect of inhibin appears to be exerted exclusively on gonadotrophs. Inhibin decreases transcription of the FSH-β gene and reduces FSH secretion in response to GnRH. Some evidence indicates that inhibin may also exert local effects on Leydig cells to enhance testosterone production and thereby may indirectly affect hypothalamic release of GnRH.

Summary

Reproduction is essential for the survival of the species. Having two different sets of the same chromosome combined produces a stronger mix of genes and tends to eliminate deleterious genes. Hence, in higher animals there are two different sexes, one set of chromosomes is in one sex and the other set in the other sex. In this chapter the hormonal control of the male reproductive structures is discussed starting with the embryology of the male gonad and associated structures. The sequence of changes to the male reproductive system as a result of hormonal influences is followed through the cycle of life.

Oxytocin in the male

Effect of oxytocin on male reproduction

Oxytocin (OT) has traditionally been considered to be a female-only hormone. With the past decade, however, it has been found to play a major role in male sexual response and in programming a number of social and non-social behaviors in both sexes. In the male, there is conclusive evidence that OT is synthesized in the testis, epididymis, and prostate. It stimulates the formation and maturation of sperm and contraction of smooth muscles in the testes, epididymis and prostate to propel the sperm down the reproductive tract (sperms are not motile within the male reproductive system so they must be pushed along by contractions in the walls and ducts of the reproductive system) (Fig. 12.69).

In addition, OT contributes to penile erection and may regulate 5a-reductase activity and so influence steroidogenesis. One of the negative effects of steroidogenesis in older men and dogs is the enlargement of the prostate gland and the promotion of prostatic adenocarcinoma.

Effect of oxytocin on cell division

The effect on cell division varies with respect to location of the oxytocin receptor (OTR) in the cell type. If the OTR is located outside of the caveolin areas (the areas where receptors are usually located in most cells), cell proliferation is inhibited. On the other hand, if the OTR is located within the caveolin area, cell division is stimulated.

The effect of OT on cell proliferation and cancer varies, but it has not been determined if this effect is

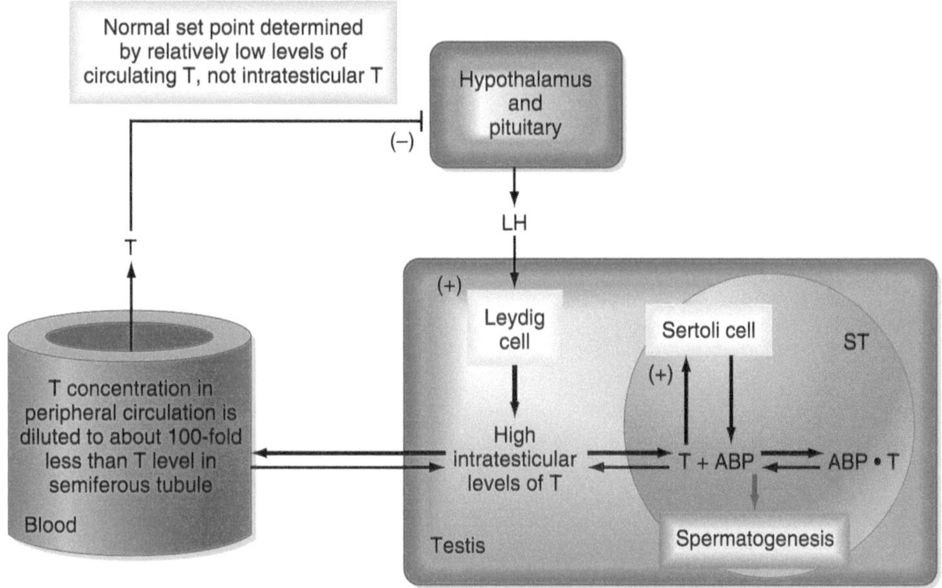

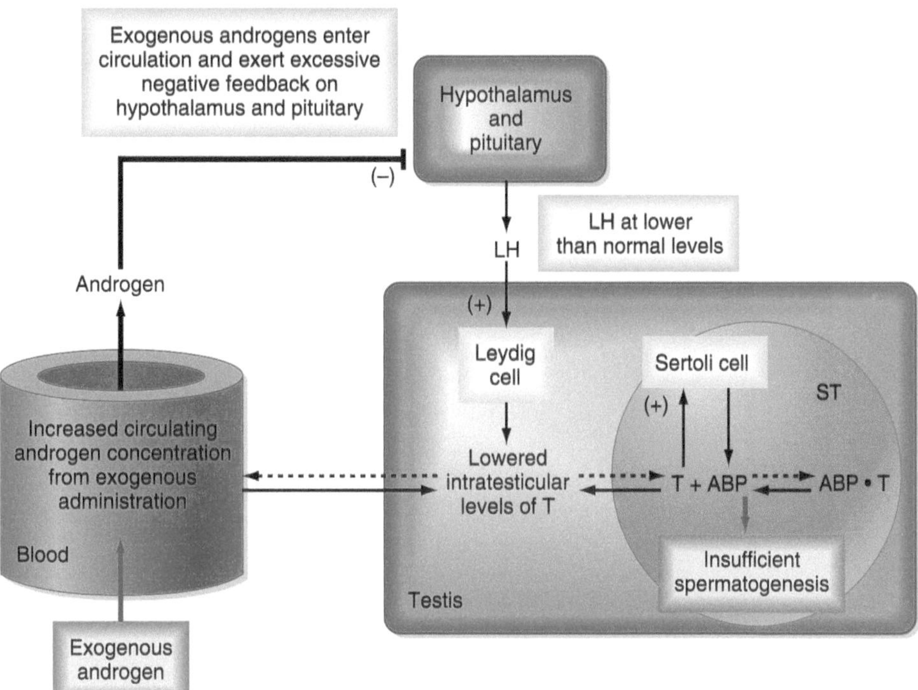

FIGURE 12.68 The effect of normal levels and high levels of exogenous androgens (as male body builders would take) on LH production. Body builders are usually sterile as a result. Source: *From Figure 44.11 in Koeppen, B. M., & Stanton, B. A. (2018).* Berne and Levy physiology *(7th ed.) (p. 796). Elsevier.*

primarily due to the location of the OTR. OT stimulates growth in osteoblasts and small- cell carcinoma of the lung. It inhibits the growth of human breast cancer cells and ovarian carcinoma cells. In the latter, it also inhibits migration and invasion (metastasis) in vitro and in vivo.

Effect on brain

OT receptors are widespread in the brain, and are found in great numbers in the hippocampus. While the exact role of OT has yet to be determined, preliminary results indicate that it may play a role in synaptic

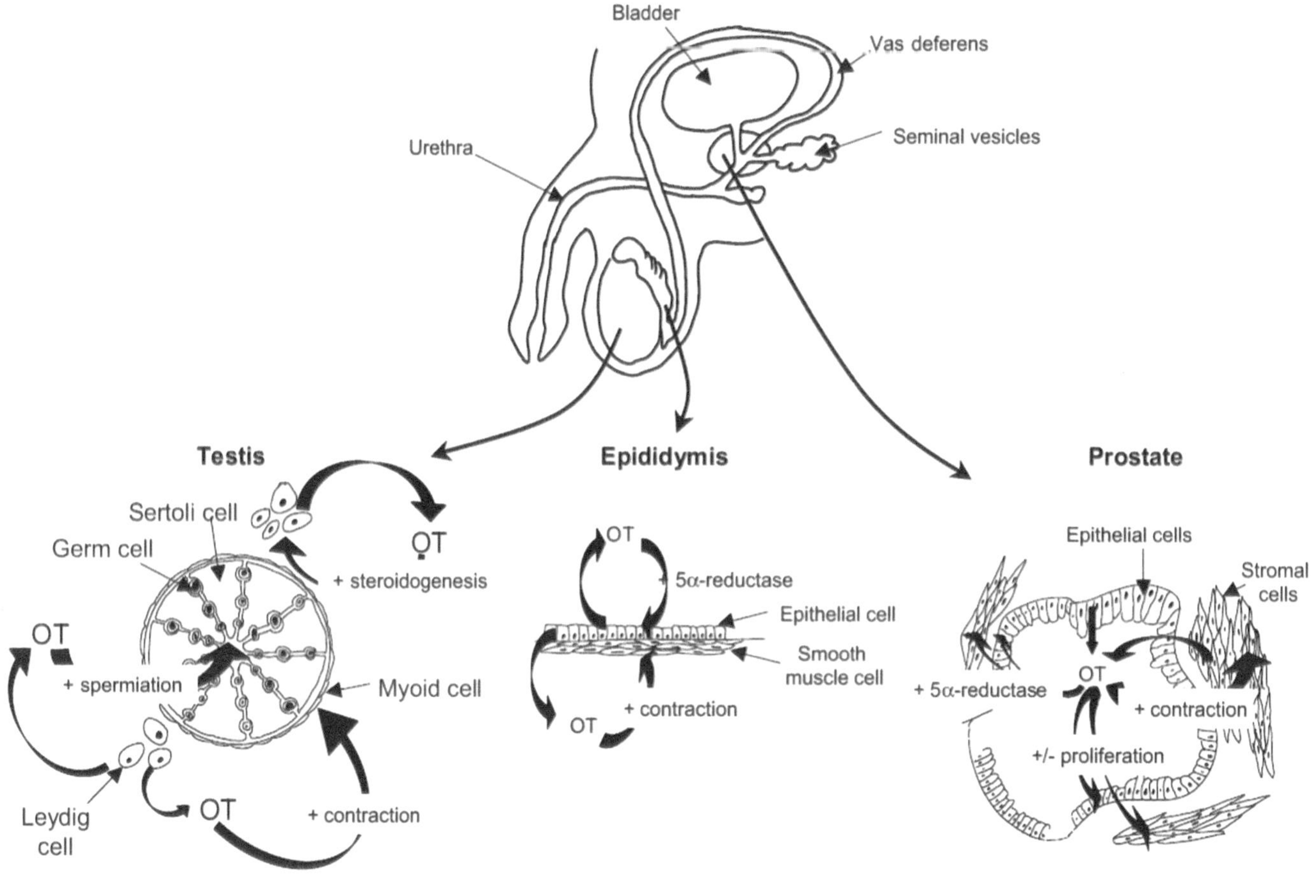

FIGURE 12.69 Effect of OT on male reproductive structures. *OT, Oxytocin.* Source: *From Thackare, H., Nicholson, D.H., & Whittington, K. (2006).* Oxytocin its role in male reproduction and new therapeutic uses. *Human Reproduction Update* 12 (4), 437–448.

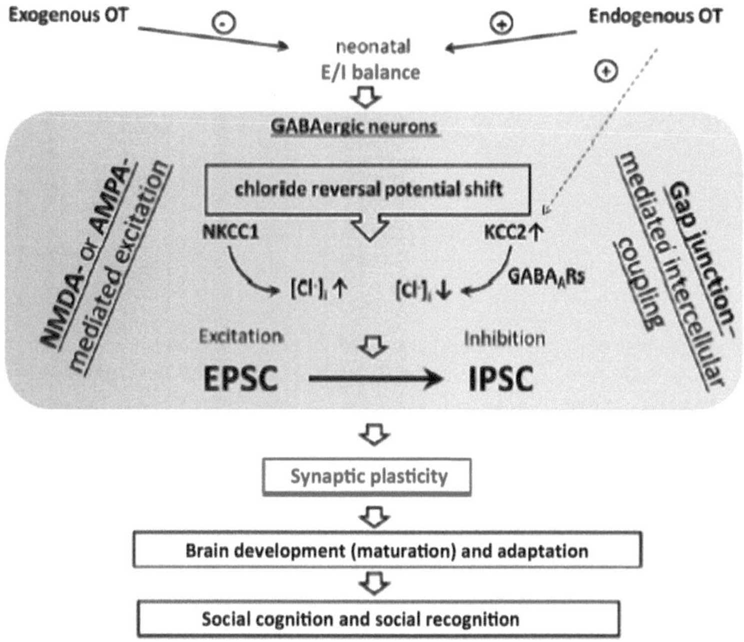

FIGURE 12.70 Oxytocin affects E/I balance in GABAergic neurons and synaptic plasticity in the developing brain. The scheme shows that GABA is an excitatory neurotransmitter early in development, but then, its features undergo changes to act as an inhibitory neurotransmitter in the brain. An increase in intracellular Cl– concentrations, induced by NKCC1, makes neurons to be excitatory. The GABAAR-mediated autoregulation is accompanied by a decrease in intracellular Cl– concentrations, leading to inhibition. This is the so-called excitation to inhibition switch in its balance. *AMPA*, α-Amino-3-hydroxy-5-methyl-4-isoxazole propionic acid; *EPSC*, excitatory postsynaptic current.; *GABA*, γ-aminobutyric acid; $GABA_A$Rs, gamma-aminobutyric acid type A receptors; *IPSC*, inhibitory postsynaptic current; *KCC2*, potassium-chloride transporter 2; *NKCC1*, sodium-potassium-chloride cotransporter 1; *NMDA*, N-methyl-D-aspartate receptor; *OT*, oxytocin. Source: *From Figure 1 in Lopatina et al., (2018).* Oxytocin and excitation/inhibition balance in social recognition. *Neuropeptides* 72, 1–11.

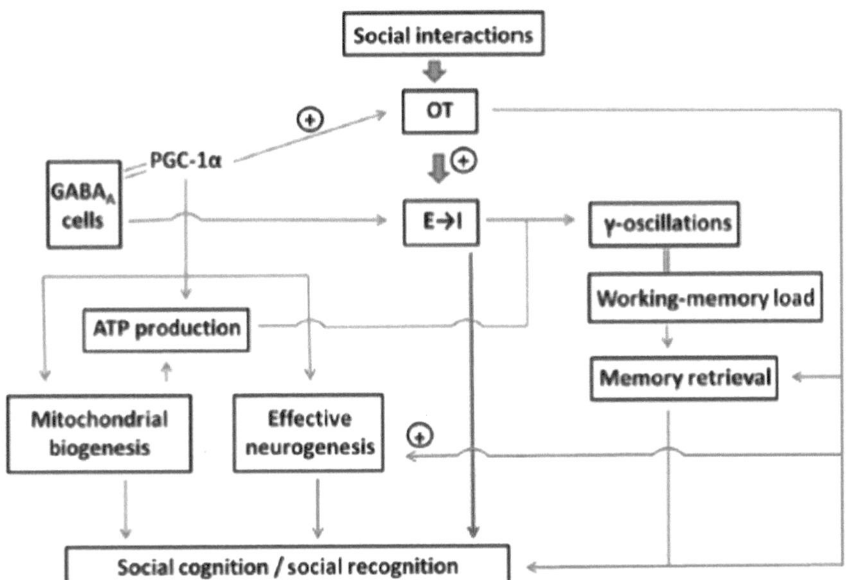

FIGURE 12.71 Schematic representation of mechanisms linking social interactions and social recognition. Social recognition is controlled by mitochondrial biogenesis, effective neurogenesis, OT action, and E/I balance. E/I balance is influenced by OT and $GABA_A$ cell activity in which PGC-1α is involved. E/I balance controls gamma-oscillations that reflect brain neuron network activity. Gamma-oscillations mark memory load and efficacy of memory retrieval. OT concentrations could be modified by social behavior and regulated by GABAergic neuronal activity. In this scheme, OT acts as a master molecule for social recognition. Impairment of the system by E/I imbalance leads to psychiatric diseases. *E/I*, excitation/inhibition; *$GABA_A$*, γ-aminobutyric acid type A; *OT*, oxytocin. Source: *From Figure 2 in Lopatina et al., (2018).* Oxytocin and excitation/inhibition balance in social recognition. *Neuropeptides* 72: 1–11.

plasticity. Such plasticity plays a significant role in social behavior (Fig. 12.70 and Fig. 12.71).

Suggested reading

Basic foundations

Achermann, J. C., & Hughes, I. A. (2017). Pediatric disorders of sex development. In S. Melmed, K. S. Polonsky, P. L. Reed, & H. M. Kronenberg (Eds.), *Williams textbook of endocrinology* (13th ed., pp. 893–963). Philadelphia, PA: Elsevier.

Mesiano, S., & Jones, E. E. (2017). The male reproductive system. In W. F. Boron, & E. L. Boulpaep (Eds.), *Medical physiology* (3rd ed., pp. 1092–1107). Philadelphia, PA: Elsevier.

Mesiano, S., & Jones, E. E. (2017). Sexual differentiation. In W. F. Boron, & E. L. Boulpaep (Eds.), *Medical physiology* (3rd ed., pp. 1072–1091). Philadelphia, PA: Elsevier.

Advanced information

Bhaskararao, G., Himabindu, Y., Nayak, S., & Sriharibabu, M. (2014). Laparoscopic gonedectomy in a case of complete androgen insensitivity syndrome. *Journal of Human Reproductive Sciences, 7*(3), 221–223. Available from https://doi.org/10.4103/0974-1208.142498.

Hughes, I. A., Werner, R., Bunch, T., & Hiort, O. (2012). Androgen insensitivity syndrome. *Seminars in Reproductive Medicine, 30*(05), 432–442. Available from https://doi.org/10.1055/s-0032-1324728.

Jung, E. J., Im, D. H., Park, Y. H., Byun, J. M., Kim, Y. N., Jeong, D. H., ... Lee, K. B. (2017). Female with 46, XY karyotype. *Obstetrics & Gynecology Science, 60*(4), 378–382.

Mascarenhas, M. N., Flaxman, S. R., Boerma, T., Vanderpoel, S., & Stevens, G. A. (2012). National, regional, and global trends in infertility prevalence since 1990: a systematic analysis of 277 health surveys. *PLOS Medicine, 9*(12), e1001356. Available from https://doi.org/10.1371/journal.pmed.1001356.

Mongan, N. P., Tadokoro-Cuccaro, R., Bunch, T., & Hughes, I. A. (2015). Androgen insensitivity syndrome. *Best Practice & Research Clinical Endocrinology & Metabolism, 29*(4), 569–580. Available from https://doi.org/10.1016/j.beem.2015.04.005.

Tadokoro-Cuccaro, R., & Hughes, I. A. (2014). Androgen insensitivity syndrome. *Current Opinion in Endocrinology, Diabetes and Obesity, 21*(6), 499–503. Available from https://doi.org/10.1097/med.0000000000000107.

C H A P T E R

13

Hormonal control of reproduction in the female: the menstrual cycle

Case study and in the clinic

Secondary amenorrhea

Signs and symptoms

A 27-year-old woman presents with secondary amenorrhea. From her menarche at age 13, she had regular monthly menses. She went on the birth control pill from age 21 to 24. Upon stopping it at age 24, her menses returned although were somewhat irregular, but she conceived and delivered 2 years ago. She breastfed for 3 months, but upon stopping, there has not been any return of menses. Her weight has been steady. There has not been any onset of hirsutism or breast discharge.

She denies headaches, any double vision or loss of peripheral vision. Functional review was otherwise unremarkable. Family history is noncontributory.

Diagnosis

On physical examination, she has an ideal body weight. Vital signs were normal. Thyroid gland was 1.5 times normal size and diffusely firm, but she was clinically euthyroid. She had normal visual fields, funduscopic, and cranial nerve examinations. There was no galactorrhea. There was normal sexual hair but no hirsutism or acne.

1. What are the possible causes of her secondary amenorrhea? What further information is needed from her history?
2. What investigations should be done?
3. Given the results of these investigations, what is the likely diagnosis?
4. What is the likely cause of this disorder?
5. What treatment should be prescribed?

Case discussion: This is a case of premature ovarian insufficiency (POI). Walk through an approach to secondary amenorrhea (i.e., cessation of menses after the patient had them at one point). After working through the causes of amenorrhea, the diagnosis should be suspected based on history, physical exam, and other testing being negative. An additional clue here is her firm thyroid gland that suggests Hashimoto chronic thyroiditis. This suggests an autoimmune predisposition, and thus autoimmune POI is suspected.

- The differential diagnosis for secondary amenorrhea includes:
  - Physiologic causes: Pregnancy, postpartum state, and stress/acute illness.
  - Pathological causes: These can be approached on an anatomical basis:
    - Hypothalamic causes: Hypothalamic disease/infiltration/tumors or "idiopathic" hypothalamic amenorrhea due to low BMI (associated with competitive level exercise and eating disorders, for example) and thus the gonadotropins shut down to preserve calories for life-sustaining functions.
    - Pituitary causes: Pituitary tumors, disease, and infiltration. Prolactin level elevations interfering with gonadotropin release.
    - Ovarian causes: PCOS (polycystic ovarian syndrome), POI, CAH (congenital adrenal hyperplasia) (this results in a relative excess of adrenal androgens and thus interruption of menses), and genetic conditions affecting the ovaries, for example, Turner syndrome and others.
  - Secondary to a systemic illness such as renal failure, hepatic disease, medications, anemia, and thyroid disease.
  - Therefore a further history should look for additional clues as to what is causing her amenorrhea: Any gynecological procedures/

Goodman's Basic Medical Endocrinology.
DOI: https://doi.org/10.1016/B978-0-12-815844-9.00013-0

(cont'd)

infections (that would cause an outflow tract obstruction), a full past medical history, and functional review to screen for other systemic diseases. In addition, enquiry about menarchal weight (weight at the onset of menarche), regularity of cycles, the presence of any breast discharge (high prolactin), hot flushes (POI), or onset of hair growth or acne (PCOS and CAH), the presence of headaches, double vision, loss of peripheral vision, loss of axillary hair (all signify possible pituitary pathology). Asking about any hypothyroidism symptoms would also be important as well as inquiring about exercise and eating habits if she is underweight to establish a diagnosis if hypothalamic amenorrhea is suspected. Any evidence of eating disorders, purging, etc., are also important pieces of information to help establish the possible cause of this presentation.

The top causes would include pregnancy, PCOS, POI, "idiopathic" hypothalamic amenorrhea, prolactin elevation, and thyroid disease.

- *Investigations are driven by the clinical history, physical exam, and clinical suspicion. This patient's firm thyroid gland might raise suspicion of a second associated autoimmune condition affecting the ovaries and resulting in POI.*
- The following real-life approach in the clinic would be:
- *Once a pregnancy test is done and is negative, then one would approach this patient as to whether she is estrogenized or not. If, clinically, the patient is estrogenized, that is, has appropriate skin caliber, and bleeds upon doing a progesterone withdrawal challenge, the etiology of her amenorrhea is more likely PCOS. If she is hypoestrogenized and does not bleed after progesterone withdrawal, then likely etiologies include POI and hyperprolactinemia (pituitary and hypothalamic disease should also be considered here).*
- *Tests to be ordered include pregnancy test, serum prolactin, thyroid-stimulating hormone (TSH), luteinizing hormone (LH), and follicle-stimulating hormone (FSH). If pregnancy test is negative, do progestin withdrawal test (if she bleeds after progestin, she is estrogenized).*
- *LH and FSH are helpful if elevated, as that would suggest ovarian insufficiency/failure and premature menopause. Elevated prolactin would be expected to result in low gonadotropins.*
- *Case findings: Pregnancy test "negative," serum FSH 80 IU/L, LH 41 IU/L, prolactin 10 μg/L, serum TSH normal. No bleeding response to progestin withdrawal.*

  Most likely diagnosis: POI (elevated LH and FSH suggest intact pituitary reserve, appropriately being elevated to compensate for the low estrogen state and lack of menses. The ovaries are the culprit here as the cause of the low estrogen state as they are failing to respond to high LH and FSH → thus ovarian failure or menopause).
- Most likely etiology is an autoimmune-mediated destruction of the ovarian follicles. Consider chromosomal abnormality such as Turner's mosaic, fragile-X. Other causes of POI include exposure to toxins (postchemotherapy and total body irradiation for cancer treatment), hemochromatosis, and other infiltrative diseases of the ovaries.

Management

Estrogen and progestin replacement therapy needs to be given at a very young age for bone and overall other health benefits. After counseling, future fertility can be an option. POI course can be variable.

Prognosis

Since POI is an autoimmune condition, it can have a waxing and waning course (such as most autoimmune conditions) and thus pregnancy is not impossible, but the number of viable follicles will diminish over time. Usually, fertility treatments (such as IVF) are necessary for conception, although spontaneous pregnancy can also occur.

Eventually, as the ovaries become fully depleted of any viable follicles, then egg donor conception is considered if that is an option that is appealing to the patient.

Hormonal control of reproduction in the female: the menstrual cycle

The ovaries serve the dual function of producing eggs and the hormones that support reproductive functions. Unlike men, in whom large numbers of gametes are produced continuously from stem cells, women release only one gamete at a time from a limited pool of preformed gametes in a process that is repeated at regular monthly intervals. Each interval encompasses the time needed for the ovum to develop, for preparation of the reproductive tract to receive the fertilized ovum, and the time allotted for that ovum to become fertilized and pregnancy established. If the ovary does not receive a signal that an embryo has begun to develop, the process of gamete maturation begins anew.

The principal ovarian hormones are the steroids estradiol and progesterone, and the peptide inhibin that orchestrates the cyclic series of events that unfold in the ovary, pituitary, and reproductive tract. As the ovum develops within its follicle, estradiol stimulates the growth of the structures of the reproductive tract that receive the sperm, facilitate fertilization, and ultimately house the developing embryo. Estradiol along with a variety of peptide growth factors produced in the developing follicle acts within the follicle to stimulate proliferation and secretory functions of granulosa cells and thereby enhances its own production. Progesterone is produced by the corpus luteum that develops from the follicle after the egg is shed. It prepares the uterus for successful implantation and growth of the embryo and is absolutely required for the maintenance of pregnancy.

Ovarian function is driven by the two pituitary gonadotropins: follicle-stimulating hormone (FSH) and luteinizing hormone (LH), which stimulate ovarian steroid production, growth of the follicle, ovulation, and development of the corpus luteum. Secretion of these hormones depends on stimulatory input from the hypothalamus through the gonadotropin-releasing hormone (GnRH) and complex inhibitory and stimulatory input from ovarian steroid and peptide hormones.

Ovaries

The adult human ovaries are paired, ellipsoid structures that measure about 5 cm in their longest dimension (Fig. 13.1).

They lie within the pelvic area of the abdominal cavity each one attached to the broad ligament that extends from either side of the uterus by peritoneal folds called the mesovarium (Figs. 13.2 and 13.3).

Both the gamete- and hormone-producing functions of the ovary take place in the outer or cortical portion (Fig. 13.4).

It is within the ovarian cortex that the precursors of the female gametes, the oocytes, are stored and develop into ova (eggs). The functional unit is the ovarian follicle that initially consists of a single oocyte surrounded by a layer

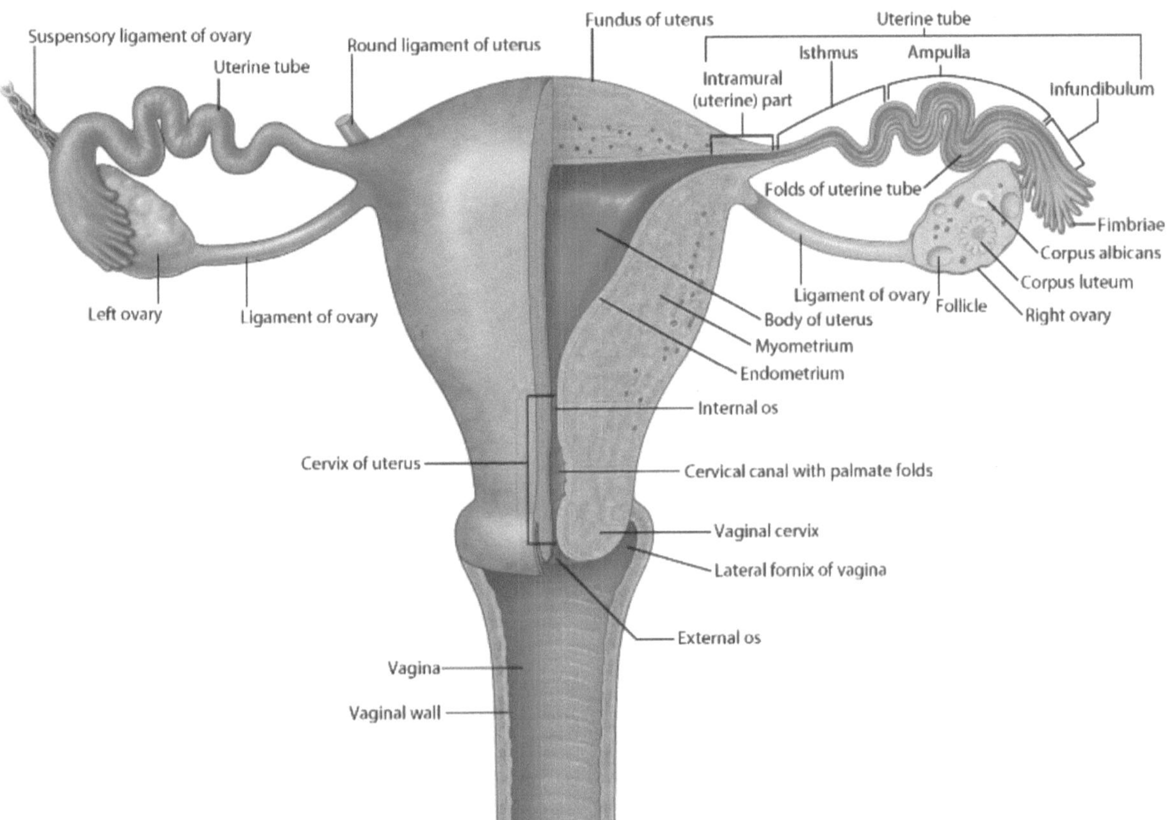

FIGURE 13.1 The uterus and ovaries. Source: *From Figure on page 242 of R. L. Drake, A. W. Vogl, A. W. M. Mitchell, R. M. Tibbitts, & P. E. Richardson. (2015).* Gray's atlas of anatomy *(2nd ed.). Elsevier.*

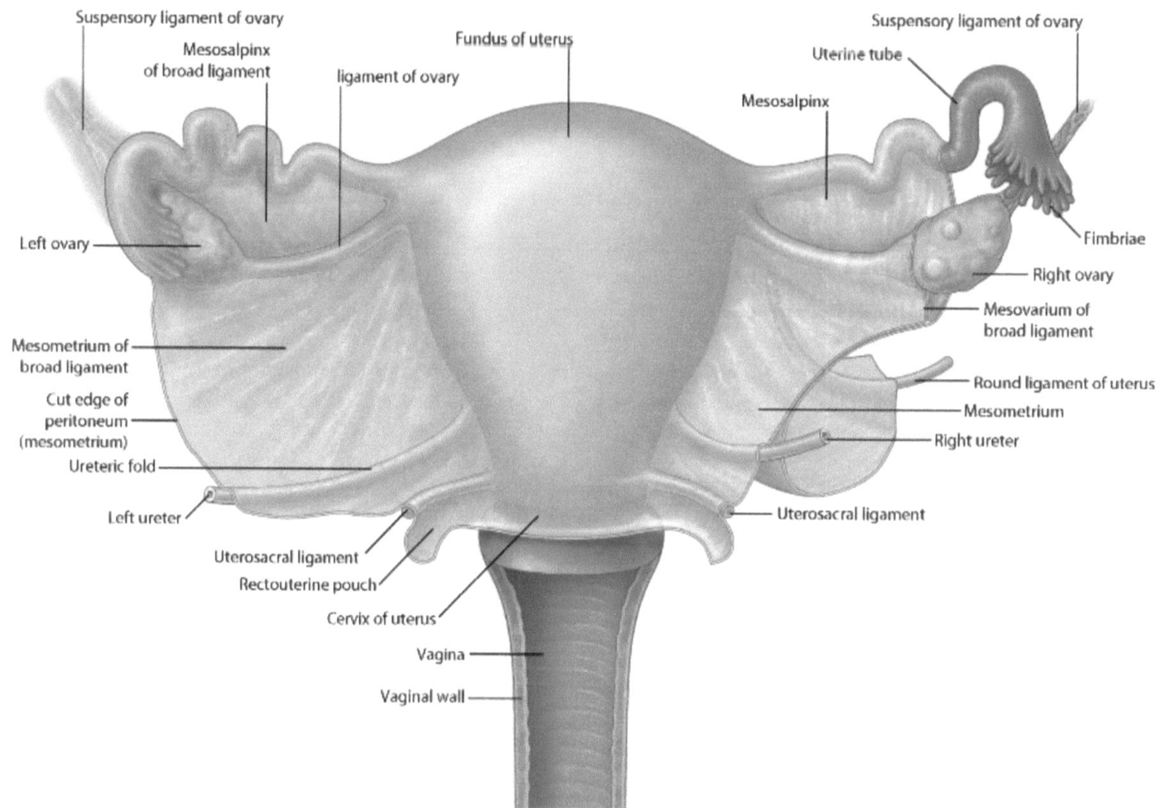

FIGURE 13.2 The uterus and the divisions of the broad ligament, which are the mesometrium, mesosalpinx, and mesovarium that are a double layer of peritoneum that wraps around each of the structures (See also Fig. 13.3.). Source: *From Figure on page 243 of R. L. Drake, A. W. Vogl, A. W. M. Mitchell, R. M. Tibbitts, & P. E. Richardson. (2015).* Gray's atlas of anatomy *(2nd ed.). Elsevier.*

FIGURE 13.3 The double folds of the peritoneum that surrounds the uterus, uterine tubes, and ovaries. They are, respectively, the mesometrium, mesosalpinx, and mesovarium. Source: *From Figure 5-58A in R. L. Drake, A. W. Vogl, & A. W. M. Mitchell. (2015).* Gray's anatomy for students *(3rd ed.) (p. 484). Elsevier.*

of granulosa cells enclosed within a basement membrane, the basal lamina, that separates the follicle from cortical stroma. When they emerge from the resting stage, follicles become ensheathed in a layer of specialized follicular cells called the cumulus oophorus (Figs. 13.5 and 13.6).

Follicles in many stages of development are found in the cortex of the adult ovary along with structures that form when the mature ovum is released by the process of ovulation. Ovarian follicles, in which the ova develop, and corpora lutea derived from them are also the sites of ovarian hormone production. The inner portion of the ovary, the ovarian medulla (Fig. 13.4), consists chiefly of vascular elements that arise from anastomoses of the uterine and ovarian arteries (Fig. 13.7).

A rich supply of unmyelinated nerve fibers also enters the medulla along with blood vessels.

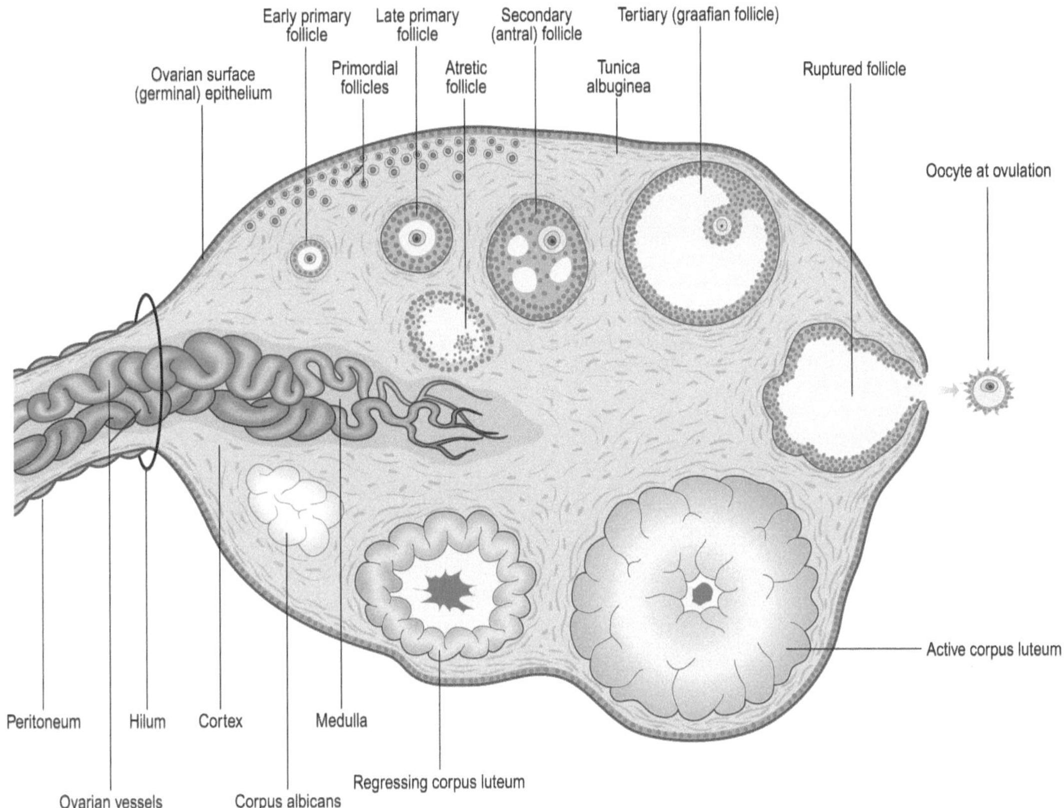

FIGURE 13.4 A schematic illustration showing a cross section of the ovary and the sequence of follicular development. Source: *From Figure 77-32 in S. Standring. (2014).* Gray's anatomy *(41st ed.) (p. 1304). Elsevier.*

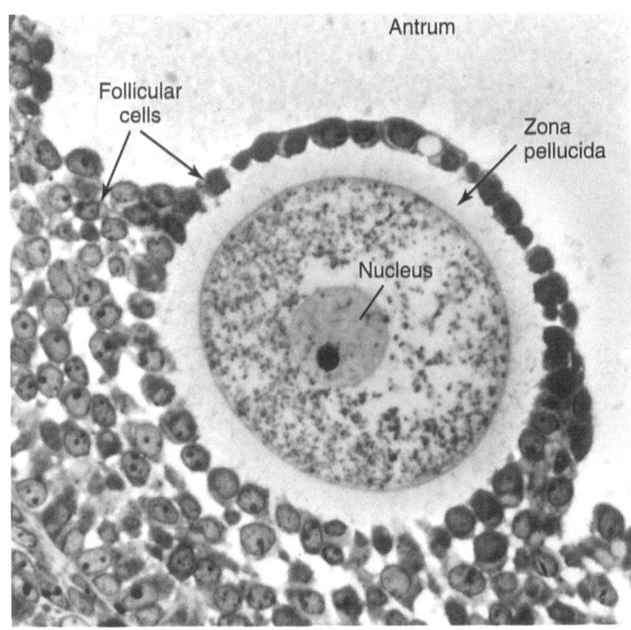

FIGURE 13.5 The thecal cells that comprise the cumulus oophorus are surrounded by a dark circle. These cells surround the follicle and project it into the lumen of the follicle. Source: *Adapted from Figure 2-8 of K. L. Moore, T. V. N. Persaud & M. G. Torchia. (2016).* The developing human *(10th ed.) (p. 21). Elsevier.*

Folliculogenesis

In contrast to the testis, which produces hundreds of millions of sperm each day, the ovary normally produces a single mature ovum about once each month. The testis must continuously renew its pool of germ cell precursors throughout reproductive life in order to sustain this rate of sperm production, whereas the ovary needs to draw only upon its initial endowment of primordial oocytes to provide the approximately 400 mature ova ovulated during the four decades of a woman's reproductive life. Although ovulation, the hallmark of ovarian activity, occurs episodically at 28-day intervals, examination of the ovary at any time during childhood or the reproductive life of a mature woman reveals continuous activity with multiple follicles at various stages in their life cycle.

Folliculogenesis begins in fetal life (Fig. 13.8).

Primordial germ cells multiply by mitosis and begin to differentiate into primary oocytes and enter meiosis between the 11th and 20th weeks after conception (Fig. 13.9).

Primary oocytes remain arrested in prophase of the first meiotic division until meiosis resumes at the time of ovulation and is not completed until the second polar

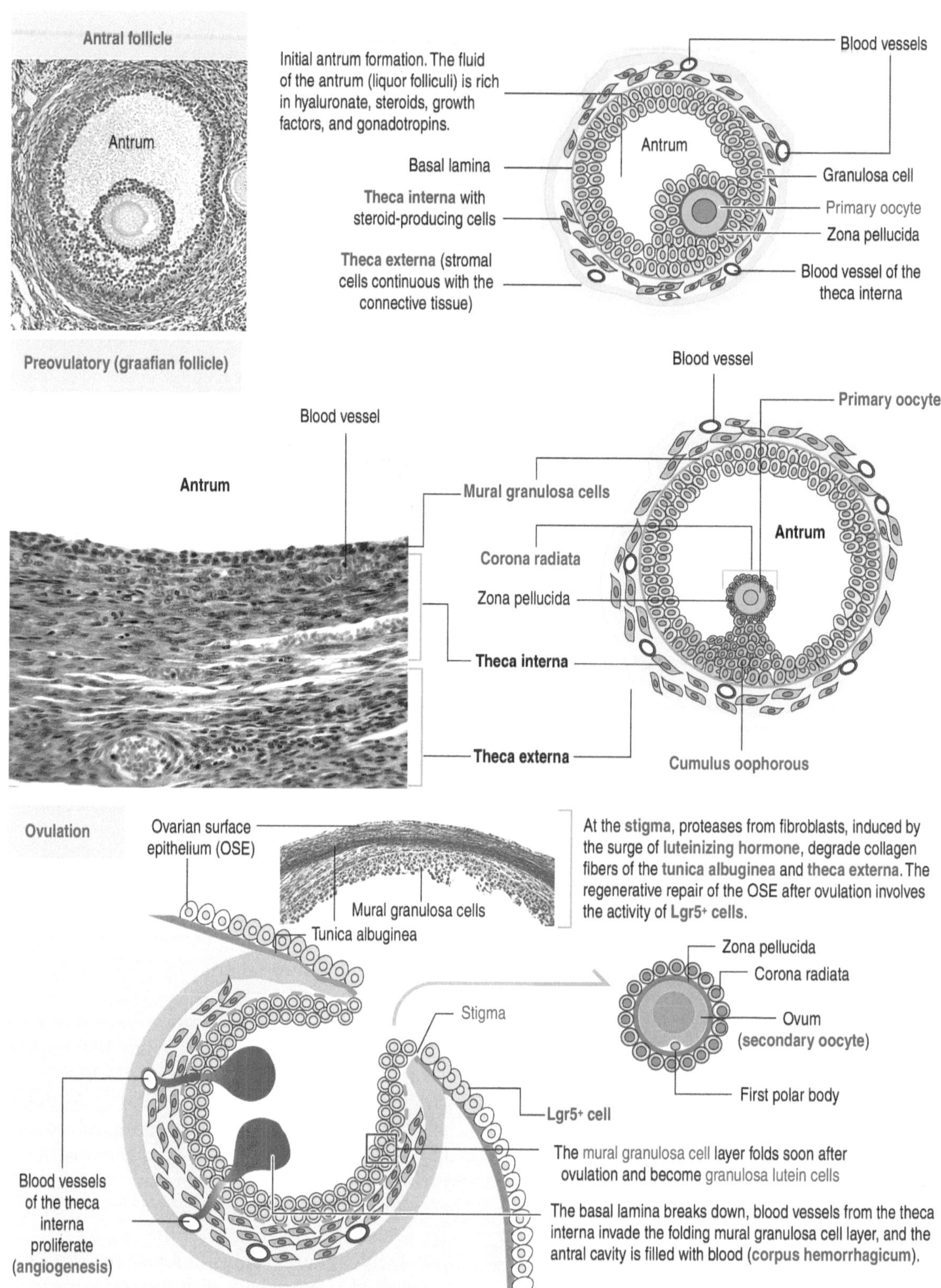

FIGURE 13.6 The cumulus oophorus within the follicle. Although not shaded as such, these cells also surround the oocyte. Source: *From Figure 22-3 in A. L. Kierszenbaum, & L. L. Tres, (2020).* Histology and cell biology: An introduction to pathology *(5th ed.) (p. 670). Elsevier.*

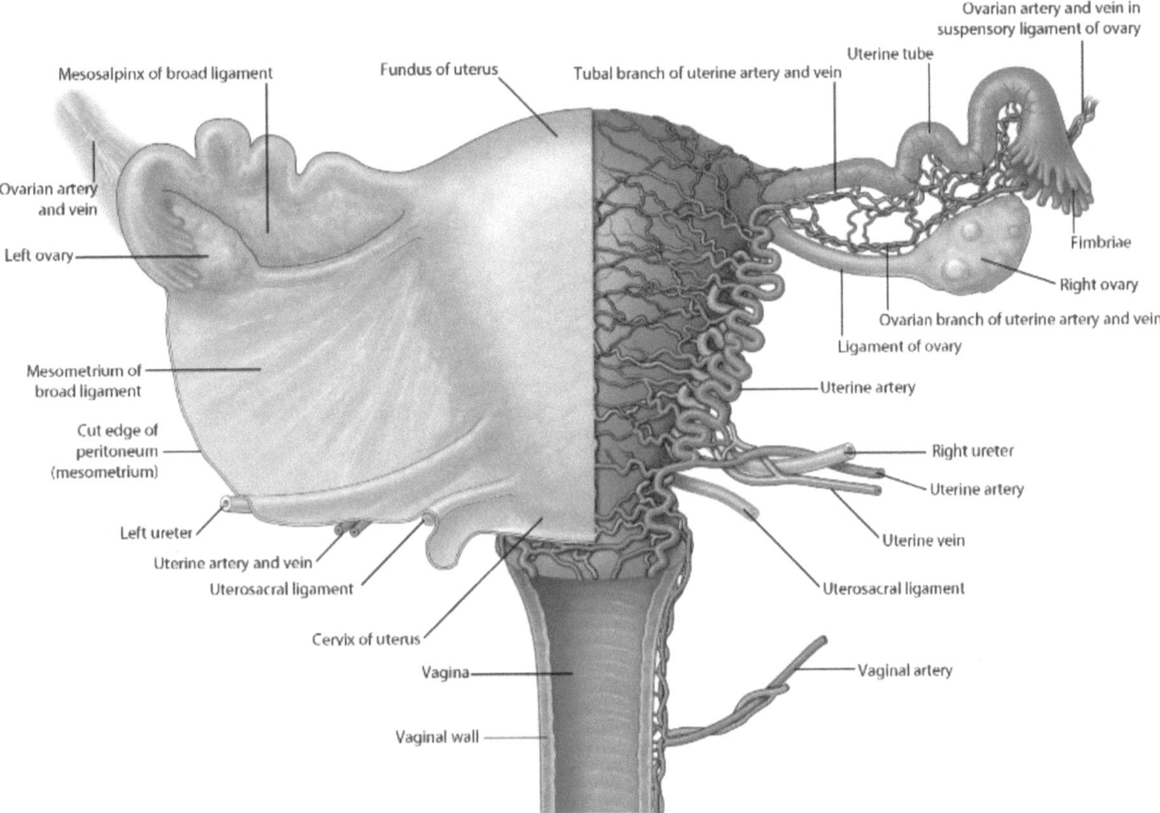

FIGURE 13.7 The vascular supply of the uterus and ovaries. Note the numerous anastomoses between the vaginal, uterine, and ovarian arteries—this ensures that all parts of the reproductive system get plenty of blood. Source: *From Figure on page 249 of R. L. Drake, A. W. Vogl, A. W. M. Mitchell, R. M. Tibbitts, & P. E. Richardson. (2015).* Gray's atlas of anatomy *(2nd ed.). Elsevier.*

body is extruded at the time of fertilization, which may be more than four decades later for some oocytes. Around the 20th-week of fetal life, there are about 6–7 million oocytes available to form primordial follicles, atresia by apoptosis (programed cell death) during the next 20 weeks reduces that amount so that the human female is born with 1 or 2 million oocytes. At no other time is there such a dramatic reduction in oocytes. Atresia continues so that at puberty, only about only 300,000–400,000 primordial follicles remain in each ovary. The majority of primordial follicles remain in a resting state for many years. By some seemingly random process, perhaps because they are relieved of inhibition or are activated by still unknown factors, some follicles enter into a growth phase and begin the 85-day journey toward ovulation—a time that spans several menstrual periods, but the vast majority become atretic and die at various stages along the way. This process begins during the fetal period and continues until menopause at around age 50, when there are no more follicles.

As primordial follicles emerge from the resting stage, the oocyte grows from a diameter of about 20 μm to about 100 μm and a layer of extracellular mucopolysaccharides and proteins called the zona pellucida forms around it (Figs. 13.5 and 13.10–13.13)

Granulosa cells change in morphology from squamous to cuboidal. This early step in the process takes 85 days. The growth of primary follicles is accompanied by migration and differentiation of mesenchymal cells to form the theca folliculi. Its inner layer, the theca interna, is composed of secretory cells with an extensive smooth endoplasmic reticulum characteristic of steroidogenic cells. The theca externa is formed by reorganization of surrounding stromal cells. At this time a dense capillary network develops around the follicle.

The oocyte completes its growth by accumulating stored nutrients and the messenger RNA and protein-synthesizing apparatus that will be activated upon fertilization. As the follicle continues to grow, granulosa cells increase in number and begin to form multiple layers. The innermost granulosa cells in the cumulus oophorus are in intimate contact with the oocyte through cellular processes that penetrate the zona pellucida and form intercellular junctions (gap junctions) with its plasma membrane (Fig. 13.14).

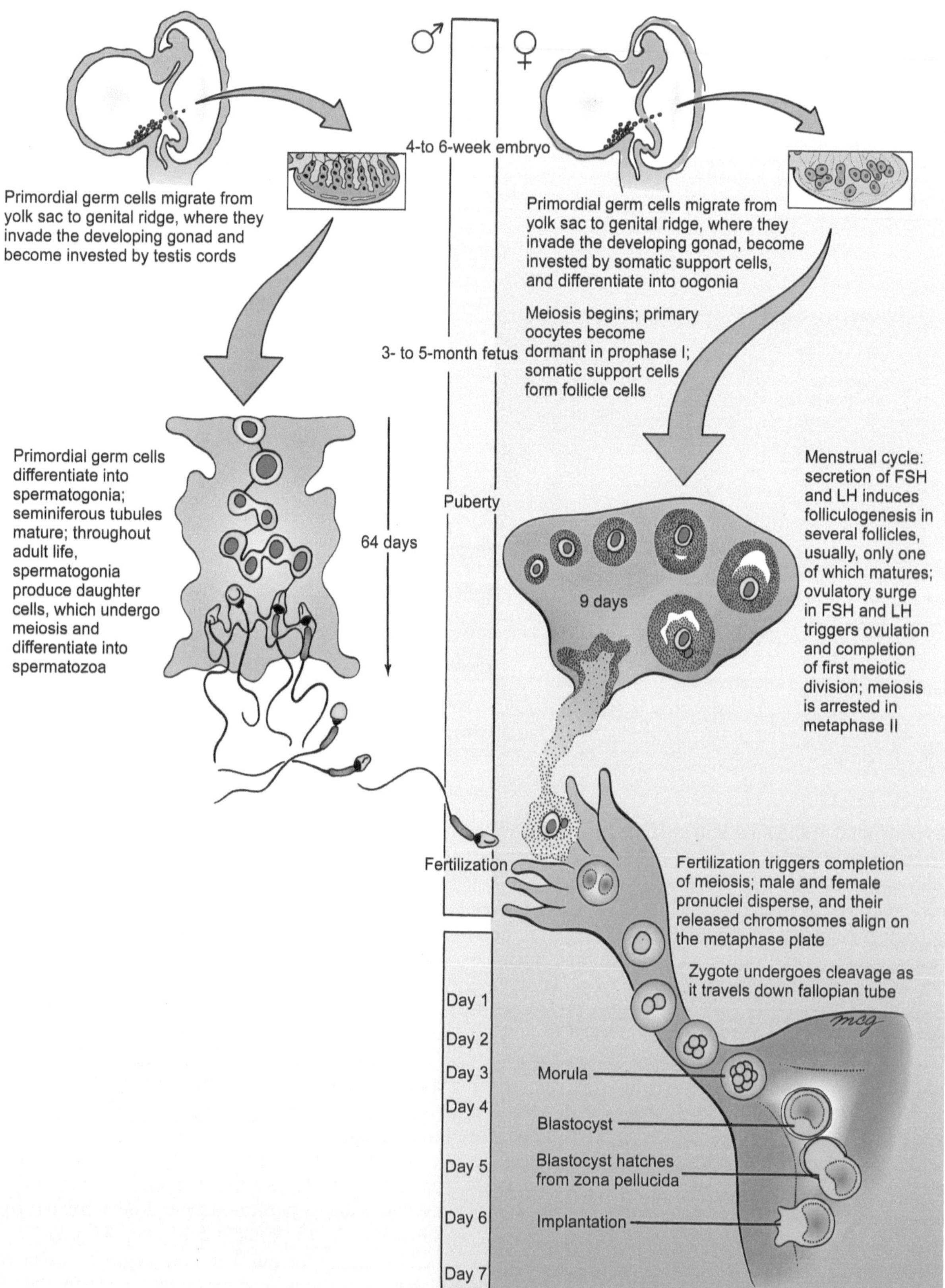

FIGURE 13.8 Time line in both male (blue background) and female (pink background) gamete formation from beginning to implantation in the uterine wall. Source: *From Unnumbered Figure at beginning of Chapter 1 in G. C. Schoenwolf, S. B. Bleyl, P. R. Brauer, & P. H. Francis-West. (2015).* Larson's human embryology *(5th ed.) (p. 15). Elsevier.*

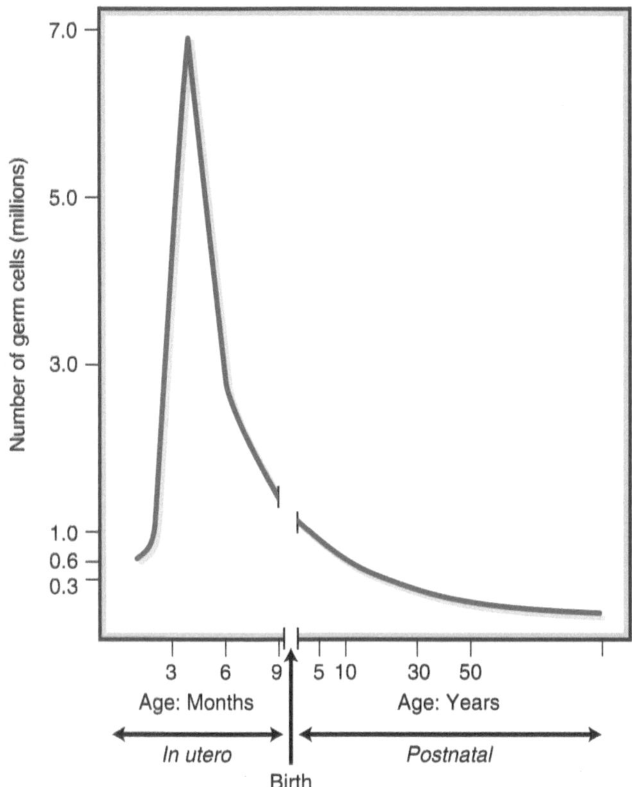

FIGURE 13.9 The number of germ cells in the ovary over the life span. Source: *From Figure 17-9 in Bulun, S. E. (2016). Chapter 17: Physiology and pathology of the female reproductive axis. In S. Malmed, K. S. Polonsky, P. R. Larsen, & H. M. Kronenberg (Eds.),* Williams textbook of endocrinology *(13th ed.) (p. 599). Elsevier.*

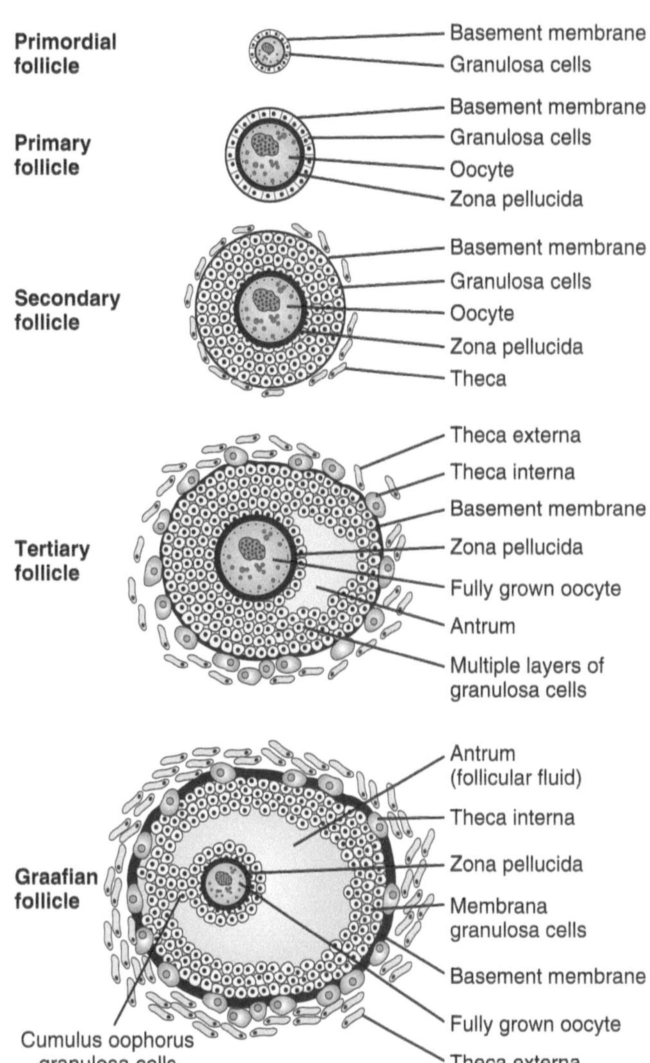

FIGURE 13.10 The sequence of development of the follicle. Source: *From Figure 17-11 in Bulun, S. E. (2016). Chapter 17: Physiology and pathology of the female reproductive axis. In S. Malmed, K. S. Polonsky, P. R. Larsen, & H. M. Kronenberg (Eds.),* Williams textbook of endocrinology *(13th ed.) (p. 601). Elsevier.*

Granulosa cells also form gap junctions with each other and function as nurse cells supplying nutrients to the oocyte that is separated from direct contact with capillaries by the basal lamina and the granulosa cells. There is bidirectional signaling between the granulosa cells and the oocyte. The granulosa cells will send transforming growth factor-β (TGF-β) and connexin 47 and 43 to the oocytes; the oocytes in return send growth and differentiation factor (GDF-9) and bone morphogenetic protein-15 (BMP-15) to the granulosa cells (Fig. 13.15).

These two substances regulate the energy metabolism and the biosynthesis of cholesterol in those cells. If connexin 43 fails to be produced, follicular development stops. If the bidirectional signal fails, then polycystic ovaries will result.

Follicular development continues with further proliferation of granulosa cells and gradual elaboration of fluid within the follicle. Follicular fluid is derived from blood plasma and contains plasma proteins, including hormones, and various proteins and steroids secreted by the granulosa cells and the ovum. Accumulation of follicular fluid brings about further enlargement of the follicle and the formation of a central fluid-filled cavity called the antrum. Follicular growth up to this stage is independent of pituitary hormones but without support from FSH (see Chapter 2: Pituitary Gland, and Chapter 12: Hormonal Control of Reproduction in the Male); further development is not possible and the follicles become atretic. Any follicle can be arrested at any stage of its development and undergoes the degenerative changes of atresia. Atresia is the fate of all the follicles that enter the growth phase before puberty, and more than 99% of the 200,000–400,000 remain at puberty. The physiological mechanisms that control this seemingly wasteful process are poorly understood.

In the presence of FSH, antral follicles continue to develop slowly for about 2 months until they reach a

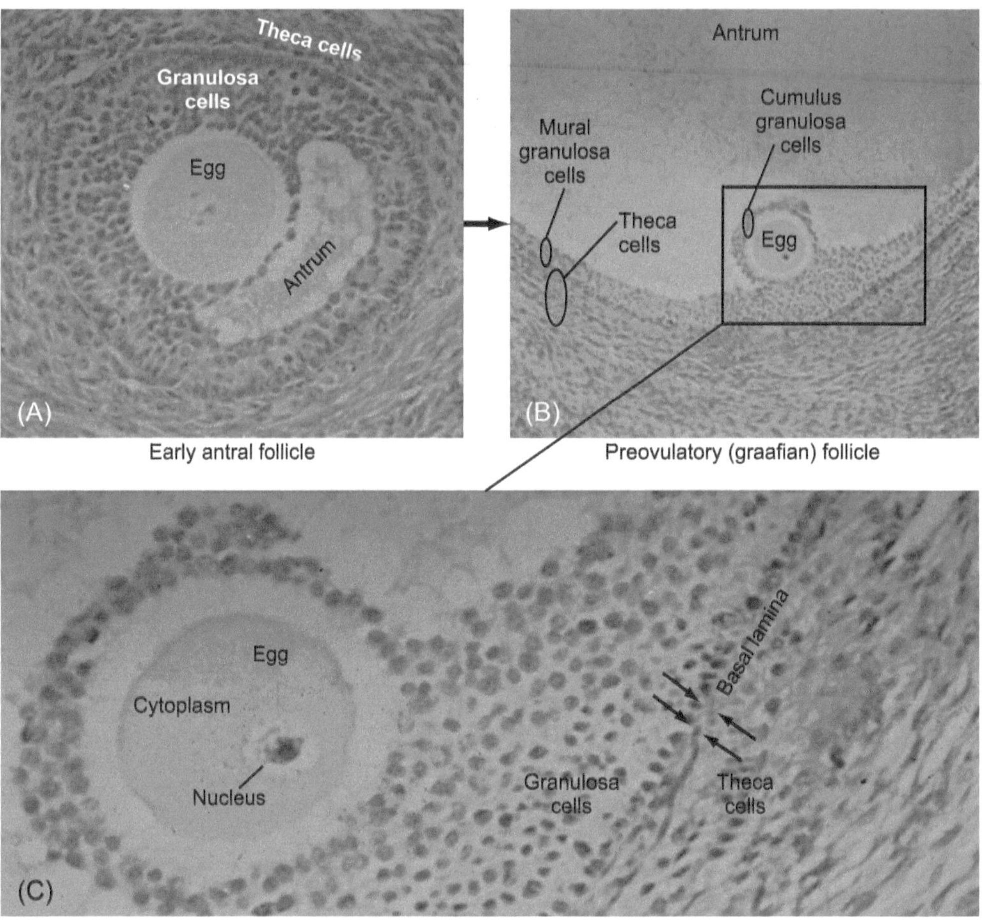

FIGURE 13.11 Micrographs showing the developing follicle and the cumulus granulosa surrounding the oocyte (egg). Source: *From Figure 17-12 in Bulun, S. E. (2016). Chapter 17: Physiology and pathology of the female reproductive axis. In S. Malmed, K. S. Polonsky, P. R. Larsen, & H. M. Kronenberg (Eds.),* Williams textbook of endocrinology *(13th ed.) (p. 602). Elsevier.*

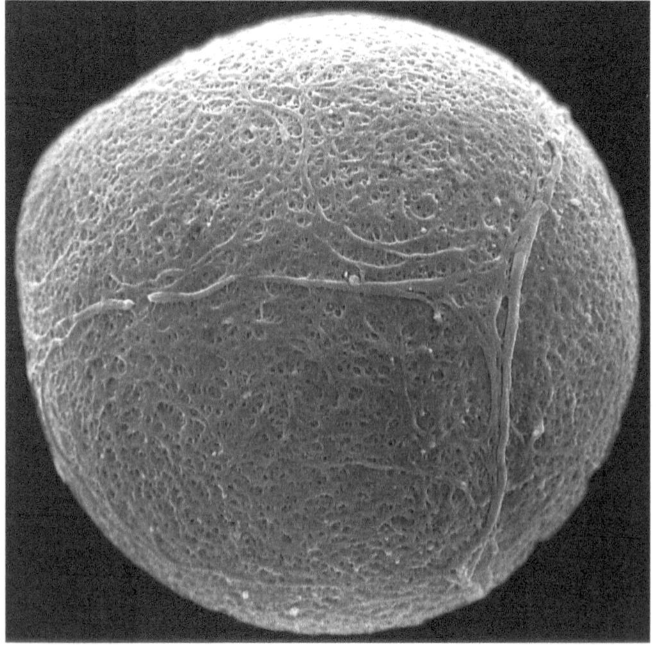

FIGURE 13.12 The zona pellucida as observed with the scanning electron microscope. The cells of the cumulus oophorus have been digested away. It is composed of many strands of mucopolysaccharide such as the strings in a ball of string. The holes where strands cross provide space for extensions of the cumulus oophorus cells to connect to the surface of the oocyte. Source: *From Figure 1-7 in G. C. Schoenwolf, S. B. Bleyl, P. R. Brauer, & P. H. Francis-West. (2015).* Larson's human embryology *(5th ed.) (p. 27). Elsevier.*

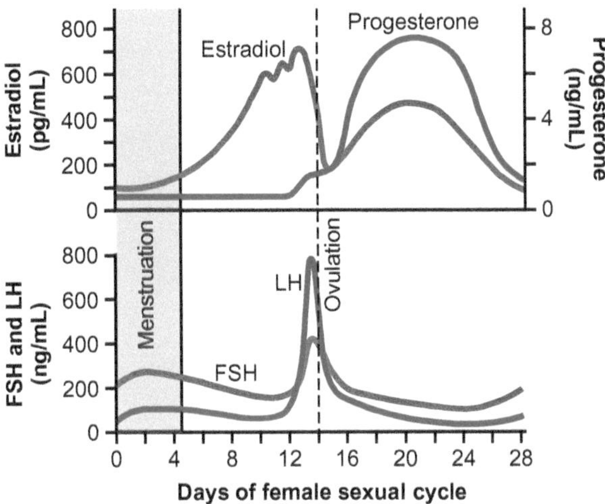

FIGURE 13.13 Approximate plasma concentrations of the gonadotropins and ovarian hormones during the normal female sexual cycle. *FSH*, follicle-stimulating hormone; *LH*, luteinizing hormone. Source: *From Figure 82-4 in Hall. (2016).* Guyton and Hall Textbook of Medical Physiology *(13th ed.) (p. 1039). Elsevier.*

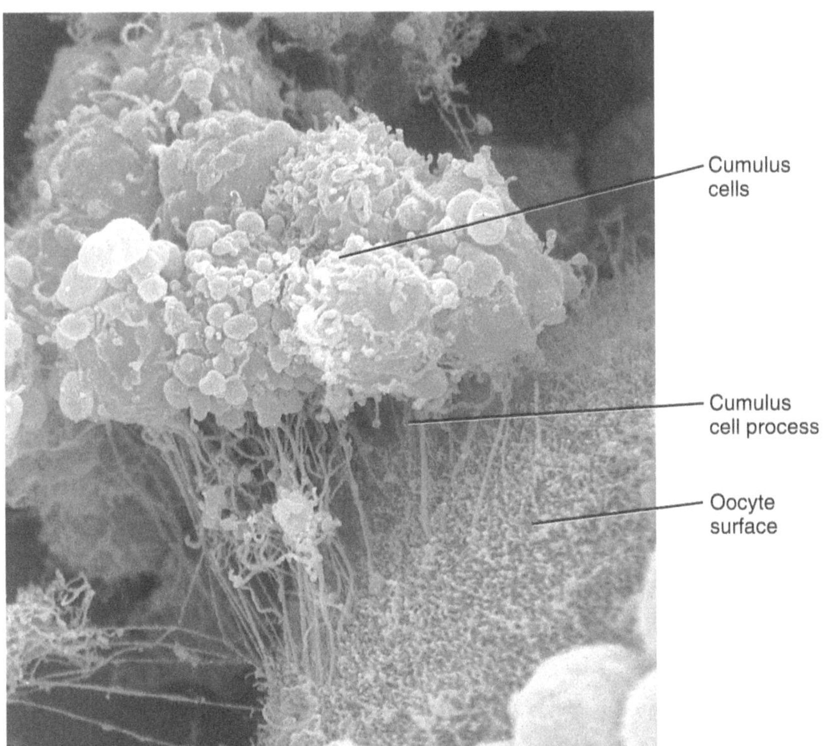

FIGURE 13.14 Cells of the cumulus oophorus extend structures through the zona pellucida (which has been digested away) to connect with the surface of the oocyte. Source: *From Figure 1-7 in G. C. Schoenwolf, S. B. Bleyl, P. R. Brauer, & P. H. Francis-West. (2015).* Larson's human embryology *(5th ed.) (p. 27). Elsevier.*

critical size. About 20 days before ovulation a group or cohort of 6–12 of these follicles enters into the final rapid growth phase, but in each cycle, normally, only one survives and ovulates, while the others become atretic and die (Figs. 13.16 and 13.17).

To review, meiosis is the process by which the number of chromosomes and the DNA content are halved. This enables two cells with a similar complement of chromosomes and DNA to join, and the resultant cell will have a normal number of chromosomes (46) and the normal amount of DNA, such as cell is referred to as genetically diploid (Figs. 13.18 and 13.19 and Table 13.1).

The chromosomes are stopped in the prophase of meiosis I by oocyte maturation inhibitor (OMI) (Fig. 13.20).

The chromosomes are not pulled apart until the preovulatory surge of FSH and LH, some 11–14 years later and only one of the follicles goes on to maturity in response to FSH and LH. This follicle is referred to

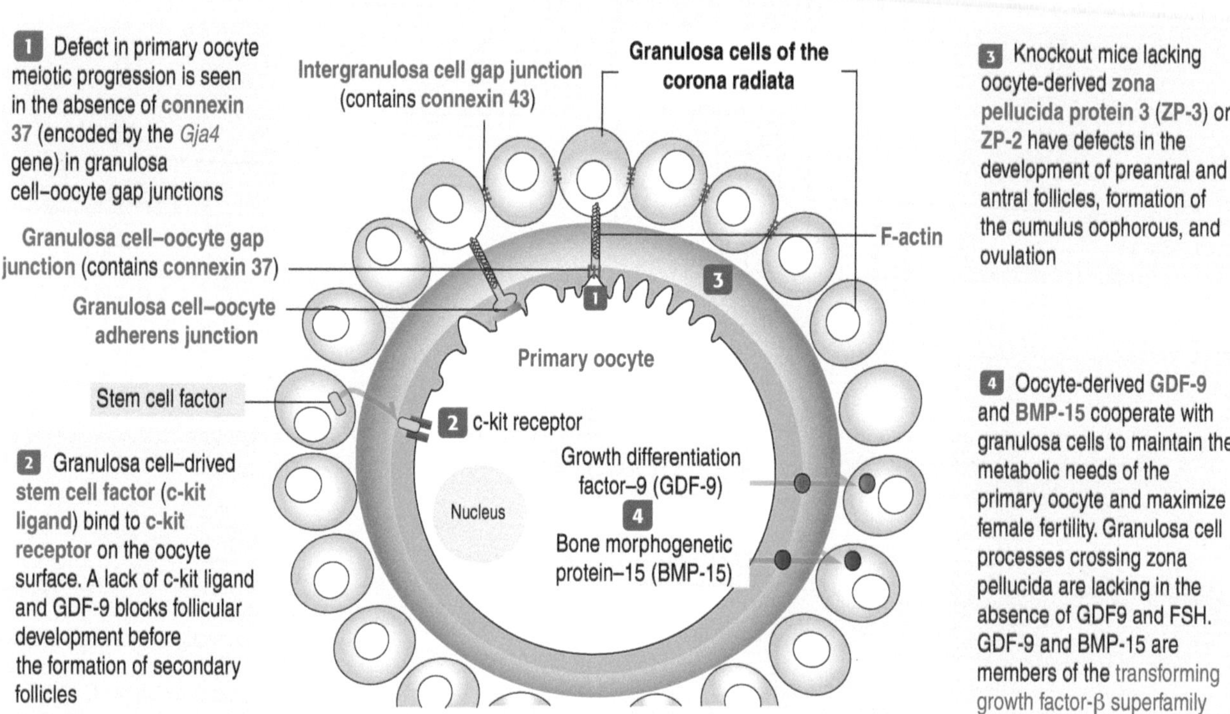

FIGURE 13.15 Bidirectional signaling in the cumulus–oocyte (granulosa cell–primary oocyte) complex. Source: *From Figure Primer 22-B in A.L. Kierszenbaum, & L.L. Tres, (2020).* Histology and cell biology: An introduction to pathology *(5th ed.) (p. 730). Elsevier.*

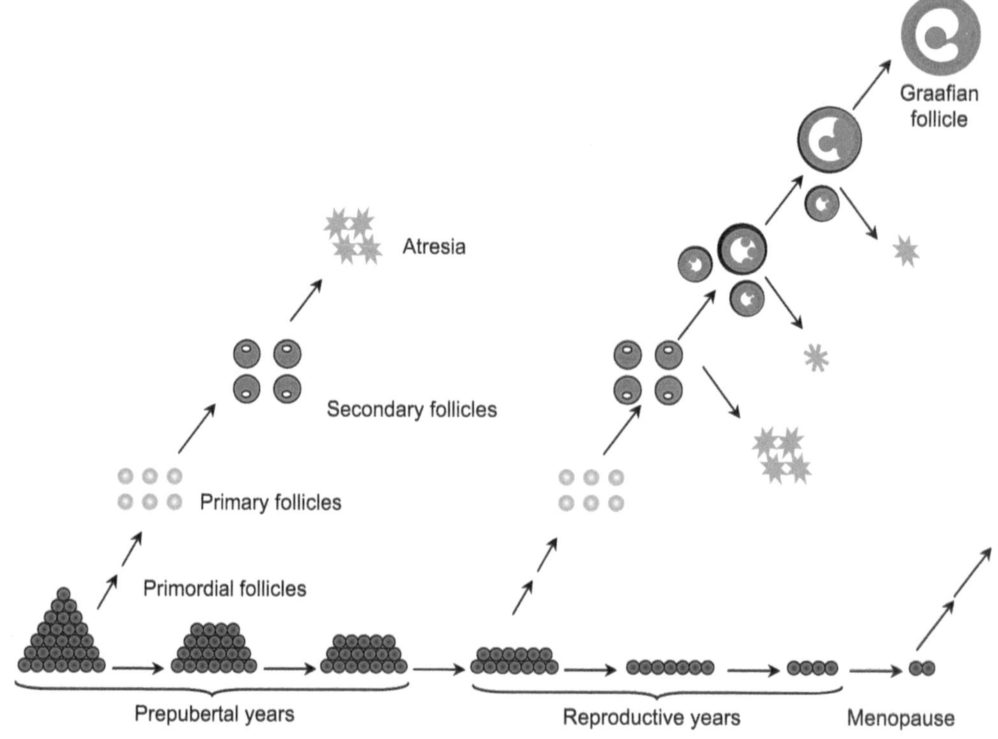

FIGURE 13.16 Follicular development at various stages of a woman's life. Source: *Adapted from McGee, E. A., & Hsueh, A. J. W. (2000).* Endocrine Reviews, 21, *200–214, with permission of the Endocrine Society.*

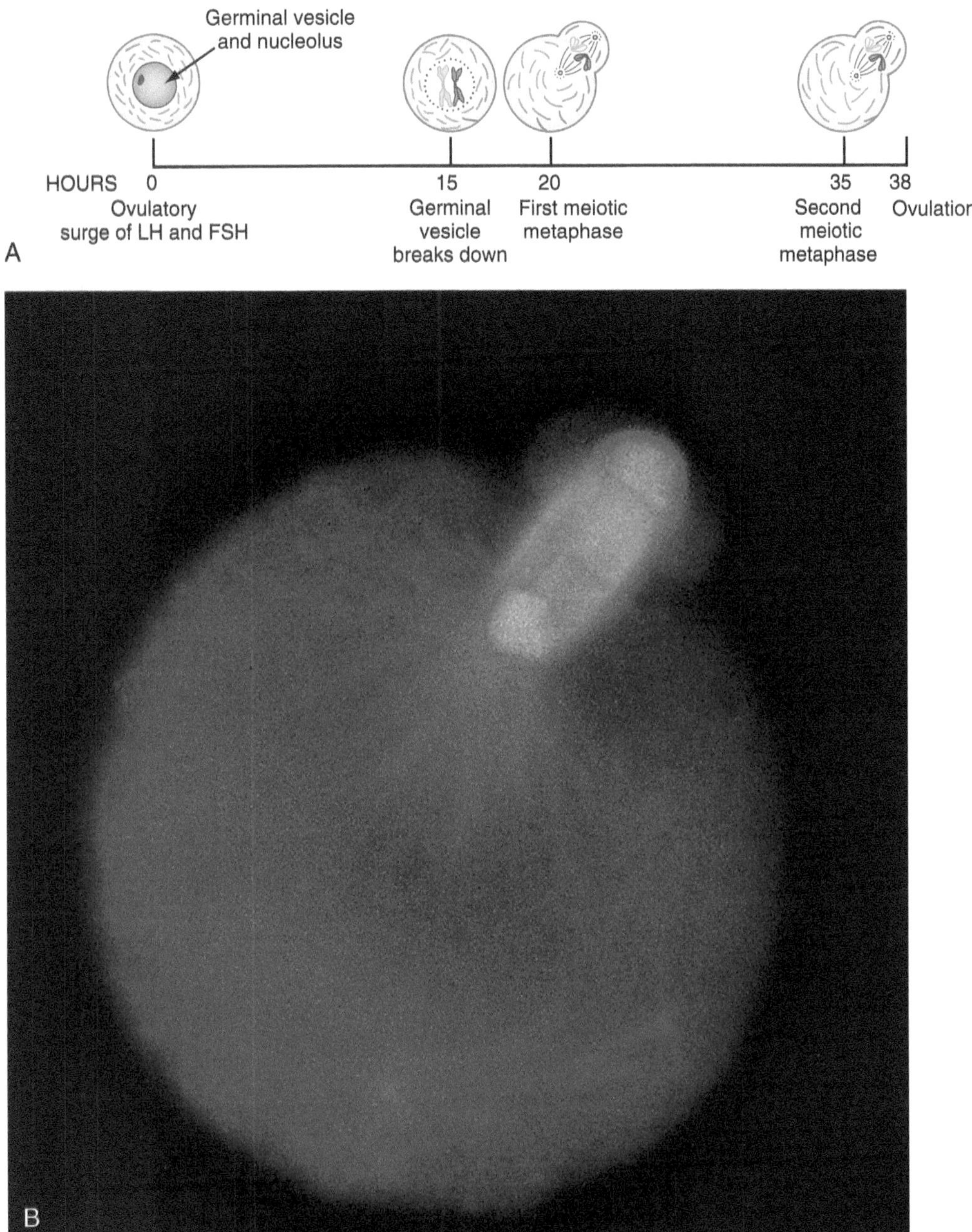

FIGURE 13.17 Meiosis sequence prior to ovulation. The germinal vesicle is another term for nucleus. It is stopped in metaphase II and will not be resumed until fertilization. Source: *From Figure 1-12A in G. C. Schoenwolf, S. B. Bleyl, P. R. Brauer, & P. H. Francis-West. (2015).* Larson's human embryology *(5th ed.) (p. 32). Elsevier.*

as the vesicular follicle or mature Graafian follicle. In response to FSH, on day 15 of the cycle, the surviving follicle resumes meiosis I. The nuclear envelope (also called the vesicular membrane) breaks down as depicted in Fig. 13.12. If separation is not complete, it is called nondisjunction and can occur at either the first or second meiotic division (Fig. 13.21).

The surviving follicle has been called the dominant follicle because it may contribute to the demise of other developing follicles. It is arrested in metaphase II by anti-Müllerian hormone (AMH). It will not resume meiosis II until after fertilization (Fig. 13.22).

As the dominant follicle matures, the fluid content in the antrum increases rapidly, possibly in response to increased colloid osmotic pressure created by partial hydrolysis of dissolved mucopolysaccharides. The ripe, preovulatory follicle reaches a diameter of 20–30 mm and bulges into the peritoneal cavity. At this time, it consists of about 60 million granulosa cells arranged in multiple layers around the periphery. The ovum and its

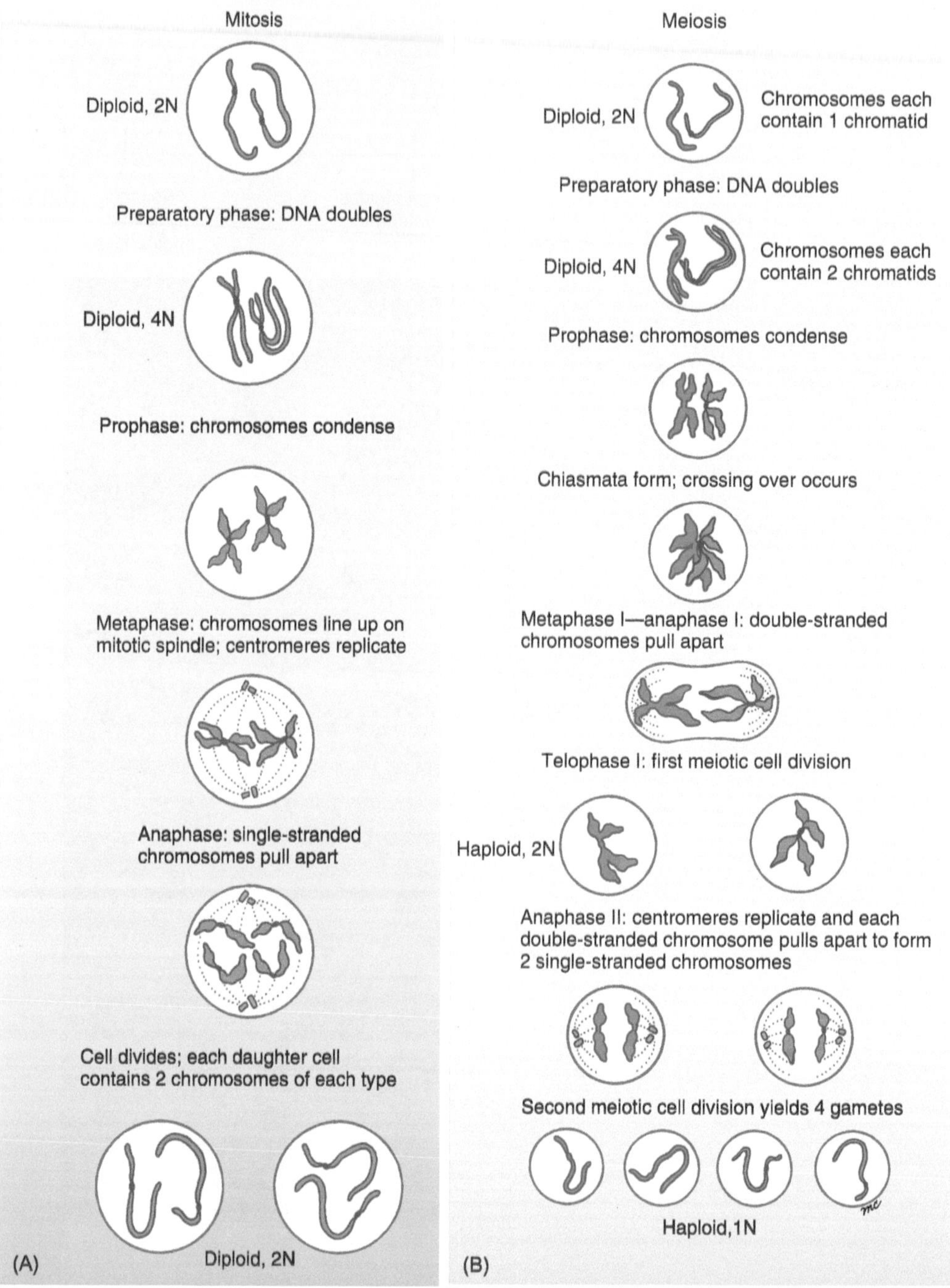

FIGURE 13.18 The comparison of the stages of mitosis and meiosis. In crossover, genetic material is exchanged. In the female, this occurs before birth in the prophase stage of meiosis. Source: *From Figure 1-2 in G. C. Schoenwolf, S. B. Bleyl, P. R. Brauer, & P. H. Francis-West. (2015).* Larson's human embryology *(5th ed.) (p. 20). Elsevier.*

surrounding layers of granulosa cells, the corona radiata, are suspended by a narrow bridge of granulosa cells (the cumulus oophorus) in a pool of more than 6 mL of follicular fluid. At ovulation a point opposite the ovum in the follicle wall, called the stigma, erodes, and the ovum with its accompanying granulosa cells (the cumulus oophorus complex) is extruded into the peritoneal cavity in a bolus of follicular fluid (Fig. 13.23).

Ovulation is not explosive but occurs relatively slowly. The extruded cumulus–oocyte is sticky and so clings to the surface of the ovary. The fimbriae of the uterine tube actively scrape it off the ovary and, with cilia on the fimbriae, move the oocyte–cumulus toward the mouth of the uterine tube (Fig. 13.24).

Following ovulation, there is ingrowth and differentiation of the remaining mural granulosa cells, thecal

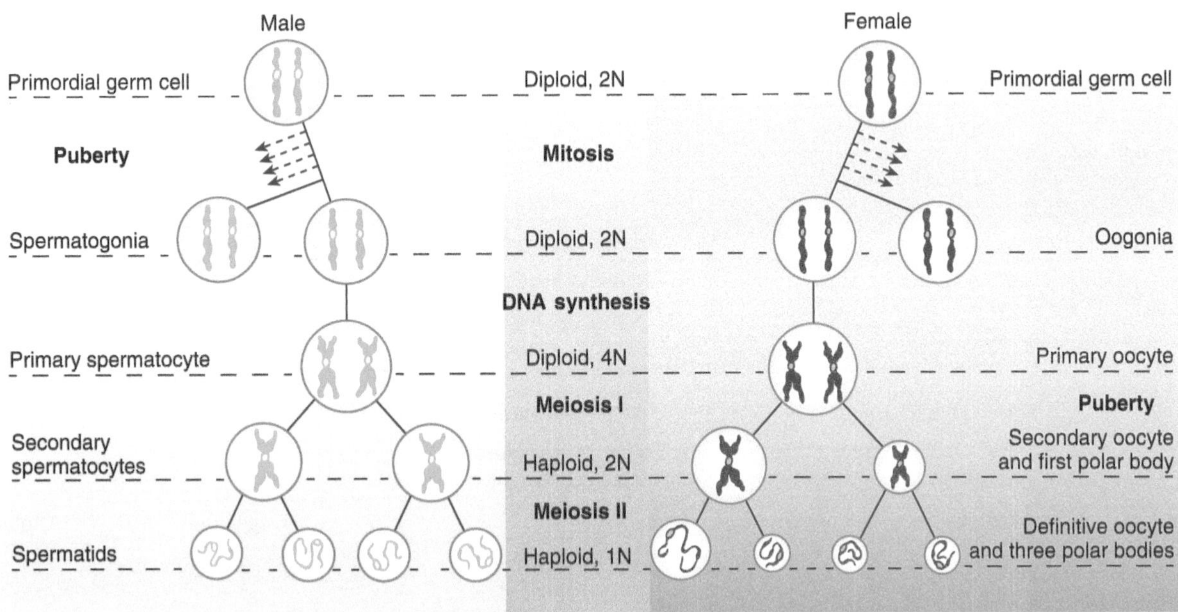

FIGURE 13.19 Terms used for the stages in the development of the gamete from a diploid to a haploid cell. Note that crossover occurs in embryonic development but does not resume until puberty. Source: *From Figure 1-3 in G. C. Schoenwolf, S. B. Bleyl, P. R. Brauer, & P. H. Francis-West. (2015).* Larson's human embryology *(5th ed.) (p. 22). Elsevier.*

cells, and some stromal cells, which fill the cavity of the collapsed follicle to form a new endocrine structure, the corpus luteum. The process by which granulosa and thecal cell are converted to luteal cells is called luteinization (meaning yellowing) and is the morphological reflection of the accumulation of lipid. Luteinization also involves biochemical changes that enable the corpus luteum to become the most active of all steroid-producing tissues per unit weight. The corpus luteum consists of large polygonal cells containing an extensive smooth endoplasmic reticulum and smaller steroid-secreting cells thought to be derived from the theca interna (Figs. 13.25 and 13.26).

Its metabolic needs are served by a rich supply of fenestrated capillaries. Unless pregnancy ensues, the corpus luteum regresses after 2 weeks, leaving a scar on the surface of the ovary.

Uterine tubes and uterus

The primitive Müllerian ducts that develop during early embryonic life give rise to the duct system that in primitive animals provides the route for ova to escape to the outside (Fig. 13.27).

In mammals, these tubes are adapted to provide a site for fertilization of ova and nurture of embryos. In female embryos the Müllerian ducts are not subjected to the destructive effects of the AMH during embryonic development (see Chapter 12: Hormonal Control of Reproduction in the Male) and, so, instead, develop into the uterine tubes, uterus, and upper portion of the vagina. Unlike the development of the sexual duct system in the male fetus, this differentiation is independent of gonadal hormones.

The paired uterine tubes (fallopian tubes) are a conduit for transfer of the ovum to the uterus (see Chapter 14: Hormonal Control of Pregnancy and Lactation). The proximal end comes in close contact with the ovary and has a funnel-shaped opening, the infundibulum, surrounded by finger-like projections called fimbriae. The uterine tube, particularly the infundibulum, is lined with ciliated cells whose synchronous beating plays an important role in egg transport. The lining of the uterine tube also contains secretory cells whose products provide nourishment for the zygote (fertilized ovum) in its 3-to 4-day journey to the uterus (Fig. 13.28).

The walls of the uterine tubes contain layers of smooth muscle cells oriented both longitudinally and circularly.

Distal portions of the Müllerian ducts fuse to give rise to the uterus. In the nonpregnant woman the uterus is a small, pear-shaped structure extending about 6–7 cm in its longest dimension.

It is capable of enormous expansion, partly by passive stretching and partly by growth, so that at the end of pregnancy, it may reach 35 cm or more in its longest dimension. Its thick walls consist mainly of smooth muscle and are called the myometrium. The secretory epithelial lining

TABLE 13.1 The events during mitotic and meiotic cell division in the germ line of both sexes. Important points are in italics.

Stage	Events	Name of cell	Condition of genome
Resting interval between mitotic cell divisions	Normal cellular metabolism occurs	♀ Oogonium ♂ Spermatogonium	Diploid, 2N
Mitosis			
Preparatory phase	DNA replication yields double-stranded chromosomes	♀ Oogonium ♂ Spermatogonium	Diploid, 4N
Prophase	Double-stranded chromosomes condense		
Metaphase	Chromosomes align along the equator; centromeres replicate		
Anaphase and telophase	Each double-stranded chromosome splits into two single-stranded chromosomes, one of which is distributed to each daughter nucleus		
Cytokinesis	Cell divides	♀ Oogonium ♂ Spermatogonium	Diploid, 2N
Meiosis I			
Preparatory phase	DNA replication yields double-stranded chromosomes	♀ Primary oocyte ♂ Primary spermatocyte	Diploid, 4N
Prophase	Double-stranded chromosomes condense; two chromosomes of each homologous pair align at the centromeres to form a four-limbed chiasma; recombination by crossing over occurs		
Metaphase	Chromosomes align along the equator; *centromeres do not replicate*		
Anaphase and telophase	One double-stranded chromosome of each homologous pair is distributed to each daughter cell		
Cytokinesis	Cell divides	♀ One secondary oocyte and the first polar body ♂ Two secondary spermatocytes	Haploid, 2N
Meiosis II			
Prophase	*No DNA replication takes place during the second meiotic division*; double-stranded chromosomes condense		
Metaphase	Chromosomes align along the equator; *centromeres replicate*		
Anaphase and telophase	Each chromosome splits into two single-stranded chromosomes, one of which is distributed to each daughter nucleus		
Cytokinesis	Cell divides	♀ One definitive oocyte and three polar bodies ♂ Four spermatids	Haploid, 1N

From Table 1-1 in G. C. Schoenwolf, S. B. Bleyl, P. R. Brauer, & P. H. Francis-West. (2015). Larson's human embryology *(5th ed.) (p. 21). Elsevier.*

is called the endometrium and varies in thickness with changes in the hormonal environment, as discussed later. The uterine tubes join the uterus at the upper, rounded end. The caudal end constricts to a narrow cylinder called the uterine cervix, whose thick wall is composed largely of dense connective tissue rich in collagen fibers and some smooth muscle. The cervical canal is lined with mucus-producing cells and usually is filled with mucus. The cervix bulges into the upper reaches of the vagina that forms the final link to the outside. The lower portion of the vagina, which communicates with the exterior, is formed from the embryonic urogenital sinus.

Meiotic prophase arrest and progression of a primary oocyte

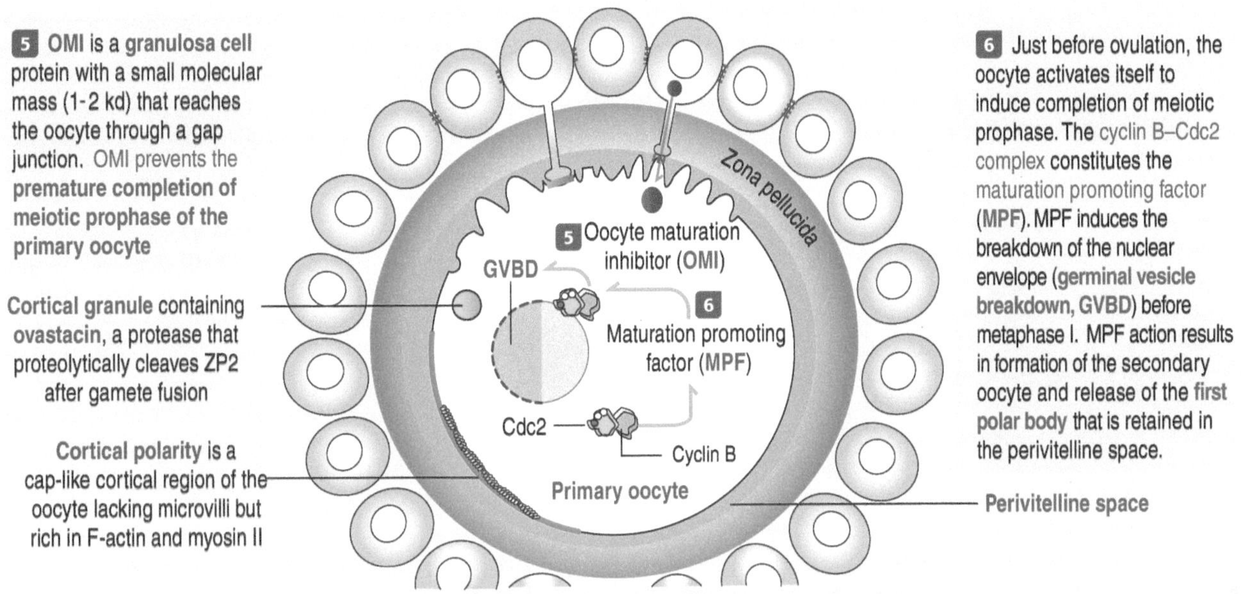

The primary oocyte overcomes meiotic arrest and continues meiosis I in response to the LH surge. This process results in GVBD, completion of meiotic prophase I, and the assembly of the meiotic spindle. As a result, the first polar body is formed and released into the perivitelline space. The secondary oocyte retains most of the cytoplasm and the first polar body degenerates within hours of formation.

Meiosis II reaches metaphase and awaits fertilization for completion and extrusion of the second polar body. A haploid state is reached

FIGURE 13.20 The arrest of meiosis in the primary oocyte is due to oocyte maturation inhibitor, a paracrine hormone secreted by the granulosa cells that surround the ovum. GVBD causes the resumption of this process in response to LH and FSH preovulatory surge. *FSH,* Follicle-stimulating hormone; *GVBD,* germinal vesicle breakdown; *LH,* luteinizing hormone. Source: *From Figure Primer 22-B in A.L. Kierszenbaum, & L.L. Tres. (2020).* Histology and cell biology: An introduction to pathology *(5th ed.) (p. 730). Elsevier.*

Ovarian hormones

The principal hormones secreted by the ovary are estrogens (estradiol-17β and estrone) and progesterone. These hormones are steroids and are derived from cholesterol by the series of reactions depicted in Figs. 13.29 and 13.30.

Their biosynthesis is intricately interwoven with the events of the ovarian cycle and is discussed in the next sections. In addition, the ovary produces a large number of biologically active peptides, most of which act within the ovary as paracrine growth factors, but at least two, inhibin and relaxin, are produced in sufficient amounts to enter the blood and produce effects in distant cells.

Estrogens

Unlike humans, most vertebrate animals mate only at times of maximum fertility of the female.

This period of sexual receptivity is called estrus, derived from the Greek word for "vehement desire." Estrogens are compounds that promote estrus and originally were isolated from follicular fluid of sow ovaries. Characteristic of steroid-secreting tissues is that little hormone is stored within the secretory cells themselves. Estrogens circulate in blood loosely bound to albumin and tightly bound to the testosterone–estrogen-binding globulin that is also called the sex hormone–binding globulin (see Chapter 12: Hormonal Control of Reproduction in the Male). Plasma concentrations of estradiol are considerably lower than those of other gonadal steroids and vary over an almost 20-fold range during the cycle.

Liver is the principal site of metabolism of the estrogens. Estradiol and estrone are completely cleared from the blood by a single passage through the liver and are inactivated by hydroxylation and conjugation with sulfate and glucuronide. About half the protein-bound estrogens in blood are conjugated with sulfate or glucuronide. Although the liver may excrete some conjugated estrogens in the bile, they are reabsorbed in the lower gut and returned to the liver in portal blood in a typical

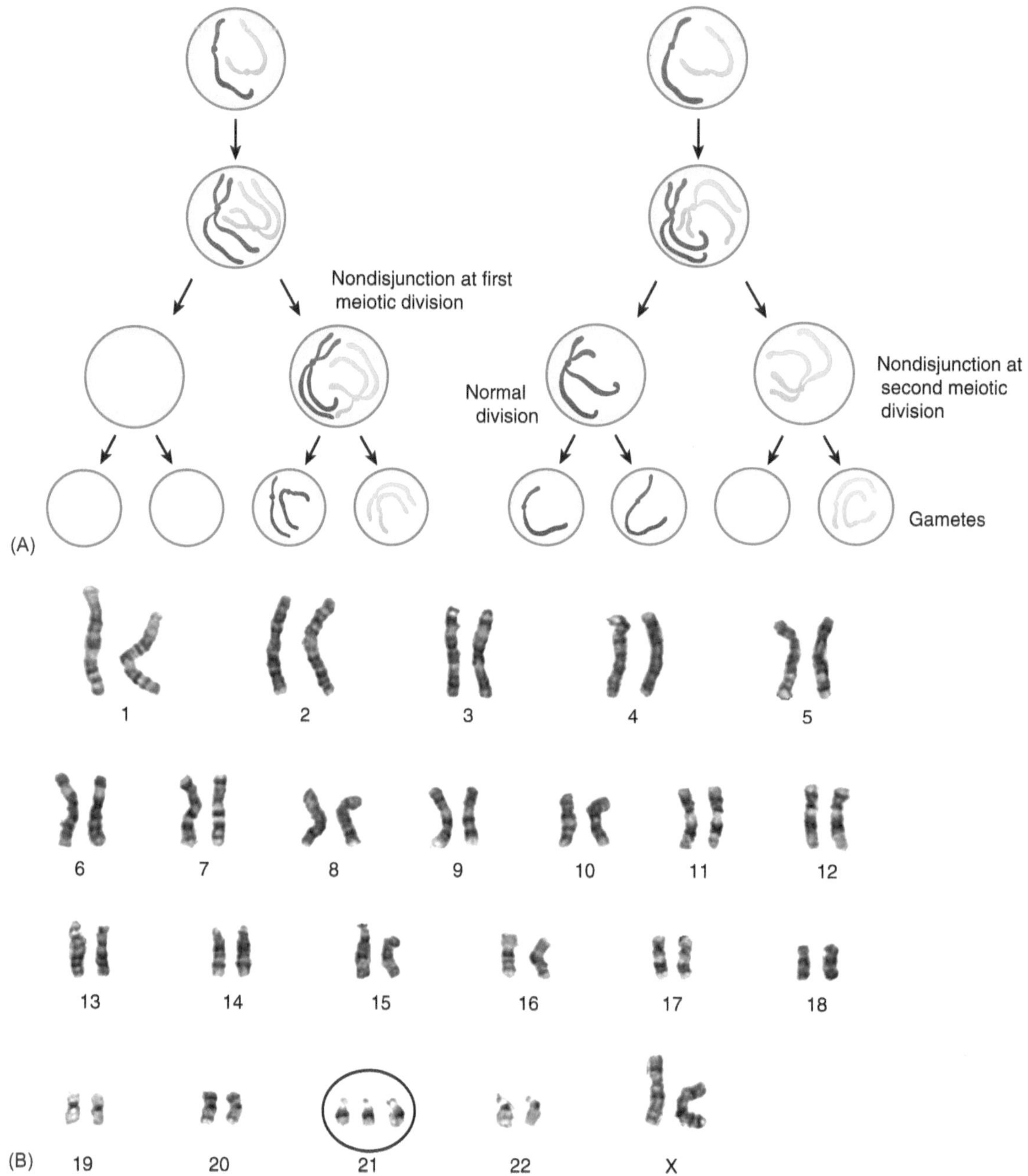

FIGURE 13.21 Nondisjunction can occur in either the first or second meiotic divisions as can be seen in (A). Illustrated in (B), below, is a karyotype of such an occurrence, in which two chromosomes of either sperm or ovum ended up in the same cell. This was joined by the gamete of the opposite sex to make a total of 3 of the number 21 chromosome, a condition called trisomy (3) 21. This is the most common trisomy resulting in survival and it is called Down syndrome. Source: *From Figure 1-8 in G. C. Schoenwolf, S. B. Bleyl, P. R. Brauer, & P. H. Francis-West. (2015).* Larson's human embryology *(5th ed.) (p. 29). Elsevier.*

enterohepatic circulatory pattern. The kidney is the chief route of excretion of estrogenic metabolites.

Progesterone

Pregnancy, or gestation, requires the presence of another ovarian steroid hormone, progesterone. In the nonpregnant woman, progesterone secretion is confined largely to cells of the corpus luteum, because it is an intermediate in the biosynthesis of all steroid hormones, small amounts may also be released from the adrenal cortex. Some progesterone is also produced by granulosa cells just before ovulation. The rate of progesterone production varies widely. Its concentration in blood ranges from virtually nil during the early

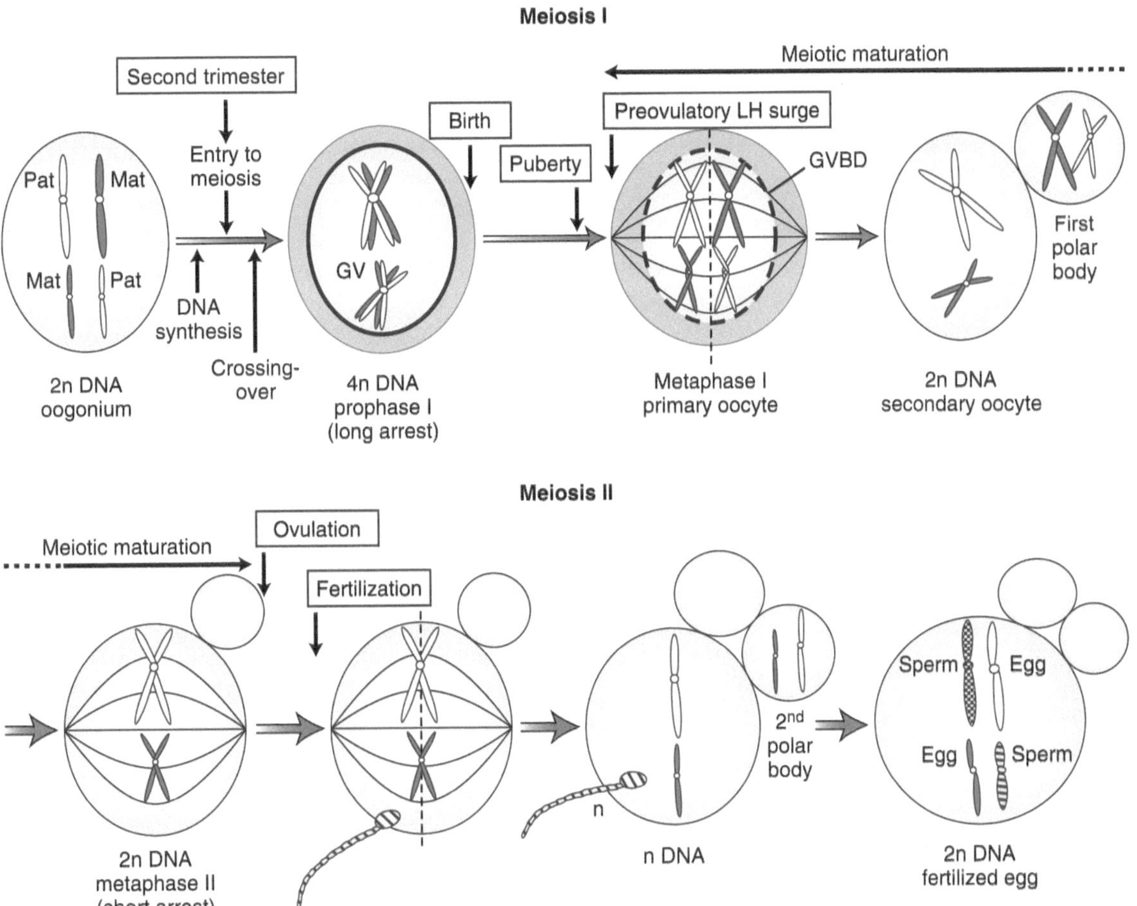

FIGURE 13.22 Meiosis I and II in the oocyte. Source: *From Figure 17-10 in Bulun, S. E. (2016). Chapter 17: Physiology and pathology of the female reproductive axis. In S. Malmed, K. S. Polonsky, P. R. Larsen, & H. M. Kronenberg (Eds.),* Williams textbook of endocrinology *(13th ed.) (p. 600). Elsevier.*

preovulatory part of the ovarian cycle to as much as 2 mg/dL after the corpus luteum has formed.

Progesterone circulates in blood in association with plasma proteins and has a high affinity for the corticosteroid-binding globulin. Liver is the principal site of progesterone inactivation, which is achieved by reduction of the A ring and the keto groups at carbons 3 and 20 to give pregnanediol that is the chief metabolite found in urine. Considerable degradation also occurs in the uterus.

Inhibin

As discussed in Chapter 12, Hormonal Control of Reproduction in the Male, inhibin is a 32 kDa disulfide-linked dimer of an α subunit and either of two β subunits, βA or βB, and enters the circulation as either inhibin A (α/βA) or inhibin B (α/βB) (Fig. 13.31).

Expression of the βA subunit is greatest in luteal cells, and expression of the βB subunit is a product of granulosa cells. Consequently, blood levels of inhibin B are highest during the periods of preovulatory growth and expansion of granulosa cells, and blood levels of inhibin A are highest during peak luteal cell function. In addition to serving as a circulating hormone, inhibin exerts paracrine actions in the ovary, and activin formed by dimerization of two β subunits also exerts important intraovarian paracrine actions. The activin-binding peptide follistatin, which blocks activin action, also plays an important intraovarian role. Although some activin is found in the circulation, its concentrations do not change during the ovarian cycle, and the source of the circulating form is primarily extraovarian.

Relaxin

The corpus luteum secretes a second peptide hormone called relaxin that was named for its ability to relax the pubic ligament of the pregnant guinea pig. In other species, including humans, it also relaxes the myometrium and plays an important role in parturition by causing softening of the uterine cervix. Relaxin is encoded in two nonallelic genes (H1 and H2) on chromosome 9.

Its peptide structure, particularly the organization of its disulfide bonds, and gene organization place it in the same family as insulin, the insulin-like growth factors (IGFs), and INSL3. Although both relaxin genes are expressed in the prostate, only the H2 gene is expressed in the ovary. A physiological role for relaxin in the nonpregnant woman has not been established.

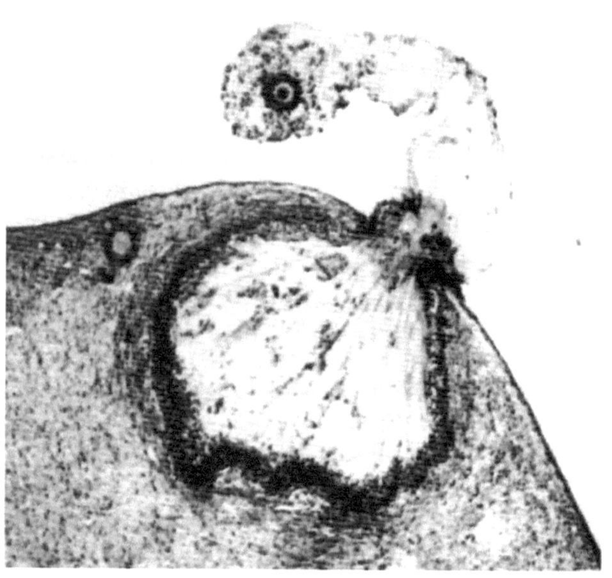

FIGURE 13.23 Ovulation in a rabbit. Follicular fluid, granulosa cells, some blood, and cellular debris continue to ooze out of the follicle even after the egg mass has been extruded. Source: *From Hafez, E. S. E., & Blandau, R. J. (1969). Gamete transport-comparative aspects. In E. S. E. Hafez, & R. J. Blandau, (Eds.),* The mammalian oviduct. *Chicago, IL: University of Chicago Press.*

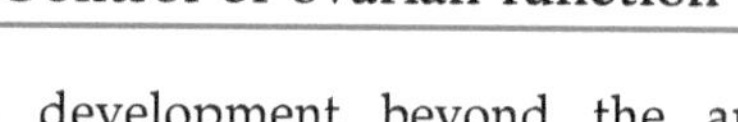

Control of ovarian function

Follicular development beyond the antral stage depends on two gonadotropic hormones secreted by the anterior pituitary gland: FSH and LH. In addition to stimulating follicular growth, gonadotropins are required for ovulation, luteinization, and steroid hormone formation by both the follicle and the corpus luteum. The relevant molecular and biochemical characteristics of these glycoprotein hormones are described in Chapter 2, Pituitary Gland, and Chapter 12, Hormonal Control of Reproduction in the Male. Follicular growth and function also depend on paracrine effects of estrogens, androgens, possibly progesterone as well as peptide paracrine factors, including IGF-II, activin, members of the TGF-β family, and others summarized in Fig. 13.32.

The sequence of rapid follicular growth, ovulation, and the subsequent formation and degeneration of the corpus luteum is repeated about every 28 days and constitutes the ovarian cycle. The part of the cycle devoted to the final rapid growth of the ovulatory follicle lasts about 14 days and is called the follicular phase. The remainder of the cycle is dominated by the corpus luteum and is called the luteal phase. It, too, lasts about 14 days. Ovulation occurs at midcycle and requires only about a day. These events are orchestrated by a complex pattern of pituitary and ovarian hormonal changes, and although ovulation and the events that surround it are the focus of these hormonal changes, preparations are underway in the background to set the stage for the next cycle in the event that fertilization does not occur.

Early growth of follicles from the primordial to the preantral stage is independent of pituitary hormones and likely is governed by paracrine factors produced by the ovum itself as well as by granulosa and thecal cells. Follicular sensitivity to gonadotropins begins at the early antral stage and gradually increases as

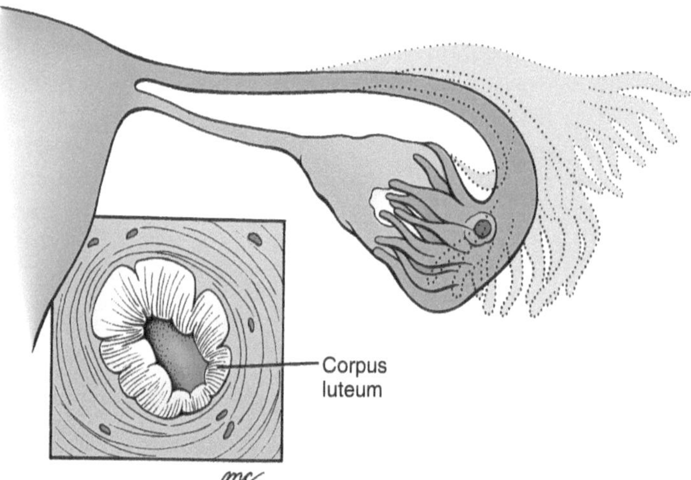

FIGURE 13.24 The fimbriae of the infundibulum of the uterine tube bend down and scrape the sticky cumulus–oocyte off the ovary. Cilia on the fimbriae then move the ovum into the opening of the uterine tube. The oocyte will remain viable (capable of being fertilized) for as long as 24 h. After that time, it cannot be fertilized. Source: *From Figure 1-13 in G. S. Schoenwolf, S. B. Bleyl, P. R. Brauer, & P. H. Francis-West. (2015).* Larson's human embryology *(5th ed.) (p. 29). Elsevier.*

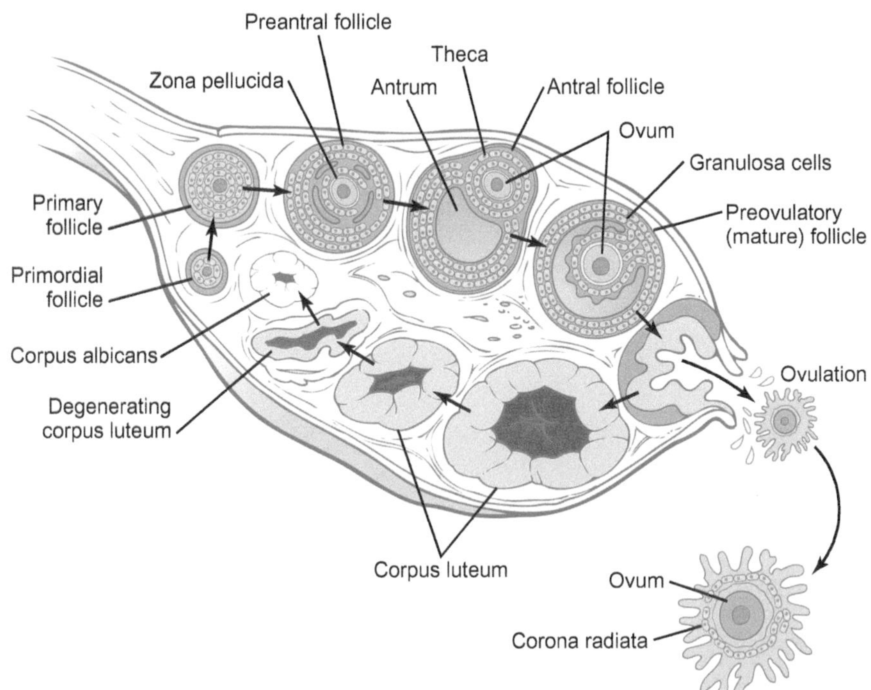

FIGURE 13.25 Stages of follicular growth in the ovary, also showing formation of the corpus luteum. Source: *From Figure 82.5 in Hall. (2016).* Guyton and Hall Textbook of Medical Physiology *(13th ed.) (p. 1040). Elsevier.*

individual follicles in each cohort slowly increase from about 0.2–2 mm in diameter, at which time they are capable of undergoing the rapid growth and development that lead to ovulation. Approximately 85 days elapse between the entry of a cohort of follicles into the gonadotropin-responsive stage and ovulation. During this time, all follicles in both ovaries are exposed to wide swings in gonadotropin concentrations, but their capacity to respond is limited by their degree of development. Ovulation occurs at the midpoint of the third cycle after the follicles reach the antral stage and have been growing in response to gonadotropins. Consequently, as the ovulatory follicle completes its final maturation, the next two cohorts already are being prepared to ovulate. The number of follicles with the potential to ovulate in each cohort is reduced by atresia at all stages of development.

Under normal circumstances, only one follicle ovulates in each cycle and appears randomly on either the right or left ovary. Usually, 6–12 follicles in each ovary are mature enough to enter into the final preovulatory growth period near the end of the luteal phase of the preceding cycle and begin to grow rapidly in response to the increase in FSH that occurs at that time. The ovulatory or "dominant" follicle from this group appears early in the follicular phase that leads to its ovulation. The physiological mechanisms for selection of a single dominant follicle are incompletely understood (see later). Recruitment of the next cohort of follicles does not begin as long as the dominant follicle or its resultant corpus luteum is present and functional.

Experimental destruction of either the dominant follicle or the corpus luteum is followed promptly by the selection and development of a new ovulatory follicle from the next cohort. Clearly at the end of the luteal phase and in the first few days of the follicular phase, multiple follicles have the potential to ovulate and can be rescued by treatment with supraphysiological amounts of FSH. This accounts for the high frequency of multiple births following some therapies for infertility. Producing multiple ova in this way is used for harvesting eggs for in vitro fertilization technologies.

Effects of follicle-stimulating hormone and luteinizing hormone on the developing follicle

Estradiol production

Granulosa cells in antral follicles are the only targets for FSH. No other ovarian cells are known to have FSH receptors. Granulosa cells of the ovulatory follicle are the major and virtually only source of estradiol in the follicular phase of the ovarian cycle and secrete estrogens in response to FSH. Until about the middle of the follicular phase, LH receptors are found only in cells of the theca interna and the stroma. LH stimulates thecal cells to produce androstenedione. Follicular synthesis of estrogen depends on complex interactions between the two gonadotropins and between theca and granulosa cells (Fig. 13.33).

Cooperative interaction of both cell types is required for physiologically relevant rates of estradiol production in the follicular phase. Neither granulosa nor theca cells express the full complement of enzymes needed for

Formation of the corpus luteum (luteinization)

Following ovulation, the follicular membrane (also called granulosa cell mural layer) of the preovulatory follicle becomes folded and is transformed into part of the corpus luteum. A surge in luteinizing hormone (LH) correlates with luteinization.

Luteinization includes the following:

(1) The lumen, previously occupied by the follicular antrum, is filled with fibrin, which is then replaced by connective tissue and new blood vessels piercing the basement membrane.

(2) Granulosa cells enlarge and lipid droplets accumulate in the cytoplasm. They become granulosa lutein cells.

(3) The spaces between the folds of the granulosa cell layer are penetrated by theca interna cells, blood vessels, and connective tissue. Theca interna cells also enlarge and store lipids. They are now theca lutein cells.

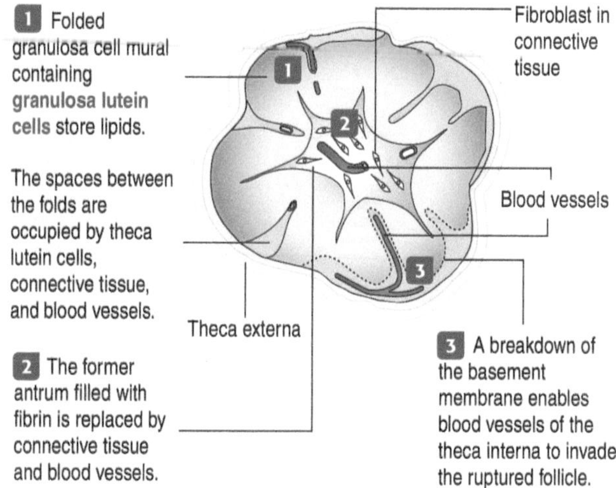

Function of the corpus luteum

The function of the corpus luteum is regulated by two gonadotropins: FSH and LH.

Follicle-stimulating hormone (FSH) stimulates the production of progesterone and estradiol by granulosa lutein cells.

LH stimulates the production of progesterone and androstenedione by theca lutein cells. Androstenedione is translocated into granulosa lutein cells for aromatization into estradiol.

During pregnancy, prolactin and placental lactogens up-regulate the effects of estradiol produced by granulosa lutein cells by enhancing the production of estrogen receptors.

Estradiol stimulates granulosa lutein cells to take up cholesterol from blood, which is then stored in lipid droplets and transported to mitochondria for progesterone synthesis.

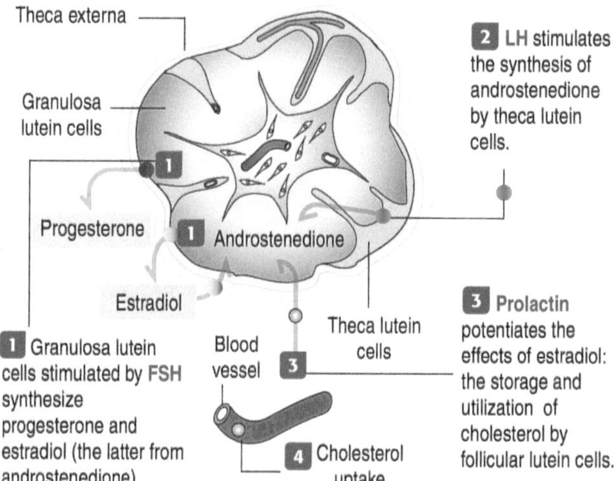

Regression of the corpus luteum (luteolysis)

If fertilization does not occur, the corpus luteum undergoes a process of regression called luteolysis.

Luteolysis involves a programmed cell death (apoptosis) sequence. It is triggered by endometrial prostaglandin F2a. The following events take place:

(1) A reduction in the blood flow within the corpus luteum causes a decline in oxygen (hypoxia).

(2) **T cells** reach the corpus luteum and produce interferon-γ, which, in turn, acts on the endothelium to enable the arrival of macrophages.

(3) Macrophages produce tumor necrosis factor ligand and the apoptotic cascade starts.

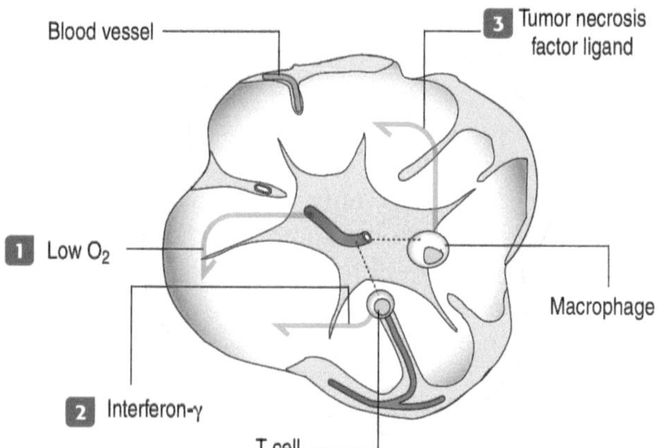

FIGURE 13.26 The life cycle of the corpus luteum. Source: *From Figure 22-6 in A.L. Kierszenbaum, & L.L. Tres. (2020).* Histology and cell biology: An introduction to pathology *(5th ed.) (p. 734). Elsevier.*

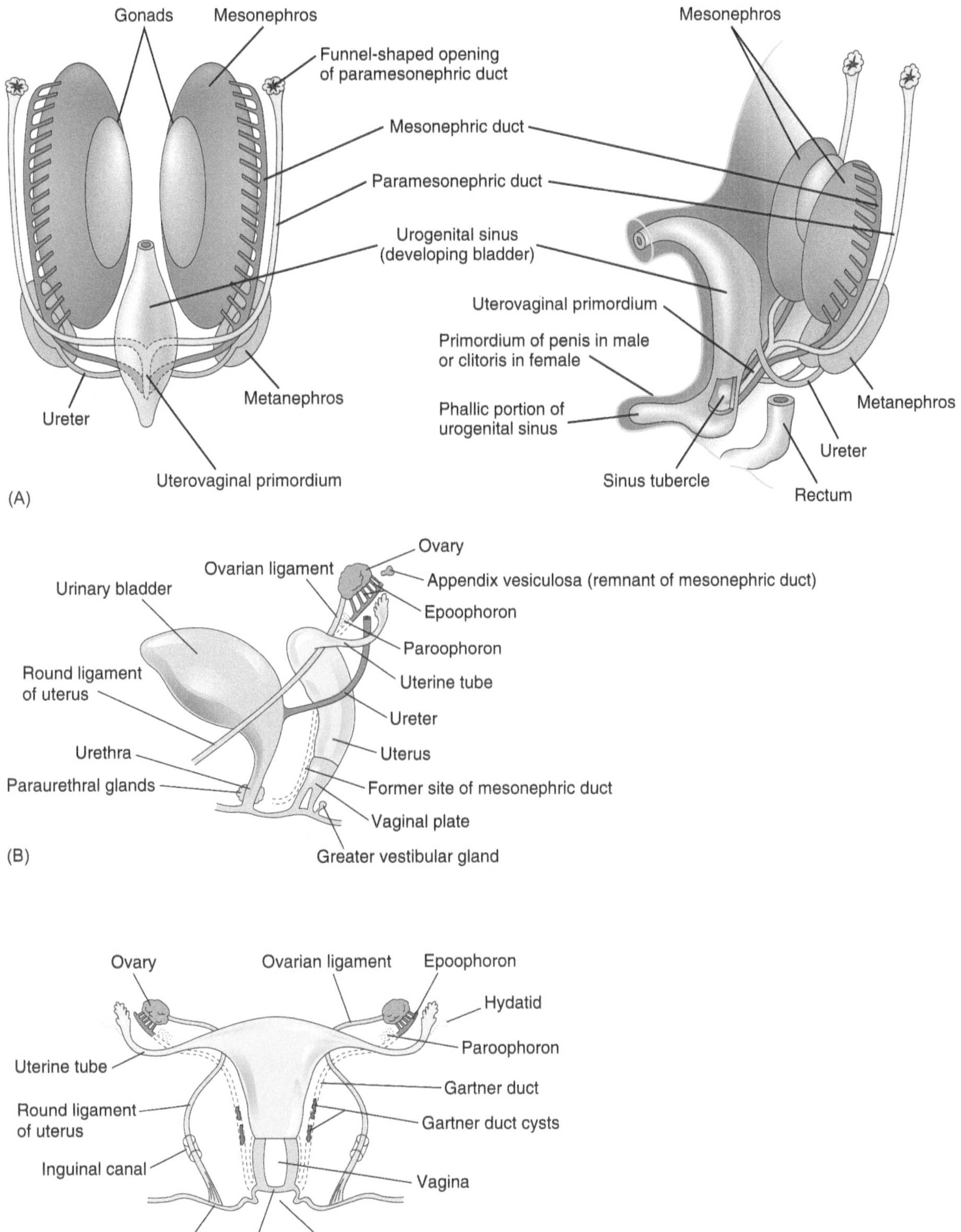

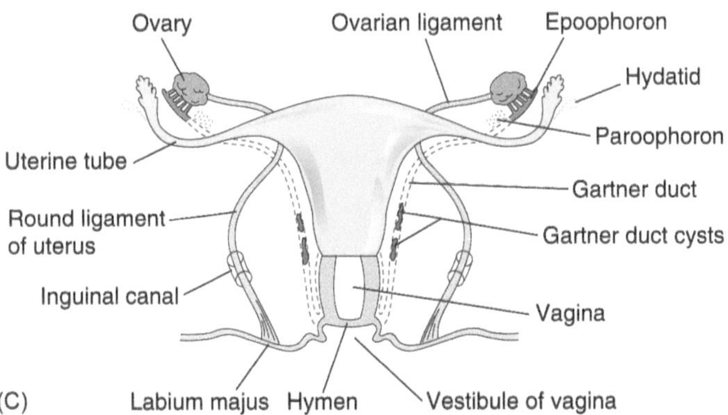

FIGURE 13.27 The formation of the uterine tubes and uterus from the paramesonephric (Müllerian) ducts. In (A), on the left, is a sketch of the structures in a 7-week-old female embryo; to the right is that of a 9-week-old female embryo; In (B), in a 12-week-old female fetus; and, in (C), in a female neonate. Source: *From Figures 12-34 and 12-33 in K. L. Moore, T. V. N. Persaud & M. G. Torcia. (2016).* The developing human *(10th ed.) (pp. 265 and 266) Elsevier.*

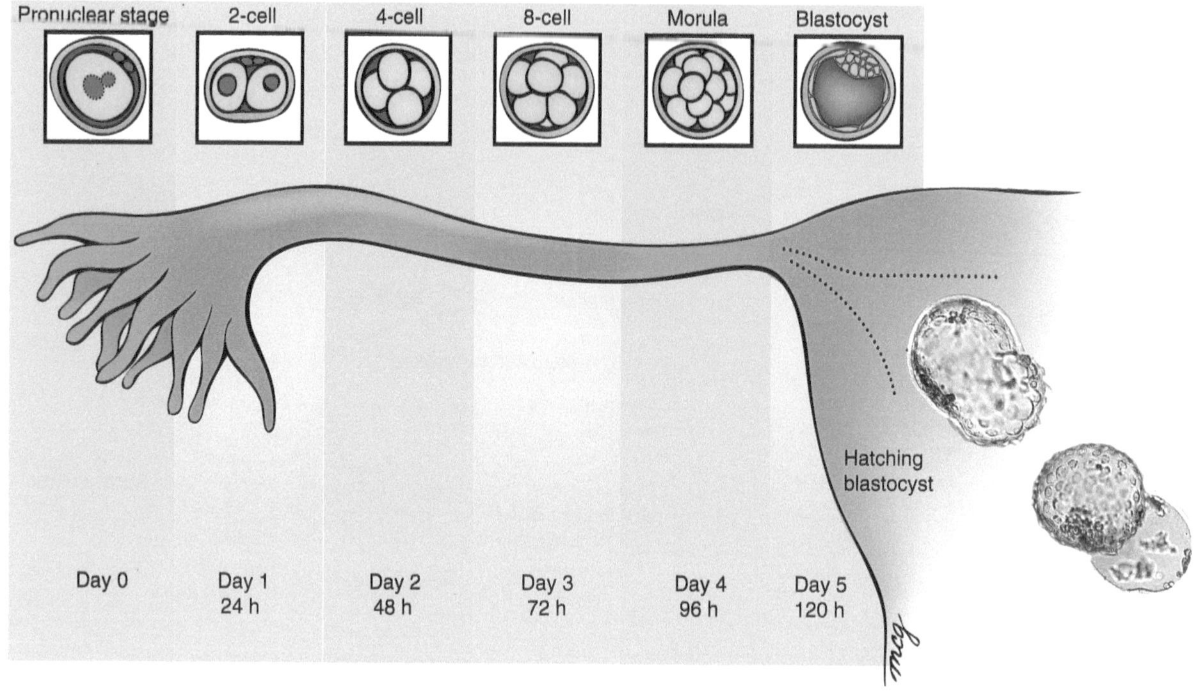

FIGURE 13.28 The movement of the fertilized embryo down the uterine tube. Source: *From Figure 1-16 in G. S. Schoenwolf, S. B. Bleyl, P. R. Brauer, & P. H. Francis-West. (2015).* Larson's human embryology *(5th ed.) (p. 36). Elsevier.*

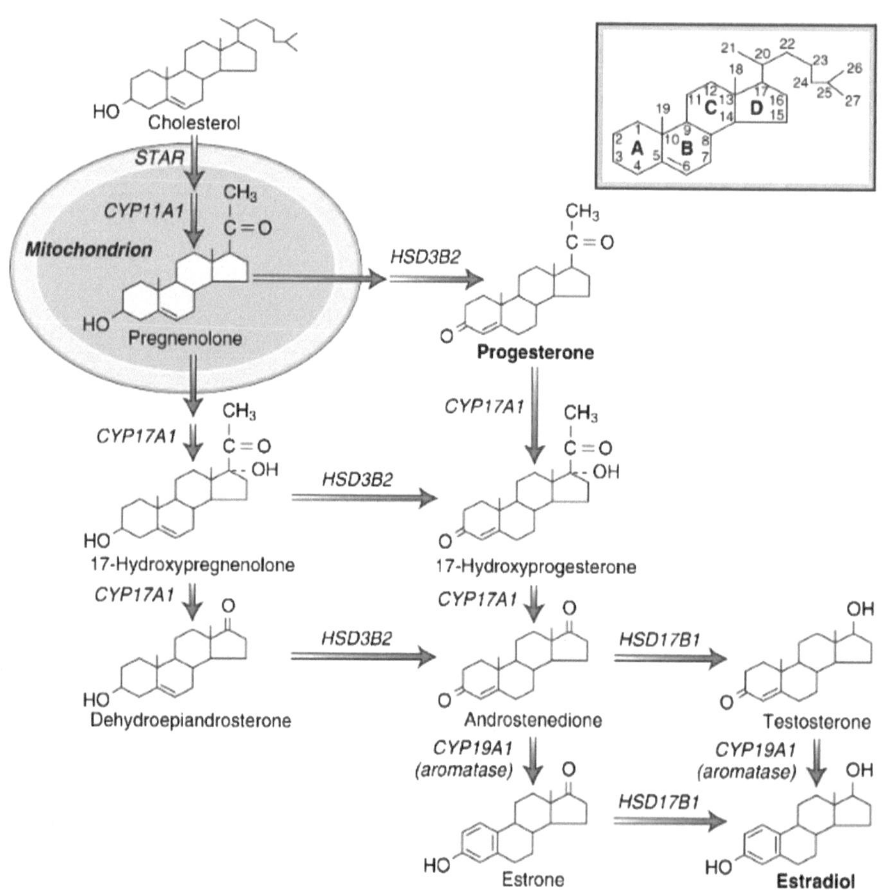

FIGURE 13.29 Steroidogenic pathway in the human ovary. The biologically active steroids progesterone and estradiol are produced primarily in the ovary of a woman of reproductive age. Estradiol production requires the activity of six steroidogenic proteins, including STAR, and six enzymatic steps. 17-Hydroxylase/17,20-lyase, the product of the CYP17A1 gene, catalyzes two enzymatic reactions. The four rings of the cholesterol molecule and its derivative steroids are identified by the first four letters in the alphabet, and the carbons are numbered in the sequence shown in the insert. CYP17A1, 17-hydroxylase/17,20-lyase; CYP19A1, aromatase; HSD17B1, 17β-hydroxysteroid dehydrogenase type 1; HSD3B2, 3β-hydroxysteroid dehydrogenase-Δ5,4 isomerase type 2; STAR, steroidogenic acute regulatory protein. Source: *From Figure 17-16 in Bulun, S. E. (2016). Chapter 17: Physiology and pathology of the female reproductive axis. In S. Malmed, K. S. Polonsky, P. R. Larsen, & H. M. Kronenberg (Eds.),* Williams textbook of endocrinology *(13th ed.) (p. 606). Elsevier.*

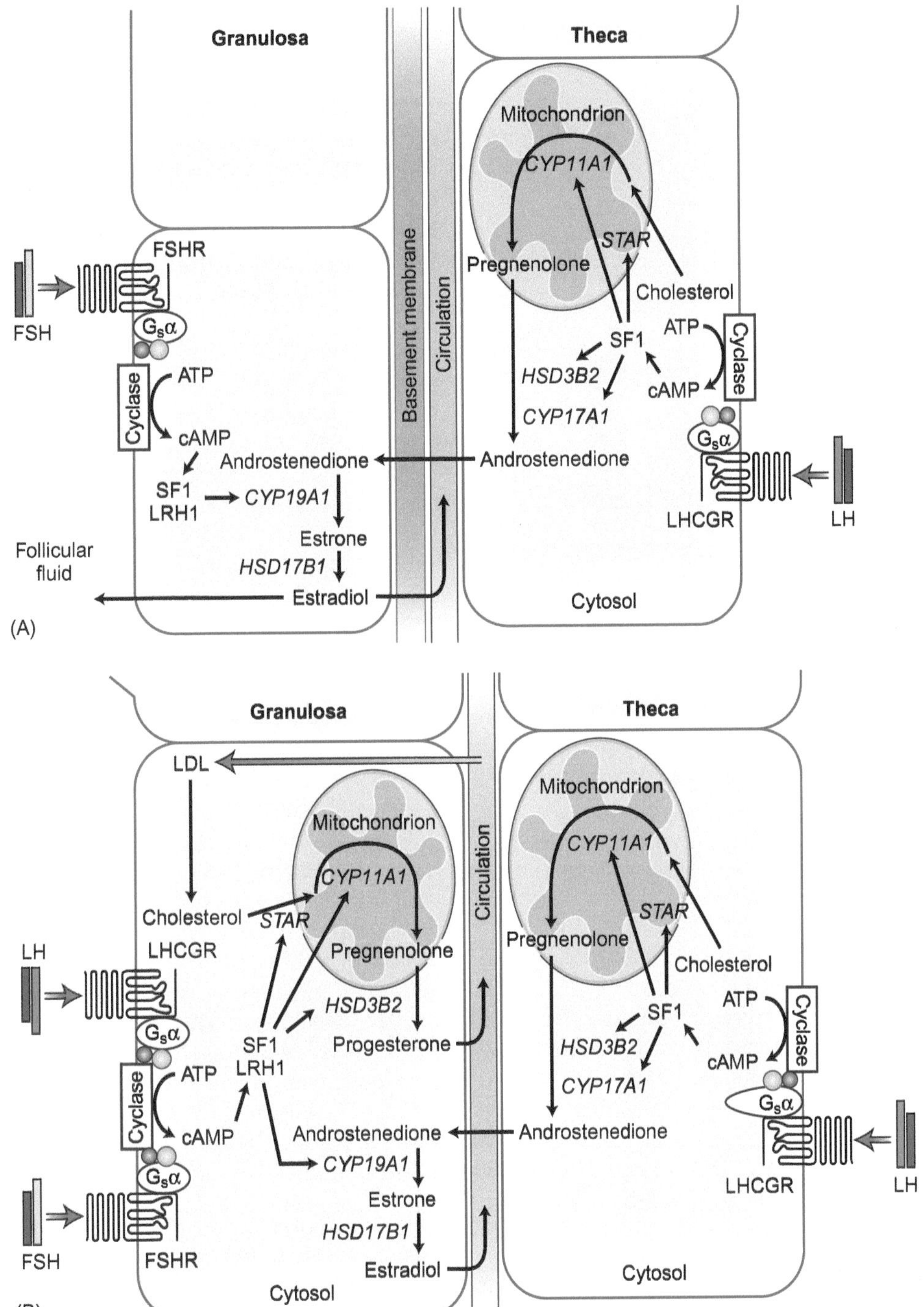

FIGURE 13.30 Two-cell hypothesis for ovarian steroidogenesis. A, The preovulatory follicle produces estradiol through a paracrine interaction between theca and granulosa cells. In response to stimulation with a gonadotropin, steroidogenic factor 1 (SF1, encoded by NR5A1, a member of the nuclear receptor family) acts as a master switch to initiate transcription of a series of steroidogenic genes in theca cells. In follicular granulosa cells, another nuclear receptor, liver homologue receptor 1 (LRH1, encoded by NR5A2), seems to primarily mediate the downstream effects of follicle-stimulating hormone (FSH) in the rodent ovary. In humans, the roles of SF1 and LRH1 in steroidogenesis in preovulatory granulosa cells are not well understood. Because granulosa cells do not have a direct connection to the circulation, CYP19A1 (aromatase) in granulosa cells depends for substrate on androstenedione that diffuses from theca cells. Two critical steps in estradiol formation are the entry of cholesterol into mitochondria facilitated by steroidogenic acute regulatory protein (STAR) in theca cells and the conversion of androstenedione to estrone catalyzed by CYP19A1 in granulosa cells. B, In the corpus luteum, granulosalutein cells are heavily vascularized, a condition that is critical for entry of abundant quantities of cholesterol into this cell type through primarily low-density lipoprotein (LDL)- cholesterol receptors and for secretion of large amounts of progesterone into the circulation. The entry of cholesterol into mitochondria (mediated by STAR) is probably the most critical steroidogenic step for progesterone formation in granulosa-lutein cells. Androstenedione produced in theca-lutein cells serves as a substrate for estrone, which is further converted to estradiol in granulosa-lutein cells. Human data suggest that LRH1 may mediate at least a portion of gonadotropin-dependent steroidogenesis in the corpus luteum. Gonadotropins, SF1, and possibly LRH1 play key roles for important steroidogenic steps in the ovary. ATP, adenosine triphosphate; cAMP, cyclic adenosine monophosphate; FSHR, FSH receptor; HSD, hydroxysteroid dehydrogenase; LHCGR, LH receptor. Source: *From Figure 17-17 in Bulun, S. E. (2016). Chapter 17: Physiology and pathology of the female reproductive axis. In S. Malmed, K. S. Polonsky, P. R. Larsen, & H. M. Kronenberg (Eds.),* Williams textbook of endocrinology *(13th ed.) (p. 608). Elsevier.*

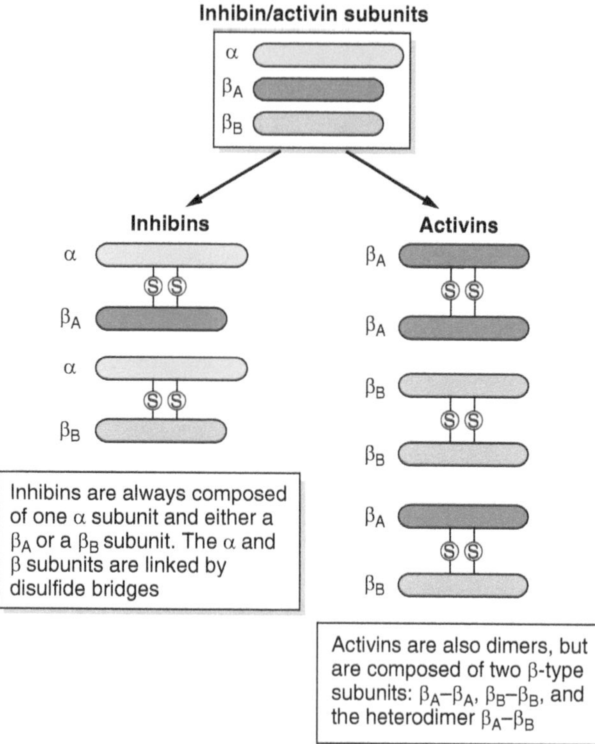

FIGURE 13.31 The inhibin and activin subunits. Source: *Redrawn from Figure 55.7 in Mesiano, S., & Jones, E. E. (2017). Chapter 55: The female reproductive system. In W. F. Boron, & E. L. Boulpaep (Eds.), Medical* physiology *(3rd ed.) (p. 1116). Elsevier.*

synthesis of estradiol. Granulosa cells are limited in their capacity to produce pregnenolone because they have little access to cholesterol delivered by the circulation in the form of low-density lipoproteins (LDL), express few LDL receptors, and have minimal levels of P450scc needed to convert cholesterol to pregnenolone. Theca cells have a direct capillary blood supply and express high levels of LDL receptors, P450scc, and P450c17. Theca cells thus can metabolize the 21 carbon pregnenolone to the 19-carbon androstenedione, but lack aromatase, and hence cannot synthesize estrogens.

Granulosa cells, on the other hand, express ample aromatase but cannot produce its 19-carbon substrate because they lack P450c17. However, granulosa cells readily aromatize androgens provided by diffusion from the theca interna. This two-cell interaction is illustrated in Fig. 13.7. The participation of two different cells, each stimulated by its own gonadotropin, accounts for the requirement of both pituitary hormones for adequate estrogen production and hence for follicular development.

Follicular development

Under the influence of FSH, granulosa cells in the follicle destined to ovulate increase by more than 100-fold, and the follicle expands about 10-fold in diameter, mainly because of the increase in follicular fluid. Differentiation of granulosa cells leads to increased expression of many genes, including the gene for the LH receptor. In early antral follicles, granulosa cells have few if any receptors for LH and are unresponsive to it.

By about the middle of the follicular phase, granulosa cells in the dominant follicle begin to express increasing amounts of LH receptors that become quite abundant just prior to ovulation. Acquisition of LH receptors in response to FSH enables these cells to respond to both FSH and LH. Induction of LH receptors and other actions of FSH on follicular development are amplified by paracrine actions of peptide growth factors and steroid hormones. In response to FSH, granulosa cells secrete IGF-II, inhibin, activin, and other growth factors, including vascular endothelial growth factor (VEGF), which greatly increase vascularization around the theca. IGF-II not only stimulates the growth and secretory capacity of granulosa cells but also acts synergistically with LH to increase synthesis of androgens by cells of the theca interna. Similarly, inhibin produced by granulosa cells in response to FSH also stimulates thecal cell production of androgens, and activin enhances FSH-induced expression of P450 aromatase in the granulosa cells. Even though theca cells lack FSH receptors, they nevertheless respond indirectly to FSH with increased production of the androgens required by the granulosa cells for estrogen secretion. Similarly, by stimulating thecal cells to produce androgens, LH augments growth and development of granulosa cells through the paracrine actions of both estrogens and androgens whose receptors are abundantly expressed in these cells (Fig. 13.34).

These events constitute a local positive feedback circuit that gives the dominant follicle progressively greater capacity to produce estradiol and makes it increasingly sensitive to FSH and LH as it matures. However, some mechanism must exist to maintain the balance between androgen production in thecal cells and their aromatization in granulosa cells, as accumulation of androgens prevents ovulation.

Cellular actions of follicle-stimulating hormone and luteinizing hormone

FSH and LH each bind to specific G-protein coupled receptors on the surface of granulosa or theca cells and activate adenylyl cyclase in the manner already described (Chapter 1: Introduction, and Chapter 12: Hormonal Control of Reproduction in the Male). Their effects are thus additive in this regard. Increased concentrations of cyclic AMP activate protein kinase A, which catalyzes phosphorylation of cyclic AMP response element–binding protein and other nuclear and cytoplasmic proteins that ultimately lead to increased transcription of genes that encode growth factors and other proteins critical for cell growth and steroid hormone production. As described for adrenal cortical (see Chapter 4: The Adrenal Glands) and Leydig cells (see Chapter 12: Hormonal Control of Reproduction in the Male), the rate-limiting step in steroid hormone synthesis requires synthesis of the steroid acute

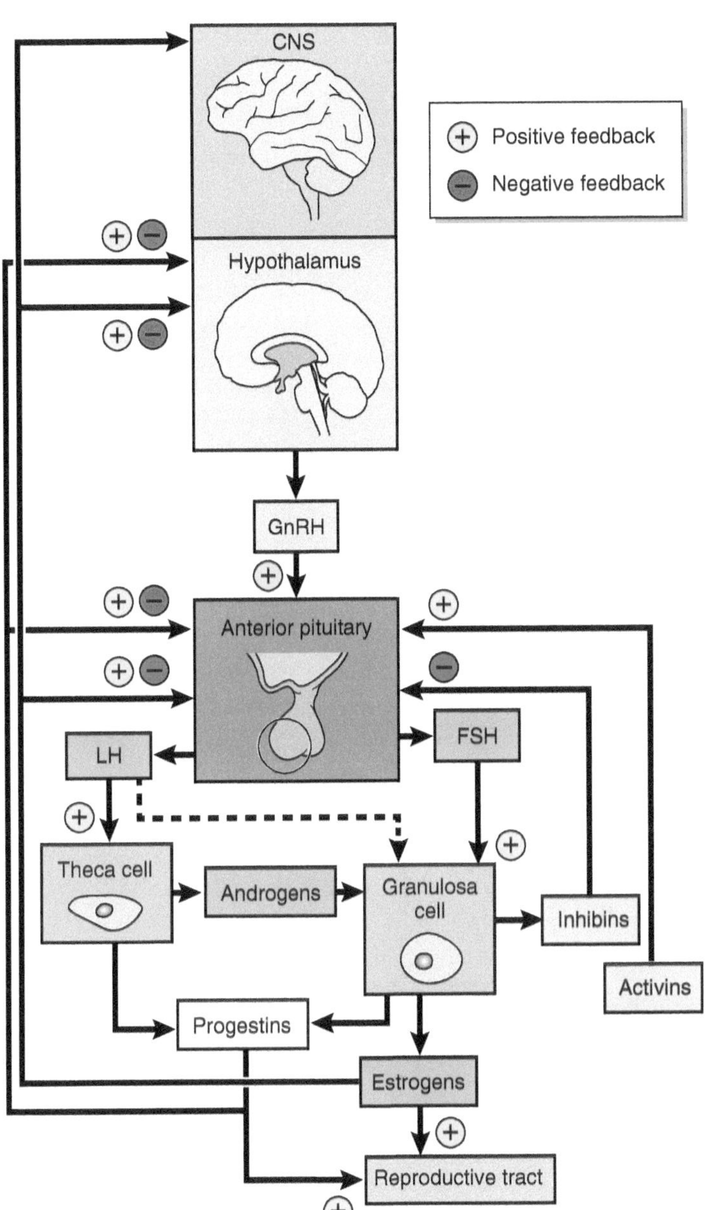

FIGURE 13.32 The major hormones that regulate ovarian function. *CNS*, Central nervous system; *FSH*, follicle-stimulating hormone; *GnRH*, gonadotropin-releasing hormone; *LH*, luteinizing hormone. Source: *Redrawn from Figure 55-3 in Mesiano, S., & Jones, E. E. (2017). The female reproductive system. In W. F. Boron, & E. L. Boulpaep (Eds.),* Medical physiology *(3rd ed.) (p. 1112). Elsevier.*

regulatory protein to deliver cholesterol to the intramitochondrial enzyme P450scc that converts it to pregnenolone (Fig. 13.7). In addition, activation of protein kinase A results in increased expression of P450c17 in theca cells and P450 aromatase in granulosa cells (Fig. 13.7). Along with increased expression of growth factors, the ripening follicle also expresses increased amounts of a protease that specifically cleaves IGF-binding protein-4 (IGFBP-4) that is present in follicular fluid and thereby increases the availability of free IGF-II. These events are summarized in Fig. 13.35.

Effects on ovulation

LH is the physiological signal for ovulation. Its concentration in blood rises sharply and reaches a peak about 16 hours before ovulation (see later). Blood levels of FSH also increase at this time, and although large amounts of FSH can also cause ovulation, the required concentrations are not achieved during the normal reproductive cycle. The events that lead to follicular rupture and expulsion of the ovum are complex and not fully understood, but the process is known to be initiated by increased production of cyclic AMP in theca and granulosa cells in response to LH and the consequent release of paracrine factors and enzymes. To date, more than 88 ovulation-related genes are known to be activated by LH at this time. Many of the changes associated with ovulation resemble changes associated with inflammation, including expression of such inflammatory cytokines as tumor necrosis factor α and interleukins 1 and 6.

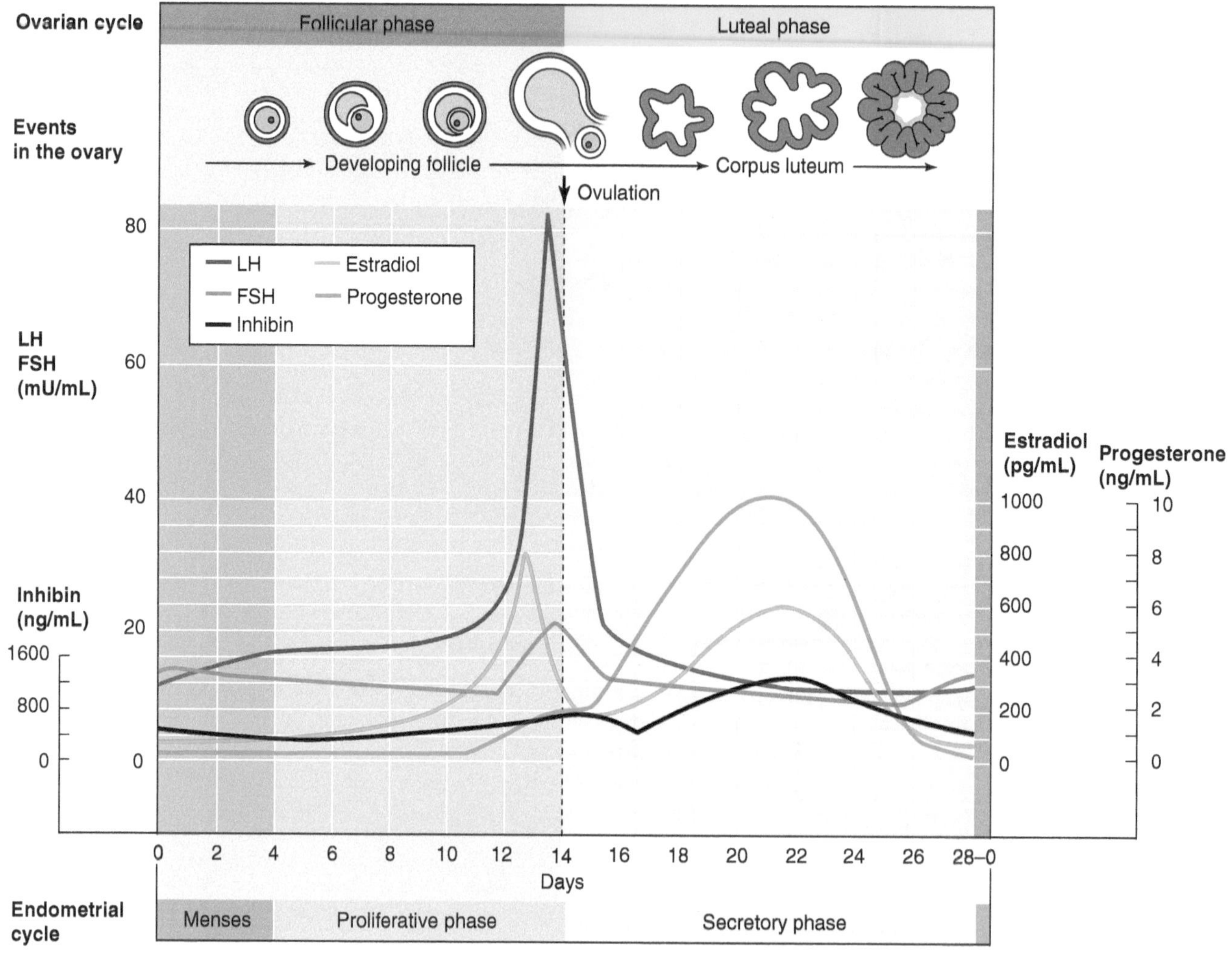

FIGURE 13.33 The estradiol and progesterone levels during the menstrual cycle. Source: *Redrawn from Figure 55-6 in Mesiano, S., & Jones, E. E. (2017). The female reproductive system. In W. F. Boron, & E. L. Boulpaep (Eds.),* Medical physiology *(3rd ed.) (p. 1115). Elsevier.*

As the follicle approaches ovulation, it accumulates follicular fluid, but despite the preovulatory swelling, intrafollicular pressure does not increase. The follicular wall becomes increasingly distensible due to activity of proteolytic enzymes that digest the collagen framework and other proteins of the intercellular matrix. Because of their newly acquired receptors, granulosa cells of the preovulatory follicle respond to LH by secreting progesterone just prior to ovulation.

Progesterone, which is essential for ovulation, acts as an autocrine stimulator of granulosa cells. In response to progesterone, granulosa cells secrete plasminogen activator, which activates the proteolytic enzyme plasmin that has accumulated in follicular fluid in the form of its inactive precursor, plasminogen. Progesterone also upregulates expression of cyclooxygenase 2 and hence the formation of prostaglandins (see Chapter 4: The Adrenal Glands). The findings that pharmacological blockade of either prostaglandin or progesterone synthesis prevents ovulation indicate that these agents play essential roles in the ovulatory process. Prostaglandins appear to activate release of lysosomal proteases in a discrete region of the follicle wall called the stigma. In addition, progesterone stimulates granulosa cells to secrete matrix metalloproteinases (MMPS) that digest collagenase and other supporting proteins in the follicular wall. One of these MMPS, called ADAMTS-1 (A Disintegrin and Metalloproteinase with ThromboSpondin repeats), increases more than 10-fold and causes the cumulus oophorous complex to expand and break loose from the granulosa cells of the follicle wall. Expansion of the cumulus oophorous complex also facilitates ovum transport in the fallopian tubes. As a result of these actions, the extracellular matrix of the theca and the surface epithelium break down and the ovum and its surrounding cumulus oophorous are extruded into the abdominal cavity.

Although little or no progesterone is produced throughout most of the follicular phase, stimulation of granulosa cells of the preovulatory follicle by LH endows them with the capacity to produce progesterone. LH upregulates expression of LDL receptors, P450scc, and doubtless other relevant proteins required for uptake of cholesterol and its conversion to pregnenolone. Because the capacity to remove the side chain at carbon 17 remains limited, 21-carbon steroids are formed faster than they can be processed to estradiol and hence are secreted as progesterone. Furthermore, as granulosa cells acquire the ability to respond to LH, they also begin to lose aromatase activity. This is reflected in the abrupt decline in estrogen production that just precedes ovulation.

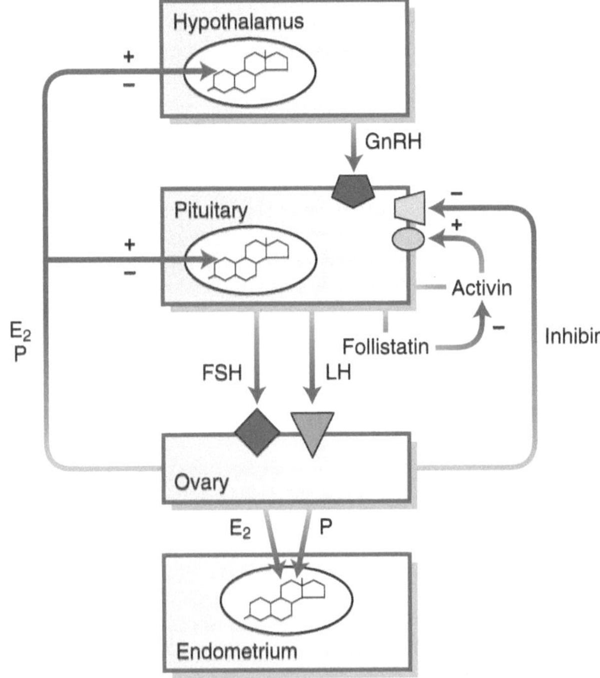

FIGURE 13.34 The hypothalamus–pituitary–ovary–endometrium axis, including feedback. Source: *From Figure 17-1B in Bulun, S. E. (2016). Chapter 17: Physiology and pathology of the female reproductive axis. In S. Malmed, K. S. Polonsky, P. R. Larsen, & H. M. Kronenberg (Eds.),* Williams textbook of endocrinology *(13th ed.) (p. 591). Elsevier.*

Effects on corpus luteum formation

LH was named for its ability to induce the formation of the corpus luteum after ovulation. However, as already mentioned, luteinization may actually begin before the follicle ruptures. Granulosa cells removed from mature follicles complete their luteinization in tissue culture without further stimulation by gonadotropin. Nevertheless, luteinization within the ovary depends on LH and is accelerated by the increased concentration of LH that precedes ovulation. The formation of the corpus luteum results largely from hypertrophy of granulosa cells whose cytoplasm increases about 10-fold as they acquire about a 100-fold increase in their capacity to produce steroid hormones. Occasionally, luteinization occurs in the absence of ovulation and results in the syndrome of luteinized unruptured follicles, which may be a cause of infertility in some women whose reproductive cycles seem otherwise normal.

The development of a vascular supply is critical for the development of the corpus luteum and its function. Although granulosa cells of the preovulatory follicle are avascular, the corpus luteum is highly vascular, and when fully developed, each steroidogenic cell appears to be in contact with at least one capillary. After extrusion of the ovum, infolding of the collapsing follicle causes the highly vascular theca interna to interdigitate with layers of granulosa cells that line the follicular wall. Under the influence of LH, granulosa cells express high levels of VEGF that

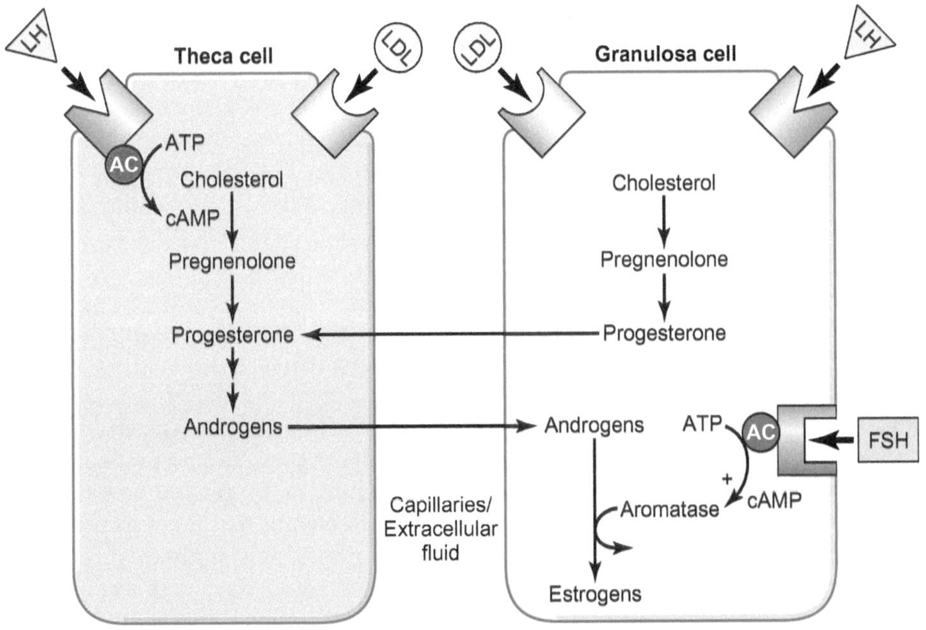

FIGURE 13.35 Interaction of follicular theca and granulosa cells for production of estrogens. The theca cells, under the control of luteinizing hormone (LH), produce androgens that diffuse into the granulosa cells. In mature follicles, follicle-stimulating hormone (FSH) acts on granulosa cells to stimulate aromatase activity, which converts the androgens to estrogens. AC, adenylate cyclase; ATP, adenosine triphosphate; cAMP, cyclic adenosine monophosphate; LDL, low-density lipoproteins. Source: *From Figure 82-8 in Hall. (2016).* Guyton and Hall Textbook of Medical Physiology *(13th ed.) (p. 1044). Elsevier.*

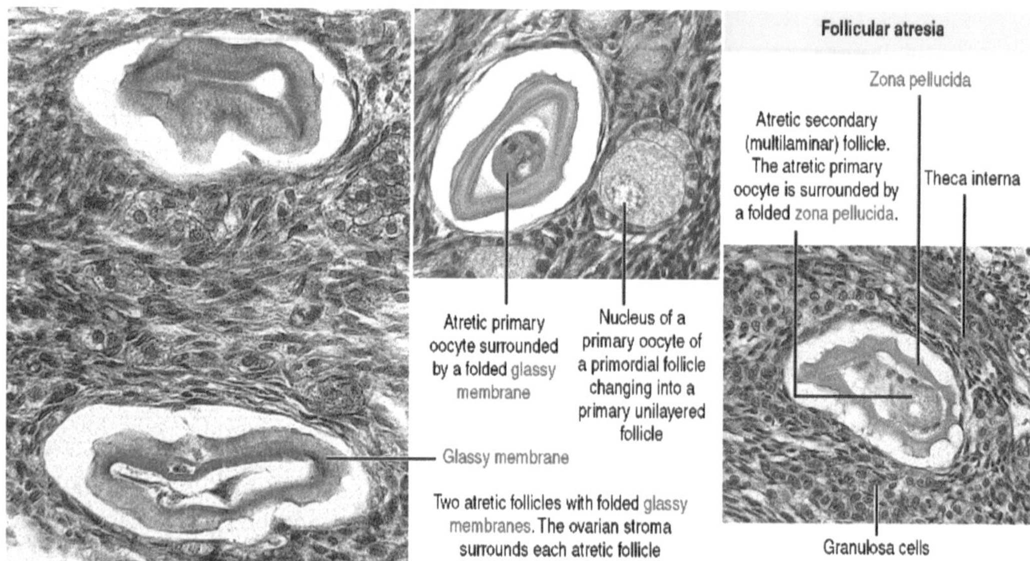

FIGURE 13.36 The interaction between the granulosa and theca lutein cells in the corpus luteum. Source: *From Figure 22-5 in A. L. Kierszenbaum & L. L. Tres (2020). Histology and cell biology: An introduction to pathology (5th ed.) (p. 733). Elsevier.*

stimulates growth and differentiation of capillary endothelial cells. It has been estimated that vascular endothelial cells make up fully half of the cells of the mature corpus luteum. The interaction between the theca lutein and granulosa lutein cells in the corpus luteum is summarized in Fig. 13.35. Although a group of about ten follicle starts to mature at the beginning of an ovulatory cycle, only one of those, the dominant follicle will mature to ovulation. The remaining follicles become atretic (Fig. 13.36).

Effects on oocyte maturation

Granulosa cells not only provide nutrients to the ovum but also prevent it from completing its meiotic division until the time of ovulation. Granulosa cells are thought to secrete a substance called OMI into follicular fluid. LH triggers resumption of meiosis at the time of ovulation perhaps by blocking production of this factor or interfering with its action.

Effects on corpus luteal function

The maintenance of steroid production by the corpus luteum depends on continued stimulation with LH. Decreased production of progesterone and premature demise of the corpus luteum is seen in women whose secretion of LH is blocked pharmacologically. In this respect, LH is said to be luteotropic. The corpus luteum has a finite life span, however, about a week after ovulation becomes progressively less sensitive to LH and finally regresses despite continued stimulation with LH. Estradiol and prostaglandin-F2α, which are produced by the corpus luteum, can hasten luteolysis and may be responsible for its demise. We do not understand the mechanisms that limit the functional life span of the human corpus luteum.

Effects on ovarian blood flow

LH also increases blood flow to the ovary and produces ovarian hyperemia. Luteinization is accompanied by production of VEGF and other angiogenic factors that increase vascularization. Blood flow may be further enhanced by release of histamine or perhaps prostaglandins. Increased ovarian blood flow increases the opportunity for delivery of steroid hormones to the general circulation and for delivery to the ovary of cholesterol-laden LDL needed to support high rates of steroidogenesis. Increased blood flow to the developing follicle may also be important for preovulatory swelling of the follicle, which depends on increased elaboration of fluid from blood plasma.

Physiological actions of ovarian steroid hormones

As just described, intraovarian actions of estradiol and progesterone are intimately connected to ovulation and formation of the corpus luteum. In general, extraovarian actions of these hormones ensure that the ovum reaches its potential to develop into a new individual. Ovarian steroids act on the reproductive tract to prepare it for fulfilling its role in fertilization, implantation, and development of the embryo, and they induce changes elsewhere that equip the female physically and behaviorally for conceiving, giving birth, and rearing the child.

Although estrogens, perhaps in concert with progesterone, drive females of subprimate species to mate, androgens, rather than estrogens, are responsible for libido in humans of either sex.

Estrogens and progesterone tend to act in concert and sometimes enhance or antagonize each other's actions. Estradiol secretion usually precedes progesterone secretion and primes target tissues to respond to progesterone. Estrogens induce the synthesis of progesterone receptors; and without estrogen priming, progesterone has little biological effect. Conversely, progesterone downregulates its own receptors and estrogen receptors in some tissues and thereby decreases responses to estrogens.

Effects on the reproductive tract

At puberty, estrogens promote growth and development of the uterine tubes, uterus, vagina, and external genitalia. Estrogens stimulate cellular proliferation in the mucosal linings as well as in the muscular coats of these structures. Even after they have matured, maintenance of size and function of internal reproductive organs requires continued stimulation by estrogen and progesterone. Prolonged deprivation after ovariectomy results in severe involution of both muscular and mucosal portions. Dramatic changes are also evident, especially in the mucosal linings of these structures, as steroid hormones wax and wane during the reproductive cycle. These effects of estrogen and progesterone are summarized in Table 13.2.

Menstruation

Nowhere are the effects of estrogen and progesterone more obvious than in the endometrium.

Estradiol secreted by the developing follicle increases the thickness of the endometrium by stimulating growth of epithelial cells in terms of both number and size. Endometrial glands form and elongate. Endometrial growth is accompanied by increased blood flow, especially through the spiral arteries, which grow rapidly under the influence of estrogens. This stage of the uterine cycle is known as the proliferative phase and coincides with the follicular phase of the ovarian cycle. Progesterone secreted by the corpus luteum causes the newly proliferated endometrial lining to differentiate and become secretory. This action is consistent with its role of preparing the uterus for nurture and implantation of the newly fertilized ovum if successful mating has occurred. The so-called uterine milk secreted by the endometrium is thought to nourish the blastocyst until it can implant. This portion of the uterine cycle is called the secretory phase and coincides with the luteal phase of the ovarian cycle (Figs. 13.37–13.39).

Maintaining the thickened endometrium depends on the continued presence of the ovarian steroid hormones. After the regressing corpus luteum loses its ability to produce adequate amounts of estradiol and progesterone, the outer portion of the endometrium degenerates and is sloughed into the uterine cavity. The mechanism for shedding the uterine lining is incompletely understood, although prostaglandin-F2α appears to play an important role, perhaps in producing vascular spasm and ischemia and in stimulating release of lysosomal proteases. Loss of the proliferated endometrium is accompanied by bleeding. This monthly vaginal discharge of blood is known as menstruation. The typical menstrual period lasts 3–5 days, and the total flow of blood seldom exceeds 50 mL. The first menstrual bleeding, called menarche, usually occurs at about age 13. Menstruation continues at monthly intervals until menopause, normally interrupted only by periods of pregnancy and lactation.

TABLE 13.2 Effects of Estrogen and Progesterone on the Reproductive Tract.

Organ	Estrogen	Progesterone
Uterine tubes	↑Celia formation and activity	↓Contractility
Muscular wall	↑Secretion	↓Secretion
	↑Contractility	
Uterus		
Endometrium	↑Proliferation	↑Differentiation and secretion
Myometrium	↑Growth and contractility	↓Contractility
Cervical glands	Watery secretion	Dense, viscous secretion
Vagina	↑Epithelial proliferation	↑Epithelial differentiation
	↑Glycogen deposition	↓Epithelial proliferation

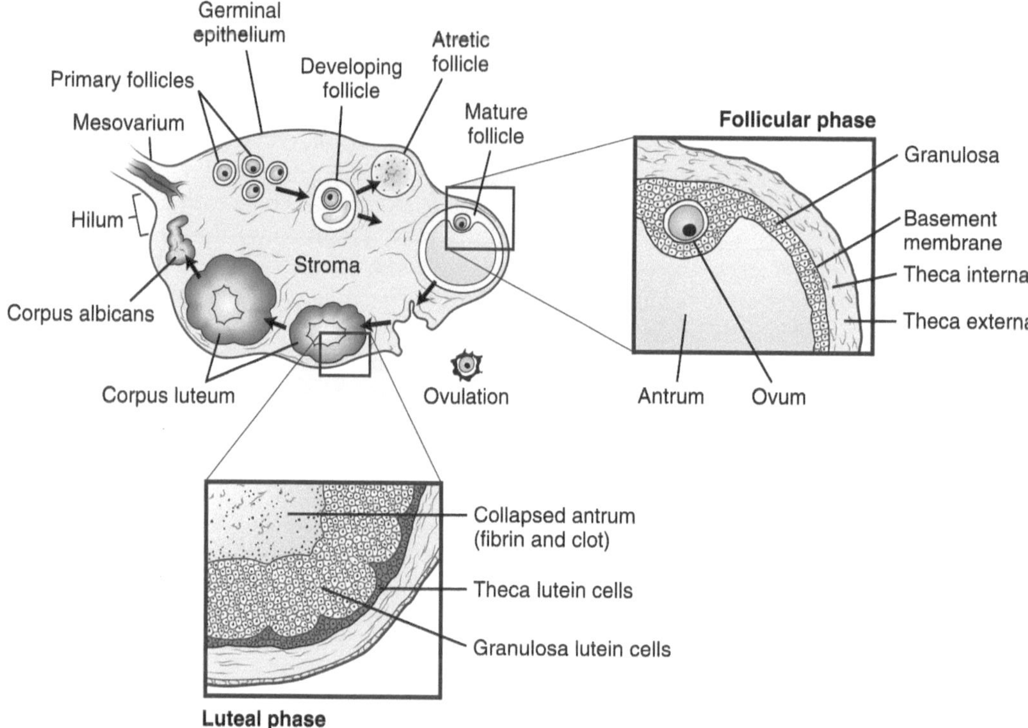

FIGURE 13.37 The mature follicle affects the follicular phase of the endometrial cycle, and the corpus luteum affects the luteal phase as the name implies. Source: *From Figure 17-6 in Bulun, S. E. (2016). Chapter 17: Physiology and pathology of the female reproductive axis. In S. Malmed, K. S. Polonsky, P. R. Larsen, & H. M. Kronenberg (Eds.),* Williams textbook of endocrinology *(13th ed.) (p. 596). Elsevier.*

In the myometrium, estradiol increases expression of contractile proteins, gap junction formation, and spontaneous contractions. In its absence, uterine muscle is insensitive to stretch or other stimuli for contraction. Further estrogen stimulation increases the irritability of uterine smooth muscle and, in particular, increases its sensitivity to oxytocin, in part as a consequence of inducing uterine oxytocin receptors (see Chapter 14: Hormonal Control of Pregnancy and Lactation). The latter phenomenon may be of significance during parturition. Progesterone counteracts these effects and decreases both the amplitude and frequency of spontaneous contractions. Withdrawal of progesterone prior to menstruation is accompanied by increased myometrial prostaglandin formation. Myometrial contractions in response to prostaglandins are thought to account for the discomfort that precedes menstruation.

Effects on the mammary glands

Development of the breasts begins early in puberty and is due primarily to estrogens that promote development of the duct system and growth and pigmentation of the nipples and areolar portions of the breast. In cooperation with progesterone, estradiol may also increase the lobuloalveolar portions of the glands, but alveolar development also requires the pituitary hormone prolactin (see Chapter 14: Hormonal Control of Pregnancy and Lactation). Secretory components, however, account for only about 20% of the mass of the adult breast. The remainder is stromal tissue and fat. Estrogens also stimulate stromal proliferation and fat deposition. It is important to recognize that the ovaries are not the only source of the estradiol that is available to the breast. Aromatization of abundant adrenal androgens, dihydroepiandrosterone, and androstenedione by breast tissues is a major source of estrogens, particularly in postmenopausal women. The responsiveness of all breast tissue elements to growth-promoting effects of estrogens is a significant factor in neoplastic breast disease. Some forms of breast cancer remain partially or completely dependent on estrogens for growth. Pharmacological blockade of aromatase or treatment with estrogen antagonists therefore has life-prolonging benefits in patients afflicted with such tumors.

Other effects of ovarian hormones

Estrogens also act on the body in ways that are not necessarily related to reproduction (Fig. 13.40).

In this regard, it is important to remember that estrogens are formed locally as well as in the ovaries and that many of these actions are not limited to women. As

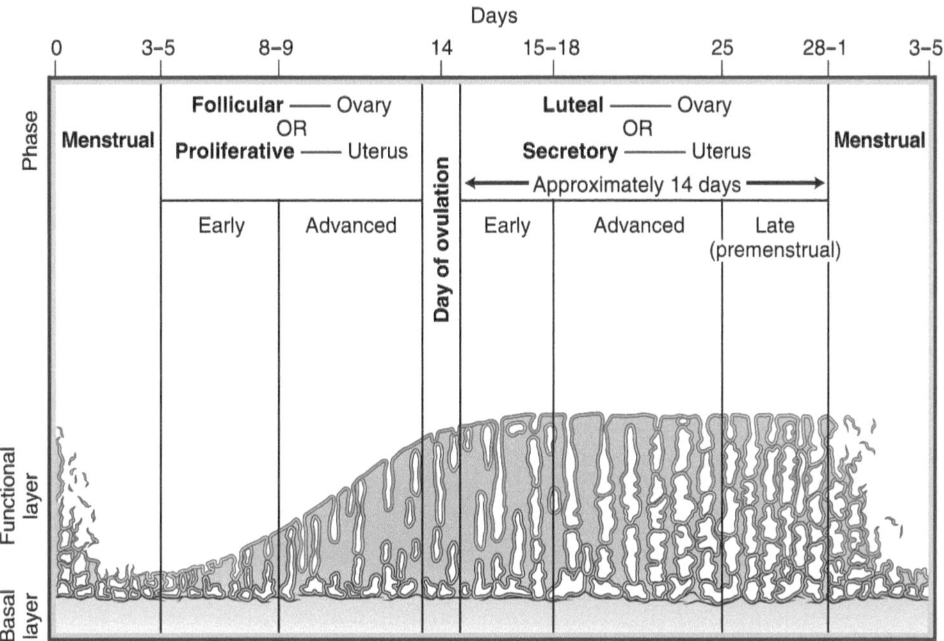

FIGURE 13.38 The menstrual cycle. See Figure 13.41 for the hormonal rise and fall. Source: *From Figure 17-21 in Bulun, S. E. (2016). Chapter 17: Physiology and pathology of the female reproductive axis. In S. Malmed, K. S. Polonsky, P. R. Larsen, & H. M. Kronenberg (Eds.),* Williams textbook of endocrinology *(13th ed.) (p. 612). Elsevier.*

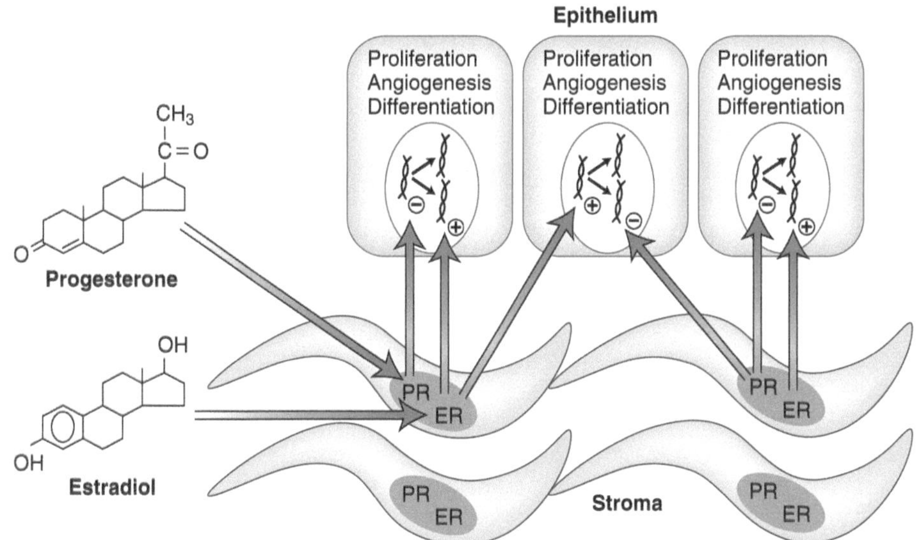

FIGURE 13.39 Effect of progesterone and estradiol on the stroma and epithelium of the endometrium of the uterus. Source: *From Figure 17-22 in Bulun, S. E. (2016). Chapter 17: Physiology and pathology of the female reproductive axis. In S. Malmed, K. S. Polonsky, P. R. Larsen, & H. M. Kronenberg (Eds.),* Williams textbook of endocrinology *(13th ed.) (p. 613). Elsevier.*

already indicated (see Chapter 11: Hormonal Control of Growth), estrogens contribute to the pubertal growth spurt by directly stimulating the growth of cartilage progenitors, closure of the epiphyseal plates, and increased growth hormone secretion. In adolescent females and males, estrogens increase bone density, and in the adult, they contribute to the maintenance of bone density by stimulating osteoblastic activity and inhibiting bone resorption. Estrogens can also cause selective changes in bone structure, especially widening of the pelvis, which facilitates passage of the infant through the birth canal.

They promote deposition of subcutaneous fat particularly in the thighs and buttocks and increase hepatic synthesis of steroid- and thyroid hormone–binding proteins. Based on epidemiological evidence, estrogens are considered to have cardiovascular protective effects, although recent studies of hormone replacement therapy in postmenopausal women have challenged this idea.

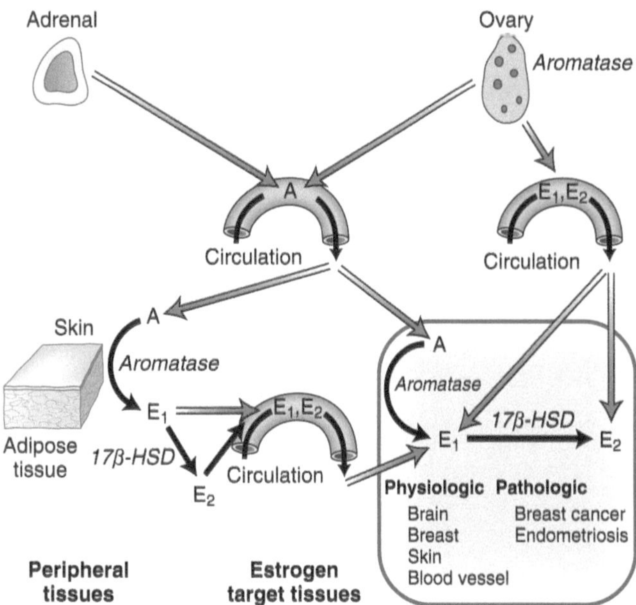

FIGURE 13.40 Effect of estrogens on other tissues. Source: *From Figure 17-19 in Bulun, S. E. (2016). Chapter 17: Physiology and pathology of the female reproductive axis. In S. Malmed, K. S. Polonsky, P. R. Larsen, & H. M. Kronenberg (Eds.),* Williams textbook of endocrinology *(13th ed.) (p. 611). Elsevier.*

Nevertheless, estrogen receptors are present in both endothelium and vascular smooth muscle, as well as cardiac muscle, and estrogens can acutely decrease vascular tone. In addition, estrogens have been found to alter plasma lipid profiles and may protect against atherogenesis. Estradiol also acts on various cells in the central nervous system and is responsible for some behavioral patterns, especially in lower animals. More recently, evidence has been brought forth that estrogens may protect cognitive functions.

Progesterone also acts on the central nervous system. In addition to its effects on regulation of gonadotropin secretion (see later), it may produce changes in behavior or mood. Progesterone has a mild thermogenic effect and may increase basal body temperature by as much as 1°F.

Because the presence of progesterone indicates the presence of a corpus luteum, a woman can readily determine when ovulation occurred and hence the time of maximum fertility, by monitoring her temperature daily. This simple, noninvasive procedure has been helpful for couples seeking to conceive a child or who are practicing the "rhythm method" of contraception. Progesterone also increases the sensitivity of the respiratory center to carbon dioxide and therefore causes mild hyperventilation. It is curious that more dramatic effects may result from withdrawal of progesterone than from administering it. Thus withdrawal of progesterone may trigger menstruation, lactation, parturition, and the postpartum psychological depression experienced by many women.

Mechanism of action

Estrogens and progesterone, like other steroid hormones, readily penetrate cell membranes and bind to receptors that are members of the nuclear receptor superfamily of transcription factors (see Chapter 1: Introduction). In addition, various rapid nongenomic effects of both hormones have been reported, but the molecular processes involved in these actions are incompletely understood. Two separate estrogen receptors, designated ERα and ERβ, are products of different genes and are expressed in many different cells in both reproductive and nonreproductive tissues of both men and women. Their DNA-binding domains are almost identical. Although some differences are present in their ligand binding domains, ERα and ERβ differ mainly in the amino acid sequences of their activation function domains. Therefore they interact with different transcriptional coactivator and other nuclear regulatory proteins to control expression of different sets of genes. Upon binding ligand, ERα and EBβ may form homo- or heterodimers before binding to DNA in estrogen-sensitive genes. The resulting synthesis of new messenger RNA is followed in turn by the formation of a variety of proteins that modify cellular activity.

Both receptors can also be activated by phosphorylation in the absence of ligand, and both receptors can modulate the transcription activating properties of other nuclear regulatory proteins without directly binding to DNA. Estrogen receptors, like most other hormone receptors, tolerate minor variations in the structures of the ligands they bind. Estrogen receptors have the interesting property of assuming different conformational changes depending upon the structure of the particular ligand that is bound. Because the conformation of the liganded receptor profoundly affects its ability to interact with other transcription regulators whose expression is cell type specific, some compounds produced in plants (phytoestrogens) or pharmaceutically manufactured antiestrogens may interfere with the expression of estrogen effects in some tissues without compromising estrogen actions in other tissues.

In addition, some compounds may activate ERα but antagonize actions of ERβ. These properties have given rise to a very important category of drugs called selective estrogen receptor modulators (SERMs), which, for example, may block the undesirable proliferative or neoplastic actions of estrogens on the breast or uterus while mimicking desirable effects on maintenance of bone density in postmenopausal women. One of these compounds, tamoxifen, which blocks estrogen action on the breast, has been used widely in treatment of estrogen-sensitive breast cancers. However, the perfect SERM has not yet been found, and aromatase inhibitors, which are more effective in suppressing breast cancers, are gaining favor and are used increasingly. Selective receptor modulation is not limited to estrogen receptors but also is seen with other nuclear receptors, including the progesterone and androgen receptors.

Two isoforms of the progesterone receptor, progesterone receptor A (PRA) and progesterone receptor B (PRB), are expressed by progesterone-responsive cells. They are products of the same gene that is transcribed from alternate promoters and translated starting at two different sites in the mRNA. PRA and PRB differ by the presence of an additional sequence of 164 amino acids at the amino terminus of PRB. This extension provides an additional region for interacting with nuclear regulatory proteins.

Liganded PRs bind to the DNA of target genes as homo- or heterodimers and in different combinations may activate different subsets of genes. When expressed together in some cells, liganded PRA can repress the activity of PRB. Both PRA and PRB expression are induced by prior exposure of cells to estrogens and can repress the activity or expression of ERα.

Regulation of the reproductive cycle

Ovulation is the central and signature event of each ovarian cycle. It follows selection and maturation of the dominant follicle and is triggered by a massive increase in blood LH concentration. This surge of LH secretion must be timed to occur when the ovum and its follicle are ready. The corpus luteum must secrete its hormones to optimize the opportunity for fertilization and establishment of pregnancy. The period after ovulation during which the ovum can be fertilized is brief, lasting less than 24 hours. If fertilization does not occur, a new follicle must be prepared. Coordination of these events requires two-way communication between the pituitary and the ovaries, and between the ovaries and the reproductive tract. Examination of the changing pattern of hormones in blood throughout the ovarian cycle provides some insight into these communications.

Pattern of hormones in blood during the ovarian cycle Fig. 13.41 illustrates daily changes in the concentrations of major hormones in a typical cycle extending from one menstrual period to the next.

The most remarkable feature of the profile of gonadotropin concentrations is the dramatic peak in LH and

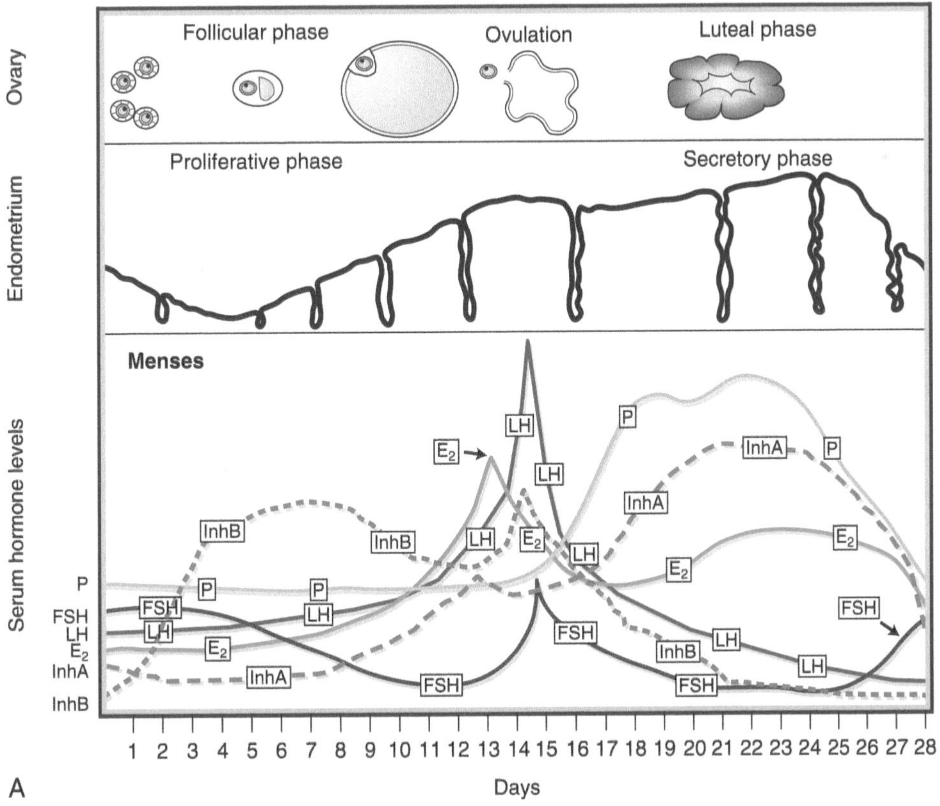

FIGURE 13.41 The changes in the follicle, endometrium thickness, and the hormone cycle during a 28-day menstrual cycle. *E2*, Estradiol; *FSH*, follicle-stimulating hormone; *inhA*, inhibin α; *inhB*, inhibin β; *LH*, luteinizing hormone; *P*, progesterone. Source: *From Figure 171 in Bulun, S. E. (2016). Chapter 17: Physiology and pathology of the female reproductive axis. In S. Malmed, K. S. Polonsky, P. R. Larsen, & H. M. Kronenberg (Eds.),* Williams textbook of endocrinology *(13th ed.) (p. 591). Elsevier.*

FSH that precedes ovulation. Except for the 2–3 days of the midcycle peak, LH concentrations remain at nearly constant low levels throughout the follicular and luteal phases. The concentration of FSH is also low through much of the cycle but begins to rise to a secondary peak late in the luteal phase, 2 or 3 days before the onset of menstruation, before declining again in the early follicular phase.

The ovarian hormones follow a different pattern. Early in the follicular phase, the concentration of estradiol is low. It then gradually increases at an increasing rate until it reaches its zenith about 12 hours before the peak in LH. Thereafter estradiol levels fall abruptly and reach a nadir just after the LH peak. During the luteal phase, there is a secondary rise in estradiol concentration that then falls to the early follicular level a few days before the onset of menstruation. Progesterone is barely or not at all detectable throughout most of the follicular phase and then begins to rise along with LH at the onset of the ovulatory peak. Progesterone continues to rise and reaches its maximum concentration several days after the LH peak.

Progesterone levels remain high for about 7 days and then gradually fall and reach almost undetectable levels a day or two before the onset of menstruation. Inhibin B concentrations are low early in the follicular phase and then rise and fall in parallel with FSH. The apparent peak that coincides with ovulation is thought to result from the absorption of inhibin B already present in high concentration in the expelled follicular fluid rather than concurrent secretion by granulosa cells. Concentrations of inhibin A reach their highest levels in the luteal phase before declining in parallel with progesterone.

Regulation of follicle-stimulating hormone and luteinizing hormone secretion

At first glance, this pattern of hormone concentrations is unlike anything seen for other anterior pituitary hormones and the secretions of their target glands. Indeed, there are unique aspects, but during most of the cycles, gonadotropin secretion is under negative feedback control similar to that seen for thyroid-stimulating hormone (see Chapter 3: Thyroid Gland), adrenal corticotropic hormone (see Chapter 4: The Adrenal Glands), and the gonadotropins in men (see Chapter 12: Hormonal Control of Reproduction in the Male). The ovulatory burst of FSH and LH secretion is brought about by a positive feedback mechanism unlike any we have considered. Secretion of FSH and LH also is controlled by GnRH that is released in synchronized pulsatile bursts from neurons whose cell bodies reside in the arcuate nuclei and the medial preoptic area of the hypothalamus (see Chapter 2: Pituitary Gland, and Chapter 12: Hormonal Control of Reproduction in the Male).

Negative feedback aspects

As we have seen, FSH and LH stimulate production of ovarian hormones (Fig. 13.7). In the absence of ovarian hormones, after ovariectomy or menopause, concentrations of FSH and LH in blood may increase as much as 5- to 10-fold. Treatment with low doses of estrogen lowers circulating concentrations of gonadotropins to levels seen during the follicular phase. When low doses of estradiol are given to subjects whose ovaries are intact, inhibition of gonadotropin secretion results in failure of follicular development. Progesterone alone, unlike estrogen, is ineffective in lowering high levels of FSH and LH in the blood of postmenopausal women, but it can synergize with estrogen to suppress gonadotropin secretion. These findings exemplify classic negative feedback. Inhibin may also provide some feedback inhibition of FSH secretion during the follicular phase and may contribute to the low level of FSH during the luteal phase, but its effects are probably small (Fig. 13.42).

In ovariectomized rhesus monkeys the normal pattern of gonadotropin concentrations can be reproduced by treating with only estradiol and progesterone. The secondary rise in FSH concentration at the end of the luteal phase most likely results from relief of feedback inhibition by estrogen, progesterone, and inhibin. Throughout the follicular and luteal phases of the cycle, steroid concentrations appear to be sufficient to suppress LH secretion.

Although the ovarian steroids and inhibin suppress FSH and LH secretion, estrogen and progesterone concentrations change during the cycle in ways that seem independent of gonadotropin concentrations. For example, estrogen rises dramatically as the follicular phase progresses, even though LH remains constant and FSH is diminishing. The mechanism for this increase in estradiol is implicit in what has already been presented and is consistent with negative feedback. Estrogen production by the maturing follicle increases without a preceding increase in gonadotropin concentration because the mass of responsive theca and granulosa cells increases as does their sensitivity to gonadotropins. In fact, the decrease in FSH during the transition from early to late follicular phase probably results from feedback inhibition by the increasing concentration of estradiol, perhaps in conjunction with inhibin B.

Although luteinizing cells do not divide, progesterone and estrogen concentrations continue to increase during the early luteal phase, well after FSH and LH have returned to basal levels.

Increasing steroid hormone production at this time reflects completion of the luteinization process.

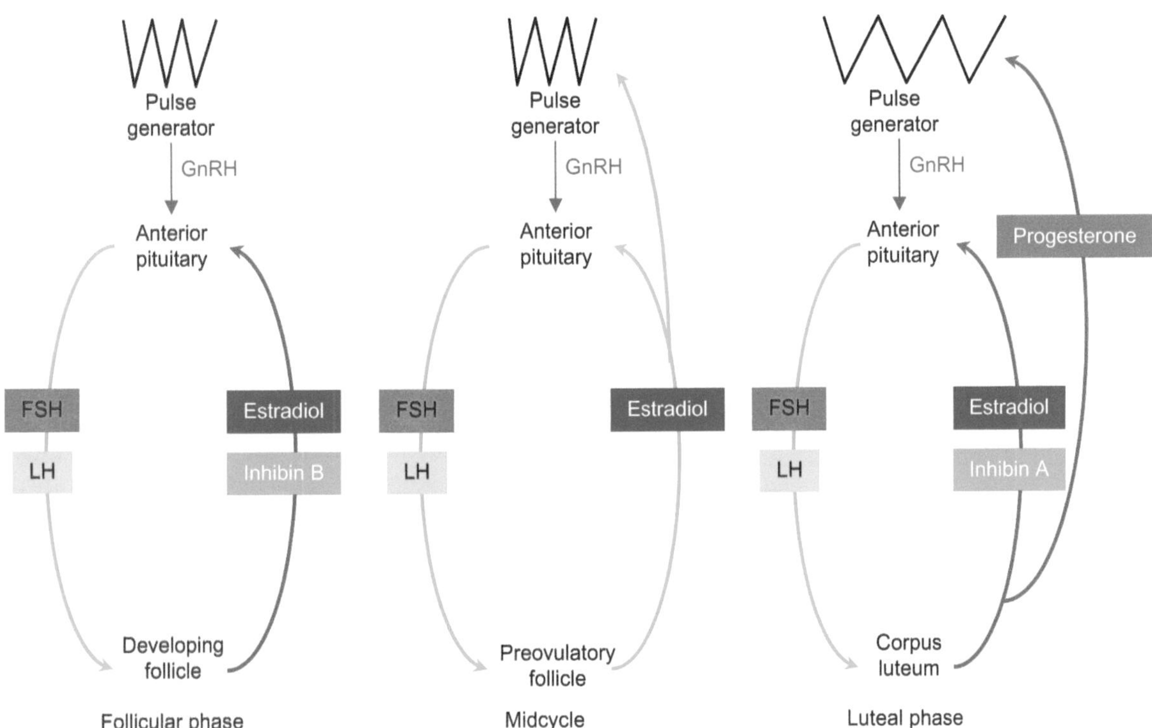

FIGURE 13.42 Ovarian–pituitary interactions at various phases of the menstrual cycle. Green arrows represent stimulation, red arrows indicate inhibitory effects.

Conversely, the gradual loss of sensitivity of luteal cells to LH accounts for the decrease in progesterone and estrogen secretion during the latter part of the luteal phase. Thus one of the unique features of the female reproductive cycle is that changes in steroid hormone production result more from changes in the number or sensitivity of competent target cells than from changes in gonadotropin concentrations (see Chapter 5: Principles of Hormone Integration).

Selection of the dominant follicle

The negative feedback aspects of regulation of the ovarian cycle play a critical role in follicular development and probably in selection of the dominant follicle, although the mechanism for selection remains speculative. The next cohort of follicles begins its preovulatory growth in response to the increased secretion of FSH that results from relief of feedback inhibition by estradiol and progesterone as the corpus luteum declines (Fig. 13.43).

Although the increase in FSH seen at this time is considerably less dramatic than the surge that precedes ovulation, it is sufficient to reach the required stimulatory threshold. Although perhaps 10 or more follicles have the potential to respond to FSH, their development is not precisely synchronized. It may be recalled that recruitment of primordial follicles from their dormant state to preantral growth is independent of gonadotropin and occurs randomly. Even small differences in development enable the most advanced follicle to respond more readily to FSH and produce estradiol and other factors that synergize with FSH to accelerate granulosa cell multiplication and development. Consequently, as this follicle grows, it becomes increasingly sensitive to FSH and secretes increasing amounts of estradiol and inhibin. Negative feedback effects of these secretions cause FSH concentrations in plasma to fall below the threshold needed to sustain the growth of the other, less developed follicles, which become atretic and die.

Increasing sensitivity of granulosa cells in the ovulatory follicle to LH and FSH presumably compensates for declining concentrations of FSH and permits continued development to the preovulatory stage.

Positive feedback aspects

The sustained increase in estradiol in the late follicular phase triggers the massive burst of LH secretion that just precedes ovulation. This LH surge can be duplicated experimentally in monkeys and women given sufficient estrogen to raise their blood levels above a critical threshold level for 2–3 days. This compelling evidence implicates increased estrogen secretion by the ripening follicle as the causal event that triggers the massive release of

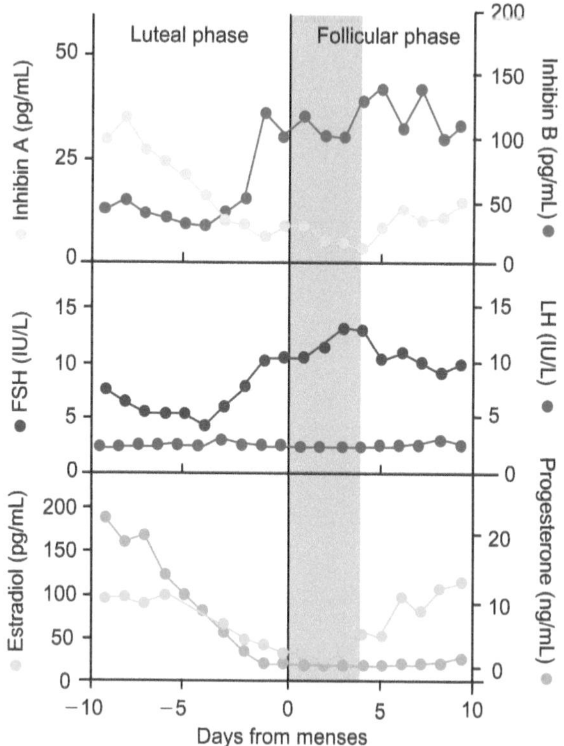

FIGURE 13.43 Mean plasma concentrations of reproductive hormones at the luteal–follicular transition. The data are similar to those shown in Fig. 13.10 but are normalized around the start of menstruation instead of the LH peak value and highlight the changes in FSH concentrations associated with development and selection of the ovulatory follicle. *FSH*, Follicle-stimulating hormone; *LH*, luteinizing hormone. Source: *Adapted from Welt, C. K., Martin, K. A., Taylor, A. E., Lambert-Messerlian, G. M., Crowley, W. F. Jr., Smith J. A., et al. (1997). Frequency modulation of follicle-stimulating hormone (FSH) during the luteal-follicular transition: Evidence for FSH control of inhibin B in normal women.* The Journal of Clinical Endocrinology and Metabolism, 82, *2645–2652.*

LH and FSH from the pituitary (Fig. 13.11, midcycle). It can be considered positive feedback because LH stimulates estrogen secretion, which in turn stimulates more LH secretion in a self-generating explosive pattern. Progesterone concentrations begin to rise about 6 hours before ovulation. This change is probably a response to the increase in LH rather than its cause. It is significant that when given in large doses progesterone blocks the estrogen-induced surge of LH that may account for the absence of repeated LH surges during the luteal phase, when the concentrations of estrogen might be high enough to trigger the positive feedback effect (Fig. 13.11, luteal phase). This action of progesterone, which may contribute to the decline in the LH surge, also contributes to its effectiveness as an oral contraceptive agent. In this regard, progesterone also inhibits follicular growth. Synthetic progestins are the basic ingredient of hormonal contraceptives and may be administered alone or in combination with estrogens.

Synthetic compounds devised for this use bind to progesterone receptors but are considerably more resistant to hepatic degradation than their natural counterparts. Most synthetic progestins are derivatives of androgens. In addition to blocking the LH surge, progestins stimulate the production of a thick cervical mucus that provides a barrier to the entry of sperm into the uterine cavity.

Neural control of gonadotropin secretion

It is clear that secretion of gonadotropins is influenced to a large measure by ovarian steroid hormones. It is equally clear that secretion of these pituitary hormones is controlled by the central nervous system. Gonadotropin secretion ceases after the vascular connection between the anterior pituitary gland and the hypothalamus is interrupted or after the arcuate nuclei of the medial basal hypothalamus are destroyed. Less drastic environmental inputs, including rapid travel across time zones, stress, anxiety, and other emotional changes, can also affect reproductive function in women, presumably through neural input to the medial basal hypothalamus. As discussed in Chapter 12, Hormonal Control of Reproduction in the Male, secretion of gonadotropins requires the operation of a hypothalamic pulse generator that produces intermittent stimulation of the pituitary gland by GnRH.

Sites of feedback control

The ovarian steroids might produce their positive or negative feedback effects by acting at the level of the hypothalamus or the anterior pituitary gland, or both. The GnRH pulse generator in the medial basal hypothalamus drives gonadotropin secretion regardless of whether negative or positive feedback prevails. Gonadotropin secretion falls to zero after bilateral destruction of the arcuate nuclei in rhesus monkeys and cannot be increased by either ovariectomy or treatment with the same amount of estradiol that evokes a surge of FSH and LH in normal animals. When such animals are fitted with a pump that delivers a constant amount of GnRH in brief pulses every hour, the normal cyclic pattern of gonadotropin is restored and the animals ovulate each month.

Identical results have been obtained in women suffering from Kallman's syndrome in which there is a developmental deficiency in GnRH production by the hypothalamus (Fig. 13.44).

In both cases, administration of GnRH in pulses of constant amplitude and frequency was sufficient to produce normal ovulatory cycles. Because both positive and negative feedback aspects of gonadotropin secretion can be produced even when hypothalamic input is clamped at constant frequency and amplitude, these effects of estradiol must be exerted at the level of the pituitary.

Although changes in amplitude and frequency of GnRH pulses are not necessary for the normal pattern

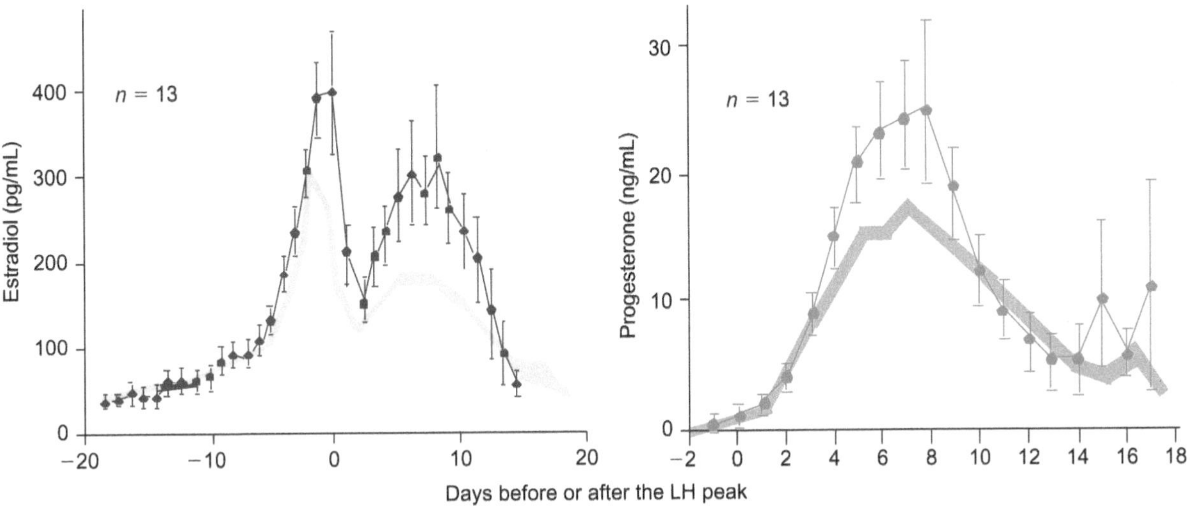

FIGURE 13.44 Results of ovulation induction employing a physiological frequency of GnRH administration to hypogonadotropic hypogonadism in women upon ovarian steroid secretion. Normal values are represented by the light green and pink shaded areas. *GnRH,* Gonadotropin-releasing hormone. Source: *From Crowley, W. F. Jr., Filicori, M., Spratt, D. J., et al. (1985). The physiology of gonadotropin-releasing hormones (GnRH) secretion in men and women.* Recent Progress in Hormone Research, 41, 473.

of gonadotropin secretion during an experimental or therapeutic regimen, variations in frequency and amplitude nevertheless occur physiologically in a way that complements and reinforces the intrinsic pattern already described. During the normal reproductive cycle, GnRH pulses are considerably less frequent in the luteal phase than in the follicular phase. Slowing the frequency of GnRH pulses from one per hour to one per 3 hours decreases LH secretion and increases FSH secretion (Fig. 13.45).

This effect of pulse frequency may contribute to the rise and fall in plasma FSH concentrations in the luteal–follicular transition despite minimal changes in LH concentrations. Progesterone may slow the frequency of GnRH pulses by stimulating hypothalamic production of endogenous opioids or perhaps by direct effects on kisspeptinergic neurons in the arcuate nuclei (see Chapter 12: Hormonal Control of Reproduction in the Male).

In addition to its negative feedback effects on the gonadotropes, estradiol may decrease the amplitude of GnRH pulses while increasing their frequency, but these effects are small and not always observed. Thus feedback effects of estradiol appear to be exerted primarily but not exclusively on the pituitary, and those of progesterone primarily but probably not exclusively on the hypothalamus.

We do not yet understand the intrapituitary mechanisms responsible for the negative and positive feedback effects of estradiol. As seen with the ovary, changes in hormone secretion may be brought about by changes in the sensitivity of target cells, as well as by changes in concentration of a stimulatory hormone. Women and experimental animals are more responsive to a test dose of GnRH at midcycle than at any other time. An increase in the number of receptors for GnRH at this time has been reported, and there is evidence that the high concentrations of estradiol that precede the LH surge upregulate GnRH receptors and stimulate LH synthesis and storage.

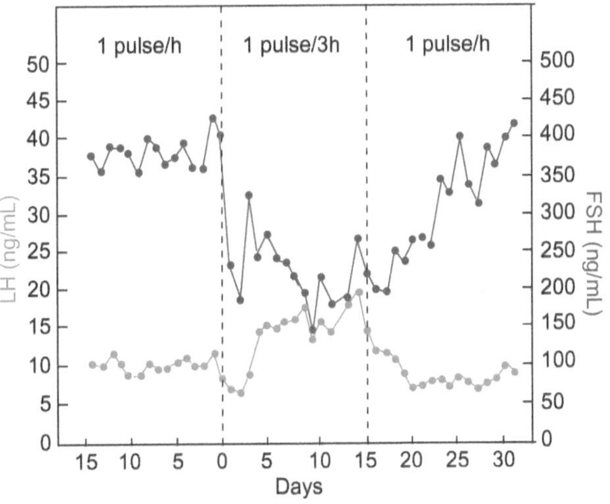

FIGURE 13.45 The effects of frequency of GnRH pulses on FSH and LH secretion. After destruction of the GnRH pulse generator in the arcuate nuclei, monkeys were fitted with pumps that delivered intermittent 6 min pulses of GnRH at the frequencies indicated. *GnRH,* Gonadotropin-releasing hormone. Source: *From Wildt, L., Häusler, A., Marshall, G., Hutchison, J. S., Plant, T. M., Belchetz, P. E., et al. (1981). Frequency and amplitude of gonadotropin-releasing hormone stimulation and gonadotropin secretion in the Rhesus monkey.* Endocrinology, 109, 376–379.

Timing of reproductive cycles

Although the pacemaker for rhythmic release of GnRH resides in the hypothalamus, the timekeeper for the slower monthly rhythm of the ovarian cycle resides in the ovary. As already indicated, the corpus luteum has a built-in life span of about 12 days and involutes despite continued stimulation with LH. A new cohort of follicles cannot arise so long as the corpus luteum remains functional. Its demise appears to relieve inhibition of FSH secretion and follicular growth. Thus the interval between the LH surge and the emergence of the new cohort of follicles is determined by the ovary. The principal event around which the menstrual cycle revolves is ovulation that depends on an ovulatory surge of LH. The length of the follicular phase may be somewhat variable and may be influenced by extraovarian events, but the timing of the LH surge resides in the ovary. It is only when the developing follicle signals its readiness to ovulate with sustained high blood levels of estradiol that the pituitary secretes the ovulatory spike of gonadotropin. Hence throughout the cycle, it is the ovary that notifies the pituitary and hypothalamus of its readiness to proceed to the next stage.

The beginning and end of cyclic ovarian activity, called menarche and menopause, occur on a longer timescale. The events associated with the onset of puberty were considered in Chapter 12, Hormonal Control of Reproduction in the Male. Although we still do not know what biological phenomena signal readiness for reproductive development and the end of the juvenile period, it appears that the timekeeper for this process resides in the central nervous system that initiates sexual development and function by activating the GnRH pulse generator. Termination of cyclic ovarian activity coincides with the disappearance or exhaustion of primordial follicles, but during the final decade of a woman's reproductive life, there is a paradoxical doubling of the rate of loss of follicles by atresia. Aging of the GnRH pacemaker may be a factor in this acceleration of follicular loss, as studies in normally cycling women indicate that both the amplitude of LH pulses and the interval intervening between pulses increases with increased age.

Summary

In this chapter the hormonal control of the female reproductive structures is discussed starting with the embryology of the female gonad and associated structures. The sequence of changes to the female reproductive system, including the menstrual cycle as a result of hormonal influences, is followed throughout the cycle of life.

Suggested readings

Basic foundations

Allen, R. H., Kaunitz, A. M., & Hickey, M. (2016). Hormonal contraception. In S. Melmed, K. S. Polonsky, P. R. Larsen, & H. M. Kronenberg (Eds.), *Williams textbook of endocrinology* (13th ed., pp. 664–693). Philadelphia, PA: Elsevier.

Bulun, S. E. (2016). Physiology and pathology of the female reproductive axis. In S. Melmed, K. S. Polonsky, P. R. Larsen, & H. M. Kronenberg (Eds.), *Williams textbook of medical physiology* (13th ed., pp. 590–663). Philadelphia, PA: Elsevier.

Mesiano, S., & Jones, E. E. (2017). The female reproductive system. In W. F. Boron, & E. L. Boulpaep (Eds.), *Medical physiology* (3rd ed., pp. 1108–1128). Philadelphia, PA: Elsevier.

Advanced information

Blorba, V. V., Zandman-Goddard, G., & Shoenfeld, Y. (2018). Prolactin and autoimmunity. *Frontiers in immunology, 9*, 73. Available from https://doi.org/10.3389/fimmu.2018.00073.

Harper-Harrison, G., & Shanahan, M. M. (2018). *Hormone replacement therapy. StatPearls*. Treasure Island, FL: Stat Pearls Publisher.

Harsh, V., & Clayton, A. H. (2018). Sex differences in the treatment of sexual dysfunction. *Current psychiatry reports, 20*(3), 18. Available from https://doi.org/10.1007/s11920-018-0883-1.

Muñoz-Mayorga, D., Guerra-Araiza, C., Torner, L., & Morales, T. (2018). Tau phosphorylation in female neurodegeneration: Role of estrogens, progesterone, and prolactin. *Frontiers in Endocrinology, 9*, 133. Available from https://doi.org/10.3389/fendo.2018.00133.

Nuzzi, R., Scalabrin, S., Becco, A., & Panzica, G. (2018). Gonadal hormones and retinal disorders: A review. *Frontiers in Endocrinology, 9*, 66. Available from https://doi.org/10.3389/fendo.2018.00066.

Pugeat, M., Plotton, I., de la Perrière, A. B., Raverot, G., Déchaud, H., & Raverot, V. (2018). Management of endocrine disease: Hyperandrogenic states in women: Pitfalls in laboratory diagnosis. *European Journal of Endocrinology, 178*(4), R141–R154. Available from https://doi.org/10.1530/eje-17-0776.

Scully, E. P. (2018). Sex differences in HIV infection. *Current HIV/AIDS Reports, 15*(2), 136–146. Available from https://doi.org/10.1007/s11904-018-0383-2.

CHAPTER

14

Hormonal control of pregnancy and lactation

Case study: Pregnancy and Crohn disease

She was the life of the party, and what parties they were! Good conversation with a limited number of guests. The talk, food, and beverage went well into the wee hours of the morning. It did not stop when she married. Indeed, the parties became even better. Her partner had his PhD and was working on a postdoctoral fellowship. She was working on her thesis research for her PhD in another department. Life was great. The only skeleton in the closet was that she had Crohn disease. But it was in remission now, no signs of it at all, although she was careful about the food she ate and she did not drink alcoholic beverages.

With her research almost finished, she began to think of her future and that of her husband. They both loved children and she decided that it was time to begin a family. At a party, she announced her decision and at another her pregnancy.

Then, without warning, her Crohn disease came back—with a vengeance. Two months into her pregnancy she had a miscarriage. For the next 5 months, she bravely fought a losing battle. She did manage to defend her thesis from her hospital bed. She got her PhD.

The disease spread from her intestinal tract to her lungs, kidneys, joints, and skin (Fig. 14.1).

More surgeries were needed to remove necrotic tissue. Total parenteral nutrition had to be started to sustain life. The destruction of her lungs continued. At the end, she succumbed to pneumonia. At autopsy, it was found she had only 25 cm of small intestine left.

Her husband, devastated, gave up his fellowship and moved 1000 miles away. He took up a new profession and eventually remarried. He has several children now, but he has never forgotten his first wife and the battle she waged.

Goodman's Basic Medical Endocrinology.
DOI: https://doi.org/10.1016/B978-0-12-815844-9.00014-2

(cont'd)

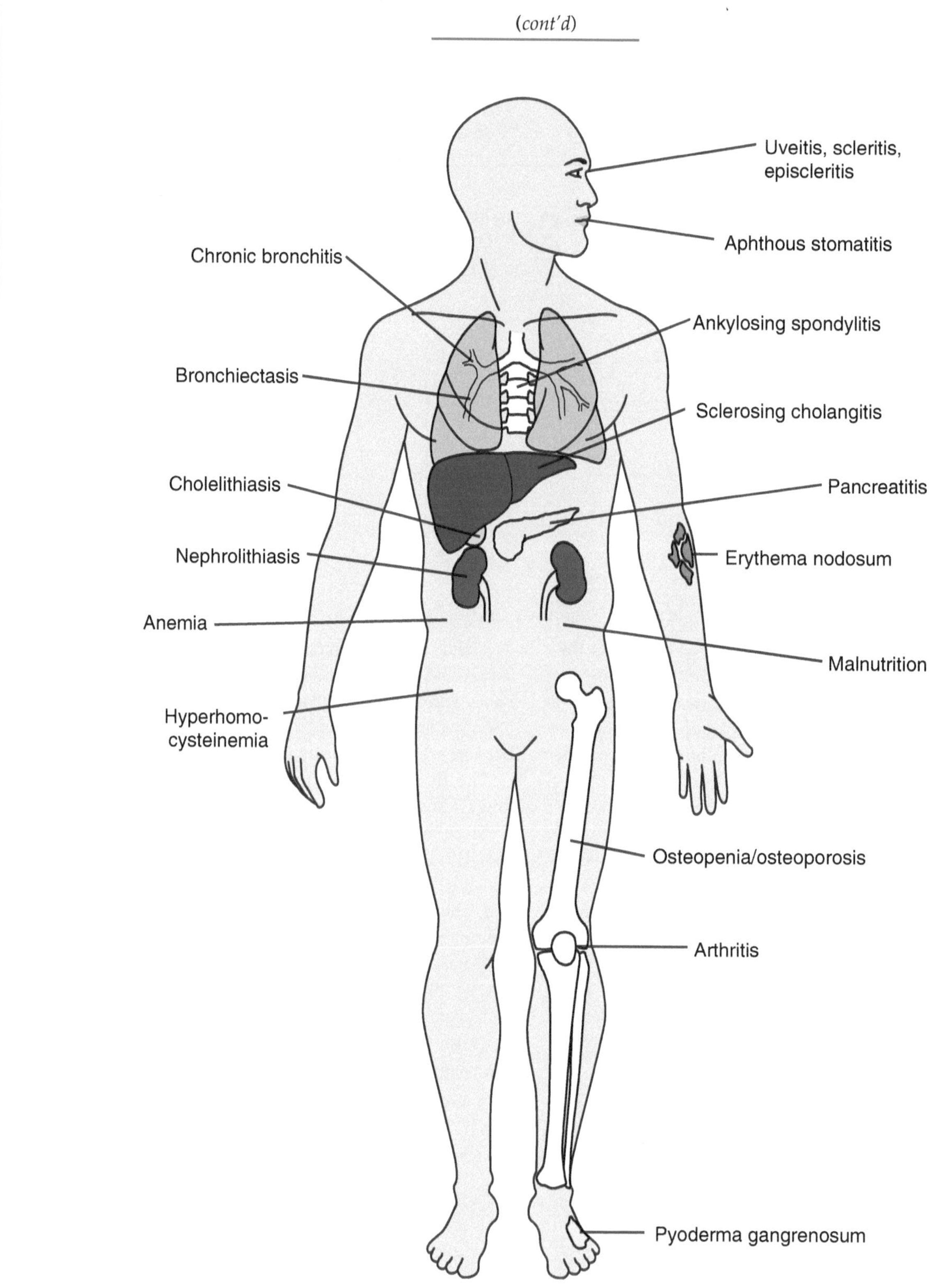

FIGURE 14.1 The extraintestinal locations of Crohn disease. Source: *Figure 19.70 in D. S. Stayer and E. Rubin (2015).* Rubin's pathology *(7th ed., p. 802). Wolters Kluwer.*

In the clinic: Crohn disease

Crohn disease is not an autoimmune disorder

Epidemiology

Male-to-female ratio in adults is almost equal (1 to 1.3), but in children, it is more prevalent in males than females. Most cases occur in the 15- to 30-year-old age group, although cases do occur in childhood and in the elderly, although in the latter group one wonders if chronic digestive problems were misdiagnosed at an earlier age. The prevalence in the United States and Canada is approximately 200 cases per 100,000 people.

Etiology

1. Microorganisms: Crohn disease can be described as an inappropriate immune response either to a yet-to-be-proven pathogen or to some other stimulus. A prevailing hypothesis is that the microorganism involved is *Mycobacterium avium paratuberculosis* (MAP), an obligate intracellular acid-fast bacterium similar to that seen in Fig. 14.2.

Crohn disease is similar to Johne's disease of cattle that is caused by MAP, a similarity that was first recognized in 1913. These organisms are resistant to the antibiotics that affect *Mycobacterium tuberculosis*, although they are destroyed by clarithromycin and rifabutin. MAP is not killed by the pasteurization of milk and has been shown to be present in water after treatment with chlorination. The conundrum is that the normal human population can also harbor the organism without any sign of disease.

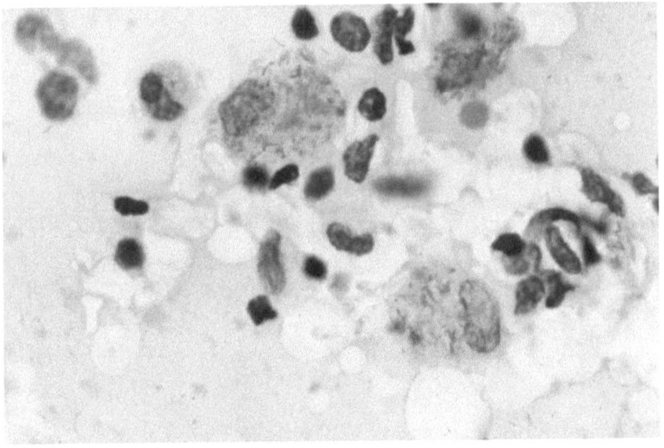

FIGURE 14.2 *Mycobacterium avium complex* (subspecies not identified in this image) shown by acid-fast stain (red) to be inside the macrophages. The bacteria survive and even multiply inside these cells. Source: *Figure 12.8 in Jaffe, Arber, Campo, Harris, & Quintanilla-Martinez (2017). Chapter 12: Bone marrow findings in inflammatory, infectious and metabolic disorders. In N. S. Rosenthal (Ed.),* Hematopathology *(2nd ed., p. 239). Elsevier.*

2. Genetics: There are a large number of candidate genes for this disorder. Most notably is nucleotide-binding oligomerization domain 2 (NOD2) which is found on chromosome 16 and is responsible for the innate immune response. Mutations in this gene would then alter the antibacterial response of the innate immune system, causing the defense to be turned over to the backup system, the adaptive immune response. Crohn disease may involve multiple genetic defects.
3. Environment: The Hruska postulate infers that susceptibility to MAP increases if a person was not breast-fed. It is also not commonly found in countries where intestinal parasites are common and water is often not chlorinated. It is most prevalent in North America and Europe where hygiene and sanitation are of paramount importance. Crohn disease is also prevalent among smokers and those who inhale second-hand smoke. Antibiotics taken in childhood are another risk factor. Of interest is that germ-free animals do not have the disorder but, if genetically susceptible, will acquire it when normal flora is introduced.
4. The immune response.

Innate immunity: There are two types of response to bacterial (and fungal and viral) invasion: innate and adaptive immunity. Both are involved in Crohn disease. As the name implies, the cells that are involved in innate immunity do not increase their response or cell numbers to repeated exposure to the same infectious agent. These cells recognize pathogen-associated molecular patterns with pattern recognition receptors (PRRs) on their cell membranes. These receptors are constitutive, that is, they are present all the time. These cells, macrophages, neutrophils, and dendritic cells (DCs) can detect extracellular bacteria (viruses, fungi, and parasites) through these PRRs especially ones called Toll-like receptors (Toll is German for "wonderful," or "great") and NOD-like receptors (Figs. 14.3 and 14.4).

Cells of the innate immune system do not produce antibodies but they do phagocytize bacteria. These innate immune cells amplify the immune response by releasing cytokines and chemokines, both of which are paracrine hormones. The cytokines induce changes in other cells, while the chemokines attract more immune cells. Together, the cytokines and chemokines initiate a response called inflammation (Fig. 14.5).

Inflammation was first defined in Roman times by Aulus Cornelius Celsus as *rubor et calor cum tumor et dolor* (redness and heat with swelling and pain). Rudolf Virchow in the 1800s added *functio laesa* [disordered (cell) function] (Fig. 14.6).

(*cont'd*)

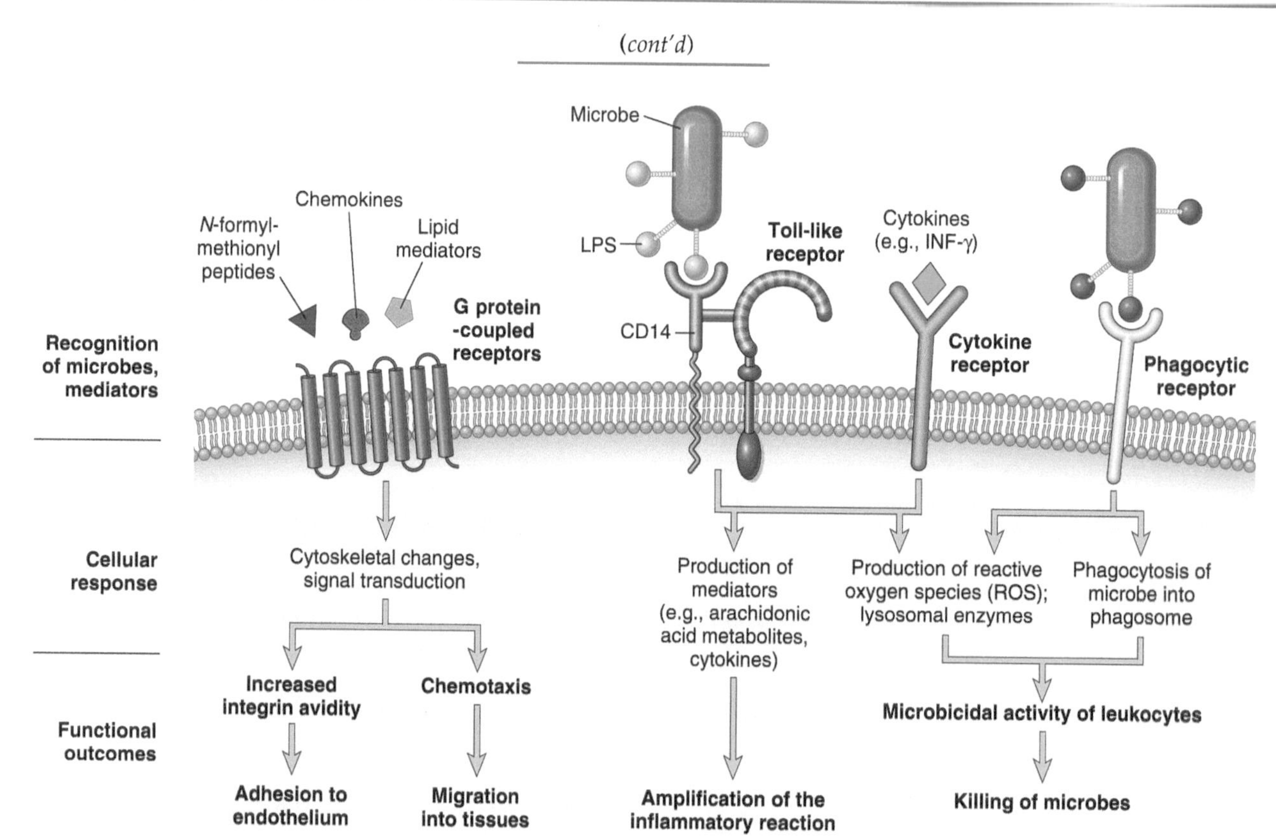

FIGURE 14.3 Toll-like receptors are one of the PRRs that this neutrophil has on the surface of its cell (NOD receptors are not illustrated). These along with other receptors and combined with other cytokines and chemokines activate the neutrophil as well as macrophages and DCs to initiate the inflammatory response. *DC*, Dendritic cell; *NOD*, nucleotide-binding oligomerization domain; *PRR*, pattern recognition receptors. Source: *Figure 3.7 in Kumar, Abbas, & Aster (2015).* Robbins and cotran pathologic basis of disease *(9th ed., p. 70). Elsevier.*

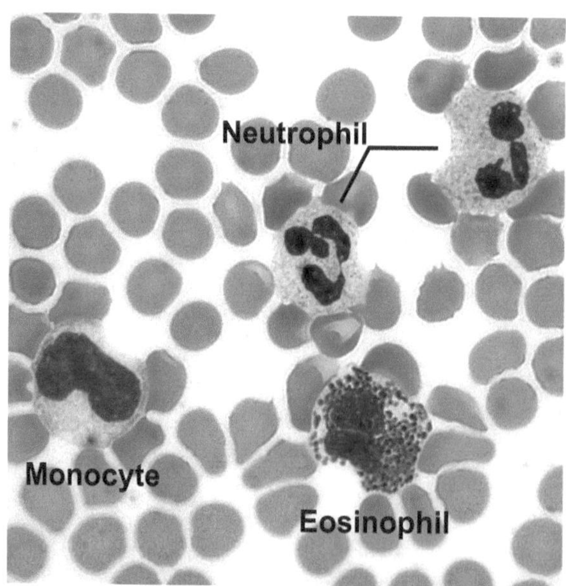

FIGURE 14.4 Blood smear demonstrating some of the cells involved in the innate immune response. Shown are normal neutrophils, a monocyte which will become a macrophage in the tissue, and an eosinophil. Source: *From Figure 8.1 in Bennett, Dolin, & Blaser (2015). Chapter 8: Granulocytic phagocytes. In F. R. DeLeo, & W. M. Nauseef (Eds.),* Mandell, Douglas and Bennett's principles and practice of infectious diseases *(8th ed., p. 79). Elsevier.*

(cont'd)

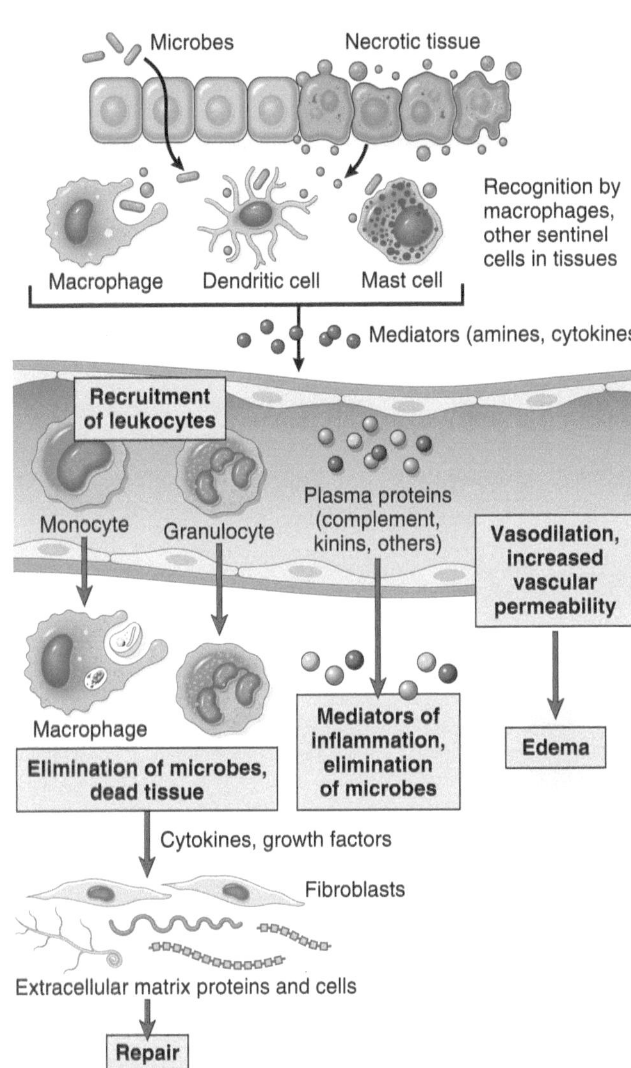

FIGURE 14.5 Sequence of events in inflammation. Source: *Figure 3.1 in Kumar, Abbas, & Aster (2015).* Robbins and Cotran pathologic basis of disease *(9th ed., p. 70). Elsevier.*

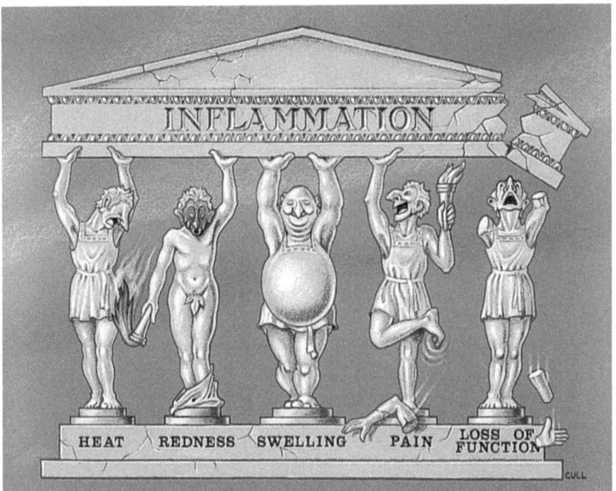

FIGURE 14.6 The five cardinal signs of inflammation. Although the illustration depicts this as being in Roman times, only the first four are from that era as loss of function was added in the 1800s by Rudolf Virchow, the founder of modern pathology. Source: *From Figure 2.1 in Damjanov (2017).* Pathology for the health professions *(5th ed., p. 24). Elsevier.*

This is the innate immune response as it is nonspecific and is the response for any pathogen or perceived tissue threat. In this response, capillaries dilate (whichcauses redness, and on the body surface can be felt as a warm area) and become more permeable to fluid (causing swelling) and to neutrophils (Figs. 14.7–14.10), macrophages, and other cells of inflammation such as eosinophils, NK (natural killer) and innate lymphoid cells (a more recently discovered cell related to NK cell).

The cells are essential for the activation of bradykinin, carried on the alpha-2 globulin, which depolarizes nociceptors, causing pain which is amplified by prostaglandins. Bradykinin also causes vasodilation and increased capillary permeability.

Adaptive immunity: Innate immunity provides a shotgun approach with each pellet nonspecific for its target, whereas adaptive immunity involves a bullet (an antibody) made for a specific target (Figs. 14.11 and 14.12).

The link between the two is the DC which, after processing by phagocytosis, can present a portion of a bacterial protein to a T-lymphocyte.

There are several forms of T lymphocytes: T-cytotoxic, T-helper (TH), and T-regulator. The TH has several subsets (TH1, TH2, etc.) all of which release different types of cytokines, paracrine hormones that affect normal cells.

There is a protein on the surface of cells. These "present" an antigen on the surface of the cell which is then "read" by a T-lymphocyte (T-cell) (Fig. 14.13).

Two types of presenter proteins are formed from the major histocompatibility genes and are designated major histocompatibility complex (MHC)-I and MHC-II. All nucleated cells have MHC-I . (Red blood cells have no nucleus and so do not have an MHC complex on their surfaces. Platelets also have no nucleus but they are the shed edges of megakaryocytes which do have a nucleus.) Only special cells in the immune system and B lymphocytes normally have the MHC-II complex. However, any cell of embryonic epithelial origin can be induced to form MHC-II complexes by interferon gamma (INFγ), which would normally only occur in inflammation. Many types

(cont'd)

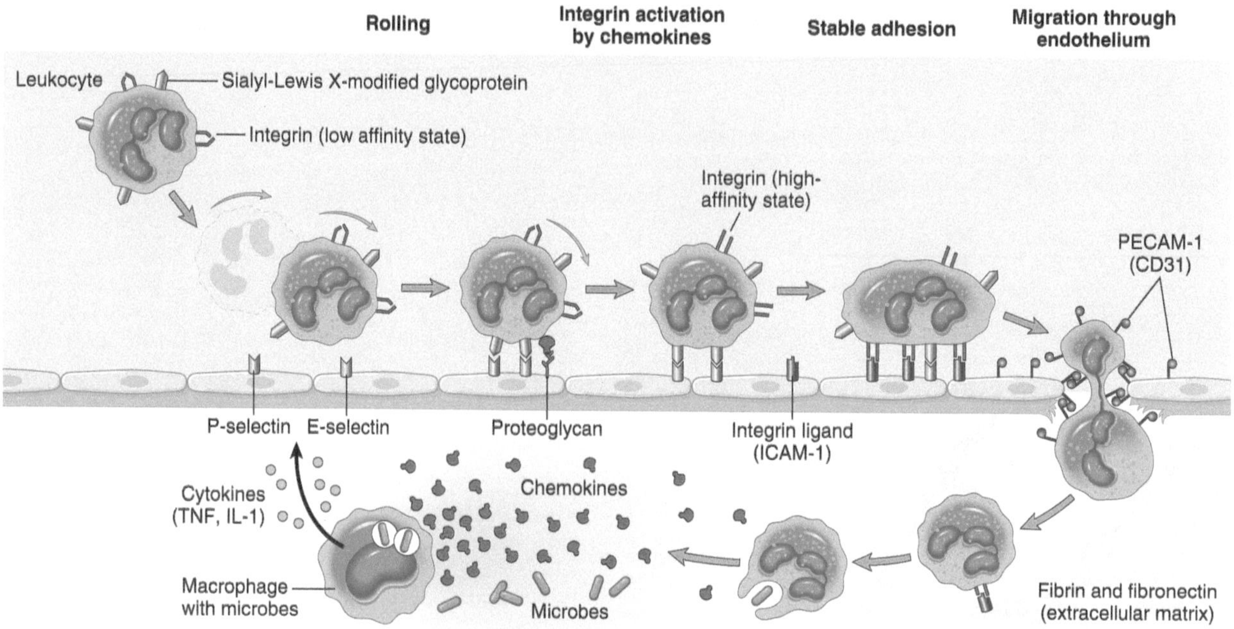

Rolling
Integrin activation by chemokines
Stable adhesion
Migration through endothelium
Leukocyte
Sialyl-Lewis X-modified glycoprotein
Integrin (low affinity state)
Integrin (high-affinity state)
PECAM-1 (CD31)
P-selectin
E-selectin
Proteoglycan
Integrin ligand (ICAM-1)
Cytokines (TNF, IL-1)
Chemokines
Macrophage with microbes
Microbes
Fibrin and fibronectin (extracellular matrix)

FIGURE 14.7 The penetration of neutrophils through a capillary wall in the innate immune response. The neutrophils first roll, then become activated by cytokines, and finally adhere to the endothelium. They then pierce the endothelium and move toward the chemokine which is where the invading microbes are located. Source: *Figure 3.4 in Kumar, Abbas, & Aster (2015).* Robbins and Cotran pathologic basis of disease *(9th ed., p. 75). Elsevier.*

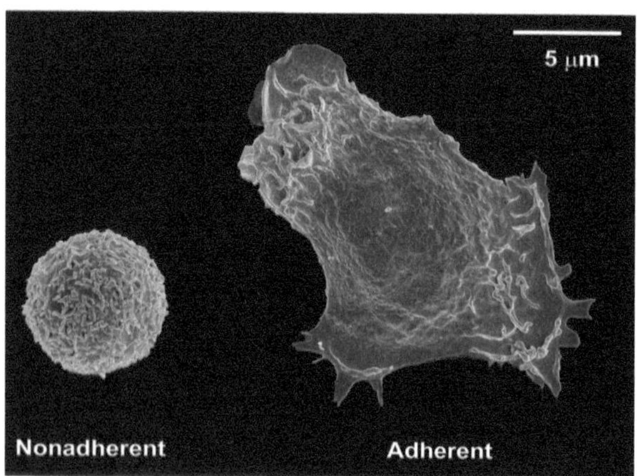

FIGURE 14.8 Scanning electron micrographs of nonadherent (circulating free in the blood) and adherent (attached to the capillary endothelial cell) neutrophils. Source: *Figure 8.4 in Bennett, Dolin, & Blaser (2015). Chapter 8: Granulocytic phagocytes. In F. R. DeLeo, & W. M. Nauseef (Eds.),* Mandell, Douglas and Bennett's principles and practice of infectious diseases *(8th ed., p. 82). Elsevier.*

of cancer cells also have them because most carcinomas and related neoplasms, such as brain tumors, are derived from cells originating from embryonic epithelium. It is not known why these cancer cells express the MHC-II complex.

One of these cytokines is INFγ that stimulates the formation of immunoproteasomes within the cell and the MHC-II complex on the cell surface of any cell derived from embryonic epithelial tissue. Proteasomes are normally found in all tissues. They degrade defective ribosomal products down to amino acids again so they can be reused to make new proteins (up to 30% of all proteins synthesized by a cell are defective). Immunoproteasomes are proteasomes that do not degrade a protein down to amino acids but, instead, degrade it little or not at all. This enables the fragment of the bacteria or defective protein from the cell to be incorporated into an MHC-II complex being formed in the rough endoplasmic reticulum (Fig. 14.14).

(cont'd)

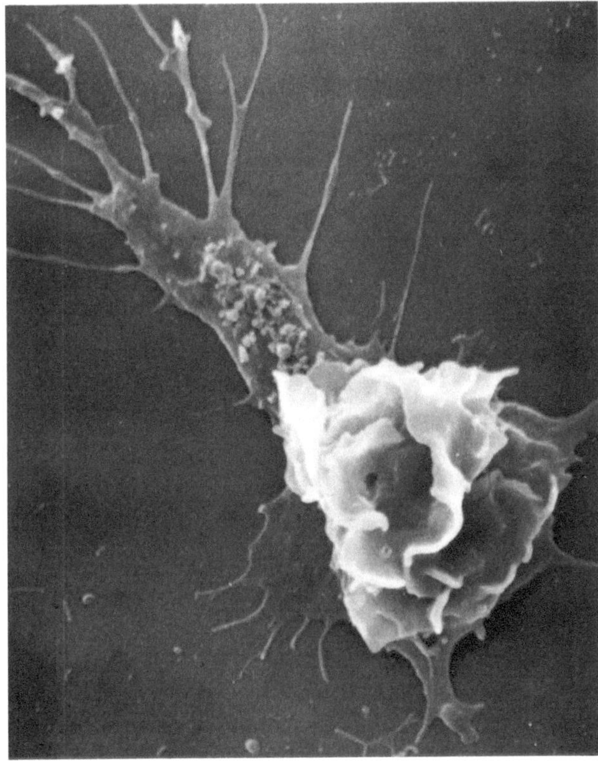

FIGURE 14.9 Scanning electron micrograph of a moving neutrophil. The cell is moving toward the upper left. This is the way it would look when it is moving within tissues. Source: *Figure 3.5 in Kumar, Abbas, & Aster (2015).* Robbins and Cotran pathologic basis of disease *(9th ed., p. 77). Elsevier.*

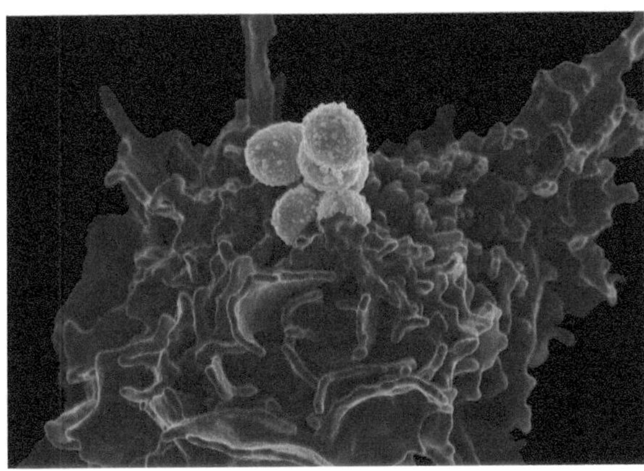

FIGURE 14.10 Scanning electron micrograph showing five *Staphylococcus aureus* (in blue) bacteria attached to a neutrophil and waiting to be phagocytized. Source: *Figure 8.5 in Bennett, Dolin, & Blaser (2015). Chapter 8: Granulocytic phagocytes. In F. R. DeLeo, & W. M. Nauseef (Eds.),* Mandell, Douglas and Bennett's principles and practice of infectious diseases *(8th ed., p. 83). Elsevier.*

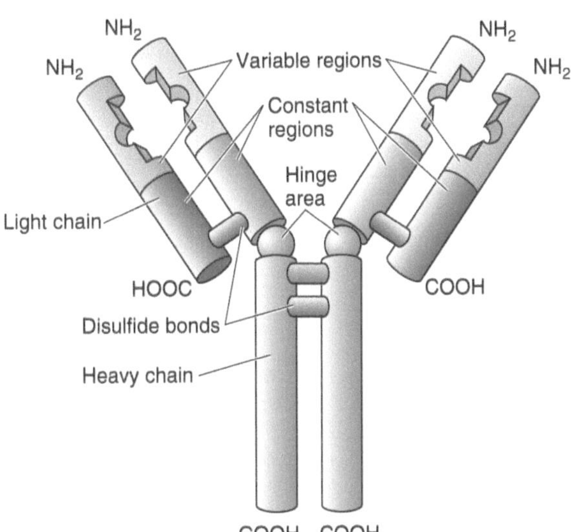

FIGURE 14.11 Structure of an antibody. The yellow ends are specific for an antigen. Source: *Figure 12.1 in Gartner, L. P. (2017).* Textbook of histology *(4th ed., p. 316). Elsevier.*

The MHC-II with the protein is shunted to the surface of the cell where it interacts with the CD4 + TH1, TH2, TH17, and T follicular helper lymphocytes (Fig. 14.15).

All of these cells produce cytokines and interleukins which stimulate macrophages to digest the bacteria (Fig. 14.16).

T_H2 lymphocytes also interact with MHC-II but they activate B-lymphocytes. The activated B-lymphocytes are divided into B-memory cells and plasma cells. The plasma cells produce antibodies specifically against the protein presented on the MHC-II complex (Fig. 14.17).

If an antigen is presented on an MHC-I complex, this attracts a CD8 + T-cell that is cytotoxic and will cause the cell to undergo self-destruction which is called apoptosis (Fig. 14.18).

In summary, two different events can occur when T cells combine with MHC complexes (Fig. 14.19). Both types of effects are seen in Crohn disease.

Pathology

Crohn disease is a focal rather than a systemic disorder. The first focal lesions are small aphthous ulcers anywhere in the gastrointestinal (GI) tract, but most commonly in the distal ileum. These ulcers are small (less than 3 mm in diameter) surrounded by a halo of erythema. These are due to the inappropriate immune

(cont'd)

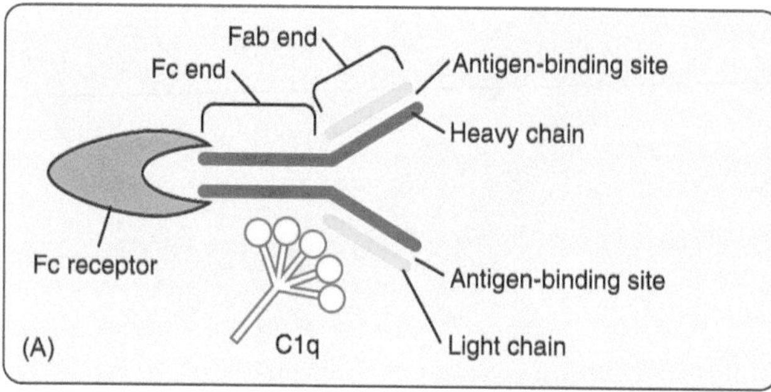

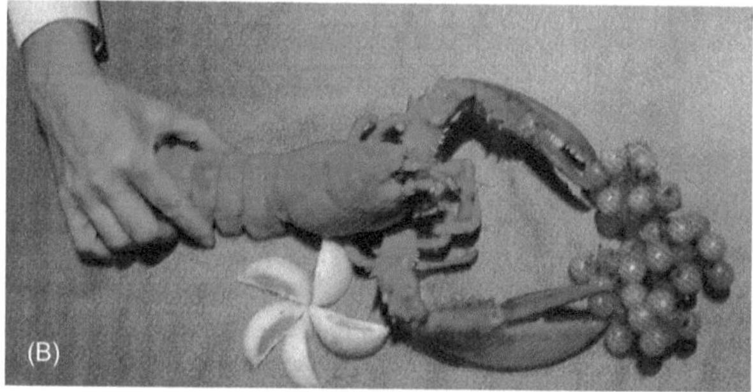

FIGURE 14.12 Using a lobster as an analogy, the antigenic binding site of the antibody binds to the antigen (the grapes in the case of the lobster). The C1q (represented by a lemon in the lobster picture) is a complement and the location indicates the binding site for a complement on the antibody. Source: *Figure 5.1 in Bennett, Dolin, & Blaser (2015). Chapter 5: Adaptive immunity: Antibodies and immunodeficiencies. In H. H. Birdsall (Ed.),* Mandell, Douglas and Bennett's principles and practice of infectious diseases *(8th ed., p. 35). Elsevier.*

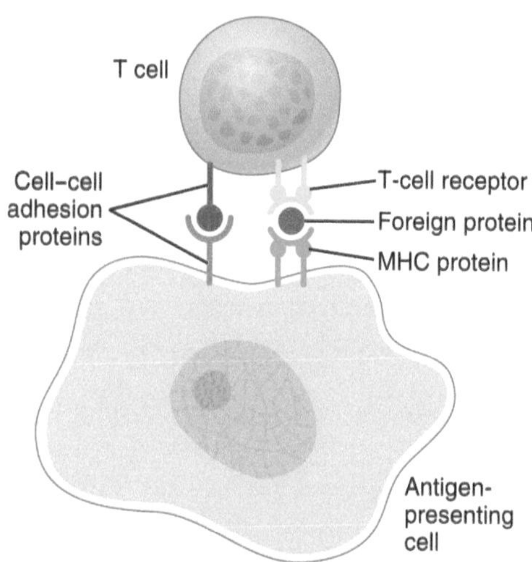

FIGURE 14.13 Presentation to a T lymphocyte of an antigen (foreign protein in this image) by an major histocompatibility complex (MHC) on the surface of an antigen-presenting cell. The foreign protein could be a part of a microorganism. Source: *Figure 35.7 in Hall, J. (2015).* Guyton and Hall textbook of medical physiology *(13th ed., p. 472). Elsevier.*

response to bacteria. If an ileostomy is performed, the ulcers disappear. They will come back if the pathway is restored and the ileum re-exposed to the normal intestinal flora. Over time, these ulcers will coalesce to form lines—longitudinal and transverse of ulcerous lesions. In between the tissue is edematous, leading to the cobblestone appearance of the intestinal lumen (Figs. 14.20–14.22).

Crohn disease tends to skip areas along the intestinal tract, in contrast to ulcerative colitis which starts at the distal colon and works up without skipping (Fig. 14.23).

Granulomas are also found, although it is not pathognomonic for Crohn disease. These are typically extensions of the aphthous ulcers. Within the granulomas, giant cells can be found, but unlike the granulomas of tuberculosis, there is no central necrosis. Granulomas can also be found in this disorder in extraintestinal tissue. The presence of granulomas is suggestive of a tuberculosis-like infection, lending support to the MAP hypothesis as a causative agent.

Another characteristic not seen in other disorders is fat wrapping. The affected part of the intestine has an overgrowth of adipose tissue on the serosal surface (Figs. 14.23 and 14.24). The presence of the fat may exacerbate the inflammatory response by the release of cytokines. It has also been observed that the increased ratio of visceral to subcutaneous fat may be a risk factor for the extension and/or complications of the disease.

Unlike ulcerative colitis, Crohn disease is transmural, destroying the normal architecture (Fig. 14.25) of the small intestine by the altered immune response, whose sequence is partly illustrated in Fig. 14.26.

Most cases of Crohn disease begin in the distal ileum of the small intestine and spread from there. Uncommonly, it may start elsewhere in the GI tract proximal to the ligament of Treitz (junction of the duodenum with the jejunum). Once started, it can and does affect other intestinal tissues and extraintestinal tissues, most commonly the joints.

(cont'd)

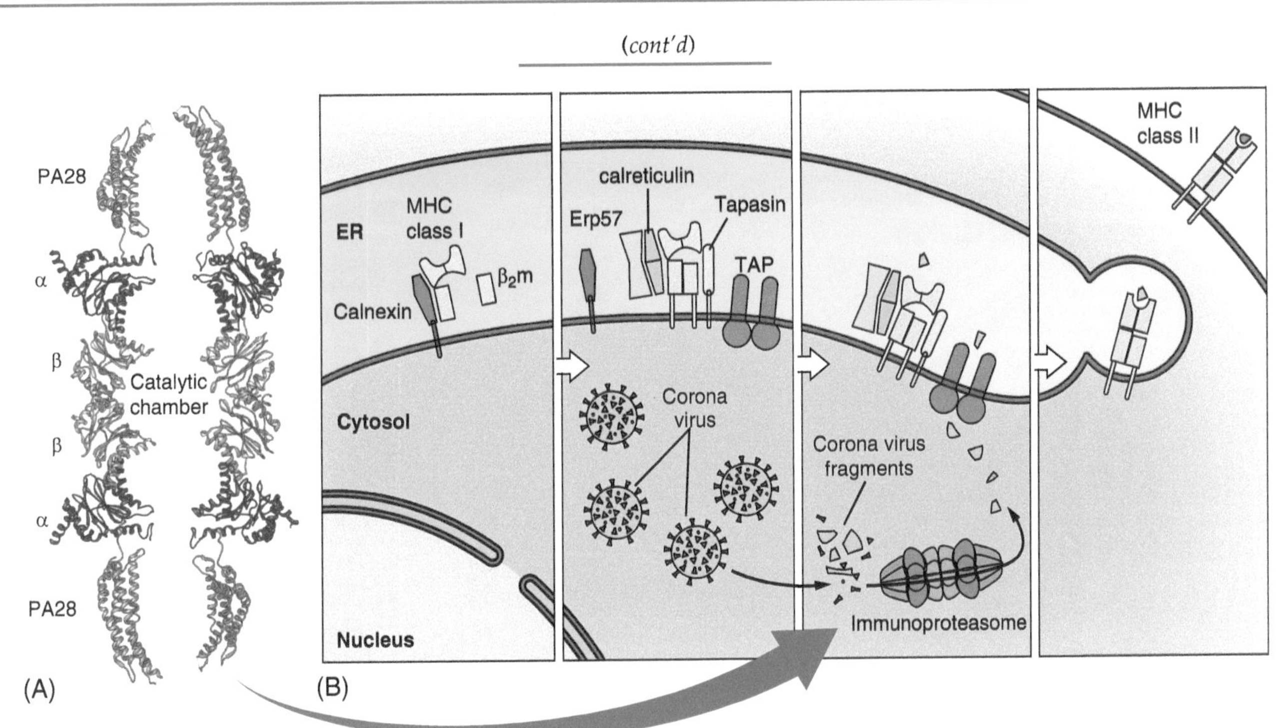

FIGURE 14.14 The pathway of DRiPs as well as pathogens through the immunoproteasome and into the MHC-I or MHC-II complex. On the left is a molecular structure of an immunoproteasome. *DRiP*, Defective ribosomal product. Source: *Figures 6.6 and 6.8 in Murphy, K., Weaver, C. (2017).* Janeway's immunobiology *(9th ed., pp. 218 and 220). WW Norton.*

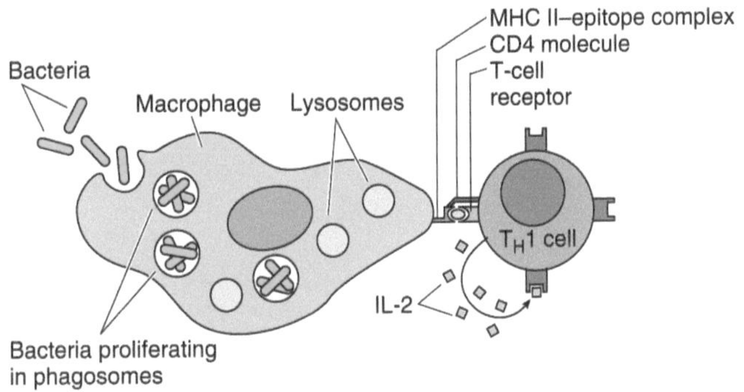

FIGURE 14.15 Macrophage expressing MHC-II complex and TH1 cell connecting to it. *TH*, T-helper. Source: *From Figure 12.4 in Gartner, L. P. (2017).* Textbook of histology *(4th ed., p. 328). Elsevier.*

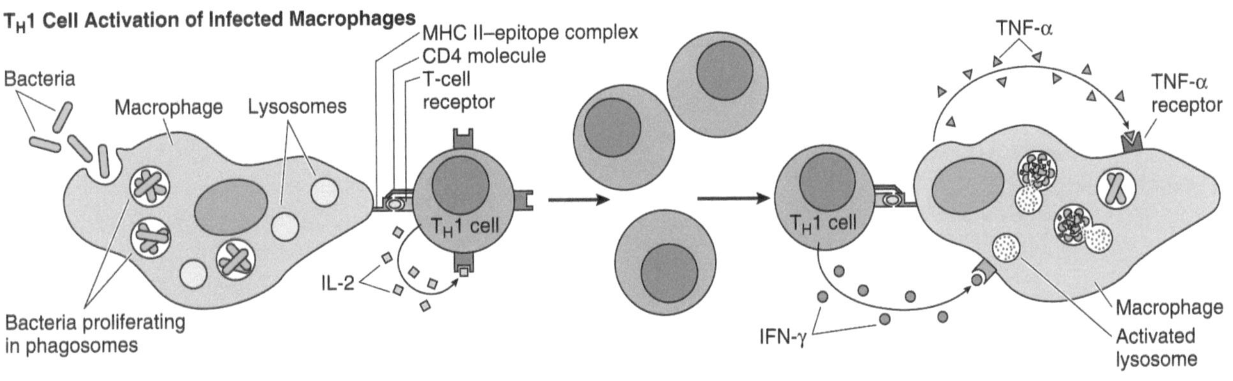

FIGURE 14.16 The activation of a macrophage to destroy the bacteria it has engulfed. Source: *Figure 12.4 in Gartner, L. P. (2017).* Textbook of histology *(4th ed., p. 328.). Elsevier.*

(*cont'd*)

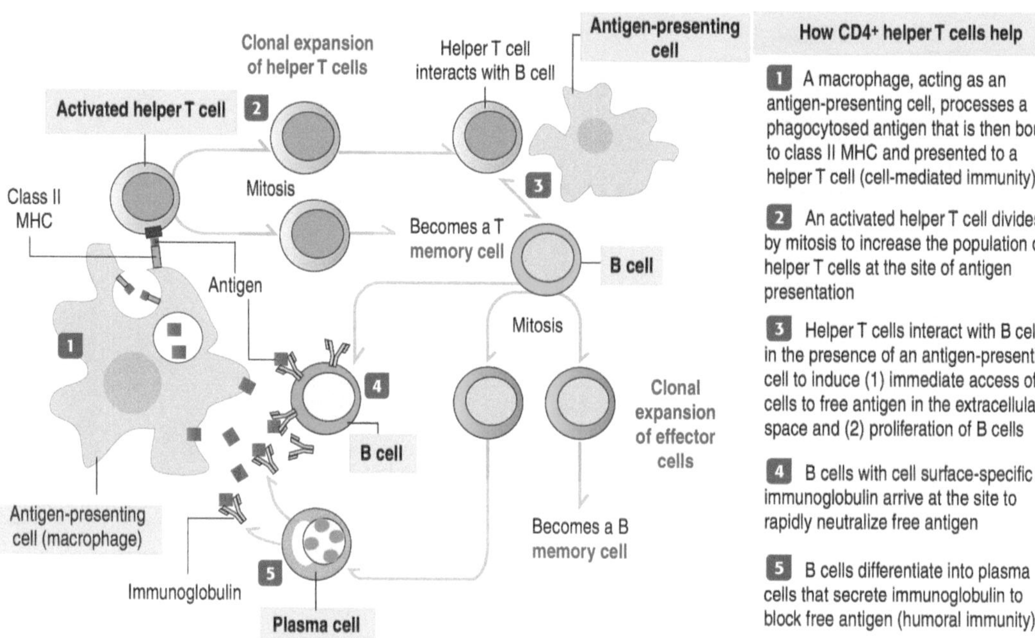

FIGURE 14.17 The sequence of events when a T_H2 helper cell combines with the MHC-II receptor displaying an antigen. Source: *Figure 10.8 in Kierszenbaum, A., & Tres, L. L. (2016).* Histology and cell biology: An introduction to pathology *(4th ed., p. 320). Elsevier.*

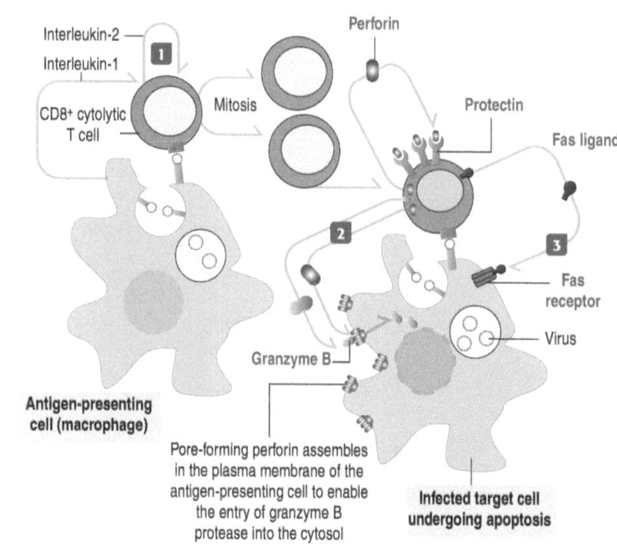

FIGURE 14.18 The sequence of events when a CD8+ cytotoxic T-cell combines with the MHC-I receptor displaying an antigen. Source: *Figure 10.9 in Kierszenbaum, A., & Tres, L. L. (2016).* Histology and cell biology: An introduction to pathology *(4th ed., p. 321). Elsevier.*

(cont'd)

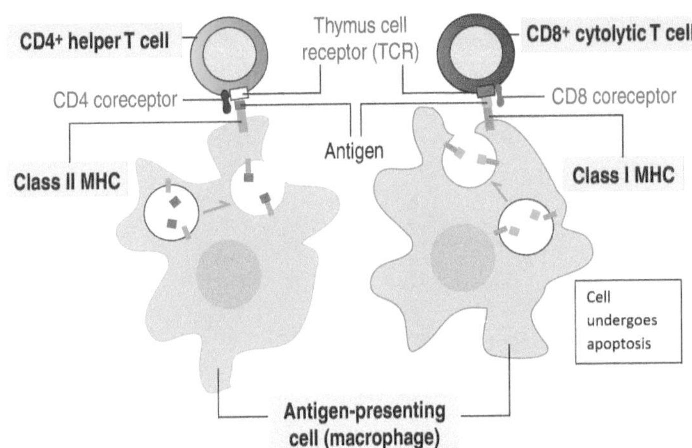

FIGURE 14.19 The expression of MHC-I and MHC-II leads to two different effects because they attract two different types of T lymphocyte. The CD8+ cell will cause the macrophage to self-destruct, while the CD4+ cell will stimulate other macrophages to destroy the engulfed antigen. Source: *Figure 10.6 in Kierszenbaum, A., & Tres, L. L. (2016).* Histology and cell biology: An introduction to pathology *(4th ed., p. 318). Elsevier.*

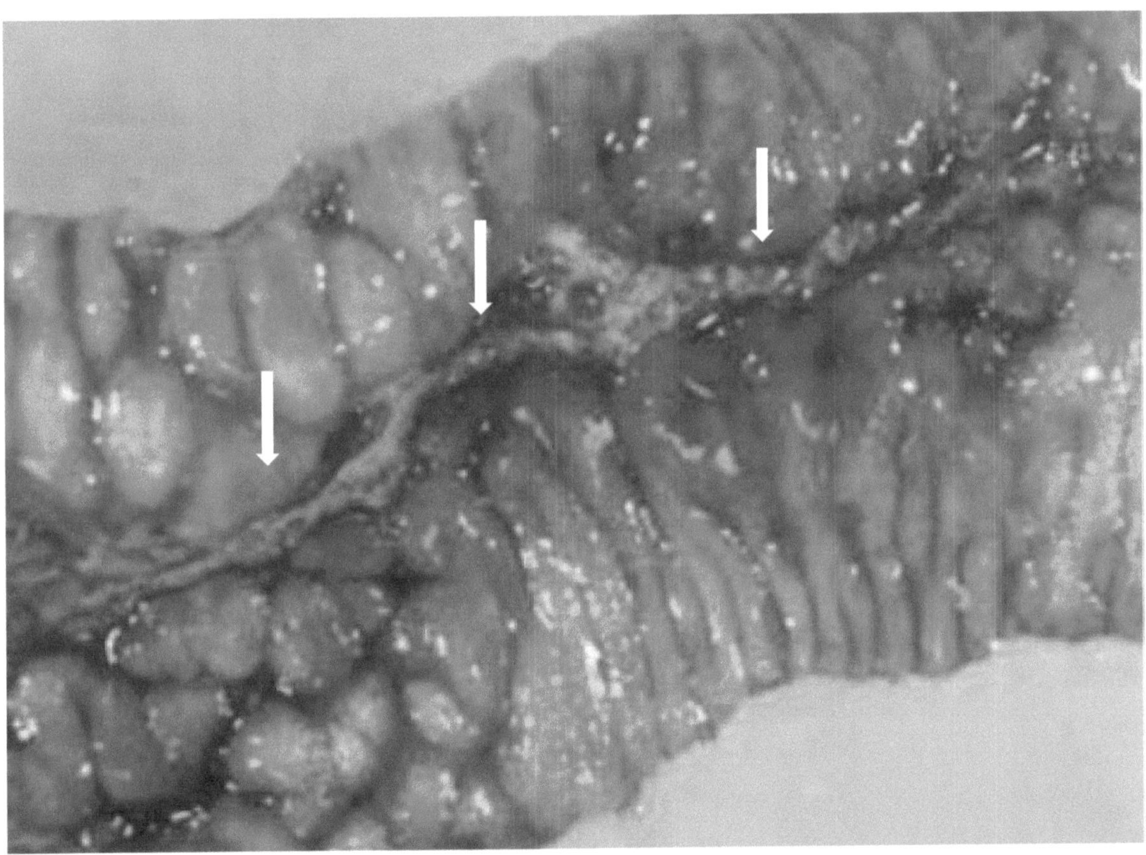

FIGURE 14.20 The edematous ileum gives a cobblestone (left) appearance to the mucosa. A longitudinal ulcer is also evident (*arrows*). On the lower right below the ulcer is the normal intestinal epithelium. Source: *From Figure 19.71B in Stayer (2015).* Rubin's pathology *(7th ed., p. 803). Wolters Kluwer.*

(cont'd)

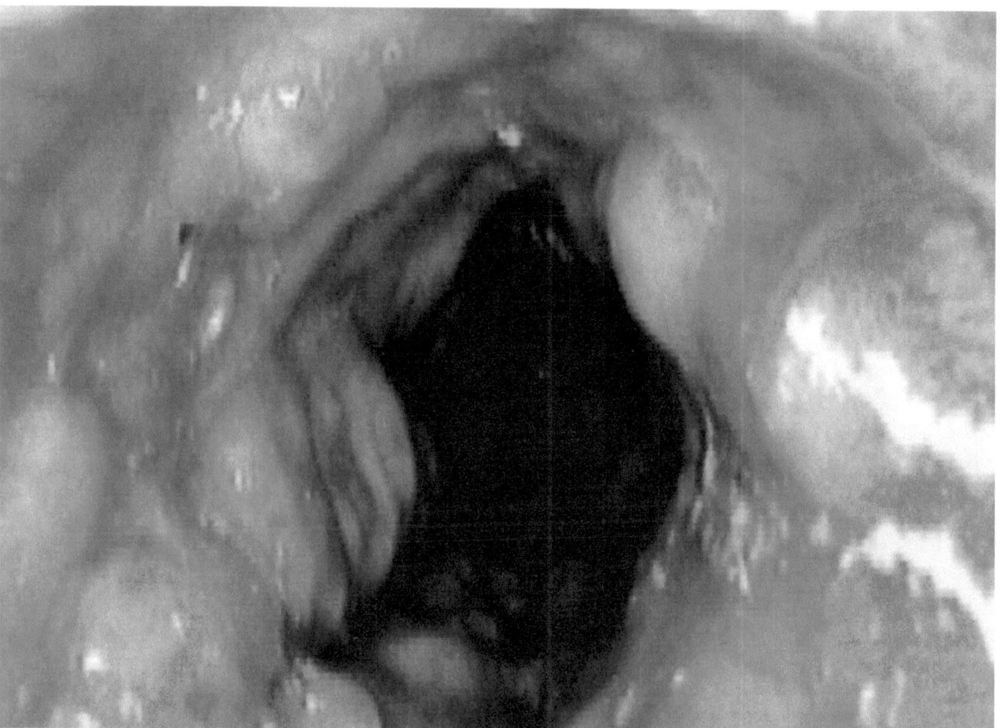

FIGURE 14.21 Illustrative of more advanced disease with erythema and edema causing the cobblestone (bumpy) appearance. Source: *Figure 117B in Feldman, Friedman, & Brandt (2016). Chapter 115: Crohn's disease. In B. E. Sands, & C. A. Siegel (Eds.),* Sleisenger and Fordtran's gastrointestinal and liver disease *(10th ed., p. 2007). Elsevier.*

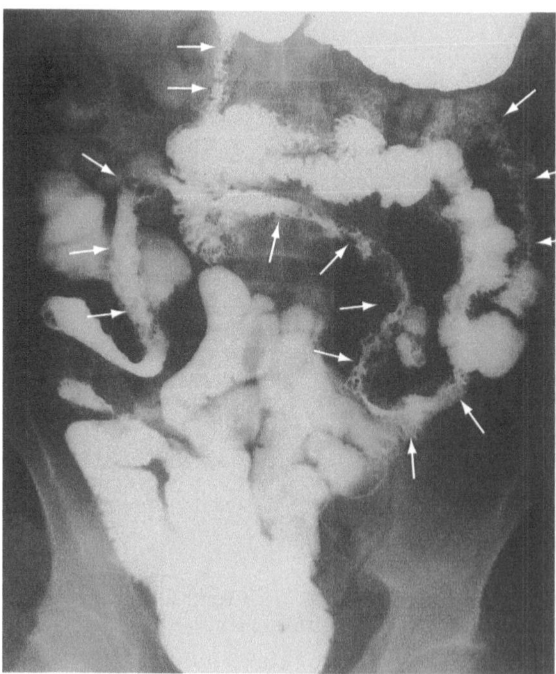

FIGURE 14.22 Multiple areas of the narrowed small bowel are evident. On the left, the arrows point to the edematous portion of the bowel that results in the cobblestone appearance typical of this disorder. Source: *From Figure 115.4 in Feldman, Friedman, & Brandt (2016). Chapter 115: Crohn's disease. In B. E. Sands, & C. A. Siegel (Eds.),* Sleisenger and Fordtran's gastrointestinal and liver disease *(10th ed., p. 2001). Elsevier.*

(*cont'd*)

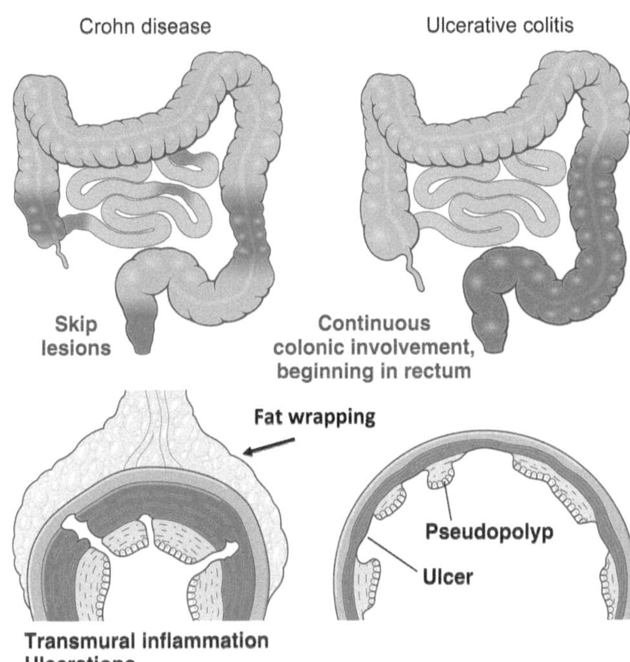

FIGURE 14.23 Crohn disease and ulcerative colitis, similar diseases but different pathologies. Both diseases are combined under the umbrella term, irritable bowel disease. Source: *From Figure 17.32 in Kumar, Abbas, & Aster (2015). Chapter 17: The gastrointestinal tract. In J. R. Turner (Ed.),* Robbins and Cotran, pathologic basis of disease *(9th ed., p. 797). Elsevier.*

Signs and symptoms: Perianal disease may anticipate the onset of intestinal disease by up to 4 years in 24% of patients. The intestinal manifestations of disease are insidious in its origins and may persist for years as intermittent colicky pain as large food particles move through constricted areas of the small intestine. Intestinal obstruction is not uncommon in the later stages of the disease. The patient may lose weight, have anorexia, frequent stools including bouts of diarrhea (the latter is more indicative of colonic involvement). Signs of malabsorption may appear such as macrocytic anemia due to lack of B_{12} uptake by the distal ileum; microcytic anemia may also occur due to blood loss. The extraintestinal extensions of the disease can involve almost every organ in the thoracic and abdominal cavities.

Diagnosis: There is no single test for Crohn disease. A careful history will be the best platform from which other tests can be done to confirm the diagnosis. The other tests would include imaging radiographs of the large and small intestine, endoscopy, and histopathology. While serology testing is used to help distinguish ulcerative colitis from Crohn disease, it is not sensitive enough to use as a primary diagnostic tool.

Management: There is no cure for Crohn disease. The primary goal is to induce a remission and treat the disease palliatively. This will improve the patient's quality of life. Aminosalicylates, antibiotics, glucocorticoids, thiopurine antimetabolites, and methotrexate are all used. Nutritional counseling and surgical intervention are also important.

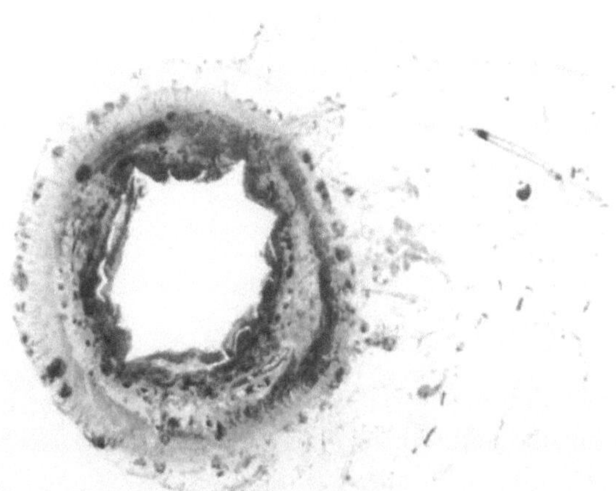

FIGURE 14.24 Fat wrapping. Whole mount of a section of the ileum shows a thick layer of fat surrounding the ileum in this case of Crohn disease. Source: *Figure 4 in Sheehan, A. L., Warren, B. F., Gear, M. W. L., & Shepherd, N. A. (1992). Fat-wrapping in Crohn's disease: Pathological basis and relevance to surgical practice.* British Journal of Surgery, *79, 955–958.*

(cont'd)

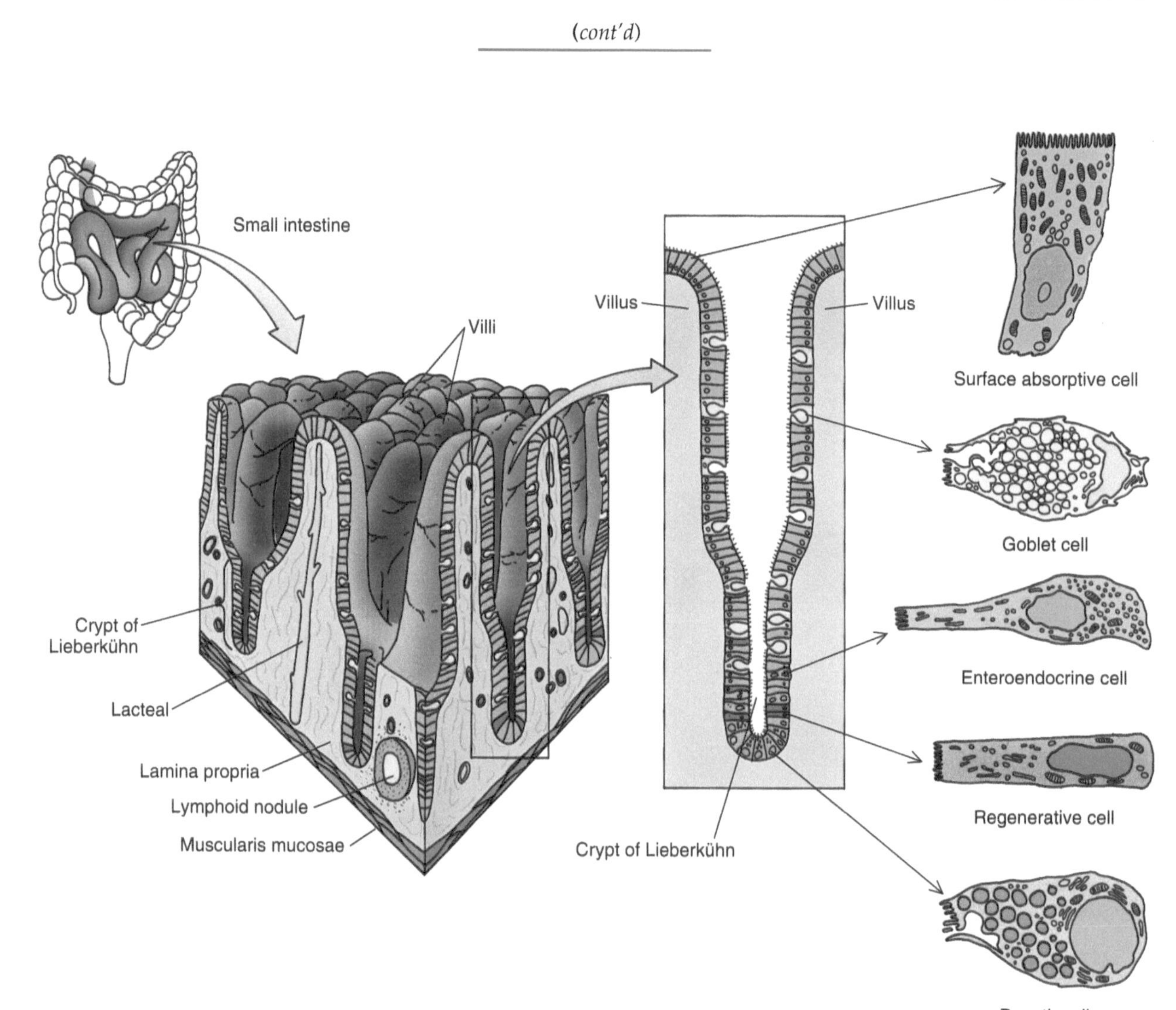

FIGURE 14.25 The normal small intestinal structure. Source: *Figure 17.13 in Gartner (2017).* Textbook of histology *(4th ed., p. 454). Elsevier.*

Management: Pregnancy: Most women will have no problems during pregnancy. However, if the disease is aggressive, it will invade and affect the uterus and therefore the developing child. If this happens, a miscarriage or spontaneous abortion will occur.

Prognosis: There is a greater risk of cancer if the disease has spread beyond the ileum. Otherwise, the risk is no greater than the general population. Over time, about 10% of the patients will be disabled by their disease. In all probability, there is a slightly higher mortality rate than the general population.

(cont'd)

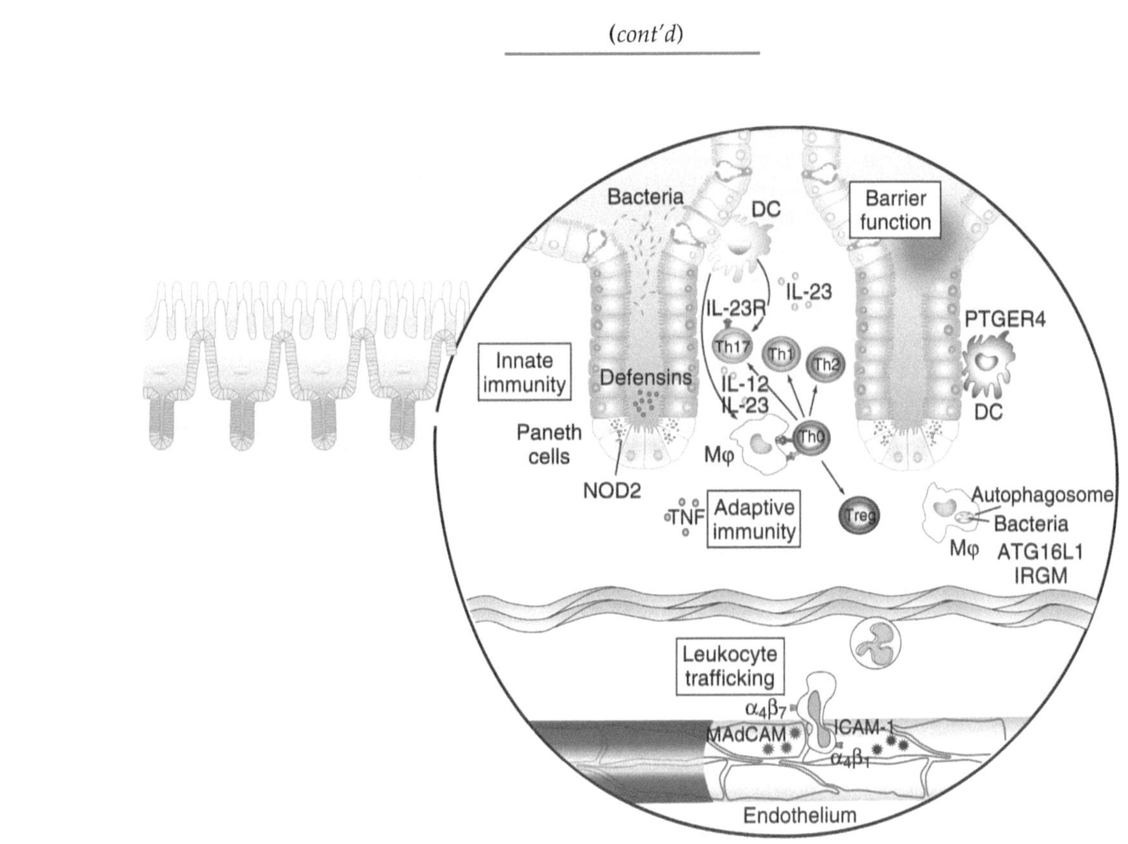

FIGURE 14.26 Sequence of events in the pathogenesis of Crohn disease. Bacteria are normally kept in check by defensins produced by paneth cells as a part of innate immunity. However, the NOD2 is defective in this image, so the bacterial invade the intestinal cell wall and enter the extracellular space where they are engulfed by a DC that bridges the gap between innate and adaptive immunity. DCs produce interleukins that attract macrophages (Mϕ), which ingest the bacteria and also stimulate, via T cells, other macrophages to ingest and destroy the bacteria. At the same time, neutrophils (innate immunity) get through the capillary wall and produce cytokines and other autocrines and paracrines. Source: *Figure 115.1 in Feldman, Friedman, & Brandt (2016). Chapter 115: Crohn's disease. In B. E. Sands, & C. A. Siegel (Eds.),* Sleisenger and Fordtran's gastrointestinal and liver disease *(10th ed., p. 1996). Elsevier.*

Hormonal control of pregnancy and lactation

Introduction

In the case study and in the clinic sections a disorder was presented that bridges the gap from the traditional hormones covered in the preceding chapters of this book to the autocrine and paracrines produced by cells of the immune system. This area of research is relatively new and still needs a lot of work before diseases such as Crohn disease and other disorders of the immunes system can be fully understood.

It is fitting, then, that the last chapter of this book covers the hormones of pregnancy and touches on some of the autocrines and paracrines that occur during the normal events in pregnancy and embryonic and fetal development.

Successful reproduction depends not only on the union of eggs and sperm but also on the survival of adequate numbers of the new generation to reach reproductive age and begin the cycle again. In some species, parental involvement in the reproductive process ends with fertilization of the ova; thousands or even millions of embryos may result from a single mating, with just a few surviving long enough to procreate. Higher mammals, particularly humans, have adopted the alternative strategy of producing only few or a single fertilized ovum at a time (Fig. 14.27).

Prolonged parental care during the embryonic and neonatal periods substitutes for huge numbers of unattended offspring as the means for increasing the likelihood of survival. Estrogen and progesterone prepare the maternal body for successful internal fertilization and hospitable acceptance of the embryo. Ovarian hormones (Figs. 14.28 and 14.29) and subsequently hormones arising from the placenta direct maternal adaptations that enable the mother to meet day-to-day challenges while ensuring optimal conditions

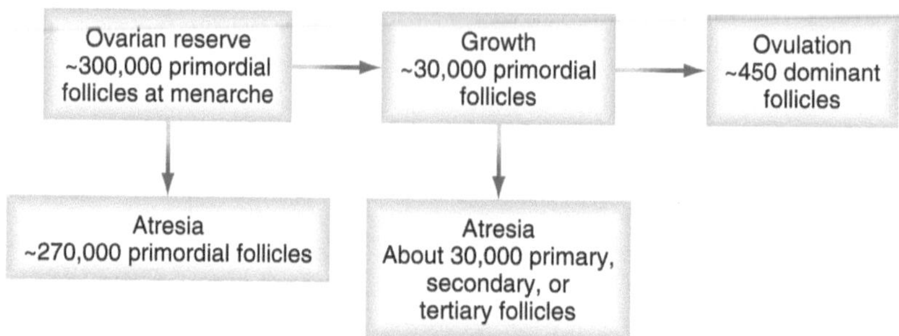

FIGURE 14.27 The fate of the ovarian follicles that survive to menarche (beginning of reproductive period in females). Most of the follicles become atretic (disintegrate) but 450 survive. These develop the fastest during a reproductive cycle and inhibit the other nine that are also developing. Each female of reproductive age could technically have 450 children if every one of her dominant follicles were fertilized after ovulation (the record is 27 pregnancies but because there were multiple births, there were 69 children). Source: *Figure 44.16 in Koeppen, B. M., & Stanton, B. A. (2018).* Berne and Levy physiology *(7th ed., p. 800). Elsevier.*

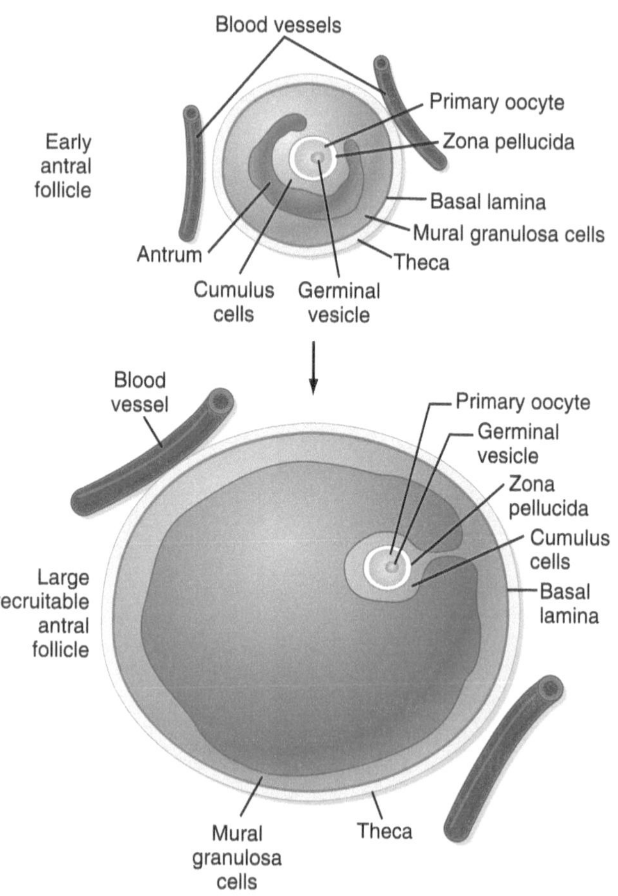

FIGURE 14.28 The theca and granulosa cells are responsible for ovarian hormones (see Fig. 14.29). Source: *Figure 44.17 in Koeppen, B. M., & Stanton, B. A. (2018).* Berne and Levy physiology *(7th ed., p. 801). Elsevier.*

for fetal development. The conceptus then takes charge. After lodging firmly within the uterine lining and gaining access to the maternal circulation, it secretes protein and steroid hormones that ensure continued maternal acceptance, and it directs maternal functions to provide for its development. Simultaneously, the conceptus withdraws whatever nutrients it needs from the maternal circulation. At the appropriate time the fetus signals its readiness to depart the uterus and initiates the birth process. While in utero, placental hormones prepare the mammary glands to produce the milk needed for nurture after birth. Finally, suckling stimulates continued milk production.

Fertilization and implantation

Gamete transport

Fertilization takes place in a distal portion of the uterine (fallopian) tube called the ampulla (Figs. 14.30 and 14.31), some distance from the site of sperm deposition in the female reproductive tract.

Yet the ovum is reached in approximately 5 minutes (however, in some cases, it may take as long as one hour) after ejaculation due primarily to the propulsion of the sperm by the contractions of the female reproductive tract during orgasm. The normal ejaculate contains 150–600 million sperm but only 50–100 reach the ampulla where fertilization takes place. Sperm usually remain fertile within the female reproductive tract for 1 to 2 days, but as long as 4 days is possible. Access to the upper reaches of the reproductive tract by sperm is heavily influenced by ovarian steroid hormones.

Estradiol is secreted in abundance late in the follicular phase of the ovarian cycle and prepares the reproductive tract for efficient sperm transport (Fig. 14.30). Glycogen deposited in the vaginal mucosa under its influence provides a substrate for the production of lactate, which lowers the pH of vaginal fluid. An acidic environment increases the motility of sperm, which is essential for their passage through the cervical canal. In addition, the copious watery secretion produced by cells lining the cervical canal under the influence of

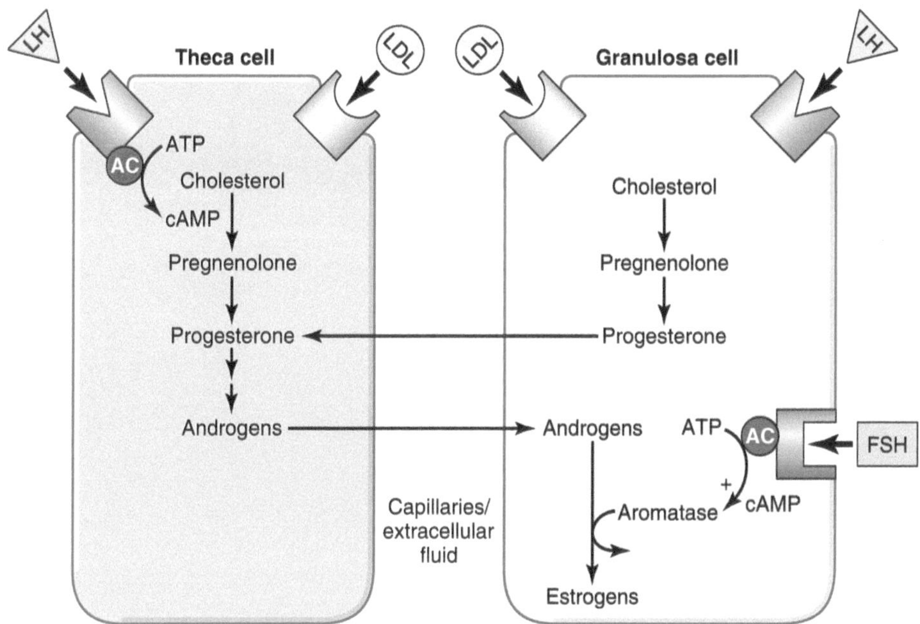

FIGURE 14.29 The production of hormones by the thecal and granulosa cells in the ovarian follicle. *AC*, Adenyl cyclase; *cAMP*, cyclic adenosine monophosphate. *Source: Figure 82.8 in Hall (2016).* Guyton and Hall textbook of medical physiology *(13th ed., p. 1044). Elsevier.*

estrogen increases access to the uterine cavity. When estrogen is absent or when its effects are opposed by progesterone, the cervical canal is filled with a viscous mucus that resists sperm penetration. Vigorous contractions of the uterus propel sperm toward the uterine tubes. Prostaglandins present in seminal plasma and oxytocin released from the pituitary in response to intercourse stimulates the contraction of the highly responsive estrogen-dominated myometrium.

Role of the uterine tubes

The uterine tubes are uniquely adapted for facilitating the transport of sperm toward the ovary and transporting the ovum in the opposite direction toward its rendezvous with sperm. It is also within the uterine tubes that sperm undergo capacitation, a process which enables them to penetrate the zona pellucida with their acrosomal enzymes. The zona pellucida is a mucopolysaccharide-and-protein protective barrier that surrounds the oocyte (Figs. 14.32 and 14.33).

Capacitation is an activation process that involves both enhancement of flagellar activity and the biochemical and structural changes in the plasma membrane of the sperm head that prepares sperm to undergo the acrosomal reaction (Fig. 14.34).

The acrosome is a membranous vesicle that is positioned at the tip of the sperm head. It is filled with several hydrolytic enzymes. Contact of the sperm head with the zona pellucida that surrounds the ovum initiates fusion of the acrosomal membrane with the plasma membrane and the exocytotic release of enzymes that digest a path through the zona pellucida clearing the way for sperm to reach the ovum (Figs. 14.35 and 14.36).

The acrosome reaction and the events that produce it are highly reminiscent of the sequelae of the hormone-receptor interactions and involve activation of membrane calcium channels, tyrosine phosphorylation, phospholipase C, and other intracellular signaling mechanisms. Initiation of the acrosomal reaction is facilitated by progesterone secreted by the mass of cumulus cells that surround the oocyte. The sperm plasma membrane contains progesterone receptors that trigger the influx of calcium within seconds. These membrane-associated receptors differ from the classical nuclear receptors.

In response to estrogens or perhaps other local signals associated with impending ovulation, muscular activity in the distal portion of the uterine tube brings the infundibulum into close contact with the surface of the ovary. At ovulation, the ovum, together with its surrounding granulosa cells (cumulus oophorus while in the ovary), is released into the peritoneal cavity and is swept into the ostium of the uterine tube by the vigorous, synchronous beating of cilia on the fimbriae at the end of the infundibulum (Fig. 14.37).

Development of cilia in the epithelial lining and their synchronized rhythmic activity are consequences of earlier exposure to estrogens. Movement of the egg mass through the ampulla toward the site of fertilization near the ampulla–isthmus junction depends principally on currents set up in tubal fluid by the beating of cilia and to a lesser extent by contractile activity of the ampulla wall to produce a churning motion (Figs. 14.38–14.40).

Propulsion of sperm through the isthmus toward the ampulla is accomplished largely by muscular contractions

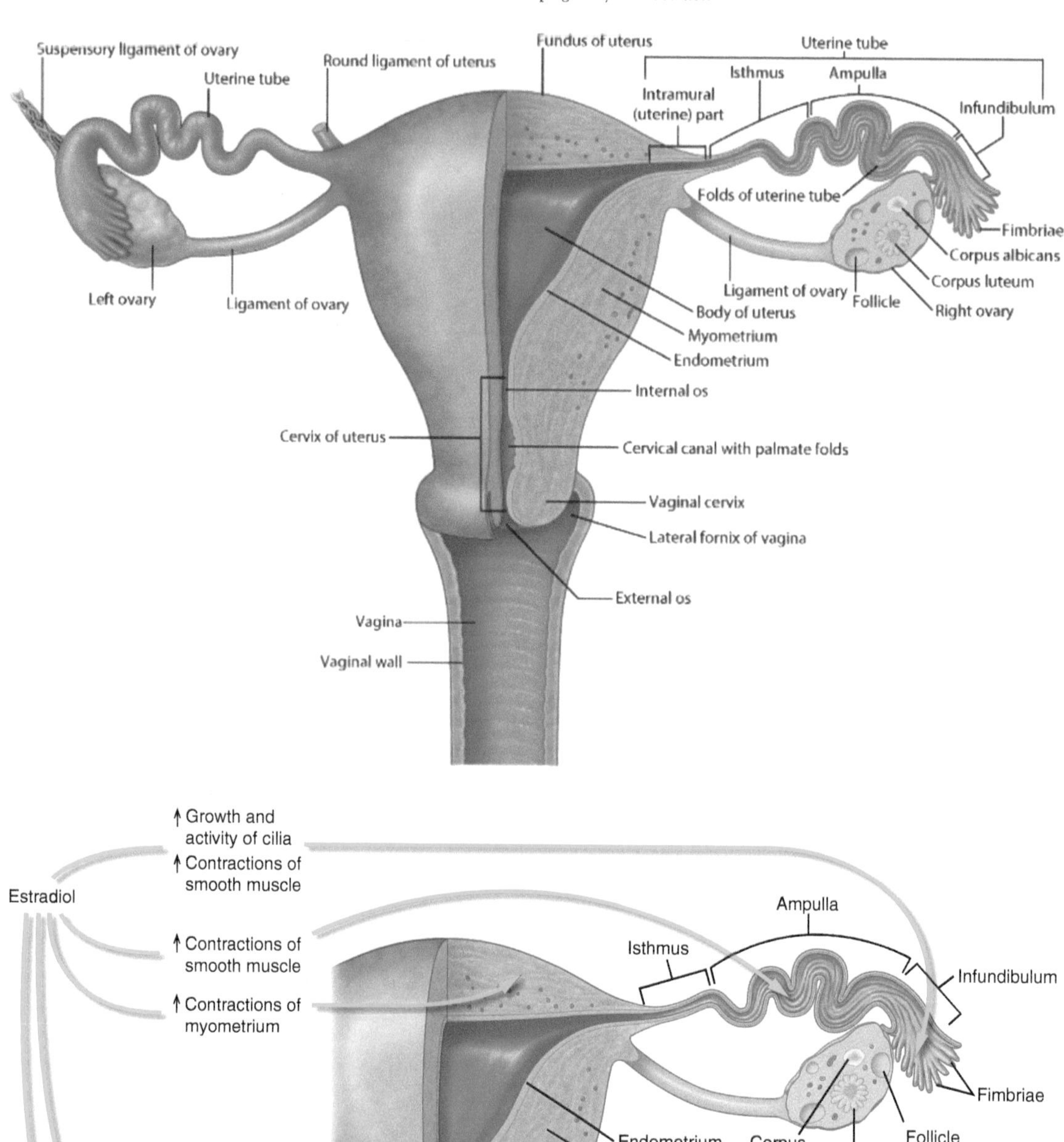

FIGURE 14.30 The uterus, uterine tube, and ovary. Source: *Figure in Drake, Vogl, Mitchell, Tibbitts, & Richardson (2015).* Gray's Atlas of anatomy *(2nd ed., p. 242). Elsevier.*

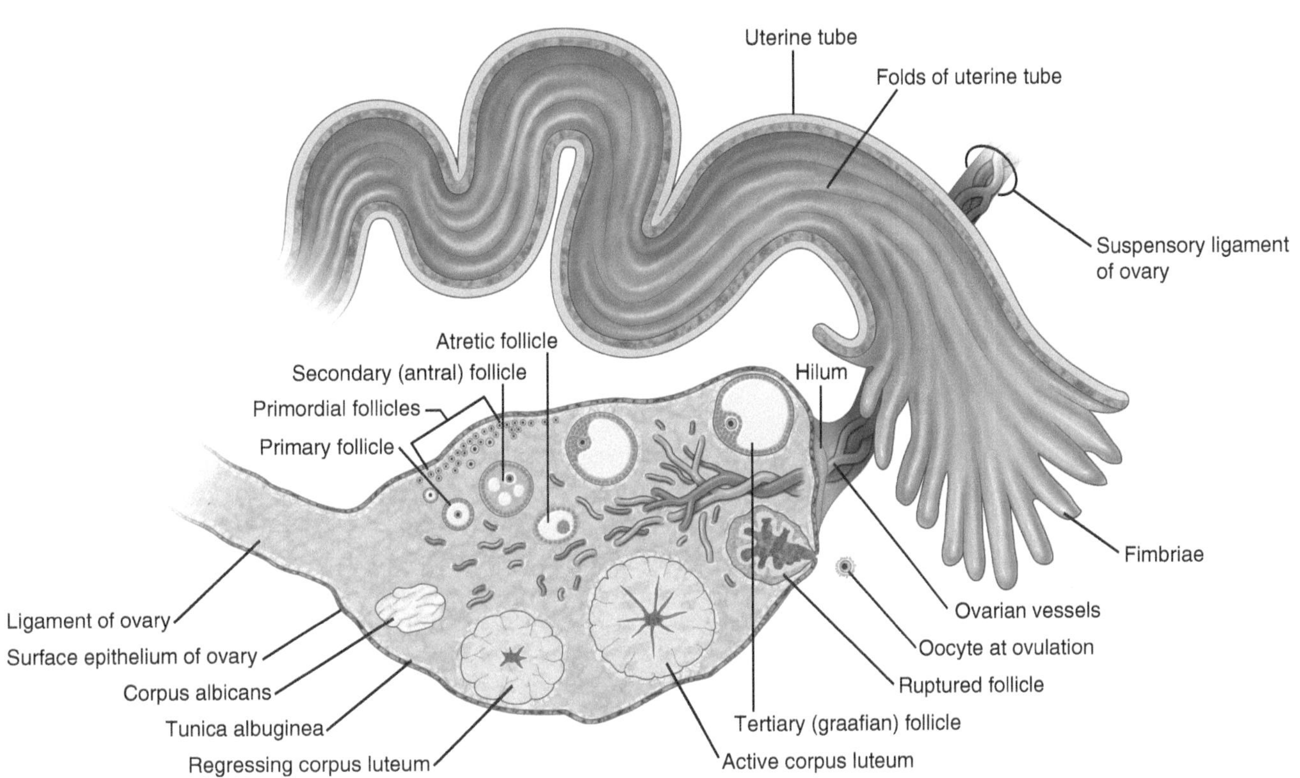

FIGURE 14.31 The uterine tube (ampulla and infundibulum portions only) and ovary in detail. Source: *Figure in Drake, Vogl, Mitchell, Tibbitts, & Richardson (2015).* Gray's Atlas of anatomy *(2nd ed., p. 242). Elsevier.*

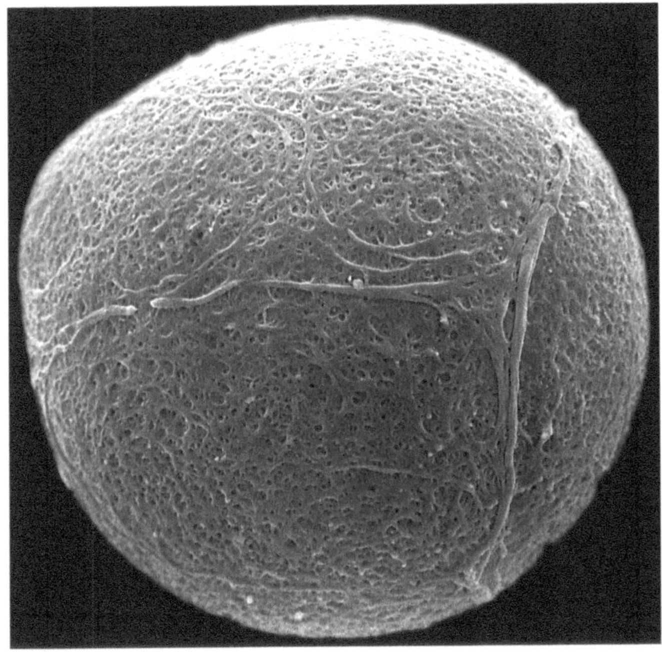

FIGURE 14.32 The zona pellucida is composed of proteins and mucopolysaccharides. It surrounds and protects the underlying oocyte. The overlying cells have been stripped away. Source: *Figure 1.7A in Schoenwolf, Bleyl, Brauer, & Francis-West (2015).* Larsen's human embryology *(5th ed., p. 27). Elsevier.*

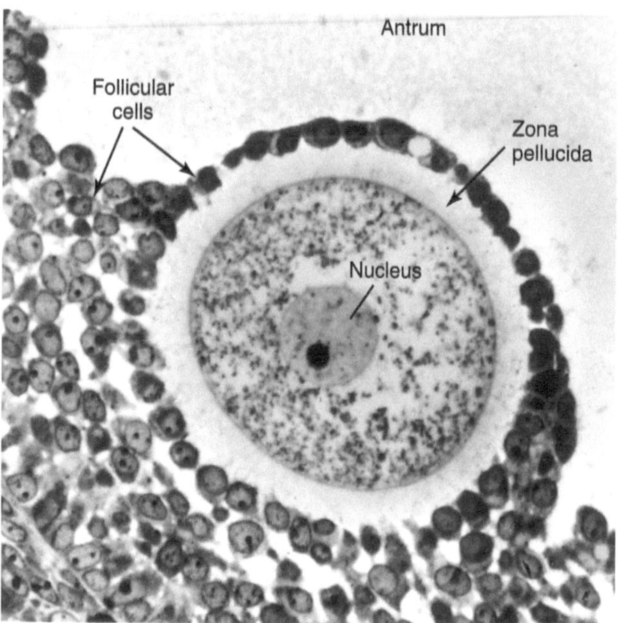

FIGURE 14.33 A cross section of the oocyte showing the zona pellucida. This image was taken before ovulation while the oocyte was still part of the ovarian follicle. The cumulus oophorus (mound-bearing egg) are supportive cells that surround the oocyte and have extensions that go through the zona pellucida and into the oocyte. Source: *Figure 2.8 in Moore, Persaud, & Torchia (2016).* The developing human *(10th ed., p. 21). Elsevier.*

of the uterine tubal wall. Circular smooth muscles of the isthmus are innervated with sympathetic fibers and have both α-adrenergic receptors, which mediate contraction, and β-adrenergic receptors, which mediate relaxation. Under the influence of estrogen the α receptors predominate. Subsequently, as estrogenic effects are opposed by progesterone, the β receptors prevail, and isthmic smooth muscles relax. This reversal in the response to adrenergic stimulation may account for the ability of the uterine tube to facilitate sperm transport through the isthmus toward the ovary and, subsequently, to promote passage of the embryo in the opposite direction toward the uterus (Fig. 14.41).

After fertilization the uterine tube retains the embryo for about 3 days and nourishes it with secreted nutrients before facilitating its entry into the uterine cavity. These complex events, orchestrated by the interplay of estrogen, progesterone, and autonomic innervation, require participation of the smooth muscle of the walls of the uterine tube as well as secretory and ciliary activity of the epithelial lining. As crucial as these mechanical actions may be, however, the uterine tube does not contribute in an indispensable way to fertility of the ovum or sperm or to their union, as modern techniques of in vitro fertilization bypass it with no ill effects.

The period of fertility is short; from the time the ovum is shed until it can no longer be fertilized is only about 6–24 hours. As soon as a sperm penetrates the ovum, meiosis II is completed and the second polar body is extruded and the pronuclei, one from the sperm and one from the oocyte, get ready to fuse (Fig. 14.42).

Once the pronuclei fuse, the fertilized ovum begins to divide (Fig. 14.43).

By the time the fertilized egg enters the uterine cavity, it has reached the blastocyst stage and consists of about 100 cells (Figs. 14.44 and 14.45).

Timing of the arrival of the blastocyst in the uterine cavity is determined by the balance between antagonistic effects of estrogen and progesterone on the contractility of the uterine tube wall. Under the influence of estrogen, circularly oriented smooth muscle of the isthmus is contracted and bars passage of the embryo to the uterus. As the corpus luteum organizes and increases its capacity to secrete progesterone, β-adrenergic receptors gain ascendancy, muscles of the isthmus relax, and the embryonic group is allowed to pass into the uterine cavity. Ovarian steroids can thus "lock" the ovum or embryo in the uterine tube or cause its delivery prematurely into the uterine cavity.

Implantation and the formation of the placenta

The blastocyst floats freely in the uterine cavity for about a day before it implants, normally on about the fifth day after ovulation (Fig. 14.46).

From the time the ovum is shed until the blastocyst implants, metabolic needs are met by secretions of the uterine tube and the endometrium. Experience with in vitro fertilization indicates that there is about a 3-day period of uterine receptivity in which implantation leads to full-term pregnancy. It should be recalled that this period of endometrial sensitivity coincides with the period of maximal progesterone output by the corpus luteum (Fig. 14.47).

In the late luteal phase of the menstrual cycle the outer layer of the endometrium differentiates to form the decidua. Decidualized stromal cells enlarge and transform from elongated spindle shape to a rounded morphology with an accumulation of glycogen. Decidualization requires high concentrations of progesterone and may be enhanced by the activity of cytokines and relaxin. Decidual cells express several proteins that may facilitate implantation but the precise roles of these proteins either in implantation or pregnancy have not been determined definitively. One such protein is the hormone prolactin, which continues to be secreted throughout pregnancy. Another is the insulin-like growth factor (IGF)-I binding protein.

At the time of implantation the blastocyst consists of an inner mass of cells destined to become the fetus and an outer rim of cells called the trophoblast. It is the trophoblast that forms the attachment to maternal decidual tissue and gives rise to the fetal membranes and the

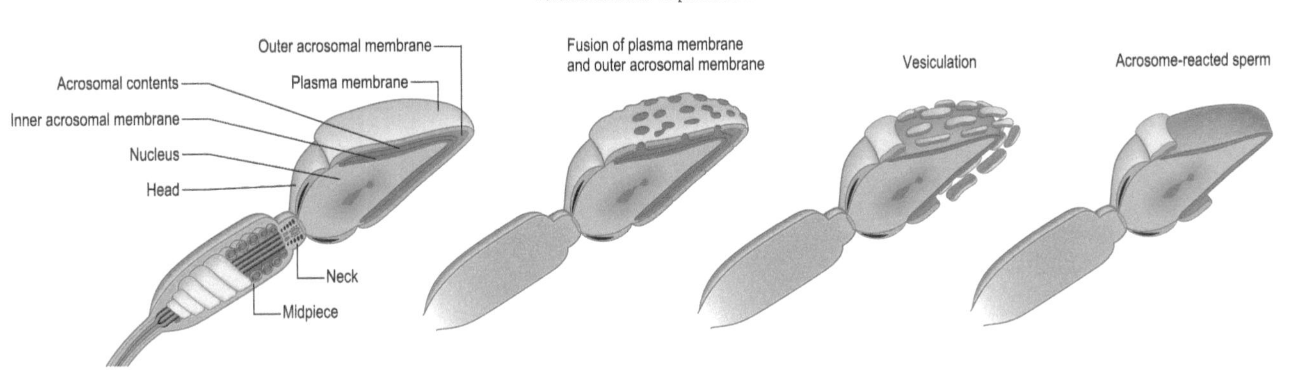

FIGURE 14.34 The sequence of events in capacitation. Source: *From Figure 8.4 in Standring (2015).* Gray's anatomy *(41st ed., p. 166). Elsevier.*

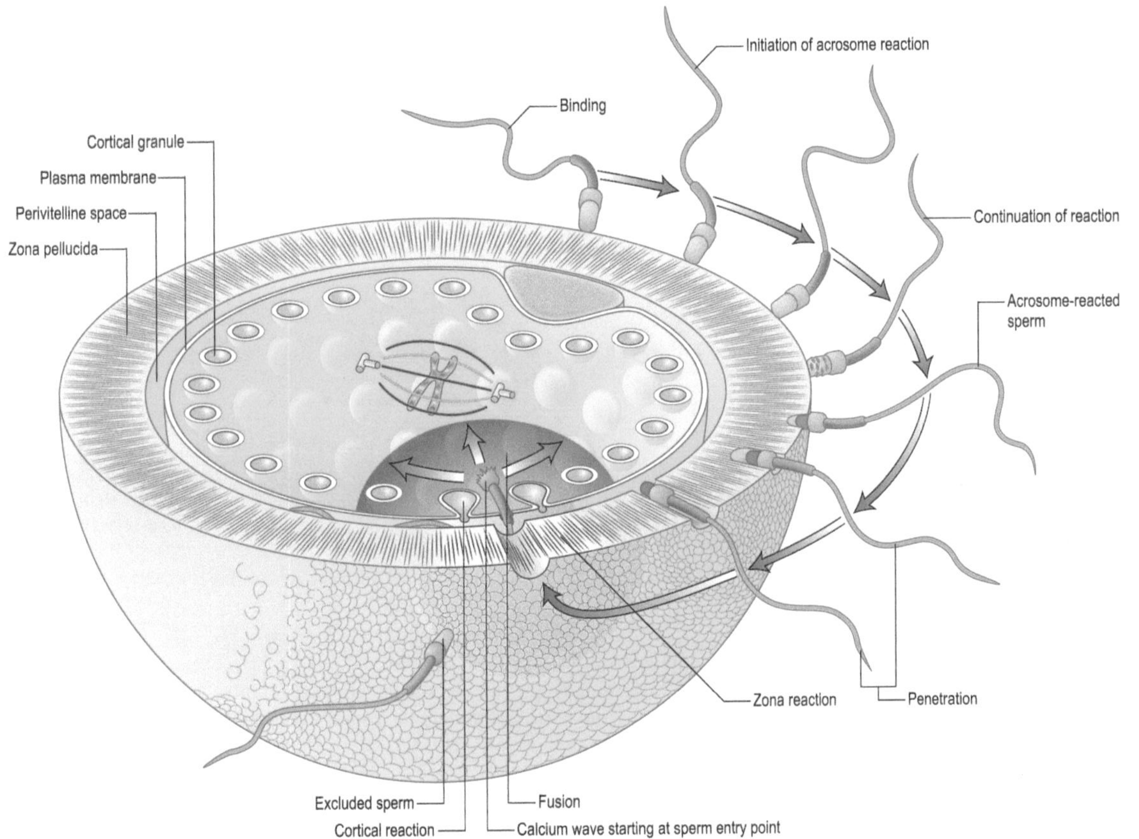

FIGURE 14.35 The fertilization of an oocyte after capacitation. Once inside the oocyte, a wave of calcium changes the permeability of the zona pellucida so that other sperm cannot enter. Should other sperm happen to enter, they are destroyed. Source: *From Figure 8.4 in Standring (2015).* Gray's anatomy *(41st ed., p. 166). Elsevier.*

definitive placenta. The implantation occurs in three steps: apposition, adhesion, and invasion (Fig. 14.48).

Cells of the trophoblast proliferate and form the multinucleated syncytiotrophoblast whose specialized functions enable it to destroy adjacent decidual cells and allow the blastocyst to penetrate deep into the uterine endometrium. Killed decidual cells are phagocytosed by the trophoblast as the embryo penetrates the subepithelial connective tissue and eventually becomes completely enclosed within the endometrium. Products released from degenerating decidual cells produce hyperemia and increased capillary permeability. Local extravasation from damaged capillaries forms small pools of blood that are in direct contact with the trophoblast and provide nourishment to the embryo until the definitive placenta forms.

The syncytiotrophoblast and an inner cytotrophoblast layer of cells soon completely surround the inner cell mass and send out solid columns of cells that further

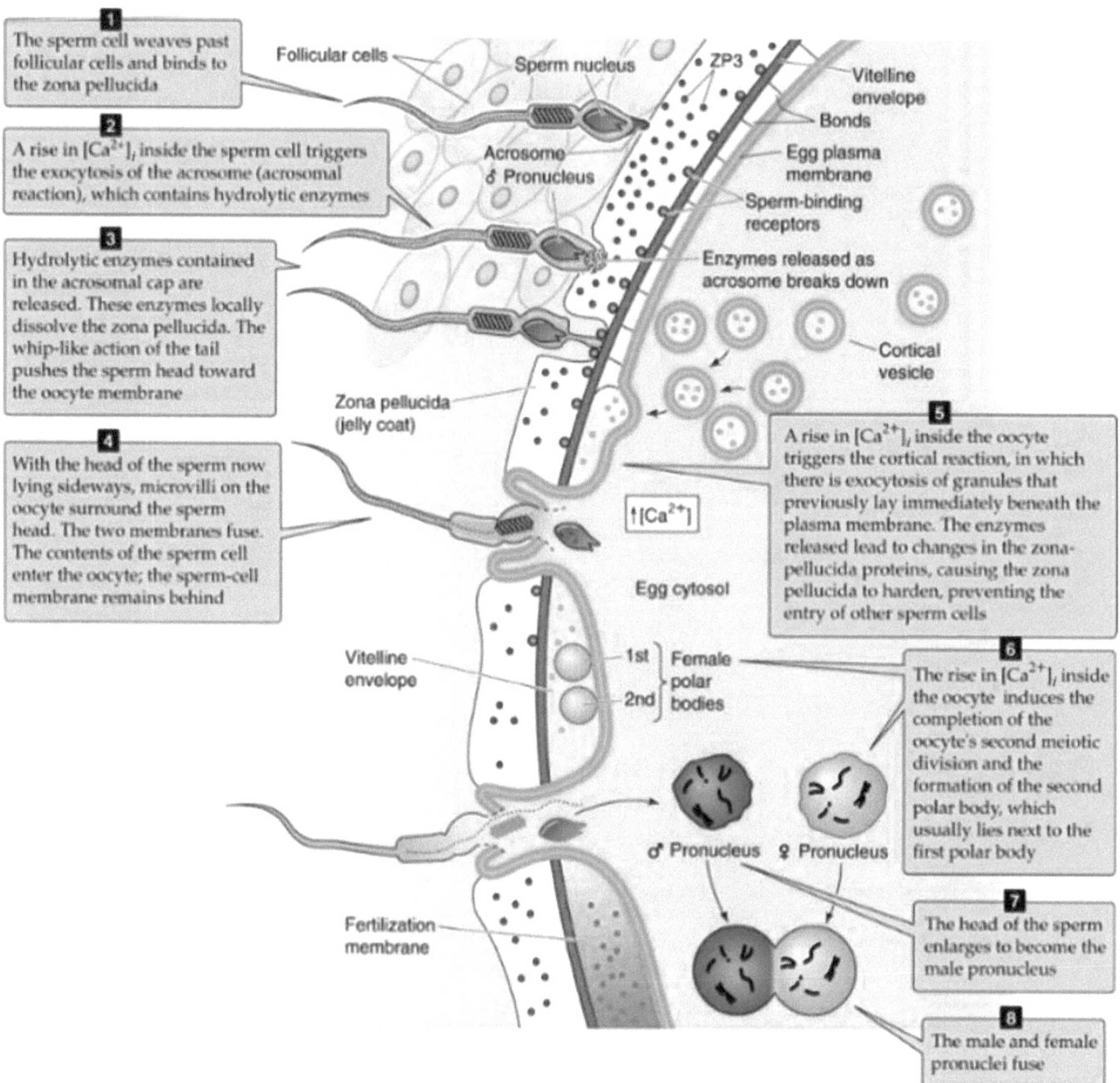

FIGURE 14.36 Events after fertilization. The release of calcium changes the zona pellucida and no other sperm usually enters the oocyte. Once in the oocyte, the sperm pronucleus waits for the oocyte pronucleus to complete meiosis II. After meiosis II has been completed the pronuclei of the sperm and oocyte fuse. Source: *Figure 51.1 in Boron, & Boulpaep (2017). Chapter 56: Fertilization, pregnancy and lactation. In S. Mesiano, & E. E. Jones (Eds.),* Medical physiology *(3rd ed., p. 1131). Elsevier.*

erode the endometrium and anchor the embryo. These columns of cells differentiate into the placental villi. As they digest the endometrium, pools of extravasated maternal blood become more extensive and fuse into a complex labyrinth that drains into venous sinuses in the endometrium. These pools expand and eventually receive an abundant supply of arterial blood. By the third week the villi are invaded by fetal blood vessels as the primitive circulatory system begins to function (Fig. 14.49).

Although much uncertainty remains regarding details of implantation in humans, it is perfectly clear that progesterone secreted by the ovary at the height of luteal function is indispensable for all these events to occur. Removal of the corpus luteum at this time or the blockade of progesterone secretion or progesterone receptors prevents implantation. Progesterone is indispensable for the maintenance of decidual cells, quiescence of the myometrium, and the formation of the dense, viscous cervical mucus that essentially seals off the uterine cavity from the outside. It is noteworthy that the implanting trophoblast and the fetus are genetically distinct from the mother and yet the maternal immune system does not reject the implanted embryo as a foreign body. Progesterone plays a decisive role in immunological acceptance of the embryo. It promotes tolerance by regulating the accumulation of lymphocyte types in the

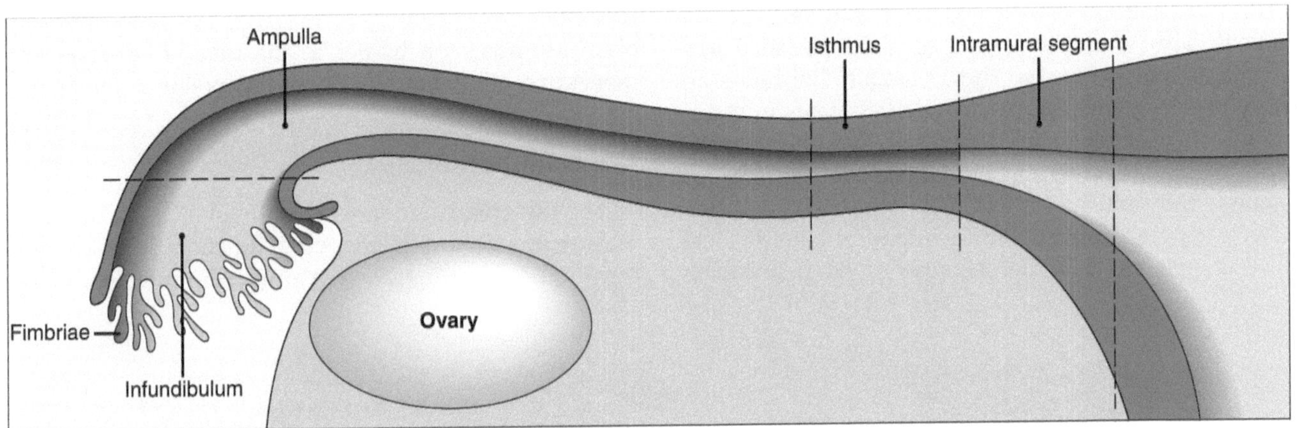

FIGURE 14.37 Schematic image of the fimbriae at the end of the infundibulum of the uterine tube. Source: *From Figure 3.19A in Lobo, Gershenson, Lentz, & Valea (2017). Chapter 3: Reproductive anatomy: Gross and microscopic, clinical correlations. In F. A. Valea (Ed.),* Comprehensive gynecology *(7th ed., p. 59). Elsevier.*

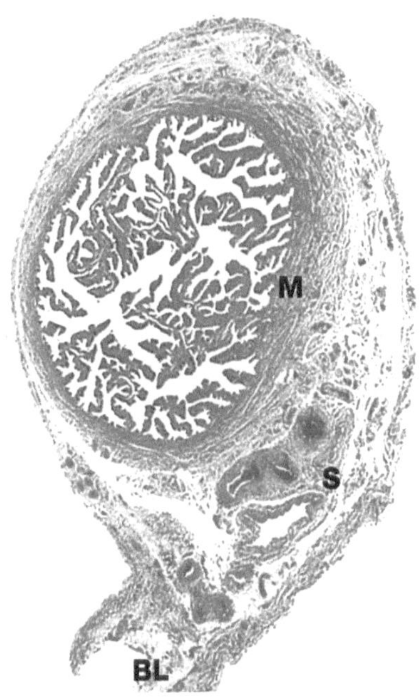

FIGURE 14.38 Section through the ampulla at 10×. Note the many folds within the ampulla. These produce a greater surface area to provide sperm and ova with nutrients. *BL*, Broad ligament of the uterus; *M*, circular muscle layer (the longitudinal layer is not visible at this magnification); *S*, serosa (visceral peritoneum). Source: *Figure 19.14A in Young, O'Dowd, & Woodford (2014).* Wheater's functional histology *(6th ed., p. 360). Elsevier.*

uterine cavity, by suppressing lymphocyte toxicity, and inhibiting the production of cytolytic cytokines. The importance of progesterone for implantation and retention of the blastocyst is underscored by the development of a progesterone antagonist (RU486, mifepristone) that prevents implantation or causes an already implanted conceptus to be shed along with the uterine lining.

The placenta

The placenta is a complex multifunctional organ that (1) anchors the developing fetus to the uterine wall; (2) provides the maternal/fetal interface for the exchange of nutrients, respiratory gases, and fetal wastes; and (3) directs maternal homeostatic adjustments to meet changing fetal needs by secreting hormones and other substances into the maternal circulation. It is a disk-shaped organ that measures about 22 cm in diameter and has an average thickness of about 2.5 cm at the end of pregnancy (Figs. 14.50–14.55).

The surface facing the developing fetus is called the chorionic plate. It is penetrated near its center by the umbilical artery and veins, which branch repeatedly to perfuse the functional units, the tree-like placental villi, with fetal blood. The villi are rooted in the chorionic plate and extend toward the basal plate, which comprises maternal decidual cells and extravillous syncytiotrophoblast.

The mature placenta contains 60–70 villous trees, each of which, through repeated branching of the secondary and tertiary villi, gives rise to more than 100,000 intermediate and terminal villi. The villi, whose combined length is estimated to be 90 km, contain increasingly finer branches of arterioles and venules that terminate as clusters of grape-like outgrowths comprised largely of sinusoidal dilated capillaries. The entire villous tree is ensheathed in a continuous layer of syncytiotrophoblast, which overlays a discontinuous layer of the cytotrophoblastic cells. The chorionic plate is fused at its edges with the basal plate to form a hollow cavity, the intervillous space, which is perfused with maternal blood that enters through multiple spiral arteries that branch off the radial arteries in the myometrium and exits by way of the uteroplacental veins (Fig. 14.56).

The syncytiotrophoblast is endowed with versatile biosynthetic capacity and is the source of the placental peptide and steroid hormones. These placental hormones are largely responsible for orchestrating adjustments in maternal physiology as pregnancy progresses. The plasma membranes of the syncytiotrophoblast contain a rich array of channels and transport molecules that enable efficient exchange of nutrients and waste products between fetal and maternal blood. Either because of its permeability properties or its enzymatic makeup, the syncytiotrophoblast also acts as a barrier to the transfer of some hormones and other molecules from the mother to the fetus.

Placental hormones

The placenta is the most recently evolved of all mammalian organs, and its endocrine function is most highly developed in primates. It is unique among endocrine

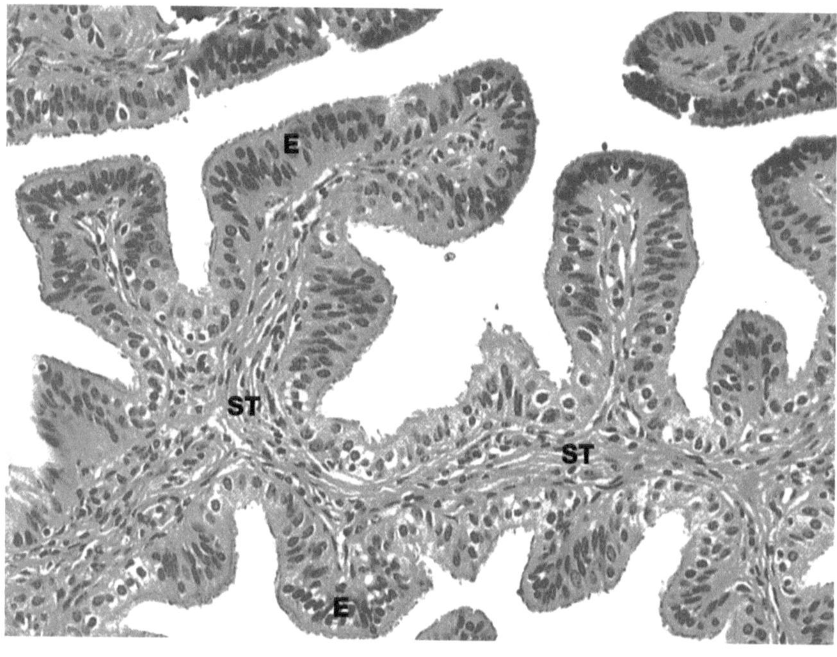

FIGURE 14.39 Medium (20×) power of the mucosal folds in Fig. 14.33. ST includes blood vessels; E includes goblet cells that produce mucus and ciliated cells that move the sperm and ovum. *E*, Epithelum; *ST*, stromal (supporting) tissue. Source: *Figure 19.14B in Young, O'Dowd, & Woodford (2014).* Wheater's functional histology *(6th ed., p. 360). Elsevier.*

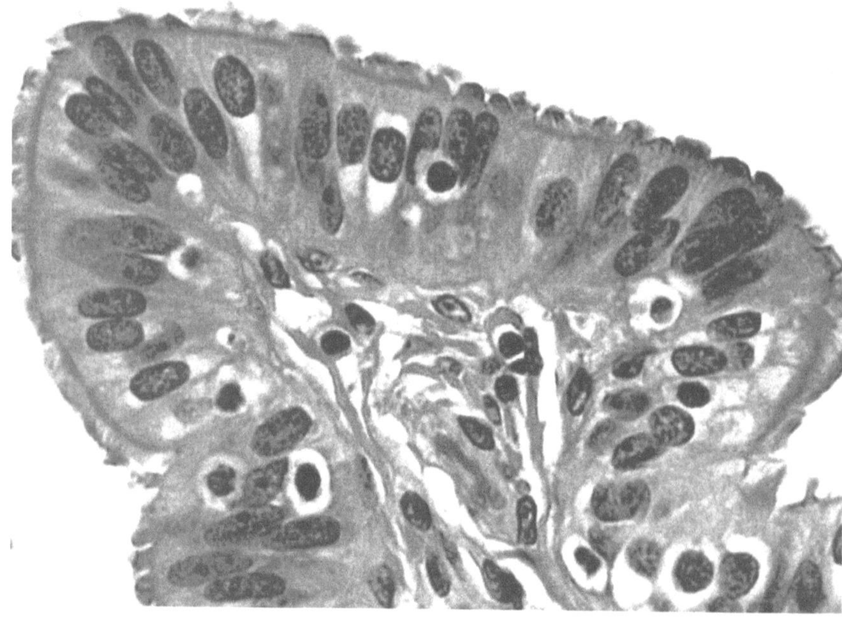

FIGURE 14.40 High power (43×) through a mucosal fold of the antrum. Note the cilia (the fuzzy structures) on the surface of the columnar cells. Some cells are secretory only, and a few are just supporting (intercalated) cells. Source: *Figure 19.14C in Young, O'Dowd, & Woodford (2014).* Wheater's functional histology *(6th ed., p. 360). Elsevier.*

glands in that, as far as is known, its secretory activity is autonomous and not subject to regulation by maternal or fetal signals. In experimental animals such as the rat, pregnancy is terminated if the pituitary gland is removed during the first half of gestation or if the ovaries, and consequently, the corpora lutea are removed at any time. In primates the pituitary gland and ovaries are essential only for a brief period after fertilization. After about 7 weeks the placenta produces enough progesterone to maintain pregnancy. In addition, it also produces large amounts of estrogens, human chorionic gonadotropin (hCG) (Fig. 14.57) and human chorionic somatomammotropin (hCS), which is also called human placental lactogen (Fig. 14.58).

It also secretes a form of growth hormone (human growth hormone variant) that is the product of a different gene than expressed in the pituitary (see Chapter 2: Pituitary Gland), thyroid-stimulating hormone (TSH), adrenocorticotropic hormone (ACTH), gonadotropin-releasing hormone (GnRH), corticotropin-releasing hormone (CRH), and a long list of other biologically active peptides. During pregnancy, there is the unique situation of hormones secreted by one individual, the fetus, regulating the physiology of another, the mother. By extracting needed nutrients and adding hormones to the maternal circulation the placenta redirects many aspects of maternal function to accommodate the growing fetus.

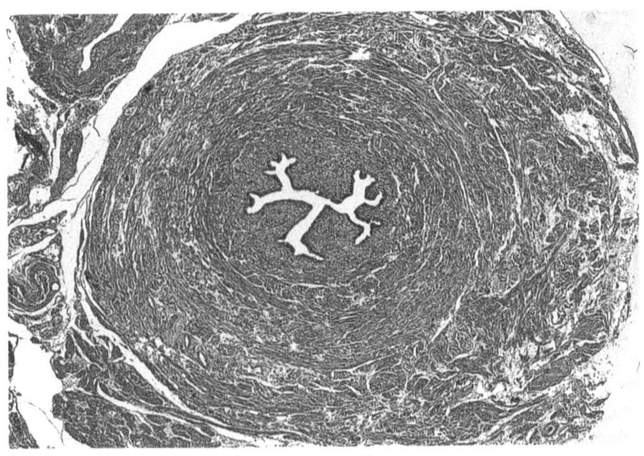

FIGURE 14.41 A cross section through the isthmus at 10 ×. This section shows the thick layers of smooth muscles innervated by the sympathetic division of the autonomic nervous system. Source: *From Figure 3.19C in Lobo, Gershenson, Lentz, & Valea (2017). Chapter 3: Reproductive anatomy: Gross and microscopic, clinical correlations. In F. A. Valea (Ed.),* Comprehensive gynecology *(7th ed., p. 59). Elsevier.*

Human chorionic gonadotropin

As already discussed (see Chapter 13: Hormonal Control of Reproduction in the Female: The Menstrual Cycle) the functional life of the corpus luteum in infertile cycles ends by the 12th day after ovulation. About 2 days later the endometrium is shed, and menstruation begins. For pregnancy to develop the endometrium must be maintained, and therefore the ovary must be notified that fertilization has occurred. The signal to the ovary in humans is a luteotropic substance secreted by the conceptus and called hCG. hCG rescues the corpus luteum (i.e., extends its life span) and stimulates it to continue secreting progesterone and estrogens, which in turn maintain the endometrium in a state favorable for implantation and placentation (Fig. 14.59).

Continued secretion of luteal steroids and inhibin notifies the pituitary gland that pregnancy has begun and inhibits secretion of the gonadotropins that would otherwise stimulate development of the next cohort of follicles.

Pituitary gonadotropins remain virtually undetectable in maternal blood throughout pregnancy as a result of the negative feedback effects of high circulating concentrations of estrogens and progesterone. Secretion of relaxin by the corpus luteum increases in early pregnancy becomes maximum at around the end of the first trimester and then declines somewhat but continues throughout pregnancy. Relaxin may synergize with progesterone in early pregnancy to suppress contractile activity of uterine smooth muscle and, in concert with estrogens, may have a role in orchestrating adaptive changes in maternal circulation (see later).

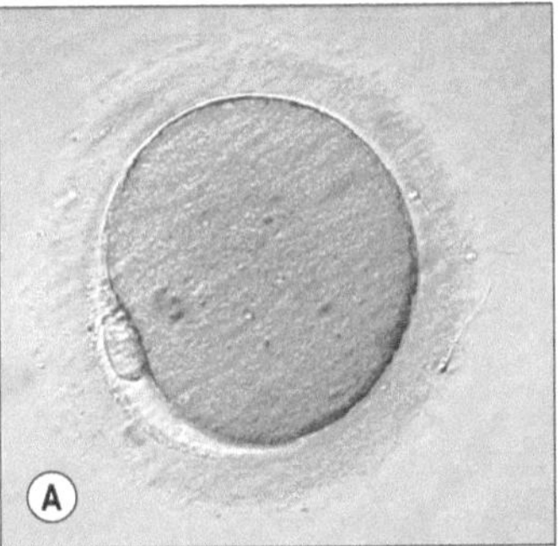

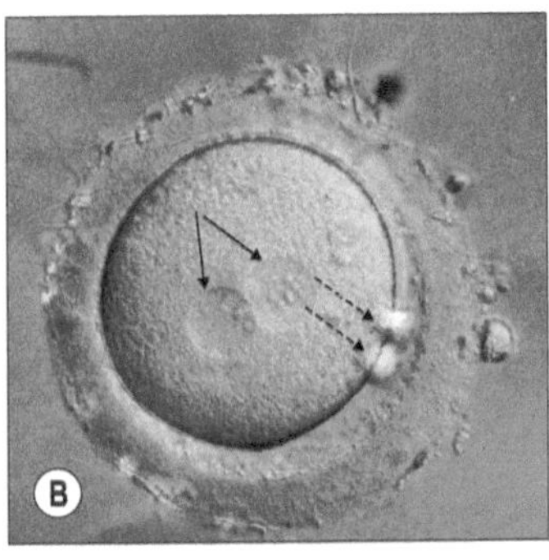

FIGURE 14.42 An unfertilized human secondary oocyte (A) before fertilization and (B) after fertilization in which the two pronuclei, one from the oocyte and the other from the sperm (*solid black arrows*) can be seen and two polar bodies (*dashed arrows*) lie just under the zona pellucida. Source: *Figure 8.5 in Standring (2015).* Gray's anatomy *(41st ed., p. 166). Elsevier.*

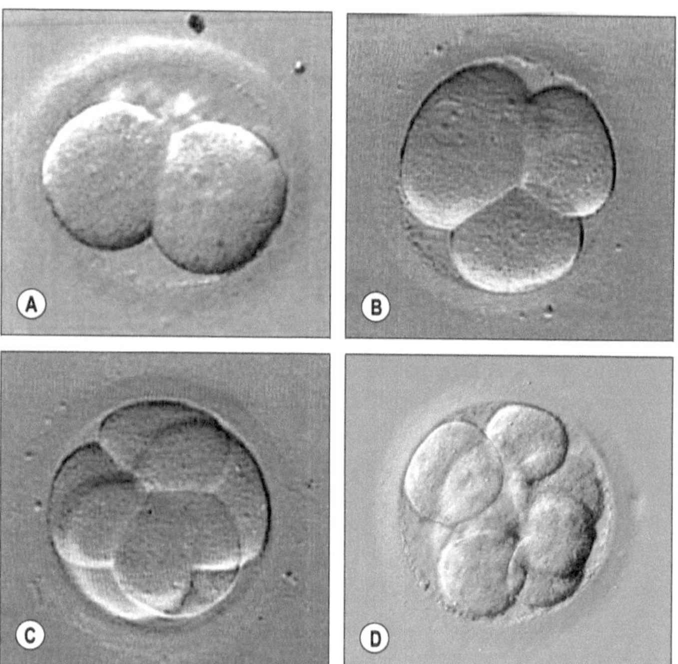

FIGURE 14.43 The first cleavage divisions of the fertilized ovum: (A) two, (B) three, (C) five, and (D) eight cells. The cells divide unevenly hence the odd number of cells. Source: *Figure 8.6 in Standring (2015).* Gray's anatomy *(41st ed., p. 167). Elsevier.*

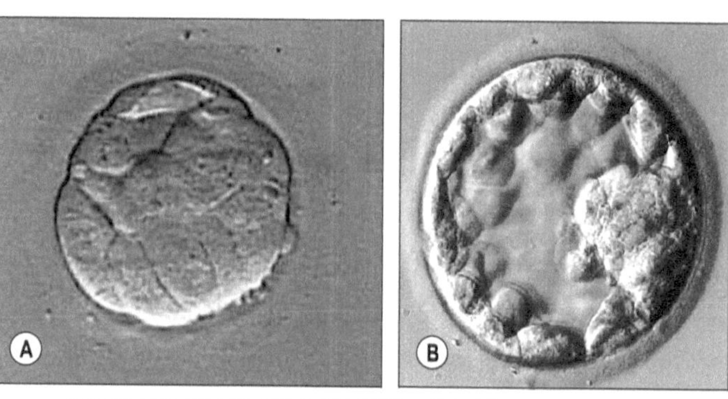

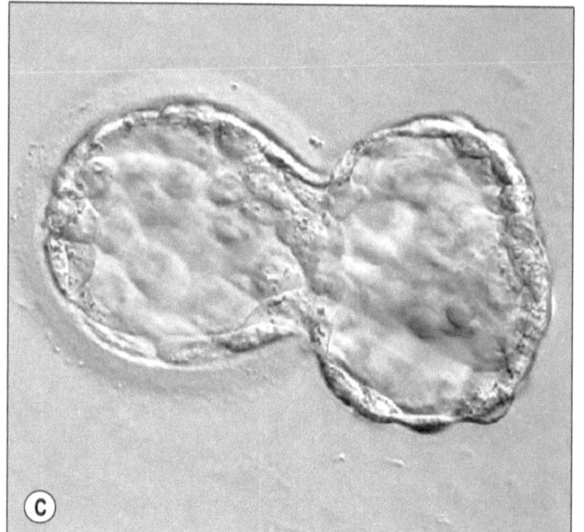

FIGURE 14.44 A morula is the term used when the number of cells reach 12. Part (A) shows a morula. When the morula forms a hollow center (B), it is called a blastocyst. (C) The blastocyst is "hatching" from the zona pellucida. It expands as it hatches. Source: *Figure 8.7 in Standring (2015).* Gray's anatomy *(41st ed., p. 167). Elsevier.*

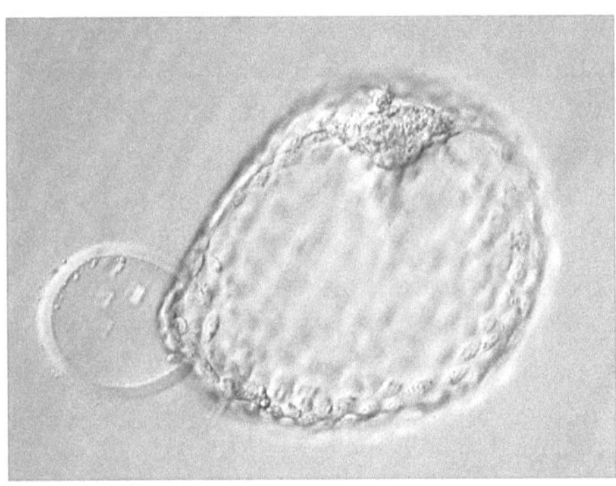

FIGURE 14.45 A newly "hatched" blastocyst leaves behind an empty zona pellucida. Source: *Figure 8.8 in Standring (2015).* Gray's anatomy *(41st ed., p. 167). Elsevier.*

hCG is a glycoprotein that is closely related to the pituitary glycoprotein hormones (see Chapter 2: Pituitary Gland). Although there are wide variations in the carbohydrate components, the peptide backbones of the glycoprotein hormones are closely related and consist of a common α subunit and activity-specific β subunits. In humans, seven genes or pseudogenes code for hCG β, but only two or three of them are expressed. The β subunit of hCG is almost identical to the β subunit of luteinizing hormone (LH), differing only by a 32-amino acid extension at the carboxyl terminus of hCG. It is not surprising, therefore, that hCG and LH act through a common receptor and that hCG has LH-like bioactivity. hCG contains considerably more carbohydrate, particularly sialic acid residues, than its pituitary counterparts, which accounts for its

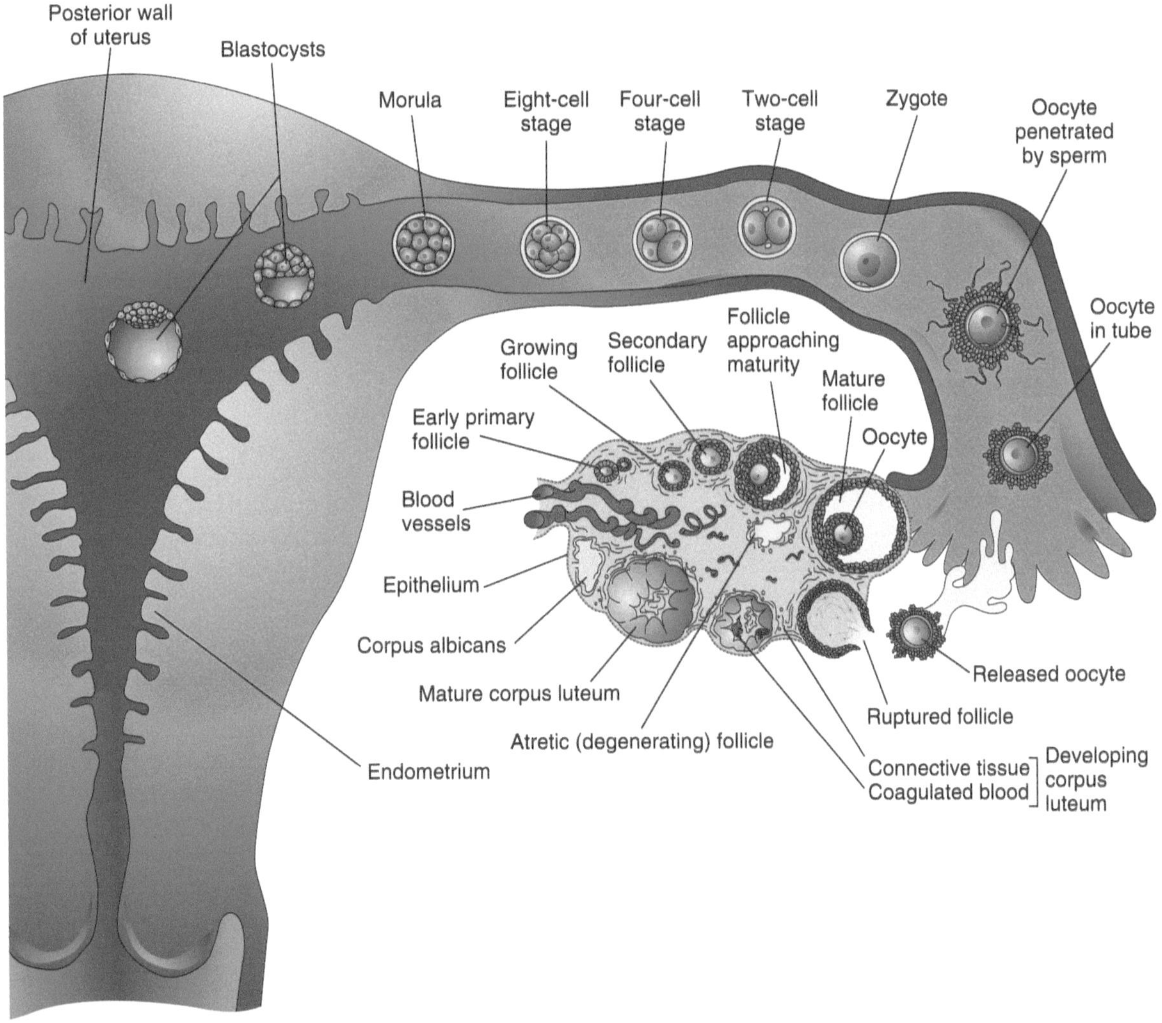

FIGURE 14.46 Summary of events until implantation on the posterior wall of the uterus (usual place for implantation). Source: *Figure 2.20 in Moore, Persuad, & Torchia (2016).* The developing human *(10th ed., p. 36). Elsevier.*

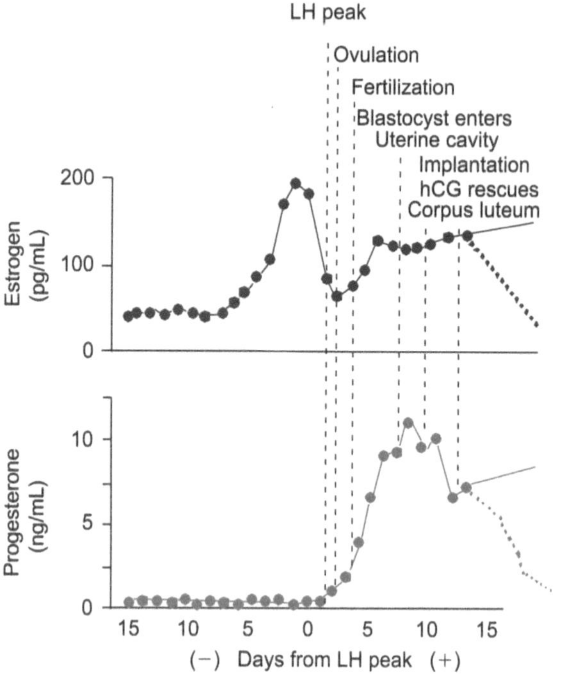

FIGURE 14.47 Relation between events of early pregnancy and steroid hormone concentrations in maternal blood. Estradiol and progesterone concentrations are redrawn from data given in Fig. 13.10. By the 10th day after the luteinizing hormone (LH) peak, there is sufficient hCG to maintain and increase estrogen and progesterone production, which would otherwise decrease (*dotted lines*) at this time. *hCG*, Human chorionic gonadotropin; *LH*, Luteinizing hormone.

extraordinary stability in blood. The half-life of hCG is more than 30 hours, as compared to just a few minutes for the pituitary glycoprotein hormones. The long half-life facilitates rapid build-up of adequate concentrations of this vital signal produced by a few vulnerable cells.

Trophoblast cells of the developing placenta begin to secrete hCG early, with detectable amounts already present in blood by about the eighth day after ovulation, when luteal function under the influence of LH is still at its height. Production of hCG increases dramatically during the early weeks of pregnancy (Fig. 14.60).

Blood levels continue to rise, and during the third month of pregnancy, reach peak values that are perhaps 200–1000 times that of LH at the height of the ovulatory surge. Presumably because of its high concentration, hCG is able to prolong the functional life of the corpus luteum, whereas LH, at the prevailing concentrations in the luteal phase of an infertile cycle, cannot. In addition, hCG concentrations remain constantly high, whereas LH concentrations rise and fall every 3 hours with each pulse of secretion. High concentrations of hCG at this early stage of fetal development are also critical for male sexual differentiation, which occurs before the fetal pituitary can produce adequate amounts of LH to stimulate testosterone synthesis by the developing testis (see Chapter 12: Hormonal Control of Reproduction in the Male). Stimulation of the fetal adrenal gland by hCG may augment estrogen production later in pregnancy (see later). Finally, it is the appearance of hCG in large amounts in urine that is used as a diagnostic test for pregnancy. Because its biological activity is like that of LH, urine containing hCG induces ovulation when injected into estrous rabbits in the classical rabbit test. This test has been replaced by a simple sensitive immunological test for hCG in urine that can detect pregnancy even before the next expected menstrual period.

Secretion of significant amounts of progesterone by the corpus luteum diminishes after about the eighth week of pregnancy despite continued stimulation by hCG. Measurements of progesterone in human ovarian venous blood indicate that the corpus luteum remains functional throughout most of the first trimester, and although some capacity to produce progesterone persists throughout pregnancy, continued presence of the ovary is not required for a successful outcome. Well before the decline in luteal steroidogenesis, placental production of progesterone becomes adequate to maintain pregnancy.

Human chorionic somatomammotropin

The other placental protein hormone that is secreted in large amounts is hCS. Like hCG, hCS is produced by the syncytiotrophoblast and becomes detectable in maternal plasma early in pregnancy. Its concentration in maternal plasma increases steadily from about the third week after fertilization and reaches a plateau by the last month of pregnancy (Fig. 14.6) when the placenta produces about 1 g of hCS each day. The concentration of hCS in maternal blood at this time is about 100 times higher than that normally seen for other protein hormones in women or men. hCS has a short half-life and, despite its high concentration at parturition, is undetectable in plasma after the first postpartum day.

Despite its abundance and its ability to produce a variety of biological actions in the laboratory, the physiological role of hCS has not been established definitively. hCS has strong prolactin-like activity and can induce lactation in test animals, but lactation normally does not begin until long enough after parturition for hCS to be cleared from maternal blood. However, it is likely that hCS promotes mammary growth in preparation for lactation. It is also likely that hCS contributes to the availability of nutrients for the developing fetus by operating like GH to mobilize maternal fat and decrease maternal glucose consumption (see Chapter 8: Hormonal Regulation of Fuel Metabolism). In this context, hCS may be at least partially responsible for the decreased glucose tolerance, the so-called gestational diabetes, experienced by many women during pregnancy (see later). Although the secretion of hCS is directed predominantly into maternal

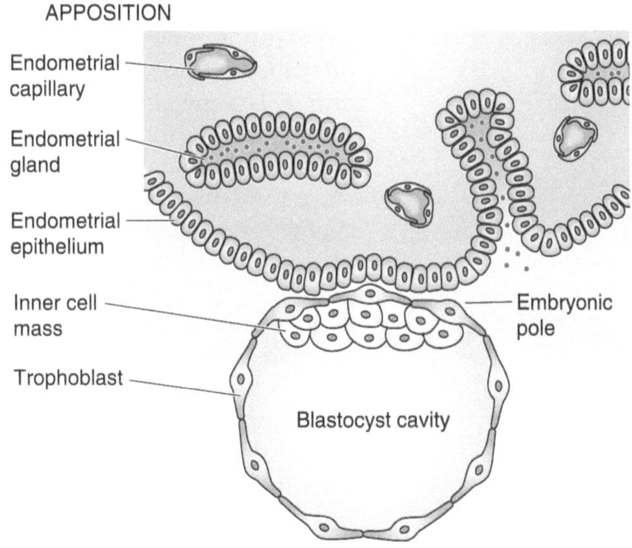

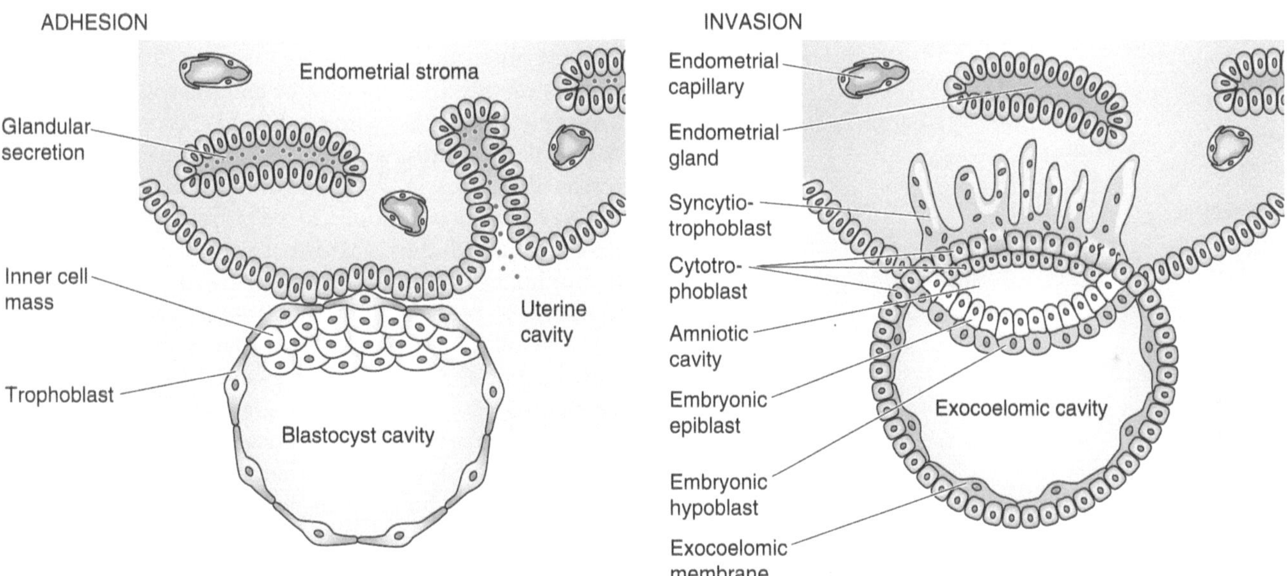

FIGURE 14.48 The implantation sequence: apposition, adhesion, and invasion. Source: *Figure 56.4 in Boron, & Boulpaep (2017). Chapter 56: Fertilization, pregnancy and lactation. In S. Mesiano, & E. E. Jones (Eds.),* Medical physiology *(3rd ed., p. 1135). Elsevier.*

blood, appreciable concentrations also are found in fetal blood in midgestation. Receptors for hCS are present in human fetal fibroblasts and myoblasts, and these cells release IGF-II when stimulated by hCS. As already discussed (see Chapter 11: Hormonal Control of Growth), fetal growth is independent of GH, but the role of hCS in this regard is unknown.

Despite these observations, evidence from genetic studies makes it unlikely that hCS is indispensable for the successful outcome of pregnancy. hCS is a member of the growth hormone-prolactin family (see Chapter 2: Pituitary Gland) and shares large regions of structural homology with both of these pituitary hormones. In humans, five genes of this family are clustered on chromosome 17, including three that encode hCS and two that encode GH. Two of the hCS genes are expressed and code for identical secretory products. The third hCS gene appears to be a pseudogene whose transcription does not produce fully processed messenger RNA. No adverse consequences for pregnancy, parturition, or early postnatal development were seen in some cases in which a stretch of DNA that contains both hCS genes and one human growth hormone gene was missing from both chromosomes. No immunoassayable hCS was present in maternal plasma, but it is possible that the remaining hCS gene or pseudogene was expressed under these circumstances or that recombination

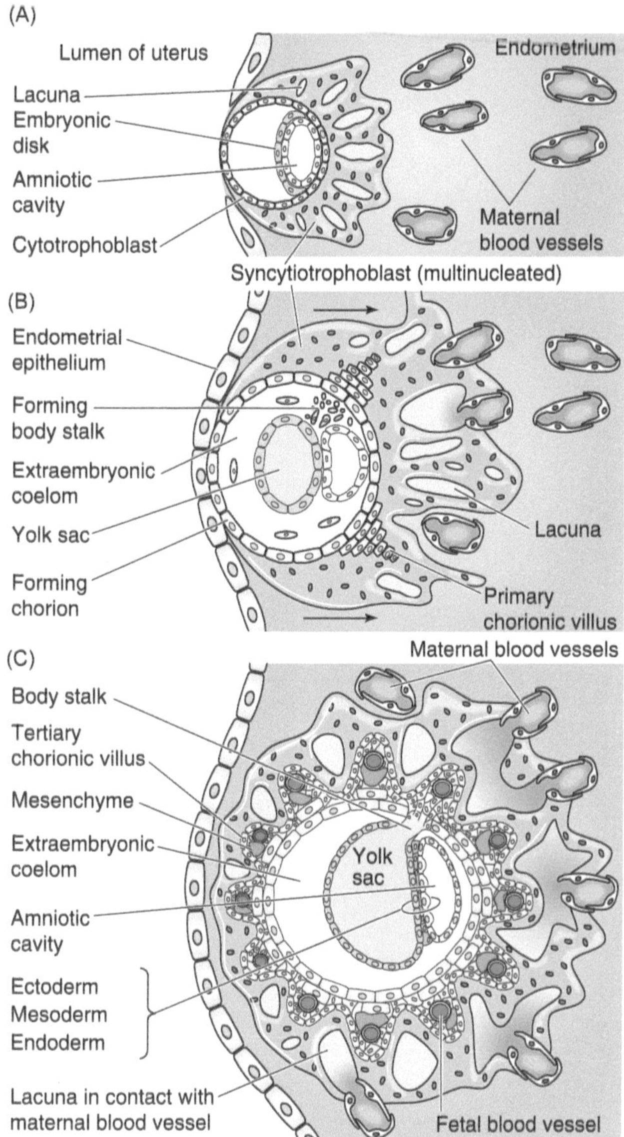

FIGURE 14.49 Sequence of development of the placenta: (A) 8, (B) 12–15, and (C) 20 days after fertilization. Source: *Figure 56.5 in Boron, & Boulpaep (2017). Chapter 56: Fertilization, pregnancy and lactation. In S. Mesiano, & E. E. Jones (Eds.),* Medical physiology *(3rd ed., p. 1137). Elsevier.*

of remaining fragments of these genes produced a chimeric protein with hCS-like activity. Regardless of whether or not hCS is indispensable for normal gestation, important functions often are governed by redundant mechanisms, and it is likely that hCS contributes in some way to a successful outcome of pregnancy.

Progesterone

As progesterone secretion by the corpus luteum declines, the trophoblast becomes the major producer of progesterone. Placental production of progesterone increases as pregnancy progresses, so that during the final months upward of 250 mg may be secreted per day. This huge amount is more than 10 times the daily production by the corpus luteum at the height of its activity and maybe even greater in women bearing more than one fetus. The placenta has little capacity to synthesize cholesterol and must import it from the maternal circulation in the form of low-density lipoproteins (LDL). In late pregnancy, progesterone production consumes an amount of cholesterol equivalent to about 25% of the daily turnover in a normal nonpregnant woman.

Production of progesterone by the placenta is not subject to regulation by any known extra placental factors other than the availability of substrate. As in the adrenals and gonads, the rate of conversion of cholesterol to pregnenolone by P450 side-chain cleavage (P450scc) determines the rate of progesterone production. In the adrenals and gonads, ACTH and LH stimulate the synthesis of the steroid acute regulatory (StAR) protein, which is required for transfer of cholesterol from cytosol to the mitochondrial matrix where P450scc resides (see Chapter 4: The Adrenal Glands). The placenta does not express StAR protein. Access of cholesterol to the interior of mitochondria is thought to be provided by a similar protein, called MLN64, that is constitutively expressed in the trophoblast. Consequently, placental conversion of cholesterol to pregnenolone bypasses the step that is regulated in all other steroid hormone-producing tissues. Ample expression of 3β-hydroxysteroid dehydrogenase allows rapid conversion of pregnenolone to progesterone. All the pregnenolone produced is either secreted as progesterone or exported to the fetal adrenal glands to serve as substrate for adrenal steroidogenesis (Fig. 14.7).

Estrogens

The human placenta is virtually the only site of estrogen production after the corpus luteum declines. However, the placenta cannot synthesize estrogens from cholesterol or use progesterone or pregnenolone as substrate for estrogen synthesis. The placenta does not express P450c17, which cleaves the C20,21 side chain to produce the requisite 19 carbon androgen precursor. Reminiscent of the dependence of granulosa cells on thecal cell production of androgens in ovarian follicles (see Chapter 13: Hormonal Control of Reproduction in the Female: The Menstrual Cycle), estrogen synthesis by the trophoblast depends on import of 19 carbon androgen substrates, which are secreted by the adrenal glands of the fetus and, to a lesser extent, the mother (Fig. 14.61). The trophoblast expresses an abundance of P450 aromatase, whose activity is sufficient to aromatize all the

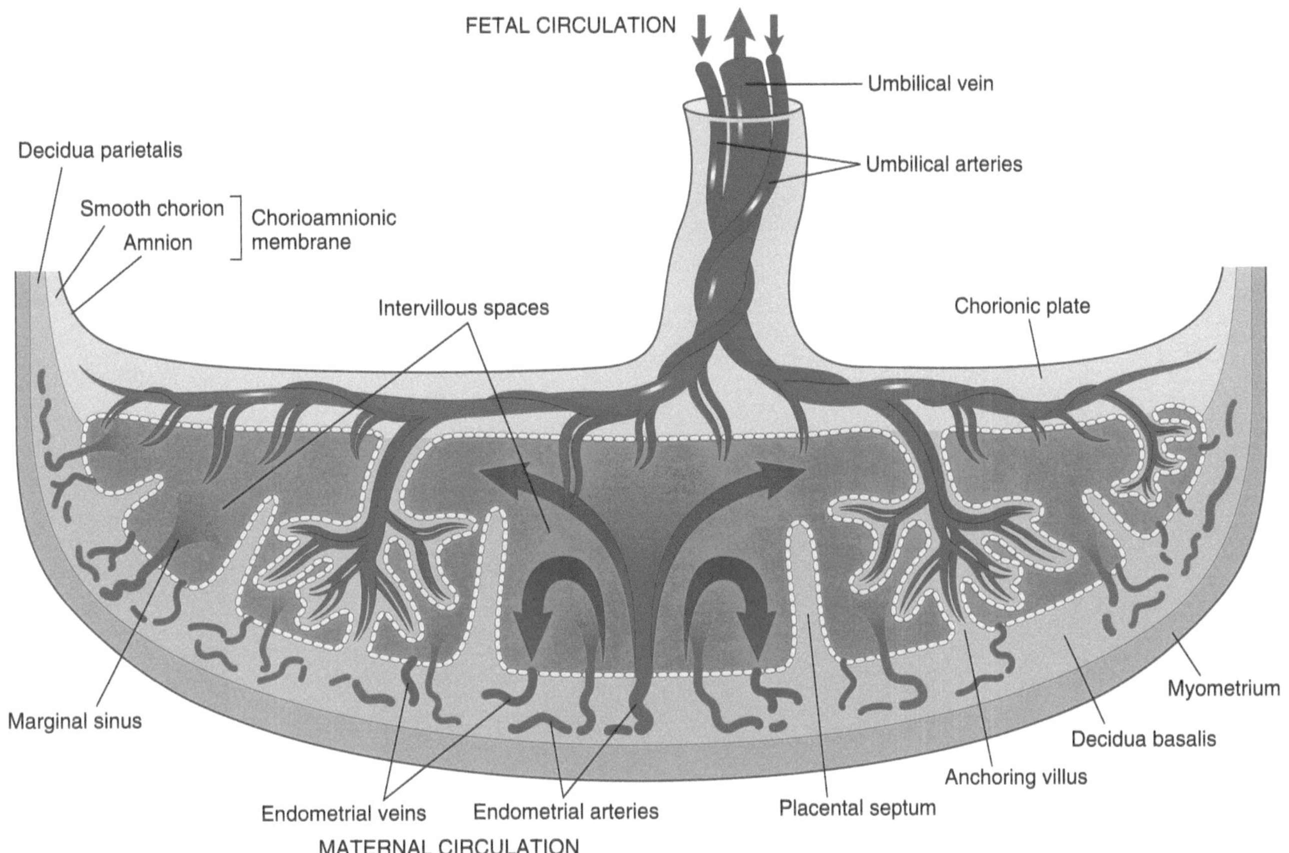

FIGURE 14.50 A schematic drawing of the human placenta. Maternal blood pools in the intervillous spaces. Oxygen and nutrients diffuse into the fetal veins, while carbon dioxide and metabolic products diffuse out of the umbilical arteries and into the same intervillous space. Maternal veins carry the blood from the intervillous spaces. Blood going toward the fetal heart is carried, by definition, in veins, whereas blood coming from the fetal heart is carried in arteries. This is one example in which blood higher in oxygen is carried in veins and blood low in oxygen is carried in arteries. Source: *Figure 22.47 in Kumar, Abbas, & Aster (2015). Chapter 22: The female genital tract. In L. H. Ellenson, & E. C. Pirog (Eds.),* Robbins and Cotran pathologic basis of disease *(9th ed., p. 1035). Elsevier.*

available substrate. The cooperative interaction between the fetal adrenal and the placenta has given rise to the term fetoplacental unit as the source of estrogen production in pregnancy.

The placental estrogens are estradiol, estrone, and estriol, which differ from estradiol by the presence of an additional hydroxyl group on carbon 16. Of these, estriol is by far the major estrogenic product. Its rate of synthesis may exceed 45 mg/day by the end of pregnancy. Despite its high rate of production, however, concentrations of unconjugated estriol in blood are lower than those of estradiol (Fig. 14.6) due to its high rate of metabolism and excretion. Although estriol can bind to estrogen receptors, it contributes little to overall estrogenic bioactivity as it is only about 1% as potent as estradiol and 10% as potent as estrone in most assays. However, estriol is almost as potent as estradiol in stimulating uterine blood flow. It is possible that the fetus uses this elaborate mechanism of estriol production to ensure that uterine blood flow remains adequate for its survival (Fig. 14.62).

The role of the fetal adrenal cortex

The fetal adrenal glands play a central role in placental steroidogenesis and hence maintenance of pregnancy and may also have a role in provoking the onset of labor at the end of pregnancy. The adrenal glands of the fetus differ significantly in both morphology and function from the adrenal glands of the adult. They are bounded by a thin outer region, called the definitive cortex, which will become the zona glomerulosa and a huge, inner "fetal zone," which regresses and disappears shortly after birth. The transitional zone at the interface of the two zones gives rise to the fasciculata and reticularis of the adult (see Chapter 4: The Adrenal Glands). In mid-pregnancy the fetal adrenals are large—larger in fact than the kidneys—and the fetal zone constitutes 80% of its mass.

Growth, differentiation, and secretory activity of the fetal adrenals are controlled by ACTH, whose actions are augmented by a variety of fetal growth factors including

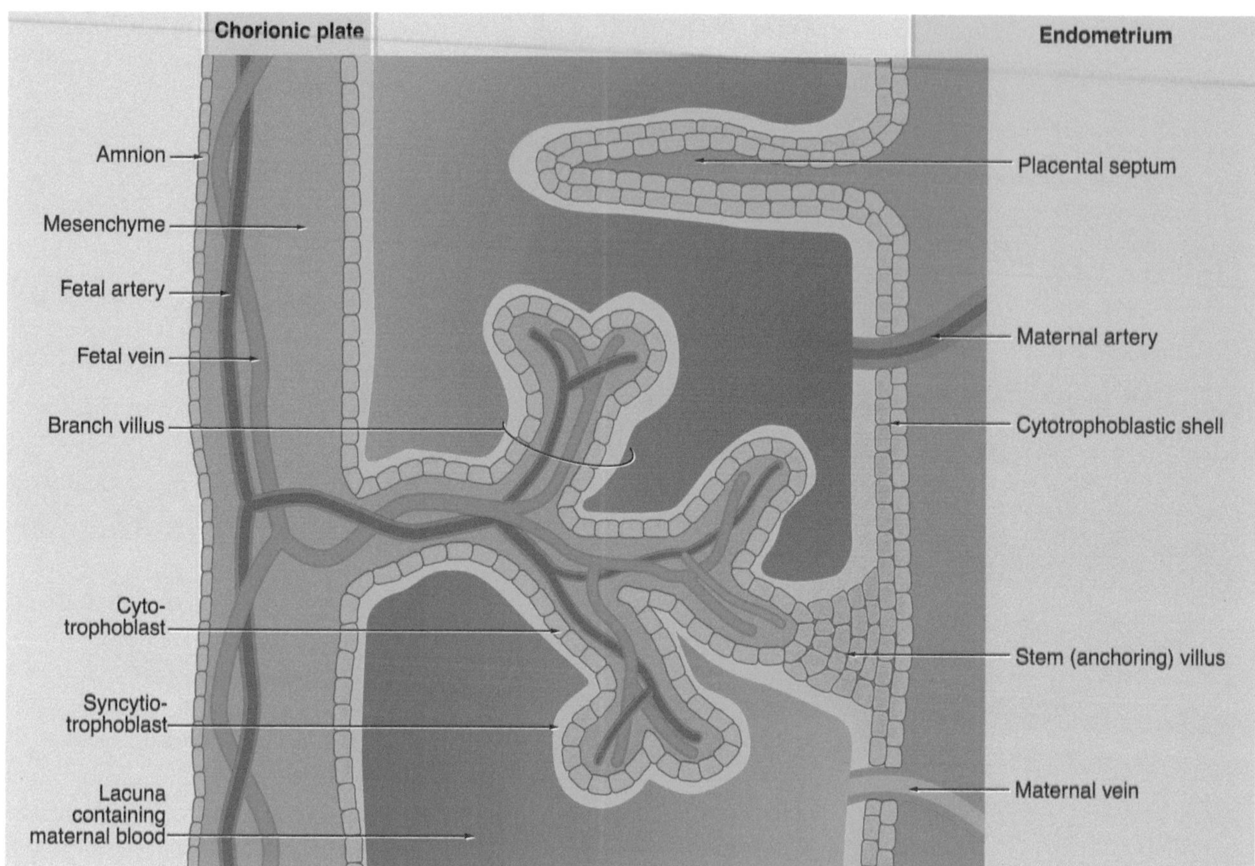

FIGURE 14.51 A schematic diagram of a section of the placenta. The lacuna is also called the intervillous space. Usually, lacuna is reserved for the spaces early in placental development and intervillous spaces in a more mature placenta (see Fig. 14.50). Source: *Figure 19.29 in Young, O'Dowd, & Woodford (2014).* Wheater's functional histology *(6th ed., p. 372). Elsevier.*

IGF-II. The fetal pituitary is the main source of ACTH, but the placenta also secretes some ACTH. In addition, the placenta secretes CRH, which not only stimulates the fetal pituitary to secrete ACTH but also directly stimulates steroidogenesis by the fetal adrenal glands.

The chief product of the fetal zone is the 19-carbon androgen dehydroepiandrosterone (DHEA), which is secreted as the biologically inert sulfate ester (DHEAS). Sulfation protects against masculinization of the genitalia in female fetuses and prevents aromatization in extragonadal fetal tissues. The fetal zone produces DHEAS at an increasing rate that becomes detectable by about the eighth week of pregnancy; well before, cortisol and aldosterone are produced by the definitive and transitional zones. At term, secretion of DHEAS may reach 200 mg/day. The cholesterol substrate for DHEAS production is synthesized in both the fetal liver and fetal adrenals. It is likely that pregnenolone released into the fetal circulation by the placenta also provides substrate.

Much of the DHEAS in the fetal circulation is oxidized at carbon 16 in the fetal liver to form 16α-DHEAS and then exported to the placenta. The placenta is highly efficient at extracting 19-carbon steroids from both maternal and fetal blood. It is rich in sulfatase and converts 16α-DHEAS to 16α-DHEA prior to aromatization to form estriol. Because synthesis of estriol reflects the combined activities of the fetal adrenals, the fetal liver, and the placenta, its rate of production, as reflected in maternal estriol concentrations, has been used as an indicator of fetal well-being. DHEAS that escapes 16α-hydroxylation in the fetal liver is converted to androstenedione or testosterone in the placenta after hydrolysis of the sulfate bond and then aromatized to form estrone and estradiol.

The role of progesterone and estrogens in maintaining pregnancy

As its name implies, progesterone is essential for maintaining all stages of pregnancy, and pharmacologic blockade of its actions at any time terminates the pregnancy. Progesterone sustains pregnancy by opposing the forces that conspire to increase uterine contractility and expel the fetus. One of these forces is physical stretch of the myometrium by the growing fetus. Stretch or tension coupled with estrogens and progesterone promotes

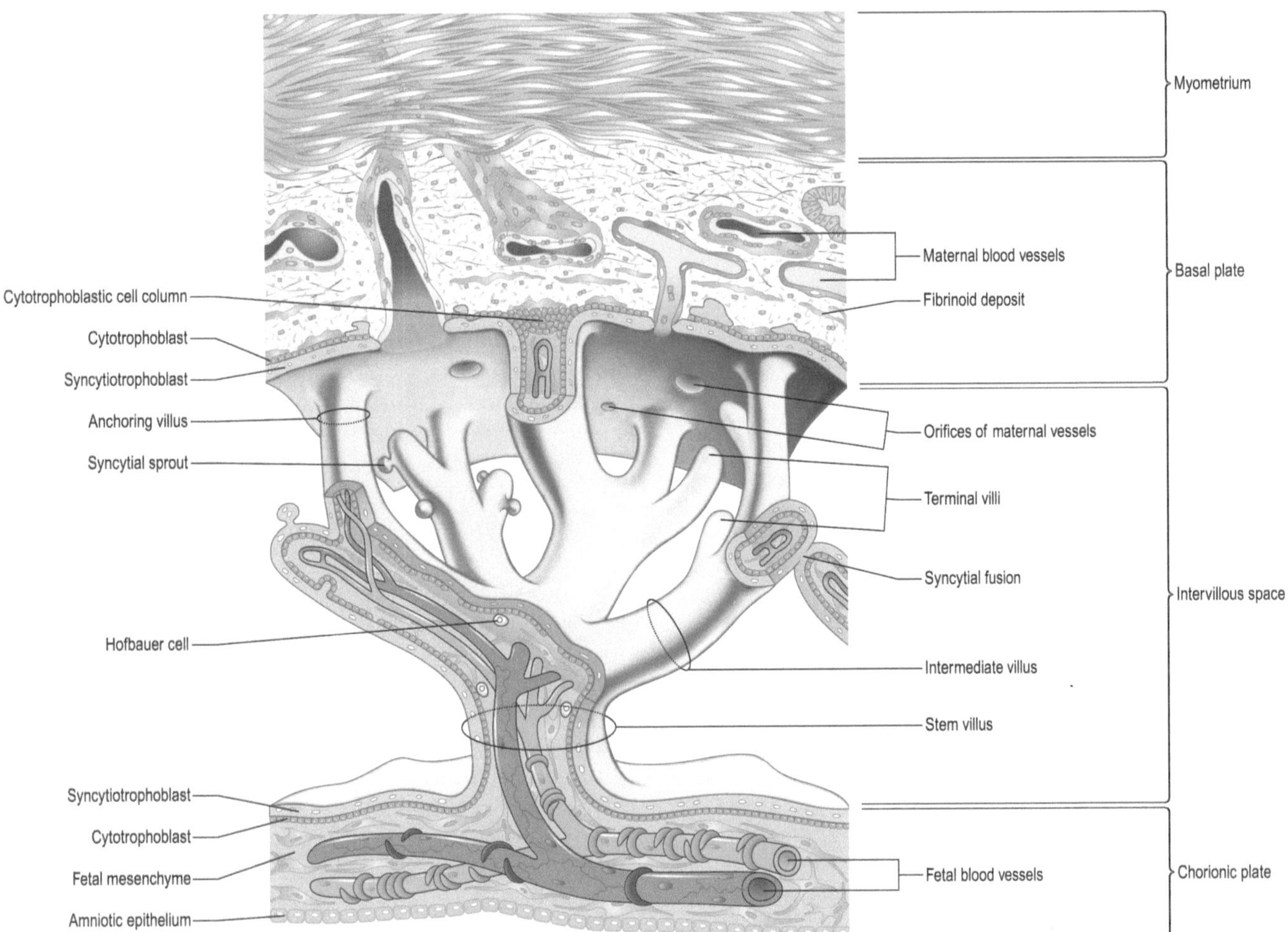

FIGURE 14.52 Detailed structure of a villus and its connections. Source: *Figure 9.7 in Standring (2015).* Gray's anatomy *(41st ed., p. 175). Elsevier.*

myometrial growth and hypertrophy in parallel with the growth of the conceptus. Estrogens promote expression of genes that code for contractile proteins, gap junction proteins that electrically couple myometrial cells, oxytocin receptors, receptors for prostaglandins, ion channels, and doubtlessly many other proteins that directly or indirectly tend to increase contractility.

Throughout pregnancy, estrogens act through a positive feedback mechanism not only to increase their own production but also to increase synthesis of progesterone, which suppresses their excitatory effects (Fig. 14.63).

Estrogens accelerate progesterone synthesis by increasing the delivery of cholesterol to the trophoblast through increased uterine blood flow and by upregulating LDL receptors and P450scc. Pregnenolone and LDLs that cross the placenta and enter the fetal circulation serve as substrate for adrenal production of DHEAS. DHEAS is then converted by the placenta to estrogens in what amounts to a positive feedback system that progressively increases estrogen production in parallel with progesterone production (Fig. 14.64).

Maternal adaptations to pregnancy

In the approximately 265 days that elapse between fertilization and delivery of a full-term infant the mother provides all the resources required to transform a single pluripotential cell to a complete new individual weighing about 3.5 kg and comprises more than 600 billion highly specialized cells. Throughout pregnancy maternal homeostatic control mechanisms ensure a hospitable environment of constant temperature; oxygen supply; waste disposal; and availability of nutrients, minerals, and vitamins. Supporting the growth and development of the fetus and the placenta with its extraordinary metabolic activity imposes significant challenges to maternal homeostasis and requires adjustments in the function of virtually every organ system.

Maternal adaptations to pregnancy are driven largely by hormones secreted into the maternal circulation by the placenta. Changes in maternal physiology must accommodate the metabolic needs of the fetus without substantially compromising her ability to make homeostatic adjustments that ensure her survival and survival of the fetus in the face of changing environmental demands. Physiological changes during pregnancy must also prepare the mother to withstand the arduous birthing process and to provide sustenance for her newborn baby. It is important to note that all the regulatory and feedback mechanisms that maintain homeostasis in the nonpregnant woman remain operative during pregnancy, but the sensitivity to physiological signals or the set points of feedback systems are modified.

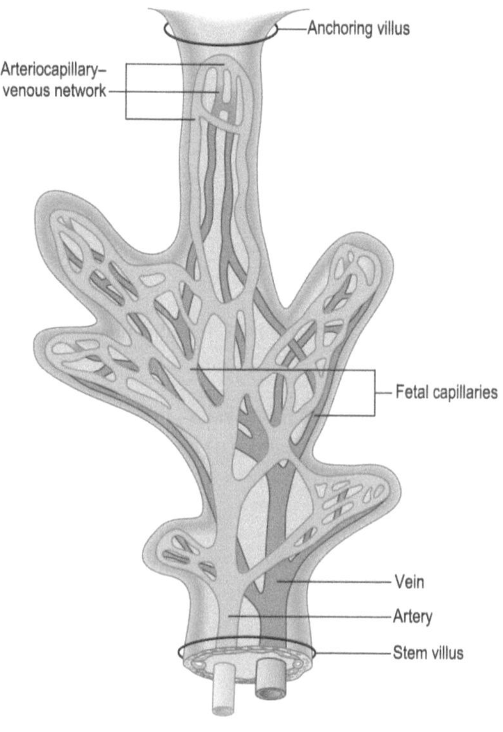

FIGURE 14.53 Details of the extensive capillary network in a placental villus. Source: *Figure 9.8A in Standring (2015).* Gray's anatomy *(41st ed., p. 176). Elsevier.*

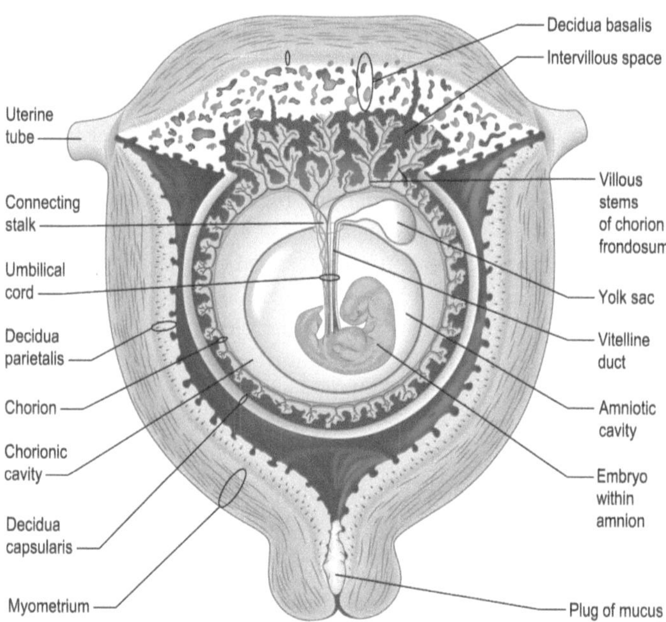

FIGURE 14.54 The orientation of the embryo and placenta in the second month of pregnancy. At this point the developing human is called an embryo. From the fourth month to term the developing human is called a fetus. This shows an implantation into the fundus of the uterus, which is unusual. Most implantations are on the anterior, posterior, or lateral walls of the uterus. Source: *Figure 9.2 in Standring (2015).* Gray's anatomy *(41st ed., p. 172). Elsevier.*

Cardiovascular adaptations

Maternal and fetal blood do not mix or come in direct contact. Passage of nutrients and gases takes place across a diffusion barrier comprising a layer of syncytiotrophoblast, basal lamina, and endothelial cells in the terminal placental villi. In late pregnancy the diffusion barrier is about 5 μm thick and has a surface area of about 12 square meters. Maintaining steep concentration gradients between maternal and fetal blood is essential for rapid active and passive exchange across this diffusion barrier. The capacity for nutrient and gas exchange must be adequate to satisfy not only the needs of the growing fetus but also of the highly metabolically active placenta, which extracts its required nutrients as they diffuse across the syncytiotrophoblast before reaching the fetal blood that perfuses the villi. Metabolic demands of the placenta in late pregnancy are nearly equal to demands of the fetus. Consequently, very high rates of maternal blood flow must perfuse the intervillous spaces to ensure adequate fetal nutrition and oxygen supply.

Uterine blood flow increases more than twentyfold from the midluteal phase of the menstrual cycle to late pregnancy, a rate that corresponds to more than 20% of the maternal cardiac output. This high rate of flow results mainly from a profound decrease in vascular resistance. Arterioles in the gravid uterus are maximally dilated under basal conditions and are insensitive to vasoconstrictor agents. In addition, resting cardiac output increases by about 50% and mean arterial pressure decreases somewhat,

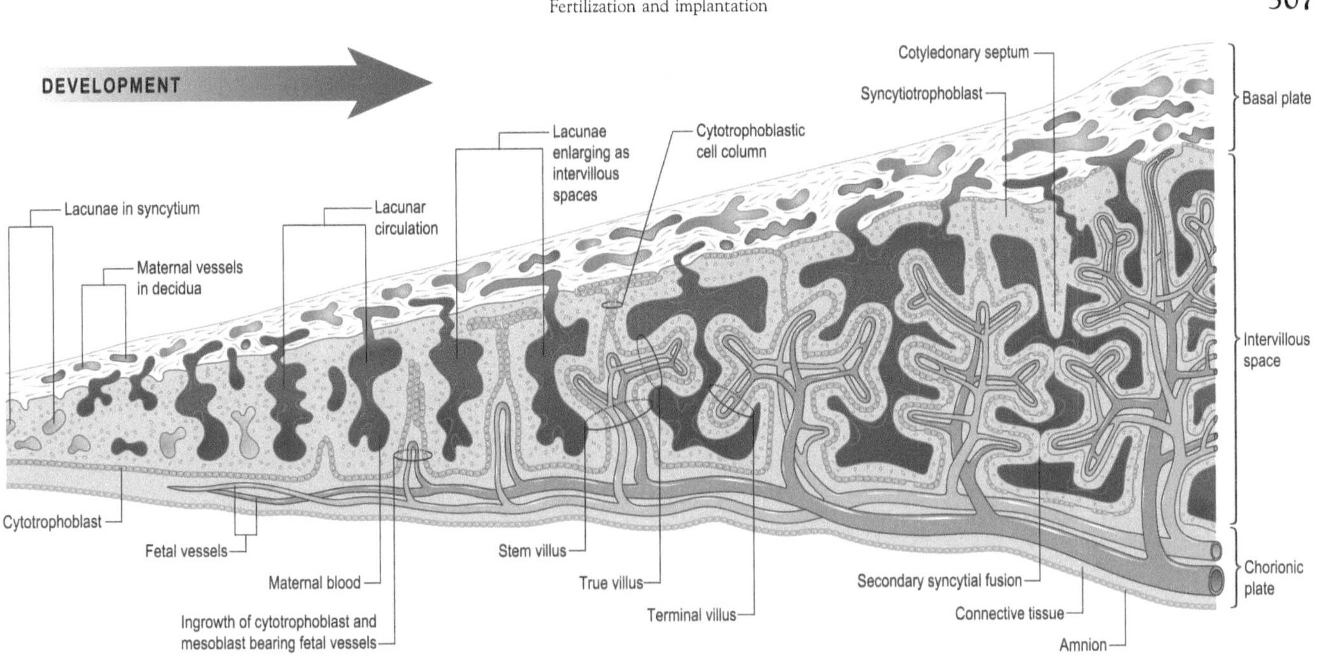

FIGURE 14.55 The placenta as it develops over 9 months. Note that the spaces are initially called lacunae and then later intervillous spaces. Source: *Figure 9.5 in Standring (2015).* Gray's anatomy *(41st ed., p. 173). Elsevier.*

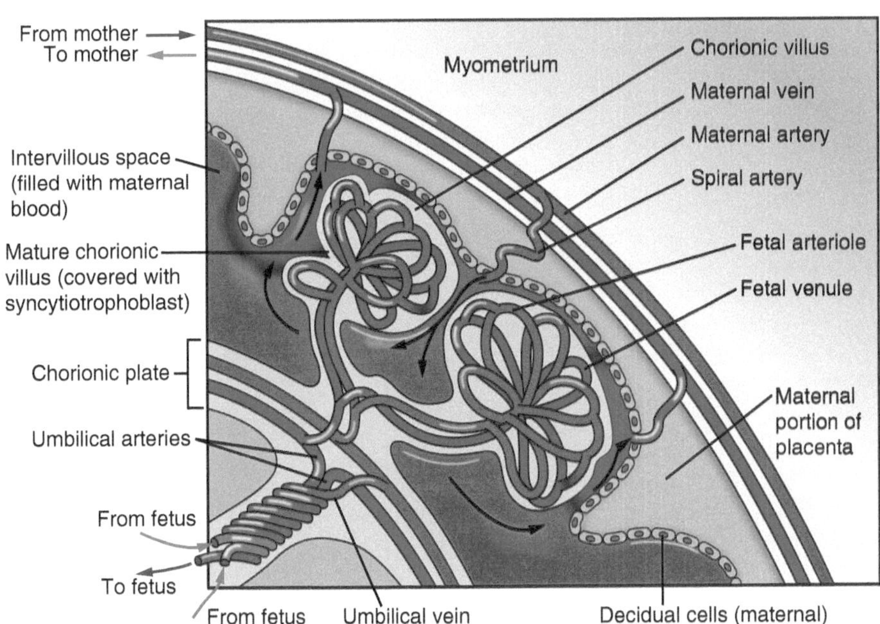

FIGURE 14.56 Placental blood flow. Note that the maternal arterial flow is to the center of the villus and venous maternal return is from either side of the villus. The villus is stylized in this diagram. Source: *Redrawn from Figure 56.6 in Boron, & Boulpaep (2017). Chapter 56: Fertilization, pregnancy and lactation. In S. Mesiano, & E. E. Jones (Eds.),* Medical physiology *(3rd ed., p. 1138). Elsevier.*

indicative of an overall decrease in peripheral vascular resistance.

The decrease in vascular resistance is not limited to the shunt-like behavior of the uterine-placental circulation but is due also to a decrease in tone of arterioles and larger arteries of the mesenteric, limb, cutaneous, and especially the renal (see later) circulations (Fig. 14.65).

In these vascular beds vasoconstrictor responses to angiotensin II and norepinephrine are attenuated, but despite these changes, baroreceptor reflexes remain operative and maintain blood pressure constant over a wide range of changing environmental demands, though at a lower set point.

The basis for the decrease in vascular resistance remains a topic of active research. Infusion of estrogens in nonpregnant human and animal subjects acutely decreases vascular resistance and produces changes that are similar, though less pronounced, to those seen in normal pregnancy. Human vascular endothelial cells express both α and β estrogen receptors, which when stimulated

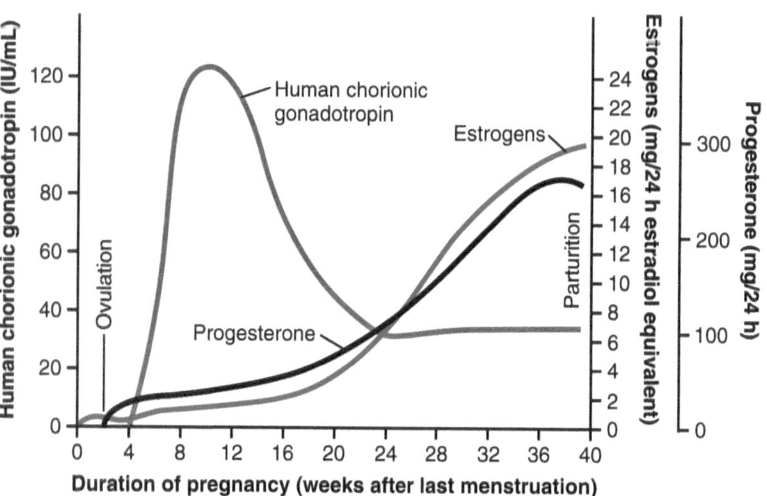

FIGURE 14.57 Secretion of hCG, progesterone, and estrogen by the placenta. *hCG*, Human chorionic gonadotropin. Source: *Figure 83.7 in Hall, J. (2016).* Guyton and Hall textbook of medical physiology *(13th ed., p. 1060). Elsevier.*

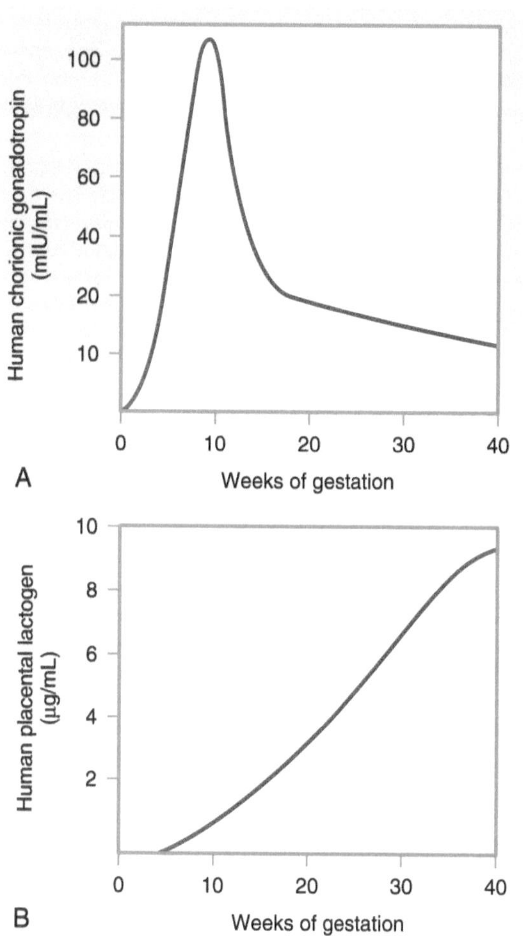

FIGURE 14.58 Human placental lactogen during pregnancy. Source: *Figure 44.34A in Koeppen, B. M., & Stanton, B. A. (2018).* Berne and Levy physiology *(7th ed., p. 821). Elsevier.*

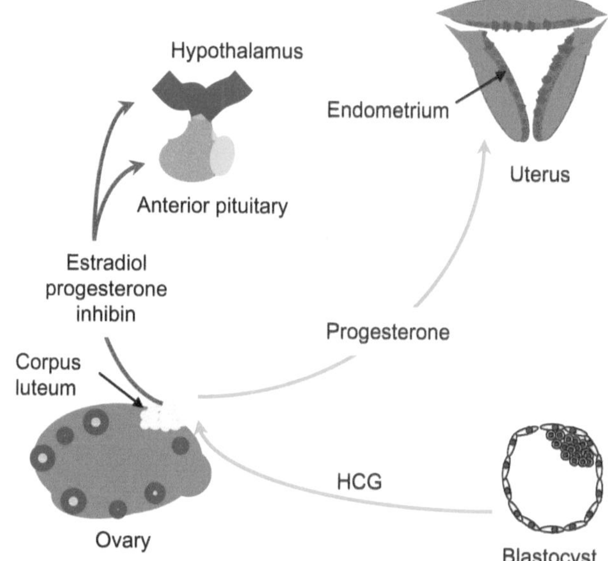

FIGURE 14.59 Maternal effects of hCG. *hCG*, Human chorionic gonadotropin.

rapidly initiate production of vasodilating agents such as nitric oxide and prostacyclin (prostaglandin I2; see Chapter 4: The Adrenal Glands). Some studies suggest a similar action of progesterone, alone or in the presence of high levels of estrogens. Recently, studies in rodents have focused on the vasodepressor effects of relaxin (see Chapter 13: Hormonal Control of Reproduction in the Female: The Menstrual Cycle), which is secreted by the corpus luteum throughout pregnancy. Its concentrations in blood increase in the early days of pregnancy in

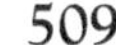

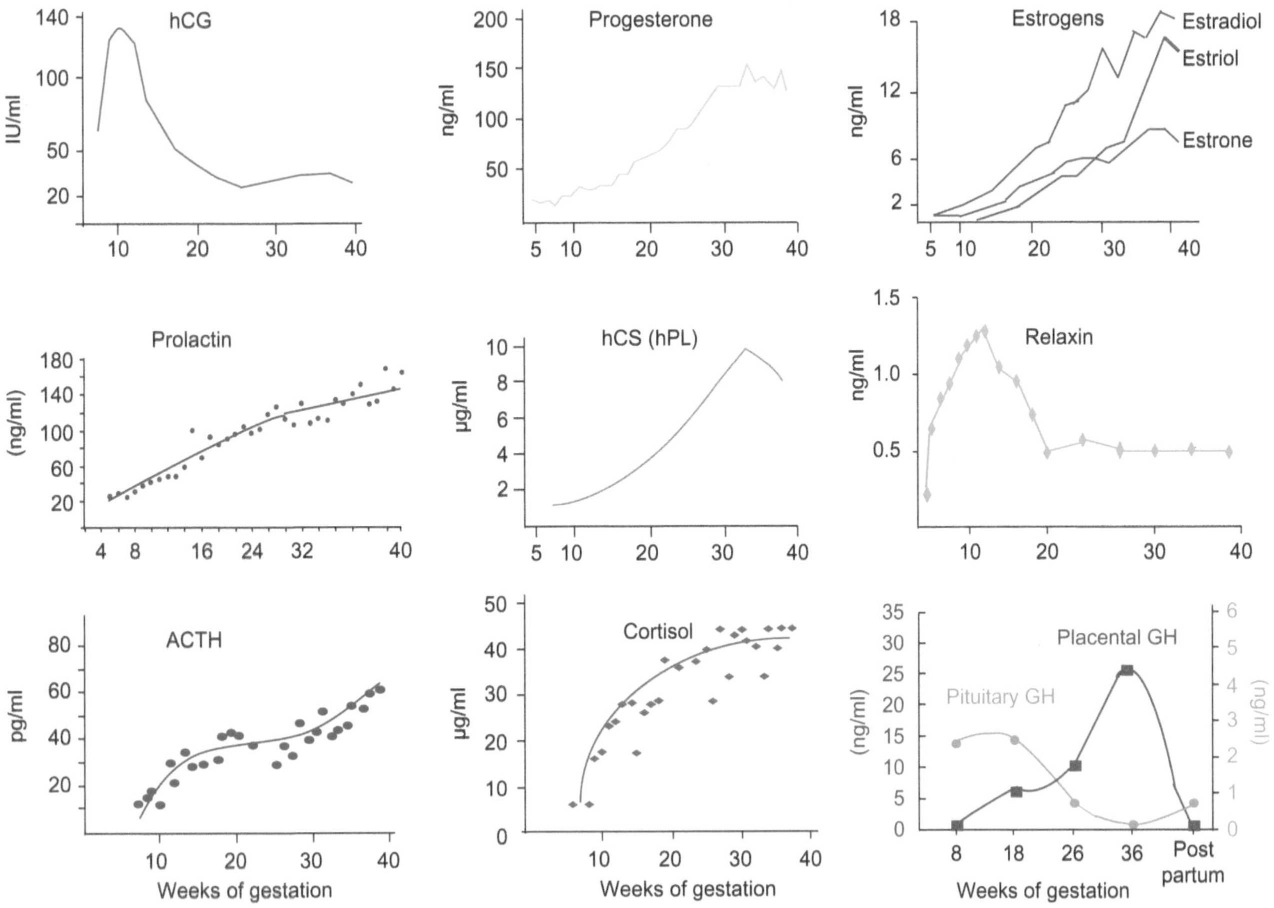

FIGURE 14.60 Changes in plasma concentrations of pregnancy-related hormones during normal gestation. Source: *Data for hCG, progesterone, estrogens, and hCS from Freinkel, N., & Metzger, B. E. (1992). Metabolic changes in pregnancy. In J. D. Wilson, & D. W. Foster (Eds.),* Williams textbook of endocrinology *(8th ed.). Philadelphia, PA: Saunders. Graph for prolactin redrawn from Rigg, L. A., Lein, A., & Yen, S. C. C. (1977). Pattern of increase in circulating prolactin levels during human gestation.* American Journal of Obstetrics and Gynecology, *129, 454–456. Graph for relaxin redrawn from data of Johnson, M. R., Abbas, A. A., Allman, A. C., Nicolaides, K. H., & Lightman, S. L. (1994). The regulation of plasma relaxin levels during human pregnancy.* Journal of Endocrinology, *142, 261–265. Graphs for cortisol and ACTH are redrawn from data of Carr, R. B., Parker, C. R., Jr., Madden, J. D., MacDonald, P. C., & Porter, J. C. (1981). Maternal plasma adrenocorticotropin and cortisol relationships throughout human pregnancy.* American Journal of Obstetrics and Gynecology, *39, 416–422. Data for GH are reproduced from Fuglsang, J., Skjaerbaek, C., Espelund, U., Frystyk, S., Fisker, A., Flyvbjerg, A., et al. (2005). Ghrelin and its relationship to growth hormones during pregnancy.* Clinical Endocrinology (Oxford), *62, 554–559.*

response to hCG (Fig. 14.60). Administration of relaxin to rodents reproduces many of the changes in renal and mesenteric blood flow seen in early pregnancy. In these animals, relaxin stimulates endothelial cell production of nitric oxide, especially in the renal and mesenteric vascular beds, but comparable results have not been found in humans.

Renal adaptations

The decline in resistance of the renal vasculature is remarkable. Renal blood flow increases by as much as 70%, and glomerular filtration increases by about 50%. The resulting increase in the amount of sodium filtered might lead to profound sodium loss in nonpregnant women. In pregnancy, however, there is net retention of about 100 mg of sodium each day between the 8th and 20th weeks of pregnancy, resulting in a 40%–50% increase in blood volume (Fig. 14.65). As discussed in Chapter 9, Regulation of Salt and Water Balance, blood volume is regulated by the renin, angiotensin, aldosterone, antidiuretic hormones (ADH), which increase salt and water retention when plasma volume is low, and by the atrial natriuretic factor (ANF), which promotes salt and water loss when vascular volume is increased. Maternal homeostatic mechanisms respond to pregnancy in much the same way as they would to a decrease in blood volume. Hormonal signals to increase sodium conservation are activated early in pregnancy, at about the same time that peripheral resistance begins to decline.

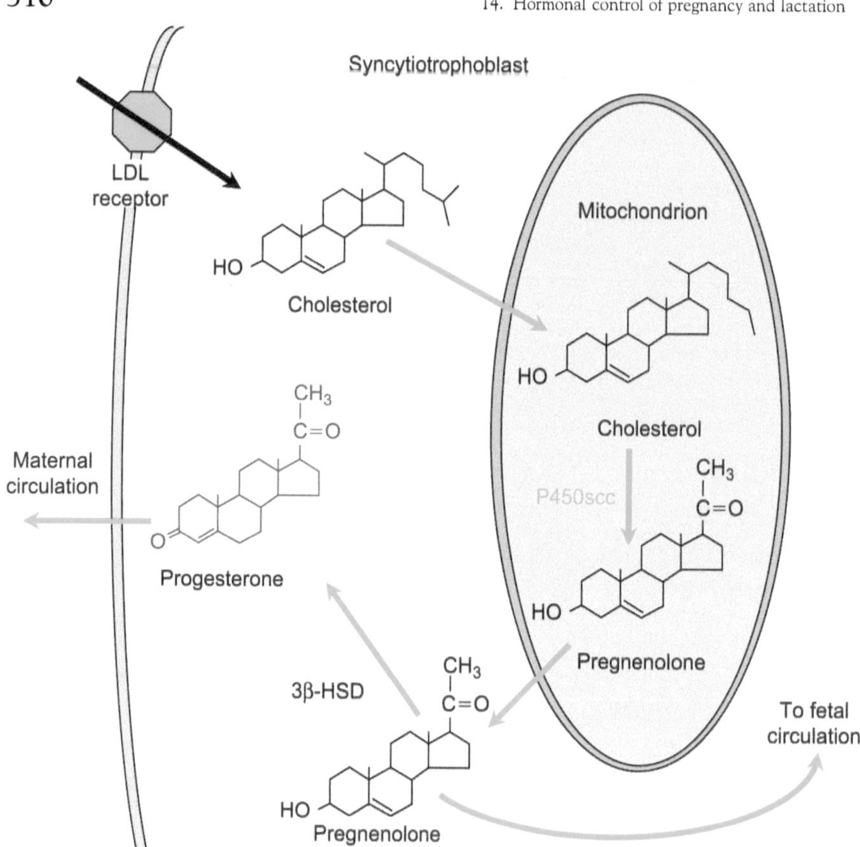

FIGURE 14.61 Progesterone synthesis by the trophoblast. Cholesterol is taken up via *LDL* receptors and transferred to the inner mitochondrial matrix by constitutively expressed protein(s) where its C22–C27 side chain is removed by *P450scc*. Pregnenolone exits the mitochondria and is oxidized to progesterone by *3β HSD*. *3β HSD*, 3β-Hydroxysteroid dehydrogenase; *LDL*, low-density lipoprotein; *P450scc*, P450 side-chain cleavage.

It is possible that the decrease in arterial pressure and the increase in compliance of the thoracic vasculature unloads the volume receptors or that estrogen and progesterone decrease the sensitivity of these stretch receptors. Alternatively, these hormones may act directly on neurons in the vasomotor center to adjust the set point for volume regulation. In any event, the renin–angiotensin–aldosterone system is activated, while volume-lowering mechanisms involving ANF are blunted. However, acute deviations from the pregnancy-adjusted set point of plasma volume trigger normal increases or decreases in renin, aldosterone, ADH, and ANF secretion, which continue to regulate vascular volume throughout pregnancy at the higher set point.

The expansion of plasma volume is accompanied by changes in the composition of the blood. Although erythrocyte formation increases, expansion of the red cell mass does not keep pace with the increase of plasma volume, and the hematocrit declines. The resulting "anemia of pregnancy" is not a reflection of compromised capacity for red blood cell formation (erythropoiesis), which increases normally in response to hemorrhage or relocation to high altitude. Red blood cell formation is driven by the hormone erythropoietin, which is secreted by renal interstitial cells. These cells monitor oxygen tension and increase hormone secretion when oxygen tension falls. The lower hematocrit may reflect an increase in sensitivity of these cells to prevailing levels of oxygen. Alternatively, the increase in renal blood flow may deliver sufficient oxygen to compensate for red cell dilution and the increased oxygen demand imposed by the increased workload of the kidney.

Expansion of plasma volume also dilutes the plasma proteins, especially albumin, whose synthesis by the liver does not keep pace with the increase in plasma volume. Albumin synthesis is driven by plasma oncotic pressure, which is monitored by hepatocytes. The sustained lower concentration of albumin indicates that the feedback mechanism that regulates hepatic albumin production is reset to a lower level, probably in response to placental steroids. Although estrogens stimulate hepatic production of clotting factors and binding proteins for thyroxine and steroid hormones, the low concentrations of these proteins have little effect on plasma colloid osmotic pressure. The importance of lowered plasma oncotic pressure for maintenance of normal pregnancy is not known, but the reduction in blood viscosity that results from lower protein and red cell concentrations contributes to the decrease in vascular resistance.

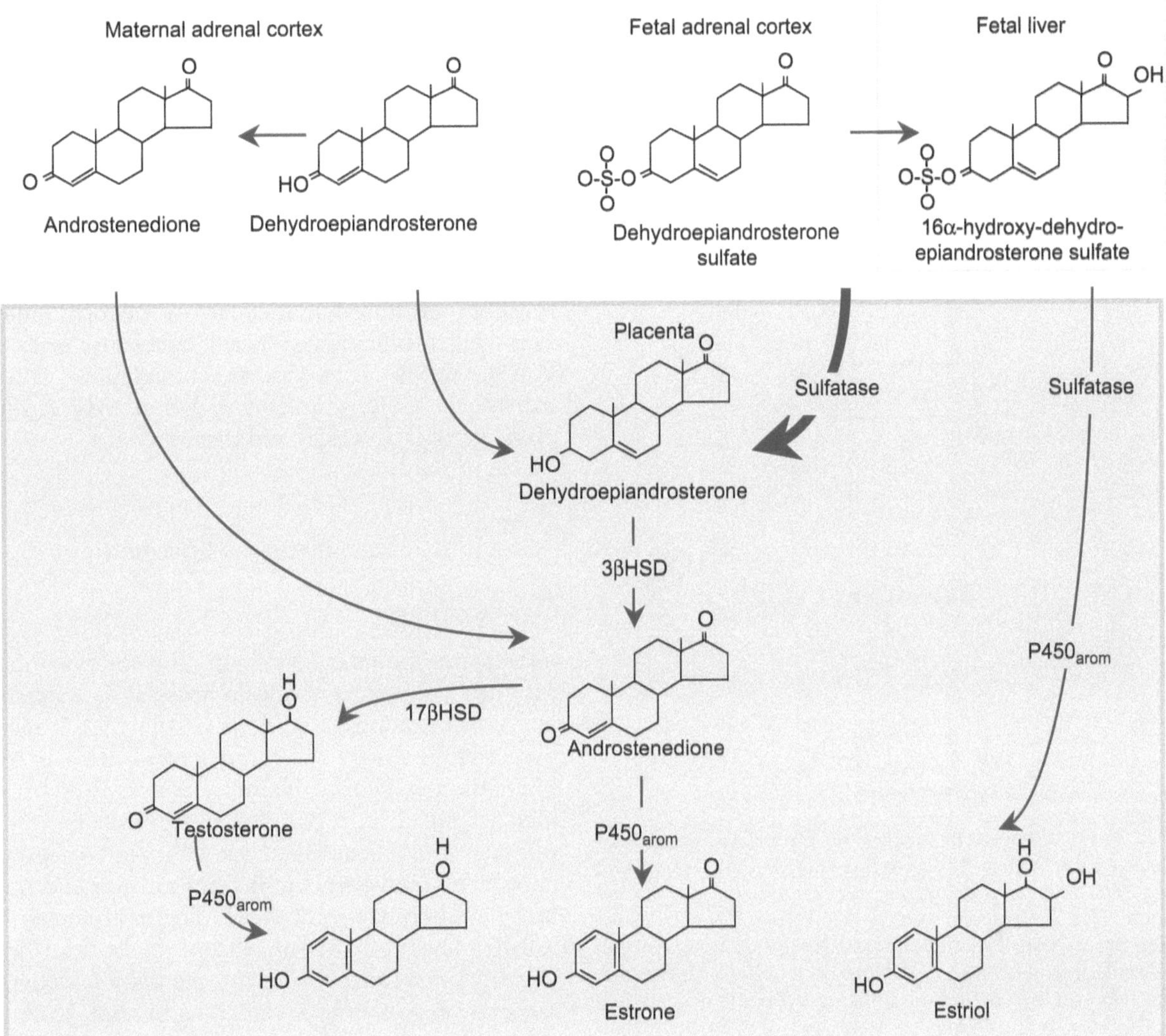

FIGURE 14.62 Biosynthesis of estrogens during pregnancy. Note that androgens formed in either the fetal or maternal adrenals are the precursors for all three estrogens, and that the placenta cannot convert progesterone to androgens. Hydroxylation of dehydroepiandrosterone sulfate on carbon 16 by the fetal liver gives rise to estriol, which is derived almost exclusively from fetal sources. Fetal androgens are secreted as sulfate esters and must first be converted to free androgens by the abundant placental sulfatase before conversion to estrogens by the enzyme *P450arom*. *17HSD*, 17-Hydroxysteroid dehydrogenase; *3β-HSD*, 3β-hydroxysteroid dehydrogenase; *P450arom*, P450aromatase.

Osmoregulation and thirst

Osmolality of body fluids is monitored by hypothalamic osmoreceptors, which regulate both water intake (thirst) and renal conservation of water through adjustments in the rate of ADH secretion (see Chapter 9: Regulation of Salt and Water Balance). Under basal conditions the concentration of sodium in the plasma of pregnant women is 3–5 mEq/L lower than in plasma of nonpregnant women, and plasma osmolality is nearly 10 mOsmol lower. Although the set point of negative feedback regulation is lowered, pregnancy does not interfere with the ability to increase or decrease ADH secretion in response to water deprivation or water loading. In accordance with increased sensitivity of the osmolar receptors, at any level of osmolality the rate of ADH secretion is greater in pregnant than in nonpregnant women (Fig. 14.11). Pregnancy shifts the relationship between osmolality and thirst to a similar extent. Thus osmolal regulation remains intact during pregnancy but operates at a lower set point.

The factors that bring about changes in sensitivity of the osmoreceptor system have not been identified and understanding of the underlying mechanism is incomplete. A similar but less pronounced shift in the relationship between ADH secretion and plasma osmolality is seen in nonpregnant women during the luteal phase of the menstrual cycle. Progesterone, relaxin, or some other product

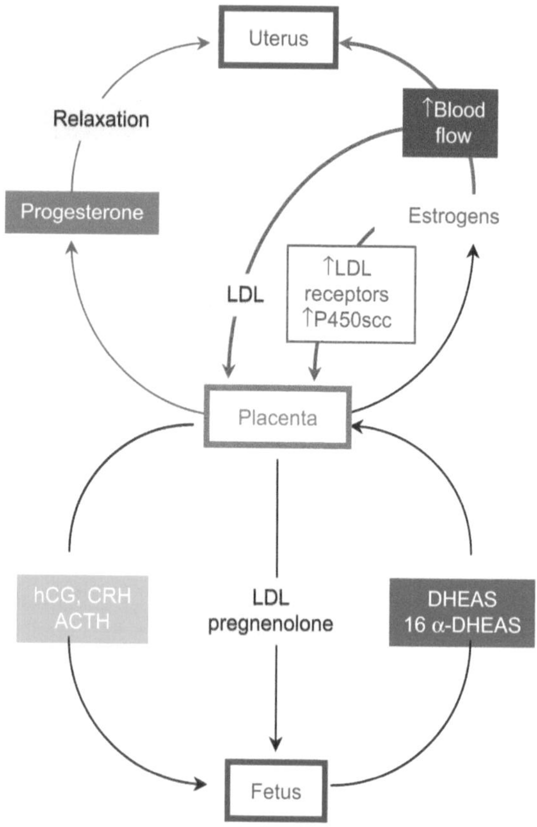

FIGURE 14.63 Effects of estrogens on the production of placental steroid hormones. By increasing uterine blood flow, and inducing *LDL* and *P450scc* enzyme, estrogens increase placental production of pregnenolone, which is used as a substrate for androgen production in the fetal adrenals. Uptake of LDL from the maternal circulation may also transfer cholesterol to the fetal circulation. *16α-DHEAS*, 16α-Hydroxy-dehydroepiandrosterone sulfate; *ACTH*, adrenocorticotropic hormone; *CRH*, corticotropin-releasing hormone; *DHEAS*, dehydroepiandrosterone sulfate; *hCG*, human chorionic gonadotropin; *P450scc*, P450 side-chain cleavage.

of the corpus luteum that continues to circulate at high levels throughout pregnancy may thus be responsible for adjusting osmoregulation. In nonpregnant individuals, the relationship between arginine vasopressin (AVP) secretion and osmolarity changes with changes in plasma volume. A leftward shift in the AVP/osmolality relationship similar to that shown in Fig. 14.66 occurs in hypovolemia (reduced plasma volume), whereas hypervolemia tends to shift the relationship in the opposite direction.

Thus it seems that the hypervolemia of pregnancy appears as hypovolemia to the volume regulating mechanisms that govern AVP secretion. Changes in the set points for volume and osmolal regulation cause regulatory centers to interpret the increase in plasma volume and the decrease osmolality in pregnancy as normal and to defend these altered states.

Fig. 14.67 summarizes the cardiovascular and renal changes produced in the first trimester and continued throughout gestation.

Hormonal signals arising in the trophoblast and/or the ovary and acting directly on vascular smooth muscle and the osmoreceptors initiate the series of changes that ultimately increase placental perfusion. It is likely, but not established that these peripheral effects are reinforced by complementary effects on regulatory centers in the brain. The adaptive value of most of these changes appears to reside in ensuring the adequacy of uteroplacental perfusion while maintaining sufficient circulatory reserve to service the needs of the mother. The adaptive value of the increase in GFR is unknown, but it may facilitate the excretion of fetal wastes and dietary toxins.

Respiratory adjustments

Gas exchange

Despite the rapid growth and intense metabolic activity of the placenta, little increase in maternal oxygen consumption is evident in the first 3 months of pregnancy because the fetoplacental mass is so small. Thereafter, oxygen consumption and CO_2 production increase steadily in parallel with increasing fetal mass to reach a level that is about 20% above the nonpregnant level. However, the flow of air into and out of the lungs (pulmonary ventilation) begins to increase in the luteal phase of the menstrual cycle and increases steadily after conception until the baby is delivered. By the end of gestation, alveolar ventilation is about 40% greater than the prepregnant rate. Breathing in excess of metabolic demand is called hyperventilation and is evident throughout pregnancy. With hyperventilation, there is excessive excretion of carbon dioxide (CO_2) and a reduction in plasma CO_2 and bicarbonate, and a slight alkalinization of the blood. Because hemoglobin is nearly saturated with oxygen at rates of pulmonary ventilation seen in nonpregnant women, hyperventilation adds little to the oxygen content of blood.

The hyperventilation of pregnancy is attributable to the high circulating concentrations of progesterone, which produces similar effects within a few hours after progesterone is given to nonpregnant subjects of either sex. Arterial CO_2 is monitored by chemoreceptors in the brain stem and carotid bodies. Progesterone increases ventilatory drive by increasing the sensitivity of these chemoreceptors to CO_2. As seen with other pregnancy-related adjustments to homeostatic mechanisms, the set point is decreased but the ability to adjust alveolar ventilation upward or downward in response to changes in arterial or inspired CO_2 is not compromised. Resetting the steady-state level of CO_2 in maternal blood facilitates the transfer

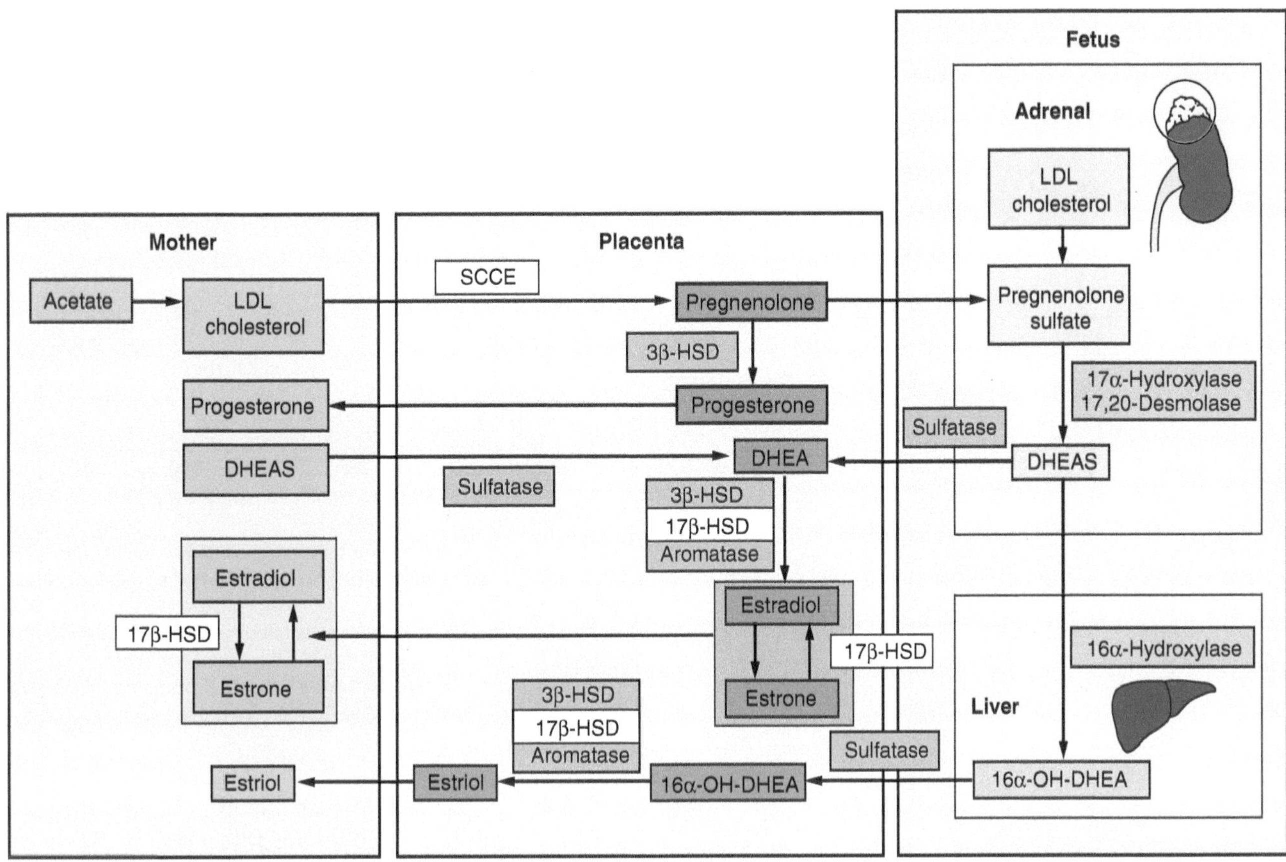

FIGURE 14.64 Interactions of hormones in the mother–placenta–fetus unit. *HSD*, Hydroxysteroid dehydrogenase; *SCCE*, side-chain-cleavage enzyme. Source: *Redrawn from Figure 56.9 in Boron, & Boulpaep (2017). Chapter 56: Fertilization, pregnancy and lactation. In S. Mesiano, & E. E. Jones (Eds.),* Medical physiology *(3rd ed., p. 1142). Elsevier.*

of CO_2 from the fetal to the maternal circulation and indirectly facilitates the oxygenation of fetal blood.

Metabolic adjustments

The energy cost to the mother of the 9 months of pregnancy is about 85,000 calories (~300 cal/day), which must be derived from the diet or fat reserves. Only about one-third of this energy consumption supports fetal growth and metabolic activities. About one-third supports placental biosynthetic and transfer processes, and most of the remainder fuels the additional workload imposed on the maternal heart, respiratory muscles, and kidneys, with a small fraction fueling the growth of the uterus and breasts.

Adipose tissue increases in the early months of pregnancy as a result of increased food intake and hyperresponsiveness of the pancreatic bets cells to nutrient intake. Fuel reserves built up at this time anticipate later metabolic demands of the mature placenta, the rapidly growing fetus, and the even later demands of lactation. Consistent with the increase in maternal adipose tissue, plasma concentrations of leptin increase during pregnancy. Leptin also is secreted by the placenta, but despite its increasing blood concentrations, food intake continues to increase throughout gestation along with the increasing metabolic requirements of the placenta and fetus. This has led to the idea that pregnancy decreases sensitivity to leptin. The role of leptin in pregnancy is unknown.

In the early months of pregnancy, insulin sensitivity is normal or perhaps slightly increased over prepregnant levels, but insulin resistance develops as gestation advances. Plasma concentrations of insulin double as insulin secretion increases in compensation for decreased sensitivity. In most women, glucose concentrations are maintained within the normal range. The secretory capacity of the beta cells increases along with a 10%–15% increase in their mass and can satisfy the insulin requirements in most women, but limited compensatory capacity in some women results in transient diabetes mellitus (gestational diabetes). Even when compensated, the rate of disposition of ingested nutrients is diminished. Greater and longer-lasting elevations in maternal blood glucose concentration after each meal facilitate the transfer of glucose from the maternal to the fetal

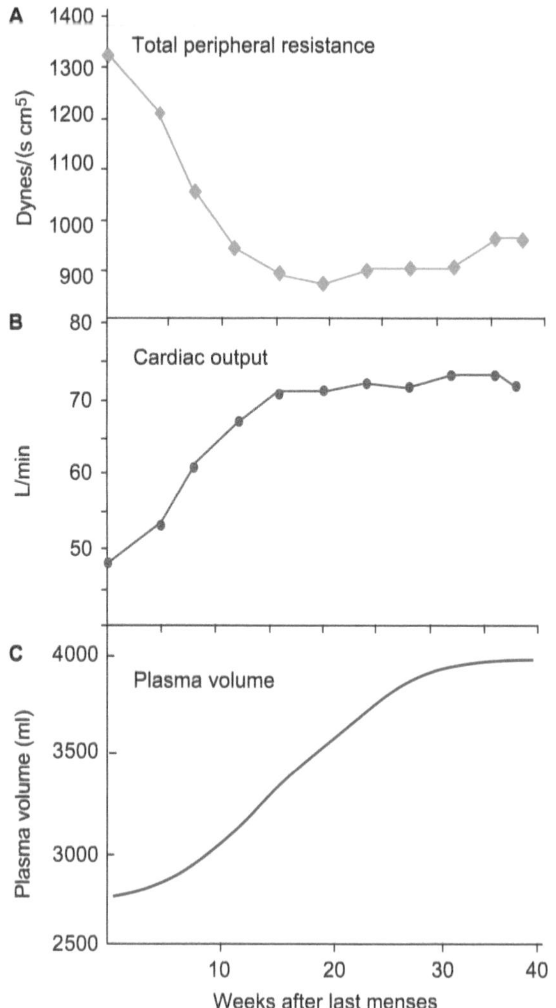

FIGURE 14.65 Changes in peripheral resistance (A), cardiac output (B), and plasma volume in normal pregnancies (C). Source: *Data in panels (A) and (B) redrawn from Robson, S. H., Hunter, S., Boys, R. J., & Dunlap, W. (1989). Serial study of factors influencing changes in cardiac output during human pregnancy.* American Journal of Physiology, 256, *H1060–H1065.*

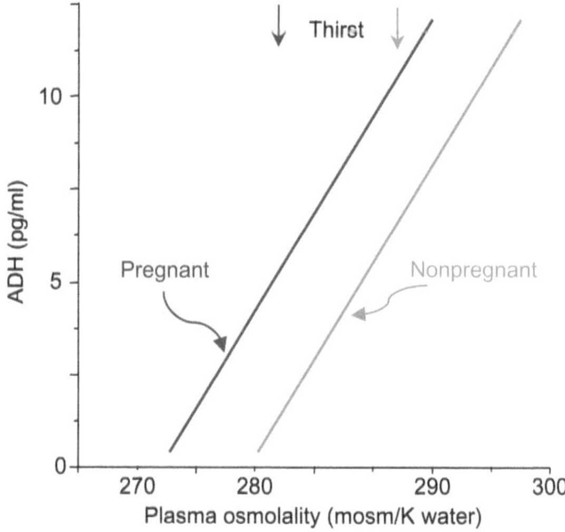

FIGURE 14.66 Relationship between plasma osmolality and ADH concentrations in eight women before and at the end of the third month of pregnancy. Arrows indicate plasma osmolality at which a conscious desire to drink (thirst) was experienced. Source: *Drawn from the data of Davison, J. M., Shiells, E. A., Philips, P. R., & Lindheimer, M. D. (1988). Serial evaluation of vasopressin release and thirst in human pregnancy.* Journal of Clinical Investigation, 81, *798–806.*

circulation. Placental uptake of glucose is independent of insulin and depends upon facilitated diffusion driven by the favorable concentration between maternal and fetal plasma.

Although direct evidence in humans is scant, most of the pregnancy-induced changes in maternal metabolism are likely to be driven by placental hormones. Increased concentrations of progesterone and hCS are thought to stimulate hypothalamic neurons that regulate appetite (see Chapter 8: Hormonal Regulation of Fuel Metabolism). The decrease in insulin sensitivity may be caused, at least in part, by the high concentrations of placental GH present in maternal plasma in the second half of gestation (Fig. 14.6). Placental GH binds to the same receptors as the pituitary form and, like its pituitary counterpart, decreases insulin sensitivity both by direct actions and through increased lipolysis. Unlike the intermittent pulses of GH secreted by the pituitary, placental GH is secreted tonically so that maternal tissues are exposed to constant high levels of hormone. HCS also binds to GH receptors. It is likely that both hormones contribute to the decrease in insulin sensitivity. Both hormones and perhaps prolactin contribute to beta-cell hypertrophy and increased secretion of insulin. Lactogens and GH stimulate the growth of rodent beta cells and enhance their responsiveness to nutrient stimulation.

Calcium balance

By the end of gestation the fetal skeleton accumulates about 30 g of calcium, mainly during the final months when as much as 300 mg of calcium is transferred from the mother each day. However, neither the concentration of ionized calcium in maternal blood nor the density of calcium in her bones decreases. Virtually, all the calcium delivered to the fetus is derived from dietary sources. Intestinal absorption of calcium doubles in response to increased plasma 1,25 dihydroxycholecalciferol (calcitriol, vitamin D hormone, 1,25(OH)2D3; see Chapter 10: Hormonal Regulation of Calcium Balance), augmented perhaps, by prolactin and hCS. Plasma concentrations of 1,25(OH)2D3 begin to increase soon after conception to about twice the prepregnant level by the 12th week and remain doubled for the remainder of pregnancy. Intestinal absorption of calcium increases

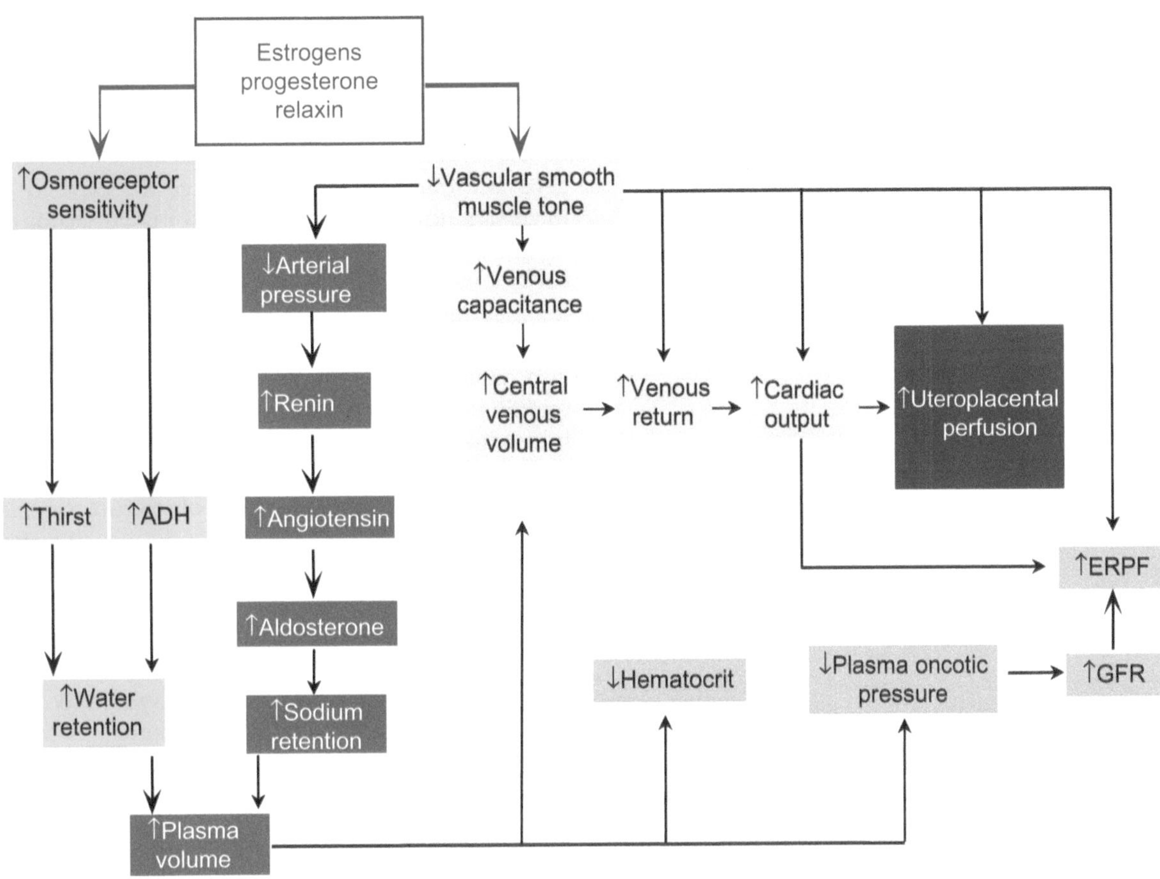

FIGURE 14.67 Summary of cardiovascular and renal changes in pregnancy. *ERPF*, Effective renal plasma flow; *GFR*, glomerular filtration rate.

long before it can be sequestered in the fetal skeleton, but hypercalcemia is prevented by increased renal calcium excretion and perhaps modest deposition in maternal bones.

In men and nonpregnant women, parathyroid hormone (PTH) is the signal for increased formation of 1,25 (OH)2D3 in the kidneys (see Chapter 10: Hormonal Regulation of Calcium Balance). However, in pregnancy, plasma concentrations of PTH decline as 1,25(OH)2D3 increases and remain low until the final months of gestation. The increased concentration of 1,25(OH)2D3 may inhibit PTH secretion through negative feedback effects on PTH synthesis (Fig. 14.68).

Increased formation of 1,25(OH)2D3 appears to result from upregulation of the renal 1α-hydroxylase enzyme by PTH-related peptide (PTHrP) secreted by both the maternal and fetal components of the placenta and by the high levels of estrogens, hCS, and prolactin. Although bone turnover is accelerated, the high concentrations of estrogen, and perhaps IGF-I and hCS may prevent net bone loss during pregnancy. In addition, the somewhat elevated levels of plasma calcium increase calcitonin secretion, but there is no evidence that calcitonin defends against bone loss in human pregnancy.

Maternal adaptations to pregnancy are summarized in Fig. 14.69.

Parturition

The process of birth, or parturition, is the expulsion of a viable baby from the uterus at the end of pregnancy and is the culmination of all the processes discussed in this and the previous two chapters. A surprising array of strategies has been adopted by different mammalian species to regulate parturition. Humans and the great apes have evolved mechanisms that appear to be unique. The scarcity of experimental models that employ similar strategies as humans therefore has hampered efforts to study underlying mechanisms of timing and initiating parturition in humans. Consequently, our understanding of the processes that bring about this climactic event in human reproductive physiology is still incomplete.

Successful delivery of the baby can take place only after the myometrium acquires the capacity for forceful, coordinated contractions and the cervix softens and becomes distensible (called ripening) so that uterine contractions can drive the baby through the cervical canal. These changes reflect the triumph of the excitatory effects

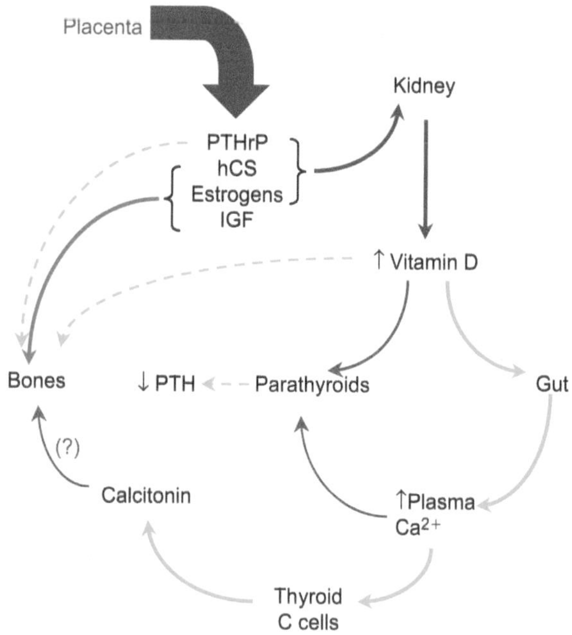

FIGURE 14.68 The influence of placental hormones on maternal calcitropic hormones and calcium balance during pregnancy. Green arrows indicate stimulation; red arrows indicate inhibition. The effects of hCS, estrogens, and IGF on bone (*blue arrow*) offset the calcium mobilizing effects of PTHrP, vitamin D, and PTH (*dashed green arrows*). *hCS*, Human chorionic somatomammotropin; *IGF*, insulin-like growth factor II; *PTH*, parathyroid hormone; *PTHrP*, parathyroid hormone–related peptide.

of estrogens over the suppressive effects of progesterone that prevailed hitherto. Indeed, in most mammals, parturition is heralded by a decline in progesterone production coincident with an increase in estrogen production. In humans and higher primates, there is neither an abrupt increase in plasma concentrations of estrogens nor a fall in progesterone at the onset of parturition. Rather, multiple gradual changes, gaining momentum over days or weeks, tip the precarious estrogen/progesterone balance in favor of estrogen dominance.

In normal deliveries, it is the fetus, which essentially has controlled events during the rest of pregnancy, that signals its readiness to be born, but maternal factors including limited distensibility of the uterus also play a role. In sheep the triggering event for parturition is an ACTH-dependent increase in cortisol production by the fetal adrenals. In this species, cortisol stimulates expression of P450c17 in the placenta and thereby shifts production of steroid hormones away from progesterone and toward estrogens. Although there is neither a stimulation of P450c17 expression in the human placenta nor a fall in progesterone in humans, the dialog between the fetal adrenals and the placenta nevertheless plays the decisive role in orchestrating the events that lead up to human parturition.

The role of corticotropin-releasing hormone

As already mentioned, CRH produced in the placenta drives steroid synthesis in the fetal zone of the adrenal glands. Although the ability to secrete 19 carbon androgens is acquired early in gestation, the capacity to produce significant amounts of cortisol is not acquired until about the 30th week of gestation. An abundant supply of cortisol in the final weeks of pregnancy is indispensable for maturation of the lungs, the GI tract, and other systems and prepares the fetus for extra uterine life. Cortisol also antagonizes the suppressive effects of progesterone on CRH production in the placenta and hence increases transcription of the CRH gene. Consequently, placental production of CRH increases about 100-fold in the final weeks of gestation. This effect of cortisol on placental expression of CRH is opposite to its negative feedback effects on CRH production in the hypothalamus. Instead of suppressing CRH production, fetal production of cortisol initiates a positive feedback loop (Fig. 14.70).

It may be recalled that CRH not only stimulates the fetal pituitary to secrete ACTH but also directly stimulates steroidogenesis in the fetal adrenal cortex. Consequently, there is an increasing drive to the adrenal to increase the production of cortisol and DHEAS. Accelerated secretion of DHEAS accounts for the steep rise in estrogen concentrations in maternal blood in the last weeks of pregnancy shown in Fig. 14.60.

CRH also stimulates the formation of prostaglandins Fα and E by fetal membranes by direct actions and by indirect actions mediated by cortisol. These prostaglandins not only participate in or initiate events that lead to rupture of the fetal membranes, softening of the uterine cervix, and contraction of the myometrium, but they also stimulate placental production of CRH and thereby establish a second positive feedback loop (Fig. 14.71).

Prostaglandins also stimulate CRH secretion by the fetal hypothalamus, increasing ACTH secretion and providing further drive for cortisol secretion and the consequent further stimulation of CRH secretion. We might expect cortisol to oppose prostaglandin formation in the fetus as it does in extrauterine tissues (see Chapter 4: The Adrenal Glands), but in fetal membranes cortisol paradoxically increases expression of the prostaglandin synthesizing enzyme, COX2, and inhibits expression of the principal prostaglandin degrading enzyme. Prostaglandin synthesis also is increased indirectly by cortisol, which stimulates the maturing fetal lungs to produce surfactant proteins and phospholipids (see Chapter 4: The Adrenal Glands). When these compounds escape into amniotic fluid, they produce a mild inflammation of the fetal membranes and stimulate macrophages to secrete inflammatory cytokines and prostaglandins.

As pregnancy progresses concentrations of CRH increase exponentially in maternal plasma, but ACTH and free cortisol concentrations increase only about fourfold. Discordance between CRH concentrations and pituitary and adrenal secretory activity is due largely to the CRH binding protein (CRH-BP), which is present in plasma of pregnant as well as nonpregnant women. In addition, pituitary responsiveness to CRH is decreased during pregnancy possibly because of downregulation of CRH receptors in corticotropes.

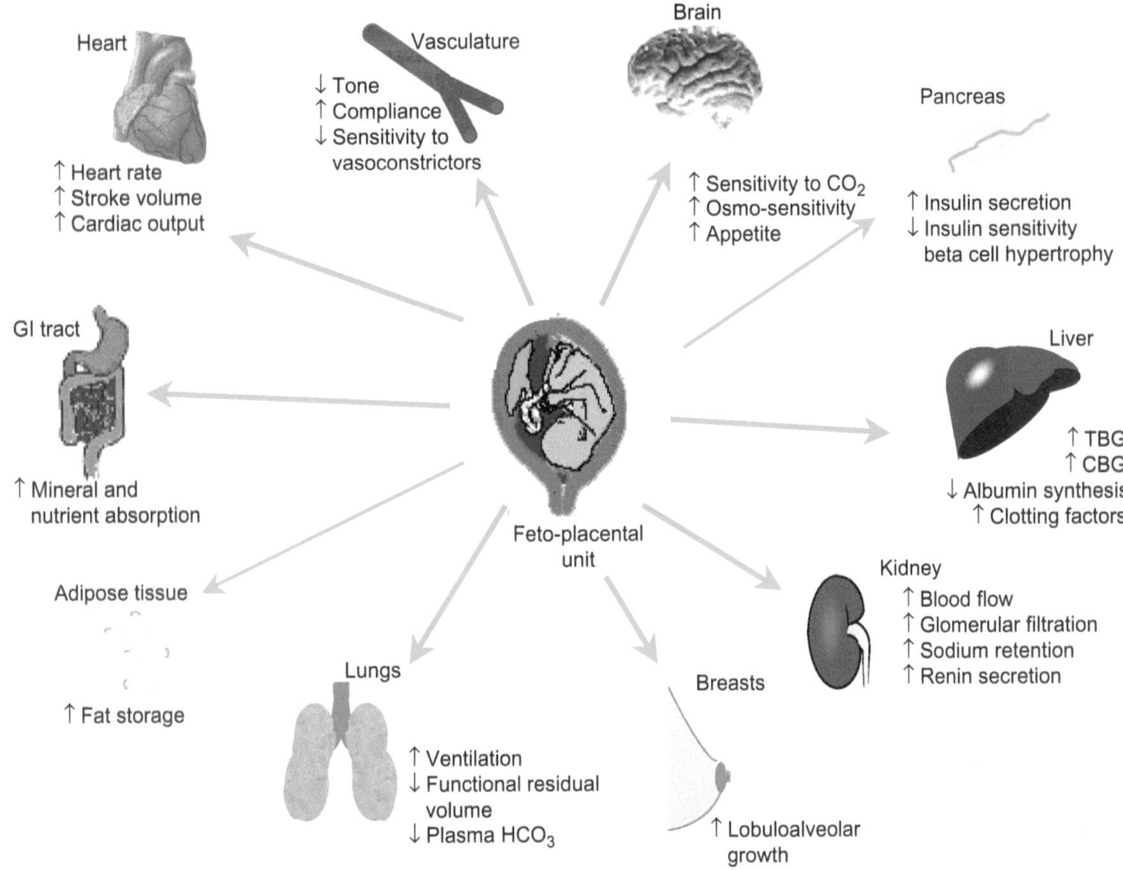

FIGURE 14.69 Summary of maternal adaptations to pregnancy.

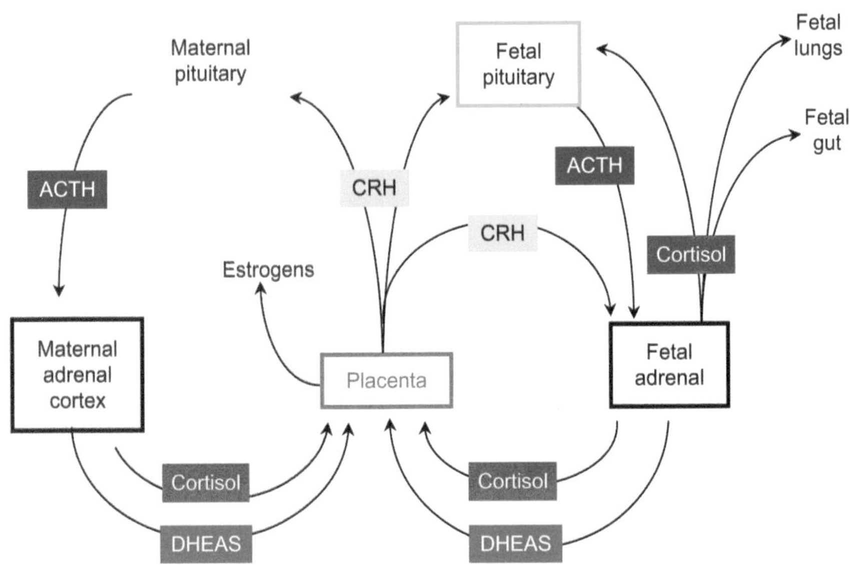

FIGURE 14.70 Effects of cortisol produced in the maternal and fetal adrenals in late pregnancy. By stimulating placental secretion of *CRH*, cortisol initiates direct and indirect (via the fetal and maternal pituitaries) positive feedback loops that enhance its own secretion and increases secretion of *DHEA-S*. In this way, cortisol induced maturation of the fetus occurs simultaneously with increased production of estrogens, which prepare the uterus for parturition. *ACTH*, adrenocorticotropic hormone; *CRH*, corticotropin-releasing hormone; *DHEA-S*, dehydroepiandrosterone sulfate.

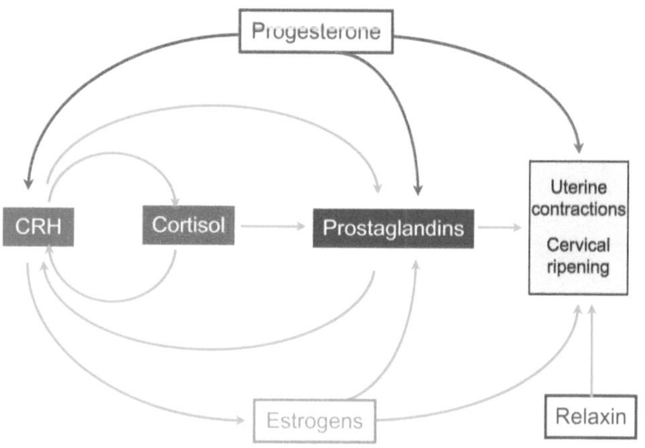

FIGURE 14.71 Positive feedback cycles that contribute to the initiation of parturition. Green arrows indicate stimulation; red arrows indicate inhibition. See the text for details. *CRH*, Corticotropin-releasing hormone.

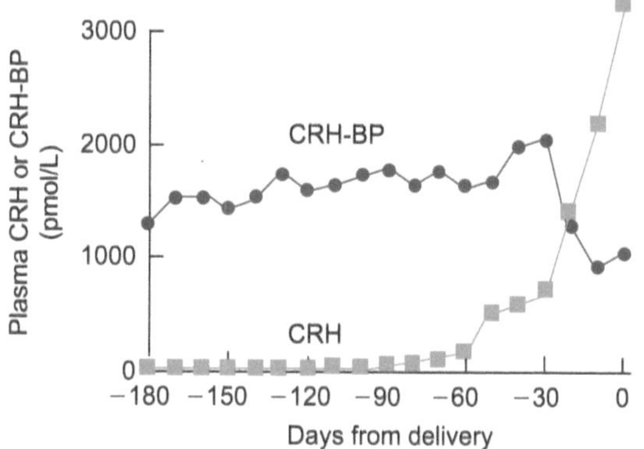

FIGURE 14.72 Changes in plasma concentrations of CRH and its binding protein (CRH-BP) in the days leading up to parturition. *CRH*, Corticotropin-releasing hormone; *CRH-BP*, corticotropin-releasing hormone-binding protein. Source: *From McLean, M., Bisits, A., Davies J., Woods, R. Lowry, P., & Smith, R. (1995). A placental clock controlling the length of human pregnancy.* Nature Medicine, 1, 460–463.

However, despite the somewhat blunted sensitivity to CRH, ACTH secretion follows the normal diurnal rhythmic pattern and increases appropriately in response to stress (see Chapter 4: The Adrenal Glands). Until about 3–4 weeks before parturition, concentrations of CRH-BP in maternal plasma vastly exceed those of CRH and there is little or no free CRH (Fig. 14.72).

For reasons that are not understood, CRH-BP concentrations fall dramatically at the same time that CRH concentrations rise most rapidly so that they exceed the binding capacity of CRH-BP. Free CRH in maternal plasma stimulates prostaglandin production in the myometrium and cervix and increases contractility and cervical ripening.

Although the increase in cortisol in fetal plasma in the last weeks of gestation is essential for maturation of the pulmonary and gastrointestinal systems in preparation for postnatal life, exposure of the fetus to maternal glucocorticoids earlier in gestation has deleterious effects. Excessive glucocorticoids may retard the growth of the placenta and the fetus and may "program" the fetus for increased susceptibility to hypertension and type 2 diabetes in adulthood. The enzyme 11β-hydroxysteroid dehydrogenase type 2 (11βHSD-2) in the syncytiotrophoblast provides a barrier to passage of cortisol from the maternal to the fetal circulation by converting it to the inactive steroid, cortisone (see Chapter 4: The Adrenal Glands). Deficiency of placental 11βHSD-2 is associated with low birth-weight and increased incidence of health problems in later life. Prostaglandins produced in the final weeks of gestation increase the abundance and activity of the type 1 isoform of 11βHSD in the chorioallantoic membranes. This isoform catalyzes the conversion of cortisone to cortisol, which not only supports fetal maturation but also contributes to further formation of prostaglandins in yet another positive feedback loop.

Though there appears to be no single event that precipitates parturition, the various processes that are set in motion weeks earlier gradually build up to overwhelm progesterone dominance and unleash excitatory forces that expel the fetus. Because circulating concentrations of progesterone do not decline until after delivery of the placenta, the concept of "functional progesterone withdrawal" has been advanced to account for the decline in progesterone effectiveness in the final days of gestation. Underlying changes in expression of progesterone receptors, cofactor distribution and interactions, and local changes in progesterone metabolism have been proposed to explain its declining influence. In any event, uterine changes in preparation for parturition brought about by prostaglandins, probably relaxin, and perhaps local paracrine factors include release of matrix metalloproteinases that digest the collagen framework of the cervix and increase its distensibility. Cessation of uterine growth that accommodated the expanding mass of the fetus and placenta at earlier stages of gestation renders the myometrium less compliant and more resistant to stretch. The contractile apparatus gains strength and irritability due to increased synthesis of contractile proteins and changes in its complement of potassium and calcium channels. Connectivity between myocytes increases with the expression of connexins and the formation of gap junctions. These changes enable the myometrium to contract forcefully and synchronously, empowering it to dilate the cervix and expel the fetus.

The role of oxytocin

Oxytocin is a neurohormone secreted by nerve endings in the posterior lobe of the pituitary gland in response to neural stimuli received by cell bodies in the paraventricular and supraoptic nuclei of the hypothalamus (see Chapter 2: Pituitary Gland). It stimulates powerful slow and prolonged contractions of the myometrium at the end of pregnancy, when uterine muscle is highly sensitive to it. Oxytocin sometimes is used clinically to induce labor. As parturition approaches, responsiveness to oxytocin increases in parallel with estrogen-induced increases in oxytocin receptors in both the endometrium and myometrium.

Oxytocin is not the physiological trigger for parturition, however, as its concentration in maternal blood normally does not increase until after labor has begun. It is secreted in a neuroendocrine reflex in response to stretching of the uterine cervix as described in Chapter 1, Introduction, but it probably has little role in initiating parturition. As a consequence of its stimulation of myometrial contraction, oxytocin protects against hemorrhage after expulsion of the placenta. Intense contraction of the newly emptied uterus acts as a natural tourniquet to control loss of blood from the dilated endometrial spiral arteries after the placenta separates from the uterine lining.

Lactation

The mammary glands are specialized secretory structures derived from the skin. As the name implies, they are unique to mammals. The glandular portion is arranged in lobules comprised of branched tubules, the lobuloalveolar ducts, from which multiple evaginations or alveoli emerge in an arrangement resembling a bunch of grapes. The alveoli are the sites of milk production and consist of single layers of secretory epithelial cells surrounded by a meshwork of contractile myoepithelial cells (Fig. 14.73).

Many lobuloalveolar ducts converge to form a lactiferous duct, which carries the milk to the nipple. Each mammary gland contains 10–15 lobules, each with its own lactiferous duct opening separately to the outside. In the inactive, nonlactating gland, alveoli are present only in rudimentary form, and the entire glandular portion consists almost exclusively of lobuloalveolar ducts. The mammary glands have an abundant vascular supply and are innervated with sympathetic nerve fibers and a rich supply of sensory fibers to the nipples and areolae.

Growth and development of the mammary glands

Prenatal growth and development of the mammary glands are independent of sex hormones and genetic sex. Until the onset of puberty, there are no differences in the male and female breast. With the onset of puberty the duct system grows and branches and the surrounding stromal and fat tissues proliferate in response to estrogens. Following estrogen priming, progesterone promotes growth and branching of the lobuloalveolar tissue, but for these steroids to be effective, prolactin, growth hormone, IGF-I, and cortisol must also be present. Lobuloalveolar growth and regression occur to some degree during each ovarian cycle. There is pronounced growth, differentiation, and proliferation of alveoli during pregnancy, when estrogen, progesterone, prolactin, and hCS circulate in high concentrations.

Milk production

Developmental changes in alveolar epithelial cells during pregnancy prepare the glands for full lactation after parturition. Some capacity to synthesize and secrete casein, and lactose is acquired by midgestation, but full production of milk is prevented by the high-circulating concentrations of progesterone and to a lesser extent, estrogens. During pregnancy and in the immediate postpartum period the alveoli are "leaky" and allow passage of small molecules into and out of the alveolar lumens between epithelial cells. One of the final events that mark full development of the secretory apparatus after parturition is the formation of tight junctions between these cells and the separation of luminal and extracellular fluids. All the constituents of milk, except water, thereafter are secreted by epithelial cells by multiple simultaneous active secretory processes.

Once the secretory apparatus has developed, production of milk depends primarily on continued episodic stimulation with high concentrations of prolactin, but adrenal glucocorticoids and insulin are also important in a permissive sense that needs to be defined more precisely. All these hormones and hCS are present in abundance during the late stages of pregnancy, yet lactation does not begin until after parturition. High concentrations of progesterone and estrogens in maternal blood inhibit lactation by interfering with the actions of prolactin, including its ability to upregulate its receptors in the mammary epithelium. With parturition the precipitous fall in progesterone levels relieves this inhibition, and prolactin receptors in alveolar epithelium may increase as much as 20-fold. The fall in progesterone concentrations triggers the onset of milk production. Initially, the mammary glands secrete only a watery fluid called colostrum, which is rich in protein but poor in lactose and fat. It takes about 2–5 days for the mammary glands to secrete mature milk with a full complement of nutrients. It is not clear if this delay reflects a slow acquisition of secretory capacity or a regulated sequence of events timed to coincide with the infant's capacity to utilize nutrients.

Milk secreted by the mammary glands provides nourishment to offspring during the immediate postnatal period and for varying times thereafter, depending on culture and custom. Milk provides all the basic nutrition, vitamins, minerals, fats, carbohydrates, and proteins

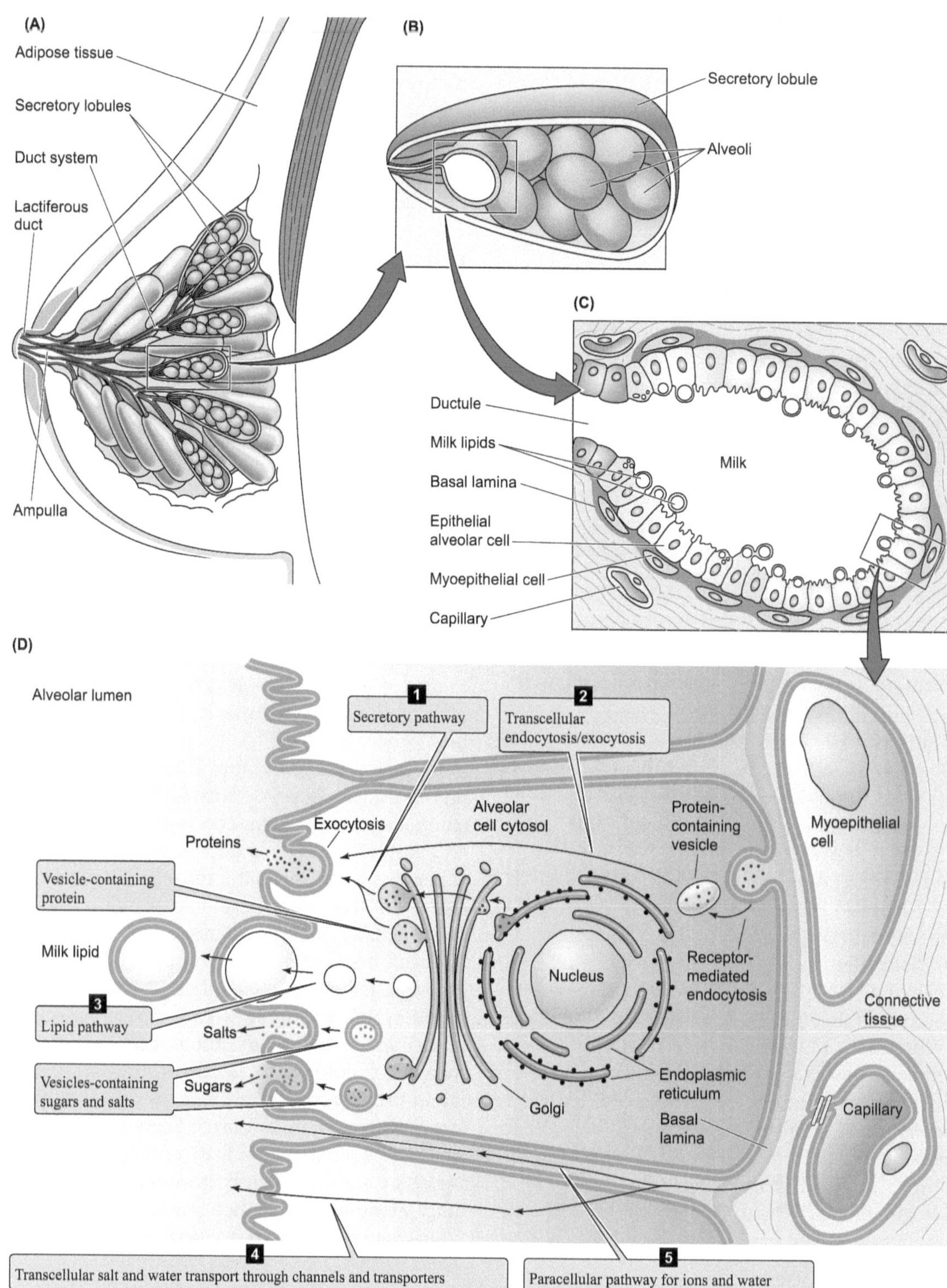

FIGURE 14.73 The breast and the production of milk: (A) lactating breast, (B) secretory lobule, (C) alveolus, and (D) epithelial alveolar cell. Source: *Figure 56.11 in Boron, & Boulpaep (2017). Chapter 56: Fertilization, pregnancy and lactation. In S. Mesiano, & E. E. Jones (Eds.),* Medical physiology *(3rd ed., p. 1147). Elsevier.*

TABLE 14.1 Composition of human colostrum, human milk and cow's milk per deciliter (100 mL) of fluid.

Component	Human colostrum	Human milk	Cow's milk
Total protein (g)	2.7	0.9	3.3
Casein (% of total protein)	44	44	82
Total fat (g)	2.9	4.5	3.7
Lactose (g)	5.7	7.1	4.8
Caloric content (kcal)	54	70	69
Calcium (mg)	31	33	125
Iron (μg)	10	50	50
Phosphorus (mg)	14	15	96
Cells (macrophages, neutrophils, and lymphocytes)	$7–8 \times 10^6$	$1–2 \times 10^6$	–

The notable difference is that none of the immune cells that enable a child to survive infections are in cow's milk (they have been destroyed or filtered out). Also of note is the higher fat content of cow's milk, which tends to make infants fed with that fluid heavier and more prone to weight problems later in life.
Reproduced from Table 56.7 in Boron, & Boulpaep (2017). Chapter 56: Fertilization, pregnancy and lactation. In S. Mesiano, & E. E. Jones (Eds.), Medical physiology *(3rd ed., p. 1148). Elsevier.*

needed by the infant until the teeth erupt. In addition, milk contains maternal immunoglobulins that are absorbed intact by the immature intestine and provide passive immunity to common pathogens. The extraordinarily versatile cells of the mammary alveoli simultaneously synthesize large amounts of proteins, fat, and lactose and secrete these constituents by different mechanisms, along with a large volume of aqueous medium whose ionic composition differs substantially from blood plasma. Human milk consists of about 1% protein, principally in the form of casein and lactalbumin, about 4% fat, and about 7% lactose (Table 14.1).

Each liter of milk also contains about 300 mg of calcium. After lactation is established the well-nourished woman suckling a single infant may produce about a liter of milk per day and as much as 3 L/day if suckling twins. It should be apparent therefore that, in addition to events in the mammary glands, regulation of milk production must extend to extramammary compensatory adjustments in intermediary metabolism (see Chapters 6–8), salt and water balance (see Chapter 9: Regulation of Salt and Water Balance), and calcium balance (see Chapter 10: Hormonal Regulation of Calcium Balance). Prolactin, acting through hypothalamic receptors, stimulates appetite and increases dietary intake, which largely compensates for the transfer of energy-rich fuels from the mother to the baby through the milk. The large amounts of calcium needed for mineralization of the infant skeleton, however, are derived largely from the maternal skeleton.

Lactation and maternal calcium balance

Each liter of human milk contains about 10 mmol of calcium, about a third of which is present as free ionic Ca^{2+}. Most of the remainder is complexed with casein and other proteins. In comparison, extracellular fluid contains about 1 mmol of ionized Ca^{2+} per liter, and intracellular fluid contains about 100 nmol/L. We still do not understand how mammary epithelial cells accomplish the formidable task of transporting such large amounts of calcium transcellularly against a substantial concentration gradient. Calcium secretion into milk is independent of vitamin D and differs from the vitamin D–sensitive mechanisms employed by intestinal and renal cells. Several steps are required for calcium to reach the alveolar lumens: calcium must enter the alveolar cells at their basolateral surfaces and then cross to the apical membranes without disrupting cellular calcium balance and then be transferred into the lumens. The molecular apparatus that transfers interstitial calcium across the basolateral membranes has not been identified. Some of the calcium enters the alveolar lumens in secretory vesicles complexed to lipid or casein. Calcium ATPases pump calcium into the Golgi stacks, where it binds to casein as it is packaged in vesicles. The remainder may reach the apical surface by diffusion through the cisternae of the endoplasmic reticulum and is pumped across the apical membrane by additional calcium ATPases.

The lactating mammary gland ensures its supply of calcium by coopting control of the calcium concentration in extracellular fluid (Fig. 14.74).

The mammary glands behave like endocrine organs and secrete PTHrP into the circulation. PTHrP otherwise is a local paracrine factor secreted by many tissues and is not found in blood except in pregnancy or in certain malignancies when its concentration is well below 1% of that seen during lactation. It may be recalled that PTHrP

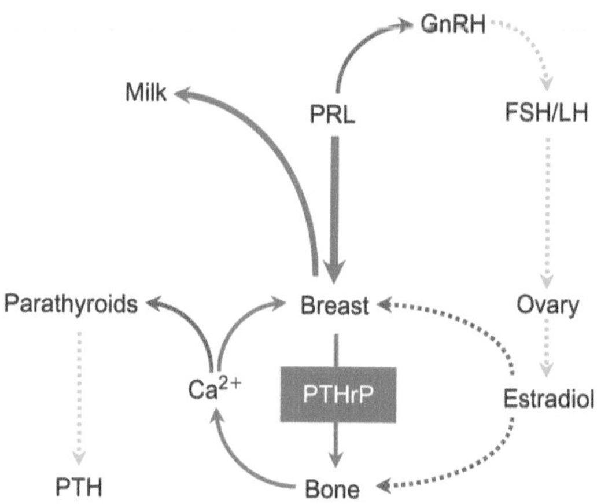

FIGURE 14.74 Relation of hormonal events in lactation to calcium metabolism. Secretion of prolactin inhibits hypothalamic secretion of the *GnRH* and stimulates secretion of the *PTHrP*. PTHrP actions on bone, unopposed by estrogens, increase calcium (Ca^{2+}) concentrations in blood and inhibit PTH secretion. Dashed arrows indicate stimulatory (green) or inhibitory (red) pathways that are blocked. *GnRH*, Gonadotropin-releasing hormone; PTH, parathyroid hormone; *PTHrP*, parathyroid hormone–related peptide.

binds to the same receptors on osteoblasts as PTH and thus stimulates the absorption of bone minerals (see Chapter 10: Hormonal Regulation of Calcium Balance). Its effectiveness in this regard is enhanced by the virtual absence of estrogens due to the suppression effects of prolactin on gonadotropin secretion (see later). During lactation, ionized calcium concentrations in plasma are at the high end of the normal range. As a result, PTH secretion is suppressed, and its plasma concentrations decline to low levels. Plasma concentrations of calcitriol (1,25 (OH)2D3), which were elevated in pregnancy, return to nonpregnant levels. Hence, intestinal uptake of calcium is not accelerated. Though substantial, calcium loss from the maternal skeleton is reversible and replenished within several months after weaning and has no impact on the development of osteoporosis later in life.

The factors that regulate synthesis of PTHrP and stimulate its secretion are not known. It is possible that secretion of PTHrP is a constitutive property of the fully differentiated alveolar epithelium, or alternatively, that synthesis and secretion are directly upregulated by prolactin or some downstream product of prolactin action. The basolateral membranes of alveolar epithelial cells contain the same calcium-sensing receptor (CaR) as found in parathyroid and renal tubular cells, and can thus monitor extracellular calcium concentrations (see Chapter 10: Hormonal Regulation of Calcium Balance). As with PTH secretion by parathyroid cells (see Chapter 10: Hormonal Regulation of Calcium Balance), detection of elevated levels of calcium by the CaR results in inhibition of PTHrP secretion. The CaR also regulates the activity of the apical calcium ATPase and increases the rate of calcium transport into the alveolar lumen to match the plasma concentration of calcium. The calcium receptor thus regulates the availability of calcium to the alveolar epithelium and simultaneously adjusts the rate of calcium transfer into milk to match its availability.

Mechanism of prolactin action

Prolactin acts on alveolar epithelial cells to stimulate expression of genes for milk proteins such as casein and lactalbumin, enzymes needed for the synthesis of lactose and triglycerides, and the proteins that govern the various steps in the different secretory processes. The prolactin receptor is a large peptide with a single membrane–spanning domain. It is closely related to the GH receptor and transmits its signal by activating tyrosine phosphorylation of intracellular proteins as described for the GH receptor (see Chapter 11: Hormonal Control of Growth). Binding of prolactin causes two receptor molecules to dimerize and activate the cytosolic enzyme, JAK-2. Some of the proteins thus phosphorylated belong to the STAT family (for signal transduction and activation of transcription), which then dimerize and migrate to the nucleus where they activate transcription of specific genes. Prolactin may also signal through activation of a cytosolic tyrosine kinase related to the src oncogene and by activating membrane ion channels. The signaling cascades set in motion the various events that accompany the growth of the secretory alveoli and production of milk.

Neuroendocrine mechanisms

Continued lactation requires more than just the right complement of hormones. Milk must also be removed regularly by suckling. Failure to empty the mammary alveoli brings lactation to a halt within about a week and results in involution of the lobuloalveolar structures. Involution results not only from prolactin withdrawal but also from inhibitory factors in milk that block secretion if allowed to remain in alveolar lumens. Suckling triggers two neuroendocrine reflexes critical for the maintenance of lactation: surges of prolactin secretion and the so-called milk let-down reflex.

Milk let-down reflex

Because each lactiferous duct has only a single opening to the outside and alveoli are not readily collapsible, application of negative pressure at the nipple does not cause milk to flow. The milk let-down reflex, also called the milk ejection reflex, permits the suckling infant to obtain milk (Fig. 14.75).

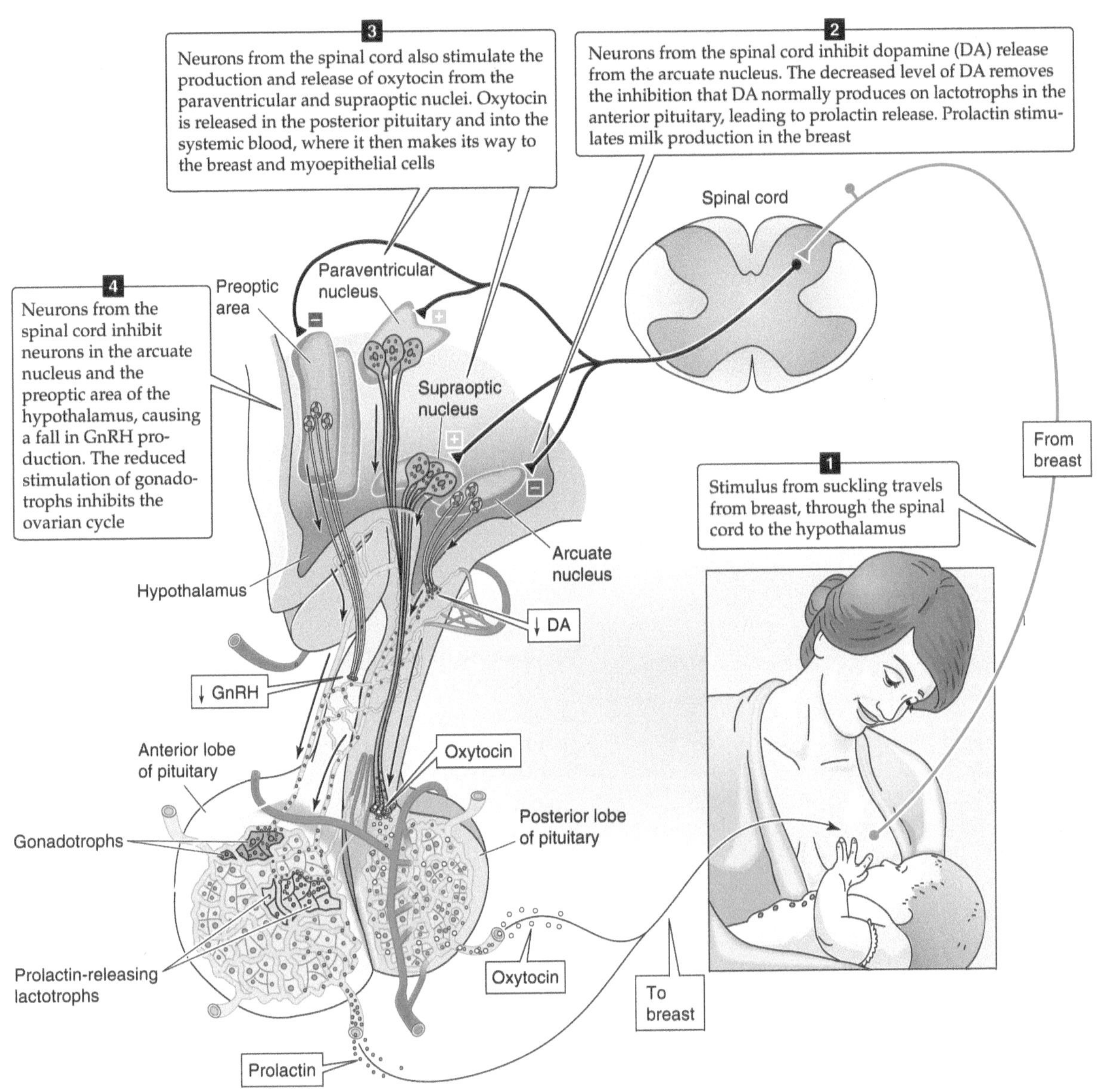

FIGURE 14.75 The suckling reflex and the hormones involved. Source: *Figure 56.12 in Boron, & Boulpaep (2017). Chapter 56: Fertilization, pregnancy and lactation. In S. Mesiano, & E. E. Jones (Eds.),* Medical physiology *(3rd ed., p. 1147). Elsevier.*

This neuroendocrine reflex involves the hormone oxytocin, which is secreted in response to suckling. Oxytocin stimulates contraction of myoepithelial cells that surround each alveolus creating positive pressure of about 10–20 mm mercury in the alveoli and the communicating duct system. Suckling merely distorts the valve-like folds of tissue in the nipple and allows the pressurized milk to be ejected into the infant's mouth. Sensory input from nerve endings in the nipple is transmitted to the hypothalamus by way of thoracic nerves and the spinal cord and stimulates neurons in the supraoptic and paraventricular nuclei to release oxytocin from terminals in the posterior lobe (Fig. 14.76).

These neurons can also be activated by higher brain centers, so that the mere sight of the baby or hearing it cry is often sufficient to stimulate milk let-down (Fig. 14.77).

Conversely, stressful conditions may inhibit oxytocin secretion, preventing the suckling infant from obtaining milk even though the breast is full.

Cellular actions of oxytocin

The oxytocin receptor is expressed principally in uterine smooth muscle and myoepithelial cells that surround mammary alveoli. It is a typical G protein–coupled receptor that signals through Gαq to phospholipase C-β

and the formation of inositol trisphosphate (IP3) and diacylglycerol (DAG). Inositol trisphosphate stimulates calcium release from intracellular stores, and DAG activates protein kinase C, which may phosphorylate and activate membrane calcium channels.

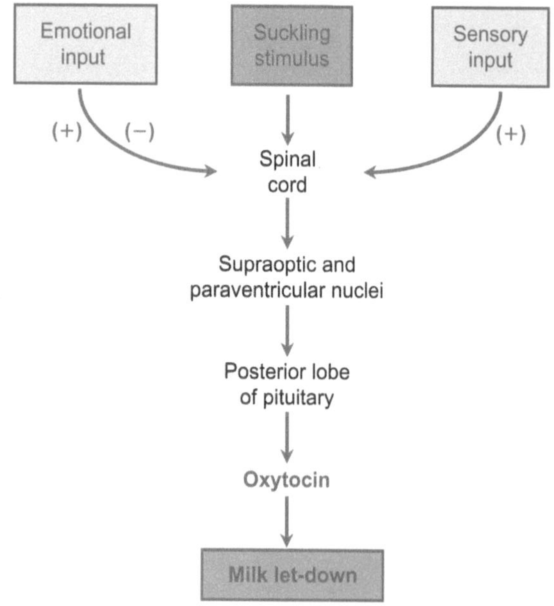

FIGURE 14.76 Control of oxytocin secretion during lactation.

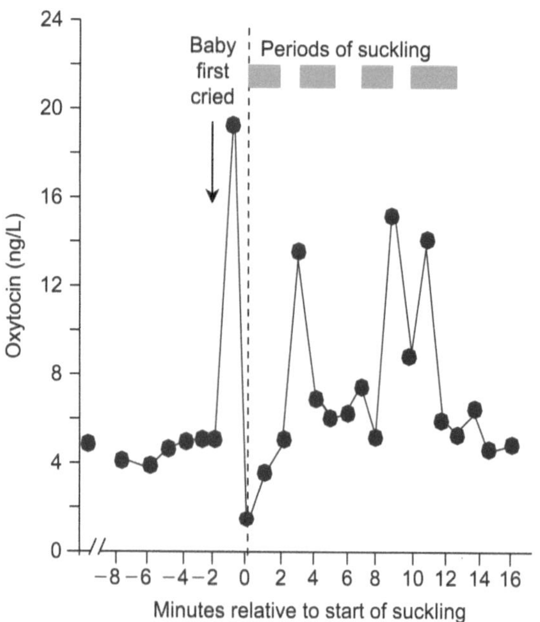

FIGURE 14.77 Relation of blood oxytocin concentrations to suckling. Note that the initial rise in oxytocin preceded the initial period of suckling. Source: *From McNeilly, A. S., Robinson, I. C. A., Houston, M. J., & Howie, P. W. (1983). Release of oxytocin and prolactin in response to suckling.* British Medical Journal, 286, 257.

Increased intracellular calcium binds to calmodulin and activates myosin light chain kinase, which initiates contraction of myoepithelial or myometrial cells.

Control of prolactin secretion

Suckling is also an important stimulus for the secretion of prolactin. During suckling the prolactin concentration in blood may increase by 10-fold or more within just a few minutes (Fig. 14.78).

Although suckling evokes secretion of both oxytocin and prolactin, the two secretory reflexes are processed separately in the central nervous system, and the two hormones are secreted independently. Emotional signals that release oxytocin and produce milk let-down are not followed by prolactin secretion. It is unlikely that prolactin secreted during suckling can act quickly enough to increase milk production to meet current demands. Rather, such episodes of secretion are important for producing the milk needed for subsequent feedings. Milk production thus is related to the frequency of suckling, which gives the newborn some control over its nutritional supply, and is an extension into the postnatal period of the self-serving control over maternal function that the fetus exercised in utero.

Increased secretion of prolactin and even milk production do not require a preceding pregnancy. Repeated stimulation of the nipples can induce lactation in some women who have never borne a child. In some cultures, postmenopausal women act as wet nurses for infants whose mothers produce inadequate amounts of milk. This fact underscores the lack of involvement of the

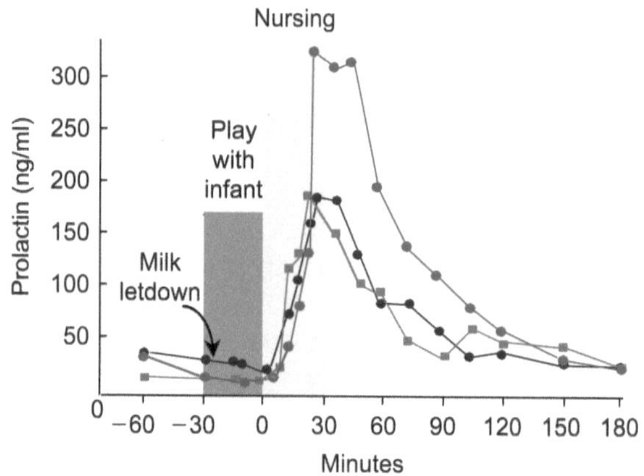

FIGURE 14.78 Plasma prolactin concentrations during nursing and anticipation of nursing. Note that although anticipation of nursing apparently resulted in oxytocin secretion, increased prolactin secretion did not occur until after suckling began. Source: *From Noel, G. L., Suh, H. K., & Franz, A. G. (1974). Prolactin release during nursing and breast stimulation in postpartum and non-postpartum subjects.* The Journal of Clinical Endocrinology and Metabolism, 38, 413.

ovarian steroids in lactation once the glandular apparatus has formed.

Prolactin is unique among the anterior pituitary hormones in the respect that its secretion is increased rather than decreased when the vascular connection between the pituitary gland and the hypothalamus is interrupted. Prolactin secretion is controlled primarily by an inhibitory hypophysiotropic hormone, dopamine (Fig. 14.23). Dopamine is synthesized by sequential hydroxylation and decarboxylation of tyrosine and is an intermediate in the synthetic pathway for epinephrine and norepinephrine (see Fig. 4.26). Surgical transection of the pituitary stalk increases plasma prolactin concentrations in peripheral blood (hyperprolactinemia) and may lead to the onset of lactation. Suckling evokes prolactin secretion through a neural pathway that inhibits dopamine release into the hypophyseal portal circulation by dopaminergic neurons whose cell bodies are located in the arcuate nuclei. It has been shown experimentally that abrupt relief from dopamine inhibition is followed by a surge of prolactin secretion. It is possible that prolactin secretion is also under positive control by a yet-to-be-identified prolactin-releasing factor. Experimentally and in some pathological states, thyrotropin-releasing hormone (TRH) increases prolactin secretion, but in spite of its potency as in this regard, it is unlikely that TRH is a physiological regulator of prolactin secretion. Normally, TSH and prolactin are secreted independently. TSH secretion does not increase during lactation, but occasionally prolactin secretion is increased in hypothyroid individuals.

Lactotrophs express estrogen receptors. Estradiol acts at the genomic level to increase the production of prolactin and stimulates proliferation and hypertrophy of lactotrophs. The high concentrations of estrogens are probably responsible for the increased number of lactotrophs in the pituitary and their high prolactin content during pregnancy. Estrogens may therefore increase prolactin secretion by increasing its availability. Although it decreases the sensitivity of lactotrophs to the inhibitory effects of dopamine, estradiol does not act directly as a prolactin-releasing factor. Paradoxically, estradiol increases dopamine synthesis in the hypothalamus and therefore increases its availability for secretion (Fig. 14.79).

To date, there is no known product of prolactin action that feeds back to regulate prolactin secretion. The effects of suckling and estrogen on prolactin secretion are open loops. Experiments in animals suggest that prolactin itself may act as its own "short-loop" feedback inhibitor by stimulating dopaminergic neurons in the arcuate nucleus. It is not certain that such an effect is applicable to humans. If prolactin is a negative effector of its own secretion, it is not clear what mechanisms override feedback inhibition to allow prolactin to rise to high levels during pregnancy.

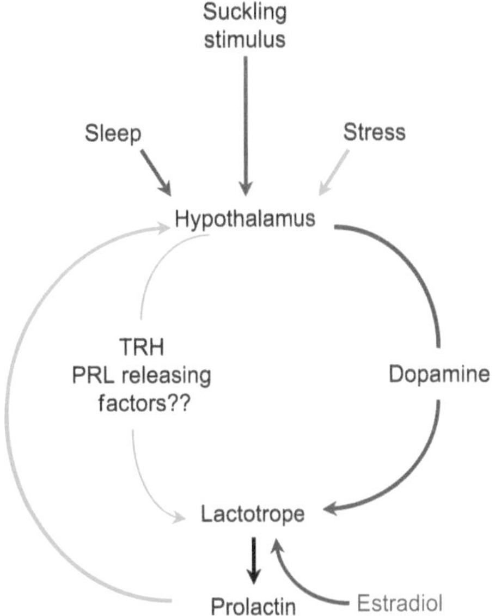

FIGURE 14.79 Control of prolactin secretion. Red arrows indicate inhibition and green arrows indicate stimulation. A physiological role for *TRH* and other postulated releasing hormones has not been established. Estradiol stimulates prolactin synthesis and may interfere with the inhibitory action of dopamine. *TRH*, Thyrotropin-releasing hormone.

Cellular regulation of prolactin secretion

As in most other endocrine cells, secretory activity of lactotrophs is enhanced by increased cytosolic concentrations of calcium and cAMP (Fig. 14.80).

Dopamine binds to G protein–coupled receptors and inhibits prolactin secretion through several temporally distinct mechanisms. Initial inhibitory effects are detectable within seconds and result from activation of G protein–gated potassium channels and the resulting hyperpolarization of the plasma membrane. Hyperpolarization deactivates voltage-sensitive calcium channels, blocking calcium entry, and intracellular calcium concentrations' decline. Minutes later, there is a decrease in cAMP, which leads to decreased transcription of the prolactin gene. Estrogens are thought to decrease responsiveness to dopamine by uncoupling dopamine receptors from G-proteins. On a longer time scale, dopamine antagonizes the proliferative effects of estrogen by mechanisms that are not understood.

Prolactin in blood

Prolactin is secreted continuously at low basal rates throughout life regardless of sex. Its concentration in

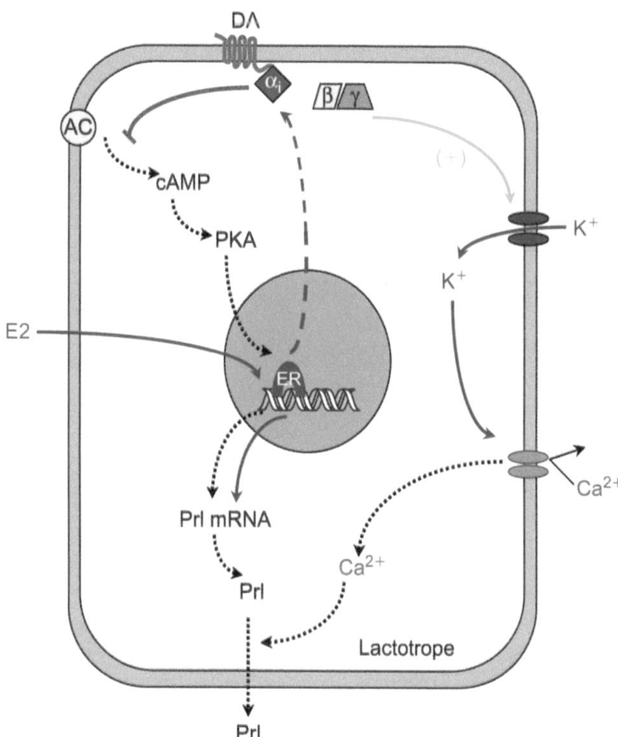

FIGURE 14.80 Cellular events in the regulation of prolactin secretion. Steps in basal synthesis and secretion are indicated by the dotted black arrows. The effects of dopamine are shown by the red arrows, and the effects of estradiol are shown in light blue. TRH (not shown) increases prolactin secretion through activation of its heptihelical receptor, which is coupled through Gαq to phospholipase Cβ and caused release of inositol trisphosphate, diacylglyceride, and increased intracellular calcium. *AC*, Adenylate cyclase; *cAMP*, cyclic adenosine monophosphate; *E2*, estradiol; *ER*, estrogen receptor; *Gi*$_\alpha$ *and* β/γ, the subunits of the heterotrimeric inhibitory G protein; *PKA*, protein kinase A; *PRL*, prolactin; *TRH*, thyrotropin-releasing hormone.

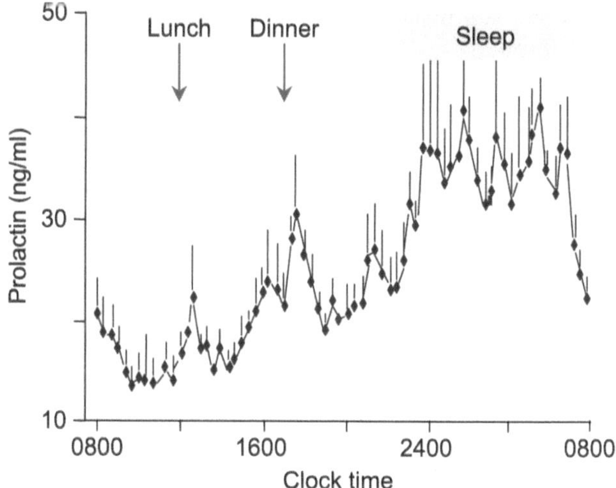

FIGURE 14.81 Around-the-clock prolactin concentrations in eight normal women. Acute elevation of prolactin level occurs shortly after onset of sleep and begins to decrease shortly before awakening. Source: *From Yen, S. C., & Jaffe, R. B. (1999). Prolactin in human reproduction. In S. C. Yen, & R. Jaffe (Eds.),* Reproductive physiology *(4th ed., p. 268). Philadelphia, PA: Saunders.*

blood increases during nocturnal sleep in a diurnal rhythmic pattern. Basal values are somewhat higher in women than in men and prepubertal children, presumably reflecting the effects of estrogens. Episodic increases in response to eating and stress are superimposed on this basal pattern (Fig. 14.81).

Prolactin concentrations rise steadily in maternal blood throughout pregnancy to about 10 times the nonpregnant value (Fig. 14.6). After delivery, prolactin concentrations remain elevated, even in the absence of suckling, and slowly return to the prepregnancy range usually within less than 2 weeks. Prolactin also increases in fetal blood as pregnancy progresses and during the final weeks reaches levels that are higher than those seen in maternal plasma. The fetal kidney apparently excretes prolactin into the amniotic fluid where at midpregnancy the prolactin concentration is 5–10 times higher than that of either maternal or fetal blood. Although some of the prolactin in maternal blood is produced by uterine decidual cells, prolactin in fetal blood originates in the fetal pituitary and does not cross the placental barrier. The high prolactin concentration seen in the newborn decreases to the low levels of childhood within the first week after birth. The physiological importance of any of these changes in prolactin concentration in either prenatal or postnatal life is not understood.

Lactation and resumption of ovarian cycles

Menstrual cycles resume as early as 6–8 weeks after delivery in women who do not nurse their babies. With breast-feeding, however, the reappearance of normal ovarian cycles may be delayed for many months. This delay, called lactational amenorrhea, serves as a natural, but unreliable, form of birth control. Lactational amenorrhea is related to high plasma concentrations of prolactin, which appear to suppress the GnRH pulse generator. Delayed resumption of fertile cycles therefore is most pronounced when breast milk is not supplemented with other foods, and consequently the frequency of suckling is high. Ovarian activity is limited to varying degrees of incomplete follicular development; even in those women who ovulate, luteal function is deficient. Hyperprolactinemia often results from a small prolactin-secreting pituitary tumor (microadenoma), and is now recognized as a common cause of infertility and abnormal or absent menstrual cycles. Treatment with bromocriptine, a drug that activates dopamine receptors, suppresses prolactin secretion, and restores normal reproductive function. The delay in resumption of cyclicity results from decreased amplitude and frequency of GnRH release by the hypothalamic GnRH pulse generator (see Chapter 13: Hormonal Control of Reproduction in the Female: The Menstrual Cycle). Pulsatile administration of GnRH to lactating women promptly restores ovulation and normal corpus luteal function.

Summary

Higher mammals nurture their developing offspring internally where it can be better protected. This growth is regulated by both maternal and fetal hormones. This chapter discusses these effects. When pregnancy is over, it is hormones that initiate labor and cause the contractions of delivery. Post partum, it is hormones that initiate lactation.

Suggested readings

Basic foundations

Anthony, K. M., Racusin, D. A., Aagaard, K., & Dildy, G. A., III (2017). Maternal physiology. In S. G. Gabbe, J. R. Niebyl, J. L. Simpson, M. B. Landon, H. L. Galan, E. R. M. Jauniaux, D. A. Driscoll, V. Berghella, & W. A. Grobman (Eds.), *Obstetrics: Normal and problem pregnancies* (7th ed., pp. 38–63). Philadelphia, PA: Elsevier.

Bulun, S. E. (2017). Physiology and pathology of the female reproductive axis. In S. Melmed, K. S. Polonsky, P. R. Larsen, & H. M. Kronenberg (Eds.), *Williams textbook of endocrinology* (13th ed., pp. 590–663). Philadelphia, PA: Elsevier.

Mesiano, S., & Jones, E. E. (2017). Fertilization, pregnancy and lactation. In W. F. Boron, & E. L. Boulpaep (Eds.), *Medical physiology* (3rd ed., pp. 1129–1150). Philadelphia, PA: Elsevier.

Additional information

Davis, W. (2015). On deaf ears, *Mycobacterium avium* paratuberculosis in pathogenesis Crohn's and other diseases. *World Journal of Gastroenterology, 21*(48), 13411–13417. Available from https://doi.org/10.3748/wjg.v21.i48.13411.

Eerdekens, A., Langouche, L., Güiza, F., Verhaeghe, J., Naulaers, G., Vanhole, C., & Van den Berghe, G. (2018). Maternal and placental responses before preterm birth: Adaptations to increase fetal thyroid hormone availability? *The Journal of Maternal-Fetal & Neonatal Medicine*, 1–12. Available from https://doi.org/10.1080/14767058.2018.1449199.

McNees, A. L., Markesich, D., Zayyani, N. R., & Graham, D. Y. (2015). *Mycobacterium paratuberculosis* as a cause of Crohn's disease. *Expert Review of Gastroenterology & Hepatology, 9*(12), 1523–1534. Available from https://doi.org/10.1586/17474124.2015.1093931.

Monif, G. R. G. (2015). The Hruska postulate of Crohn's disease. *Medical Hypotheses, 85*(6), 878–881. Available from https://doi.org/10.1016/j.mehy.2015.09.019.

Philips, E. M., Jaddoe, V. W. V., Asimakopoulos, A. G., Kannan, K., Steegers, E. A. P., Santos, S., & Trasande, L. (2018). Bisphenol and phthalate concentrations and its determinants among pregnant women in a population-based cohort in the Netherlands, 2004–5. *Environmental Research, 161*, 562–572. Available from https://doi.org/10.1016/j.envres.2017.11.051.

Rinaldi, J. C., Santos, S. A. A., Colombelli, K. T., Birch, L., Prins, G. S., Justulin, L. A., & Felisbino, S. L. (2018). Maternal protein malnutrition: Effects on prostate development and adult disease. *Journal of Developmental Origins of Health and Disease*, 1–12. Available from https://doi.org/10.1017/S2040174418000168.

Romano, M. E., Eliot, M. N., Zoeller, R. T., Hoofnagle, A. N., Calafat, A. M., Karagas, M. R., … Braun, J. M. (2018). Maternal urinary phthalate metabolites during pregnancy and thyroid hormone concentrations in maternal and cord sera: The HOME Study. *International Journal of Hygiene and Environmental Health*. Available from https://doi.org/10.1016/j.ijheh.2018.03.010.

Uzoigwe, J. C., Khaitsa, M. L., & Gibbs, P. S. (2007). Epidemiological evidence for *Mycobacterium avium* subspecies paratuberculosis as a cause of Crohn's disease. *Epidemiology and Infection, 135*(7), 1057–1068. Available from https://doi.org/10.1017/S0950268807008448.

Wagner, C. L., Baatz, J. E., Newton, D., & Hollis, B. W. (2018). Analytical considerations and general diagnostic and therapeutic ramifications of milk hormones during lactation. *Best Practice & Research Clinical Endocrinology & Metabolism, 32*(1), 5–16. Available from https://doi.org/10.1016/j.beem.2017.11.004.

Index

Note: Page numbers followed by "*f*," "*t*" and "*b*" refer to figures, tables, and boxes, respectively.

H

R

S